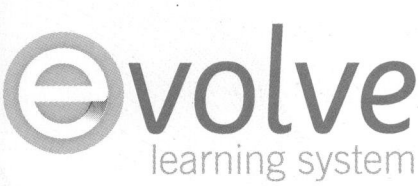

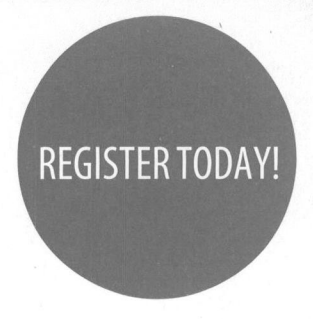

D0702043

To access your Student Resources, visit:

http://evolve.elsevier.com/Haugen/careplanning/

Register today and gain access to:

- **Online Care Planner**
  Build, edit, and print a customized care plan by choosing from 33 nursing diagnoses from the 7th edition of *Ulrich & Canale's Nursing Care Planning Guides*. Select each set of Diagnoses, Outcomes, and Interventions you wish to include in the care plan.

- **Additional Care Plans**
  Choose from 15 additional nursing diagnosis and disorder care plans for further study and guidance.

- **Animations**
  Review over 70 detailed pathophysiology animations.

ELSEVIER

7TH EDITION

ULRICH & CANALE'S nursing

care
planning guides

Prioritization, Delegation, and Critical Thinking

Nancy Haugen PhD, RN
Associate Professor and ABSN Program Chair
School of Nursing
Samuel Merritt University
Oakland, California

Sandra Galura MSN, RN, CCRN, CPAN
Clinical Nurse Educator
Post Anesthesia Care Unit
Florida Hospital
Orlando, Florida

ELSEVIER
SAUNDERS

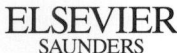

SAUNDERS

3251 Riverport Lane
St. Louis, Missouri 63043

ULRICH AND CANALE'S NURSING CARE PLANNING GUIDES:
PRIORITIZATION, DELEGATION, AND CRITICAL THINKING
IN PATIENT CARE

ISBN: 978-1-4377-0174-6

Library of Congress Cataloging in Publication Data

Haugen, Nancy.
Ulrich & Canale's nursing care planning guides: prioritization, delegation, and critical thinking/Nancy Haugen, Sandra Galura.—7th ed.
    p. ; cm.
Other title: Ulrich and Canale's nursing care planning guides
Other title: Nursing care planning guides
Rev. ed. of: Nursing care planning guides: for adults in acute, extended, and home care settings/Susan Puderbaugh Ulrich, Suzanne Weyland Canale. 6th ed. c2005.
Includes bibliographical references and index.
ISBN 978-1-4377-0174-6 (pbk.: alk. paper)
    1. Nursing—Planning—Handbooks, manuals, etc. 2. Nursing care plans—Handbooks, manuals, etc. I. Galura, Sandra. II. Ulrich, Susan Puderbaugh. Nursing care planning guides. III. Title. IV. Title: Ulrich and Canale's nursing care planning guides. V. Title: Nursing care planning guides.
    [DNLM: 1. Nursing Care. 2. Nursing Assessment. 3. Patient Care Planning. WY 100.1 H371u2011]
RT49.U47 2011
610.73—dc22
                                                                2010019582

Executive Editor: Robin Carter
Developmental Editor: Deanna Dedeke
Publishing Services Manager: Deborah L. Vogel
Senior Project Manager: Ann E. Rogers
Design Direction: Karen Pauls

Printed in the United States of America

Last digit is the print number: 9 8 7 6 5

To my husband David and my children Jeffery and Sara–
Thank you for your love and support. You are my pride and joy!
—Nancy Haugen

To my son Jacob, husband Mike, and all of my past and current students who
continue to challenge me to be the very best at whatever role I assume!
—Sandra J. Galura

About the Authors

Nancy Haugen, PhD, RN has more than 25 years of experience in nursing and nursing education. She has clinical experience in medical-surgical nursing, obstetrics, critical care, and post anesthesia care. She has also worked in health care facilities as the Director of Education, Infection Control, and Employee Health. Dr. Haugen's academic experience includes teaching in associate degree, generic baccalaureate degree, and accelerated baccalaureate degree programs. Her areas of teaching include medical-surgical nursing, health assessment, pharmacology, and pathophysiology. Dr. Haugen is currently an Associate Professor and Chair of the Accelerated BSN program at Samuel Merritt University in Oakland, California. She received her ASN and BSN from Southern Adventist University, her MN from Louisiana State University, and her PhD from the University of Florida. She is a member of Sigma Theta Tau International, Nu XI chapter.

Sandra J. Galura, MSN, RN, CCRN, CPAN, has more than 20 years of experience in critical care and post anesthesia nursing practice. She is currently a Clinical Nurse Educator for the Post Anesthesia Care Unit at Florida Hospital in Orlando, Florida. In addition, she is currently employed as adjunct faculty for Florida Hospital College of Health Sciences in Orlando. She received her BSN from Troy University in Troy, Alabama and her MSN from the University of Central Florida in Orlando. She is currently a doctoral candidate at the University of Central Florida with research focusing on immunosuppressant adherence in adult renal transplant recipients. She is active both locally and nationally in professional organizations including the American Society of PeriAnesthesia Nurses (ASPAN) and the American Association of Critical Care Nurses (AACN). She has served as a member of the Education/Research Committee and as an active member of the Clinical Practice Committee for ASPAN.

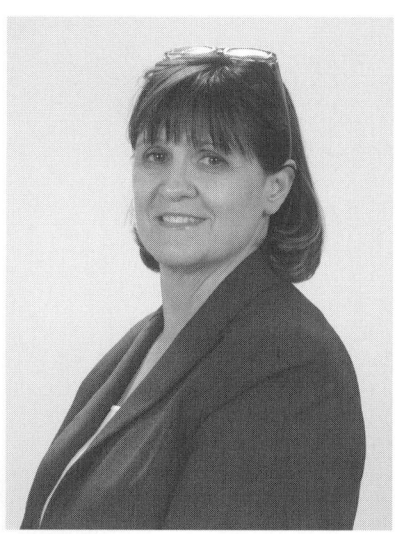

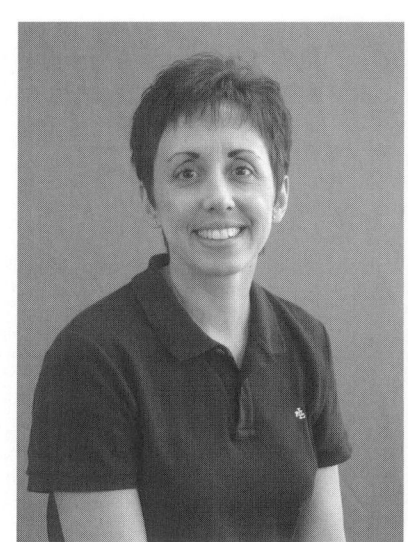

Reviewers

Mariann Montgomery, MSN, RN, CNE
Assistant Professor of Nursing
Kent State University Tuscarawas
New Philadelphia, Ohio

Rosemary Macy, RN, MS
Assistant Professor
Department of Nursing
Boise State University
Boise, Idaho

Charlotte A. Wisnewski, PhD, RN, BC
Assistant Professor
School of Nursing
University of Texas–Medical Branch
Galveston, Texas

STUDENT REVIEWERS

Sarah Hollenberg
Nursing Program
University of Missouri–St. Louis
St. Louis, Missouri

Lindsay Walsh
Nursing Program
Truman State University
Kirksville, Missouri

Preface

Ulrich and Canale's Nursing Care Planning Guides is a comprehensive reference to guide the planning of nursing care for adults with commonly recurring medical-surgical conditions. The scope of the book has been broadened to include information that is applicable to clients receiving nursing care in acute care, community, extended care, and home care settings. The book has been updated to include the most recent NANDA International (NANDA-I)–approved nursing diagnoses and Nursing Outcomes Classification (NOC) and Nursing Interventions Classification (NIC) labels.

This book contains care plans for a variety of medical-surgical conditions. Each of the care plans includes a description of the medical condition or surgery and identifies the relevant nursing diagnoses and collaborative diagnoses. For each diagnosis there is a specific etiology statement, a desired outcome, and a complete list of nursing actions. This edition maintains a continued focus on comprehensive etiology statements, comprehensive coverage of potential complications (collaborative diagnoses), and thorough client teaching. The content represents standards of nursing care and is intended to be a guide for students and practitioners to use in planning individualized client care.

Chapter 1 provides guidelines on how to manage and delegate nursing care and how to modify and individualize nursing care plans. Included in the chapter is a step by-step approach to delegating nursing actions to both patient care assistants and licensed practical or vocational nurses. Guidelines are provided for modifying and individualizing nursing care using a case study approach to demonstrate the collection of data, selection of pertinent nursing diagnoses, and individualization of etiology statements, desired outcomes, and nursing actions.

Chapter 2 addresses 33 commonly used nursing diagnoses. The key component of this unit is the inclusion of the rationale for each nursing action, which provides the nursing student and practitioner with a clear understanding of how each action helps to achieve the desired outcome for the specific nursing diagnosis. In addition to actions and rationales, the following information is included for each nursing diagnosis in this unit: NANDA-I–based definition, related factors or risk factors, defining characteristics, desired outcomes, documentation criteria, and suggested NIC interventions. This unit also facilitates the planning of care for the client with a medical-surgical condition that is not addressed in this text.

Chapter 3 focuses on care of the client having surgery. The standardized care plans on Preoperative and Postoperative Care should be used with each surgical care plan in the text. In addition, a plan of care for the client undergoing conscious sedation is provided.

Chapters 4 through 14 include care plans that provide information regarding conditions or treatment modalities. Chapters 4 through 13 are divided according to body systems. Care plans within each chapter deal with conditions that are frequently seen in health care settings. The care plans in Chapter 14 cover treatment modalities for neoplastic disorders. Each of the standardized care plans in these units can be used to plan care for a client with a condition not covered in this text.

Chapter 15 focuses on care of the elderly client. It includes the nursing diagnoses that reflect the biopsychosocial changes that commonly occur with aging and are intensified with the stressors of illness. The information is applicable to care of the elderly in all health care settings and can be used independently or in combination with care plans appropriate to the client's concurrent medical condition(s) and/or surgical situation.

Chapter 16 focuses on care at the end of life. The information is applicable to clients in acute, extended care settings, or in the home. Nursing diagnoses included in the care plan are those common to all persons facing death and can be used in conjunction with care plans pertinent to the client's specific medical diagnoses.

The content in each care plan is organized in a traditional nursing care plan format that can readily be adapted to other plan-of-care formats used by health care providers (e.g., critical paths, clinical practice guidelines). Each care plan is organized as follows:

INTRODUCTION

The introduction provides the reader with an overview of the condition including a basic definition and discussion of the pathophysiological mechanisms involved and/or a description of the surgical procedure or selected treatment modality. This overview is not intended to be a substitute for the information provided in medical-surgical nursing texts or other references but rather a quick refresher or a starting point for additional research. Within this section, the reader will also find the focus of the care plan (highlighted in bold type).

OUTCOME/DISCHARGE CRITERIA

This section includes criteria that serve as a guide for determining the client's readiness for discharge from the specific health care setting. Recognizing that client education is a vital aspect of health care, the authors use these criteria as the basis for the detailed teaching that is included at the end of each care plan.

NURSING AND COLLABORATIVE DIAGNOSES

The nursing and collaborative diagnoses describe the actual or potential health problems that a client with a particular condition may experience. Nursing diagnoses were selected from those approved by NANDA-I through 2011 and are indicated with the **NDx** symbol. In some instances the authors have included nursing diagnoses that have been modified or are not currently on the NANDA-I list. Nursing diagnoses that are not unique to a particular condition but may be relevant for a client (e.g., spiritual distress) have not consistently been included but should be considered when individualizing each care plan. Collaborative diagnoses have been included to incorporate potential complications and electrolyte imbalances for which there are not established nursing diagnostic labels. Specific etiology statements that incorporate pathophysiological and psychosocial factors are identified for the majority of the nursing and collaborative diagnosis labels. As with other portions of the standardized care plans, these etiologies need to be individualized for each client. In most instances, the authors did not include etiologies for the nursing diagnosis labels that deal directly with client teaching (i.e., deficient knowledge, ineffective health maintenance, ineffective therapeutic regimen management) because of the numerous individual variables that may affect a client's ability to learn, maintain health, and manage his/her therapeutic regimen.

In order to provide consistency in the care plans, the nursing and collaborative diagnoses statements have usually been listed in the same order. Within each care plan, an effort has been made to prioritize the diagnoses, however, individual patient circumstances may necessitate reprioritization. Priorities will need to be established by the student and practitioner based on the individual client's current needs.

CLINICAL MANIFESTATIONS

The clinical manifestations for the nursing and collaborative diagnosis provide assessment critera for the client. Clinical manifestations are differentiated between subjective and objective manifestations and provide the supporting data for selection and prioritization of the appropriate nursing diagnosis.

DESIRED OUTCOMES

The desired outcomes for the nursing and collaborative diagnoses provide criteria for evaluating client progress and the effectiveness of care provided. The student and practitioner should modify the goal and specific outcome criteria as needed to reflect what is realistic for each individual client.

Target dates for the desired outcomes have not been included since these are determined by the client's current status.

NURSING ACTIONS AND SELECTED PURPOSES/RATIONALES

This column contains nursing actions that can assist the client to achieve the desired outcomes. The actions include detailed assessments that are based on clinical manifestations associated with the diagnostic label as identified in the literature and/or defined by NANDA-I. These assessments assist the user to determine if the nursing or collaborative diagnosis is an actual problem or if the client is at risk for developing it. The nursing interventions are specific and realistic yet global enough to allow for regional and multidisciplinary variations in standards of care. The selected purposes or rationales have been included to clarify actions that may not be fundamental nursing knowledge.

SUGGESTED NOC AND NIC LABELS

Suggested NOC outcomes and NIC interventions are listed for the nursing diagnoses in each care plan. These classification systems are included to demonstrate how they are linked to nursing diagnoses and to increase awareness and use of standardized outcome criteria and nursing interventions in the care planning process.

CLIENT TEACHING/CONTINUED CARE

Although client teaching is included throughout the care plans, the majority of the teaching is found in the actions for the nursing diagnoses of deficient knowledge, ineffective health maintenance, and ineffective therapeutic regimen management. The included client teaching uses terminology that most clients can understand.

ONLINE RESOURCES

The seventh edition's companion ⊖volve website provides even more planning and study resources. The *Online Care Planner* offers access to all 33 of the nursing diagnoses care plans printed in the seventh edition in electronic format, allowing users to build care plans for specific conditions by selecting and customizing nursing diagnoses. These care plans can then be saved to another location and printed. Along with the care plans printed in the seventh edition text, additional in-depth care plans are provided on the ⊖volve website. A comprehensive list of all care plans, both print and electronic, is located inside the front cover of this book. In addition, the companion website now also features more than 130 narrated, 3-D, pathophysiology-based animations that correspond to disorders content in the text.

Ultimately, the value of a systematic approach to individualized client care is measured by its effect on the quality of care provided to the client. While overall care of a client is coordinated and planned by registered nurses, many interventions are delegated to licensed and unlicensed members of the healthcare delivery team. Within each care plan, actions that can be delegated to licensed (LPN/LVN) or unlicensed (UAP) personnel are indicated with an asterisk (*). Although actions may be indicated as delegatable, students and practitioners should consult their individual state Nurse Practice Act as well as organizational policies when deciding whether to delegate nursing interventions.

The authors hope that the seventh edition of this book will assist with the integration of the numerous aspects of client care, facilitate critical thinking and implementation of the nursing process, and provide both the student and the practitioner with a guide for planning and implementing high-quality client care.

ACKNOWLEDGMENTS

The authors of the seventh edition of *Ulrich & Canale's Nursing Care Planning Guides* would like to acknowledge the many years of contributions from the previous author team, Susan Puderbaugh Ulrich, ESN, MSN, and Suzanne Weyland Canale, BSN, MSN, from Lane Community College in Eugene, Oregon. Updating and revising a book of this scope is no small undertaking, but the fact that these two authors developed this content with such dedication and revised it so thoroughly over a period of 20 years is an even bigger accomplishment. We are honored to be able to contribute to the evolution of this book as new authors. We wish to acknowledge the former authors' contributions and sincerely thank them for their past efforts.

Contents

*For a full, detailed care plan on this topic, go to http://evolve/
elsevier.com/Haugen/careplanning/.

1

Prioritization, Delegation, and Critical Thinking in Client Management

Management and provision of nursing care is an exciting, challenging, and rewarding experience. Nurses practice in a variety of care settings as critical members of a multidisciplinary health care team. The delivery of nursing care is accomplished with registered nurses (RNs), licensed vocational nurses (LVNs)/licensed practical nurses (LPNs), and unlicensed assistive personnel. As a manager of care, the RN is responsible for both clinical decision-making and proper delegation of client care to other members of the care delivery team. While each member of the team plays an important role in the care of the client, it is the RN's responsibility to determine which interventions can be safely delegated to specific team members.

PRIORITIZATION

The nurse is responsible for prioritizing and individualizing a client's plan of care. Prioritization is defined as "deciding which needs or problems require immediate action and which ones could be delayed until a later time because they are not urgent" (Silvestri, 2004, p. 65). The RN must identify problems, formulate interventions to address those problems, and prioritize interventions that must be accomplished quickly to achieve optimum client outcomes. However, planning care that is prioritized, individualized, and comprehensive can be challenging due to lack of time and lack of adequate resources. Hansten and Jackson (2004) identify criteria for evaluating and weighing tasks or processes to be prioritized:

1. Is the task or process life threatening or potentially life threatening if not completed?
2. Would another client be endangered if the task is left for later?
3. Is the task or process essential to client or staff safety?
4. Is the task or process essential to the client's plan of care?

Three levels of priority setting (Alfaro-Lefevre, 2004) also aid the nurse in prioritizing nursing care:

1. ABCs—airway, breathing, and/or circulation
2. Mental status changes, unrelated medical issues, acute pain, acute elimination issues, and/or abnormal lab values
3. Health problems such as long-term issues (e.g., coping, rest)

A fourth level, Maslow's hierarchy of needs, spans the continuum of the most crucial needs necessary for survival to self-actualization and can also be used to aid in priority setting. Physiological needs, necessary for the continued function of the human body, often require the greatest attention when prioritizing client care. However, attention to safety needs such as the prevention of accidents and adverse client outcomes must be considered a high priority as long as the client's physiological needs have been stabilized.

DELEGATION

Both the National Council of State Boards of Nursing (NCSBN) and the American Nurses Association (ANA) define delegation as "the process for a nurse to direct another person to perform nursing tasks and activities" (ANA and NCSBN, 2005, p. 1). Nurses responsible for delegation must be aware of many variables aside from the client's condition. To safely and appropriately delegate nursing care, the nurse must have an understanding of the appropriate state's Nurse Practice Act, which identifies which tasks may be delegated, when the tasks may be delegated, and to whom the tasks may be delegated.

The first step in the delegation process is the assessment of the client. In addition, to safely delegate, the nurse must assess the qualifications of each member of the health care delivery team. Once the nurse determines the client's condition and the tasks to be delegated, the nurse then identifies the team member to whom the task will be delegated based on an understanding of their qualifications and skills. Once the tasks to be delegated are determined, the nurse must communicate the actions to the delegate, including what to do, when to do it, and to whom it should be done. Delegates should also be informed of the circumstances under which they should ask for assistance. Clear communication is critical, so that delegates have a complete understanding of the delegated task, as well as of the conditions that require the assistance of an RN. The Five Rights of Delegation (ANA and NCSBN, 2005) summarize the process and include the following:

1. The right task
2. Under the right circumstance
3. To the right person
4. With the right directions and communication
5. Under the right supervision and evaluation

While the RN is responsible for the safe delegation of nursing tasks to the appropriate team member, responsibility and accountability for the safe completion of interventions are not delegated and remain the ultimate responsibility of the RN. The nurse must monitor the implementation of the task and determine whether the task was completed appropriately and in a timely manner. After completion of delegated tasks, the nurse must evaluate both the delegation process and client outcomes. Questions that should be answered in evaluating this process include the following:

Was the task delegated to the appropriate individual?

Did the delegate perform the task correctly and in a timely manner?

Was the expected client outcome achieved?

Was the client satisfied with the care received?

Was the communication between the nurse and the delegate appropriate to accomplish the required intervention?

What if anything did not go as planned, and what could have prevented this from occurring?

The algorithm on the facing page may be used to assist the nurse in the delegation process (Fig. 1-1):

CRITICAL THINKING

To deliver prioritized, individualized, and safe nursing care, the professional nurse must be able to think critically by analyzing information. This information is obtained from multiple sources to determine the best plan of action that safely and effectively meets the client's basic physiological needs. Critical thinking is composed of attitudes, knowledge, and skills.

The attitude of inquiry enables the professional nurse to recognize the existence of a client problem and seek out both assessment and collaborative data that describe the encountered problem. Knowledge enables the professional nurse to weigh the accuracy of different kinds of evidence as the client's plan of care is altered to address prioritized problems. Finally, skill enables the professional nurse to apply both inquiry and knowledge in the delivery of safe patient care.

The nursing process (assess, diagnose, plan, implement, evaluate) provides a framework by which the professional nurse can connect clinical events and data obtained from a variety of sources with the appropriate interventions to safely manage and evaluate client care.

This book is intended to facilitate the care planning process, as well as to identify interventions that may be delegated to members of the nursing care team and to adults with common and recurring medical-surgical conditions. Within each care plan are nursing and collaborative diagnoses with etiological factors, desired outcomes with measurable behavioral criteria, and independent and dependent nursing actions and delegable actions with selected purposes or rationales. Safe, comprehensive care can be planned in a minimal amount of time using this book.

CREATING AN INDIVIDUALIZED, PRIORITIZED PLAN OF CARE

To be most effective, the standardized nursing care plan must be adapted to the client's individual needs. A process for planning individualized, prioritized client care follows:

1. Read the nurse's admission assessment/history information and the medication administration record of the assigned client.

2. Review the history, current diagnostic test results, nurses' notes for the last 48 hours, progress notes of health care providers (e.g., physician, dietitian, physical and occupational therapists, pain management specialist, social worker, discharge planner), and current consultation reports.

3. Interview the client, and complete an assessment using the tool provided by your nursing school or health care facility.

4. Read about the client's diagnosis and nursing care in a current medical-surgical nursing text.

5. Select the appropriate standardized care plan(s) from this text, and read the introductory information at the beginning of the care plan(s).

6. Select the nursing and collaborative diagnoses that are appropriate for your client and supported by assessment findings; choose the etiological factors that are relevant, and modify them as appropriate.

7. Modify the desired outcomes so that they are measurable and realistic for your client; establish appropriate target dates.

8. Select and prioritize the nursing actions that are relevant to the client's immediate care needs; add to or modify the actions to meet the needs of your client; include specific medications and treatments as well as client preferences and other actions that will facilitate the achievement of the desired client outcomes.

9. Determine if the client is stable and to which team member nursing interventions may be delegated.

10. Communicate delegable actions to the appropriately qualified individual.

11. Evaluate the delegation process, the quality of the delegated task, and client outcomes.

The following situation is used to illustrate how these standardized nursing care plans can be used by the student and the practitioner in planning individualized client care:

Mary G. is a 30-year-old woman hospitalized following a spinal cord injury suffered in a motor vehicle collision (MVC). She has been bedridden for the past 3 weeks due to a thoracic spine injury at the T-10 level that has resulted in paraplegia with improving upper body strength, with movement of upper extremities, and with diminished respiratory capacity and endurance. She has two children between the ages of 3 to 6 years. Both Mary and her husband have been trying to prepare the children for Mary's physical disability. They have no other family members living nearby.

1. **Read the nurse's admission assessment/history information and the medication administration record of the assigned client.**

    It is determined that Mary is a 30-year-old married woman. Her religious preference is Protestant. Her diagnosis is spinal cord transection at T-10. She is receiving morphine sulfate, 15 mg every 2 hours (q2h); Dialose, 100 mg/day; and milk of magnesia, 30 mL orally (p.o.) every evening.

2. **Review the history, current diagnostic test results, nurses' notes for the last 48 hours, progress notes of health care providers (e.g., physician, dietitian, physical and occupational therapists, pain management specialist, social worker, discharge planner), and consultation reports.**

Decision Tree for Delegation to Nursing Assistive Personnel

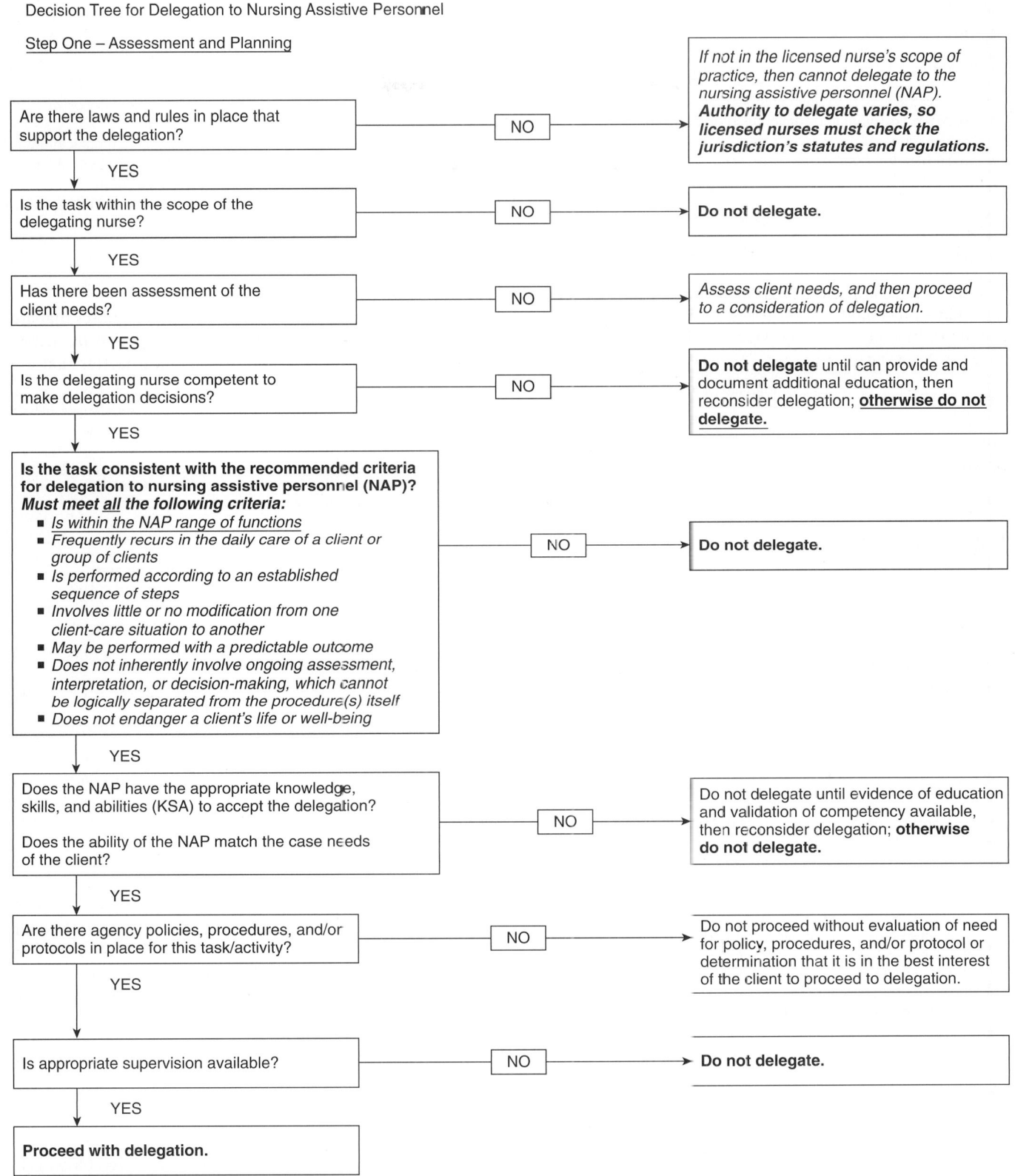

Figure 1-1 National Council of State Boards of Nursing Decision Tree for Delegation to Nursing Assistive Personnel. (From the American Nurses Association and the National Council of State Boards of Nursing: *Joint statement on delegation* [2005]. Available at: www.ncsbn.org/Joint_statement.pdf. Accessed June 9, 2009.)

Continued

NDx = NANDA-I Diagnosis　　**D** = Delegatable Action　　● = UAP　　✦ = LVN/LPN　　⊝▶ = Go to ⊝volve for animation

Step Two – Communication

Communication must be a two-way process.

The nurse:	The NAP:	Documentation:

■ Assesses the assistant's understanding
 ○ How the task is to be accomplished
 ○ When and what information is to be reported, including:
  ✓ Expected observations to report and record
  ✓ Specific client concerns that would require prompt reporting
■ Individualizes for the NAP and client situation
■ Addresses any unique client requirements and characteristics, and clear expectations of:
 ○ Assesses the assistant's understanding of expectations, providing clarification if needed
 ○ Communicates his or her willingness and availability to guide and support assistant
 ○ Assures appropriate accountability by verifying that the receiving person accepts the delegation and accompanying responsibility
	■ **Asks questions regarding the delegation and seeks clarification of expectations if needed**
	■ Informs the nurse if the assistant has not done a task/function/activity before, or has only done infrequently
	■ Asks for additional training or supervision
	■ Affirms understanding of expectations
	■ Determines the communication method between the nurse and the NAP
	■ Determines the communication and plan of action in emergency situations
		Timely, complete, and accurate documentation of provided care:
		■ Facilitates communication with other members of the health care team
		■ Records the nursing care provided

Step Three – Surveillance and Supervision

The purpose of surveillance and monitoring is related to nurse's responsibility for client care within the context of a client population. The nurse supervises the delegation by monitoring the performance of the task or function and assures compliance with standards of practice, policies, and procedures. Frequency, level, and nature of monitoring vary with needs of client and experience of assistant.

The nurse considers the:	The nurse determines:	The nurse is responsible for:
■ Client's health care status and stability of condition ■ Predictability of responses and risks ■ Setting where care occurs ■ Availability of resources and support infrastructure ■ Complexity of the task being performed	■ The frequency of onsite supervision and assessment based on: ○ Needs of the client ○ Complexity of the delegated function/task/activity ○ Proximity of nurse's location	■ Timely intervening and follow-up on problems and concerns. Examples of the need for intervening include: ○ Alertness to subtle signs and symptoms (which allows nurse and assistant to be proactive before a client's condition deteriorates significantly) ○ Awareness of assistant's difficulties in completing delegated activities ○ Providing adequate follow-up to problems and/or changing situations is critical aspect of delegation

Step Four – Evaluation and Feedback

Evaluation is often the forgotten step in delegation.

In considering the effectiveness of delegation, the nurse addresses the following question:
■ Was the delegation successful? ○ Was the task/function/activity performed correctly? ○ Was the client's desired and/or expected outcome achieved? ○ Was the outcome optimal, satisfactory, or unsatisfactory? ○ Was communication timely and effective? ○ What went well? What was challenging? ○ Were there any problems or concerns? If so, how were they addressed? ■ Is there a better way to meet the client need? ■ Is there a need to adjust the overall plan of care, or should this approach be continued? ■ Were there any "learning moment" for the assistant and/or the nurse? ■ Was appropriate feedback provided to the assistant regarding the performance of the delegation? ■ Was the assistant acknowledged for accomplishing the task/activity/function?

Figure 1-1, cont'd National Council of State Boards of Nursing Decision Tree for Delegation to Nursing Assistive Personnel.

From the history it is determined that Mary had a motor vehicle collision 3 weeks ago. She is experiencing back pain related to nerve root irritation at the site of her spinal cord injury. She has been bedridden since the time of her accident. The physician's progress notes indicate that Mary's paraplegia is permanent, and the goal of care is to optimize her current physiological state and keep her comfortable.

Diagnostic test results reveal that Mary's red blood cell (RBC) count, hemoglobin (Hgb), hematocrit (Hct), and serum protein levels are decreased.

The nurses' notes reveal that Mary needs assistance with all activities. She is able to feed herself but is only consuming 10% of her meals. She had a bowel movement this morning following digital stimulation. Mary has an indwelling urinary catheter, and her intake and output are balanced. She has been crying frequently and states that neither she nor her husband are coping well with her disability.

3. **Interview the client and complete an assessment using the tool provided by your nursing school or health care facility.**

   The interview and physical assessment reveal that Mary has persistent reddened areas on her left hip and coccyx; diminished breath sounds bilaterally in both lung bases, shallow respirations of 24 breaths/min; crackles (rales) in both lungs; and a cough that is productive of yellow, foul-smelling sputum. She has normal bowel sounds and states that she usually has a bowel movement every other day following digital stimulation. Mary is alert, oriented, and able to move her upper extremities. She has no movement in her lower extremities, but she is able to transfer herself with assistance to a wheelchair. She complains of pain in her back.

4. **Read about the client's diagnosis and nursing care in a current medical-surgical nursing text.**

   Review **Spinal Cord Injury** and **Impaired Physical Mobility. NDx**

5. **Select the appropriate standardized care plan(s) from this text and read the introductory information at the beginning of the care plan(s).**

   Based on the physician's statement that Mary's primary treatment plan is focused on optimizing her current physical condition and pain control, it is determined that the appropriate care plans for Mary are **Spinal Cord Injury** and **Impaired Physical Mobility. NDx**

6. **Select and prioritize the nursing and collaborative diagnoses that are appropriate for your client. Choose the** etiological factors that are relevant and modify them as appropriate.

   It is determined that there are numerous diagnoses and etiological factors from the care plan on **Spinal Cord Injury.** Examples of some of the nursing diagnoses within this care plan are as follows. The etiological factors have been modified to reflect Mary's situation.

   a. **Ineffective Breathing Pattern NDx**
      related to:
      1. The depressant effect of narcotic (opioid) analgesics loss of abdominal and intercostal muscle function (innervation of these muscles at the thoracic level)
   b. **Ineffective Airway Clearance NDx**
      related to:
      1. Decreased mobility, decreased effectiveness of cough resulting from diminished lung/chest wall expansion, depressant effect of narcotic (opioid) analgesics
   c. **Acute/Chronic Pain:** back-, rib-, and pelvic-related nerve root irritation at the site of spinal cord injury metastases
   d. **Ineffective Coping NDx** related to ongoing grieving associated with spinal cord injury and its effect on body function

7. **Determine which nursing interventions may be delegated to the appropriately qualified individual within the nursing care team.**

   The process for individualization of etiologies and delegation of nursing actions is demonstrated using the nursing diagnosis of **Risk for Constipation NDx** as a prototype.

STANDARDIZED	INDIVIDUALIZED
Risk for Constipation NDx related to: (Etiologies from the care plan on Impaired Physical Mobility NDx) a. Diminished defecation reflex associated with: 　1. Suppression of urge to defecate because of lack of privacy and reluctance to use bedpan 　2. Decreased gravity filling of lower rectum resulting from horizontal positioning	**Risk for Constipation NDx** related to: a. Diminished defecation reflex associated with: 　1. Lack of awareness of stool in rectum associated with sensory loss below the level of injury 　2. Decreased gravity filling of lower rectum resulting from horizontal positioning 　3. Loss of central nervous system control over defecation reflex
b. Weakened abdominal muscles associated with generalized loss of muscle tone resulting from prolonged immobility and lack of innervation	b. Loss of autonomic nervous system function below the level of injury during a period of spinal shock
c. Decreased gastrointestinal motility associated with decreased activity and the increased sympathetic nervous system activity that occurs with anxiety	c. Decreased activity

8. **Modify the desired outcomes so that they are measurable and realistic for your client. Establish appropriate target dates.**

The process for individualization of a desired outcome is demonstrated using the nursing diagnosis of **Risk for Constipation NDx** as a prototype.

NDx = NANDA-I Diagnosis   **D** = Delegatable Action   ● = UAP   ◆ = LVN/LPN   ⊜▶ = Go to ⊜volve for animation

STANDARDIZED

(Outcome from the care plan on Immobility)
The client will not experience constipation as evidenced by:
a. Usual frequency of bowel movements
b. Passage of soft, formed stool
c. Absence of abdominal distention and pain, feeling of rectal fullness or pressure, and straining during defecation

INDIVIDUALIZED

Mary will not experience constipation as evidenced by:
a. Passing soft, formed stool at least every other day
b. Absence of abdominal distention and abdominal pain

STANDARDIZED

(Outcome from the care plan on End-of-Life Care)
The client will maintain a bowel routine that provides optimal comfort.

INDIVIDUALIZED

Same as previous example.

9. **Select the nursing actions that are relevant to the client's care. Add to or modify the actions to meet the needs of your client. Include specific medications and treatments as well as client preferences and other actions that will facilitate the achievement of the desired client outcomes.**

The process for individualization of nursing actions is demonstrated below using the nursing diagnosis of **Risk for Constipation NDx** as a prototype.

STANDARDIZED

a. Assess for signs and symptoms of constipation (e.g., decrease in frequency of bowel movements; passage of hard, formed stools; anorexia; abdominal distention and pain; feeling of fullness or pressure in rectum; straining during defecation).
b. Assess bowel sounds. Report a pattern of decreasing bowel sounds.
c. Implement measures to prevent constipation:
    1. Encourage client to defecate whenever the urge is felt.
    2. Place client in high-Fowler's position for bowel movements unless contraindicated.
    3. Encourage client to relax, provide privacy, and have call signal within reach during attempts to defecate (measures to promote relaxation enable client to relax the levator ani muscle and external anal sphincter, which facilitates evacuation of stool).
    4. Encourage client to establish a regular time for defecation, preferably within an hour after a meal.
    5. Instruct client to increase intake of foods high in fiber (e.g., bran, whole-grain breads and cereals, fresh fruits and vegetables) unless contraindicated.
    6. Instruct client to maintain a minimum fluid intake of 2500 mL/day unless contraindicated.
    7. Encourage client to drink hot liquids upon arising in the morning in order to stimulate peristalsis.
    8. Encourage client to perform isometric abdominal strengthening exercises unless contraindicated.
    9. If client is taking analgesics for pain management, encourage the use of nonnarcotic rather than narcotic (opioid) analgesics when appropriate.
    10. Increase activity as allowed.
    11. Administer laxatives or cathartics and/or enemas if ordered.

INDIVIDUALIZED

a. Assess Mary every shift for signs and symptoms of constipation (e.g., no bowel movement for three days; passage of hard, formed stools; increased anorexia; abdominal distention).
b. Assess bowel sounds. Report a pattern of decreasing bowel sounds.
c. Implement measures to prevent Mary's constipation:
    1. Encourage Mary to use regular rectal stimulation to have a regular bowel movement.
    2. Place Mary on bedpan in high-Fowler's position for bowel movements.
    3. Turn on soft music, provide privacy, and have call signal within reach during attempts to defecate.

    4. Encourage Mary to attempt digital rectal stimulation about 30 minutes after breakfast.
    5. Offer bran cereal and fresh fruit for breakfast; encourage Mary to select foods high in fiber for lunch and dinner.
    6. Encourage Mary to increase her fluid intake; offer 200 mL of apple juice, orange juice, or water every hour while she is awake.
    7. Offer hot tea with breakfast.

    8. Omit—not appropriate for a patient with spinal cord injury.
    9. Omit—Mary needs the narcotic analgesic for effective pain management.

    10. Increase passive and active ROM as indicated.
    11. Administer milk of magnesia, 30 mL p.o. each evening; and Dialose, 100 mg p.o. each morning.

d. Consult physician about checking for an impaction and digitally removing stool if client has not had a bowel movement in three days, if client is passing liquid stool, or if other signs and symptoms of constipation are present.

e. Consult appropriate health care provider if signs and symptoms of constipation persist and appear to be an ongoing problem.

d. Consult physician about checking for an impaction and digitally removing stool if Mary has not had a bowel movement for four days and other signs and symptoms of constipation are present.

e. Consult appropriate health care provider if signs and symptoms of constipation occur and appear to be an ongoing problem.

SAMPLE INDIVIDUALIZED CARE PLAN

Individualized Care Plan for Mary for the Nursing Diagnosis of Risk for Constipation

DATA

Mary states had a bowel movement this morning

Normal bowel sounds

Physician's orders: milk of magnesia, 30 mL p.o. each evening; Dialose, 100 mg p.o. every morning

Bedridden for 3 weeks

Consuming only 10% of meals

Mary states usually has bowel movement every other day (q.o.d.) about 30 minutes after breakfast

Activity: bed rest; requires assistance with all activities

Receiving morphine sulfate every 2 hours

NURSING DIAGNOSIS

Risk for Constipation **NDx** related to:

a. Diminished defecation reflex associated with decreased nervous system responses in spinal cord injury state and decreased gravity filling of lower rectum resulting from horizontal positioning

b. Decreased ability to respond to urge to defecate associated with weakened abdominal muscles and impaired physical mobility

c. Decreased gastrointestinal motility associated with decreased activity, use of morphine sulfate, and increased sympathetic nervous system activity that occurs with anxiety and pain

d. Decreased intake of fluids and foods high in fiber

DESIRED OUTCOME

Mary will not experience constipation as evidenced by:

a. Passing a soft, formed stool at least q.o.d.

b. Absence of abdominal distention

NURSING ACTIONS

a. Assess Mary every shift for signs and symptoms of constipation (e.g., no bowel movement for 3 days; passage of hard, formed stool; increased anorexia; abdominal distention; abdominal pain.

b. Assess bowel sounds. Report a pattern of decreasing bowel sounds.

c. Implement measures to prevent Mary's constipation. **D** ● ✦
  1. Place Mary on bedpan in high-Fowler's position for bowel movements. **D** ● ✦
  2. Turn on soft music, provide privacy, and have call signal within reach during attempts to defecate. **D** ● ✦
  3. Encourage Mary to attempt to digital rectal stimulation about 30 minutes after breakfast. **D** ✦
  4. Offer bran cereal and fresh fruit for breakfast; encourage Mary to select foods high in fiber for lunch and dinner. **D** ✦
  5. Encourage Mary to increase her fluid intake; offer 200 mL of apple juice, orange juice, or water every hour while she is awake. **D** ✦
  6. Offer hot tea with breakfast. **D** ✦
  7. Administer milk of magnesia, 30 mL p.o. each evening, and Dialose, 100 mg p.o. each morning. **D** ✦

d. Consult physician about checking for an impaction and digitally removing stool if Mary has not had a bowel movement for 4 days and other signs and symptoms of constipation are present.

e. Consult appropriate health care provider if signs and symptoms occur and appear to be an ongoing problem.

See Bibliography at the back of the book.

NDx = NANDA-I Diagnosis   **D** = Delegatable Action   ● = UAP   ✦ = LVN/LPN   ⊜▶ = Go to ⊜volve for animation

2

Selected Nursing Diagnoses, Interventions, Rationales, and Documentation

---

Nursing Diagnosis | ## ACTIVITY INTOLERANCE NDx

Definition: Insufficient physiological or psychological energy to endure or complete required or desired daily activities

CLINICAL MANIFESTATIONS

Subjective	**Objective**
Verbal report of fatigue or weakness	Abnormal heart rate or blood pressure response to activity; exertional discomfort or dyspnea; electrocardiographic changes reflecting dysrhythmias or ischemia; unable to speak with physical activity

RISK FACTORS

- Bedrest or immobility
- Generalized weakness
- Sedentary lifestyle
- Imbalance between oxygen supply/demand

DESIRED OUTCOMES

The client will demonstrate an increased tolerance for activity as evidenced by:
a. Verbalization of feeling less fatigued and weak
b. Ability to perform activities of daily living without exertional dyspnea, chest pain, diaphoresis, dizziness, and significant changes in vital signs

DOCUMENTATION

- Activity level
- Statements of weakness and fatigue
- Exertional dyspnea, chest pain, diaphoresis, or dizziness
- Vital signs before, during, and after activity
- Therapeutic interventions
- Client teaching

NOC OUTCOMES

Activity tolerance; discomfort level; endurance; fatigue level; psychomotor energy; self-care status; self-care: activities of daily living; vital signs; energy conservation

NIC INTERVENTIONS

Activity therapy; energy management; oxygen therapy; nutrition management; sleep enhancement; cardiac care; cardiac rehabilitation; teaching regarding prescribed activity

---

NURSING ASSESSMENT	**RATIONALE**
Assess for signs and symptoms of activity intolerance: • Statements of fatigue or weakness • Exertional dyspnea, chest pain, diaphoresis, or dizziness • Abnormal heart rate response to activity (e.g., increase in rate of 20 beats/min above resting rate, rate not returning to preactivity level within 3 minutes after stopping activity, change from regular to irregular rate) • A significant change (15 to 20 mm Hg) in blood pressure with activity	*Early recognition of signs and symptoms of activity intolerance allows for prompt intervention.*
Assess complete blood cell count (CBC) and report abnormal values.	*Anemia results in decreased oxygen-carrying capacity of the blood.*

THERAPEUTIC INTERVENTIONS	RATIONALE

Independent Actions

Implement measures to promote rest and/or conserve energy (e.g., maintain prescribed activity restrictions, minimize environmental activity and noise, provide uninterrupted rest periods, assist with care, and limit the number of visitors). **D** ● ✦

Cells use oxygen and fat, protein, and carbohydrate to produce the energy needed for all body activities. Rest and activities that conserve energy result in a lower metabolic rate, which preserves nutrients and oxygen for necessary activities.

Discourage smoking and excessive intake of beverages high in caffeine such as coffee, tea, and colas.

Both nicotine and excessive caffeine intake can increase cardiac workload and myocardial oxygen utilization, thereby decreasing the amount of oxygen necessary for energy production.

Implement measures to improve respiratory status (e.g., encourage use of incentive spirometer; elevate head of bed; assist with turning, coughing, and deep breathing) if ineffective breathing pattern, ineffective airway clearance, or impaired gas exchange is contributing to client's activity intolerance. **D** ✦

Altered respiratory function can lead to inadequate tissue oxygenation, which results in less efficient energy production and a reduced ability to tolerate activity. Improving respiratory status increases the amount of oxygen available for energy production. It also eases the work of breathing, which reduces energy expenditure.

Instruct client to report a decreased tolerance for activity and to stop any activity that causes chest pain, shortness of breath, dizziness, or extreme fatigue or weakness.

These symptoms indicate that insufficient oxygen is reaching the tissues and that activity has been increased beyond a therapeutic level.

Dependent/Collaborative Actions

Implement measures to increase cardiac output (e.g., administer positive inotropic agents, vasodilators, or antidysrhythmics as ordered; elevate the head of the bed) if decreased cardiac output is contributing to the client's activity intolerance.

Sufficient cardiac output is necessary to maintain an adequate blood flow and oxygen supply to the tissues. Adequate tissue oxygenation promotes more efficient energy production, which subsequently improves client's activity tolerance.

Implement measures to reduce fever if present (e.g., administer tepid sponge bath, administer antipyretics as ordered). **D** ✦

An elevated temperature increases the metabolic rate with subsequent depletion of available energy and a decrease in the ability to tolerate activity.

Maintain oxygen therapy as ordered.

An oxygen deficiency results in anaerobic metabolism, which is less efficient than the aerobic mechanism of energy supply. Supplemental oxygen helps to alleviate hypoxia and restore the more efficient aerobic metabolism, thereby improving energy levels and activity tolerance.

Implement measures to maintain an adequate nutritional status (e.g., provide a diet high in essential nutrients, provide dietary supplements as indicated, and administer vitamins and minerals as ordered).

Metabolism is the process by which nutrients are transformed into energy. If nutrition is inadequate, energy production is decreased, which subsequently reduces one's ability to tolerate activity.

Implement measures to treat anemia if present (e.g., administer prescribed iron, folic acid, and/or vitamin B_{12}; administer packed red blood cells as ordered). **D**

Anemia reduces the oxygen-carrying capacity of the blood. Resolution of anemia increases oxygen availability to the cells, which increases the efficiency of energy production and subsequently improves activity tolerance.

Increase client's activity gradually as allowed and tolerated. **D** ● ✦

A gradual increase in activity helps prevent a sudden increase in cardiac workload and myocardial oxygen consumption and the subsequent imbalance between oxygen supply and demand. Progressive activity also helps strengthen the myocardium, which enhances cardiac output and improves activity tolerance.

Consult physician if signs and symptoms of activity intolerance persist.

Notifying the physician allows for modification of the treatment plan.

Nursing Diagnosis | **AIRWAY CLEARANCE, INEFFECTIVE** NDx

Definition: Inability to clear secretions or obstructions from the respiratory tract to maintain a clear airway

CLINICAL MANIFESTATIONS

Subjective	Objective
Verbal report of shortness of breath	Dyspnea, orthopnea; diminished breath sounds; adventitious breath sounds (crackles, rhonchi, wheezes); cough, ineffective or absent sputum production; difficulty vocalizing; wide-eyed; restlessness; changes in respiratory rate and rhythm; cyanosis

RISK FACTORS

- **Environmental:** Smoking; smoke inhalation; second-hand smoke
- **Obstructed airway:** Airway spasm; retained secretions; excessive mucus; presence of artificial airway; foreign body in airway; secretions in the bronchi; exudates in the alveoli
- **Physiological:** Neuromuscular dysfunction; hyperplasia of the bronchial walls; chronic obstructive pulmonary disease; infection; asthma; allergic/reactive airways

DESIRED OUTCOMES

The client will maintain clear, open airways as evidenced by:
a. Normal breath sounds
b. Normal rate and depth of respirations
c. Absence of dyspnea

DOCUMENTATION

- Breath sounds
- Rate, depth, and ease of respirations
- Characteristics of cough
- Description of sputum
- Therapeutic interventions
- Client teaching

NOC OUTCOMES

Aspiration prevention; mechanical ventilation response: respiratory status: airway patency; respiratory status: ventilation

NIC INTERVENTIONS

Respiratory monitoring; airway management; airway suctioning; chest physiotherapy; cough enhancement

NURSING ASSESSMENT

Assess for signs and symptoms of ineffective airway clearance:
- Abnormal breath sounds
- Rapid, shallow respirations
- Dyspnea
- Nonproductive cough

RATIONALE

Early recognition of signs and symptoms of ineffective airway clearance allows for prompt intervention.

THERAPEUTIC INTERVENTIONS

RATIONALE

Independent Actions
Implement measures to decrease pain if present:
- Splint chest or abdominal incisions with pillow when coughing and deep breathing. **D** ✦

Instruct and assist client to change position, deep breathe, and cough or "huff" every 1 to 2 hours. **D** ✦

Pain often interferes with a client's willingness to move, cough, and deep breathe. Pain reduction enables the client to increase activity and cough and deep breathe more effectively, all of which promote effective airway clearance.

Repositioning helps mobilize secretions. Deep breathing helps clear the airways by loosening secretions and promoting a more effective cough. Coughing or "huffing" (i.e., a forced expiration technique) accelerates airflow through the airways, which helps mobilize and clear mucus and foreign matter from the respiratory tract.

Continued...

THERAPEUTIC INTERVENTIONS	RATIONALE
Discourage smoking.	*Irritants present in smoke increase mucus production, impair ciliary function, and can cause inflammation and damage to the bronchial walls. This results in narrowed airways and stasis of pulmonary secretions.*
Perform oral suctioning if needed. **D** ✦	*Suctioning removes secretions from the large airways. It also stimulates coughing, which helps clear airways of mucus and foreign matter.*

Dependent/Collaborative Actions

Implement measures to decrease pain: • Administer prescribed analgesics before planned activity. **D** ✦	*Pain often interferes with a client's willingness to move, cough, and deep breathe. Pain reduction enables the client to increase activity and cough and deep breathe more effectively, all of which promote effective airway clearance.*
Increase activity as allowed and tolerated. **D** ● ✦	*Activity helps to mobilize secretions and promotes deeper breathing. Deep breathing can help loosen secretions and enhance the effectiveness of coughing.*
Implement measures to thin secretions and maintain adequate moisture of the respiratory mucous membranes: • Maintain a fluid intake of 2500 mL/day, if tolerated. • Humidify inspired air. **D** ✦	*Adequate hydration and humidified inspired air help thin secretions, which facilitates the mobilization and expectoration of secretions. These actions also reduce dryness of the respiratory mucous membrane, which helps enhance mucociliary clearance.*
Assist with the administration of mucolytics (e.g., acetylcysteine) and diluting or hydrating agents (e.g., water, saline) via nebulizer as ordered.	*Mucolytics and diluents or hydrating agents are mucokinetic substances that reduce the viscosity of mucus, thus making it easier for the client to mobilize and clear secretions from the respiratory tract.*
Administer expectorants if ordered (e.g., guaifenesin, dornase alfa). **D** ✦	*Expectorants reduce the viscosity of sputum, making it easier to be removed by coughing or suctioning.*
Administer the following medications if ordered: • Bronchodilators • Methylxanthines (e.g., theophylline, aminophylline, oxtriphylline) • Sympathomimetic (adrenergic) agents (e.g., albuterol, terbutaline, metaproterenol, salmeterol) • Anticholinergic agents (e.g., ipratropium) • Corticosteroids • Prednisone • Methylprednisolone • Beclomethasone • Flunisolide • Triamcinolone • Budesonide • Leukotriene modifiers • Montelukast • Zafirlukast **D** ✦	*These medications increase the patency of the airways and enhance bronchial airflow. Methylxanthines and sympathomimetics produce bronchodilation by relaxing the bronchial smooth muscle. Anticholinergic agents block cholinergic reflex constriction of the bronchioles and decrease mucus production. Corticosteroids and leukotriene modifiers reduce inflammation in the airways, which results in decreased bronchial hyperactivity and constriction and mucus production.*
Administer central nervous system depressants judiciously.	*Central nervous system depressants depress the cough reflex, which can result in stasis of secretions.*
Assist with or perform postural drainage therapy if ordered.	*Postural drainage therapy techniques (e.g., vibration, percussion, postural drainage) use the forces of motion and gravity to mobilize secretions from the periphery of the lungs to the larger central airways where they can be removed by coughing or suctioning.*
Consult the appropriate health care provider (e.g., physician, respiratory therapist) if signs and symptoms of ineffective airway clearance persist.	*Notifying the appropriate health care provider allows for modification of the treatment plan.*

Nursing Diagnosis ANXIETY NDx

Definition: Vague, uneasy feeling of discomfort or dread accompanied by an autonomic response (the source is often nonspecific or unknown to the individual); a feeling of apprehension caused by anticipation of danger. It is an altering signal that warns of impending danger and enables the individual to take measures to deal with a threat.

CLINICAL MANIFESTATIONS

Subjective	**Objective**
Behavioral: Expressed concerns due to change in life events	**Behavioral:** Diminished productivity; scanning and vigilance; poor eye contact; restlessness; glancing about; extraneous movement (e.g., foot shuffling, hand/arm movements); insomnia; fidgeting
Affective: Expression of painful and persistent increased helplessness; uncertainty; increased wariness; feelings of inadequacy	**Affective:** Regretful; irritability, anguish; scared; jittery; overexcited; rattled; focus on self; fearful; distressed; worried, apprehensive; anxious
Physiological: Reported dry mouth; nausea, fatigue	**Physiological:** Voice quivering; trembling/hand tremors; shakiness; urinary urgency; increased pulse; pupil dilation; increased reflexes; abdominal pain; sleep disturbance; tingling in extremities; cardiovascular excitation; increased perspiration; facial tension; anorexia; heart pounding; diarrhea; weakness; facial flushing; superficial vasoconstriction; twitching; faintness; respiratory difficulties; increased blood pressure
Cognitive: Reported fear of unspecific consequences; awareness of physiological symptoms	**Cognitive:** Blocking of thought; confusion; preoccupation; forgetfulness; rumination; impaired attention; decreased perceptual field; tendency to blame others; difficulty concentrating; diminished ability to problem solve; diminished ability to learn

RISK FACTORS

- Exposure to toxins
- Threat to or change in role status
- Unconscious conflict about essential values/goals of life
- Familial association/hereditary
- Unmet needs
- Interpersonal transmission/contagion
- Situational/maturational crises
- Threat of death
- Threat to or change in health status
- Threat to or change in interaction patterns
- Threat to or change in role function
- Threat to self-concept
- Threat to or change in environment
- Stress
- Threat to or change in economic status
- Substance abuse

DESIRED OUTCOMES

The client will experience a reduction in anxiety as evidenced by:
  a. Verbalization of feeling less anxious
  b. Usual sleep pattern
  c. Relaxed facial expression and body movements
  d. Stable vital signs
  e. Usual perceptual ability and interaction with others

DOCUMENTATION

- Verbalization of feeling anxious
- Sleep pattern
- Facial expression and body movement
- Vital signs
- Focus on self
- Client's perception of precipitating factors
- Therapeutic interventions
- Client/family teaching

NOC OUTCOMES

Anxiety level; anxiety self-control; concentration; coping; hyperactivity level

NIC INTERVENTIONS

Anxiety reduction; calming technique; emotional support; presence

NURSING ASSESSMENT

Assess for signs and symptoms of anxiety:
- Verbalization of feeling anxious
- Insomnia
- Tenseness
- Shakiness
- Restlessness
- Diaphoresis
- Tachycardia
- Elevated blood pressure
- Self-focused behaviors

RATIONALE

Early recognition of signs and symptoms of anxiety allows for prompt intervention.

NDx = NANDA-I Diagnosis   **D** = Delegatable Action   ● = UAP   ✦ = LVN/LPN   ⊖▶ = Go to ⊖volve for animation

Continued...

THERAPEUTIC INTERVENTIONS	RATIONALE

Independent Actions

Encourage verbalization of feelings and concerns and assist client to identify specific stressors that may be causing anxiety. Provide feedback.

Verbalization of feelings and concerns helps the client identify factors that are causing anxiety. Providing feedback helps the client clarify and validate feelings and concerns and identify techniques that can reduce anxiety.

Orient client to environment, equipment, and routines. **D ✦ ●**

Familiarity with the environment and usual routines reduces the client's anxiety about the unknown, provides a sense of security, and increases his/her sense of control, all of which help decrease anxiety.

All care providers should properly introduce themselves and identify their role. If possible, maintain consistency in staff assigned to his/her care.

Introduction to staff familiarizes the client with those individuals who will be working with him/her, which provides the client with a feeling of stability, which reduces the anxiety that typically occurs with change.

Assure client that staff members are nearby. Respond to call signal as soon as possible.

Close contact and a prompt response to requests provide a sense of security and facilitate the development of trust, thus reducing the client's anxiety.

All care providers should maintain a calm, supportive, confident manner when interacting with the client. **D ✦ ●**

A sense of calmness and confidence conveys to the client that someone is in control of the situation, which helps reduce anxiety.

Reinforce physician's explanations and clarify misconceptions the client has about the diagnostic tests, disease condition, treatment plan, surgical procedure, and/or prognosis.

Factual information and an awareness of what to expect help decrease the anxiety that arises from uncertainty.

Implement measures to reduce respiratory distress if present:
- Elevate the head of the bed.
- Encourage the client to breathe deeply and more slowly.

Improvement of respiratory status helps relieve anxiety associated with the feeling of not being able to breathe.

Implement measures to reduce pain if present:
- Instruct and assist with relaxation techniques.

Pain can create or increase anxiety because it is often perceived as a threat to well-being. Pain also causes sympathetic nervous system stimulation with subsequent feelings of tenseness and increased anxiety.

Provide a calm, restful environment. **D ●**

A calm, restful environment facilitates relaxation and promotes a sense of security, which reduces anxiety.

When appropriate, assist the client to meet spiritual needs (e.g., arrange for a visit from the clergy).

Spiritual support is a source of comfort and security for many people and can help reduce the client's anxiety.

Encourage significant others to project a caring, concerned attitude without obvious anxiousness.

Anxiety is easily transferable from one person to another. If significant others convey empathy, provide reassurance, and do not appear anxious, they can help reduce the client's anxiety.

Include significant others in orientation and teaching sessions and encourage their continued support of the client.

Significant others can help reduce the client's anxiety by reinforcing information that he/she has difficulty understanding or recalling. In addition, the presence of significant others often provides the client with a sense of support and security, which helps to reduce anxiety.

Provide information based on current needs of client at a level he/she can understand. Encourage the client to ask questions and to seek clarification of information provided.

Providing the client with information that he/she is not ready to process or cannot understand tends to increase anxiety. Making the client feel comfortable enough to ask questions or clarify information helps to reduce anxiety.

Include significant others in orientation and teaching sessions and encourage their continued support of the client.

Significant others can help reduce the client's anxiety by reinforcing information that he/she has difficulty understanding or recalling. In addition, the presence of significant others often provides the client with a sense of support and security, which helps reduce anxiety.

Dependent/Collaborative Actions

Administer oxygen therapy as ordered. **D ✦**

Improvement of respiratory status helps relieve anxiety associated with the feeling of not being able to breathe.

Administer prescribed analgesics if pain is present. **D ✦**

Pain can create or increase anxiety because it is often perceived as a threat to well-being. Pain also causes sympathetic nervous system stimulation with subsequent feelings of tenseness and increased anxiety.

THERAPEUTIC INTERVENTIONS	RATIONALE
Administer prescribed antianxiety agents if indicated. **D** ✦	*Medications are sometimes prescribed to help reduce the client's anxiety. Benzodiazepines (e.g., lorazepam, diazepam, alprazolam, chlordiazepoxide) are the drugs of choice for management of short-term anxiety. These drugs augment the inhibitory effect of gamma-aminobutyric acid (GABA) on cell membrane responses to excitatory neurotransmitters.*
Initiate a social service referral and/or assist client to identify and contact appropriate community resources if indicated.	*Concerns about factors such as finances, follow-up medical care, and home maintenance can be a source of great anxiety. Facilitating contact with the appropriate resources can help reduce the client's anxiety and provide ongoing support.*
Consult appropriate health care provider (e.g., psychiatric nurse practitioner, psychologist, psychiatrist, physician) if above actions fail to control anxiety.	*Notifying the appropriate health care provider allows for modification of the treatment plan.*

Nursing Diagnosis ASPIRATION, RISK FOR NDx

Definition: At risk for entry of gastrointestinal secretions, oropharyngeal secretions, solids, or fluids into tracheobronchial passages

CLINICAL MANIFESTATIONS

Subjective	Objective
Report of shortness of breath, difficulty swallowing	Rhonchi; dull percussion note over affected lung area; cough; tachypnea; tachycardia; presence of tube feeding in tracheal aspirate; dyspnea, cough, excessive drooling

RISK FACTORS

- Reduced level of consciousness
- Depressed cough and gag reflexes
- Presence of tracheostomy or endotracheal tube
- Incompetent lower esophageal sphincter
- Gastrointestinal tubes
- Tube feedings
- Medication administration
- Situations hindering elevation of upper body
- Increased intragastric pressure
- Increased gastric residual
- Decreased gastrointestinal motility
- Delayed gastric emptying
- Impaired swallowing
- Facial, oral, neck surgery or trauma
- Wired jaws

DESIRED OUTCOMES

The client will not aspirate secretions or foods/fluids as evidenced by:
  a. Clear breath sounds
  b. Resonant percussion note over lungs
  c. Absence of cough, tachypnea, and dyspnea

DOCUMENTATION

- Breath sounds
- Percussion note over lungs
- Respiratory rate and effort
- Presence of cough
- Pulse rate
- Color of tracheal aspirate
- Therapeutic interventions
- Client/family teaching

NOC OUTCOMES

Aspiration prevention; body positioning: self initiated; gastrointestinal function; nausea and vomiting control; respiratory status; risk control; swallowing status

NIC INTERVENTIONS

Aspiration precautions; respiratory monitoring; swallowing therapy; airway suctioning

Continued...

NURSING ASSESSMENT	RATIONALE
Assess for and report signs and symptoms of aspiration of secretions or foods/fluids: • Rhonchi • Dull percussion note over affected lung area • Cough • Tachypnea • Dyspnea • Tachycardia • Presence of tube feeding in tracheal aspirate	*Early recognition of signs and symptoms of aspiration allows for prompt intervention.*
Assist with diagnostic studies to determine if aspiration is occurring during swallowing (e.g., videofluoroscopy).	*Aspiration of foods/fluids during swallowing process is evident on studies such as videofluoroscopy. Knowing when aspiration occurs during the swallowing process aids in the development of an individualized plan of care to prevent further aspiration.*
Monitor chest radiograph results. Report findings of pulmonary infiltrate.	*Evidence of pulmonary infiltrate on chest radiograph results can indicate that aspiration has occurred.*

THERAPEUTIC INTERVENTIONS	RATIONALE

Independent Actions

Implement measures to prevent aspiration if client has a depressed or absent gag reflex, severe dysphagia, and/or decreased level of consciousness:	*The risk for aspiration is high when mechanisms to protect the client's airway (e.g., gag reflex, swallowing reflex) are impaired or the client has a decreased level of consciousness.*
• Withhold oral foods/fluids. **D** ✦	*Withholding oral foods/fluids eliminates the possibility of aspiration of same.*
• Place client in a side-lying position unless contraindicated. **D** ● ✦	*Placing the client in a side-lying position allows oral secretions to accumulate in the mouth where they can be expectorated or removed by suctioning rather than flow into the pharynx where they can enter the larynx and be aspirated.*
• Perform oral hygiene and/or oropharyngeal suctioning as often as needed to remove excess secretions. **D** ✦	*Removing excess secretions from the mouth and pharynx prevents them from entering the larynx and being aspirated.*
Implement measures to prevent vomiting (e.g., eliminate noxious sights and odors). **D** ✦	*When the client vomits, gastric contents move up the esophagus, through the pharynx, and into the mouth. While vomitus is in the pharynx, it can spill into the larynx resulting in aspiration.*
If client is receiving tube feedings, check tube placement before each feeding or on a routine basis if tube feeding is continuous. **D** ✦	*Verification of feeding tube placement ensures that the tube feeding solution goes into the alimentary tract rather than the lungs.*
Implement measures to prevent aspiration when client is eating and drinking:	*When the client is eating and drinking, there is a high risk for aspiration before the swallowing reflex is triggered (i.e., the larynx and pharynx are at rest and the airway is open at this time), during swallowing if the larynx does not close completely, and after swallowing when the larynx opens again.*
• Place client in high Fowler's position unless contraindicated. **D** ● ✦	*This position uses gravity to facilitate movement of foods/fluids through the pharynx into the esophagus where the risk for aspiration is greatly reduced.*
• Instruct client to avoid laughing or talking when swallowing.	*Normally, when the swallowing reflex is triggered, the folds of the larynx that form its three valves contract so that aspiration does not occur as foods/fluids pass from the back of the mouth through the pharynx. When the client talks and laughs, air is forced through the trachea and the larynx opens. Instructing the client to avoid talking and laughing when swallowing reduces the risk of the airway being open when food/fluid is in the pharynx.*

THERAPEUTIC INTERVENTIONS	RATIONALE
• Encourage client to concentrate on eating and drinking and allow ample time for meals and snacks.	*If the client becomes distracted and/or is rushed during meals or snacks, swallowing and breathing attempts can become uncoordinated. This results in the larynx being open when the food/fluid is in the pharynx, which greatly increases the risk for aspiration.*
• Instruct client to dry swallow, cough twice, or clear his or her throat after swallowing if indicated.	*If the client has a swallowing impairment such as decreased pharyngeal peristalsis, food/fluid can remain in the pharyngeal recesses after the swallowing reflex has occurred. Dry swallowing, coughing, or clearing the throat helps ensure that the pharynx is clear after swallowing, which reduces the risk for aspiration.*
Instruct and assist the client to perform oral hygiene after meals.	*Good oral hygiene after meals results in removal of remaining food particles that could enter the larynx and be aspirated into the lungs.*
Dependent/Collaborative Actions Administer antiemetics as ordered. **D** ✦	*When the client vomits, gastric contents move up the esophagus, through the pharynx, and into the mouth. While vomitus is in the pharynx, it can spill into the larynx resulting in aspiration.*
Implement measures to reduce the risk of regurgitation (i.e., maintain gastric decompression as ordered, provide small meals rather than large ones, evaluate patient clinical tolerance of tube feedings if gastric residual greater than 200 to 250 mL), maintain client in high Fowler's position for at least 30 minutes after meals and tube feedings, administer upper gastrointestinal stimulants as ordered. **D** ✦	*As gastric secretions or foods/fluids accumulate in the stomach, upward pressure is placed on the lower esophageal sphincter (LES). If the pressure increases significantly and/or the client has an incompetent LES, regurgitation can occur. Contents that move up through the esophagus into the pharynx can spill into the larynx, resulting in aspiration.*
Perform actions to improve swallowing if indicated (e.g., select foods/fluids appropriate to client's swallowing ability, reinforce exercises to strengthen and develop muscles used in swallowing).	*Improving the ability to swallow helps ensure that foods/fluids do not enter the larynx when the client is eating or drinking.*

Nursing Diagnosis BREATHING PATTERN, INEFFECTIVE NDx

Definition: Inspiration and/or expiration that does not provide adequate ventilation

CLINICAL MANIFESTATIONS

Subjective	Objective
Verbal reports of shortness of breath	Dyspnea; orthopnea; respiratory rate (adults [ages ≥14 years], <11 or >24 breaths/min; infants, <25 or >60 breaths/min; ages 1 to 4 years, <20 or >30 breaths/min; ages 5 to 14 years, <14 or >25 breaths/min); depth of breathing (tidal volume: adults, 500 mL at rest; infants, 6 to 8 mL/kg); decreased inspiratory/expiratory pressure; decreased minute ventilation; decreased vital capacity; nasal flaring; use of accessory muscles to breathe; assumption of three-point position; altered chest excursion; pursed-lip breathing; prolonged expiration phases; increased anterior-posterior chest diameter; decreased pulse oximetry readings

RISK FACTORS

- Hyperventilation
- Hypoventilation syndrome
- Bony deformity
- Pain
- Perception/cognitive impairment

- Anxiety
- Decreased energy/fatigue
- Neuromuscular dysfunction
- Musculoskeletal impairment
- Chest wall deformity

- Obesity
- Spinal cord injury
- Body position
- Neurological immaturity
- Respiratory muscle fatigue

Continued...

DESIRED OUTCOMES

The client will maintain an effective breathing pattern as evidenced by:
a. Normal rate and depth of respirations
b. Symmetrical chest excursion
c. Absence of dyspnea

NOC OUTCOMES

Respiratory status: airway patency; respiratory status: ventilation; respiratory status: gas exchange; vital signs

DOCUMENTATION

- Rate, depth, and ease of respirations
- Chest excursion
- Oximetry results
- Therapeutic interventions
- Client teaching

NIC INTERVENTIONS

Respiratory monitoring; ventilation assistance; anxiety reduction

NURSING ASSESSMENT

Assess for signs and symptoms of an ineffective breathing pattern (e.g., shallow respirations, tachypnea, limited chest excursion, dyspnea, use of accessory muscles when breathing).

Monitor for and report a significant decrease in oximetry results.

RATIONALE

Early recognition of signs and symptoms of an ineffective breathing pattern allows for prompt intervention.

Oximetry is a noninvasive method of measuring arterial oxygen saturation. The results assist in evaluating respiratory status.

THERAPEUTIC INTERVENTIONS

Independent Actions
Implement measures to reduce chest or abdominal pain if present (e.g., splint incision with pillow during coughing and deep breathing). **D** ✦

Implement measures to decrease fear and anxiety (e.g., assure client that breathing deeply will not dislodge tubes or cause incision to break open, interact with client in a confident manner).

Implement measures to increase strength and activity tolerance if client is weak and fatigued (e.g., provide uninterrupted rest periods, maintain optimal nutrition). **D** ✦

Place client in a semi- to high-Fowler's position unless contraindicated. Position with pillows to prevent slumping. **D** ● ✦

If client must remain flat in bed, assist with position change at least every 2 hours. **D** ● ✦

Instruct client to deep breathe or use incentive spirometer every 1 to 2 hours. **D** ✦

Instruct client in and assist with diaphragmatic and pursed-lip breathing techniques if appropriate. NOTE: Diaphragmatic breathing is most often indicated for clients who have had thoracic surgery or clients who have chronic airflow limitation (e.g., emphysema) or neuromuscular conditions that cause fixation or weakening of the diaphragm.

RATIONALE

A client with chest or upper abdominal pain often guards respiratory efforts and breathes shallowly in an attempt to prevent additional discomfort.

Fear and anxiety may cause a client to breathe shallowly or to hyperventilate. Decreasing fear and anxiety allows the client to focus on breathing more slowly and taking deeper breaths.

An increase in strength and activity tolerance enables the client to breathe more deeply and participate in activities to improve breathing pattern.

A semi- to high-Fowler's position allows for maximal diaphragmatic excursion and lung expansion. Prevention of slumping is essential because slumping causes the abdominal contents to be pushed up against the diaphragm and restricts lung expansion.

Compression of the thorax and subsequent limited chest wall and lung expansion occur when the client lies in one position. Frequent repositioning promotes maximal chest wall and lung expansion.

Deep breathing and use of an incentive spirometer promote maximal inhalation and lung expansion. Deep inhalation also stimulates surfactant production, which lowers alveolar surface tension and subsequently increases lung compliance and ease of inflation.

Diaphragmatic breathing promotes greater movement of the diaphragm and decreases the use of accessory muscles for inspiration. Use of this technique eases the work of breathing and ultimately promotes an increased efficiency of alveolar ventilation. Pursed-lip breathing causes a mild resistance to exhalation, which creates positive pressure in the airways. This pressure helps prevent airway collapse and subsequently promotes more complete alveolar emptying.

THERAPEUTIC INTERVENTIONS	RATIONALE
Instruct client to breathe slowly if hyperventilating.	*Hyperventilation is an ineffective breathing pattern that can eventually lead to respiratory alkalosis. The client can often slow breathing rate if he/she concentrates on doing so.*

Dependent/Collaborative Actions

Administer prescribed analgesics before planned activity. **D ✦**	*Pain reduction enables the client to breathe more deeply.*
Assist with positive airway pressure techniques (e.g., continuous positive airway pressure [CPAP], bilevel positive airway pressure [BiPAP], flutter/positive expiratory pressure [PEP] device) if ordered.	*Positive airway pressure techniques increase intrapulmonary (i.e., alveolar) pressure, which helps reexpand collapsed alveoli and prevent further alveolar collapse.*
Instruct client in and assist with segmental or localized breathing exercises if appropriate (may be indicated for clients with painful respiratory conditions or clients who have had thoracic or abdominal surgery).	*Segmental or localized breathing exercises improve expansion of apical and/or basal areas of the lung by having the client focus on selectively expanding these areas of the chest.*
Increase activity as allowed and tolerated. **D ✦**	*During activity, especially ambulation, the client usually takes deeper breaths, thus increasing lung expansion.*
Administer central nervous system depressants judiciously. Hold medication and consult physician if respiratory rate is less than 12/min.	*Central nervous system depressants cause depression of the respiratory center in the brainstem, which can result in a decreased rate and depth of respiration.*
Consult appropriate health care provider (e.g., physician, respiratory therapist) if ineffective breathing pattern continues.	*Notifying the appropriate health care provider allows for modification of treatment plan.*

Nursing Diagnosis ## CARDIAC OUTPUT, DECREASED NDx

Definition: Inadequate blood pumped by the heart to meet metabolic demands of the body

CLINICAL MANIFESTATIONS

Subjective	Objective
Behavioral/Emotional: Verbalization of anxiety; restlessness	**Altered Heart Rate/Rhythm:** Dysrhythmias; palpitations; electrocardiogram (ECG) changes
	Altered Preload: Jugular vein distention (JVD); fatigue; edema; murmurs; increased/decreased central venous pressure (CVP); increased/decreased pulmonary artery wedge pressure (PAWP); weight gain
	Altered Afterload: Cold/clammy skin; shortness of breath/dyspnea; oliguria; prolonged capillary refill; decreased peripheral pulses; variations in blood pressure (BP) readings; increased/decreased systemic vascular resistance (SVR); increased/decreased pulmonary vascular resistance (PVR); skin color changes
	Altered Contractility: Crackles; cough; orthopnea/paroxysmal nocturnal dyspnea; cardiac output (CO) <4 L/min; cardiac index <2.5 L/min; decreased ejection fraction, stroke volume index (SVI), left ventricular stroke work index (LVSWI); S_3 or S_4 sounds

RISK FACTORS

- Altered heart rate/rhythm
- Altered stroke volume
- Altered preload
- Altered afterload
- Altered contractility

Continued...

DESIRED OUTCOMES

The client will maintain adequate CO as evidenced by:
  a. BP within normal range for client
  b. Apical pulse regular and 60 to 100 beats/min
  c. Absence of gallop rhythms
  d. Absence of fatigue and weakness
  e. Unlabored respirations at 12 to 20 breaths/min
  f. Clear, audible breath sounds
  g. Usual mental status

DOCUMENTATION

- Vital signs
- Heart sounds
- Activity tolerance
- Breath sounds
- Ease of respirations
- Mental status
- Peripheral pulses
- Capillary refill time
- Skin color and temperature
- Urine output
- Presence of edema
- Presence of JVD
- Hemodynamic measurements (e.g., CO, pulmonary artery pressure [PAP], pulmonary capillary wedge pressure [PCWP], CVP)
- Therapeutic interventions
- Client teaching
- Dysrhythmias

NOC OUTCOMES

Cardiac pump effectiveness; cardiopulmonary status; circulation status; fluid overload severity; tissue perfusion: abdominal organs, cardiac, cellular, cerebral, and peripheral; vital signs

NIC INTERVENTIONS

Cardiac care: acute; invasive hemodynamic monitoring; hemodynamic regulation; cardiac precautions; dysrhythmia management; oxygen therapy; hypovolemia management; hypervolemia management; electrolyte management: hypomagnesemia; electrolyte management: hyperkalemia; cardiac care: rehabilitative

NURSING ASSESSMENT

Assess for and report signs and symptoms of decreased CO:
- Variations in BP (may be increased because of compensatory vasoconstriction; may be decreased when compensatory mechanisms and pump fail)
- Tachycardia
- Presence of gallop rhythm
- Fatigue and weakness
- Dyspnea, tachypnea
- Crackles (rales)
- Restlessness, change in mental status
- Dizziness, syncope
- Diminished or absent peripheral pulses
- Cool extremities
- Pallor or cyanosis of skin
- Capillary refill time greater than 2 to 3 seconds
- Oliguria
- Edema
- JVD
- Hemodynamic abnormalities such as decreased CO and increased PAP, PCWP, and CVP

Monitor ECG readings and report significant abnormalities.

Monitor chest radiograph results. Report findings of cardiomegaly, pulmonary vascular congestion, pleural effusion, or pulmonary edema.

RATIONALE

Early recognition of signs and symptoms of decreased CO allows for prompt intervention.

ECG readings provide data regarding functioning of the heart's electrical conduction system. Altered generation or transmission of electrical impulses often causes an abnormal heart rate or rhythm that can lead to decreased CO.

Chest radiograph films provide data regarding the size of the heart, volume of blood in the pulmonary vessels, and fluid accumulation in the pleural space, pulmonary interstitium, and alveoli. Cardiomegaly often results in decreased CO, whereas pulmonary vascular congestion, pleural effusion, and pulmonary edema are often a result of decreased CO.

NURSING ASSESSMENT	RATIONALE
Monitor serum electrolytes, cardiac enzymes, troponin, and brain natriuretic peptide (BNP) levels.	*Alterations in serum electrolytes such as potassium and magnesium can precipitate cardiac dysrhythmias that may significantly alter CO/tissue perfusion. Serum troponin level alterations can indicate myocardial tissue damage, while serum BNP levels can indicate congestive heart failure. The presence of either situation can influence optimum CO.*

THERAPEUTIC INTERVENTIONS	RATIONALE

Independent Actions

Implement measures to reduce cardiac workload:	*Cardiac workload is the effort the heart expends to pump blood. The work of the heart is determined largely by the volume of blood distending the ventricles at the end of diastole (preload) and the amount of tension the ventricle must pump against to eject blood (afterload). Decreasing cardiac workload reduces the work that the compromised heart must perform in order to pump an adequate amount of blood. This results in increased CO.*
• Place client in a semi- to high-Fowler's position. **D** ● ✦	*Elevation of client's upper body reduces cardiac workload by decreasing venous return from the periphery and subsequently reducing preload.*
• Instruct client to avoid activities that create a Valsalva response (e.g., straining to have a bowel movement, holding breath while moving up in bed).	*When a client exhales after the Valsalva maneuver, the intrathoracic pressure falls, causing a sudden increase in venous return and a subsequent increase in preload and cardiac workload. The rebound increase in heart rate and BP that occurs after the Valsalva maneuver also causes an increase in cardiac workload.*
• Perform actions to promote physical and emotional rest (e.g., maintain a calm, quiet environment; limit the number of visitors; maintain activity restrictions). **D** ✦	*Physical rest reduces cardiac workload by lowering the body's energy requirements and subsequent need for oxygen. Promoting emotional rest reduces cardiac workload by preventing the increase in heart rate and BP that accompanies stress-induced sympathetic nervous system stimulation.*
• Perform actions to promote adequate tissue oxygenation (e.g., encourage deep breathing exercises and use of incentive spirometer). **D** ✦	*When tissue oxygenation is adequate, the heart does not need to work as hard to supply oxygen to the tissues; thus, more oxygen is available for myocardial use.*
• Discourage smoking.	*Nicotine stimulates catecholamine output, which increases heart rate and causes vasoconstriction and subsequently increases cardiac workload. Smoking also reduces oxygen availability because hemoglobin has a greater affinity for the carbon monoxide in smoke than for oxygen. This increases cardiac workload as the heart tries to compensate for the reduced oxygen levels.*
• Discourage excessive intake of beverages high in caffeine such as coffee, tea, and colas	*Excessive caffeine can increase cardiac workload because caffeine is a myocardial stimulant and can increase the rate and force of myocardial contractions.*
• Provide small meals rather than large ones.	*Large meals can increase cardiac workload because they require a greater increase in blood supply to the gastrointestinal tract to aid digestion.*

Dependent/Collaborative Actions

Implement measures to prevent hypovolemia (e.g., maintain a minimal fluid intake of 1000 mL/day unless ordered otherwise, consult physician before giving diuretics if excessive weight loss has occurred or client develops postural hypotension, administer blood and/or colloid or crystalloid solutions as ordered).	*Hypovolemia reduces venous return to the heart, which subsequently decreases the amount of blood in the ventricles at the end of diastole (preload). This results in a decrease in stroke volume and CO.*
Maintain oxygen therapy as ordered. **D** ✦	*When tissue oxygenation is adequate, the heart does not need to work as hard to supply oxygen to the tissues; thus, more oxygen is available for myocardial use.*

Continued...

THERAPEUTIC INTERVENTIONS	RATIONALE
Perform actions to prevent or treat fluid volume excess (e.g., maintain prescribed fluid and dietary sodium restrictions, administer diuretics as ordered).	*Preventing or treating excess fluid volume reduces vascular volume, which decreases preload and afterload and subsequently reduces cardiac workload.*
Increase activity gradually as allowed and tolerated. **D** ●	*A gradual increase in activity prevents a sudden increase in cardiac workload. A graded activity program also helps strengthen and tone the myocardium, which ultimately increases CO.*
Administer the following medications if ordered:	
• Positive inotropic agents (e.g., digitalis preparations, dobutamine, dopamine, inamrinone, milrinone)	*Positive inotropic agents increase CO by improving myocardial contractility.*
• Nitrates (e.g., nitroglycerin, isosorbide dinitrate)	*Nitrates decrease cardiac workload and myocardial oxygen demands by relaxing peripheral veins and, to a lesser extent, arterioles. This reduces venous return to the heart (preload) and peripheral vascular resistance (afterload). Nitrates also dilate nonsclerosed coronary arteries, which improves coronary blood flow and myocardial oxygen supply.*
• Direct-acting vasodilators (e.g., sodium nitroprusside, hydralazine) or centrally acting or alpha-adrenergic inhibitors (e.g., clonidine, prazosin, doxazosin)	*Vasodilators reduce cardiac workload by dilating the arterioles and subsequently decreasing peripheral vascular resistance (afterload). Certain vasodilators also dilate the veins, which decreases venous return and lowers diastolic ventricular filling pressure (preload).*
• Angiotensin-converting enzyme (ACE) inhibitors (e.g., captopril, enalapril, lisinopril, benazepril, fosinopril, quinapril) or angiotensin II receptor antagonists (e.g., losartan, valsartan)	*ACE inhibitors/angiotensin II receptor antagonists block the formation/effect of angiotensin II (a potent vasoconstrictor), which subsequently also causes a decrease in aldosterone output. The reduction in angiotensin II and aldosterone results in a decrease in total peripheral vascular resistance and reduced sodium and water retention, which leads to decreased cardiac workload.*
• Beta-adrenergic blocking agents (e.g., propranolol, metoprolol, atenolol, nadolol, sotalol)	*Beta-adrenergic blockers reduce cardiac workload by blocking sympathetic nervous system stimulation of beta-receptors in the heart.*
• Anticholinergic agents (e.g., atropine)	*CO is dependent on stroke volume and heart rate. Anticholinergics increase the heart rate (i.e., have a positive chronotropic effect) and are used to increase CO in clients with bradydysrhythmias.*
• Antidysrhythmics (e.g., flecainide, lidocaine, disopyramide, procainamide, amiodarone, esmolol, sotalol, adenosine)	*Antidysrhythmics improve CO by correcting automaticity and/or conduction abnormalities in the heart. By slowing the heart rate and/or decreasing irregularity of the heart rate, the diastolic filling time is prolonged, resulting in an increased preload and stroke volume.*
• Calcium channel blocking agents (e.g., nifedipine, verapamil, diltiazem, nicardipine, amlodipine)	*Calcium channel blockers dilate the coronary arteries, thus improving coronary blood flow and myocardial oxygen supply. They also reduce cardiac workload by dilating peripheral arteries and subsequently reducing afterload. Certain calcium channel blockers (e.g., diltiazem, verapamil) also have an antidysrhythmic effect, which subsequently increases CO by helping restore normal heart rate and rhythm.*
Consult physician if signs and symptoms of decreased CO persist or worsen.	*Notifying the physician allows for modification of treatment plan.*

Nursing Diagnosis **COMFORT, READINESS FOR ENHANCED** NDx

For a full, detailed care plan on this topic, go to http://evolve.elsevier.com/Haugen/careplanning/.

Nursing Diagnosis **CONFUSION, RISK FOR ACUTE** NDx

Definition: At risk for set of reversible disturbances of consciousness, attention, cognition, and perception that develops over a short period

CLINICAL MANIFESTATIONS

Subjective	Objective
Report of visual, auditory hallucinations	Exaggerated emotional responses; fluctuations in level of consciousness/cognition; alterations in normal sleep/wake cycle; increased agitation/restlessness; altered perceptive ability (inappropriate responses); lack of ability to initiate or follow through with goal-directed or purposeful behavior

RISK FACTORS

- Medication reaction/drug-to-drug interaction
- Substance abuse
- Delirium
- Metabolic imbalances
- Chronic illness exacerbation
- Elderly
- Dementia
- Hypoxemia
- Pain
- Sleep deprivation

DESIRED OUTCOMES

The client will regain usual reality orientation and level of consciousness as evidenced by:
a. Ability to participate independently in activities of daily living
b. Decrease in agitation/restlessness
c. Improvement in sleep/wake cycles
d. Appropriate responses to environmental stimuli

DOCUMENTATION

- Level of consciousness/orientation
- Electrolyte values
- Oxygenation
- Vital signs
- Safety risk
- Restraint use

NOC OUTCOMES

Cognitive orientation; neurological status: consciousness; fatigue level; anxiety level; agitation level; sleep; electrolyte and acid-base balance; respiratory status: gas exchange; blood glucose level

NIC INTERVENTIONS

Delirium management; electrolyte monitoring; electrolyte management; acid-base management; oxygen therapy; peripheral sensation management

NURSING ASSESSMENT	RATIONALE
Assess for signs and symptoms of acute confusion (e.g., changes in level of consciousness, changes in baseline behavior, increased agitation, hallucinations, and impaired perceptive ability).	*Early recognition of signs and symptoms of acute confusion allows for prompt intervention.*
Assess vital signs for evidence of poor perfusion (e.g., hypotension, tachycardia, tachypnea).	*Poor perfusion to vital organs such as the brain, which can be exacerbated by hypotension or extreme tachycardia, can alter normal cognitive states, leading to confusion.*
Monitor serum glucose levels, drug levels for abnormalities. Monitor pulse oximetry for hypoxemia.	*Altered metabolic parameters (e.g., hypoglycemia and hypoxia) can contribute to confusion and as a priority must be ruled out as potential causes of confusion. Failure to rule out possible metabolic causes of confusion can lead to serious adverse patient outcomes.*
Assess for contributing factors (e.g., substance abuse/withdrawal, episodes of high fever, exposure to toxic substances, drug-to-drug interactions, chronic illness exacerbations, sleep alterations, diet/nutritional alterations).	*Because of the reversible nature of acute confusion, contributing factors should be identified and corrected to return the patient to his/her normal state of cognition.*

THERAPEUTIC INTERVENTIONS	RATIONALE
Independent Actions Implement measures to maintain a safe patient care environment (e.g., supervision/sitter, family member assistance, side rails). **D** ✦ *Note: the use of restraints should be limited because this may worsen the situation by increasing agitation.*	*A confused patient is at risk for injury. Measures must be implemented that protect the patient from injury. Restraints must be used with extreme caution (e.g., behavior that is indicative of violence) because use may increase the risk of patient injury.*

NDx = NANDA-I Diagnosis   **D** = Delegatable Action   ● = UAP   ✦ = LVN/LPN   ⊖▶ = Go to ⊖volve for animation

Continued...

THERAPEUTIC INTERVENTIONS	RATIONALE
Implement measures that assist with client orientation (e.g., clock/calendar within visual field of the client). **D ● ✦**	The use of orientation aids will assist the patient in establishing an awareness of self and the environment.
Establish routines as much as possible when providing care and be as consistent as possible in following the routine. **D ● ✦**	A consistent routine aids in task completion and helps reduce confusion. A consistent, stable environment reduces confusion and frustration.
Implement measures that reduce sensory overload to the patient: **D ● ✦** • Cluster nursing care to provide adequate rest periods. • Maintain a calm environment, eliminating any unnecessary noise. • Provide undisturbed periods of rest.	Reducing sensory overload by limiting environmental noise and stimulation will help prevent the patient from becoming more confused.
Implement measures that foster an awareness of self and environment: **D ● ✦** • Address patient by name. • Mention the date, time, and place frequently during the day.	Fostering a sense of self and environment will aid in regaining/maintaining usual reality orientation.
Provide simple instructions allowing patient adequate time to respond, communicate, and make decisions. **D ● ✦**	These actions help to decrease confusion, reduce frustration, and promote task completion.
Encourage family members to share stories, discuss familiar people and events, and assist with orientation. **D ✦**	Sharing familiar events promotes a sense of continuity and creates a sense of overall security and comfort in a confused patient.

Dependent/Collaborative Actions

Administer short-acting sleep aids as ordered to facilitate undisturbed periods of rest. **D ✦**	Undisturbed rest periods will help restore cognitive orientation in acutely confused patients without metabolic alterations.
Administer psychotropics cautiously to control restlessness, hallucinations, and agitation. **D ✦**	Medication to reduce restlessness, hallucinations, and agitation can help calm a confused patient. It is most important that metabolic alterations are ruled out as the cause of the confusion/agitation and restlessness before medication administration.
Notify physician of continued or intensifying confusion, concerning drug-to-drug interactions, and abnormal laboratory results.	Notifying the appropriate health care provider allows for modification of the treatment plan.

Nursing Diagnosis ## CONSTIPATION NDx

Definition: A decrease in normal frequency of defecation accompanied by difficult or incomplete passage of stool and/or passage of excessively hard, dry stool

CLINICAL MANIFESTATIONS

Subjective	Objective
Report of straining with defecation; pain with defecation; increased abdominal pressure; feeling of rectal fullness or pressure; inability to pass stool; headache; indigestion; verbalization of abdominal pain and tenderness, and nausea	Change in bowel pattern; bright red blood with stool; presence of soft, pastelike stool in rectum; distended abdomen; dark, black, or tarry stool; percussed abdominal dullness; decreased volume of stool; decreased frequency; dry, hard, formed stool; palpable rectal mass; abdominal pain; anorexia; change in abdominal growling (borborygmi); atypical presentation in older adults (e.g., change in mental status, urinary incontinence; unexplained falls, elevated body temperature); severe flatus; hypoactive or hyperactive bowel sounds; palpable abdominal mass; abdominal tenderness with or palpable muscle resistance; nausea and/or vomiting; oozing liquid stool

RISK FACTORS

- **Functional:** Recent environmental changes; habitual denying/ignoring of urge to defecate; insufficient physical activity; irregular defecation habits; inadequate toileting (e.g., timeliness, positioning for defecation, privacy); abdominal muscle weakness.
- **Psychological:** Depression; emotional stress; mental confusion
- **Pharmacological:** Anticonvulsants; antilipemic agents; laxative overdose; calcium carbonate; aluminum-containing antacids; nonsteroidal anti-inflammatory agents; opiates; anticholinergics; diuretics; iron salts; phenothiazines; sedatives; sympathomimetics; bismuth salts; antidepressants; calcium channel blockers
- **Mechanical:** Rectal abscess or ulcer; pregnancy; rectal anal fissures; tumors; megacolon (Hirschsprung's disease); electrolyte imbalance; rectal prolapse; prostate enlargement; neurological impairment; rectal anal stricture; rectocele; postsurgical obstruction; hemorrhoids; obesity
- **Physiological:** Poor eating habits; decreased motility of gastrointestinal tract; inadequate dentition or oral hygiene; insufficient fiber intake; insufficient fluid intake; change in usual foods and eating pattern; dehydration

DESIRED OUTCOMES

The client will maintain usual bowel elimination pattern as evidenced by:
a. Usual frequency of bowel movements
b. Passage of soft, formed stool
c. Absence of abdominal distention and pain, feeling of rectal fullness or pressure, and straining during defecation

DOCUMENTATION

- Occurrence of last bowel movement
- Characteristics of stool
- Abdominal distention or report of pain
- Reports of fullness or pressure in rectum
- Reports of straining at stool
- Bowel sounds
- Therapeutic interventions
- Client teaching

NOC OUTCOMES

Bowel elimination; gastrointestinal function; hydration; nausea and vomiting severity; symptom control

NIC INTERVENTIONS

Constipation/impaction management

NURSING ASSESSMENT	RATIONALE
Ascertain client's usual bowel elimination habits.	*Knowledge of the client's usual bowel elimination habits is essential in determining whether constipation is present, because the frequency of defecation varies among individuals.*
Assess for signs and symptoms of constipation: • Decrease in frequency of bowel movements • Passage of hard, formed stools • Anorexia • Abdominal distention and pain • Feeling of fullness or pressure in rectum • Straining during defecation	*Early recognition of signs and symptoms of constipation allows for prompt intervention.*
Assess bowel sounds. Report a pattern of decreasing bowel sounds.	*Bowel sounds are produced by peristaltic activity. A pattern of decreasing bowel sounds indicates a decrease in bowel motility, which can lead to and be present with constipation.*

THERAPEUTIC INTERVENTIONS	RATIONALE
Independent Actions Encourage client to defecate whenever the urge is felt. **D** ● ✦	*If the client feels the urge to defecate but suppresses it by contracting the external anal sphincter, the defecation reflex will subside after a few minutes and not recur for several hours or until additional feces enter the rectum. Repeated inhibition of the defecation reflex results in progressive weakening of the reflex. In addition, when the defecation reflex is inhibited, feces remain in the colon longer and water continues to be absorbed from the feces, making the stool drier, harder, and subsequently more difficult to evacuate.*

Continued...

THERAPEUTIC INTERVENTIONS	RATIONALE
Assist client to toilet or bedside commode or place in high-Fowler's position on bedpan for bowel movements unless contraindicated. **D** ● ✦	*A sitting position aids in the expulsion of stool by taking advantage of gravity. This position also enhances the client's ability to perform the Valsalva maneuver, which increases intra-abdominal pressure and forces the fecal contents downward and into the rectum where the defecation reflex is then elicited.*
Encourage client to relax, provide privacy, and have call signal within reach during attempts to defecate. **D** ✦	*If the client is able to relax during attempts to defecate, he/she will be able to relax the levator ani muscle and external anal sphincter, thus facilitating the passage of stool.*
Encourage client to establish a regular time for defecation, preferably within an hour after a meal. **D** ✦	*Attempting to have a bowel movement within an hour after a meal, particularly breakfast, takes advantage of mass peristalsis, which occurs only a few times a day and is strongest after meals. Mass peristalsis is stimulated by the gastrocolic reflex, which is initiated by the presence of foods/fluids in the stomach and duodenum.*
Instruct client to increase intake of foods high in fiber (e.g., bran, whole grain breads and cereals, fresh fruits and vegetables) unless contraindicated.	*Foods high in fiber provide bulk to the fecal mass and keep the stool soft because of the ability of fiber to absorb water. The increased bulkiness (i.e., mass) of the stools stimulates peristalsis, which promotes more rapid movement of stool through the colon. Also, the shorter the time that feces remain in the intestine, the less water is absorbed from it, which helps prevent the formation of hard, dry stools that are difficult to expel.*
Encourage client to drink hot liquids (e.g., coffee, tea) upon arising in the morning. **D** ✦	*Ingestion of hot fluids can stimulate peristalsis.*

Dependent/Collaborative Actions

Instruct client to maintain a minimal fluid intake of 2500 mL/day unless contraindicated.	*Inadequate fluid intake reduces the water content of feces, which results in hard, dry stool that is difficult to evacuate.*
Increase activity as allowed and tolerated. **D** ● ✦	*Ambulation stimulates peristalsis, which promotes the passage of stool through the intestines.*
When appropriate, encourage the use of nonnarcotic rather than narcotic (opioid) analgesics for pain management.	*Narcotic analgesics slow peristalsis, which delays transit of intestinal contents. This delay also results in increased absorption of fluid from the fecal mass with the subsequent formation of hard, dry stool.*
Administer laxatives or cathartics (e.g., stool softeners, bulk-forming agents, irritants/stimulants, lubricants, saline/osmotic agents) as ordered. **D** ✦	*Laxatives/cathartics act in a variety of ways to soften the stool, increase stool bulk, stimulate bowel motility, and/or lubricate the fecal mass and thereby promote the evacuation of stool.*
Administer cleansing and/or oil retention enemas if ordered. **D** ● ✦	*A cleansing enema stimulates peristalsis and evacuation of stool by distending the colon with a large volume of solution and/or by irritating the colonic mucosa. An oil retention enema facilitates the passage of stool by softening the fecal mass and lubricating the rectum and anal canal.*
Consult physician about checking for an impaction and digitally removing stool if the client has not had a bowel movement in 3 days, if he/she is passing liquid stool, or if other signs and symptoms of constipation are present.	*An impaction prohibits the normal passage of feces. Digital removal of an impacted fecal mass may be necessary before normal passage of stool can occur.*
Consult appropriate health care provider if diarrhea persists.	*Notifying the appropriate health care provider allows for modification of the treatment plan.*

CONTAMINATION NDx/CONTAMINATION, RISK FOR NDx

Definition: Accentuated risk for or actual environmental contaminants in doses sufficient to cause adverse health effects

CLINICAL MANIFESTATIONS

Subjective	Objective
Verbalization of exposure to potentially toxic agents	*Note*: Health effects will depend upon the type of contaminant and may include all body systems. Principal routes of exposure include inhalation, absorption, ingestion, and injection.
	Types of contaminants include incapacitating agents, chemical agents (organophosphates), nerve agents (sarin), cyanide agents, vesicant/blister agents (nitrogen mustards), pulmonary/choking agents (chlorine), riot control agents (pepper spray/tear gas). Objective assessment data will reflect the offending agent and route of absorption.
Pesticides/Chemicals/Biologicals: Complaints of a "stomachache"; cramping; blurred vision; joint and muscle aches; difficulty breathing; flu symptoms; verbalization of nausea; hallucinations	Cardiac dysrhythmias; hypertension/hypotension; diarrhea; nausea; muscle weakness; confusion; seizures; decreased level of consciousness; cough; labored breathing; cyanosis; skin lesions (rash, pustules, scabs)
Radiation: Report of nausea; visual changes; difficulty breathing; verbalization of weakness; fatigue; skin irritation; abdominal pain	Symptoms of radiation sickness (i.e., weakness, hair loss, changes in blood chemistries, hemorrhage, diminished organ function); paresthesias; confusion; lethargy; changes in level of consciousness; skin irritation; itching; blistering; burns; erythema; ulcerations
Waste: Verbalization of nausea; abdominal cramps	Anorexia; diarrhea; weight loss; jaundice; weakness; fever
Pollution: Verbalization of difficulty breathing; chest pain; headaches; shortness of breath	Reddened conjunctiva; tearing; wheezing; pulmonary congestion; nasal congestion

RISK FACTORS

- **External:** Chemical contamination of food and/or water; bioterrorism; disasters; insufficient or absent use of decontamination protocol; inappropriate or no use of protective clothing; living in poverty; poor sanitation; climate conditions
- **Internal:** Gestational age during exposure; developmental stage; gender; nutritional factors; the presence of preexisting disease

DESIRED OUTCOMES

The client will experience minimal health alterations.

DOCUMENTATION

- Therapeutic interventions
- Decontamination protocol
- Isolation precautions

NOC OUTCOMES

Respiratory status: gas exchange; physical injury severity; anxiety level; fear level; community disaster readiness

NIC INTERVENTIONS

Triage: disaster; infection control; anxiety reduction; crisis intervention; environmental risk protection; bioterrorism preparedness

NURSING ASSESSMENT

Assess vital signs, including temperature, noting signs and symptoms of inhalation, absorption, ingestion, or injection of environmental contaminants by performing frequent, prioritized multisystem assessment.
- Monitor airway and respiratory status (e.g., rate and depth of breathing, adventitious breath sounds, pulse oximetry).

- Monitor cardiac rhythm.

RATIONALE

Early recognition of signs and symptoms of contamination allows for prompt intervention.

Effects of contaminants can be delayed 2 to 24 hours. Rapid onset of pulmonary symptoms indicates a poor prognosis. Early detection allows for aggressive treatment of symptoms.
Cardiac monitoring should be implemented for any patients exhibiting irregularity (i.e., symptomatic bradycardia, symptomatic tachycardia) to allow for prompt intervention.

NDx = NANDA-I Diagnosis   **D** = Delegatable Action   ● = UAP   ✦ = LVN/LPN   ⊝▶ = Go to ⊝volve for animation

Continued...

NURSING ASSESSMENT	RATIONALE
• Assess neuromuscular status.	*Variable routes of exposure to nerve agents may result in symptoms that may not appear for 30 minutes to 18 hours. Vaporized nerve agents are most toxic, with symptoms appearing within seconds. Diagnosis and treatment are based on observations of signs and symptoms.*
• Assess integumentary system.	*Contaminants absorbed through the skin or eyes produce immediate symptoms. Prompt assessment allows for early implementation of interventions.*
• Monitor serum chemistry and complete blood cell count (CBC) results, reporting abnormalities.	*Monitoring lab values allows for the assessment of hematological and multisystem consequences of exposure to contaminants.*

THERAPEUTIC INTERVENTIONS	RATIONALE

Independent Actions
Actual exposure:

Provide protective clothing for all health care providers caring for the exposed client (e.g., disposable scrubs, waterproof shoe covers, gowns with seams taped, hat, mask, goggles, double gloves taped at the wrist). **D** ● ✦	*Health care providers must protect themselves from contamination and control further spread.*
Institute decontamination protocols:	
• Remove and isolate clothing for decontamination. Clothing exposed to radiation must be sealed in an airtight container and labeled appropriately.	*Prompt removal of contaminated clothing prevents further exposure of skin to contaminants, prevents further absorption of contaminants, and facilitates effective decontamination. Removing clothing can reduce contamination 80% to 90%.*
• Wash intact skin or damaged skin with soap and water. **D** ● ✦	*Washing exposed skin reduces the amount of contaminants absorbed.*
• Irrigate exposed/injured eyes copiously with water. **D** ✦	*Irrigation of eyes reduces the amount of contaminants absorbed.*
• Implement appropriate isolation precautions (universal, airborne, droplet, and contact isolation). **D** ✦	*Appropriate isolation precautions will assist in reducing the further spread of contaminants and protect health care providers caring for the exposed client.*
Explain decontamination protocols and the need for isolation to patient and family to help alleviate anxiety.	*Providing factual information to the patient and family concerning treatment will help in reducing anxiety associated with fear.*
Encourage patient to verbalize feelings, perceptions, and fears. **D** ✦	*Verbalization of fears or concerns can assist the health care practitioner in identifying knowledge deficits amenable to education while alleviating apprehension on the part of the client.*

Dependent/Collaborative Actions

Establish intravenous access for the administration of medications. **D** ✦	*Many of the drugs used to treat environmental contamination are administered intravenously requiring establishment of access.*
Administer oxygen, bronchodilators, corticosteroids for pulmonary symptoms. **D** ✦	*The use of supplemental oxygen will improve the client's arterial oxygen level, which may become compromised with the development of pulmonary edema. Bronchodilators and corticosteroids will assist with treating inflammatory changes occurring with pulmonary pathology, improving oxygenation and ventilation.*
Wash exposed skin with 0.5% sodium hypochlorite solution for 10 minutes. **D** ✦	*Use of this solution is helpful with gross contamination of the skin, rendering offending contaminants harmless.*
Administer activated charcoal as quickly as possible for gastrointestinal decontamination. **D** ✦	*Activated charcoal should be administered as soon as possible because it absorbs almost all commonly ingested drugs and chemicals except iron, lithium, ethanol, and potassium. Emesis and gastric lavage should be avoided.*

THERAPEUTIC INTERVENTIONS	RATIONALE
Administer drugs for treatment of nerve agent poisoning (e.g., atropine, pralidoxime, and diazepam). **D** ✦	*Atropine administration is indicated for clients exhibiting muscarinic cholinergic excess (e.g., drying of bronchial secretions and decreasing adverse effects including salivation, lacrimation, urination, defecation, and emesis). Pralidoxime administration is indicated for all patients requiring atropine and in those with or at risk for nicotinic cholinergic (decreased atropine requirements) and treatment of muscle fasciculations and weakness (nicotinic signs of poisoning). Diazepam or other benzodiazepines are indicated in patients with signs of severe toxicity or seizures.*
Administer drugs for the treatment of cyanide poisoning (e.g., intranasal amyl nitrate, sodium nitrite, sodium thiosulfate). **D** ✦	*Amyl nitrite is administered as an inhalant, followed by sodium nitrite and sodium thiosulfate, which are given intravenously. The nitrites are given to convert hemoglobin in the red blood cell to methemoglobin, which attracts the cyanide away from the cytochrome oxidase and allows the cell to continue the process of aerobic metabolism. Thiosulfate is given to facilitate detoxification of cyanide by the body's own cyanide clearance system.*
Administer antibiotics for secondary bacterial infections. **D** ✦	*Clients exhibiting signs and symptoms of infection (e.g., fever, chills, sweating, increased white blood cell count, pus in open wounds require the administration of antibiotics to help the body and normal defenses overcome infections.*

Risk for exposure:

Conduct surveillance for environmental contamination. Notify agencies authorized to protect the environment of contaminants in the area.	*Assessment of the client's community and immediate environment can assist with the identification of contaminants that could threaten individual and community health status.*
Assist individuals to modify the environment to minimize risk or assist in relocating to a safer environment.	*Nurses can assist individuals and communities in incorporating environmentally responsible ways in dealing with activities of daily living.*
Collaborate with other agencies to schedule mass casualty and disaster readiness drills.	*In the event a disaster that predisposes a community to contaminants becomes a reality, local health care providers and the community at large must be prepared to respond appropriately.*

⊖▶ Nursing Diagnosis **COPING, INEFFECTIVE** NDx

For a full, detailed care plan on this topic, go to http://evolve.elsevier.com/Haugen/careplanning/.

⊖▶ Nursing Diagnosis **DECISION-MAKING, READINESS FOR ENHANCED** NDx

For a full, detailed care plan on this topic, go to http://evolve.elsevier.com/Haugen/careplanning/.

Nursing Diagnosis **DIARRHEA** NDx

Definition: Passage of loose, unformed stools

CLINICAL MANIFESTATIONS

Subjective	Objective
Report of urgency, abdominal pain and cramping	Hyperactive bowel sounds; at least 3 loose liquid stools per day

Continued...

RISK FACTORS

- **Situational:** Alcohol abuse; toxins; laxative abuse; radiation; tube feedings; adverse effects of medications; contaminants; travel
- **Psychosocial:** High stress levels and anxiety
- **Physiological:** Inflammation; malabsorption; infectious processes; irritation; parasites

DESIRED OUTCOMES

The client will have fewer bowel movements and more formed stool.

DOCUMENTATION

- Frequency of defecation
- Characteristics of stool
- Complaints of abdominal cramping
- Bowel sounds
- Therapeutic interventions
- Client teaching

NOC OUTCOMES

Bowel continence; bowel elimination; fluid balance; symptom severity; gastrointestinal function

NIC INTERVENTIONS

Diarrhea management

NURSING ASSESSMENT	RATIONALE
Ascertain client's usual bowel elimination habits	*Knowledge of the client's usual bowel elimination habits helps determine the severity of the diarrhea.*
Assess for and report signs and symptoms of diarrhea (e.g., frequent loose stools; urgency; abdominal cramping; hyperactive bowel sounds).	*Early recognition of signs and symptoms of diarrhea allows for prompt intervention.*
Assess for factors that may be causing diarrhea (e.g., antimicrobial agents, laxative use, tube feedings, gastrointestinal disorder, change in dietary intake, intestinal infection).	*Knowing the cause of the diarrhea is a critical component in identifying the appropriate treatment.*

THERAPEUTIC INTERVENTIONS	RATIONALE

Independent Actions

As diet advances, gradually progress from fluids to small meals. **D ● ✦**

Gradual introduction of small amounts of fluid and then food helps prevent a sudden increase in peristalsis and diarrhea.

Instruct the client to avoid the following foods/fluids:

- Those known to aggravate diarrhea such as spicy foods, alcohol, coffee, and fatty foods

  These substances are thought to increase intestinal motility and may also cause excessive mucus secretion, which increases the liquidity of the intestinal contents.

- Those that are extremely hot or cold

  Extremes in temperature of ingested foods/fluids often stimulate peristalsis.

- Those high in lactose such as milk and milk products

  Diarrhea may temporarily deplete the gastrointestinal enzyme lactase, which is essential for the hydrolysis and subsequent absorption of lactose. The nonabsorbed lactose has an osmotic effect and draws water into the colon, which results in more liquid stool. The lactose also serves as a base for bacterial fermentation in the colon. The lactic and fatty acids produced by this fermentation process irritate the colon, with a subsequent increase in bowel motility and diarrhea.

- Those foods high in fiber such as whole-grain cereals, raw fruits and vegetables

  Fiber increases bulk of the stool because of its ability to absorb water. The increased mass (i.e., bulk) of the stools stimulates peristalsis. Limiting fiber intake decreases the water content of the stool, which results in drier, firmer, and less bulky stools. The decrease in bulk (i.e., mass) results in less stimulation of peristalsis, and the dryness of the stools slow intestinal transit time.

THERAPEUTIC INTERVENTIONS	RATIONALE
• Those foods made with synthetic, nonabsorbable sugars (e.g., sorbitol) that are found in many dietetic foods.	*Synthetic, nonabsorbable sugars are not well absorbed from the gastrointestinal tract and tend to draw water into the intestine by osmosis. This excess water in the intestine increases fluidity and volume of stool.*
Implement measures to reduce fear and anxiety: • Provide client teaching. • All care providers are to interact with the client in a calm manner.	*Parasympathetic activity may dominate in some stressful situations and cause increased gastrointestinal motility and diarrhea.*
Encourage the client to rest. **D** ✦	*Physical activity stimulates peristalsis.*
Dependent/Collaborative Actions	
Limit oral intake to clear liquids and replacement solutions as ordered. **D** ✦ • Pedialyte • Resol • Rehydrate • Administer prescribed antianxiety agents. **D** ✦	*Peristalsis is stimulated by the presence of foods/fluids in the stomach and duodenum. Restricting oral intake to clear liquids and/or replacement solutions during the acute phase of diarrhea not only allows the bowel to rest but also helps prevent malnutrition and fluid and electrolyte imbalances.*
If the client is receiving tube feeding, administer the solution at room temperature. Consult physician about reducing the rate of administration and/or the concentration of the tube feeding solution if diarrhea occurs. **D** ✦	*Tube feeding can increase peristalsis if the solution is given while cold or if large amounts are given too quickly. Full-strength tube feeding solution has relatively high osmolality, which subsequently draws water into the intestine and causes an osmotic diarrhea. Reducing the concentration of the feeding solution lessens the risk for osmotic diarrhea.*
Consult physician regarding measures to remove fecal impaction if present (e.g., digital removal of stool, oil retention enema).	*When a fecal impaction is present, the secretory activity of the bowel increases in an attempt to lubricate and promote evaluation of the impacted feces. The liquid portion of the feces above the mass then leaks around the impaction, resulting in a continuous oozing of diarrheal stool.*
Administer the following antidiarrheal agents if ordered: **D** ✦ • Opioids (e.g., paregoric) or synthetic opioids (e.g., loperamide, diphenoxylate hydrochloride)	*Opioids and synthetic opioids decrease gastrointestinal motility, which delays the passage of intestinal contents and subsequently allows more time for water to be reabsorbed from the feces. This results in fewer bowel movements and more formed stool.*
• Bulk-forming agents (e.g., methylcellulose, psyllium hydrophilic mucilloid, polycarbophil)	*Bulk-forming agents absorb water in the bowel, resulting in a more formed stool.*
• Adsorbents/protectants (e.g., attapulgite [Kaopectate], bismuth subsalicylate [Pepto-Bismol]).	*Adsorbents/protectants act locally to coat the walls of the gastrointestinal tract and absorb toxins that are stimulating gut motility and/or secretions.*
Consult appropriate health care provider if diarrhea persists.	*Notifying the appropriate health care provider allows for modification of the treatment plan.*

Nursing Diagnosis   **FALLS, RISK FOR** NDx**/INJURY, RISK FOR** NDx

Definition: Increased susceptibility to falling that may cause physical harm

CLINICAL MANIFESTATIONS

Subjective	Objective
Expressed concern for safety during ambulation; stated history of previous falls	Unsteadiness when ambulating; use of ambulation aids; visual field deficits; confusion; orthostatic hypotension; medication therapy (e.g., antihypertensives, diuretics, hypnotics, antianxiety agents, narcotics, antidepressants); anemias, arthritis

Continued...

RISK FACTORS

- Weakness and fatigue
- Dizziness or syncope
- Cluttered environment
- Diminished mental status
- Medications

- Musculoskeletal weakness
- Impaired balance
- Orthostatic hypotension
- Presence of acute illness

- Visual field deficits
- Age 65 or older
- History of falls
- Use of assistive devices

DESIRED OUTCOMES

The client will remain free from falls.

DOCUMENTATION

- Patient safety level
- Safety precautions/interventions
- Restraint

NOC OUTCOMES

Falls prevention behavior; risk detection; knowledge: fall prevention

NIC INTERVENTIONS

Environmental management; fall prevention

NURSING ASSESSMENT

Assess client's risk for falls using standardized assessment tool (e.g., Fall Risk Assessment).

Assess client's balance and mobility skills.

Evaluate client's medications to determine whether they place the client at increased risk for falls.

RATIONALE

A client's risk for falls increases with the number of risk factors. Determining the client's risk for falls allows implementation of the appropriate preventive measures.

Determining the client's baseline status allows for the implementation of the appropriate preventive measures

Some medications may cause excessive drowsiness, altered mental states, or physiological changes such as orthostatic hypotension that can increase the risk of falls in clients. Early identification of such medications allows for implementation of appropriate preventive measures.

THERAPEUTIC INTERVENTIONS

Independent Actions

Implement measures to prevent falls: **D** ● ✦
- Orient client to surroundings (room; nurse call system).
- Place articles within easy reach of the client.
- Reduce clutter in client's immediate environment.
- Assist unsteady client with ambulation.
- Have client wear safe footwear when ambulating (e.g., nonskid shoes/slippers).
- Ensure adequate lighting in client's room.
- Encourage client to use ambulation aids and glasses.
- Keep bed in lowest position.
- Use side rails of appropriate height and length.

Monitor client's ability to transfer to and from a bed, wheelchair, and toilet. **D** ● ✦
- Use proper technique when transferring a patient to and from a bed, wheelchair, and toilet.

Involve family to aid with activities of daily living and prevention of falls.

Dependent/Collaborative Actions

Collaborate with health care providers to monitor and minimize side effects of medications that increase the risk of falls.

Implement the use of restraints as ordered.

RATIONALE

Physical hazards in the client's immediate environment increase the risk for accidental injury. Falls are usually a result of both intrinsic (illness, drug therapy) and extrinsic or environmental factors. Extrinsic factors are much easier to modify and eliminate.

Older adults are more likely to fall in the bedroom and the bathroom, with most falls occurring when transferring from beds, chairs, and toilets.

In the acute care environment, frequent observation of clients at risk for falls is necessary to reduce the risk for falls.

Intrinsic factors increasing the risk of falls may be modified or eliminated if identified and discussed with the appropriate health care provider.

Avoid the use of restraints if at all possible. If restraints must be used, choose the least restrictive device and follow institutional policy for the monitoring and documentation of the client's condition.

THERAPEUTIC INTERVENTIONS	RATIONALE
Consult physical therapy for strengthening, exercises, gait training, and help with balance to increase mobility.	*Collaboration with other disciplines is an important part of a client's plan of care. Additional resources provided during the hospital stay as well as in preparation for discharge can assist the client in gaining the strength, mobility, and endurance to reduce the risk for falls.*
Notify physician of client falls.	*Notifying the appropriate health care provider allows for modification of the treatment plan.*

Nursing Diagnosis **FLUID VOLUME, DEFICIENT** NDx

Definition: Decreased intravascular volume, interstitial and/or intracellular fluid

CLINICAL MANIFESTATIONS

Subjective	Objective
Report of thirst; weakness	Decreased urine output; increased urine concentration; sudden weight loss (except in third spacing); decreased venous filling; increased body temperature; decreased pulse volume/pressure; change in mental status; elevated hematocrit (Hct); decreased skin/tongue turgor; dry skin/mucous membranes; increased pulse rate; decreased blood pressure (BP)

RISK FACTORS
- Active fluid volume loss
- Failure of regulatory mechanisms

DESIRED OUTCOMES

The client will not experience a deficient fluid volume as evidenced by:
a. Normal skin turgor
b. Moist mucous membrane
c. Stable weight
d. BP and pulse within normal range for client and stable with position change
e. Capillary refill time less than 2 to 3 seconds
f. Usual mental status
g. Blood urea nitrogen (BUN) and Hct within normal range
h. Balanced intake and output

DOCUMENTATION
- Vital signs
- Condition of skin and mucous membranes
- Weight
- Capillary refill time
- Appearance of neck veins when client is supine
- Mental status
- Intake and output
- Presence of nausea, vomiting, or other contributing factors
- Intravenous fluid therapy
- Client teaching

NOC OUTCOMES

Fluid balance; hydration; kidney function; vital signs; acute confusion level

NIC INTERVENTIONS

Fluid management; fluid monitoring; fluid resuscitation; hypovolemia management; intravenous therapy

NURSING ASSESSMENT	RATIONALE
Assess for signs and symptoms of deficient fluid volume: • Decreased skin turgor • Dry mucous membranes, thirst • Weight loss of 2% or greater over a short period • Postural hypotension and/or low BP • Weak, rapid pulse	*Early recognition of signs and symptoms of deficient fluid volume allow for prompt intervention.*

Continued...

NURSING ASSESSMENT	RATIONALE
• Capillary refill time greater than 2 to 3 seconds • Neck veins flat when client is supine • Change in mental status • Decreased urine output Assess BUN/Hct for abnormal elevations.	*Net fluid volume deficits result in decreased renal blood flow, decreased glomerular filtration, acute tubular necrosis and resulting elevated blood urea nitrogen (BUN) levels. Hypovolemia results in hemoconcentration resulting in elevated hematocrit (Hct) levels.*

THERAPEUTIC INTERVENTIONS	RATIONALE
Independent Actions Implement measures to reduce nausea and vomiting if present: • Instruct client to ingest food/fluid slowly. • Eliminate noxious sights and odors.	*Nausea often causes the client to have decreased fluid volume intake. Persistent vomiting results in excessive loss of fluid.*
Implement measures to control diarrhea if present: • Discourage intake of spicy foods and foods high in fiber or lactose.	*Persistent or severe diarrhea results in excessive loss of gastrointestinal fluid.*
Implement measures to reduce fever if present: **D ● ✦** • Sponge bath client with tepid water. • Remove excessive clothing or bedcovers.	*Fever may be accompanied by diaphoresis, which can result in excessive loss of fluid.*
Carefully measure drainage: **D ✦** • Nasogastric • Wound • Urine	*Accurate intake/output records must be maintained to ensure fluid loss is replaced appropriately.*
Maintain a fluid intake of at least 2500 mL/day unless contraindicated. **D ✦**	*Adequate fluid intake needs to be provided in order to ensure adequate hydration.*
Dependent/Collaborative Actions Administer antiemetics as ordered. **D ✦**	*Nausea often causes the client to have decreased fluid volume intake. Persistent vomiting results in excessive loss of fluid.*
Administer antidiarrheal agents as ordered. **D ✦**	*Persistent or severe diarrhea results in excessive loss of gastrointestinal fluid.*
Administer antipyretics as ordered. **D ✦**	*Fever may be accompanied by diaphoresis, which can result in excessive loss of fluid*
Administer and maintain intravenous replacement fluids as ordered. **D ✦**	*Replacing fluid volume that is lost helps prevent/treat deficient fluid volume.*
Consult physician if signs and symptoms of deficient fluid volume persist or worsen.	*Notifying the physician allows for modification of the treatment plan.*

⊖► Nursing Diagnosis FLUID VOLUME, EXCESS NDx

Definition: Increased isotonic fluid retention

CLINICAL MANIFESTATIONS

Subjective	Objective
Verbal reports of shortness of breath	Jugular venous distention; decreased hemoglobin and hematocrit (Hct); weight gain over short period; dyspnea; intake exceeds output; pleural effusion; orthopnea; S₃ heart sound; pulmonary congestion; change in respiratory pattern; change in mental status; blood pressure (BP) changes; pulmonary artery pressure changes; oliguria; specific gravity changes; azotemia; altered electrolytes; restlessness; anxiety; abnormal breath sounds (crackles); edema, may progress to anasarca; increased central venous pressure (CVP); positive hepatojugular reflex

RISK FACTORS
- Compromised regulatory mechanism
- Excess fluid intake
- Excess sodium intake

DESIRED OUTCOMES

The client will not experience excess fluid volume as evidenced by:
a. Stable weight
b. BP within normal range
c. Absence of S$_3$ heart sound
d. Normal pulse volume
e. Balanced intake and output
f. Usual mental status
g. Normal breath sounds
h. Blood urea nitrogen (BUN) and Hct within normal limits
i. Absence of dyspnea, orthopnea, peripheral edema, and distended neck veins
j. CVP within normal range

DOCUMENTATION
- BP
- Weight
- Heart sounds
- Pulse volume
- Intake and output
- Mental status
- Breath sounds, ease of respirations
- Presence of edema and neck vein distention
- CVP readings
- Therapeutic interventions
- Client teaching

NOC OUTCOMES

Cardiopulmonary status; fluid balance; fluid overload severity; kidney function; respiratory status; vital signs; weight: body mass

NIC INTERVENTIONS

Fluid management; fluid monitoring; hypervolemia management

NURSING ASSESSMENT

Assess for signs and symptoms of excess fluid volume:
- Weight gain of 2% or greater in a short period
- Elevated BP (BP may not be elevated if fluid has shifted out of the vascular space)
- Presence of an S$_3$ heart sound
- Bounding pulse
- Intake greater than output
- Change in mental status
- Crackles (rales), diminished or absent breath sounds
- Dyspnea, orthopnea
- Peripheral edema
- Distended neck veins
- Elevated CVP

Monitor chest radiograph results. Report findings of pulmonary vascular congestion, pleural effusion, or pulmonary edema.

Monitor BUN, Hct, and electrolytes for abnormalities.

RATIONALE

Early recognition of signs and symptoms of excess fluid volume allows for prompt intervention.

Chest radiograph films provide data about pulmonary vascular status and fluid accumulation in the pleural space, pulmonary interstitium, and alveoli.

Fluid volume excess results in a decreased Hct because of hemodilution and a decreased BUN. Electrolyte values will be altered in the presence of excess fluid volume.

THERAPEUTIC INTERVENTIONS

RATIONALE

Independent Actions
Encourage client to rest periodically in a recumbent position if tolerated. **D** ✦

Lying flat promotes venous return, which leads to increased cardiac output and renal blood flow. This increases the glomerular filtration rate and promotes diuresis.

Dependent/Collaborative Actions
Maintain fluid restrictions as ordered. **D** ✦

Fluid restriction helps to reduce total body water and prevent the accumulation of excess fluid.

Continued...

THERAPEUTIC INTERVENTIONS	RATIONALE
Restrict sodium intake as ordered. **D** ✦	*Excess fluid volume is an isotonic retention of both sodium and water. Restricting sodium intake will result in less sodium and subsequently less water being reabsorbed by the kidneys.*
If client is receiving intravenous fluids that contain a sizeable amount of sodium (0.9% normal saline, lactated Ringer's), consult physician about a change in the solution or rate of infusion.	*Excess fluid volume can result from overzealous or prolonged intravenous administration of sodium-containing fluids, particularly ones that contain sizable amounts of sodium.*
If client is receiving numerous and/or large-volume intravenous medications, consult pharmacist about ways to prevent excessive fluid administration (stop primary infusion during administration of intravenous medications, dilute medications in the minimum amount of solution).	*Limiting the amount of intravenous solution infused at any one time and maximizing the concentration of intravenous medications help prevent an additional fluid burden in the person who has or is at risk for fluid volume overload.*
Administer diuretics as ordered. **D** ✦	*Most diuretics inhibit sodium reabsorption in the renal tubules. This results in decreased water reabsorption and subsequent excretion of excess fluid.*
Consult physician if signs and symptoms of excess fluid volume persist or worsen.	*Notifying the physician allows for modification of the treatment plan.*

Nursing Diagnosis   # GAS EXCHANGE, IMPAIRED NDx

Definition: Excess or deficit in oxygenation and/or carbon dioxide (CO_2) elimination at the alveolar-capillary membrane

CLINICAL MANIFESTATIONS

Subjective	Objective
Verbalization of visual disturbances; headache upon awakening	Decreased CO_2; tachycardia; hypercapnia; restlessness; somnolence; irritability; hypoxia; confusion; dyspnea; abnormal arterial blood gases; cyanosis (in neonates only); abnormal skin color (pale, dusky); hypoxemia; abnormal rate, rhythm, depth of breathing; diaphoresis; nasal flaring; low partial pressure of oxygen (O_2) in arterial blood (PaO_2); low pulse oximetry

RISK FACTORS

- Ventilation/perfusion imbalance
- Alveolar-capillary membrane changes

DESIRED OUTCOMES

The client will experience adequate gas (O_2/CO_2) exchange as evidenced by:
a. Usual mental status
b. Unlabored respirations at 12 to 20 breaths/min
c. Oximetry results within normal range
d. Arterial blood gas (ABG) values within normal range
e. Normal breath sounds
f. Normal rate and depth of respirations
g. Absence of dyspnea

DOCUMENTATION

- Respiratory rate
- Difficulty breathing
- Mental status
- Oximetry results
- Route and rate of O_2 administration
- Therapeutic interventions
- Client teaching

NOC OUTCOMES

Respiratory status: ventilation; acute confusion level; gas exchange; activity tolerance; airway patency; tissue perfusion: pulmonary vital signs

NIC INTERVENTIONS

Respiratory monitoring; O_2 therapy; airway management; chest physiotherapy; cough enhancement; acid-base management

NURSING ASSESSMENT	RATIONALE
Assess for and report signs and symptoms of impaired gas (O_2/CO_2) exchange: • Restlessness, irritability • Confusion, somnolence • Tachypnea, dyspnea • Decreased PaO_2 and/or increased partial pressure of CO_2 in arterial blood ($PaCO_2$)	*Early recognition of signs and symptoms of impaired gas exchange allows for prompt intervention.*
Monitor for and report a significant decrease in oximetry results.	*Oximetry is a noninvasive method of measuring arterial O_2 saturation. The results assist in evaluating respiratory status.*

THERAPEUTIC INTERVENTIONS	RATIONALE

Independent Actions

Place client in a semi- to high-Fowler's position unless contraindicated. Position with pillows to prevent slumping. If client is experiencing dyspnea or orthopnea, position overbed table so he/she can lean on it if desired. **D** ● ✦	*These positions allow for increased diaphragmatic excursion and maximum lung expansion, which promotes optimal alveolar ventilation and O_2/CO_2 exchange.*
Instruct client to change position, deep breathe, and cough or "huff" every 1 to 2 hours.	*Frequent repositioning helps mobilize secretions and aids lung expansion. Deep breathing helps loosen secretions and promotes a more effective cough. It also promotes maximum lung expansion and stimulates surfactant production. Coughing or "huffing" (a forced expiration technique) mobilizes secretions and facilitates removal of these secretions from the respiratory tract. These actions promote optimal alveolar ventilation and O_2/CO_2 exchange.*
Reinforce correct use of incentive spirometer every 1 to 2 hours. **D** ✦	*Incentive spirometer use promotes slow, deep inhalation, which improves lung expansion and helps clear airways by loosening secretions and promoting a more effective cough. These actions enhance alveolar ventilation and the exchange of O_2/CO_2.*
Implement measures to reduce chest or abdominal pain if present (e.g., splint incision with pillow during coughing and deep breathing). **D** ● ✦	*A client with chest or abdominal pain often guards respiratory efforts and breathes shallowly in an attempt to prevent additional discomfort. Pain reduction enables the client to breathe more deeply, which enhances alveolar ventilation and O_2/CO_2 exchange.*
Implement measures to decrease fear and anxiety (e.g., assure client that breathing deeply will not dislodge tubes or cause incision to break open, interact with client in a confident manner). **D** ● ✦	*Fear and anxiety may cause a client to breathe shallowly or to hyperventilate. Decreasing fear and anxiety allows the client to focus on breathing more slowly and taking deeper breaths, which subsequently enhances alveolar ventilation and the exchange of O_2/CO_2.*
Instruct client in, and assist with, diaphragmatic breathing and pursed-lip breathing techniques if appropriate. NOTE: Diaphragmatic breathing is most often indicated for clients who have had thoracic surgery or clients who have chronic airflow limitation (e.g., emphysema) or neuromuscular conditions that cause fixation or weakening of the diaphragm.	*Diaphragmatic breathing promotes greater movement of the diaphragm and decreases the use of the accessory muscles for inspiration. Use of this technique eases the work of breathing and ultimately promotes an increased efficiency of alveolar ventilation. Pursed-lip breathing causes a mild resistance to exhalation, which creates positive pressure in the airways. This pressure helps prevent airway collapse and subsequently promotes more complete alveolar emptying.*
Discourage smoking. **D** ✦	*Smoking impairs gas exchange because it:* • *Reduces effective airway clearance by increasing mucus production and impairing ciliary function* • *Decreases O_2 availability (hemoglobin binds with the carbon monoxide in smoke rather than with O_2)* • *Causes damage to the bronchial and alveolar walls* • *Causes vasoconstriction and subsequently reduces pulmonary blood flow.*

Continued...

THERAPEUTIC INTERVENTIONS	RATIONALE
Dependent/Collaborative Actions	
Implement measures to facilitate removal of pulmonary secretions (e.g., suction, postural drainage, percussion, vibration) if ordered.	*Excessive secretions and/or client's inability to clear secretions from the respiratory tract lead to stasis of secretions, which can impair O_2/CO_2 exchange. Suction and chest physiotherapy techniques may be necessary to facilitate removal of pulmonary secretions and thereby promote adequate gas exchange.*
Assist with positive airway pressure techniques (e.g., continuous positive airway pressure [CPAP], bilevel positive airway pressure [BiPAP], flutter/positive expiratory pressure [PEP] device) if ordered.	*Positive airway pressure techniques increase intrapulmonary (alveolar) pressure, which helps reexpand collapsed alveoli and prevent further alveolar collapse so that gas exchange can take place.*
Maintain O_2 therapy as ordered. **D** ● ✦	*Supplemental O_2 increases the concentration of O_2 in the alveoli, which increases the diffusion of O_2 across the alveolar-capillary membrane.*
Maintain activity restrictions as ordered. Increase activity gradually as allowed and tolerated. **D** ● ✦	*Restricting activity lowers the body's O_2 requirements and thus increases the amount of O_2 available for gas exchange. A gradual increase in activity conserves energy and thereby lessens O_2 utilization, yet promotes mobilization.*
Administer medications that may be ordered to improve client's respiratory status (e.g., bronchodilators, analgesics, antibiotics, corticosteroids, anticoagulants, diuretics). **D** ✦	*Medication therapy is an integral part of treating many respiratory conditions that impair alveolar gas exchange (e.g., bronchodilators improve bronchial airflow and subsequently increase O_2/CO_2 exchange; analgesics can reduce pain and promote deeper breathing and increased activity; antibiotics help resolve certain respiratory infections; corticosteroids reduce inflammation in the lungs and improve bronchial airflow; anticoagulants treat thromboemboli of the pulmonary vessels and subsequently improve pulmonary perfusion; diuretics reduce fluid accumulation in the pulmonary interstitium and alveoli, which subsequently improves gas exchange).*
Administer central nervous system depressants judiciously. Hold medication and consult physician if respiratory rate is less than 12 breaths/min.	*Central nervous system depressants cause depression of the respiratory center and cough reflex. This can result in hypoventilation and stasis of secretions with subsequent impaired gas exchange.*
Consult appropriate health care provider (e.g., physician, respiratory therapist) if signs and symptoms of impaired gas exchange persist or worsen.	*Notifying the appropriate health care provider allows for modification of treatment plan.*

Nursing Diagnosis ## GLUCOSE LEVEL, BLOOD, RISK FOR UNSTABLE NDx

Definition: Risk for variation of blood glucose/sugar levels from the normal range

CLINICAL MANIFESTATIONS

Subjective	Objective
Hypoglycemia: Reports of hunger; lightheadedness and weakness	**Hypoglycemia:** Confusion; difficulty speaking; shakiness; sweating; below-normal blood glucose levels
Hyperglycemia: Report of frequent hunger; blurred vision; weight loss; dry mouth	**Hyperglycemia:** Frequent urination; elevated blood glucose levels

RISK FACTORS

- Type I and II diabetes, prediabetes, poor diet and nutrition
- Obesity
- Sedentary lifestyle
- Family history of diabetes
- Giving birth to a baby weighing >9 lb
- High-density lipoprotein (HDL) cholesterol <35 mg/dL
- High triglyceride levels
- High blood pressure
- Age >45 years
- History of gestational diabetes
- Ethnic background of Hispanic, black, Native American, and Asian
- Metabolic syndrome
- Deficient knowledge of diabetes management

DESIRED OUTCOMES

The client will not experience unstable glucose levels as evidenced by:
a. Serum fasting serum glucose levels of 70 to 110 mg/dL
b. 2-hour postprandial serum glucose readings of:
   0 to 50 years <140 mg/dL
   50 to 60 years <150 mg/dL
   ≥60 years <160 mg/dL
c. Glycosylated hemoglobin levels (hemoglobin A_{1c}) <7%
d. Demonstrated ability to accurately monitor blood glucose
e. Demonstrated ability to accurately administer insulin
f. Identification of self-care measures if blood glucose is too high or too low

DOCUMENTATION

- Blood glucose levels
- Diet and nutrition
- Therapeutic interventions
- Client and family teaching

NOC OUTCOMES

Healthy diet; stable blood glucose levels; diabetes self-management; medication adherence; health-promoting behaviors

NIC INTERVENTIONS

Blood glucose monitoring; vital signs monitoring; monitor for signs and symptoms of blood glucose changes; facilitate adherence to diet and exercise regimen; encourage patient self-management of blood glucose levels

NURSING ASSESSMENT

Assess for and report signs and symptoms of variations in blood glucose levels:
- Anxiety
- Confusion
- Irritability
- Lethargy or behavior changes
- Drowsiness or fatigue
- Polydipsia
- Nausea
- Vomiting
- Dry mouth
- Blurred vision
- Cold, clammy skin
- Shakiness
- Nervousness
- Fainting

Obtain blood glucose levels and hemoglobin A_{1c} levels and report abnormalities.

Assess self-management skills related to blood glucose levels.

Monitor hemoglobin A_{1c} levels.

Evaluate client's medication regimen for medications that can alter blood glucose levels.

RATIONALE

Early recognition of signs and symptoms of abnormal blood glucose levels allows for prompt intervention.

Blood glucose levels and hemoglobin A_{1c} levels indicate the effectiveness of monitoring and treatment.

Assessment determines need for education and support in self-management of blood glucose levels.

Provides the health care team with a 2- to 3-month overview of how well the client has controlled glucose levels. These data are helpful in discharge planning.

Some medication can cause hyperglycemia or hypoglycemia.

THERAPEUTIC INTERVENTIONS

Independent Actions
Monitor intake and output. **D** ● ✦

RATIONALE

Individuals at risk for blood glucose alterations are at a significant risk for dehydration.

Continued...

THERAPEUTIC INTERVENTIONS	RATIONALE
Client and family teaching and discharge planning on control of blood glucose level through:	*Education has been shown to improve control of blood glucose levels and client self-monitoring, and client sense of control over disease.*
• Diet	*Adherence to a diabetic diet can be used to help regulate blood glucose levels.*
• Exercise	*A regular exercise routine has been shown to control blood glucose levels and decrease the amount of adipose tissue.*
• Medication administration	*Improves client's sense of control over the disease process and maintenance of blood glucose levels*
• Self-monitoring of blood glucose	*Reduces incidences of hyperglycemia or hypoglycemic episodes and reduces complications of disease*
• Recognition and treatment of signs and symptoms of hyperglycemia and hypoglycemia	*Allows for prompt intervention and decreases large variations in blood glucose levels*
• Smoking cessation	*Smoking has been associated with worsening glucose control and insulin resistance.*

Dependent/Collaborative Actions

Monitor blood glucose levels at meals and at bedtime. More frequent monitoring of blood glucose levels (e.g., every 4 to 6 hours) is required when client is to have nothing by mouth (NPO). Refer to facility policy for frequency. **D** ● ✦	*Frequent blood glucose testing is important for maintenance of appropriate blood glucose levels. When the client is NPO, this is important to prevent significant declines in blood glucose levels.*
Monitor blood glucose levels every hour in a client who is receiving continuous intravenous insulin. **D** ✦	*Blood glucose levels change quickly and may require immediate intervention.*
Administer oral hypoglycemics and insulin as needed. (Note: Always check blood glucose levels before insulin administration.) **D** ✦	*Timely administration of insulin assists in maintaining appropriate blood glucose levels and prevents progression to diabetes ketoacidosis.*
Administer ½ cup of fruit juice for hypoglycemia if client is able to take fluids. Administer 50% dextrose in water (D50W) or intramuscular glucagon if client is unable to take oral carbohydrates. (NOTE: Review hospital policy for variations.)	*Early treatment of hypoglycemia can prevent more severe hypoglycemia. D50W is an alternative to oral carbohydrates when the patient is unable to take fluids.*
Refer client for dietary counseling and diabetic education.	*Dietary counseling and diabetic education are interventions that can increase client knowledge of the disease process. Knowledge of disease process can facilitate adherence to treatment plans.*
Refer client and family to community resources.	*Provides for continuum of care.*

Nursing Diagnosis   GRIEVING* NDx

Definition: A normal complex process that includes emotional physical, spiritual, social, and intellectual responses and behaviors by which individuals families, and communities incorporate an actual, anticipated, perceived loss into their daily lives.

CLINICAL MANIFESTATIONS

Subjective	Objective
Report of sorrow, guilt, pain; changes in dream patterns	Changes inactivity level; anger; blame, detachment; disorganization; difficulty in expressing the loss; denial of loss, changes in sleep patterns

RISK FACTORS

• Loss of an object (e.g., people, posessions, job status, home, ideals, parts and processes of the body)

---

*This diagnostic label includes anticipatory grieving and grieving after the actual loss.

DESIRED OUTCOMES

The client will demonstrate beginning progression through the grieving process as evidenced by:
  a. Verbalization of feelings about the loss
  b. Usual sleep pattern
  c. Participation in treatment plan and self-care activities
  d. Use of available support systems

DOCUMENTATION

- Verbalization of feelings about the loss
- Participation in activities
- Eating pattern
- Sleep pattern
- Interaction with others
- Measures used to adapt to loss
- Client/family teaching

NOC OUTCOMES

Resolves feelings about loss; maintains personal grooming habits; reports adequate sleep and nutrition; involvement in social activities; progresses through grief stages

NIC INTERVENTIONS

Grief work facilitation; emotional support; presence; support system enhancement

NURSING ASSESSMENT	RATIONALE
Assess for signs and symptoms of grieving: • Expression of distress about the loss • Change in eating habits • Inability to concentrate • Insomnia • Anger • Sadness • Withdrawal from significant others • Denial of loss	*Assessment of signs and symptoms of grieving helps the nurse determine the phase of grieving the client is experiencing. This knowledge aids in the development of effective strategies that can assist the client to progress through the phases of grieving.*
Assess for factors that may hinder and facilitate client's acknowledgment of the loss.	*In order for grief work to begin. the client needs to acknowledge the loss. An awareness of factors that may hinder and facilitate this acknowledgment assists in the development of effective strategies to accomplish this goal.*

THERAPEUTIC INTERVENTIONS	RATIONALE
Independent Actions Assist client to acknowledge the loss (e.g., encourage conversation about the loss including how or why it occurred and its impact on his/her future).	*The client needs to acknowledge the loss in order for grief work to begin.*
Discuss the grieving process and assist client to accept the phases of grieving as an expected response to an actual and/or anticipated loss.	*An awareness of the feelings and behaviors commonly associated with each phase of the grieving process assists the client to accept his/her responses to the loss.*
Allow time for client to progress through the phases of grieving (phases vary among theorists but progress from shock and alarm to acceptance).	*Grieving is a process that occurs in phases or stages that progress over time. Some phases may not be experienced by the client, and some may overlap or recur. The amount of time necessary to reach resolution of grief is very individual, may take months to years, and must be allowed to occur in order to reduce the risk for dysfunctional grieving.*
Provide an atmosphere of care and concern (e.g., provide privacy, be available and nonjudgmental, display empathy and respect). **D** ● ✦	*A supportive, nonthreatening environment provides the basis for a constructive, therapeutic relationship between the client and nurse. This allows the client to express feelings of grief and work toward its resolution.*
Implement measures to promote trust (e.g., answer questions honestly, provide requested information). **D** ● ✦	*A feeling of trust in the caregiver promotes the development of a therapeutic relationship in which the client can feel free to verbalize feelings. This facilitates the progression of grief work.*
Encourage the verbal expression of anger and sadness about the loss experienced. Recognize displacement of anger and assist client to see the actual cause of angry feelings and resentment. Establish limits on abusive behavior if demonstrated. **D** ● ✦	*The verbal expression of feelings of anger and sadness facilitates movement toward resolution of grief. Displacement of angry feelings needs to be acknowledged so that grieving can progress but should not be allowed to interfere with the therapeutic process.*
Encourage client to express feelings in whatever ways are comfortable (e.g., writing, drawing, conversation). **D** ● ✦	*Expression of feelings helps the client integrate both positive and negative aspects of the loss and move toward its acceptance.*

NDx = NANDA-I Diagnosis   **D** = Delegatable Action   ● = UAP   ✦ = LVN/LPN   ⊖▶ = Go to ⊖volve for animation

Continued...

THERAPEUTIC INTERVENTIONS	RATIONALE
Assist client to use techniques that have helped him/her cope in previous situations of loss.	*Techniques that have previously facilitated the client's adjustment to situations of loss are often effective when used to help him/her cope with the current loss.*
Support behaviors suggesting successful grief work (e.g., verbalizing feelings about loss, focusing on ways to adapt to loss, learning needed skills, developing or renewing relationships).	*Positive feedback about behaviors that suggest successful grief work reinforces those behaviors and promotes positive adaptation to loss.*
Explain the phases of the grieving process to significant others. Encourage their support and understanding.	*When significant others are knowledgeable about the phases of the grieving process, they are more likely to understand and accept the client's behavior and assist him/her to move toward resolution of grief.*
Facilitate communication between the client and significant others. Be aware that they may be in different phases of the grieving process.	*Effective communication between the client and significant others enhances the client's ability to express feelings and successfully move through the phases of grieving.*

Dependent/Collaborative Actions

THERAPEUTIC INTERVENTIONS	RATIONALE
Provide information about counseling services and support groups that might assist client in working through grief.	*Counseling and support groups can assist the client in working through grief by:* • *Providing insight into his/her responses to the loss* • *Decreasing the feelings of aloneness and isolation that frequently accompany a loss* • *Helping identify methods or skills that can be used to help cope with the loss*
When appropriate, assist client to meet spiritual needs (e.g., arrange for a visit from clergy).	*Spiritual support can be a source of strength and solace to the client and can facilitate resolution of grief.*
Consult appropriate health care provider (e.g., psychiatric nurse practitioner, grief counselor, physician) if signs of dysfunctional grieving (e.g., persistent denial of losses, excessive anger or sadness, emotional lability) occur.	*Notifying the appropriate health care provider allows for modification of the treatment plan.*

⊖▶ **Nursing Diagnosis** | # HEALTH BEHAVIORS, RISK-PRONE NDx

For a full, detailed care plan on this topic, go to http://evolve.elsevier.com/Haugen/careplanning/.

⊖▶ **Nursing Diagnosis** | # INFECTION, RISK FOR NDx

Definition: At increased risk for being invaded by pathogenic organisms

CLINICAL MANIFESTATIONS*

Subjective	Objective
Verbalization of chills; loss of energy; loss of appetite; reports of pain frequency, urgency, or burning with urination	Elevated temperature; increased heart rate; abnormal breath sounds; productive cough of purulent, green, or rust-colored sputum Cloudy urine Increase WBC count in urinalysis; presence of bacteria Heat, swelling, and/or unusual drainage in an area Increase WBC count for significant change in differential

*Clinical manifestations vary depending on the site of infection.

RISK FACTORS

- Inadequate primary defenses (broken skin, traumatized tissue, decrease in ciliary action, stasis of body fluids, change in pH of secretions, altered peristalsis)
- Inadequate secondary defenses (decreased hemoglobin, leukopenia, suppressed inflammatory response)
- Immunosuppression
- Inadequate acquired immunity
- Trauma
- Tissue destruction and increased environmental exposure
- Chronic disease
- Malnutrition
- Invasive procedures
- Pharmaceutical agents (e.g., immunosuppressants)
- Rupture of amniotic membranes
- Insufficient knowledge to avoid exposure to pathogens

DESIRED OUTCOMES

The client will remain free of infection as evidenced by:
a. Absence of fever and chills
b. Pulse rate within normal limits
c. Usual mental status
d. Normal breath sounds
e. Cough productive of clear mucus only
f. Voiding clear urine without reports of frequency, urgency, and burning
g. Absence of heat, pain, redness, swelling, and unusual drainage in any area
h. White blood cell (WBC) and differential counts within normal range for client
i. Negative results of cultured specimens

DOCUMENTATION

- Temperature
- Pulse rate
- Presence of chills
- Mental status
- Breath sounds
- Characteristics of urine, sputum, and wound drainage
- Evidence of inflammation in any area
- Evidence of unusual drainage from any area
- Therapeutic interventions
- Client/family teaching

NOC OUTCOMES

Infection free

NIC INTERVENTIONS

Infection control; infection protection; incision site care; tube care; wound care; nutrition management

NURSING ASSESSMENT	RATIONALE
Assess for and report signs and symptoms of infection (be aware that some signs and symptoms vary depending on the site of infection, the causative agent, and the age and immune status of the client): <ul><li>Elevated temperature</li><li>Chills</li><li>Increased pulse rate</li><li>Malaise, lethargy, acute confusion</li><li>Loss of appetite</li><li>Abnormal breath sounds</li><li>Productive cough of purulent, green, or rust-colored sputum</li><li>Cloudy urine</li><li>Reports of frequency, urgency, or burning when urinating</li><li>Urinalysis showing a WBC count greater than 5, positive leukocyte esterase or nitrites, or presence of bacteria</li><li>Heat, pain, redness, swelling, or unusual drainage in any area</li><li>Elevated WBC count and/or significant change in differential</li></ul>	*Early recognition of signs and symptoms of infection allows for prompt intervention.*
Obtain specimens (e.g., urine, wound drainage, vaginal drainage, sputum, blood) for culture as ordered. Report positive results.	*Cultures are done to identify the specific organism(s) causing the infection. Culture results provide information that helps determine the most effective treatment.*

Continued...

THERAPEUTIC INTERVENTIONS	RATIONALE

Independent Actions

Maintain a fluid intake of at least 2500 mL/day unless contraindicated. **D** ✦	Adequate hydration helps prevent infection by: • *Helping maintain adequate blood flow and nutrient supply to the tissues* • *Promoting urine formation and subsequent voiding, which flushes pathogens from the bladder and urethra* • *Thinning respiratory secretions so that they can more easily be removed by coughing or suctioning (respiratory secretions provide a good medium for growth and colonization of microorganisms)*
Use good hand hygiene and encourage client to do the same. **D** ● ✦	*Good hand hygiene removes transient flora, which reduces the risk of transmission of pathogens. Use of products such as an antibacterial soap, a chlorhexidine solution, or an alcohol-based handrub agent can actually inhibit the growth of or kill microorganisms, which further reduces infection risk.*
Adhere to the appropriate precautions established to prevent transmission of infection to the client (e.g., standard precautions, transmission-based precautions on other clients, neutropenic precautions). **D** ● ✦	*Adhering to the appropriate precautions that have been established to help prevent the transmission of microorganisms reduces the client's risk of infection.*
Use sterile technique during invasive procedures (e.g., urinary catheterizations, venous and arterial punctures, injections, tracheal suctioning, wound care and dressing changes). **D** ✦	*Use of sterile technique reduces the possibility of introducing pathogens into the body.*
Anchor catheters/tubings (e.g., urinary, intravenous, wound drainage) securely. **D** ✦	*Catheters/tubings that are not securely anchored have some degree of in-and-out movement. This movement increases the risk of infection because it allows for the introduction of pathogens into the body. It can also cause tissue trauma, which can result in colonization of microorganisms.*
Change equipment, tubings, and solutions used for treatments, such as intravenous infusions, respiratory care, irrigations, and enteral feedings according to hospital policy.	*The longer that equipment, tubings, and solutions are in use, the greater the chance of colonization of microorganisms, which can then be introduced into the body.*
Maintain a closed system for drains (e.g., wounds, chest tubes, urinary catheters) and intravenous infusions whenever possible.	*Each time a drainage or infusion system is opened, pathogens from the environment have an opportunity to enter the body. Maintaining a closed system decreases this risk, which reduces the possibility of infection.*
Change peripheral intravenous line sites according to hospital policy. **D** ✦	*Peripheral intravenous line sites are changed routinely to reduce persistent irritation of one area of a vein wall and the resultant colonization of microorganisms at that site.*
Protect client from others with infections. **D** ● ✦	*Protecting the client from others with infections reduces his/her risk of exposure to pathogens.*
Implement measures to maintain healthy, intact skin (e.g., keep skin lubricated, clean, and dry; instruct or assist client to turn every 2 hours; keep bed linens dry and wrinkle-free). **D** ● ✦	*Healthy, intact skin reduces the risk for infection by:* • *Providing a physical barrier against the introduction of pathogens into the body* • *Removing many of the microorganisms on the surface of the skin by means of the constant shedding of the epidermis* • *Inhibiting the growth of some bacteria on the surface of the skin (sebum contains fatty acids, which create a slightly acidic environment that inhibits the growth of some bacteria)*
Implement measures to reduce stress (e.g., reduce fear, anxiety, and pain; help client identify and use effective coping mechanisms). **D** ✦	*Stress causes an increased secretion of cortisol. Cortisol interferes with some immune responses, which subsequently increases the client's susceptibility to infection.*
Maintain an optimal nutritional status.	*Adequate nutrition is needed to maintain normal function of the immune system.*
Instruct and assist client to perform good perineal care routinely and after each bowel movement. **D** ✦	*The perineal area contains a large number of organisms. Routine cleansing of the area reduces the risk of colonization of organisms and subsequent perineal, urinary tract, and/or vaginal infection.*

THERAPEUTIC INTERVENTIONS	RATIONALE
Instruct and assist client to perform good oral hygiene as often as needed. **D** ✦	*Frequent oral hygiene helps prevent infection by removing most of the food, debris, and many of the microorganisms that are present in the mouth. It also helps maintain the integrity of the oral mucosa, which provides a physical and chemical barrier to pathogens.*
Implement measures to prevent urinary retention (e.g., instruct client to urinate when the urge is felt, promote relaxation during voiding attempts.	*A client experiencing urinary retention is at increased risk for urinary tract infection because:* • *The urine that accumulates in the bladder creates an environment conducive to the growth and colonization of microorganisms.* • *Voiding does not occur so microorganisms are not flushed from the mucous lining of the urethra; these microorganisms can colonize and ascend into the bladder.*
Implement measures to prevent stasis of respiratory secretions (e.g., assist client to turn, cough, and deep breathe; increase activity as allowed and tolerated; perform tracheal suctioning if indicated). **D** ✦	*Respiratory secretions provide a good medium for growth of microorganisms. By preventing stasis, there is less chance of colonization of the microorganisms and a decreased risk for development of respiratory tract infection.*
Instruct client to receive immunizations (e.g., influenza vaccine, pneumococcal vaccine) if appropriate.	*Immunizations are often recommended to reduce the possibility of some infections in high-risk clients (e.g., those clients who are immunosuppressed, elderly, or have a chronic disease).*

Dependent/Collaborative Actions

Administer vitamins and minerals as ordered. **D** ✦	*Adequate nutrition is needed to maintain normal function of the immune system.*
Provide appropriate wound care (e.g., use dressing materials that maintain a moist wound surface, assist with debridement of necrotic tissue, use dressing materials that absorb excess exudate, protect granulating tissue from trauma and contamination, maintain patency of wound drains). **D** ✦	*Proper wound care facilitates wound healing and reduces the number of pathogens that enter or are present in the wound, which reduces the risk of the wound becoming infected.*
Administer bethanechol as ordered). **D** ✦	*Relaxes the bladder sphincter muscles and stimulates urination.*
Consult appropriate health care provider regarding initiation of antimicrobial therapy if indicated. Question orders that do not seem appropriate (e.g., prolonged use of antimicrobials, excessively high dose of an antimicrobial, unnecessary use of broad-spectrum or multiple antimicrobials).	*Most antimicrobials disrupt cell wall synthesis, which halts the growth of, or kills microorganisms. This can effectively reduce the client's risk for infection. Antimicrobial orders that seem inappropriate should be questioned because they can result in the elimination of normal flora and/or the development of drug-resistant microorganisms, which actually increase the client's risk for infection.*

Nursing Diagnosis **MOBILITY, PHYSICAL, IMPAIRED** NDx

Definition: State in which there is limited independent purposeful physical movement of the body or one or more extremities

CLINICAL MANIFESTATIONS

Subjective	**Objective**
Verbalization of pain; discomfort; fatigue	Decreased reaction time; difficulty moving; engages in substitution for movement; supporting the affected limb; exertional dyspnea; contractures; limited ability to perform gross and fine motor skills; limited range of motion (ROM); intentional movement-induced tremor; postural instability; uncoordinated movements

Continued...

RISK FACTORS

- Sedentary lifestyle
- Limited cardiovascular endurance
- Joint stiffness or contracture
- Pain and/or discomfort
- Depression and/or anxiety

- Neuromuscular impairment
- Prescribed movement restrictions
- Decreased muscle strength and/or mass
- Activity intolerance

- Cognitive impairment
- Lack of knowledge regarding the value of physical activity
- Loss of bone mass
- Sensoriperceptual impairments

DESIRED OUTCOMES

The client will improve mobility as evidenced by:
a. Increased physical activity
b. Movement of affected limb or limbs
c. Participation in activities of daily living (ADLs)
d. Demonstration of appropriate use of assistive devices to improve movement

DOCUMENTATION

- ADLs
- Muscle strength
- Distance ambulated
- Passive or active ROM
- Therapeutic interventions
- Client/family teaching

NOC OUTCOMES

Activity tolerance; cardiovascular status; fall prevention behavior; endurance; prevention of contractures; increase strength in body or affected limb; willingness to participate in activities

NIC INTERVENTIONS

Positioning; ambulation; pain relief; active and/or passive ROM

NURSING ASSESSMENT	RATIONALE
Assess client's movement ability and activity tolerance. Use a tool such as the *Assessment Tool for Safe Patient Handling and Movement* or the *Functional Independence Measures (FIM)*.	Assessment of mobility is used to best determine how to facilitate movement. Assessment of activity tolerance provides a baseline for patient strength and endurance with movement.
Assess for cause of immobility.	It is important to determine if the cause of immobility is physical or psychological, and to plan interventions to improve mobility.
Assess circulation, motion, and feeling in digits.	Circulation may be compromised by edema of extremities, which can lead to tissue necrosis and/or contractures.
Assess skin integrity.	Routine examination of the skin provides for early detection and intervention of pressure sores. Pressure sores develop quickly in patients who are immobile.
Assess emotional response to immobility.	Determine client's acceptance of temporary or permanent limitations. This impacts implementation of therapeutic interventions.
Assess need for assistive devices.	Determine client's needs for assistive devices as well as proper use of wheelchairs, walkers, canes, etc., to reduce incidence of falls.

THERAPEUTIC INTERVENTIONS	RATIONALE
Independent Actions Encourage and implement strength training activities: • Active and/or passive ROM • Ambulation • Use of trapeze for pull-ups • ADLs **D** ● ✦	Inactivity contributes to muscle weakening. Contractures can develop as early as 8 hours of immobility. These activities maintain and increase the client's strength and ability to move.
Use assistive devices to help client with movement: • Crutches • Gait belt • Walker **D** ● ✦	Assistive devices help the caregivers decrease the potential for falls and/or injuries.
Cluster treatments and care activities to allow for uninterrupted periods of rest. **D** ● ✦	Increases client's tolerance and strength for activities.
Encourage patient with positive reinforcement during activities. **D** ● ✦	A positive approach to activities supports the client's accomplishment, engagement in new activities, and improves self-esteem.
Implement falls protocol.	Client safety is a priority.
Maintain the bed in low position and keep side rails up. **D** ● ✦	Reduces prolonged pressure on tissues, decreasing potential for tissue ischemia and pressure sores.

THERAPEUTIC INTERVENTIONS	RATIONALE
For bedridden patients, turn and reposition every 2 hours. **D ● ✦**	*Turning clients allows for appropriate circulation to tissues.*
Position client with appropriate devices (wedges, pillows, kinetic bed, air bed, gel mattress). **D ● ✦**	*Reduces prolonged pressure on tissues, decreasing potential for tissue ischemia and pressure sores*
Use sequential compression devices or antiembolic stockings. **D ● ✦**	*Improves venous circulation and helps to prevent thrombophlebitis in lower extremities*
Implement measures to maintain healthy, intact skin (e.g., keep skin lubricated, clean, and dry; instruct or assist client to turn every 2 hours; keep bed linens dry and wrinkle-free). **D ● ✦**	*Healthy, intact skin reduces the risk of pressure sores and infection.*
Maintain an optimal nutritional status. Increase protein intake.	*Adequate nutrition is needed to maintain adequate energy level.*
Increase fluid intake to 2000 to 3000 mL/day unless contraindicated.	*Increased fluid maintains adequate hydration and helps prevent constipation and hardening of the stool.*
Encourage coughing and deep breathing exercises and use of incentive spirometry.	*Prevents buildup of secretions and promotes lung expansion.*
Initiate bowel program.	*Prolonged immobility can lead to constipation.*
Assist client with acceptance of immobility.	*Helps patient accept limitations and focus on a new quality of life.*

Dependent/Collaborative Actions

Consult appropriate health care provider: Dietitian, physician, and occupational therapist.	*These individuals provide specific activities and exercise programs to improve strength and mobility.*
Administer pain medications before activities. **D ✦**	*Reduces muscle stiffness and tension, allowing the client to participate in activities.*

Nursing Diagnosis

NUTRITION: LESS THAN BODY REQUIREMENTS, IMBALANCED NDx

Definition: Intake of nutrients insufficient to meet the body's metabolic needs

CLINICAL MANIFESTATIONS

Subjective	Objective
Reports of lack of appetite; fatigue; irritability; poor self-esteem; verbalization of sore mucous membranes	Loss of weight with adequate food intake; body weight 20% or more under ideal weight; sore, inflamed buccal cavity; capillary fragility; pale conjunctiva and mucous membranes; poor muscle tone; excessive hair loss; amenorrhea; decreased blood urea nitrogen (BUN) and elevated creatinine levels; decreased albumin and prealbumin levels; decreased hematocrit (Hct), decreased hemoglobin (Hgb), and decreased white blood cells

RISK FACTORS

- Inability to ingest or digest food or absorb nutrients because of biological, psychological, or economic factors

DESIRED OUTCOMES

The client will maintain an adequate nutritional status as evidenced by:
  a. Weight within normal range for the client
  b. Normal BUN and serum albumin, prealbumin, Hct, Hgb, and lymphocyte levels
  c. Usual strength and activity tolerance
  d. Healthy oral mucous membrane

DOCUMENTATION

- Weight
- Activity tolerance
- Condition of oral mucous membrane
- Type of diet and amount consumed
- Therapeutic interventions
- Client/family teaching

Continued...

NOC OUTCOMES	NIC INTERVENTIONS
Appropriate appetite; positive body image; bowel elimination; compliance with prescribed diet; adequate hydration; weight maintenance behavior	Nutritional monitoring; nutritional counseling; nutritional management; nutrition therapy; weight gain assistance; weight management

NURSING ASSESSMENT	RATIONALE
Assess for and report signs and symptoms of malnutrition: • Weight significantly below client's usual weight or below normal for client's age, height, and body frame • Increased BUN and low serum albumin, prealbumin, Hct, Hgb, and lymphocyte levels • Weakness and fatigue • Sore, inflamed oral mucous membrane • Pale conjunctiva	*Early recognition of signs and symptoms of malnutrition allows for prompt intervention.*
Monitor percentage of meals and snacks client consumes. Report a pattern or inadequate intake.	*An awareness of the amount of foods/fluids the client consumes alerts the nurse to deficits in nutritional intake. Reporting an inadequate intake allows for prompt intervention.*
Perform or assist with anthropometric measurements such as skinfold thickness, body circumferences (e.g., hip, waist, mid-upper arm), and bioelectrical impedance analysis if indicated. Report results that are lower than normal.	*Anthropometric measurements provide information about the amount of muscle mass, body fat, and protein reserves the client has. These assessments assist in evaluating the client's nutritional status.*

THERAPEUTIC INTERVENTIONS	RATIONALE

Independent Actions

Implement measures to prevent vomiting if indicated (e.g., eliminate noxious sites and odors). **D** ● ✦	*Vomiting results in actual loss of nutrients.*
Implement measures to control diarrhea if present (e.g., discourage intake of spicy foods and foods high in fiber or lactose). **D** ● ✦	*Increased intestinal motility that occurs with or causes diarrhea results in a decreased absorption of nutrients in the bowel. In addition, diarrhea causes an actual loss of nutrients.*
Implement measures to improve oral intake:	
• Perform actions to reduce nausea, pain, fear, and anxiety if present. **D** ● ✦	*Decreases client's appetite and oral intake.*
• Perform actions to relieve gastrointestinal distention if present (e.g., encourage and assist client with frequent ambulation) unless contraindicated. **D** ● ✦	*Distention of the gastrointestinal tract (especially the stomach and duodenum) can result in stimulation of the satiety center and subsequent inhibition of the feeding center in the hypothalamus. This effect, along with the discomfort that occurs with distention, decreases appetite.*
• Increase activity as allowed and tolerated. **D** ● ✦	*Activity usually promotes a general feeling of well-being, which can result in improved appetite.*
• Maintain a clean environment and a relaxed, pleasant atmosphere. **D** ● ✦	*Noxious sites and odors can inhibit the feeding center in the hypothalamus. Maintain a clean environment helps prevent this from occurring. In addition, maintaining a relaxed, pleasant atmosphere can help reduce the client's stress and promote a feeling of well-being which tends to improve appetite and oral intake.*
• Encourage a rest period before meals if indicated. **D** ● ✦	*The physical activity of eating requires some expenditure of energy. Fatigue can reduce the client's desire and ability to eat.*
• Provide oral hygiene before meals. **D** ● ✦	*Oral hygiene moistens the oral mucous membrane, which may make it easier to chew and swallow. It also freshens the mouth and removes unpleasant tastes. This can improve the taste of foods/fluids, which helps stimulate appetite and increase oral intake.*
• Serve foods/fluids that are appealing to the client and adhere to personal and cultural (e.g., religious, ethnic) preferences whenever possible. **D** ● ✦	*Foods/fluids that appeal to the client's senses (especially sight and smell) and are in accordance with personal and cultural preferences are most likely to stimulate appetite and promote interest in eating.*

THERAPEUTIC INTERVENTIONS	RATIONALE
• Serve frequent, small meals rather than large ones if client is weak, fatigues easily, and/or has a poor appetite. **D** ● ✦	*Providing small rather than large meals can enable a client who is weak or fatigues easily to finish a meal. Also, a client who has a poor appetite is often more willing to attempt to eat smaller meals because they seem less overwhelming than larger ones. If smaller meals are served, the number of meals per day should be increased to help ensure adequate nutrition.*
• Encourage significant others to bring in client's favorite foods unless contraindicated and eat with him/her if client desires.	*A client's favorite foods/fluids tend to stimulate his/her appetite more than institutional foods/fluids. The presence of significant others during meals helps create a familiar social environment that can stimulate appetite and improve oral intake.*
• If client is experiencing dyspnea, place him/her in a high-Fowler's position and provide supplemental oxygen therapy during meals if indicated.	*Because a person cannot swallow and breathe at the same time, relief of dyspnea increases the likelihood of maintaining a good oral intake. In addition, relieving dyspnea decreases the client's anxiety about and preoccupation with breathing efforts and increases the ability to focus on eating and drinking.*
• Perform actions to compensate for taste alterations if present (e.g., add extra sweeteners to foods unless contraindicated, encourage client to experiment with different flavorings and seasonings, provide alternative sources of protein if meats such as beef or pork taste bitter or rancid).	*Enhancing the taste of foods/fluids and providing nutritious alternatives to those that taste unpleasant to the client help to stimulate appetite and improve oral intake.*
• Allow adequate time for meals; reheat foods/fluids if necessary. **D** ● ✦	*A client who feels rushed during meals tends to become anxious, lose his/her appetite, and stops eating. Appetite is also suppressed if foods/fluids normally served hot or warm become cold and do not appeal to the client.*
• Limit fluid intake with meals unless the fluid has a high nutritional value. **D** ● ✦	*When the stomach becomes distended, its volume receptors stimulate the satiety center in the hypothalamus, and the client reduces his/her oral intake. Drinking liquids with meals distends the stomach and may cause satiety before an adequate amount of food is consumed.*
Ensure that meals are well balanced and high in essential nutrients.	*The client must consume a diet that is well balanced and high in essential nutrients in order to meet his/her nutritional needs. Dietary supplements are often needed to help accomplish this.*
Allow the client to assist in the selection of foods/fluids that meet nutritional needs. **D** ● ✦	*The client who is actively involved in menu planning is more likely to adhere to the diet plan. In addition, the involvement increases his/her sense of control, which promotes a feeling of well-being and can lead to an increased oral intake.*

Dependent/Collaborative Actions

Administer medications that may be ordered to improve client's nutritional status (e.g., antiemetics, antidiarrheals, gastrointestinal stimulants, and vitamins and minerals). **D** ✦	*Medications may relieve vomiting, diarrhea, and distention of the gastric tract, which decreases the discomfort that occurs with each of these signs and symptoms. Vitamins and minerals are needed to maintain metabolic functioning. If the client's dietary intake does not provide adequate amounts of them, oral and/or parenteral supplements may be necessary.*
Obtain a dietary consult if necessary.	*A dietitian is best able to evaluate whether the foods/fluids selected will meet the client's nutritional needs.*
Perform a calorie count if ordered. Report information to the dietitian and physician.	*A calorie count provides information about the caloric and nutritional value of the foods/fluids the client consumes. The information obtained helps the dietitian and physician determine whether an alternative method of nutritional support is needed.*
Consult the physician about an alternative method of providing nutrition (e.g., parenteral nutrition, tube feeding, etc.) if the client does not consume enough food or fluids to meet nutritional needs.	*If the client's oral intake is inadequate, an alternative method of providing nutrients needs to be implemented.*

| Nursing Diagnosis | **ORAL MUCOUS MEMBRANE, IMPAIRED** NDx |

Definition: Disruption of the lips and/or soft tissue of the oral cavity

CLINICAL MANIFESTATIONS

Subjective	Objective
Report sensitive tongue; bad taste in the mouth; oral pain/discomfort; self-report of difficulty eating or swallowing; self-report of diminished or absent taste	Purulent drainage or exudates; gingival recession, pockets deeper than 4 mm; enlarged tonsils beyond what is developmentally appropriate; smooth, atrophic geographic tongue; mucosal denudation; presence of pathogens; difficult speech; gingival or mucosal pallor; xerostomia (dry mouth); vesicles, nodules, or papules; white patches/plaques, spongy patches, or white curdlike exudate; oral lesions or ulcers; halitosis; edema; hyperemia; desquamation; coated tongue; stomatitis; bleeding; macroplasia; gingival hyperplasia; fissures, cheilitis; red or bluish masses (e.g., hemangiomas)

RISK FACTORS

- Chemotherapy
- Chemical (e.g., alcohol, tobacco, acidic foods, drugs, regular use of inhalers or other noxious agents)
- Depression
- Immunosuppression
- Aging-related loss of connective, adipose, or bone tissue
- Barriers to professional care
- Cleft lip or palate
- Medication side effects
- Lack of or decreased salivation
- Trauma
- Pathological conditions: oral cavity (radiation to head or neck)
- Nothing by mouth (NPO) for more than 24 hours
- Mouth breathing
- Malnutrition or vitamin deficiency
- Dehydration
- Infection
- Ineffective oral hygiene
- Mechanical (e.g., ill-fitting dentures, braces, tubes [endotracheal/nasogastric], surgery in oral cavity)
- Decreased platelets
- Immunocompromised
- Radiation therapy
- Barriers to oral self-care
- Diminished hormone levels (women)
- Stress
- Loss of supportive structures

DESIRED OUTCOMES

The client will maintain a healthy oral cavity as evidenced by:
  a. Absence of inflammation and discomfort
  b. Pink, moist, intact mucosa

DOCUMENTATION

- Client reports of oral dryness and/or discomfort
- Condition of oral mucous membranes
- Therapeutic interventions
- Client teaching

NOC OUTCOMES

Oral hygiene; tissue integrity of skin and mucous membranes; hydration; nutritional status

NIC INTERVENTIONS

Oral health maintenance; oral health restoration; oral health promotion

NURSING ASSESSMENT	RATIONALE
Assess for and report signs and symptoms of impaired oral mucous membrane (e.g., reports of oral dryness and discomfort, coated tongue, inflamed and/or ulcerated oral mucosa).	*Early recognition of signs and symptoms of impaired oral mucous membrane allows for prompt intervention.*
Culture oral lesions as ordered. Report positive results.	*A positive culture reveals the organisms present in a lesion, which provides direction for the treatment plan.*

THERAPEUTIC INTERVENTIONS	RATIONALE

Independent Actions

Assist client to perform oral hygiene as often as needed (e.g., after meals and at bedtime, at least every 2 hours if NPO). **D** ● ✦	*Good oral hygiene helps maintain health of the oral mucous membrane by removing food particles and debris that harbor or promote the growth of pathogenic organisms that can cause inflammation and infection. Brushing the teeth also stimulates circulation to the gums.*

THERAPEUTIC INTERVENTIONS	RATIONALE
Assist client to perform oral hygiene using a soft bristle toothbrush or sponge-tipped swab and to floss teeth gently. **D** ● ✦	*Use of appropriate oral hygiene devices and techniques helps to effectively remove food particles and debris from client's mouth without causing trauma to the oral mucous membrane.*
Avoid use of mouthwashes containing alcohol and oral care products that contain lemon and glycerin. **D** ● ✦	*Mouthwashes containing alcohol and oral care products containing lemon and glycerin have a drying and irritating effect on the oral mucous membrane. Excessive use of the lemon-glycerin products also increases acidity in the mouth, which results in further irritation of the oral mucosa.*
Encourage client to rinse mouth frequently with water. **D** ● ✦	*Frequent rinsing of the mouth helps alleviate dryness, which reduces the risk for cracking and breakdown of the oral mucosa. Rinsing also helps prevent inflammation and infection in the mouth by removing food particles and debris that can harbor or promote the growth of pathogenic organisms.*
Lubricate client's lips frequently. **D** ● ✦	*Lubricating the client's lips helps keep them moist, which helps prevent drying and cracking of the lips.*
Encourage client to breathe through nose rather than mouth. **D** ✦	*Air inspired through the nose is humidified by the layer of mucus that coats the lining of the nasal cavity. Air inspired through the mouth lacks this moisture and is drying to the oral mucous membrane.*
Encourage client not to smoke or chew tobacco.	*Smoking dries the oral mucous membrane. Irritation and subsequent inflammation can occur when tobacco is in contact with the oral mucosa.*
Encourage a fluid intake of at least 2500 mL/day unless contraindicated. **D** ● ✦	*Adequate hydration helps keep the oral mucosa moist, which reduces the risk of cracking and breakdown.*
Encourage client to suck on hard candy if allowed. **D** ✦	*Sucking on hard candy stimulates salivation, which helps alleviate dryness of the oral mucosa and the subsequent risk of cracking and breakdown. Saliva also helps maintain oral mucosal health by washing away food particles and debris that harbor or promote the growth of pathogenic organisms and by directly destroying some of the bacteria present in the mouth.*
Assist client to select foods of moderate temperature and those that are soft and bland. **D** ● ✦	*Foods that are extremely hot or cold; hard, crusty, or rough; spicy; and/or acidic may cause thermal, mechanical, or chemical trauma to the oral mucosa.*
Encourage client to maintain an optimal nutritional status.	*Adequate nutrition is needed to maintain the high cellular turnover of the oral mucous membrane. Good nutrition also promotes optimal function of the immune system, which reduces the client's risk of oral cavity infection.*
Inspect client's dentures. Note if they are rough, cracked, or ill-fitting.	*Rough, cracked, or ill-fitting dentures can cause mechanical trauma and subsequent inflammation and breakdown of the oral mucosa. The discomfort in the affected area(s) can result in a decreased oral intake, which further compromises the health of the oral mucosa.*

Dependent/Collaborative Actions

Administer topical anesthetics, oral protective agents, analgesics, and antimicrobials if ordered. **D** ✦	*Topical anesthetics, oral protective agents, and analgesics promote comfort if the oral mucous membrane is inflamed or if breakdown is present. The increased comfort can result in an improved oral intake, which helps maintain health of the oral mucosa. Antimicrobials prevent or treat infection of the oral mucosa.*
Consult appropriate health care provider if dryness, irritation, discomfort, and/or breakdown of the oral cavity persist or worsen. Consult the physician about an alternative treatment plan	*Notifying the appropriate health care provider allows for modification of the treatment plan.*
Consult a dentist if dentures are rough, cracked, or ill-fitting.	*Notifying a dentist to improve fit and condition of dentures will help improve the health of the oral mucosa.*

NDx = NANDA-I Diagnosis   **D** = Delegatable Action   ● = UAP   ✦ = LVN/LPN   ⊖▶ = Go to ⊖volve for animation

Nursing Diagnosis **PAIN, ACUTE** NDx

Definition: Unpleasant sensory and emotional experience arising from actual or potential tissue damage or described in terms of such damage (International Association for the Study of Pain); sudden or slow onset of any intensity from mild to severe with an anticipated or predictable end and a duration of less than 6 months

CLINICAL MANIFESTATIONS

Subjective	Objective
Verbal or coded report of pain; verbal report of sleep disturbance; self-focus; narrowed focus (altered time perception, impaired thought processes)	Autonomic responses (e.g., facial mask diaphoresis; changes in blood pressure (BP), respiration, pulse rate; pupillary dilatation); expressive behavior (e.g., restlessness, moaning, crying, vigilance, irritability, sighing); changes in appetite and eating; protective gestures; guarding behavior; eyes lack luster, fixed or scattered movement, beaten look, grimace; reduced interaction with people and environment; autonomic change in muscle tone (may span from listless to rigid); distraction behavior (e.g., pacing, seeking out other people and/or activities, repetitive activities)

RISK FACTORS

- Injury agents (biological, chemical, physical, psychological)

DESIRED OUTCOMES

The client will experience diminished pain as evidenced by:
  a. Verbalization of decrease in or absence of pain
  b. Relaxed facial expression and body positioning
  c. Increased participation in activities
  d. Stable vital signs

DOCUMENTATION

- Verbal description of pain
- Rating of pain intensity
- Facial expression
- Body movement and position
- Vital signs
- Participation in activities
- Factors that precipitate, aggravate, and alleviate pain
- Therapeutic interventions
- Client/family teaching

NOC OUTCOMES

Pain control; comfort status: physical discomfort level; pain level; stress level

NIC INTERVENTIONS

Pain management; environmental management: comfort; analgesic administration

NURSING ASSESSMENT	RATIONALE
Assess for signs and symptoms of pain (e.g., verbalization of pain, grimacing, reluctance to move, restlessness, diaphoresis, increased BP, tachycardia).	*Early recognition of signs and symptoms of pain allows for prompt intervention and improved pain control.*
Assess client's perception of the severity of pain using a pain intensity rating scale.	*An awareness of the severity of pain being experienced helps determine the most appropriate intervention(s) for pain management. Use of a pain intensity rating scale gives the nurse a clearer understanding of the pain being experienced and promotes consistency when communicating with others about the client's pain experience.*
Assess the client's pain pattern (e.g., location, quality, onset, duration, precipitating factors, aggravating factors, alleviating factors).	*Knowledge of the client's pain pattern assists in the identification of effective pain management interventions.*

NURSING ASSESSMENT	RATIONALE
Ask the client to describe previous pain experiences and methods used to manage pain effectively.	Many variables affect a client's response to pain (e.g., age, sex, coping style, previous experience with pain, culture, cause of pain). Knowledge of the client's usual response to pain and methods previously used to manage pain effectively enables the nurse to evaluate the client's pain more accurately and facilitates the identification of effective strategies for pain management.

THERAPEUTIC INTERVENTIONS	RATIONALE

Independent Actions

Implement measures to reduce fear and anxiety (e.g., assure client that his/her need for pain relief is understood, plan methods for achieving pain control with client, provide a calm environment).	Fear and anxiety can decrease the client's threshold and tolerance for pain and thereby heighten the perception of pain. In addition, pain management methods are not as effective if the client is tense and unable to relax.
Implement measures to promote rest (e.g., minimize environmental activity and noise). **D** ● ✦	Fatigue can decrease the client's threshold and tolerance for pain and thereby heighten the perception of pain. If the client is well rested, he/she often experiences decreased pain and increased effectiveness of pain management measures.
Provide or assist with nonpharmacological methods for pain relief. Examples include: • Relaxation techniques (e.g., progressive relaxation exercises, meditation, guided imagery) • Distraction measures (e.g., listening to music, conversing, watching television, playing cards, reading) • Position change	Nonpharmacological pain management includes a variety of interventions. It is believed that most of these are effective because they stimulate closure of the gating mechanism in the spinal cord and subsequently block the transmission of pain impulses. In addition, some interventions are thought to stimulate the release of endogenous analgesics (e.g., endorphins) that inhibit the transmission of pain impulses and/or alter the client's perception of pain. Many of the nonpharmacological interventions also help decrease pain by promoting relaxation.

Dependent/Collaborative Actions

Administer analgesics before activities and procedures that can cause pain and before pain becomes severe. **D** ✦	The administration of analgesics before a pain-producing event helps minimize the pain that will be experienced. Analgesics are also more effective if given before pain becomes severe because mild to moderate pain is controlled more quickly and effectively than severe pain.
Administer the following medications as ordered: **D** ✦ • Opioid (narcotic) analgesics • Nonopioid (nonnarcotic) analgesics such as acetaminophen and salicylates and other nonsteroidal anti-inflammatory agents (e.g., ketorolac, ibuprofen, naproxen) • Anesthetic agents (e.g., bupivacaine, etidocaine).	Pharmacologic therapy is an effective method of reducing or relieving pain. Opioid analgesics act mainly by altering the client's perception of pain and emotional response to the pain experience. Nonopioid analgesics are thought to interfere with the transmission of pain impulses by inhibiting prostaglandin synthesis. Anesthetics help control pain by inhibiting the initiation and conduction of pain impulses along the sensory pathways at and near the infusion site.
Provide or assist with nonpharmacologic methods for pain relief such as cutaneous stimulation measures (e.g., pressure, massage, heat and cold applications, transcutaneous electrical nerve stimulation [TENS], acupuncture).	It is believed that most of these are effective because they stimulate closure of the gating mechanism in the spinal cord and subsequently block the transmission of pain impulses.
Consult physician about an order for patient-controlled analgesia (PCA) if indicated.	The use of PCA allows the client to self-administer analgesics within parameters established by the physician. This method facilitates pain management by ensuring prompt administration of the drug when needed, providing more continuous pain relief, and increasing the client's control over the pain.
Consult appropriate health care provider (e.g., physician, pharmacist, pain management specialist) if above measures fail to provide adequate pain relief.	Notifying the appropriate health care provider allows for modification of the treatment plan.

NDx = NANDA-I Diagnosis   **D** = Delegatable Action   ● = UAP   ✦ = LVN/LPN   Ⓔ▶ = Go to Ⓔvolve for animation

Nursing Diagnosis **SELF-CARE, READINESS FOR ENHANCED** NDx

Definition: A pattern of performing activities for oneself that helps to meet health-related goals and can be strengthened

Related to:

CLINICAL MANIFESTATIONS

Subjective	Objective
Expresses desire to advance independence in maintaining life; enhance independence in maintaining health; enhance independence in maintaining personal development; enhance independence in maintaining well-being; enhance knowledge of strategies for self-care	Not applicable

DESIRED OUTCOMES

The client will have enhanced self-care as evidenced by:
a. Identification and performance of desired self-care activities
b. Expressed desire to improve self-care habits
c. Ability to evaluate effectiveness of self-care habits

DOCUMENTATION

- Client/family teaching

NOC OUTCOMES

Adherence behavior; health-seeking behavior; health promotion; information processing; knowledge: decision process; health behavior; health promotion; participation in health care decisions; self-care status

NIC INTERVENTIONS

Active listening; family integrity promotion; self-care assistance; self-respect facilitation; support system enhancement; spiritual growth facilitation; self-care teaching

NURSING ASSESSMENT	RATIONALE
Assess client's current self-care habits.	*Assessment of the client's current self-care activities provides the basis for planning further self-care activities.*
Assess client's confidence in ability to perform more self-care habits.	*It is important to determine whether the client has the confidence to perform new self-care activities. Confidence in one's ability to change behaviors impacts the success in maintaining change.*

THERAPEUTIC INTERVENTIONS	RATIONALE
Independent Actions	
Encourage client in pursuit of enhanced self-care activities.	*Encouragement will support the client to begin and maintain self-care activities.*
Collaborate with the client to set realistic goals.	*Developed goals should include short- and long-term goals. Short-term goals are more achievable and provide the client confidence to reach the long-term goals. Goals should be specific and realistic, with consideration for the patient's ability.*
Provide positive reinforcement when behaviors are met.	*Positive reinforcement promotes a sense of self-efficacy in the client.*
Promote family involvement in developing self-care activities.	*Self-care activities help improve a client's health and decrease the incidence of repeated hospitalizations. The client's family plays a significant role in promoting success of self-care behaviors.*
Implement culturally sensitive interventions.	*Recognize the impact of culture on self-care. A client's cultural background influences self-care activities and adherence to them.*
Provide client with information to enhance self-care behaviors.	*Specific self-care needs are based on the type of disease process and/ or symptoms experienced by the client.*
Inform client of community resources available to support and enhance self-care.	*Client should know what community resources are available to enhance self-care behaviors.*
Use a variety of teaching strategies to enhance self-care behaviors.	*Learning is enhanced when a variety of teaching methods are used.*

THERAPEUTIC INTERVENTIONS	RATIONALE
Evaluate effectiveness of self-care behaviors.	*This helps the client realize the progress made and verifies the client's ability to maintain self-care behaviors and/or identify new behaviors.*
Educate client and family to evaluate the effectiveness of self-care activities.	*This helps the client determine when and/or if progress is being made and improves the client's confidence in his/her ability to improve well-being.*

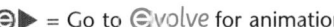 **Nursing Diagnosis** ## SELF-CONCEPT, DISTURBED* NDx

For a full, detailed care plan on this topic, go to http://evolve.elsevier.com/Haugen/careplanning/.

Nursing Diagnosis ## SKIN INTEGRITY, IMPAIRED, RISK FOR NDx

Definition: At risk for skin being adversely altered

CLINICAL MANIFESTATIONS

Subjective	Objective
Verbalization of areas of decreased sensation	Pallor, redness, and breakdown of skin covering bony prominences, dependent areas, pruritic areas, perineum, and areas of decreased sensation

RISK FACTORS

- **External:** Radiation; physical immobilization; hypothermia or hyperthermia; chemical substance; mechanical factors (e.g., shearing forces, pressure, restraint); humidity; excretions and/or secretions; moisture; extremes of age
- **Internal:** Medication; skeletal prominence; immunologic factors; developmental factors; altered sensation; altered pigmentation; altered metabolic state; altered circulation; alterations in skin turgor (changes in elasticity); alterations in nutritional state (e.g., obesity, emaciation); psychogenetic

DESIRED OUTCOMES

The client will maintain skin integrity as evidenced by:
  a. Absence of redness and irritation
  b. No skin breakdown

DOCUMENTATION

- Appearance of skin
- Therapeutic interventions
- Client/family teaching

NOC OUTCOMES

Skin integrity; intact mucous membranes

NIC INTERVENTIONS

Pressure ulcer prevention; skin surveillance; bathing; pressure management; skin care: topical treatments; positioning; bedrest care

NURSING ASSESSMENT	RATIONALE
Determine client's risk for skin breakdown using a risk assessment tool (e.g., Norton Scale, Braden Scale, Gosnell Scale).	*Prompt identification of the client's risk for skin breakdown leads to earlier implementation of actions to maintain skin integrity. Use of a risk assessment tool aids in the identification of factors that could cause skin breakdown.*
Inspect the skin (especially bony prominences, dependent areas, pruritic areas, perineum, and areas of decreased sensation and/or edema) for pallor, redness, and breakdown.	*Early recognition of signs of impaired skin integrity allows for prompt intervention.*

*This diagnostic label includes the nursing diagnosis of disturbed body image and situational low self-esteem.

NDx = NANDA-I Diagnosis **D** = Delegatable Action ● = UAP ◆ = LVN/LPN ⊖▶ = Go to ⓔvolve for animation

Continued...

THERAPEUTIC INTERVENTIONS	RATIONALE

Independent Actions

Implement measures to prevent prolonged and/or excessive pressure on any area of the skin: **D ● ✦**

- Assist client to turn at least every 2 hours unless contraindicated.
- Instruct or assist client to shift weight at least every 30 minutes.
- Position client properly using supportive devices such as pillows and pads as needed.
- Keep bed linens wrinkle-free.
- Ensure that external devices such as braces, casts, and restraints are applied properly.
- Ensure that client is not lying on tubings.
- Use pressure-reducing or pressure-relieving devices (e.g., gel or foam cushions, alternating pressure mattress, air-fluidized bed) if indicated.

Prolonged and/or excessive pressure on the skin obstructs capillary blood flow to that area. The resultant hypoxia, impaired flow of nutrients, and accumulation of waste products in the area of obstructed blood flow make that tissue more susceptible to breakdown. Measures that prevent the excessive pressure or ensure that pressure is relieved often enough to avoid obstruction of capillary blood flow help maintain skin integrity.

Gently massage around reddened areas at least every 2 hours. **D ● ✦**

Massage stimulates circulation to the skin and underlying tissues. The improved blood flow helps maintain skin integrity by increasing the supply of oxygen and nutrients available to the cells and by removing waste products of metabolism. To avoid damaging the capillaries, massage should be gentle rather than deep, and massage over reddened areas should be avoided.

Implement measures to prevent shearing (e.g., keep head of bed as flat as possible, gatch knees slightly when head of bed is elevated 30 degrees or higher, limit length of time client is in semi-Fowler's position to 30-minute intervals). **D ● ✦**

When one tissue layer slides past another in an opposite direction (i.e., shearing), the capillaries in the affected area are kinked, stretched, or severed. This compromises the area's blood supply and increases the risk of tissue breakdown. A client in a semi-Fowler's position is likely to slide down in the bed. When this occurs, his/her skin tends to remain stationary while the underlying tissues and skeletal structures shift position, resulting in shearing.

Implement measures to reduce friction between the skin and another surface (e.g., apply a protective covering such as a hydrocolloid or transparent membrane dressing to susceptible areas of the skin, apply thin layer of a dry lubricant such as powder or cornstarch to bottom sheet or client's skin, lift and move client carefully using turn sheet and adequate assistance, adequately secure restraints and tubings, pat skin dry rather than rub). **D ● ✦**

The outermost layers of skin can be damaged when dragged along or rubbed against another surface. Reducing friction helps prevent skin surface irritation and abrasion.

Keep client's skin clean. **D ● ✦**

Keeping the skin clean removes many of the surface microorganisms, which, if allowed to accumulate, increase the risk of irritation or infection and subsequent skin breakdown.

Use a mild soap when bathing client. **D ● ✦**

Sebum, which is secreted by the skin, helps maintain skin integrity by preventing excess evaporation of moisture, keeping the skin soft and pliable, and destroying some of the bacteria on the skin's surface. Using a mild rather than a harsh, alkaline soap helps ensure that some sebum remains on the skin after bathing.

Implement measures to keep skin free of excessive moisture:

- Thoroughly dry skin after bathing and as often as needed, paying special attention to skinfolds and opposing skin surfaces (e.g., axillae, perineum, beneath breasts). **D ● ✦**
- Keep bed linens dry. **D ✦**
- Protect skin surrounding wound from drainage (e.g., change dressing when damp, apply a drainage collection device if needed). **D ✦**
- If use of absorbent products such as pads or undergarments is necessary, select those that effectively absorb moisture and keep it away from the skin.

Excessive moisture on the skin or prolonged exposure of the skin to moisture softens the epidermal cells and makes them less resistant to damage. Moisture also harbors microorganisms that can cause irritation or infection, and it increases the possibility of friction between the skin and the surface it is against. Removing excessive moisture and protecting the skin from prolonged contact with moisture reduces the risk of skin irritation and subsequent breakdown.

THERAPEUTIC INTERVENTIONS	RATIONALE
Increase activity as allowed and tolerated. **D** ● ✦	*Activity stimulates circulation, which helps maintain skin integrity by increasing the flow of oxygen and nutrients to the skin and underlying tissues. In addition, increasing activity reduces the risk of prolonged pressure occurring on any area as a result of decreased mobility.*
Maintain an optimal nutritional status.	*An inadequate nutritional status results in muscle atrophy, a decrease in the amount of subcutaneous tissue, and skin that is thin and less elastic. Subsequently, the skin and tissue are more vulnerable to injury because they are less able to withstand minor trauma. In addition, a malnourished client is more susceptible to the effects of pressure because there is less padding between the skin and underlying bone.*
Implement measures to prevent drying of the skin: • Encourage a fluid intake of 2500 mL/day unless contraindicated. • Apply a moisturizing lotion and/or emollient to the skin at least once a day. **D** ● ✦	*Dry skin is more prone to cracking and has decreased elasticity, which make it susceptible to damage.* • *An adequate fluid intake helps ensure that the skin remains well hydrated.* • *Moisturizing lotion and some emollients provide a source of moisture to the skin. Emollients also form a protective barrier on the epidermis, which reduces the evaporation of moisture.*
Protect skin from contact with urine and feces (e.g., perform actions to prevent incontinence and/or diarrhea, keep perineal area clean and dry, apply a protective ointment or cream to perineal area). **D** ● ✦	*Urine and feces are irritants that can cause inflammation and breakdown of the skin. In addition, the moisture in urine and feces softens epidermal cells and increases friction between opposing skin surfaces and between the skin and bed linen.*
If edema is present, handle edematous areas carefully and implement measures to reduce fluid accumulation in dependent areas (e.g., instruct client in and assist with range of motion exercises, elevate affected extremities whenever possible).	*Edematous areas have an increased risk for skin breakdown because the oxygen and nutrient supply to the skin is compromised by the increased distance that exists between the capillaries and the cells. Handling edematous areas carefully and implementing measures to reduce edema decrease the risk for skin breakdown.*
If the client is experiencing pruritus, implement measures to reduce the itching sensation (e.g., apply cool compress to pruritic area), keep his/her nails trimmed, and apply mittens if necessary. **D** ● ✦	*The client experiencing pruritus is likely to scratch the affected areas, which irritates the skin and can cause excoriation. Implementing measures to reduce the itching sensation helps prevent scratching. Trimming the client's nails and applying mittens if necessary reduce the risk of trauma to the skin if he/she does scratch the pruritic areas.*

Dependent/Collaborative Actions

Administer antihistamines as prescribed. **D** ✦	*Administering antihistamines can decrease itching.*
Notify appropriate health care provider (e.g., physician, enterostomal therapist, wound care specialist) if skin breakdown occurs.	*Notifying the appropriate health care provider allows for modification of treatment plan.*

Nursing Diagnosis ## SLEEP PATTERN, DISTURBED NDx

Definition: Time-limited disruption of sleep (natural, periodic suspension of consciousness) amount and quality

CLINICAL MANIFESTATIONS

Subjective	Objective
Verbal complaints of difficulty falling asleep; verbal complaints of not feeling well rested; dissatisfaction with sleep	Awakening earlier than desired; prolonged awakenings; sleep maintenance insomnia; self-induced impairment of normal pattern; sleep onset greater than 30 minutes; early morning insomnia; increased proportion of stage 1 sleep; less than age-normed total sleep time; three or more nighttime awakenings; decreased proportion of stages 3 and 4 sleep (e.g., hyporesponsiveness, excess sleepiness, decreased motivation); decreased proportion of rapid eye movement (REM) sleep (e.g., REM rebound, hyperactivity, emotional lability, agitation and impulsivity, atypical polysomnographic features); decreased ability to function

Continued...

RISK FACTORS

- **Psychological:** Ruminative presleep thoughts; daytime activity pattern; thinking about home; body temperature; temperament; dietary; childhood onset; inadequate sleep hygiene; sustained use of anti-sleep agents; circadian asynchrony; frequently changing sleep-wake schedule; depression; loneliness; frequent travel across time zones; daylight/darkness exposure; grief; anticipation; shift work; delayed or advanced sleep phase syndrome; loss of sleep partner, life change; preoccupation with trying to sleep; periodic gender-related hormonal shifts; biochemical agents; fear; separation from significant others; social schedule inconsistent with chronotype; aging-related sleep shifts; anxiety; medications; fear of insomnia; maladaptive conditioned wakefulness; fatigue; boredom
- **Environmental:** Noise; unfamiliar sleep furnishings; ambient temperature, humidity; lighting; other-generated awakening; excessive stimulation; physical restraint; lack of sleep privacy/control; interruptions for therapeutics, monitoring, lab tests; sleep partner; noxious odors
- **Parental:** Mother's sleep-wake pattern; parent-infant interaction; mother's emotional support
- **Physiological:** Urinary urgency, incontinence; fever; nausea; stasis of secretions; shortness of breath; position; gastroesophageal reflux

DESIRED OUTCOMES

The client will attain optimal amounts of sleep as evidenced by:
- a. Statements of feeling well rested
- b. Ability to perform normal daily activities

DOCUMENTATION

- Statements of difficulty falling asleep, interruptions in sleep, and/or not feeling well rested
- Therapeutic interventions
- Client teaching

NOC OUTCOMES

Rest; sleep; personal well-being

NIC INTERVENTIONS

Sleep enhancement; energy management

NURSING ASSESSMENT	RATIONALE
Assess for signs and symptoms of a disturbed sleep pattern (e.g., statements of difficulty falling asleep, sleep interruptions, or not feeling well rested).	*Early recognition of signs and symptoms of a disturbed sleep pattern allows for prompt intervention.*
Determine client's usual sleep habits.	*Knowledge of the client's usual sleep-wake cycle and routines that help induce and maintain sleep helps the nurse plan interventions aimed at preventing a sleep pattern disturbance.*

THERAPEUTIC INTERVENTIONS	RATIONALE

Independent Actions

Discourage long periods of sleep during the day unless signs and symptoms of sleep deprivation exist or daytime sleep is usual for client. **D** ● ✦	*Long periods of sleep during the day are often a change in the client's usual sleep-wake cycle and cause desynchronization of his/her circadian rhythm. This can result in a poorer quality of sleep.*
Implement measures to reduce fear and anxiety (e.g., maintain a calm, confident manner when working with client; assist client to identify specific stressors and ways to cope with them).	*Fear and anxiety stimulate the sympathetic nervous system, which increases alertness and makes it difficult for the client to fall asleep. Sympathetic nervous system stimulation is also believed to shorten the duration of nonrapid eye movement (NREM) and REM sleep, which results in a poorer quality of sleep.*
Encourage participation in relaxing diversional activities during the evening. **D** ● ✦	*Involvement in relaxing activities in the evening helps the client fall asleep more easily.*
Discourage intake of foods/fluids high in caffeine (e.g., chocolate, coffee, tea, colas) in the evening. **D** ● ✦	*Caffeine acts as a central nervous system stimulant and can interfere with relaxation and subsequent sleep induction. Caffeine also acts as a diuretic, which can cause an interruption in sleep if the client awakens in response to the urge to urinate.*
Offer client an evening snack that includes milk unless contraindicated. **D** ● ✦	*Milk contains the amino acid l-tryptophan, which is believed to help induce and maintain sleep.*
Allow client to continue usual sleep practices (e.g., position; time; presleep routines such as reading, watching television, listening to music, and meditating) whenever possible. **D** ● ✦	*Adherence to usual sleep practices promotes mental and physical relaxation that assists the client to maintain his/her usual sleep-wake cycle.*

THERAPEUTIC INTERVENTIONS	RATIONALE
Reduce environmental distractions (e.g., close door to client's room; use night light rather than overhead light whenever possible; lower volume of paging system; keep staff conversations at a low level and away from client's room; close curtains between clients in a semi-private room or ward; keep beepers and alarms on low volume; provide client with "white noise" such as a fan, soft music, or tape-recorded sounds of the ocean or rain; have sleep mask and earplugs available for client if needed). **D** ● ✦	*Environmental activity, noise, and light can interfere with the client's ability to fall asleep and stay asleep. Reducing stimuli helps prevent a sleep pattern disturbance.*
Encourage client to avoid drinking alcohol in the evening.	*Although alcohol can induce drowsiness, which promotes sleep induction, it is known to interfere with REM sleep. Alcohol also inhibits the release of antidiuretic hormone (ADH), which can cause an interruption in sleep if the client awakens in response to the urge to urinate.*
Encourage client to avoid smoking before bedtime. **D** ● ✦	*Nicotine is a stimulant that can interfere with sleep by making it difficult for the client to relax and fall asleep and to stay asleep.*
Implement measures to reduce interruptions during sleep (e.g., restrict visitors, group care whenever possible) so that client is able to sleep undisturbed for 70- to 100-minute intervals. **D** ✦	*One sleep cycle takes about 70 to 100 minutes to complete. Each time the cycle is interrupted, it begins again with NREM stage 1 sleep so the client loses portions of NREM and/or REM sleep. When the client is deprived of NREM sleep, lethargy and depression occur. Loss of REM sleep results in irritability and anxiety. Reducing the frequency of sleep interruptions helps ensure that the client progresses through all the sleep stages and does not experience a sleep pattern disturbance.*

Dependent/Collaborative Actions

THERAPEUTIC INTERVENTIONS	RATIONALE
If possible, administer medications that can interfere with sleep (e.g., steroids, diuretics) early in the day rather than late afternoon or evening. **D** ✦	*Administering these medications as early as possible during the day helps prevent nighttime insomnia and/or frequent awakenings.*
Administer prescribed sedative-hypnotics if indicated. **D** ✦	*Sedative-hypnotics are central nervous system depressants that promote sleep by reducing anxiety, shortening sleep induction, and/or reducing arousal level (wakefulness). These medications should be used for only a short time because they interfere with the length of REM sleep and can actually create a disturbance in the client's sleep-wake cycle.*
Consult appropriate health care provider if signs and symptoms of sleep deprivation (e.g., irritability, lethargy, agitation, inability to concentrate) occur and persist or worsen.	*Notifying the appropriate health care provider allows for modification of treatment plan.*

Nursing Diagnosis # SWALLOWING, IMPAIRED NDx

Definition: Abnormal functioning of the swallowing mechanism related to deficits in oral, pharyngeal, or esophageal structure or function

---

Continued...
CLINICAL MANIFESTATIONS

Subjective	Objective
Esophageal phase impairment: Verbalization of heartburn or epigastric pain; unexplained irritability surrounding mealtime; complaints of "something stuck"	**Pharyngeal phase impairment:** Altered head positions; inadequate laryngeal elevation; food refusal; unexplained fevers; delayed swallow; recurrent pulmonary infections; gurgly voice quality; nasal reflux; choking, coughing, or gagging; multiple swallows; abnormality in pharyngeal phase by swallow study **Oral phase impairment:** Lack of tongue action to form bolus; weak suck resulting in inefficient nippling; incomplete lip closure; food pushed out of mouth; slow bolus formation; premature entry of bolus; piecemeal deglutition; lack of chewing; food falls from mouth; nasal reflux; inability to clear oral cavity; long meals with little consumption; coughing, choking, gagging before a swallow; abnormality in oral phase of swallow study; pooling in lateral sulci; sialorrhea or drooling **Esophageal phase impairment:** Acidic-smelling breath; vomitus on pillow; repetitive swallowing or ruminating; regurgitation of gastric contents or wet burps; bruxism; nighttime coughing or awakening; observed evidence of difficulty in swallowing (e.g., stasis of food in oral cavity, coughing or choking); hyperextension of head, arching during or after meals; abnormality in esophageal phase by swallow study; odynophagia; hematemesis; vomiting

RISK FACTORS

- **Congenital deficits:** Upper airway anomalies; failure to thrive or protein-energy malnutrition; conditions with significant hypotonia; respiratory disorders; history of tube feeding; behavioral feeding problems; self-injurious behavior; neuromuscular impairment (e.g., decreased or absent gag reflex, decreased strength or excursion of muscles involved in mastication, perceptual impairment, facial paralysis); mechanical obstruction (e.g., edema, tracheostomy tube, tumor); congenital heart disease; cranial nerve involvement

- **Neurological problems:** Upper airway anomalies; laryngeal abnormalities; achalasia; gastroesophageal reflux disease; acquired anatomic defects; cerebral palsy; internal traumas; tracheal, laryngeal, esophageal defects; traumatic head injury; developmental delay; external traumas; nasal or nasopharyngeal cavity defects; oral cavity or oropharynx abnormalities; premature infants

DESIRED OUTCOMES:

The client will experience an improvement in swallowing as evidenced by:
  a. Verbalization of same
  b. Absence of food in oral cavity after swallowing
  c. Absence of coughing and choking when eating and drinking

DOCUMENTATION

- Verbalization of difficulty swallowing
- Stasis of food in oral cavity
- Coughing or choking when eating or drinking
- Consistency of foods/fluids client is able to swallow without difficulty
- Therapeutic interventions
- Client/family teaching

NOC OUTCOMES

Swallowing status; chewing ability; oral cavity clearance; food acceptance

NIC INTERVENTIONS

Swallowing therapy; aspiration precautions; positioning; risk assessment

NURSING ASSESSMENT	RATIONALE
Assess for signs and symptoms of impaired swallowing (e.g., statements of difficulty swallowing, stasis of food in oral cavity, coughing or choking when eating or drinking).	*Early recognition of signs and symptoms of impaired swallowing allows for prompt intervention.*

NURSING ASSESSMENT	RATIONALE
Assist with studies to evaluate client's swallowing (e.g., videofluoroscopy) if ordered.	*Swallowing is a complex act that consists of voluntary and involuntary neuromotor components. Studies that evaluate the client's ability to swallow help identify the specific physiological dysfunction, which aids in planning effective interventions.*

THERAPEUTIC INTERVENTIONS	RATIONALE

Independent Actions

If client has viscous oral secretions, implement measures to liquefy these secretions (e.g., encourage a fluid intake of 2500 mL/day unless contraindicated, administer a papain product before meals as ordered). **D** ● ✦

Thick oral secretions interfere with movement of food in the mouth. Liquefying these secretions makes it easier for a bolus of food to be formed and moved to the back of the mouth. Liquefying the secretions also helps ensure that the bolus formed is moist so that it stays intact and triggers an effective swallowing reflex.

If client's mouth is dry, implement measures to moisten mouth before meals and snacks (e.g., provide good oral care, stimulate salivation by having client suck on hard candy unless contraindicated, encourage use of a saliva substitute such as Salivart). **D** ● ✦

A moist mouth helps lubricate food, which makes it easier to chew, form into a bolus, and manipulate toward the back of the mouth. A formed, moist bolus more effectively triggers the swallowing reflex and moves more easily through the esophagus.

Instruct and assist client to select foods/fluids that are appropriate for his/her swallowing ability. Some general guidelines include:

Impaired swallowing can result from structural or neurological problems. The types of foods/fluids a client can swallow effectively vary depending on the particular swallowing difficulty.

- Avoiding foods that tend to fall apart in the mouth (e.g., applesauce, cake, muffins) and those that consist of small food particles (e.g., rice, peas, corn, nuts) if client has impaired tongue control

Clients with impaired tongue movement have difficulty keeping foods that tend to fall apart in the mouth or consist of small pieces in a bolus that can be transferred to the back of the mouth. Some small pieces of food may fall to the back of the mouth, but because the food is not in a bolus, it will not trigger a strong swallowing reflex.

- Avoiding foods that are sticky (e.g., peanut butter, soft bread, honey)

Sticky foods are difficult to move through the mouth because they tend to adhere to various structures, especially the hard palate. It is also difficult to form these foods into the distinct bolus needed to trigger the swallowing reflex.

- Moistening dry foods with gravy or sauces (e.g., catsup, sour cream, salad dressing)

Moist foods are more easily formed into a bolus and moved through the mouth and esophagus.

- Selecting thick rather than thin fluids or adding a thickening agent (e.g., "Thick-It," gelatin, baby cereal) if client has a delayed swallowing reflex and/or poor tongue control

Thin fluids pass rapidly through the mouth and can pour over the back of the tongue without triggering an effective swallow. Thick fluids remain more cohesive and are able to stimulate the swallowing reflex more effectively.

Place client in a high-Fowler's position for meals and snacks unless contraindicated. **D** ● ✦

A high-Fowler's position uses gravity to aid in the flow of foods/fluids through the esophagus.

If client has difficulty chewing and maneuvering a bolus of food to the back of the mouth, instruct him/her to tilt head down when chewing and forming a bolus, then raise chin slightly when ready to swallow.

Tilting the head down allows client more time to chew and form a bolus because the food is in the front of the mouth where it does not trigger the swallowing reflex. Raising the chin facilitates movement of the bolus to the back of the mouth so that the swallowing reflex can be triggered. NOTE: Caution client to avoid tilting head back when swallowing since this position increases the risk for aspiration.

Serve foods/fluids that are hot or cold instead of room temperature. **D** ● ✦

Foods/fluids that are hot or cold trigger a more effective swallowing reflex because they have a greater stimulatory effect on the sensory receptors in the mouth.

If client has motor and sensory dysfunction of one side of the mouth or face, instruct and assist him/her to tilt head toward the unaffected side when eating and drinking and to place food in the unaffected side of the mouth.

When foods/fluids are directed toward the unaffected side of the mouth, the client is able to more effectively chew and use his/her tongue to form a bolus and move it to the back of the mouth. The unaffected side of the mouth also has more tension in the buccal musculature so foods/fluids are more likely to get to the back of the mouth rather than collect between the cheek and the mandible. Sensory receptors on the unaffected side also trigger a stronger swallowing reflex than those on the affected side.

NDx = NANDA-I Diagnosis   **D** = Delegatable Action   ● = UAP   ✦ = LVN/LPN   ⊖▶ = Go to ⓔvolve for animation

Continued...

THERAPEUTIC INTERVENTIONS	RATIONALE
Encourage client to concentrate on the act of swallowing. Provide verbal cueing as needed.	*The client can achieve a more effective swallow by focusing on chewing and moving foods/fluids to the back of the mouth where the swallowing reflex is triggered.*
Instruct client to avoid putting too much food/fluid in mouth at one time. **D** ● ✦	*Overfilling the mouth makes it difficult for the client to form a distinct bolus and effectively move it to the back of the mouth where it triggers the swallowing reflex.*
Encourage client to perform exercises to strengthen tongue and facial muscles if indicated (e.g., drinking through a straw; opening mouth and moving tongue anteriorly, posteriorly, and laterally; pushing tongue upward against resistance using an object such as a tongue blade, Popsicle, or sucker).	*Strong tongue and facial muscles increase the client's ability to chew food, form a bolus, and direct the bolus to the back of the mouth where it triggers the swallowing reflex.*

Dependent/Collaborative Actions

Consult speech pathologist about methods for dealing with client's specific swallowing impairment.	*Consulting with persons who are knowledgeable about the management of swallowing difficulties aids in the development of an individualized plan of care to improve the client's swallowing.*
Implement measures to reduce oral and pharyngeal discomfort if indicated (e.g., administer topical and/or systemic analgesics as ordered). **D** ✦	*Oral and pharyngeal discomfort can interfere with the client's ability and willingness to adequately chew food and swallow effectively.*
Consult appropriate health care provider (e.g., physician, speech pathologist) if swallowing difficulties persist or worsen.	*Notifying the appropriate health care provider allows for modification of treatment plan.*

Nursing Diagnosis   # TISSUE PERFUSION, INEFFECTIVE* NDx

Definition: Decrease in oxygen resulting in failure to nourish the tissues at the capillary level

CLINICAL MANIFESTATIONS

Subjective	Objective
Gastrointestinal: Verbalization of nausea; abdominal pain or tenderness **Peripheral:** Report of altered sensations **Cerebral:** Report of difficulty in swallowing **Cardiopulmonary:** Report of chest pain; sense of "impending doom"	**Renal:** Altered blood pressure (BP) outside acceptable parameters; hematuria; oliguria or anuria; elevation in blood urea nitrogen (BUN)/creatinine ratio **Gastrointestinal:** Hypoactive or absent bowel sounds; abdominal distention **Peripheral:** Edema; positive Homans' sign; altered skin characteristics (hair, nails, moisture); weak or absent pulses; skin temperature changes; skin discolorations; diminished arterial pulsations; skin color pale on elevation, color does not return on lowering of leg; delayed healing; claudication; BP changes in extremities; bruits **Cerebral:** Speech abnormalities; altered mental status; changes in motor response; behavioral changes; extremity weakness or paralysis **Cardiopulmonary:** Altered respiratory rate outside acceptable parameters; use of accessory muscles; capillary refill greater than 3 seconds; abnormal arterial blood gas values; chest pain; bronchospasm; dyspnea; dysrhythmias; nasal flaring; chest retraction

---

*NANDA International identifies five types of ineffective tissue perfusion: renal, cerebral, cardiopulmonary, gastrointestinal, peripheral. A client can experience more than one type of ineffective tissue perfusion, and the actions for the various types are often similar. The information presented here focuses on ineffective tissue perfusion in general rather than a specific type.

RISK FACTORS

- Hypovolemia
- Interruption of arterial flow
- Hypervolemia
- Exchange problems
- Interruption of venous flow
- Mechanical reduction of venous and/or arterial blood flow
- Hypoventilation
- Impaired transport of the oxygen across alveolar and/or capillary membrane
- Mismatch of ventilation with blood flow
- Decreased hemoglobin concentration in blood
- Enzyme poisoning
- Altered affinity of hemoglobin for oxygen

DESIRED OUTCOMES

The client will maintain adequate systemic tissue perfusion as evidenced by:
a. BP within normal range
b. Usual mental status
c. Extremities warm with absence of pallor and cyanosis
d. Palpable peripheral pulses
e. Capillary refill time less than 2 to 3 seconds
f. Absence of edema
g. Absence of exercise-induced pain
h. Urine output at least 30 mL/h

DOCUMENTATION

- BP
- Mental status
- Skin color and temperature
- Peripheral pulses
- Capillary refill time
- Presence of edema
- Exercise-induced pain
- Urine output
- Therapeutic interventions
- Client teaching

NOC OUTCOMES

Circulation status; tissue perfusion: cellular

NIC INTERVENTIONS

Circulatory care: arterial insufficiency; circulatory care: venous insufficiency; cardiac care: acute; hypovolemia management

NURSING ASSESSMENT	RATIONALE
Assess for and report signs and symptoms of diminished tissue perfusion (e.g., decreased BP, restlessness, confusion, cool extremities, pallor or cyanosis of extremities, diminished or absent peripheral pulses, slow capillary refill, edema, claudication, angina, oliguria).	*Early recognition of signs and symptoms of diminished tissue perfusion allows for prompt intervention.*
Assess results of radiographic studies as ordered (e.g., arteriograms, computed tomography [CT] scans).	*These studies highlight areas with decreases in tissue perfusion.*

THERAPEUTIC INTERVENTIONS	RATIONALE
Independent Actions	
Maintain a minimum fluid intake of 2500 mL/day unless contraindicated.	*Adequate hydration is essential for maintenance of a vascular volume sufficient to maintain adequate tissue perfusion.*
Instruct client to change from a supine to an upright position slowly if he/she has postural hypotension.	*Changing from a supine to a sitting or standing position slowly allows time for the baroreceptors to adjust to the change in the distribution of blood associated with an upright position; this helps keep the BP at a level sufficient to maintain adequate tissue perfusion.*
Discourage positions such as crossing legs, pillows under knees, and use of knee gatch. **D** ● ✦	*These positions exert pressure on vessels in the lower extremities, which compromises blood flow.*
Encourage client to avoid sitting or standing for prolonged periods. **D** ● ✦	*Prolonged sitting or standing causes venous stasis.*
If client is on bedrest, instruct and assist with range-of-motion exercises at least three times per day and active foot and leg exercises every 1 to 2 hours. **D** ● ✦	*When a client is on bedrest, blood pools in the extremities as a result of decreased muscle activity. Range-of-motion exercises help reduce venous stasis. The rhythmic muscle contractions that occur during active foot and leg exercises cause intermittent compression of the veins, which improves venous return.*
Encourage and assist client with ambulation as soon as allowed and tolerated. **D** ● ✦	*Ambulation causes rhythmic contractions of the leg muscles. This creates a pumping effect on the leg veins, which subsequently increases venous return.*

NDx = NANDA-I Diagnosis **D** = Delegatable Action ● = UAP ✦ = LVN/LPN ⊖▶ = Go to ⊖volve for animation

Continued...

THERAPEUTIC INTERVENTIONS	RATIONALE
Implement measures to prevent vasoconstriction:	*Vasoconstriction narrows vessel lumens, which results in diminished blood flow through the affected vessels. Vasoconstriction may also increase afterload, which can decrease cardiac output and systemic tissue perfusion.*
• Perform actions to reduce stress. **D** ● ✦	*Stress stimulates the sympathetic nervous system, which results in vasoconstriction.*
• Discourage smoking. **D** ● ✦	*Nicotine increases catecholamine output, which subsequently causes vasoconstriction.*
• Perform actions to keep client from getting cold (e.g., maintain a comfortable room temperature, provide adequate clothing and blankets). **D** ● ✦	*When the body is cold, peripheral vasoconstriction occurs in an attempt to contain body heat.*

Dependent/Collaborative Actions

Administer intravenous fluids and/or blood if ordered.	*Intravenous fluids and/or blood help maintain vascular volume, which is essential for adequate tissue perfusion.*
If client's activity is limited and/or venous insufficiency is a problem, consult physician about an order for antiembolism stockings or an intermittent pneumatic compression device. **D** ✦	*Antiembolism stockings and intermittent pneumatic compression devices promote venous return by exerting either constant pressure or intermittent pressure on the vessels in the lower extremities.*
Implement measures to improve cardiac output (e.g., administer positive inotropic agents, vasodilators, and/or antidysrhythmics if ordered; promote rest) if decreased cardiac output is contributing to inadequate tissue perfusion.	
Administer the following medications if ordered:	
• Antiplatelet agents and/or anticoagulants **D** ✦	*Antiplatelet agents and anticoagulants may be used to prevent or treat clots that may obstruct blood flow.*
• Hemorrheologic agents (e.g., pentoxifylline) **D** ✦	*Pentoxifylline is a hemorrheologic agent that improves microcirculation by decreasing blood viscosity and improving red blood cell flexibility.*
• Peripheral vasodilators (e.g., isoxsuprine, cilostazol) **D** ✦	*These medications dilate cerebral and peripheral blood vessels, making them useful in treatment of cerebral vascular insufficiency and peripheral vascular disease.*
• Antihypertensives **D** ✦	*Antihypertensives reduce systemic vascular resistance, which subsequently improves systemic tissue perfusion.*
Consult appropriate health care provider if signs and symptoms of diminished tissue perfusion persist or worsen.	*Notifying the appropriate health care provider allows for modification of treatment plan.*

| Nursing Diagnosis | **URINARY ELIMINATION, IMPAIRED*** NDx |

Definition: Dysfunction in urine elimination

CLINICAL MANIFESTATIONS

Subjective	Objective
Functional: Verbalization of need to void	**Functional:** Loss of urine before reaching toilet; may be incontinent only in early morning
Overflow: Verbalization of voluntary leakage of small volumes of urine; nocturia	**Overflow:** Bladder distention; high postvoid residual volume; observed involuntary leakage of small volumes of urine
Reflex: Verbalization of no sensation to void; sensation of urgency without voluntary inhibition of bladder contraction; sensations associated with full bladder (e.g., restlessness, abdominal discomfort); inability to voluntarily inhibit voiding; loss of urine with activities that place pressure on the bladder	**Reflex:** Inability to voluntarily inhibit voiding; incomplete emptying of bladder with lesions above sacral and pontine micturition center
Urge: Reports urinary urgency; reports involuntary loss of urine with bladder contractions and spasms; reports inability to reach toilet in time to avoid urine loss	**Stress:** Loss of urine with activities that place pressure on the bladder (i.e., coughing, sneezing, laughing, running)

*NANDA International identifies five types of urinary incontinence: functional, overflow, reflex, urge, and stress. A client can experience a combination of types of incontinence, and the actions for various types often are similar. The information presented here focuses on incontinence in general rather than a specific type.

RISK FACTORS

- **Functional:** Changes in environmental factors; impaired cognition/vision; neuromuscular limitations; psychological factors; weakened supporting pelvic structures
- **Overflow:** Bladder outlet obstruction; fecal impaction; urethral obstruction; detrusor external sphincter dyssynergia; detrusor hypocontractility; severe pelvic prolapse; side effects of medications—anticholinergics, calcium channel blockers, decongestants
- **Reflex:** Tissue damage; neurological impairment above level of sacral or pontine micturition center
- **Urge:** Alcohol intake; atrophic urethritis/vaginitis; bladder infections; caffeine intake; decreased bladder capacity; fecal impaction; use of diuretics; detrusor hyperactivity with impaired bladder contractility
- **Stress:** Degenerative changes in pelvic muscles; weak pelvic muscles; high intra-abdominal pressure; intrinsic urethral sphincter deficiency

DESIRED OUTCOMES

The client will experience urinary continence.

DOCUMENTATION:

- Episodes of urinary incontinence
- Statements of being unable to control urinary elimination
- Therapeutic interventions
- Client teaching

NOC OUTCOMES

Symptom control; urinary continence; urinary elimination; knowledge: disease process

NIC INTERVENTIONS

Urinary incontinence care; prompted voiding; self-care assistance: toileting; urinary habit training; urinary bladder training; pelvic muscle exercise

NURSING ASSESSMENT	RATIONALE
Assess for and report urinary incontinence.	*Early recognition of signs and symptoms of urinary incontinence allows for prompt intervention.*
Monitor client's pattern of fluid intake and urination (e.g., times and amounts of fluid intake, types of fluids consumed, times and amounts of voluntary and involuntary voiding, reports of sensation of need to void, activities preceding incontinence).	*Knowledge of the client's fluid intake and urination pattern assists in the identification of factors that may be causing urinary incontinence. This information helps the nurse plan individualized interventions that promote urinary continence.*
Assist with urodynamic studies (e.g., urethral pressure profile, uroflowmetry, cystometrogram) if ordered.	*Urodynamic studies may be done to determine the cause(s) of urinary incontinence. The studies provide information about the motor and sensory function of the bladder and urethra.*

THERAPEUTIC INTERVENTIONS	RATIONALE

Independent Actions

Offer bedpan or urinal, or assist client to bedside commode or bathroom every 2 to 4 hours if indicated. **D ● ✦**	*Urinary incontinence occurs when the pressure in the bladder becomes greater than the pressure exerted by the urinary sphincters. Emptying the bladder before the pressure becomes too great reduces the risk of incontinence.*
Allow client to assume a normal position for voiding (usually sitting for females and standing for males) unless contraindicated. **D ● ✦**	*A sitting or standing position uses gravity to facilitate bladder emptying. The more completely the bladder is emptied, the less risk there is of incontinence.*
Implement measures to reduce delays in toileting (e.g., have call signal within client's reach and respond promptly to requests for assistance; have bedpan, urinal, or bedside commode readily available to client; provide easy access to bathroom; provide client with easy-to-remove clothing such as pajamas with Velcro closures or an elastic waistband). **D ● ✦**	*If client is having difficulty controlling urination, any delay in toileting increases the risk of incontinence. Measures that enable the client to use a bedpan, urinal, bedside commode, or toilet in a timely manner help reduce the risk of incontinence.*
Instruct client to perform pelvic floor muscle exercises (e.g., stopping and starting stream during voiding; squeezing buttocks together, then relaxing the muscles) if appropriate.	*Pelvic floor muscle exercises help strengthen the pelvic floor muscles and improve the tone of the external urinary sphincter. As this is achieved, the risk for incontinence decreases.*

Continued...

THERAPEUTIC INTERVENTIONS	RATIONALE
Instruct client to space fluids evenly throughout the day rather than drinking a large quantity at one time.	*Drinking a large amount of fluid at one time results in rapid filling of the bladder, which increases pressure in the bladder and the subsequent risk of incontinence.*
Limit oral fluid intake in the evening. **D** ● ✦	*As the client's bladder fills and pressure in the bladder increases during sleep, he/she is less likely to be aware of and/or able to respond to the urge to urinate. By limiting fluid intake in the evening, bladder filling during the night is decreased, which reduces the risk of incontinence.*
Instruct client to avoid drinking alcohol and beverages containing caffeine such as colas, coffee, and tea.	*Alcohol and caffeinated beverages increase urine formation because of their mild diuretic effect. With increased urine formation, bladder filling increases, causing a rise in pressure in the bladder, which subsequently increases the risk of incontinence. Alcohol and caffeine also act as chemical irritants to the bladder and contribute to urge incontinence.*

Dependent/Collaborative Actions
Administer the following medications if ordered:

• Cholinergic (parasympathomimetic) agents (e.g., bethanechol) **D** ✦	*If incontinence results from incomplete bladder emptying, cholinergic (parasympathomimetic) drugs may be prescribed to stimulate contraction of the detrusor muscle (smooth muscle of the bladder). This enhances bladder emptying and reduces the risk of incontinence.*
• Anticholinergics (e.g., tolterodine, oxybutynin) **D** ✦	*Hyperactivity of the bladder detrusor muscle can cause a sudden increase in pressure in the bladder and result in incontinence, especially if there is decreased bladder outlet resistance. Anticholinergics may be prescribed to reduce bladder detrusor muscle activity and thereby reduce the risk of incontinence.*
Consult appropriate health care provider if urinary incontinence persists.	*Notifying the appropriate health care provider allows for modification of treatment plan.*

Nursing Diagnosis **URINARY RETENTION** NDx

Definition: Incomplete emptying of the bladder

CLINICAL MANIFESTATIONS

Subjective	Objective
Verbalization of sensation of bladder fullness or difficulty urinating	Bladder distention; small, frequent voiding or absence of urine output; dribbling of urine; residual urine; overflow incontinence

RISK FACTORS

- High urethral pressure caused by weak detrusor
- Inhibition of reflex arc
- Strong urinary sphincter
- Blockage of urine

DESIRED OUTCOMES

The client will not experience urinary retention as evidenced by:
a. Voiding at normal intervals
b. No reports of bladder fullness and suprapubic discomfort
c. Absence of bladder distention and dribbling of urine
d. Balanced intake and output

DOCUMENTATION

- Frequency of urination and amount voided each time
- Reports of bladder fullness and/or suprapubic discomfort
- Bladder distention
- Evidence or statements of dribbling of urine
- Patency of urinary catheter if present
- Intake and output
- Therapeutic interventions
- Client teaching

NOC OUTCOMES	NIC INTERVENTIONS
Urinary elimination	Urinary retention care; fluid management; bladder training; intermittent catheterization

NURSING ASSESSMENT	RATIONALE
Assess for signs and symptoms of urinary retention: • Frequent voiding of small amounts (25-60 mL) of urine • Reports of bladder fullness or suprapubic discomfort • Bladder distention • Dribbling of urine • Output less than intake	*Early recognition of signs and symptoms of urinary retention allows for prompt intervention.*
Assist with urodynamic studies (e.g., urethral pressure profile, uroflowmetry, cystometry) if ordered.	*Urodynamic studies may be indicated when neurogenic dysfunction is the suspected cause of urinary retention. The studies provide information about the motor and sensory function of the bladder and urethra.*

THERAPEUTIC INTERVENTIONS	RATIONALE

Independent Actions

Instruct client to urinate when the urge is first felt. **D** ● ✦	*If the client feels the urge to urinate but suppresses it by contracting the external urinary sphincter, the urge will subside and not recur until the bladder fills more. If the client repeatedly suppresses the urge to urinate and the bladder fills too much or is chronically distended, the micturition reflex becomes less sensitive and does not effectively stimulate urination when the bladder fills.*
Implement measures to promote relaxation during voiding attempts (e.g., provide privacy, hold a warm blanket against abdomen, encourage client to read). **D** ● ✦	*If the client is relaxed when trying to urinate, he/she is better able to relax the pelvic floor muscles and external urinary sphincter and allow voiding to occur.*
If client is having difficulty voiding, run water, place his/her hands in warm water, and/or pour warm water over perineum unless contraindicated. **D** ✦ ●	*These measures have been found to trigger the micturition reflex and thereby promote voiding. They also promote a sense of relaxation, which facilitates voiding.*
Allow client to assume a normal position for voiding (usually sitting for females and standing for males) unless contraindicated. **D** ● ✦	*A sitting or standing position uses gravity to facilitate bladder emptying. Allowing the client to assume a normal voiding position also promotes relaxation, which facilitates voiding.*
Instruct and assist client to lean upper body forward and/or gently press downward on the lower abdomen when attempting to void unless contraindicated. **D** ● ✦	*Leaning forward or gently pressing downward on the lower abdomen increases pressure on the bladder. This pressure helps create a sensation of bladder fullness, which stimulates the micturition reflex.*

Dependent/Collaborative Actions

Administer cholinergic (parasympathomimetic) drugs (e.g., bethanechol) if ordered. **D** ✦	*Cholinergic (parasympathomimetic) drugs promote urination by stimulating contraction of the bladder detrusor muscle.*
Administer prescribed analgesic if client has pain.	*Pain blocks the client's ability to relax and subsequently relax the pelvic floor muscles and external urinary sphincter and allow voiding to occur.*
If an indwelling urinary catheter is present, implement measures to ensure its patency (e.g., keep tubing free of kinks, keep collection bag below bladder level, irrigate catheter if indicated). **D** ● ✦	*Maintaining patency of the indwelling catheter prevents urinary retention.*
Consult appropriate health care provider if signs and symptoms of urinary retention persist.	*Notifying the appropriate health care provider allows for modification of treatment plan.*

See Bibliography at the back of the book.

NDx = NANDA-I Diagnosis   **D** = Delegatable Action   ● = UAP   ✦ = LVN/LPN   ⊖▶ = Go to ⊖volve for animation

3

Nursing Care of the Client Having Surgery

CONSCIOUS SEDATION

In the acute care setting, many clients undergo invasive procedures using conscious sedation. Conscious sedation does not require the presence of an anesthesiologist. The physician is most often credentialed in conscious sedation based on the policies and procedures of the health care facility. The role of the nurse in conscious sedation focuses on the administration of the ordered sedative/narcotic agents and the physiological monitoring of the client's response to both the medications and the procedure. Common opioids used in conscious sedation include morphine, meperidine (Demerol), and fentanyl (Sublimaze). Opioids are administered in combination with sedatives to reduce the incidence of pain and improve the client's tolerance of the procedure. Common sedatives used for conscious sedation include diazepam (Valium) and midazolam (Versed).

The American Society of Anesthesiologists (2004, p. 1) defines conscious sedation as "a drug-induced depression of consciousness during which patients respond purposefully to verbal commands, either alone or accompanied by light tactile stimulation. No interventions are required to maintain a patent airway, and spontaneous ventilation is adequate. Cardiovascular function is usually maintained." When used safely, conscious sedation provides moderate sedation/analgesia while maintaining adequate cardiopulmonary function, protective reflexes, and the ability to respond appropriately to stimulation.

This care plan focuses on the care of the adult client who is receiving or has received conscious sedation for an invasive procedure. Because of the nature of ongoing assessment, intervention, and evaluation of the client's tolerance to medications and procedure, delegation rarely occurs. Much of the information is applicable to clients having conscious sedation in an outpatient setting (e.g., physician's office, surgical care center).

OUTCOME/DISCHARGE CRITERIA

The client will:
1. Maintain optimum respiratory function
2. Remain free from injury
3. Remain free from pain
4. Remain oriented to person, place, and time
5. Return to baseline cognition

⊖▶ **Nursing Diagnosis** ## ACTUAL/RISK FOR IMPAIRED RESPIRATORY FUNCTION*

Definition: Actual or risk for an **ineffective breathing pattern NDx** or inspiration/expiration that does not provide adequate ventilation. Actual or risk for **impaired gas exchange NDx** or a deficiency in oxygenation and/or excess in carbon dioxide elimination at the alveolar-capillary membrane level.

CLINICAL MANIFESTATIONS

Subjective	Objective
Verbal reports of difficulty breathing	Altered rate/depth of respirations (apnea, dyspnea, tachypnea); use of accessory muscles to breathe; abnormal arterial blood gas values; diaphoresis; irritability; restlessness; tachycardia; cyanosis

*This diagnostic label includes the following nursing diagnoses: ineffective breathing pattern and impaired gas exchange.

Continued...

RISK FACTORS

- Administration of pharmacological agents with potential to depress normal respiratory function (opioids, benzodiazepines)
- Altered level of consciousness
- Airway obstruction

DESIRED OUTCOMES

The client will maintain effective respiratory function as evidenced by:
- a. Self-report of ability to breathe comfortably
- b. Baseline rate and depth of respirations
- c. Pulse oximetry/arterial blood gas values within baseline values
- d. Usual mental status
- e. Absence of apnea/dyspnea

NOC OUTCOMES

Respiratory status: ventilation

NIC INTERVENTIONS

Ventilation assistance; respiratory monitoring

NURSING ASSESSMENT

NURSING ASSESSMENT	RATIONALE
Assess rate, depth, and effort of respirations every 5 to 15 minutes during and after the administration of conscious sedation. Report signs and symptoms of ineffective respiratory function: • Tachypnea • Bradypnea • Apnea • Restlessness • Diaphoresis • Irritability	*Early recognition of signs and symptoms of ineffective respiratory function allows for prompt intervention.*
Monitor continuous pulse oximetry during the procedure and postprocedure until client has returned to baseline status.	*Early recognition of low arterial oxygen saturation (SaO_2) values allows for prompt intervention. Pulse oximetry provides an indirect measure of SaO_2.*
Monitor for signs of airway obstruction.	*Occlusion of the airway by the tongue can occur in an unconscious client. Loss of consciousness in a patient undergoing conscious sedation is an untoward side effect and should be reported to the physician immediately.*
Assess arterial blood gas values as indicated.	*Allows for a more direct assessment of a client's oxygenation status including carbon dioxide level*

THERAPEUTIC INTERVENTIONS

THERAPEUTIC INTERVENTIONS	RATIONALE
Independent Actions Implement measures to decrease fear and anxiety: • Assure client during the procedure.	*Fear and anxiety associated with the procedure may cause the client to breathe shallow or hyperventilate. Decreasing anxiety may allow client to focus on breathing more slowly and regularly.*
If the procedure allows, position the client to facilitate optimum breathing: • Side-lying position	*A side-lying position will prevent the tongue from falling back and occluding the client's posterior pharynx.*
If the procedure allows, instruct the client to deep breathe periodically during the procedure.	*Periodic deep breathing allows for ventilation of carbon dioxide that may accumulate if the client's ventilations become too shallow.*
Postprocedure, encourage the client to deep breathe at intervals to assist with recovery: • "Stir-up regimen"	*After the conclusion of the procedure and conscious sedation, stimulating the patient to deep breathe at intervals assists in returning the patient to a more conscious state as well as enhances the elimination of carbon dioxide.*
Monitor for the recurrence of respiratory depression if narcotic/sedative reversal agents were administered.	*Extended monitoring of the client's respiratory status is necessary if reversal agents were administered, because the half-life of administered sedatives/opioids may outlast the effects of reversal agents.*

THERAPEUTIC INTERVENTIONS	RATIONALE
Dependent/Collaborative Actions Administer supplemental oxygen as ordered.	*Administer supplemental oxygen as needed to keep SaO_2 >95%. Administer oxygen with caution to clients with chronic obstructive pulmonary disease (COPD) because this action may take away their hypoxic stimulus to breathe.*

Implement measures to reverse apnea:
• Ventilate the patient with an Ambu bag that delivers a fraction of inspired oxygen (FIO_2) of 100%.
• Administer narcotic/sedative reversal agents as ordered.
  • Naloxone (Narcan)
  • Flumazenil (Romazicon)
• Prepare to assist with intubation/mechanical ventilation if apnea is not corrected.
	Apnea is an adverse effect of sedative/narcotic conscious sedation. While preparing to administer the appropriate reversal agents, the nurse should assist with proper ventilation of the client until spontaneous respiratory effort returns or the client is intubated.

Notify the appropriate health care provider of continued signs and symptoms of ineffective respiratory function.	*Notifying the appropriate health care provider allows for modification of the treatment plan.*

Nursing Diagnosis · RISK FOR INJURY NDx

Definition: At risk of injury as a result of environmental conditions interacting with the client's adaptive and defensive resources

CLINICAL MANIFESTATIONS

Subjective	Objective
Verbalization of auditory, visual, or sensory hallucinations	Confusion; agitation; altered level of consciousness; immobility

RISK FACTORS

• Altered level of consciousness after administration of pharmacological agents (opioids, sedatives)

DESIRED OUTCOMES

The client will be free of injury related to perioperative disorientation.

NOC OUTCOMES

Risk control

NIC INTERVENTIONS

Environmental management: safety; positioning: intraoperative

NURSING ASSESSMENT	RATIONALE
Assess the client's responses to procedural sedation, noting the level of sedation and/or adverse effects of sedation: • Vital signs • Pulse oximetry • Level of consciousness • Cardiac rate and rhythm • Comfort level/tolerance of procedure	*Early recognition of a client's response to sedation and/or the adverse effects of sedation allows for the implementation of the appropriate safety interventions to protect the client from injury.*
Assess environmental conditions surrounding the sedated client.	*Early identification of environmental factors that may contribute to injury in the sedated client allows for implementation of the appropriate safety precautions.*

Continued...

THERAPEUTIC INTERVENTIONS	RATIONALE

Independent Actions
Before procedure, ensure the availability of essential monitoring equipment/emergency cart:
• Oxygen and delivery sources
• Suction apparatus
• Noninvasive blood pressure device
• Electrocardiograph
• Pulse oximeter
• Narcotic and sedative reversal agents
  • Naloxone (Narcan)
  • Flumazenil (Romazicon)
	In the event of an adverse reaction to pharmacological agents used for conscious sedation, or an adverse reaction to a procedure, the appropriate emergency equipment must be available and in proper working order.

Ensure the bed is locked, in the lowest possible position, and appropriate devices are present to secure patient during the procedure: • Side rails • Safety straps	*If the procedure is done bedside, ensure the client's bed is in the locked and lowest possible position that does not interfere with the procedure. Side rails and safety straps may be necessary to properly secure the client, preventing injury.*
Ensure proper positioning of the client during the procedure in order to prevent injury: • Maintain proper body alignment. • Avoid pressure on bony prominences.	*During a procedure requiring conscious sedation, a client's mobility may be limited.* *Maintaining proper body alignment and padding bony prominences will help to protect the client from injury.*
Document the dosage, route, and effects of all administered medications and intravenous (IV) fluids.	*Documentation of interventions promotes continuity of care and improves communication among health care team members. Knowledge of procedural agents administered is beneficial for nurses participating in the safe recovery of a patient after conscious sedation.*
Dependent/Collaborative Actions Establish and maintain an appropriate-sized IV line. The type of access chosen will depend upon established policies and physician preferences.	*A secure IV access is needed as a route to administer narcotic/ sedative reversal agents or emergency medications in the event of an untoward reaction to the administered pharmacological agents or procedure.*
Assist with securing a client's airway in the event of an adverse reaction to pharmacological agents: • Obtain appropriate airway adjuncts to maintain patent airway (oral, nasal airway). • Administer oxygen via appropriate delivery device. • Provide oral pharyngeal suction as necessary to protect from aspiration. • Assist with endotracheal intubation to secure airway if protective reflexes are lost.	*Respiratory depression/arrest is possible with the administration of pharmacological agents used in conscious sedation. The nurse must be prepared to assist in securing the airway if the patient becomes unconscious and loses protective reflexes.*
Administer appropriate narcotic/sedative reversal agents in the event the client is rendered unconscious: • Naloxone (Narcan) • Flumazenil (Romazicon)	*In the event that a client becomes unconscious with a compromised airway due to loss of protective reflexes, reversal can be obtained with the appropriate reversal agents.*

Nursing Diagnosis ACUTE PAIN NDx

Definition: An unpleasant sensory and emotional experience arising from actual or potential tissue damage or described in terms of such damage; sudden or slow onset of any intensity from mild to severe with an anticipated or predictable end and a duration of less than 6 months

CLINICAL MANIFESTATIONS

Subjective	Objective
Verbal reports of discomfort	Crying; muscle tension or rigidity; diaphoresis; elevated blood pressure; increased heart rate; increased respiratory rate

RISK FACTORS
- Physical injury agents related to a medical procedure

DESIRED OUTCOMES

The client will report pain to be relieved or controlled at a satisfactory level.

NOC OUTCOMES

Pain level

NIC INTERVENTIONS

Pain management

NURSING ASSESSMENT	**RATIONALE**

Assess the client for signs and symptoms of pain frequently during the course of the procedure:
- Verbalization of pain
- Grimacing
- Restlessness
- Increased blood pressure
- Tachycardia

Early recognition of signs and symptoms of pain allows for prompt intervention.

THERAPEUTIC INTERVENTIONS	**RATIONALE**

Independent Actions
Implement measures to reduce fear and anxiety:
- Assure client that a nurse will be present during the entire procedure to assess and ensure that adequate sedation and pain relief are provided.

Position the patient for comfort as the procedure allows:
- Pad bony prominences. **D** ✦
- Provide joint support as needed. **D** ✦

Dependent/Collaborative Actions
Administer opioid narcotics as ordered.

Consult appropriate health care provider if above measures fail to provide adequate pain relief.

Fear and anxiety can decrease the client's threshold and tolerance for pain and thereby heighten the perception of pain.

Proper positioning of limbs and support of bony prominences may assist in alleviating pain associated with lying prolonged in one position during a procedure.

Opioid analgesics act mainly by altering the client's perception of pain and emotional response to the pain experience. It is important for the nurse to address pain needs because sedation will not relieve pain.

Notifying the appropriate health care provider allows for modification of the treatment plan.

Nursing Diagnosis ## ACUTE CONFUSION NDx

Definition: Abrupt onset/at risk for reversible disturbances of consciousness, attention cognition, and perception that develop over a short period

CLINICAL MANIFESTATIONS

Subjective	**Objective**
Verbalization of hallucinations	Fluctuation in consciousness; level of consciousness; increased agitation; increased restlessness; exaggerated emotional responses

RISK FACTORS
- Medication reaction/interaction
- Anesthesia/surgery
- Severe pain

DESIRED OUTCOMES

a. Decrease in agitation/restlessness
b. Appropriate responses to environmental stimuli

NOC OUTCOMES

Cognitive ability

NIC INTERVENTIONS

Delirium management

NDx = NANDA-I Diagnosis **D** = Delegatable Action ● = UAP ✦ = LVN/LPN ⊖▶ = Go to ⊖volve for animation

Continued...

NURSING ASSESSMENT	RATIONALE
Assess the client for signs and symptoms of acute confusion: • Fluctuations in consciousness • Hallucinations • Increased agitation • Increased restlessness	*Early recognition of signs and symptoms of confusion allows for prompt intervention.*
Assess for and report possible physiological alterations: • Hypoglycemia • Hypoxia • Hypotension • Adverse effects of medications	*Acute confusion is a clinical manifestation of a variety of physiological alterations. To reduce the risk of injury/untoward outcomes, it is critical that any physiological alteration is ruled out as a contributing factor. Prompt attention to these physiological factors may shorten the duration of the confusion.*
Monitor continuous pulse oximetry.	*Provides a rapid, indirect measure of oxygenation*

THERAPEUTIC INTERVENTIONS	RATIONALE

Independent Actions

Reorient the patient as indicated:
* Address the client by a familiar name. **D** ✦

Use of reality orientation can help improve the cognition of a client.

Communicate clearly and provide simple explanations to the client. **D** ✦

Simple explanations are more readily understood by a confused client.

Provide the patient with ongoing information and reassurance as needed. **D** ✦

Actions may help to reduce the frustration/anxiety that may accompany confusion.

Implement measures to protect the client from injury:
* Keep side rails up. **D** ✦
* Provide constant surveillance. **D** ✦

A confused client is at risk for injury.
Protective measures help to ensure risk reduction. These measures should be continued until return of the client's baseline cognition.

Dependent/Collaborative Actions

Administer medications for anxiety/agitation as ordered.

Confusion may be treated with medications.
The client must be monitored for side effects of these medications.

Use soft physical restraints as needed only if client is at an increased risk for injury and if all other interventions fail to correct confusion.

A confused client is at risk for injury.
Protective measures help to ensure risk reduction. These measures should be continued until return of the client's baseline cognition.

ADDITIONAL CARE PLANS

RISK FOR ASPIRATION
Related to medication administration altering normal level of consciousness

ANXIETY
Related to the unfamiliar environment and procedure

KNOWLEDGE DEFICIT
Related to poor recall secondary to medication effects

PREOPERATIVE CARE

The preoperative phase begins when the client decides to have surgery, and ends when the client enters the operating room area. Although surgical procedures are performed in a variety of settings (e.g., hospitals, day surgery centers, physicians' offices), the basic preoperative client care is similar. The goals of preoperative care are to prepare the client physically and psychologically for the surgery and the postoperative period. Thorough preoperative preparation reduces the client's postoperative fear and anxiety and the risk of postoperative complications. In order to individualize this care plan, the client's psychological and physiological status, the surgical setting, the length of time before the surgical procedure, the type of anesthesia to be used, and the planned surgical procedure must be considered.

This care plan focuses on the adult client who is scheduled for a surgical procedure. It should be used in conjunction with each surgical care plan.

PREOPERATIVE GOALS

The client will:
- Share thoughts and feelings about the impending surgery and its anticipated effects
- Verbalize an understanding of the surgical procedure, preoperative care, and postoperative sensations and care
- Demonstrate the ability to perform activities designed to prevent postoperative complications

---

Nursing Diagnosis **FEAR** NDx**/ANXIETY** NDx

Definition: Fear/anxiety related to a change in health status, situational crisis, and fear of the unknown

CLINICAL MANIFESTATIONS

Subjective	Objective
Expressed concern due to surgical procedure; scared, rattled, distressed; apprehensive; fearful; sense of impending doom; fear of consequences	Preoccupation; impaired attention; difficulty concentrating; forgetfulness; increased pulse; increased blood pressure; increased respiratory rate, trembling hands/facial tension

RISK FACTORS

- Unfamiliar environment and separation from significant others
- Anticipated loss of control associated with effects of anesthesia
- Lack of understanding of diagnostic tests and planned surgical procedure
- Financial concerns associated with the surgery and recovery period
- Potential embarrassment or loss of dignity associated with body exposure
- Risk of disease if blood transfusions are necessary
- Anticipated pain
- Surgical findings
- Changes in appearance, body functioning, and usual lifestyle and roles
- Possibility of death

DESIRED OUTCOMES

The client will experience a reduction in fear and anxiety as evidenced by:
  a. Verbalization of feeling less anxious
  b. Usual sleep pattern
  c. Relaxed facial expression and body movements
  d. Stable vital signs
  e. Usual perceptual ability and interactions with others

NOC OUTCOMES

Anxiety level; anxiety self-control; fear level; fear self-control

NIC INTERVENTIONS

Anxiety reduction; calming technique; emotional support; presence; teaching: preoperative

NURSING ASSESSMENT

Assess client for signs and symptoms of fear and anxiety:
- Verbalization of feeling anxious
- Insomnia
- Tenseness
- Shakiness
- Restlessness
- Diaphoresis
- Tachycardia
- Elevated blood pressure
- Self-focused behaviors

RATIONALE

Early recognition of signs and symptoms of anxiety allows for prompt intervention.

Continued...

NURSING ASSESSMENT	RATIONALE
Gather the following assessment data from the client during the preoperative period: • Level of understanding of planned surgical procedure • Perceptions about the surgery and its anticipated results • Significance of the surgical procedure and hospitalization • Previous surgical and hospital experiences • Availability of adequate support systems • Arrangements made for responsibilities such as job, child care, meal preparation, and home maintenance if needed during the recovery period	*Assessment of the client's baseline knowledge and understanding of the procedure allows for the nurse to formulate individualized preoperative teaching.* *Identification of available support systems assists with the discharge planning process.*

THERAPEUTIC INTERVENTIONS	RATIONALE
Independent Actions Implement measures to reduce fear and anxiety: • Orient client to environment, equipment, and routines. **D ● ✦**	*Familiarity with the environment and routines reduces the client's anxiety about the unknown, provides a sense of security, and increases the client's sense of control, all of which help to reduce anxiety.*
• Introduce client to staff who will be participating in care; if possible, maintain consistency in staff assigned to client's care.	*Introduction of staff familiarizes the client with those individuals who will be working with him/her, which provides a sense of comfort with the environment. Consistency in staff assignment provides the client with a feeling of stability, which reduces anxiety associated with change.*
• Assure client that staff members are nearby; respond to call signal as soon as possible. **D = ● ✦**	*Close contact and a prompt response to requests provide a sense of security and facilitate the development of trust, reducing the client's anxiety.*

• Maintain a calm, supportive, confident manner when interacting with client:
  • Provide a calm, restful environment.
  • Instruct client in relaxation techniques and encourage participation in diversional activities.
	A sense of calmness and confidence conveys to the client that someone is in control of the situation, which helps reduce anxiety.

• Encourage verbalization of fear and anxiety; provide feedback: • Assist client to identify specific stressors and ways to cope with them.	*Verbalization of fears, feelings, and concerns helps the client identify factors that are causing anxiety.*

• Reinforce physician's explanations and clarify misconceptions the client has about the surgical procedure including purpose, size and location of incision, and anticipated outcome:
  • Explain all pre-surgical diagnostic tests.
  • Provide information about preoperative routines and anticipated postoperative care.
  • Provide information based on current needs of the client at a level that the client can understand; encourage questions and clarification of information provided.
  • Assure client that blood is screened carefully and that the risk for contracting blood-borne disease is minimal.
	Factual information and an awareness of what to expect help to decrease the anxiety that arises from uncertainty.

• Perform actions to help client maintain a sense of dignity:
  • Provide privacy when appropriate.
  • Avoid unnecessary body exposure during preoperative procedures.
  • Allow client to wear dentures, glasses, wig, etc., into the operating room suite if possible.
	Increasing a client's sense of control regarding his/her body can help the client to maintain a sense of dignity, which can reduce anxiety.

THERAPEUTIC INTERVENTIONS	RATIONALE

• Orient client to measures implemented to ensure safety in the surgical setting:
  • Instruct client that he/she will be marking the surgical site with the surgeon if laterality (left/right) is a feature of the surgical procedure.
  • Instruct client that before the start of any invasive medical procedure, a time-out is taken by the operating room staff to confirm the correct client, procedure, and site.
  • Instruct client that it is OK to ask questions if there is reason for concern.
	National patient safety goal requirements issued by The Joint Commission requires the implementation of safety measures designed to reduce surgical errors.
	Implementing measures such as marking the surgical site, taking a time-out in the operating room, and encouraging the active involvement of the client in the process can help reduce the risk of errors as well as reduce fear and anxiety in a patient who may be feeling a loss of control.

• Assure client that pain relief needs will be met postoperatively.	*Fear and anxiety can decrease the client's threshold for pain and heighten a client's perception of pain. Anxiety can be reduced if the client is assured that pain needs will be met after surgery.*
• Encourage significant others to project a caring, concerned attitude without obvious anxiousness. • Include significant others in orientation and teaching sessions and encourage their continued support of client.	*Anxiety is easily transferable from one person to another. If significant others covey empathy, provide reassurance, and do not appear anxious, they can help reduce a client's anxiety. In addition, significant others can help to reduce anxiety by reinforcing information that the client has difficulty understanding or recalling.*

• Enable client to maintain a sense of control by:
  • Including client in planning of preoperative care and allowing choices whenever possible
  • Explaining that the purpose of the written consent form is to indicate voluntary and informed consent, and to protect against unsanctioned surgery
  • Discussing the purpose and benefits of an advanced directive for health care and providing assistance as needed to complete the necessary documents
	Enabling the client to make health care decisions can enhance feelings of autonomy and decrease anxiety.

• When appropriate, assist client to meet spiritual needs. • Arrange for a visit from clergy.	*Spiritual support is a source of comfort and security for many people and can help reduce a client's anxiety.*

Dependent/Collaborative Actions

Implement measures to reduce fear and anxiety:

• Initiate a social service referral if indicated.	*Concerns about factors such as finances, follow-up medical care, and home maintenance can be a source of great anxiety.* *Facilitating contact with the appropriate resources can help reduce the client's anxiety and provide ongoing support.*
• Administer prescribed antianxiety agents if indicated.	*Medications are sometimes prescribed to help reduce the client's anxiety. Benzodiazepines (e.g., lorazepam, diazepam, alprazolam, chlordiazepoxide) are the drugs of choice for managing short-term anxiety.*
Consult appropriate health care provider (e.g., psychiatric nurse clinician, physician) if above actions fail to control fear and anxiety.	*Notifying the appropriate health care provider can allow for modification of the treatment plan.*

Nursing Diagnosis **DISTURBED SLEEP PATTERN** NDx

Definition: Time limited disruption of sleep (natural, periodic suspension of consciousness) amount and quantity

CLINICAL MANIFESTATIONS

Subjective	Objective
Expressed difficulty falling asleep; not feeling well rested; dissatisfaction with sleep; decreased ability to function	Changes in behavior (e.g., increasing irritability, disorientation, listlessness, restlessness, lethargy); physical signs (e.g., hand tremors, expressionless face, dark circles under eyes, frequent yawning)

Continued...

RISK FACTORS	DESIRED OUTCOMES

RISK FACTORS
- Fear
- Anxiety
- Presurgical treatments and procedures
- Unfamiliar environment

DESIRED OUTCOMES

The client will obtain optimal amounts of sleep as evidenced by statements of feeling well rested.

NOC OUTCOMES

Sleep

NIC INTERVENTIONS

Sleep enhancement

NURSING ASSESSMENT

Assess for signs and symptoms of a disturbed sleep pattern:
- Statements of difficulty falling asleep, interrupted sleep, or not feeling well rested.

RATIONALE

Early recognition of signs and symptoms of disturbed sleep patterns allows for prompt intervention.

THERAPEUTIC INTERVENTIONS

RATIONALE

Independent Actions
Implement measures to promote sleep:
- Perform actions to reduce fear and anxiety.
- Encourage participation in relaxing diversional activities during the evening.
- Satisfy basic needs such as comfort and warmth before sleep. **D** ● ✦
- Encourage client to urinate just before bedtime. **D** ● ✦
- Allow client to continue usual sleep practices (e.g., position; time; presleep routines such as reading, watching television, listening to music, and meditating) whenever possible.
- Reduce environmental distractions: **D** ● ✦
  - Close door to client's room.
  - Use night light rather than overhead light whenever possible.
  - Lower volume of paging system.
  - Keep staff conversations at a low level and away from client's room.
  - Close curtains between clients in a semiprivate room or ward.
  - Keep beepers and alarms on low volume.
  - Have earplugs available for client if needed.
- Perform actions to reduce interruptions during sleep: **D** ✦
  - Restrict visitors.
  - Group care activities such as administration of medications, treatments, physical care, and assessments whenever possible.
- Adjust evening dietary patterns to promote sleep: **D** ✦
  - Discourage intake of foods/fluids high in caffeine such as chocolate, coffee, tea, and colas in the evening.
  - Offer client an evening snack that includes milk unless contraindicated.
- Encourage client to avoid smoking before bedtime.

- Encourage client to avoid drinking alcohol in the evening.

During times of illness, adequate rest and sleep are essential to the healing process.
Primary differences exist between the client's home and the hospital setting, creating barriers to effective sleep/rest.
Within the hospital setting, nursing actions that influence a client's environment help to support normal rest and sleep habits.

To reduce interruptions during sleep, 70 to 100 minutes of uninterrupted sleep is usually needed to complete one sleep cycle).
Grouping care activities when possible gives patient uninterrupted sleep time.

Many food products contain stimulants such as caffeine that could interfere with therapeutic sleep patterns. Consuming foods high in caffeine less than 4 hours before bedtime may interfere with sleep. Milk contains L-tryptophan, which is believed to help induce and maintain sleep.
Nicotine is a stimulant and could interfere with therapeutic sleep patterns.
Alcohol interferes with rapid eye movement (REM) sleep.

Nursing Diagnosis **GRIEVING** NDx

Definition: Intellectual and emotional responses through which an individual attempts to adjust self-concept based upon a perceived personal loss

CLINICAL MANIFESTATIONS

Subjective	Objective
Expression of distress at potential loss; expression of guilt or bargaining with a higher power; denial of significance of potential loss	Inability to concentrate; insomnia; anger; sadness; withdrawal from significant others

RISK FACTORS

- Potential loss of or change in a body part and/or usual body functioning
- Appearance
- Lifestyle
- Roles

DESIRED OUTCOMES

The client will demonstrate beginning progression through the grieving process as evidenced by:
  a. Verbalization of feelings about anticipated losses and changes after surgery
  b. Usual sleep pattern
  c. Participation in preoperative care and self-care activities
  d. Use of available support systems

NOC OUTCOMES

Grief resolution

NIC INTERVENTIONS

Grief work facilitation; emotional support

NURSING ASSESSMENT

Assess for signs and symptoms of anticipatory grieving such as expression of distress about the losses or changes that may occur as a result of the surgery, change in eating habits, inability to concentrate, insomnia, anger, sadness, withdrawal from significant others.

RATIONALE

Early identification of signs and symptoms of grieving allows for the implementation of the appropriate interventions.

THERAPEUTIC INTERVENTIONS

Independent Actions
Implement measures to facilitate the grieving process:
- Assist client to acknowledge the anticipated losses.

- Discuss the grieving process and assist client to accept the phases of grieving (phases vary among theorists but progress from shock and alarm to acceptance) as an expected response to the anticipated losses:
  - Explain the phases of the grieving process to significant others; encourage their support and understanding.
- Provide an atmosphere of care and concern:
  - Provide privacy.
  - Be available and nonjudgmental.
  - Display empathy and respect.
- Perform actions to promote trust:
  - Answer questions honestly and provide requested information.

RATIONALE

Acknowledging anticipated losses allows grief work to begin, as factors that may hinder and facilitate acknowledgment can be identified.

Providing an explanation of the grieving process can assure clients that the feelings they are experiencing are normal and are a part of a process they may need to work through to facilitate emotional healing.

Providing an atmosphere of care and concern allows the client to feel free to express feelings.

An open environment and trusting relationship promotes free discussion of feelings and concerns.

NDx = NANDA-I Diagnosis   **D** = Delegatable Action   ● = UAP   ✦ = LVN/LPN   ⊖▶ = Go to ⊖volve for animation

Continued...

THERAPEUTIC INTERVENTIONS	RATIONALE
• Support behaviors suggesting successful grief work, such as verbalizing feelings about anticipated losses, expressing sorrow, and focusing on ways to adapt to anticipated losses:	*Expression of feelings can help to facilitate the grieving process; however, destructive behavior can be damaging.*
• Encourage the verbal expression of anger and sadness about the anticipated losses; recognize displacement of anger and assist client to see the actual cause of angry feelings and resentment.	
• Encourage client to express feelings in whatever ways are comfortable such as writing, drawing, and conversation.	
• Support realistic hope about changes that may result from the surgery.	*Hope should be provided within the parameters of the client's individual situation; however, false reassurance is to be avoided.*
• Provide information about counseling services and support groups that might assist client in working through grief.	*Additional resources can help to meet the ongoing needs of the client and facilitate further grief work.*
• When appropriate, assist client to meet spiritual needs:	*The spirituality of clients affects their ability to cope with loss. Individuals with a strong interconnectedness with a higher power show resilience when confronting grief.*
• Arrange for a visit from clergy.	

CLIENT TEACHING

Nursing Diagnosis **DEFICIENT KNOWLEDGE** NDx

Definition: Absence of cognitive information related to a specific topic

CLINICAL MANIFESTATIONS

Subjective	Objective
Verbalization of the problem	Exaggerated behaviors; inaccurate follow through of instruction; inaccurate performance of test; inappropriate behaviors (e.g., hysterical, hostile, agitated, apathetic)

RISK FACTORS
- Lack of understanding regarding the surgical procedure
- Routines associated with surgery
- Physical preparation for the surgical procedure
- Sensations that normally occur after surgery and anesthesia, and postoperative care

NOC OUTCOMES	NIC INTERVENTIONS
Knowledge: disease process; knowledge: treatment regimen	Teaching: preoperative; teaching: individual

NURSING ASSESSMENT	RATIONALE
Assess the client's baseline understanding of the surgical procedure, preoperative care, and postoperative sensations and care.	*Identifying the client's baseline knowledge level will allow for the development of the appropriate teaching plan.*
Assess the client's baseline literacy level.	*A client's health literacy level should be assessed before providing instruction so the appropriate teaching plan can be developed. Unless the nurse considers the client's intellectual abilities when developing the teaching plan, teaching will be unsuccessful.*

THERAPEUTIC INTERVENTIONS	RATIONALE

Desired Outcomes: The client will demonstrate:
   a. An understanding of the surgical procedure, preoperative care, and postoperative sensations and care
   b. The ability to perform activities designed to prevent postoperative complications

Independent Actions

Provide information about usual preoperative routines for the surgery to be performed, such as blood work, electrocardiogram (ECG), urinalysis, chest radiograph, insertion of urinary catheter and/or nasogastric tube, bowel and skin preparation, and removal of prosthetic devices.

Provide information about:
- Scheduled time and estimated length of surgery
- Food and fluid restrictions before surgery
- Preoperative medications and planned anesthesia
- Body position during surgical procedure
- Purpose for and estimated length of stay in preoperative holding area and postanesthesia care unit (PACU)
- Sensations that can occur after surgery such as dryness of mouth, sore throat after endotracheal intubation, and pain at surgical site

Inform client of the anticipated postoperative care:
- Equipment such as dressings, intravenous lines, drainage tubes, traction devices, antiembolism stockings, and intermittent pneumatic compression device
- Activity limitations and expectations
- Dietary modifications
- Treatments such as respiratory care, circulatory management, and wound care, and the expected frequency
- Assessments such as intake and output, lung sounds, vital signs, neurological checks, and bowel sounds, and the expected frequency
- Medications such as antiemetics, analgesics, and antimicrobials
- Pain management measures such as oral, parenteral, and/or intravenous medications; epidural analgesia; patient-controlled analgesia [PCA]; positioning; and relaxation techniques

Provide instructions about activities the client will be expected to perform postoperatively. These may include:
- Effective coughing and deep breathing techniques
- Correct use of incentive spirometer
- Active foot and leg exercises
- Correct methods for moving in bed, getting out of bed, and ambulating

Providing information about procedures enhances knowledge as well as decreases anxiety, as clients have a better understanding of what to expect during a procedure.

Allow time for questions and clarification. Provide feedback.

Allowing time for questions and clarification allows the nurse to evaluate the effectiveness of teaching and make the appropriate adjustments to the teaching plan.

Reinforce information provided by the anesthesiologist and surgeon about the surgery.

Reinforcing important information allows the nurse to both summarize key concepts and further assess the client's understanding of instructions.

POSTOPERATIVE CARE

The postoperative phase begins when the client is transferred from surgery to a postanesthesia care unit (PACU) and ends when the client has recovered from the surgical intervention. The length of the postoperative phase varies depending on factors such as the client's age and preoperative health status, the type of anesthesia used, the length and type of surgery, and the client's physiological and psychological responses postoperatively.

This care plan focuses on postoperative care of an adult client who has received general anesthesia and has been transferred from the recovery area to the clinical care unit. Much of the information is applicable to clients having surgery in an outpatient setting (e.g., physician's office, surgical care center) and to those receiving follow-up care in an extended care facility or home setting. This care plan should be used in conjunction with all surgical care plans.

OUTCOME/DISCHARGE CRITERIA

The client will
1. Tolerate prescribed diet.
2. Tolerate expected level of activity.
3. Have surgical pain controlled.
4. Have clear, audible breath sounds throughout lungs.
5. Have evidence of normal wound healing.
6. Have no signs and symptoms of infection or postoperative complications.
7. Identify ways to prevent postoperative infection.
8. Demonstrate ability to perform wound care.
9. State signs and symptoms to report to health care provider.
10. Share thoughts and feelings about the surgery, diagnosis, prognosis, and treatment plan.
11. Verbalize an understanding of, and a plan for, adhering to recommended follow-up care including future appointments with health care provider, dietary modifications, activity level, treatments, and medications prescribed.

Nursing Diagnosis ## INEFFECTIVE TISSUE PERFUSION NDx (RENAL, CEREBRAL, CARDIOPULMONARY, GASTROINTESTINAL, PERIPHERAL)

Definition: Decrease in blood circulation to the periphery that may compromise health

CLINICAL MANIFESTATIONS

Subjective	Objective
Cardiopulmonary: Report of chest pain; feelings of lightheadedness **Gastrointestinal:** Report of nausea; abdominal pain	**Cardiopulmonary:** capillary refill >3 seconds; chest pain; altered respiratory rate **Cerebral:** mental status changes **Peripheral arterial:** cold extremities; diminished arterial pulses; weak or absent pulses **Renal:** anuria; oliguria; elevated blood urea nitrogen (BUN)/creatinine **Gastrointestinal:** hypoactive or absent bowel sounds; nausea

RISK FACTORS
- Hypovolemia associated with fluid loss and decreased fluid intake
- Peripheral pooling of blood associated with decreased activity and diminished vasomotor responses resulting from the effects of anesthesia and some medications (e.g., narcotic [opioid] analgesics)

DESIRED OUTCOMES

The client will maintain adequate tissue perfusion as evidenced by:
  a. Blood pressure (B/P) within normal range for client and stable with position change
  b. Usual mental status
  c. Extremities warm with absence of pallor and cyanosis
  d. Palpable peripheral pulses
  e. Capillary refill time less than 2 to 3 seconds
  f. Urine output at least 30 mL/h

NOC OUTCOMES

Circulation status

NIC INTERVENTIONS

Circulatory care: venous insufficiency; circulatory care: arterial insufficiency; hypovolemia management

NURSING ASSESSMENT	RATIONALE
Assess for and report signs and symptoms of diminished tissue perfusion: • Significant decrease in B/P; postural hypotension • Dizziness or lightheadedness when changing to an upright position • Restlessness or confusion • Cool extremities, pallor, or cyanosis of extremities • Diminished or absent peripheral pulses • Slow capillary refill • Oliguria or anuria	• *Early recognition of signs and symptoms of diminished tissue perfusion allow for prompt intervention.*

THERAPEUTIC INTERVENTIONS	RATIONALE
Independent Actions Implement measures to maintain adequate tissue perfusion: • Instruct client to change slowly from a supine to an upright position.	*Changing from a supine to a sitting or standing position slowly allows time for autoregulatory mechanisms to adjust to the change in the distribution of blood associated with an upright position.*

• Perform actions to prevent peripheral pooling of blood and increase venous return:
  • Instruct and assist client to perform active foot and leg exercises every 1 to 2 hours while awake. **D** ✦
  • Encourage and assist with ambulation as soon as allowed and tolerated (client should be instructed to pick up feet instead of shuffling). (**D** ●)
  • Discourage positions that compromise blood flow in lower extremities such as crossing legs, pillows under knees, and sitting for long periods. **D** ✦
	When a client is on bedrest, blood pools in the extremities as a result of decreased muscle activity. Range-of-motion activity exercises help reduce venous stasis.
	Rhythmic muscle contractions that occur during active foot and leg exercises cause intermittent compression of the veins, which improves venous return.

• Perform actions to prevent vasoconstriction:
  • Implement measures to reduce stress such as explaining procedures, reducing discomfort, and maintaining a calm environment.
  • Discourage smoking.
  • Implement measures to keep client from getting cold by maintaining a comfortable room temperature and providing adequate clothing and blankets. (**D** ●)
	Vasoconstriction narrows vessel lumens, which results in diminished blood flow through the affected vessels. Nicotine increases catecholamine output, which causes vasoconstriction. When the body is cold, peripheral vasoconstriction occurs in an attempt to contain body heat.

Dependent/Collaborative Actions Implement measures to maintain adequate tissue perfusion: • Administer blood products as ordered. • Maintain a minimum fluid intake of 2500 mL/day unless contraindicated; if oral intake is inadequate or contraindicated, maintain intravenous fluid therapy as ordered. **D** ✦	*Intravenous fluids and/or blood help maintain vascular volume, which is essential for adequate tissue perfusion. Adequate hydration is essential for maintenance of a vascular volume sufficient to maintain adequate tissue perfusion.*
• Perform actions to prevent peripheral pooling of blood and increase venous return: • Consult physician about an order for antiembolism stockings or an intermittent pneumatic compression device during period of reduced activity.	*Antiembolic stockings and intermittent pneumatic compression devices promote venous return by exerting either constant pressure or intermittent pressure on the vessels in the lower extremities.*
Consult physician if signs and symptoms of diminished tissue perfusion persist or worsen.	*Notifying the appropriate health care provider allows for modification of the treatment plan.*

Nursing Diagnosis INEFFECTIVE BREATHING PATTERN NDx

Definition: Inspiration and/or expiration that does not provide adequate ventilation

CLINICAL MANIFESTATIONS

Subjective	Objective
Verbal report of dyspnea/difficulty breathing	Alterations in depth of breathing; altered chest excursion; bradypnea; decreased minute ventilation; use of accessory muscles to breathe

RISK FACTORS

- Increased rate of respirations associated with fear and anxiety
- Decreased rate and depth of respirations associated with the depressant effect of anesthesia and some medications (e.g., narcotic [opioid] analgesics, some antiemetics)
- Reluctance to breathe deeply because of pain, fear, anxiety, weakness, and fatigue
- Restricted chest expansion resulting from positioning and elevation of the diaphragm if abdominal distention is present

DESIRED OUTCOMES

The client will maintain an effective breathing pattern as evidenced by:
 a. A normal rate and depth of respirations
 b. Absence of dyspnea

NOC OUTCOMES

Respiratory status: ventilation

NIC INTERVENTIONS

Ventilation assistance; respiratory monitoring

NURSING ASSESSMENT	RATIONALE
Assess for signs and symptoms of an ineffective breathing pattern: • Shallow or slow respirations • Limited chest excursion • Tachypnea or dyspnea • Use of accessory muscles when breathing	*Early recognition of signs and symptoms of an ineffective breathing pattern allows for prompt intervention.*
Assess/monitor pulse oximetry (arterial oxygen saturation [SaO_2]), arterial blood gases (ABGs) as indicated.	*Monitoring continuous SaO_2 readings allows for the early detection of hypoxia.* *Assessment of ABGs allows for a more direct measurement of both the partial pressure of oxygen in arterial blood (PaO_2) and the partial pressure of carbon dioxide in arterial blood ($PaCO_2$), both of which reflect the adequacy of ventilation.*

THERAPEUTIC INTERVENTIONS	RATIONALE

Independent Actions

Implement measures to improve breathing pattern: **D** ● ✦
- Perform actions to reduce fear and anxiety:
  - Promote a calm, restful environment.
- Perform actions to reduce pain: **D** ✦
  - Reposition client for comfort.
  - Instruct client to support incision when moving or coughing.
- Perform actions to reduce the accumulation of gas and fluid in the gastrointestinal tract: **D** ✦
  - Maintain patency of nasogastric, gastric, or intestinal tubes if present.
- Perform actions to increase strength and improve activity tolerance:
  - Implement measures to conserve energy (e.g., organize care to allow for periods of rest; decrease noise).

Reducing fear and anxiety helps to prevent shallow and/or rapid breathing.

Reducing pain helps to increase the client's willingness to move and breathe more deeply.

Reducing the accumulation of gas in the gastrointestinal tract decreases pressure on the diaphragm, facilitating more effective ventilation.

Increasing activity tolerance enables the client to breathe more deeply and participate in activities to improve breathing pattern.

THERAPEUTIC INTERVENTIONS	RATIONALE
• Have client deep breathe or use incentive spirometer every 1 to 2 hours. **D** ✦	*Deep breathing and use of an incentive spirometer promotes maximal inhalation and lung expansion.*
• Instruct client to breathe slowly if hyperventilating.	*Hyperventilation is an ineffective breathing pattern that can lead to respiratory alkalosis. A client can often slow breathing rate by concentrating on doing so.*
• Place client in a semi- to high-Fowler's position unless contraindicated. (**D** ●)	*A semi- to high-Fowler's position allows for maximal diaphragmatic excursion and lung expansion.*
• If client must remain flat in bed, assist with position change at least every 2 hours. (**D** ●)	*Compression of the thorax and subsequent limited chest wall expansion occur when the client lies in one position. Frequent repositioning promotes maximal chest wall and lung expansion.*

Dependent/Collaborative Actions

Implement measures to improve breathing pattern:

• Increase activity as allowed and tolerated. **D** ● ✦	*During activity, especially ambulation, the client usually takes deeper breaths, thus increasing lung expansion.*

• Assist with positive airway pressure techniques if ordered.
  • Continuous positive airway pressure (CPAP)
  • Bilevel positive airway pressure (BiPAP)
  • Flutter/positive expiratory pressure ([PEP] device)
	Positive airway pressure techniques increase intrapulmonary alveolar pressure, which helps reexpand collapsed alveoli and prevent further alveoli collapse.

• Administer central nervous system depressants judiciously. • Hold medication and consult physician if respiratory rate is less than 12/min.	*Central nervous system depressants cause depression of the respiratory center in the brainstem, which can result in a decreased rate and depth of respiration.*
• Perform actions to reduce pain: • Administer analgesics before activities and procedures that can cause pain and before pain becomes severe. **D** ✦	*Reducing pain helps to increase the client's willingness to move and breathe more deeply.*

Consult appropriate health care provider if:

• Ineffective breathing pattern continues • Client develops signs and symptoms of impaired gas exchange such as restlessness, irritability, confusion, significant decrease in oximetry results, decreased PaO_2 and increased $PaCO_2$ levels	*Notifying the appropriate health care provider allows for modification of treatment plan.*

Nursing Diagnosis **INEFFECTIVE AIRWAY CLEARANCE** NDx

Definition: Inability to clear secretions or obstructions from the respiratory tract to maintain a clear airway

CLINICAL MANIFESTATIONS

Subjective	Objective
Verbal report of dyspnea/difficulty breathing	Dyspnea, orthopnea; diminished breath sounds; adventitious breath sounds (crackles, rhonchi, wheezes); cough, ineffective or absent sputum production; difficulty vocalizing; wide-eyed; restlessness; changes in respiratory rate and rhythm; cyanosis

Continued...

RISK FACTORS

- Occlusion of the pharynx in the immediate postoperative period associated with relaxation of the tongue, resulting from the effects of anesthesia and some medications (e.g., narcotic [opioid] analgesics)
- Stasis of secretions associated with (1) decreased activity, (2) depressed ciliary function resulting from the effects of anesthesia, and (3) difficulty coughing up secretions resulting from the depressant effects of anesthesia and some medications (e.g., narcotic [opioid] analgesics, some antiemetics), pain, weakness, fatigue, and the presence of tenacious secretions (can occur as a result of deficient fluid volume)
- Increased secretions associated with irritation of the respiratory tract (can result from inhalation anesthetics and endotracheal intubation)

DESIRED OUTCOMES

The client will maintain clear, open airways as evidenced by:
  a. Normal breath sounds
  b. Normal rate and depth of respirations
  c. Absence of dyspnea

NOC OUTCOMES

Respiratory status: ventilation; respiratory status: airway patency

NIC INTERVENTIONS

Respiratory monitoring; airway management; cough enhancement

NURSING ASSESSMENT	RATIONALE
Assess for signs and symptoms of ineffective airway clearance: • Abnormal breath sounds • Rapid, shallow respirations • Dyspnea • Cough	*Early recognition of signs and symptoms of an ineffective airway clearance allows for prompt intervention.*
Assess/monitor pulse oximetry (SaO_2), ABGs as indicated.	*Monitoring continuous SaO_2 readings allows for the early detection of hypoxia.* *Assessment of ABGs allows for a more direct measurement of both PaO_2 and $PaCO_2$, both of which reflect the adequacy of ventilation.*

THERAPEUTIC INTERVENTIONS	RATIONALE
Independent Actions Implement measures to promote effective airway clearance: • Position client on side and/or insert an artificial airway if necessary.	*An artificial airway helps prevent obstruction of airway by tongue.*

• Perform actions to reduce pain:
  • Reposition client for comfort. **D** ✦ ●
  • Instruct client to support incision when moving or coughing. **D** ✦
	Reducing pain helps to increase the client's willingness to move and breathe more deeply.

• Instruct and assist client to change position at least every 2 hours while in bed. **D** ● ✦	*Repositioning helps mobilize secretions.*
• Perform actions to promote the removal of secretions: • Instruct and assist client to deep breathe and cough every 1 to 2 hours. **D** ✦	*Deep breathing can help loosen secretions and enhance the effectiveness of coughing.*
• Discourage smoking.	*Irritants in smoke increase mucus production, impair ciliary function, and can cause inflammation and damage to the bronchial walls.*
• Perform suctioning if needed. **D** ✦	*Suctioning removes secretions from the large airways. It also stimulates coughing, which helps clear airways of mucus and foreign matter.*

THERAPEUTIC INTERVENTIONS	RATIONALE

Dependent/Collaborative Actions

Implement measures to promote effective airway clearance:

- Implement measures to thin tenacious secretions and reduce drying of the respiratory mucous membrane:
  - Maintain a fluid intake of at least 2500 mL/day unless contraindicated.
  - Humidify inspired air as ordered. **D** ✦
- Assist with administration of mucolytics and diluent or hydrating agents via nebulizer if ordered:
  - Acetylcysteine
  - Water, saline
- Increase activity as allowed and tolerated. **D** ● ✦
- Administer central nervous system depressants judiciously.

Consult appropriate health care provider such as a physician or respiratory therapist if:

- Signs and symptoms of ineffective airway clearance persist
- Signs and symptoms of impaired gas exchange are present:
  - Restlessness
  - Irritability
  - Confusion
  - Significant decrease in oximetry results
  - Decreased PaO_2 and increased $PaCO_2$

Adequate hydration and humidified inspired air help thin secretions, which facilitates the mobilization and expectoration of secretions.

These actions also reduce dryness of the respiratory mucous membrane, which helps enhance mucociliary clearance.

Mucolytics and diluents or hydrating agents are mucokinetic substances that reduce the viscosity of mucus, thus making it easier for the client to mobilize and clear secretions from the respiratory tract.

Activity helps to mobilize secretions and promotes deeper breathing.

Central nervous system depressants depress the cough reflex, which can result in stasis of secretions.

Notifying the appropriate health care provider allows for modification of the treatment plan.

Nursing Diagnosis RISK FOR IMBALANCED FLUID AND ELECTROLYTES*

Definition: Presence of risk factors that could lead to excessive fluid loss, electrolyte loss, or excess fluid volume resulting from compromised regulatory mechanisms

CLINICAL MANIFESTATIONS

Subjective	Objective
Deficient fluid volume: verbalization of increased thirst; headaches; muscle cramps	**Deficient fluid volume:** restlessness; weakness; postural hypotension; inability to concentrate; tachycardia; decreased urine output
Excessive fluid volume: verbalization of swelling; nausea, shortness of breath	**Excessive fluid volume:** adventitious breath sounds, blood pressure changes, oliguria, S_3 heart sound, changes in mental status, distended neck veins
Electrolyte loss: verbalization of muscle cramps; nausea; palpitations; paresthesia; dizziness	**Electrolyte loss:** confusion, altered mental status, muscle twitching/spasms, EKG changes, arrhythmias

RISK FACTORS

- **Deficient fluid volume:** restricted oral fluid intake before, during, and after surgery; blood loss; and loss of fluid associated with vomiting, nasogastric tube drainage, and/or profuse wound drainage
- **Hypokalemia, hypochloremia,** and **metabolic alkalosis:** loss of electrolytes and hydrochloric acid associated with vomiting and nasogastric tube drainage

- Excess fluid volume: vigorous fluid therapy during and immediately after surgery and an increased secretion of antidiuretic hormone (ADH; output of ADH is stimulated by trauma, pain, and anesthetic agents)

---

*This diagnostic label includes the following nursing diagnoses: deficient fluid volume and excessive fluid volume.

NDx = NANDA-I Diagnosis   **D** = Delegatable Action   ● = UAP   ✦ = LVN/LPN   ⊖▶ = Go to ⊖volve for animation

Continued...

DESIRED OUTCOMES

1. The client will not experience deficient fluid volume, hypokalemia, hypochloremia, or metabolic alkalosis as evidenced by:
   a. Clear lung sounds and being free of dyspnea
   b. Absence of an S_3 heart sound
   c. B/P and pulse within normal range for client and stable with position change
   d. Capillary refill time less than 2 to 3 seconds
   e. Normal pulse volume
   f. Urine output greater than 30 mL/h
   g. Usual mental status
   h. Balanced intake and output within 48 hours after surgery
   i. Return of peristalsis within expected time
   j. Absence of cardiac dysrhythmias, muscle weakness, paresthesias, twitching, spasms, and dizziness
   k. Serum electrolyte and blood gas values within normal range
   l. Normal skin turgor
   m. Moist mucous membranes
   n. Stable weight

2. The client will not experience excess fluid volume as evidenced by:
   a. Stable weight
   b. Stable B/P
   c. Absence of an S_3 heart sound
   d. Normal pulse volume
   e. Balanced intake and output within 48 hours after surgery
   f. Usual mental status
   g. BUN/hematocrit (Hct), and serum sodium and osmolality levels within normal range
   h. Absence of dyspnea, orthopnea, edema, and distended neck veins

NOC OUTCOMES

Fluid balance; electrolyte balance; acid-base balance

NIC INTERVENTIONS

Fluid monitoring; fluid management; fluid and electrolyte management; electrolyte management: hypokalemia; acid-base monitoring; acid-base management: metabolic alkalosis

NURSING ASSESSMENT	RATIONALE
Assess for and report signs and symptoms of deficient fluid volume:	*Early recognition of signs and symptoms of imbalanced fluid and electrolytes allows for prompt intervention.*
• Decreased skin turgor, dry mucous membranes, thirst	
• Weight loss of 2% or greater over a short period	
• Postural hypotension and/or low B/P	
• Weak, rapid pulse	
• Capillary refill time greater than 2 to 3 seconds	
• Neck veins flat when client is supine	
• Change in mental status	
• Continued low urine output 48 hours after surgery with a change in specific gravity	*The specific gravity will usually increase with an actual fluid volume deficit but may be decreased depending on the cause of the deficit*
• Elevated BUN	
Assess for and report signs and symptoms of hypokalemia:	
• Cardiac dysrhythmias	
• Postural hypotension	
• Muscle weakness	
• Nausea and vomiting	
• Continued abdominal distention	
• Hypoactive or absent bowel sounds	
• Low serum potassium level	
Assess for and report signs and symptoms of hypochloremia:	
• Dizziness	
• Paresthesias	
• Muscle twitching or spasms	
• Hypoventilation	
• Low serum chloride level	
• Elevated pH and $PaCO_2$	

NURSING ASSESSMENT	RATIONALE
Assess for and report signs and symptoms of excess fluid volume: • Weight gain of 2% or greater over a short period • Elevated B/P (B/P may not be elevated if fluid has shifted out of vascular space) • Presence of an S_3 heart sound • Bounding pulse • Intake that continues to be greater than output 48 hours postoperatively • Change in mental status • Crackles (rales), diminished or absent breath sounds • Low serum sodium level and low osmolality indicate hypoosmolar overhydration. • Decreased BUN and Hct (low Hct could also indicate blood loss) • Dyspnea, orthopnea • Edema • Distended neck veins • Chest radiograph results showing pulmonary vascular congestion, pleural effusion, or pulmonary edema	
Monitor serum electrolyte levels, hemogram, serum osmolality, and ABG values as indicated.	*Monitoring serum electrolyte levels, hemogram, and serum osmolality allows for the early detection of fluid/electrolyte imbalances.* *Assessment of ABG values allows for a more direct measurement of both pH and $PaCO_2$, which may influence electrolyte imbalances.*
Assess results of chest radiograph as indicated.	*Chest radiograph films provide data about pulmonary vascular status and fluid accumulation in the pleural space, pulmonary interstitium, and alveoli.*

THERAPEUTIC INTERVENTIONS	RATIONALE
Independent Actions Implement measures to prevent or treat deficient fluid volume, hypokalemia, hypochloremia, and metabolic alkalosis: • Perform actions to prevent nausea and vomiting: • Encourage client to take deep, slow breaths when nauseated. **D** ✦	*Nausea often causes the client to have decreased fluid volume intake. Persistent vomiting results in excessive loss of fluid.*
• If a nasogastric tube is present and needs to be irrigated frequently and/or with large volumes of solution, irrigate it with normal saline rather than water. **D** ✦	*Irrigation of a nasogastric tube with normal saline instead of water helps to prevent excess loss of gastric electrolytes.*

• Perform actions to reduce fever if present:
  • Sponge client with tepid water. **D** ●
  • Remove excessive clothing or bedcovers. **D** ●
	Fever may be accompanied by diaphoresis, which can result in excessive loss of fluid.

• Carefully measure drainage: **D** ✦
  • Wound
  • Nasogastric
	Accurate intake/output records must be maintained to ensure fluid loss is replaced appropriately.

• When oral intake is allowed and tolerated, assist client to select foods/fluids high in potassium: **D** ✦
  • Bananas
  • Orange juice
  • Potatoes
  • Raisins
  • Cantaloupe
  • Tomato juice
	Intake of foods/fluids high in potassium helps correct hypokalemia.

Implement measures to prevent or treat excess fluid volume: • Maintain fluid restrictions if ordered. **D** ✦	

NDx = NANDA-I Diagnosis   **D** = Delegatable Action   ● = UAP   ✦ = LVN/LPN   ⊖▶ = Go to ⊖volve for animation

Continued...

THERAPEUTIC INTERVENTIONS	RATIONALE

Dependent/Collaborative Nursing Actions

Implement measures to prevent or treat deficient fluid volume, hypokalemia, hypochloremia, and metabolic alkalosis:

- Perform actions to prevent nausea and vomiting:
  - Administer antiemetics and gastrointestinal stimulants as ordered. **D** ✦

Nausea often causes the client to have decreased fluid volume intake. Persistent vomiting results in excessive loss of fluid.

- Perform actions to reduce fever if present:
  - Administer antipyretics as ordered. **D** ✦

Fever may be accompanied by diaphoresis, which can result in excessive loss of fluid

- Administer fluid and electrolyte replacements if ordered.

Replacing fluid/electrolyte volume that is lost helps prevent/treat deficient fluid volume.

- Maintain a fluid intake of at least 2500 mL/day unless contraindicated. **D** ✦

Adequate fluid intake needs to be provided in order to ensure adequate hydration.

Implement measures to prevent or treat excess fluid volume:

- Administer fluid replacement therapy judiciously, especially within first 48 hours after surgery.

The stress of surgery along with anesthesia can trigger the secretion of ADH, which can lead to fluid retention/positive fluid balance. The client must be monitored for fluid volume excess until perioperative fluids are mobilized.

- If client is receiving intravenous fluids that contain sizable amounts of sodium such as 0.9% sodium chloride (NaCl) or lactated Ringer's solution, consult physician about a change in the solution or a decrease in the rate of infusion.

Excess fluid volume can result from overzealous or prolonged intravenous administration of sodium-containing fluids, particularly ones that contain sizable amounts of sodium.

- If client is receiving numerous and/or large-volume intravenous medications, consult pharmacist about ways to prevent excessive fluid administration:
- Stop primary infusion during administration of intravenous medications, dilute medication in the minimum amount of solution.

Limiting the amount of intravenous solution infused at any one time and maximizing the concentration of intravenous medications help prevent an additional fluid burden in the person who has or is at risk for fluid volume overload.

- Administer diuretics if ordered to increase excretion of water. **D** ✦

Most diuretics inhibit sodium reabsorption in the renal tubules. This results in decreased water reabsorption and subsequent excretion of excess fluid.

Consult physician if signs and symptoms of deficient fluid volume, excess fluid volume, and electrolyte imbalances persist or worsen.

Notifying the physician allows for modification of the treatment plan.

Nursing Diagnosis   IMBALANCED NUTRITION: LESS THAN BODY REQUIREMENTS NDx

Definition: Intake of nutrients insufficient to meet metabolic needs

CLINICAL MANIFESTATIONS

Subjective	Objective
Verbalization of abdominal cramping or pain; aversion toward eating; lack of interest in food; altered taste sensation; weakness/fatigue; sore, painful mucous membranes	Inadequate food intake; inability to ingest food; diarrhea; hypoactive or absent bowel sounds; weakness of muscles of mastication; weight significantly below client's usual weight; pale conjunctiva; inflamed mucous membranes

RISK FACTORS

- Inability to ingest food and/or absorb nutrients, decreased oral intake associated with prescribed dietary modifications, pain, weakness, fatigue, nausea, dislike of prescribed diet, and feeling of fullness (can occur as a result of abdominal distention)
- Inadequate nutritional replacement therapy
- Loss of nutrients associated with vomiting
- Increased nutritional needs associated with the increased metabolic rate that occurs during wound healing

DESIRED OUTCOMES

The client will maintain an adequate nutritional status as evidenced by:
  a. Weight within normal range for client
  b. Normal BUN, serum albumin, Hct, and hemoglobin (Hgb) levels and lymphocyte count
  c. Usual strength and activity tolerance
  d. Healthy oral mucous membrane

NOC OUTCOMES	NIC INTERVENTIONS
Nutritional status	Nutritional monitoring; nutrition management; nutrition therapy; diet staging

NURSING ASSESSMENT	RATIONALE
Assess for and report signs and symptoms of malnutrition: • Weight significantly below client's usual weight or below normal for client's age, height, and body frame • Weakness and fatigue • Sore, inflamed oral mucous membrane • Pale conjunctiva	*Early recognition of signs and symptoms of malnutrition allows for prompt intervention.*
Assess for return of bowel function every 2 to 4 hours.	*Once the client begins to expel flatus, the physician should be notified so oral intake can be resumed as soon as possible.*
Monitor serum albumin, prealbumin, serum total protein, serum ferritin, transferrin, Hgb, Hct, and electrolyte levels as indicated.	*Serum albumin levels less than 3.5 g/100 mL is considered an indicator of poor nutritional status. Early recognition of abnormal lab values reflective of the client's overall nutritional state allows for prompt intervention.*
When oral intake is allowed, monitor percentage of meals and snacks client consumes. Report pattern of inadequate intake.	*An awareness of the amount of foods/fluids a client consumes alerts the nurse to deficits in nutritional intake. Reporting inadequate intake allows for prompt intervention.*

THERAPEUTIC INTERVENTIONS	RATIONALE

Independent Actions

When food or oral fluids are allowed, implement measures to maintain an adequate nutritional status:
• Implement measures to prevent nausea and vomiting: **D** ● ✦
  • Eliminate noxious sights and odors from the environment.
  • Encourage the client to take deep, slow breaths when nauseated.
  • Instruct client to change positions slowly.
  • Apply a cold washcloth to the client's forehead.
	The presence of nausea can decrease the appetite. Preventing nausea and vomiting can improve the client's appetite.

• Implement measures to reduce pain: • Instruct client to support incision with movement. **D** ✦	*The presence of pain decreases the appetite.*

• Implement measures to reduce the accumulation of gas and fluid in the gastrointestinal tract and prevent constipation:
  • Encourage frequent position changes. **D** ✦
  • Encourage ambulation. **D** ✦
	The subsequent feeling of fullness that accompanies gas accumulation leads to an early feeling of satiety.

• Encourage a rest period before meals. **D** ✦	*To conserve energy for consuming meals, rest periods before eating should be encouraged.*
• Provide nursing assistance during meals. **D** ●	
• Maintain a clean environment and a relaxed, pleasant atmosphere. **D** ●	*A pleasant environment helps to promote adequate intake.*
• Provide oral hygiene before meals. **D** ●	*Good oral hygiene enhances appetite. A moist oral mucosa makes chewing and swallowing easier. Oral hygiene can also remove unpleasant tastes, improving the taste of foods/fluids.*
• Serve frequent, small meals rather than large ones if client is weak, fatigues easily, and/or has a poor appetite. **D** ✦	*Small frequent meals are better tolerated in clients with a poor appetite.*
• Encourage significant others to bring in client's favorite foods unless contraindicated. **D** ✦	*Food preferences enhance a client's appetite.*
• Allow adequate time for meals; reheat foods/fluids if necessary. **D** ●	*Research has demonstrated that it takes 35 minutes to feed the client who is willing to eat.*
• Limit fluid intake with meals (unless the fluid has high nutritional value). **D** ✦	*A high fluid intake with meals promotes a feeling of fullness and early satiety that may decrease actual food intake.*

Continued...

THERAPEUTIC INTERVENTIONS	RATIONALE
Dependent/Collaborative Nursing Actions When food or oral fluids are allowed, implement measures to maintain an adequate nutritional status: • Administer antiemetics as ordered. **D** ✦	*The presence of nausea can decrease the appetite. Preventing nausea and vomiting can improve the client's appetite.*
• Administer pain medications as ordered. **D** ✦	*The presence of pain decreases the appetite.*
• Increase activity as tolerated and allowed. **D** ●	*Activity promotes gastric emptying, which reduces feeling of gastric fullness; it also usually promotes a sense of well-being, which can improve appetite.*
• Obtain a dietary consult if necessary to assist client in selecting foods/fluids that meet nutritional needs, are appealing, and adhere to personal and cultural preferences as well as the prescribed dietary modifications.	*A dietician or nutritional support team can help clients individualize their diet within prescribed dietary restrictions. Providing food in line with client preferences can enhance adherence to prescribed diet.*
• Ensure that meals are well balanced and high in essential nutrients; offer dietary supplements if indicated.	*Dietary supplements have shown a positive relationship with weight gain, reduced mortality, and reduced length of hospitalization.*
• Administer vitamins and minerals if ordered. **D** ✦	*Vitamins and minerals are essential to many metabolic processes in the body.*
• Perform a calorie count if ordered. Report information to dietitian and physician. **D** ✦	*Information gathered from an accurate calorie count is used to determine the adequacy of a client's daily diet or the need for nutritional support.*
Consult physician about an alternative method of providing nutrition if client does not consume enough food or fluids to meet nutritional needs: • Enteral tube feedings • Parenteral nutrition	*Notifying the physician allows for modification of the treatment plan.*

Nursing Diagnosis   ACUTE PAIN NDx

Definition: Unpleasant sensory and emotional experience arising from actual or potential tissue damage or described in terms of such damage (International Association for the Study of Pain): sudden or slow onset of any intensity from mild to severe with an anticipated or predictable end and a duration of <6 months

CLINICAL MANIFESTATIONS

Subjective	Objective
Report of pain in the cognitively aware patient can be rated using an intensity scale (e.g., 0-10) to identify the current level of pain intensity	Inability to take a deep breath (e.g., splinting), guarding, elevated B/P, elevated pulse rate, diaphoresis, increase in the rate and depth of breathing

RISK FACTORS
• Tissue trauma and reflex muscle spasms associated with the surgery
• Irritation from drainage tubes
• Stress on surgical area associated with deep breathing, coughing, and/or movement.

DESIRED OUTCOMES

The client will experience diminished pain as evidenced by:
   a. Verbalization of a decrease in or absence of pain
   b. Relaxed facial expression and body positioning
   c. Increased participation in activities
   d. Stable vital signs

NOC OUTCOMES

Pain control; pain: adverse psychological response; comfort level

NIC INTERVENTIONS

Pain management; analgesic administration

NURSING ASSESSMENT	RATIONALE
Assess for and report signs and symptoms of acute pain: • Verbalization of pain • Grimacing • Reluctance to move • Restlessness • Diaphoresis • Increased B/P • Tachycardia	*Early recognition of signs and symptoms of pain allows for prompt intervention.*
Assess client's perception of the severity of pain using a pain intensity rating scale.	*An awareness of the severity of pain being experienced helps to determine the most appropriate interventions for pain management. Use of a pain intensity rating scale give the nurse a clearer understanding of the pain being experienced and promotes consistency with others about the client's pain experience.*
Assess the client's pain pattern: • Location • Quality • Onset • Duration • Precipitating factors • Aggravating factors • Alleviating factors	*Knowledge of the client's pain pattern assists in the identification of effective pain management strategies.*

THERAPEUTIC INTERVENTIONS	RATIONALE

Independent Actions

Implement measures to reduce pain:
• Perform actions to reduce fear and anxiety about the pain experience:
  • Assure client that the need for pain relief is understood.
  • Plan methods for achieving pain control with client.
	Fear and anxiety can decrease the client's threshold and tolerance for pain and thereby heighten the perception of pain. In addition, pain management methods are not as effective if the client is tense and unable to relax.

• Perform actions to promote rest: • Minimize environmental activity and noise. **D** ●	*Promoting rest helps to reduce fatigue and subsequently increase the client's threshold and tolerance for pain.*

• Provide or assist with nonpharmacological methods for pain relief: **D** ● ✦
  • Massage
  • Position change
  • Progressive relaxation exercises
  • Restful environment
  • Diversional activities such as watching television, reading, or conversing
	Nonpharmacological pain management includes a variety of interventions. It is believed that most of these are effective because they stimulate closure of the gating mechanism in the spinal cord and subsequently block the transmission of pain impulses. In addition, some interventions are thought to stimulate the release of endorphins that inhibit the transmission of nerve impulses and/or alter the client's perception of pain. Many of the nonpharmacological interventions also help to decrease pain by promoting relaxation.

• Instruct and assist client to support abdominal or chest incision with a pillow or hands when turning, coughing, and deep breathing. **D** ✦	*The action of "splinting" an incision or providing support to the incision when turning, coughing, and deep breathing helps to provide support and reduce tension on the incision.*
• If an abdominal incision is present, instruct the client to bend knees while coughing and deep breathing. **D** ✦	*Bending the knees while coughing and deep breathing helps to reduce tension on abdominal muscles and incisions.*
• Securely anchor drainage tubes. **D** ✦	*Securing drainage tubes helps to decrease tissue irritation resulting from movement of tubes.*

Dependent/Collaborative Actions

Implement measures to reduce pain:
• Administer the following medications as ordered*: **D** ✦
  • Narcotic (opioid) analgesics
  • Nonnarcotic analgesics such as acetaminophen and salicylates and other nonsteroidal anti-inflammatory agents
  • Local anesthetics (e.g., bupivacaine, etidocaine)
  • Muscle relaxants
	Pharmacological therapy is an effective method of reducing or relieving pain. All medications reduce pain by a variety of pharmacological effects.

*Delegation is dependent on the route of administration.

NDx = NANDA-I Diagnosis   **D** = Delegatable Action   ● = UAP   ✦ = LVN/LPN   ⊖▶ = Go to ℮volve for animation

Continued...

THERAPEUTIC INTERVENTIONS	RATIONALE

• Encourage client to use patient-controlled analgesia (PCA) device as instructed.
• Maintain integrity of analgesia delivery system:
  • Epidural
  • Intravenous
  • Subcutaneous
  • Transdermal
• Administer analgesics before activities and procedures that can cause pain and before pain becomes severe.* **D** ✦
	Better understanding of the pain management treatment approach can help to improve control of pain.
	Maintaining integrity of the delivery system ensures client receives full benefit of the prescribed medication.
	
	The administration of analgesics before a pain-producing event helps minimize the pain that will be experienced. Analgesics are also more effective if given before pain becomes severe because mild to moderate pain is controlled more quickly and effectively than severe pain.

Consult appropriate health care provider if above measures fail to provide adequate pain relief: • Physician • Pharmacist • Pain management specialist	*Notifying the appropriate health care provider allows for modification of the treatment plan.*

Nursing Diagnosis # ALTERED COMFORT: ABDOMINAL DISTENTION AND GAS PAIN

Definition: An unpleasant sensation of being physically ill at ease that may be localized or generalized but is not described in terms of tissue damage

CLINICAL MANIFESTATIONS

Subjective	Objective
Verbal reports of abdominal fullness or gas pain	Clutching or guarding of the abdomen; restlessness; reluctance to move; grimacing; increasing abdominal girth

RISK FACTORS

• Decreased peristalsis resulting from manipulation of the bowel during abdominal surgery and depressant effect of anesthesia and medications (opioid analgesics)
• Decreased activity

DESIRED OUTCOMES

The client will experience diminished abdominal distention and gas pain as evidenced by:
  a. Verbalization of decreased abdominal fullness and pain
  b. Relaxed facial expression and body positioning
  c. Decrease in abdominal girth

NOC OUTCOMES	NIC INTERVENTIONS
Comfort level; symptom control	Flatulence reduction

NURSING ASSESSMENT	RATIONALE
Assess for and report signs and symptoms of abdominal distention or gas pain.	*Early recognition of signs and symptoms of abdominal distention or gas pain allows for prompt intervention.*

THERAPEUTIC INTERVENTIONS	RATIONALE
Independent Actions Implement measures to reduce the accumulation of gas and fluid in the gastrointestinal tract: • Encourage and assist client with frequent position changes and ambulation as soon as allowed and tolerated. **D** ●	*Activity stimulates peristalsis and expulsion of flatus.*

*Delegation is dependent on the route of administration.

THERAPEUTIC INTERVENTIONS	RATIONALE
• Instruct the client to avoid activities such as chewing gum, drinking through a straw, and smoking.	*Activities that promote air swallowing increase abdominal gas distention.*
• Maintain patency of nasogastric, gastric, or intestinal tube if present. **D** ✦	*Maintaining the patency of tubes designed to decompress the abdomen ensures adequate evacuation of gas, reducing distention.*
• When oral intake is allowed, instruct client to avoid intake of carbonated beverages and gas-producing foods (e.g., cabbage, onions, beans).	
• Encourage client to expel flatus whenever the urge is felt. **D** ✦	

Dependent/Collaborative Actions
Implement measures to reduce the accumulation of gas and fluid in the gastrointestinal tract:

• Encourage use of nonnarcotic analgesics once the period of severe pain has subsided. **D** ✦	*Narcotic (opioid) analgesics depress gastrointestinal activity, contributing further to gas and the risk of constipation.*
• Maintain food and oral fluid restrictions as ordered. **D** ✦	
• Consult physician regarding insertion of a rectal tube or administration of a return-flow enema if indicated.	*Notifying the appropriate health care provider allows for modification of the treatment plan.*
• Administer gastrointestinal stimulants (e.g., metoclopramide, bisacodyl) if ordered. **D** ✦	*Gastrointestinal stimulants increase gastrointestinal motility.*
Consult physician if signs and symptoms of abdominal distention and gas pain persist or worsen.	*Notifying the appropriate health care provider allows for modification of the treatment plan.*

Nursing Diagnosis **NAUSEA** NDx

Definition: A subjective, unpleasant, wavelike sensation in the back of the throat, epigastrium, or abdomen that may lead to the urge or need to vomit

CLINICAL MANIFESTATIONS

Subjective	Objective
Verbal report of nausea; sour taste in the mouth	Gagging; increased salivation

RISK FACTORS
• Stimulation of visceral afferent pathways resulting from abdominal distention and/or the irritating effect of some medications on the gastric mucosa
• Stimulation of the cerebral cortex resulting from pain, stress, and/or noxious environmental stimuli
• Stimulation of the chemoreceptor trigger zone resulting from rapid movement and the effect of some medications (e.g., morphine)

DESIRED OUTCOMES
The client will experience relief of nausea and vomiting as evidenced by:
   a. Verbalization of relief of nausea
   b. Absence of vomiting

NOC OUTCOMES
Nausea and vomiting control; nausea and vomiting severity

NIC INTERVENTIONS
Nausea management; vomiting management; environmental management: comfort

NURSING ASSESSMENT	RATIONALE
Assess for nausea and vomiting.	*Early recognition of signs and symptoms of nausea and vomiting allows for prompt intervention.*

Continued...

THERAPEUTIC INTERVENTIONS	RATIONALE

Independent Actions

Implement measures to prevent nausea and vomiting:

- Perform actions to reduce the accumulation of gas and fluid in the gastrointestinal tract: **D** ✦
  - Frequent position changes
  - Early ambulation
  - Expel flatus when urge felt

As gas accumulates in the intestines, the bowel wall stretches causing feelings of fullness, pain, and cramping that can contribute to nausea.

- Consider alternative therapies for the treatment of nausea:
  - Inhalation of isopropyl alcohol
  - Continuous acupressure with bands or buttons on the wrist

Inhalation of isopropyl alcohol for clients who have undergone general anesthesia has been shown to be somewhat effective for postoperative nausea and vomiting (PONV). Acupressure was demonstrated to be a noninvasive, inexpensive, safe treatment for PONV.

- Perform nonpharmacological actions to reduce pain:
  - Proper positioning
  - Splinting of incisions

Pain is known to contribute to PONV.

- Eliminate noxious sights and odors from the environment.

Noxious stimuli can cause stimulation of the vomiting center.

Implement distraction techniques when client experiences nausea:
  - Slow, deep breaths
  - Guided imagery

Distraction techniques can help draw attention away from nausea. Slow, deep breaths in the immediate postanesthesia period can help rid the body of inhaled anesthetic agents.

- Instruct client to change positions slowly.

Rapid movement can result in chemoreceptor trigger zone stimulation and subsequent excitation of the vomiting center.

- Provide oral hygiene after each emesis. **D** ●

Oral care can help remove foul tastes associated with vomiting.

- When oral intake is allowed:
  - Advance diet slowly (usually beginning with clear liquids and progressing to solid food).

Slow advances in diet allow for gradual adjustment of the digestive tract to the presence of food.

  - Avoid serving foods with an overpowering aroma; remove lids from hot foods before entering room.

Sudden, concentrated food odors can stimulate nausea.

  - Provide small, frequent meals rather than 3 large ones.

Nausea can be prevented by ingesting small meals.

  - Instruct client to ingest foods and fluids slowly.

Eating slowly can reduce the incidence of nausea.

  - Instruct client to avoid foods/fluids that irritate the gastric mucosa (e.g., spicy foods; caffeine-containing beverages such as coffee, tea, and colas).

Foods that irritate the gastric mucosa may lead to the development of nausea.

  - Encourage client to consume foods that prevent nausea (e.g., dry, bland foods such as toast/crackers and liquids such as ginger ale).

Foods that are bland and dry are better tolerated by a nauseated client. Ginger root has been demonstrated to be an effective treatment for nausea and vomiting.

  - Instruct client to avoid foods high in fat.

Fat delays gastric emptying and may contribute to nausea.

  - Instruct client to rest after eating with head of bed elevated.

Resting in a sitting position after eating may help prevent nausea.

Dependent/Collaborative Nursing Actions

Implement measures to prevent nausea and vomiting:

- Administer antiemetics and gastrointestinal stimulants (e.g., metoclopramide) if ordered. **D** ✦

Antiemetic medications can reduce the incidence of nausea. Gastrointestinal stimulants promote peristalsis.

  - Administer medications known to cause gastric irritation (e.g., aspirin and aspirin-containing products, corticosteroids, ibuprofen) with or immediately after meals unless contraindicated.

Administering medications known to irritate the stomach with foods helps reduce the potential for nausea and enhance absorption of the medications.

Consult physician if above measures fail to control nausea and vomiting.

Notifying the appropriate health care provider allows for modification of the treatment plan.

Nursing Diagnosis **IMPAIRED ORAL MUCOUS MEMBRANE** NDx

Definition: Disruption of lips and soft tissues of oral cavity

CLINICAL MANIFESTATIONS

Subjective	Objective
Verbal report of difficulty swallowing, oral discomfort, or bad taste in the mouth	Difficult speech; decreased salivation

RISK FACTORS

- Deficient fluid volume associated with restricted oral intake and fluid loss
- Decreased salivation associated with food and fluid restrictions and the effect of anesthesia and some medications (e.g., narcotic [opioid] analgesics)

DESIRED OUTCOMES

The client will maintain a moist, intact oral mucous membrane.

NOC OUTCOMES

Oral hygiene

NIC INTERVENTIONS

Oral health maintenance; oral health promotion

NURSING ASSESSMENT	RATIONALE
Assess for dryness of the oral mucosa.	*Early recognition of signs and symptoms of a dry oral mucosa allows for prompt intervention.*

THERAPEUTIC INTERVENTIONS	RATIONALE

Independent Actions

Implement measures to relieve dryness of the oral mucous membrane: **D** ✦

- Instruct and assist client to perform oral hygiene as often as needed.
  - Avoid use of products that contain lemon and glycerin and use of mouthwashes containing alcohol.

These products have a drying and irritating effect on the oral mucous membrane.

- Encourage client to rinse mouth frequently with water. **D** ●
- Lubricate client's lips frequently. **D** ●

Frequent lubrication of the lips helps prevent drying and cracking.

- Encourage client to breathe through nose rather than mouth.

Breathing through the nose allows for the proper warming and humidification of air, which is bypassed with mouth breathing.

- Encourage client not to smoke.

Smoking dries the oral mucosa and has been linked to mucous membrane breakdown and oral cancer.

- Encourage client to suck on hard candy unless contraindicated.

Action helps to stimulate salivation, moistening the oral mucosa.

Dependent/Collaborative Actions

Implement measures to relieve dryness of the oral mucous membrane:

- Maintain intravenous fluid therapy as ordered.

Intravenous fluid therapy enhances hydration and helps to improve the condition of dry mucous membranes.

- Increase oral fluid intake as soon as allowed and tolerated. **D** ● ✦

Increasing oral fluid intake promotes hydration and stimulates salivation.

Consult physician if signs and symptoms of parotitis (e.g., pain, tenderness, and swelling at the angle of the jaw; fever) occur.

Notifying the appropriate health care provider allows for modification of the treatment plan.

Nursing Diagnosis | **ACTUAL/RISK FOR IMPAIRED TISSUE INTEGRITY** NDx

Definition: Damage to mucous membrane, corneal, integumentary, or subcutaneous tissues

CLINICAL MANIFESTATIONS

Subjective	Objective
Not applicable	Damaged or disrupted corneal, mucous membrane, integumentary, or subcutaneous tissue

RISK FACTORS

- Disruption of tissue associated with the surgical procedure
- Delayed wound healing associated with factors such as decreased nutritional status and inadequate blood supply to wound area
- Irritation of skin associated with contact with wound drainage, pressure from tubes, and use of tape
- Mechanical damage to the cornea by shearing or friction forces

DESIRED OUTCOMES

1. The client will experience normal healing of surgical wounds as evidenced by:
   a. Gradual reduction in periwound swelling and redness
   b. Presence of granulation tissue if healing is by secondary or tertiary intention
   c. Intact, approximated wound edges if healing is by primary intention
2. The client will maintain tissue integrity in areas in contact with wound drainage, tape, and tubings as evidenced by:
   a. Absence of redness and irritation
   b. No skin breakdown

NOC OUTCOMES

Wound healing: primary intention; wound healing: secondary intention; tissue integrity: skin and mucous membranes

NIC INTERVENTIONS

Skin surveillance; pressure management; positioning; wound care; incision site care

NURSING ASSESSMENT

Assess for and report signs and symptoms of impaired wound healing:
- Increasing periwound swelling
- Redness, pale or necrotic tissue in wounds healing by secondary or tertiary intention
- Separation of wound edges in wounds healing by primary intention.

Inspect skin areas that are in contact with wound drainage, tape, and tubings for signs of irritation and breakdown.

RATIONALE

Early recognition of signs of impaired skin integrity allows for prompt intervention.

THERAPEUTIC INTERVENTIONS

Independent Actions
Implement measures to promote wound healing: **D** ✦
- Perform actions to maintain an adequate nutritional status (e.g., provide well-balanced, nutritious meals, allow adequate time for meals, reheat food as needed).
- Perform actions to maintain adequate circulation to wound area:
  - Do not apply dressings tightly unless ordered.

RATIONALE

Maintaining adequate nutrition is important for tissue healing and repair. Malnourished clients are more likely to have skin that is vulnerable to injury and nonhealing.
Excessive pressure impairs circulation to the area/wound.

THERAPEUTIC INTERVENTIONS	RATIONALE

• Perform actions to protect the wound from mechanical injury:
  • Ensure that dressings are secure enough to keep them from rubbing and irritating wound.
  • Carefully remove tape and dressings when performing wound care.
  • Remind client to keep hands away from wound area.
  • Implement measures to prevent falls.
	Mechanical injury can interrupt normal skin integrity.

• Perform actions to decrease stress on wound area:
  • Instruct and assist client to support the involved area when moving.
  • Instruct and assist client to splint abdominal and chest wounds when coughing.
  • Apply an abdominal binder during periods of activity if ordered.
  • Implement measures to reduce the accumulation of gas and fluid in the gastrointestinal tract in clients who have had abdominal surgery.
  • Implement measures to prevent nausea and vomiting in clients who have had chest, back, or abdominal surgery.
	Actions such as excessive coughing, movement during periods of activity, and violent nausea and vomiting may disrupt the integrity of a fresh surgical incision. Efforts directed at supporting or splinting incisions during this activity will aid in supporting a healing surgical incision.

• Perform actions to prevent wound infection: • Use good hand hygiene. Implement measures to prevent tissue irritation and breakdown in areas in contact with wound drainage, tape, and tubings: **D** ✦	*The presence of a wound infection delays healing.*

• Perform actions to prevent wound drainage from contacting or remaining on skin:
  • Cleanse skin and change dressings when appropriate.
  • Apply a collection device over drains and incisions that are draining continuously and/or copiously.
  • Apply a protective barrier product to skin that is likely to be in frequent contact with drainage.
 	
  • Maintain patency of drainage tubes.
	Excessive moisture on the skin or prolonged exposure of the skin to moisture softens epidermal cells and makes them less resistant to damage. Moisture also harbors microorganisms that can cause irritation or infection. Removing excessive moisture and protecting the skin from prolonged contact with moisture reduces the risk of skin irritation and subsequent breakdown.
	Maintaining patent drainage tubes helps to decrease the risk of leakage around the tubes.

• When positioning clients, ensure that they are not lying on tubings.	*Pressure on the skin can compromise circulation to that area; in addition, if a drainage tubing is occluded, there is an increased risk for leakage of drainage around the tube.*
• Anchor all tubings securely to prevent excessive movement of tubes against tissues.	*Friction from tubes rubbing against skin can lead to injuries to the epidermal layer.*
• Apply a water-soluble lubricant to external nares every 2 to 4 hours.	*The lubricant helps to decrease irritation from nasogastric tube and nasal airway or cannula, which may lead to skin breakdown.*

• Perform actions to decrease skin irritation resulting from the use of tape:
  • Use only necessary amount of tape.
  • Use hypoallergenic tape whenever possible.
  • Apply skin sealant or barrier before applying tape if indicated.
  • Use Montgomery straps or tubular netting.
  • When removing tape, pull it in the direction of hair growth; use adhesive solvents if necessary.
	Skin sensitive to adhesive tape can become severely inflamed and slough when the tape is removed.
	
	The use of Montgomery straps to secure a dressing over a wound site avoids repeated application and removal of tape if frequent dressing changes are anticipated.

NDx = NANDA-I Diagnosis   **D** = Delegatable Action   ● = UAP   ✦ = LVN/LPN   ⊖▶ = Go to ⊖volve for animation

Continued...

THERAPEUTIC INTERVENTIONS	RATIONALE

Dependent/Collaborative Actions

If signs and symptoms of impaired wound healing occur:
- Perform or assist with wound care as ordered:
  - Debridement
  - Packing

Debridement removes necrotic tissue and helps to rid a potential source of infection. Wounds cannot move through the stages of healing if they become infected. Removal of nonviable tissue helps to prevent wound infection if altered skin integrity occurs.

- Prepare client for surgical revision of the wound if planned.

If tissue breakdown occurs:
- Notify appropriate health care provider (physician, wound care specialist).
- Perform care of involved areas as ordered or per standard hospital procedure.

Notifying the appropriate health care provider allows for modification of the treatment plan.

Nursing Diagnosis: # ACTIVITY INTOLERANCE NDx

Definition: Insufficient physiological or psychological energy to endure or complete required or desired daily activities

CLINICAL MANIFESTATIONS

Subjective	Objective
Verbal report of fatigue or weakness; exertional discomfort	Abnormal heart rate or B/P response to activity; dyspnea; electrocardiographic changes reflecting arrhythmias or ischemia; unable to speak with physical activity

RISK FACTORS

- Bed rest or immobility due to surgical procedure, generalized weakness, or imbalance between oxygen supply/demand

DESIRED OUTCOMES

The client will demonstrate an increased tolerance for activity as evidenced by:
  a. Verbalization of feeling less fatigued and weak
  b. Ability to perform activities of daily living without exertional dyspnea, chest pain, diaphoresis, dizziness, and significant changes in vital signs

NOC OUTCOMES

Energy conservation; rest; self-care: activities of daily living; activity tolerance

NIC INTERVENTIONS

Energy management; nutrition management; sleep enhancement; pain management

NURSING ASSESSMENT	RATIONALE

Assess for and report signs and symptoms of activity intolerance:
- Statements of fatigue or weakness
- Exertional dyspnea, chest pain, diaphoresis, or dizziness
- Abnormal heart rate response to activity (e.g., increase in rate of 20 beats/min above resting rate, rate not returning to preactivity level within 3 minutes after stopping activity, change from regular to irregular rate)
- A significant change (15-20 mm Hg) in B/P with activity.

Monitor hemogram for abnormalities.

Early recognition of signs of activity intolerance allows for prompt intervention.

Anemia can lead to decreased oxygen-carrying capacity of the blood and can contribute to activity intolerance.

THERAPEUTIC INTERVENTIONS	RATIONALE

Independent Actions

Implement measures to improve activity tolerance:

- Perform actions to promote rest and/or conserve energy: **D** ✦
  - Maintain activity restrictions as ordered.
  - Minimize environmental activity and noise.
  - Organize nursing care to allow for periods of uninterrupted rest.
  - Limit number of visitors and their length of stay.
  - Assist client with self-care activities as needed. **D** ●
  - Keep supplies and personal articles within easy reach. **D** ●
  - Instruct client in energy-saving techniques (e.g., using shower chair when showering, sitting to brush teeth or comb hair)
  - Implement measures to reduce fear and anxiety:
    - Maintain a calm, supportive manner when interacting with the client.
  - Implement measures to promote sleep:
    - Position the client for comfort. **D** ●

  - Implement measures to reduce discomfort:
  - Support incision when turning, coughing, and deep breathing.
- Perform actions to improve breathing pattern and facilitate airway clearance: **D** ✦
  - Encourage the use of incentive spirometry.
  - Encourage turning, coughing, and deep breathing.

Instruct client to:
- Report a decreased tolerance for activity.
- Stop any activity that causes chest pain, shortness of breath, dizziness, or extreme fatigue or weakness.

Dependent/Collaborative Actions

Implement measures to improve activity tolerance:
- Administer packed red blood cells if ordered.

- Increase client's activity gradually as allowed and tolerated. **D** ●

- Maintain oxygen therapy as ordered. **D** ✦

- Perform actions to maintain an adequate nutritional status: **D** ✦
  - Advance diet as tolerated/prescribed.
  - Administer dietary supplements.

Consult physician if signs and symptoms of activity intolerance persist or worsen.

Cells use oxygen and fat, protein, and carbohydrates to produce the energy needed for all body activities. Rest and activities that conserve energy result in a lower metabolic rate, which preserves nutrients and oxygen for necessary activities.

Fear and anxiety can increase a client's oxygen consumption, which can lead to increased energy consumption and activity intolerance.

Rest and activities that conserve energy result in a lower metabolic rate, which preserves nutrients and oxygen for necessary activities.

Enhancing comfort allows for rest, which conserves energy and preserves nutrients and oxygen necessary for activity.

Altered respiratory function can lead to inadequate tissue oxygenation, which results in less effective energy production and a reduced ability to tolerate activity.

Improving respiratory status increases the amount of oxygen necessary for energy production.

These symptoms indicate that insufficient oxygen is reaching the tissues and that activity has been increased beyond a therapeutic level.

Anemia reduces the oxygen-carrying capacity of the blood. Resolution of anemia increases oxygen availability to the cells, which increases the efficiency of energy production and improves activity tolerance.

A gradual increase in activity prevents a sudden increase in cardiac workload and myocardial oxygen consumption. Progressive activity helps strengthen the myocardium, enhancing cardiac output and improving activity tolerance.

Supplemental oxygen helps to alleviate hypoxia and restore more efficient aerobic metabolism, thereby improving energy levels and activity tolerance.

Metabolism is the process by which nutrients are transformed into energy. If nutrition is inadequate, energy production is decreased, which reduces the client's ability to tolerate activity.

Notifying the appropriate health care provider allows for modification of the treatment plan.

NDx = NANDA-I Diagnosis **D** = Delegatable Action ● = UAP ✦ = LVN/LPN ⊖▶ = Go to ⊖volve for animation

Nursing Diagnosis **IMPAIRED PHYSICAL MOBILITY** NDx

Definition: Limitation in independent, purposeful physical movement of the body or of one or more extremities

CLINICAL MANIFESTATIONS

Subjective	Objective
Verbal report of inability to move	Difficulty turning; exertional dyspnea; limited range of motion; decreased reaction time; mechanical barriers (e.g., casts, splints, abductor pillows, restraints)

RISK FACTORS

- Weakness and fatigue associated with tissue hypoxia, inadequate nutritional status, and difficulty resting and sleeping
- Pain and nausea
- Depressant effect of anesthesia and some medications (e.g., narcotic [opioid] analgesics, some antiemetics)
- Fear of falling, dislodging tubes, and compromising surgical wounds
- Activity restrictions imposed by the treatment plan

DESIRED OUTCOMES

The client will achieve maximum physical mobility within the limitations imposed by the surgical procedure and postoperative treatment plan.

NOC OUTCOMES

Mobility

NIC INTERVENTIONS

Exercise therapy: ambulation; environmental management

NURSING ASSESSMENT	RATIONALE
Assess for and report signs and symptoms impaired mobility: • Pain or discomfort on movement • Limited range of motion • Movement-induced shortness of breath	*Early recognition of signs of impaired mobility allows for prompt intervention.*
Assess client's degree of pain.	*Early recognition of signs and symptoms of pain allows for prompt intervention and improved pain control, which may facilitate mobility in the surgical patient.*
Assess nutritional status and energy level.	*An awareness of the client's nutritional status alerts the nurse to deficiencies that may contribute to a decreased energy level, which may decrease activity tolerance and lead to immobility.*

THERAPEUTIC INTERVENTIONS	RATIONALE

Independent Actions
Implement measures to increase mobility:
- Perform actions to reduce pain:
  - Schedule attempts to increase activity when analgesics are at peak effect. **D** ✦
- Perform actions to prevent nausea and vomiting: **D** ✦
  - Schedule attempts to increase activity when antiemetics are at peak effect.
- Encourage use of nonnarcotic analgesics rather than narcotic (opioid) analgesics once severe pain has subsided
- Perform actions to decrease client's fear of injury:
  - Implement measures to prevent falls.
  - Anchor all dressings and tubings securely to decrease risk of inadvertent removal during activity. **D** ✦
- Assure client that level of activity ordered is expected to facilitate rather than compromise wound healing and postoperative recovery.

Allowing prescribed analgesics to achieve peak effect increases the likelihood the client will have an acceptable pain level that will allow for an increase in mobility.

Movement can aggravate nausea, interfering with attempts to increase mobility.

Nonnarcotic analgesics alleviate mild pain without the sedative effects of opioid analgesics, which may interfere with mobility.
Clients who are anxious are frequently unable to tolerate exercise. Creating a safe and effective care environment will help to decrease a client's fear of injury.

Mobility promotes a general sense of well-being and improves endurance, strength, and health, reducing the risk of complications of immobility.

THERAPEUTIC INTERVENTIONS	RATIONALE
• Encourage activity and participation in self-care as allowed and tolerated; put side rails up and provide overhead trapeze if appropriate.	*Actions help to promote independent movement.*
Encourage the support of significant others. Allow them to assist client with activity unless contraindicated.	*Support systems provide clients with a sense of well-being in the hospitalized setting.*

Dependent/Collaborative Actions
Implement measures to increase mobility:
- Perform actions to improve activity tolerance:
  - Administer antiemetics. **D** ✦
  - Administer analgesics and/or nonnarcotic analgesics. **D** ✦
  - Treat anemia as indicated by administering prescribed folic acid, vitamin B$_{12}$, or packed red blood cells.
- Consult appropriate health care provider (e.g., physician, physical therapist) if client is unable to achieve expected level of mobility.

Actions that control pain and relieve nausea can improve the mobility of the client. Anemia reduces the oxygen-carrying capacity of the blood. Resolution of anemia increases oxygen availability to the cells, which increases the efficiency of energy production and subsequently improves activity tolerance.

Notifying the appropriate health care provider allows for modification of the treatment plan.

Nursing Diagnosis SELF-CARE DEFICIT

Definition: Impaired ability to perform basic personal care activities and instrumental activities of daily living

CLINICAL MANIFESTATIONS

Subjective	Objective
Verbal reports of inability to perform basic personal care activities	Inability to access bathroom; inability to wash body; inability to maintain appearance at acceptable level; inability to put on necessary items of clothing

RISK FACTORS	DESIRED OUTCOMES
• Impaired physical mobility associated with weakness, fatigue, pain, nausea, depressant effect of some medications, fear of dislodging tubes and compromising surgical wound, and activity restrictions	The client will perform self-care activities within physical limitations and postoperative activity restrictions.

NOC OUTCOMES	NIC INTERVENTIONS
Self-care: activities of daily living	Self-care assistance

NURSING ASSESSMENT	RATIONALE
Assess for physical limitation or postoperative restrictions that may interfere with a client's ability to perform self-care.	*Early recognition of signs and symptoms of physical limitations allows for prompt intervention.*

THERAPEUTIC INTERVENTIONS	RATIONALE
Independent Actions With client, develop a realistic plan for meeting daily physical needs. Assist the client with activities he/she is unable to perform independently. **D** ● ✦	*Including the client in developing a plan of care promotes autonomy and helps to establish a sense of control.*

Continued...

THERAPEUTIC INTERVENTIONS	RATIONALE
Implement measures to facilitate the client's ability to perform self-care activities: **D** ● ✦	*Pain relief facilitates range of motion, which may increase the client's ability to perform self-care.*
• Schedule care at a time when client is most likely to be able to participate (e.g., when analgesics are at peak effect, after rest periods, not immediately after meals or treatments).	
• Keep needed objects within easy reach.	
• Allow adequate time for accomplishment of self-care activities.	
• Perform actions to increase physical mobility.	
Obtain assistive devices as necessary.	*Environmental factors may interfere with the client's ability to perform self-care activities. The ability to perform self-care activities may be enhanced with adaptation of the client's care environment.*
Encourage maximum independence within physical limitations and postoperative activity restrictions. **D** ● ✦	
Inform significant others of client's abilities to perform own care. Explain the importance of encouraging and allowing client to maintain an optimal level of independence.	*The ability to perform self-care is essential for optimum self-esteem.*

⊖▶ **Nursing Diagnosis** **RISK FOR URINARY RETENTION** NDx

Definition: Incomplete emptying of the bladder

CLINICAL MANIFESTATIONS

Subjective	**Objective**
Verbal reports of inability to urinate; feelings of the need to strain to empty the bladder	Palpable distended bladder; urinary dribbling

RISK FACTORS	DESIRED OUTCOMES
• Increased tone of the urinary sphincters associated with sympathetic nervous system stimulation resulting from pain, fear, and anxiety	The client will not experience urinary retention as evidenced by:
• Decreased perception of bladder fullness associated with depressant effect of anesthesia and some medications (e.g., narcotic [opioid] analgesics)	a. Voiding at normal intervals
	b. No reports of bladder fullness and suprapubic discomfort
• Relaxation of the bladder muscle associated with depressant effect of anesthesia and some medications (e.g., narcotic [opioid] analgesics) and stimulation of the sympathetic nervous system (can result from pain, fear, and anxiety)	c. Absence of bladder distention and dribbling of urine
	d. Balanced intake and output within 48 hours after surgery

NOC OUTCOMES	NIC INTERVENTIONS
Urinary elimination	Urinary retention care

NURSING ASSESSMENT	RATIONALE
Assess for signs and symptoms of urinary retention:	*Early recognition of signs and symptoms of urinary retention allows for prompt intervention.*
• Frequent voiding of small amounts (25-60 mL) of urine	
• Reports of bladder fullness or suprapubic discomfort	
• Bladder distention	
• Dribbling of urine	

NURSING ASSESSMENT	RATIONALE
Monitor intake and output.	*Administration of anesthetic agents impairs normal bladder emptying. Adequate volume replacement is necessary to fill bladder and stimulate micturition.* *Any continued oliguria or anuria should be reported to the physician to allow for modification of the treatment plan.*

THERAPEUTIC INTERVENTIONS	RATIONALE

Independent Actions
Implement measures to prevent urinary retention:
- Instruct client to urinate when the urge is first felt.

  If the client feels the urge to urinate but suppresses it by contracting the external urinary sphincter, the urge will subside and not recur until the bladder fills more.

- Perform actions to promote relaxation during voiding attempts:

  If the client is relaxed when trying to urinate, he/she is better able to relax the pelvic floor muscles and external urinary sphincter, allowing voiding to occur.

  - Provide privacy, hold a warm blanket against abdomen, encourage client to read. **D** ●
- Perform actions that may help trigger the micturition reflex and promote a sense of relaxation during voiding attempts:
  - Run water, place client's hands in warm water, pour warm water over perineum. **D** ✦
- Allow client to assume a normal position for voiding unless contraindicated. **D** ●

  A sitting or standing position if possible uses gravity to facilitate bladder emptying.

- Instruct client to lean upper body forward and/or gently press downward on lower abdomen during voiding attempts unless contraindicated.

  Proper positioning is necessary in order to put pressure on the bladder (pressure helps create a sensation of bladder fullness, which stimulates the micturition reflex)

Dependent/Collaborative Actions
Implement measures to prevent urinary retention:
- Perform actions to reduce postoperative pain.
  - Encourage use of nonnarcotic rather than narcotic (opioid) analgesics once period of severe pain has subsided. **D** ✦

    Narcotic analgesics may decrease the perception of a full bladder and promote urinary retention. The use of nonnarcotic analgesics may reduce this effect.

- Consult physician regarding intermittent catheterization or insertion of an indwelling catheter if above actions fail to alleviate urinary retention.
- If urinary catheter is present, prevent urinary retention by maintaining patency of the catheter. **D** ✦
- Keep tubing free of kinks, irrigate as ordered.
- Consult physician if there is no urine output within 6 to 8 hours after surgery or if output continues to be less than intake 48 hours after surgery.

  For the first 48 hours postoperatively, urine output is expected to be less than intake because of factors such as blood loss and increased secretion of ADH. Consulting the appropriate health care provider allows for modification of treatment plan.

- Administer cholinergic (parasympathomimetic) drugs to stimulate bladder contraction. **D** ✦

  Cholinergic (parasympathomimetic) drugs promote urination by stimulating contraction of the bladder detrusor muscle.

Collaborative Diagnosis RISK FOR HYPOVOLEMIC SHOCK

Definition: Inadequate tissue perfusion caused by a loss of whole blood, plasma, or interstitial fluid

CLINICAL MANIFESTATIONS

Subjective	Objective
Verbal reports of feeling dizzy or lightheaded	Restlessness; agitation; confusion; changes in mental status; significant decrease in B/P; postural hypotension; rapid, weak pulse; rapid respirations; cool skin; pallor, cyanosis diminished or absent peripheral pulses; urine output less than 30 mL/h

NDx = NANDA-I Diagnosis **D** = Delegatable Action ● = UAP ✦ = LVN/LPN ⊖▶ = Go to evolve for animation

Continued...

RISK FACTORS

- Hemorrhage associated with opening of wound (can occur as a result of inadequate wound closure, stress on incision line, and/or poor wound healing), slippage of closures on ligated vessels, and/or disruption of clots at incision site
- Deficient fluid volume associated with restricted oral intake and excessive fluid loss

DESIRED OUTCOMES

The client will not develop hypovolemic shock as evidenced by:
  a. Usual mental status
  b. Stable vital signs
  c. Skin warm and usual color
  d. Palpable peripheral pulses
  e. Urine output at least 30 mL/h

NURSING ASSESSMENT

Assess for and report signs and symptoms of hypovolemic shock:
- Restlessness, agitation, confusion, or other change in mental status
- Significant decrease in B/P
- Postural hypotension
- Rapid, weak pulse
- Rapid respirations
- Cool skin
- Pallor, cyanosis
- Diminished or absent peripheral pulses
- Urine output less than 30 mL/h

Monitor Hgb, Hct, and prothrombin time (PT)/partial thromboplastin time (PTT) values.

Monitor hemodynamic values if present:
- Central venous pressure (CVP)

RATIONALE

Early recognition of signs and symptoms of hypovolemic shock allows for implementation of the appropriate interventions.

Elevated clotting times may contribute to postoperative hemorrhage and hypovolemic shock. Monitoring Hgb/Hct and PT/PTT will allow for implementation of the appropriate interventions.

If present, hemodynamic values are beneficial in guiding fluid resuscitation and preventing fluid volume overload.

THERAPEUTIC INTERVENTIONS

Independent Actions

Implement measures to prevent hypovolemic shock:
- If bleeding occurs, apply firm, prolonged pressure to area if possible.

If signs and symptoms of hypovolemic shock occur:
- Place client flat in bed with legs elevated unless contraindicated.
- Monitor vital signs frequently.

Dependent/Collaborative Actions

If signs and symptoms of hypovolemic shock occur:
- Administer oxygen as ordered. **D** ✦

- Administer blood and/or volume expanders if ordered. **D** ✦
- Prepare client for insertion of hemodynamic monitoring devices:
  - Central venous catheter
  - Intra-arterial catheter

RATIONALE

These actions prevent further loss of blood or volume, which may contribute to hypovolemic shock.

Elevation of legs facilitates the return of blood pooled in the extremities to the central circulation, improving blood flow to the vital organs.

Supplemental oxygen is beneficial because oxygen delivery to the tissues is compromised in shock states.

Blood and/or fluid volume expanders will help restore circulating volume. The agent of choice is driven by laboratory values.

Hemodynamic monitoring devices can measure preload/filling pressures, which are low in hypovolemic shock states.

Collaborative Diagnosis RISK FOR ATELECTASIS

Definition: Collapse of lung tissue caused by hypoventilated alveoli

CLINICAL MANIFESTATIONS

Subjective	Objective
Verbal reports of difficulty breathing	Diminished or absent breath sounds; dull percussion over affected area; increased respiratory rate; dyspnea; tachycardia; elevated temperature

RISK FACTORS

- Shallow respirations, stasis of secretions in the alveoli and bronchioles, and decreased surfactant production (results from inadequate deep breathing and changes in regional blood flow in the lungs)

DESIRED OUTCOMES

The client will not develop atelectasis as evidenced by:
a. Clear, audible breath sounds
b. Resonant percussion note over lungs
c. Unlabored respirations at 12 to 20 breaths/min
d. Pulse rate within normal range for client
e. Afebrile status

NURSING ASSESSMENT

Assess for and report signs and symptoms of atelectasis:
- Diminished or absent breath sounds
- Dull percussion note over affected area
- Increased respiratory rate
- Dyspnea
- Tachycardia
- Elevated temperature

Monitor pulse oximetry as indicated.

Monitor chest radiograph results.

RATIONALE

Early recognition of signs and symptoms of atelectasis allows for prompt intervention.

Pulse oximetry is an indirect measure of oxygen saturation. Monitoring pulse oximetry (SaO_2) allows for early detection of hypoxia and implementation of the appropriate interventions.

Chest radiograph provides radiographic confirmation of atelectasis.

THERAPEUTIC INTERVENTIONS

Independent Actions
Implement measures to prevent atelectasis: **D** ✦
- Perform actions to improve breathing pattern:
  - Encourage client to deep breathe.
  - Incentive spirometry
- Perform actions to promote effective airway clearance:
  - Turn, cough, and deep breathe.
- If signs and symptoms of atelectasis occur:
  - Increase frequency of position change, coughing or "huffing," deep breathing, and use of incentive spirometer.

Consult physician if signs and symptoms of atelectasis persist or worsen.

RATIONALE

Lack of movement places a client at risk for atelectasis. Changing positions frequently, coughing, and deep breathing help to expand the lungs, enhancing alveolar expansion.

Notifying the appropriate health care provider will allow for modification of the treatment plan.

NDx = NANDA-I Diagnosis   **D** = Delegatable Action   ● = UAP   ✦ = LVN/LPN   ⟳▶ = Go to ⟳volve for animation

Collaborative Diagnosis RISK FOR DEEP VEIN THROMBOSIS

Definition: A clot that forms in the vessel wall of the lower extremities

CLINICAL MANIFESTATIONS

Subjective	Objective
Verbal reports of pain or tenderness in an extremity	Increase in circumference of extremity; distention of superficial vessels in extremity; unusual warmth of extremity; positive Homans' sign (not always a reliable indicator)

RISK FACTORS

- Venous stasis associated with decreased activity, positioning during and after surgery, increased blood viscosity (can result from deficient fluid volume), and abdominal distention (the distended intestine may put pressure on the abdominal vessels)
- Hypercoagulability associated with increased release of tissue thromboplastin into the blood (occurs as a result of surgical trauma) and hemoconcentration and increased blood viscosity (can occur as a result of deficient fluid volume)
- Trauma to vein walls during surgery

DESIRED OUTCOMES

The client will not develop a deep vein thrombus as evidenced by:
  a. Absence of pain, tenderness, swelling, and distended superficial vessels in extremities
  b. Usual temperature of extremities
  c. Negative Homans' sign

NURSING ASSESSMENT

Assess for and report signs and symptoms of a deep vein thrombus:
- Pain or tenderness in extremity
- Increase in circumference of extremity
- Distention of superficial vessels in extremity
- Unusual warmth of extremity
- Positive Homans' sign (not always a reliable indicator)

RATIONALE

Early recognition of signs and symptoms of deep vein thrombosis allows for prompt intervention.

THERAPEUTIC INTERVENTIONS

RATIONALE

Independent Actions

Implement measures to prevent thrombus formation: **D** ✦
- Perform actions to prevent peripheral pooling of blood such as leg exercises:
  - Ankle rotation
  - Alternate dorsiflexion and plantar extension of both feet.

Leg and ankle exercises help promote venous return and reduce the risk of venous thromboembolism.

If signs and symptoms of a deep vein thrombus occur: **D** ✦
- Maintain client on bed rest until activity orders received.
- Elevate foot of bed 15° to 20° above heart level if ordered.
- Discourage positions that compromise blood flow (e.g., pillows under knees, crossing legs, sitting for long periods).

Avoid putting pressure on the posterior knees because this action will compress leg veins, increasing turbulent blood flow, and increase the risk of thromboembolism formation. If a thrombus is suspected, elevate the affected extremity and do not massage the area because of the danger of dislodging the thrombus.

Dependent/Collaborative Actions

Implement measures to prevent thrombus formation:
- Apply mechanical devices designed to increase venous return in the immobile patient: **D** ✦
  - Sequential compression devices
  - Thromboembolic (elastic) stockings
- Maintain a minimum fluid intake of 2500 mL/day (unless contraindicated). **D** ✦

These devices decrease venous stasis in the lower extremities and increase venous return through the deep leg veins, which are prone to the formation of a thromboembolism. These devices should remain in place until the patient is ambulatory.

Adequate hydration helps to reduce blood viscosity, which may contribute to the formation of a thromboembolism.

THERAPEUTIC INTERVENTIONS	RATIONALE

• Administer anticoagulants:
  • Low- or adjusted-dose heparin
  • Fondaparinux
  • Warfarin
  • Low-molecular-weight heparin **D** ✦
	Anticoagulants, if indicated, help to suppress the formation of clots.

If signs and symptoms of a deep vein thrombus occur: • Prepare client for diagnostic studies (e.g., venography, duplex ultrasound, impedance plethysmography).	*Additional studies may be indicated to confirm the presence of a thromboembolism so the appropriate interventions can be implemented.*

Collaborative Diagnosis | RISK FOR PULMONARY EMBOLISM

Definition: A clot that detaches from the vessel wall and circulates within the blood, becoming lodged in the pulmonary vasculature

CLINICAL MANIFESTATIONS

Subjective	Objective
Verbal reports of sudden chest pain or shortness of breath	Dyspnea; tachypnea; tachycardia; apprehension; low PaO_2

RISK FACTORS

- Venous stasis associated with decreased activity, positioning during and after surgery, increased blood viscosity (can result from deficient fluid volume), and abdominal distention (the distended intestine may put pressure on the abdominal vessels)
- Hypercoagulability associated with increased release of tissue thromboplastin into the blood (occurs as a result of surgical trauma) and hemoconcentration and increased blood viscosity (can occur as a result of deficient fluid volume)
- Trauma to vein walls during surgery

DESIRED OUTCOMES

The client will not experience a pulmonary embolism as evidenced by:
  a. Absence of sudden chest pain
  b. Unlabored respirations at 12 to 20 breaths/min
  c. Pulse rate 60 to 100 beats/min
  d. ABG values within normal range

NURSING ASSESSMENT	RATIONALE
Assess for and report signs and symptoms of a pulmonary embolism: • Sudden chest pain • Dyspnea • Tachypnea • Tachycardia • Apprehension • Low PaO_2	*Early recognition of signs and symptoms of a pulmonary embolism allows for prompt intervention.*
Monitor continuous pulse oximetry.	*Pulse oximetry is an indirect measure of oxygen saturation. Monitoring pulse oximetry (SaO_2) allows for early detection of hypoxia and implementation of the appropriate interventions.*
Monitor ABG values.	*Pulmonary embolism is suggested if ABG values indicate hypoxemia (PaO_2 <80 mm Hg) and hyperventilation (low $PaCO_2$).*
Monitor D-dimer laboratory results for abnormalities. Monitor results of perfusion scan and/or CT pulmonary angiography.	*Elevated levels of D-dimer in the blood in combination with computed tomography (CT) pulmonary angiography are indicative of pulmonary embolism.*

Continued...

THERAPEUTIC INTERVENTIONS	RATIONALE

Independent Actions
Implement measures to prevent a pulmonary embolism:
• Perform actions to prevent and treat a deep vein thrombus.
If signs and symptoms of a pulmonary embolism occur: **D** ✦
• Maintain client on strict bed rest in a semi- to high-Fowler's position.
• Do not exercise, check for Homans' sign in, or massage any extremity known to have a thrombus.
• Caution client to avoid activities that create a Valsalva response:
   • Straining to have bowel movement
   • Holding breath while moving up in bed
	The most common sources of pulmonary emboli are dislodged thrombi from the deep veins in the thighs.
	If a venous thromboembolism is suspected, actions should be implemented to prevent dislodgment of an existing thrombi.

Dependent/Collaborative Actions If signs and symptoms of a pulmonary embolism occur: • Maintain oxygen therapy as ordered. **D** ✦	*Supplemental oxygen is indicated to correct the hypoxemia associated with a pulmonary embolism. The concentration of oxygen administered should be guided by pulse oximetry and/ or ABG analysis.*

• Prepare client for diagnostic tests:
   • ABGs
   • D-dimer level
   • Ventilation-perfusion lung scan
   • Pulmonary angiography
• Administer anticoagulants: **D** ✦
   • Heparin
   • Warfarin
• Prepare client for surgical intervention:
   • Vena caval interruption device (vena cava filter)
   • Embolectomy
	Diagnosis of a pulmonary embolism is confirmed using a combination of tests.
	
	Anticoagulants, if indicated, help to suppress the formation of clots. The best action is to prevent the formation of thromboemboli in those at risk.
	A vena caval interruption device helps to prevent further pulmonary emboli.

Collaborative Diagnosis | # RISK FOR PARALYTIC ILEUS

Definition: Paralysis of the intestines resulting in blockage of the intestines

CLINICAL MANIFESTATIONS

Subjective	Objective
Verbal reports of persistent abdominal pain and cramping	Firm, distended abdomen; absent bowel sounds; failure to pass flatus; abdominal x-ray showing distended bowel

RISK FACTORS

• Manipulation of intestines during abdominal surgery, depressant effect of anesthesia and some medications (e.g., narcotic [opioid] analgesics, some antiemetics) on bowel motility, hypokalemia, and hypovolemia (can cause decreased blood supply to the intestine)

DESIRED OUTCOMES

The client will not develop a paralytic ileus as evidenced by:
  a. Absence or resolution of abdominal pain and cramping
  b. Soft, nondistended abdomen
  c. Gradual return of bowel sounds
  d. Passage of flatus

NURSING ASSESSMENT	RATIONALE
Assess for and report signs and symptoms of paralytic ileus: • Development of or persistent abdominal pain and cramping • Firm, distended abdomen • Absent bowel sounds • Failure to pass flatus	*Early recognition of signs and symptoms of a paralytic ileus allows for prompt intervention.*
Monitor results of abdominal x-ray.	*An abdominal x-ray that demonstrates distended bowel may be indicative of a paralytic ileus.*

THERAPEUTIC INTERVENTIONS	RATIONALE
Independent Actions Implement measures to prevent paralytic ileus: • Increase activity as soon as allowed and tolerated. **D** ● ✦	*Early ambulation in a postoperative client promotes the return of peristalsis.*
Dependent/Collaborative Actions Implement measures to prevent paralytic ileus: • Perform actions to maintain adequate tissue perfusion: • Administer gastrointestinal stimulants (e.g., metoclopramide) if ordered. **D** ✦	*Gastrointestinal stimulants help to maintain adequate blood supply to the bowel.*
• Perform actions to prevent hypokalemia. • Administer potassium supplements.	*Hypokalemia promotes atony of the intestinal wall, which results in a decrease in peristalsis.*
If signs and symptoms of paralytic ileus occur: **D** ✦ • Withhold all oral intake. • Insert nasogastric tube and maintain suction as ordered.	*Paralytic ileus results in cessation of normal peristalsis. The client should have nothing by mouth (NPO) with a nasogastric tube in place to facilitate gastric decompression until the ileus is resolved.*

Collaborative Diagnosis RISK FOR DEHISCENCE

Definition: Pulling apart of a surgical wound at the suture line

CLINICAL MANIFESTATIONS

Subjective	Objective
Verbal reports of something "popping" or "giving way" at the incision site	Separation of edges of the wound

RISK FACTORS
• Inadequate wound closure
• Stress on incision line associated with persistent coughing, distention, or vomiting
• Poor wound healing associated with decreased tissue perfusion of wound area, inadequate nutritional status, and infection

DESIRED OUTCOMES
The client will not experience dehiscence as evidenced by intact, approximated wound edges.

NURSING ASSESSMENT	RATIONALE
Assess for and report evidence of wound dehiscence: • Separation of edges of the wound	*Early recognition of evidence of wound dehiscence allows for prompt intervention.*
Assess for and immediately report signs and symptoms of evisceration: • Sudden profuse drainage of serosanguineous fluid from wound • Protrusion of intestinal contents	*Total separation of wound layers sometimes results in evisceration. This is an emergency situation that requires surgical intervention.*

NDx = NANDA-I Diagnosis   **D** = Delegatable Action   ● = UAP   ✦ = LVN/LPN   ⊖▶ = Go to ⊖volve for animation

Continued...

THERAPEUTIC INTERVENTIONS	RATIONALE

Independent Actions

Implement measures to promote wound healing.

Implement measures to reduce stress on the wound: **D** ✦

* Limit movement of affected area.
* If client has a chest or abdominal incision, instruct the client to avoid coughing.
* If an abdominal incision is present, place the client on bed rest in a semi-Fowler's position with knees slightly flexed.

Proper wound healing decreases the risk of dehiscence.

Decreased stress on the incision reduces the risk of wound dehiscence.

Dependent/Collaborative Actions

If dehiscence occurs:

* Cover wound with a sterile, nonadherent dressing.
* Apply skin closures (e.g., butterfly tape, Steri-Strips) to the incision line if appropriate.

Assist with resuturing the wound if indicated.

A wound that has dehisced requires a sterile, nonadherent dressing. The choice of a dry dressing or wet dressing will depend upon the presence of evisceration.

DISCHARGE TEACHING/CONTINUED CARE

Nursing Diagnosis **DEFICIENT KNOWLEDGE** NDx, **INEFFECTIVE FAMILY THERAPEUTIC REGIMEN MANAGEMENT** NDx, **OR INEFFECTIVE HEALTH MAINTENANCE** NDx*

Definition: Absence or deficiency of cognitive information related to specific topic (lack of specific information necessary for clients/significant others) to make informed choices regarding condition/treatment/lifestyle changes; pattern of regulating and integrating into family processes a program for treatment of illness and the sequelae of illness that is unsatisfactory for meeting specific health goals; inability to identify, manage, and/or seek out help to manage health

CLINICAL MANIFESTATIONS

Subjective	**Objective**
Verbalization of the problem	Inaccurate follow through of instructions; inappropriate behaviors

RISK FACTORS

* Cognitive deficiency
* Misinterpretation of information

* Lack of interest in learning
* Language/cultural barriers

NOC OUTCOMES	NIC INTERVENTIONS
Knowledge: treatment regimen	Teaching: individual; teaching: prescribed activity/exercise; teaching: prescribed medication; health system guidance

NURSING ASSESSMENT	RATIONALE
Assess client's ability and readiness to learn. Assess the client's understanding of teaching.	*Learning is more effective when the client is motivated and understands the importance of what is to be learned. Readiness to learn changes based on situations, physical and emotional challenges.*

*The nurse should select the diagnostic label that is most appropriate for the client's discharge teaching needs.

THERAPEUTIC INTERVENTIONS	RATIONALE

Desired Outcomes: The client will identify ways to prevent postoperative infection.

Independent Actions

• Instruct client in ways to prevent postoperative infection: • Continue with coughing (unless contraindicated) and deep breathing every 2 hours while awake. • Continue to use incentive spirometer if activity is limited.	*Coughing and deep breathing exercises as well as incentive spirometry help to reduce atelectasis, reexpand alveoli, and decrease the risk of a postoperative pulmonary infection. Deep breathing helps to clear airways by loosening secretions and promoting a more effective cough.*
• Increase activity as ordered.	*Activity helps to mobilize secretions and promotes deeper breathing.*
• Avoid contact with persons who have infections. • Avoid crowds during flu and cold seasons.	*During the healing process, while an individual's resistance to infection may be lowered, the client should avoid situations that increase the risk for infection. Protecting the client from others with infections reduces the risk of exposure to pathogens.*
• Decrease or stop smoking.	*Irritants in smoke increase mucus production and impair ciliary function, which can increase the risk for postoperative pulmonary infection.*
• Drink at least 10 glasses of liquid per day unless contraindicated.	*Proper hydration helps to thin pulmonary secretions, which facilitates mobilization and expectoration, reducing the risk of pulmonary infection. Proper hydration also helps maintain adequate blood flow and nutrient supply to healing tissues.*
• Maintain a balanced nutritional intake.	*Adequate nutrition is necessary for proper wound healing and maintenance of normal immune system function.*
• Maintain a proper balance of rest and activity.	*Rest helps the body to better use nutrients and oxygen for healing. Activity helps to reduce the risk of complications of prolonged immobility.*
• Maintain good personal hygiene (especially oral care, hand washing, and perineal care).	*Good personal hygiene helps to maintain the integrity of protective mucosal linings (oral), reduce the amount of harmful organisms (perineal, oral, hand), and reduce the risk of colonization of organisms and subsequent infection.*
• Avoid touching any wound unless it is completely healed.	*Touching the wound may increase the transmission of pathogens, increasing the risk for infection.*
• Maintain sterile or clean technique as ordered during wound care.	*The use of sterile technique reduces the risk of introduction of pathogens into the body.*

THERAPEUTIC INTERVENTIONS	RATIONALE

Desired Outcomes: The client will demonstrate the ability to perform wound care.

Independent Actions

Discuss the rationale for, frequency of, and equipment necessary for the prescribed wound care.	
Provide client with the necessary supplies (e.g., dressings, irrigating solution, tape) for wound care and with names and addresses of places where additional supplies can be obtained.	
Demonstrate wound care and proper cleansing of any reusable equipment. Allow time for questions, clarification, and return demonstration.	*Return demonstration allows for the nurse to determine the client's comprehension of the task. Any deficiencies in performance can be addressed with further instruction.*

Continued...

THERAPEUTIC INTERVENTIONS	RATIONALE

Desired Outcomes: The client will state signs and symptoms to report to the health care provider.

Independent Actions

Instruct the client to report the following signs and symptoms:

- Persistent low-grade or significantly elevated (38.3° C [101° F]) temperature
- Difficulty breathing
- Chest pain
- Cough productive of purulent, green, or rust-colored sputum
- Increasing weakness or inability to tolerate prescribed activity level
- Increasing discomfort or discomfort not controlled by prescribed medications and treatments
- Continued nausea or vomiting
- Increasing abdominal distention and/or discomfort
- Separation of wound edges
- Increasing redness, warmth, pain, or swelling around wound
- Unusual or excessive drainage from any wound site
- Pain or swelling in calf of one or both legs
- Urine retention
- Frequency, urgency, or burning on urination
- Cloudy or foul-smelling urine

Signs and symptoms are indicative of potential infection and should be reported to the appropriate health care provider in a timely manner to avoid complications.

Recognition of signs and symptoms of infection allows for prompt intervention.

THERAPEUTIC INTERVENTIONS	RATIONALE

Desired Outcomes: The client will verbalize an understanding of and a plan for adhering to recommended follow-up care including future appointments with health care provider, dietary modifications, activity level, treatments, and medications prescribed.

Independent Actions

Reinforce importance of keeping scheduled follow-up appointments with the health care provider.

Reinforce physician's instructions about dietary modifications. Obtain a dietary consult for client if needed.

Reinforce physician's instructions on suggested activity level and treatment plan.

Explain the rationale for, side effects of, and importance of taking medications prescribed. Inform client of pertinent food and drug interactions.

Implement measures to improve client compliance:

- Include significant others in teaching sessions if possible.

- Encourage questions and allow time for reinforcement and clarification of information provided.
- Provide written instructions on scheduled appointments with health care provider, dietary modifications, activity level, treatment plan, medications prescribed, and signs and symptoms to report.

A follow-up appointment with the health care provider is important to monitor continued recovery.

A proper diet helps to enhance proper wound healing. Reinforcing instructions helps the nurse to both assess the client's level of understanding and determine the need for further instruction.

Activity levels must be maintained to ensure the proper balance between rest that aids in healing and activity that prevents complications.

The client should be educated on how to take medications that are prescribed to be used as needed. It should be emphasized that the client should not increase the frequency or dosage of these medications without permission from the health care provider.

Involvement of significant others in patient teaching improves adherence to discharge instructions.

Information is presented with time for questions to allow for clarification of information.

Written instructions allow the client to refer to instructions as needed.

ADDITIONAL CARE PLANS

RISK FOR CONSTIPATION
Related to decreased gastrointestinal motility associated with manipulation of bowel during abdominal surgery, depressant effect of anesthesia and narcotic (opioid) analgesics, and decreased activity

DISTURBED SLEEP PATTERN
Related to fear, anxiety, discomfort, inability to assume usual sleeping position, and frequent assessments and treatments

RISK FOR INFECTION
Pneumonia related to stasis of pulmonary secretions and aspiration (if it occurs)

Wound infection related to contamination associated with introduction of pathogens during or after surgery; decreased resistance to infection associated with factors such as diminished tissue perfusion of wound area and inadequate nutritional status

Urinary tract infection related to increased growth and colonization of microorganisms associated with urinary stasis; introduction of pathogens associated with an indwelling catheter if present

RISK FOR FALLS
Related to weakness and fatigue; dizziness or syncope associated with postural hypotension resulting from peripheral pooling of blood and blood loss during surgery; central nervous system depressant effect of some medications (narcotic [opioid] analgesics, some antiemetics); presence of tubing or equipment

RISK FOR ASPIRATION
Related to decreased level of consciousness and absent or diminished gag reflex associated with depressant effect of anesthesia and narcotic (opioid) analgesics; supine positioning; increased risk for gastroesophageal reflux associated with increased gastric pressure resulting from decreased gastrointestinal motility

FEAR/ANXIETY
Related to unfamiliar environment; pain; lack of understanding of surgical procedure performed; diagnosis and postoperative treatment plan; possible change to body image and roles; and financial concerns

See Bibliography at the back of the book.

The Client with Alterations in Respiratory Function

ASTHMA

Asthma is a disorder characterized by intermittent and reversible obstruction of the airways. This airflow obstruction is caused by bronchial hyperresponsiveness and inflammation of the airway mucous membranes. Allergens enter the airway and initiate the inflammatory cascade. Mast cells found in the basement membranes of the bronchial walls degranulate and release inflammation response mediators, which cause increased capillary permeability and vasodilation, and recruitment of eosinophils, lymphocytes, and neutrophils. The response leads to the production of thick, tenacious mucus that blocks the airways. Combined with the bronchial hyperresponsiveness and capillary vasodilation and permeability, intake of air significantly decreases, and air is trapped in the lungs below the obstruction. Chronic inflammation leads to remodeling of the bronchial walls. The bronchial walls hypertrophy, and mucus-producing cells undergo hyperplasia.

Asthma attacks are variable and unpredictable, range from mild to severe, and differ from client to client. Clinical manifestations of an asthma attack include dyspnea, wheezing, chest tightness, tachycardia, sweating, cough, tightening of neck muscles, and use of accessory muscles to breathe. The client may also have an audible wheezing or whistling on exhalation. Indications that asthma is becoming worse include an increase in the frequency and severity of asthma attacks and an increased need to use bronchodilators.

There is no clear indication why some people get asthma and others, exposed to the same conditions, do not. It is possibly due to a combination of environmental and genetic factors. Triggers for an asthma attack also vary from client to client and may include airborne allergens and air pollutants, viral respiratory infections, cold air, stress, medications (i.e., nonsteroidal anti-inflammatory drugs [NSAIDs]), exercise, gastroesophageal reflex disease, smoke, and occupational factors.

This care plan focuses on care of the adult client with asthma who is hospitalized during an exacerbation of the illness. Much of the information is applicable to clients receiving follow-up care in an extended care facility or home setting.

OUTCOME/DISCHARGE CRITERIA

The client will:
1. Have improved respiratory function
2. Have vital signs within client's normal range
3. Tolerate expected level of activity
4. Verbalize an understanding of medications ordered including rationale, food and drug interactions, side effects, methods of administering, and importance of taking as prescribed
5. Demonstrate appropriate use of inhalers.

Nursing Diagnosis **IMPAIRED RESPIRATORY FUNCTION***

Definition: Inspiration and/or expiration that does not provide adequate ventilation; inability to clear secretions or obstructions from the respiratory tract to maintain a clear airway

Ineffective breathing pattern NDx
Related to:
- Increased rate of respirations associated with fear and anxiety, and feeling of "air hunger"
- Decreased depth of respirations associated with weakness, fatigue, fear, anxiety

---

*This diagnostic label includes the following nursing diagnoses: ineffective breathing pattern, ineffective airway clearance, and impaired gas exchange.

Ineffective airway clearance NDx
Related to:
- Narrowing of the airways associated with:
  - Excessive mucus production, inflammation, and bronchospasm
  - Bronchial wall remodeling with bronchial hypertrophy and hyperplasia of mucus-secreting cells
- Stasis of secretions associated with:
  - Difficulty coughing up secretions resulting from fatigue, weakness, and presence of tenacious secretions if fluid intake is inadequate
  - Impaired ciliary function resulting from loss of ciliated epithelium (occurs with inflammation, destruction, and fibrosis of bronchial walls)

Impaired Gas Exchange NDx
Related to:
- Narrowing or obstruction of the small airways

CLINICAL MANIFESTATIONS

Subjective	Objective
Reports of restlessness; irritability; somnolence; chronic cough; chest tightness	Rapid shallow respirations; abnormal breath sounds—wheezing; cough; use of accessory muscles when breathing; significant decrease in oximetry results; abnormal arterial blood gas values; reduced activity tolerance

RISK FACTORS
- Genetics
- Smoking
- Allergies
- Environmental factors

DESIRED OUTCOMES

The client will maintain adequate respiratory function as evidenced by:
  a. Usual rate and depth of respiration
  b. Decreased dyspnea
  c. Usual or improved breath sounds
  d. Usual mental status
  e. Oximetry results within normal range for client
  f. Arterial blood gas values within normal range for client

NOC OUTCOMES

Respiratory status; airway patency; respiratory status: ventilation; respiratory status: gas exchange

NIC INTERVENTIONS

Respiratory monitoring; airway management; chest physiotherapy; cough enhancement; oxygen therapy; medication administration; ventilation assistance; cough enhancement; fear and anxiety reduction

NURSING ASSESSMENT	RATIONALE
Assess for signs and symptoms of impaired respiratory function:	*Early recognition of signs and symptoms of ineffective breathing patterns allows for prompt intervention.*
• Rapid, shallow respirations	*Rapid, shallow respirations do not provide adequate ventilatory*
• Dyspnea, orthopnea	*support. Difficulty with breathing and the need to sit up to*
• Use of accessory muscles when breathing	*breathe, as well as use of accessory muscles, lead to client fatigue and further decline in respiratory status.*
• Abnormal breath sounds (e.g., wheezes, crackles)	*Changes in the characteristics of breath sounds may be due to airway obstruction, mucus plugs, or retained secretions in larger airways. Wheezing is associated with bronchospasms.*
• Cough effectiveness	*Muscle fatigue/weakness may impair effective clearance of secretions.*
• Restlessness, irritability	• *Restlessness, irritability, and change in mental status or level*
• Confusion, somnolence	*of consciousness indicate an oxygen deficiency and require immediate treatment.*
• Central cyanosis (a late sign)	• *The bluish discoloration of the skin and mucous membranes occur in the presence of deoxygenated hemoglobin. This occurs when arterial oxygen saturation falls below 85% to 90%.*

NDx = NANDA-I Diagnosis   **D** = Delegatable Action   ● = UAP   ✦ = LVN/LPN   ⊖▶ = Go to ⊖volve for animation

Continued...

NURSING ASSESSMENT	RATIONALE
Assess arterial blood gas and pulse oximetry values and report abnormal findings.	• *Oximetry is a non-invasive method of measuring arterial oxygen saturation. The results assist in evaluating respiratory status. Decreasing PaO_2 and increasing CO_2 are indicators or respiratory problems.* • *Allows for evaluation of client's current oxygenation status, so that appropriate supplemental oxygen therapy can be implemented.*

THERAPEUTIC INTERVENTIONS	RATIONALE

Independent Actions

Implement measures to improve respiratory status. Place client in a semi-Fowler's position. **D ● ✦**	*Positioning in semi-Fowler's position promotes optimal gas exchange by enabling chest expansion and diaphragm excursion.*
Instruct client in breathing exercises focusing on hypoventilation, breath holding after exhalation, and breathing through the nose.	*These techniques help clients decrease the need for beta$_2$-agonists and inhaled corticosteroids.*
Instruct client in exercises involving shoulder rotations and arm lifts performed in sync with breathing.	*This technique helps to expand the lungs.*
Discourage smoking.	*The irritants in smoke increase mucus production, impair ciliary function, and can cause inflammation and damage to the bronchial and alveolar walls; the carbon monoxide decreases oxygen availability.*
Maintain activity restrictions and increase activity as allowed and tolerated.	*Conservation of energy through activity restrictions allows energy to be focused on breathing. Increasing activity as tolerated helps to mobilize secretions and promotes deeper breathing.*
Perform actions to reduce fear and anxiety (e.g., assure client that staff members are nearby; respond to call signal as soon as possible; provide calm, restful environment; instruct in relaxation techniques). **D ● ✦**	*The experience of anxiety during an asthma attack can exacerbate the attack.*
Maintain client fluid intake of at least 2500 mL/day unless contraindicated. **D ✦**	*Maintaining adequate hydration decreases the viscosity of secretions and improves ciliary action in removing secretions.*

Dependent/Collaborative Actions

Implement measures to improve respiratory status. Administer beta-$_2$ adrenergic agonists inhaled during an acute attack and oral for ongoing therapy. **D ✦**	*Beta-$_2$ agonists are the treatment of choice for an asthma attack because they relax airway smooth muscles and decrease bronchoconstriction.*
Administer and monitor oxygen as ordered.	*Provides support for the respiratory system until it is able to function appropriately.*
Administer Heliox (a helium/oxygen mixture).	*The combination of helium and oxygen is lighter than air and easier to breathe when gas flow is compromised by bronchospasms.*
Administer corticosteroids both inhaled and oral.	*Corticosteroids decrease airway inflammation and thereby improve bronchial airflow.*
Consult appropriate health care providers (respiratory therapist and physician) if signs and symptoms of impaired respiratory function persist or worsen.	*Notifying the appropriate health care professionals allows for a multifaceted approach to treatment.*

Nursing Diagnosis ACTIVITY INTOLERANCE NDx

Definition: Insufficient physiological or psychological energy to endure or complete required or desired daily activities

Related to:

• Tissue hypoxia associated with impaired gas exchange
• Inadequate nutrition status
• Difficulty resting and sleeping associated with dyspnea, excessive coughing, fear, anxiety, frequent assessment and treatments, and side effects of medication therapy (e.g., some bronchodilators, corticosteroids)
• Increased energy expenditure associated with strenuous breathing efforts and persistent coughing

CLINICAL MANIFESTATIONS

Subjective	Objective
Verbal report of fatigue or weakness	Abnormal heart rate or blood pressure (B/P) response to activity; exertional discomfort or dyspnea; electrocardiographic changes reflecting dysrhythmias or ischemia; unable to speak with physical activity

RISK FACTORS

- Smoking
- Malnutrition
- Allergens
- Insomnia

DESIRED OUTCOMES

The client will demonstrate an increased tolerance for activity as evidenced by:
  a. Verbalization of feeling less fatigued and weak
  b. Ability to perform ADL without exertional dyspnea, chest pain, diaphoresis, dizziness, and significant changes in vital signs

NOC OUTCOMES

Activity tolerance; endurance, fatigue level; vital signs; asthma: self-management

NIC INTERVENTIONS

Activity therapy; energy management; oxygen therapy; nutrition management; sleep enhancement; cardiac care; cardiac rehabilitation; teaching regarding prescribed activity

NURSING ASSESSMENT	RATIONALE
Assess for signs and symptoms of activity intolerance: • Statements of fatigue or weakness • Exertional dyspnea, chest pain, diaphoresis, or dizziness • Abnormal heart rate response to activity (e.g., increase in rate of 20 beats/min above resting rate, rate not returning to preactivity level within 3 minutes after stopping activity, change from regular to irregular rate) • Significant change (15-20 mm Hg) in B/P with activity	*Early recognition of signs and symptoms of activity intolerance allows for prompt intervention.*

THERAPEUTIC INTERVENTIONS	RATIONALE
Independent Actions Implement measures to promote rest and/or conserve energy (e.g., maintain prescribed activity restrictions, minimize environmental activity and noise, provide uninterrupted rest periods, assist with care, keep supplies and personal articles within easy reach, limit the number of visitors, use shower chair when showering, sit to brush teeth or comb hair). **D** ● ✦	*Cells use oxygen and fat, protein, and carbohydrates to produce the energy needed for all body activities. Rest and activities that conserve energy result in a lower metabolic rate, which preserves nutrients and oxygen for necessary activities.*
Implement measures to promote sleep (e.g., elevate head of bed and support arms on pillows to facilitate breathing, maintain oxygen therapy during sleep, discourage intake of fluids high in caffeine in the evening, reduce environmental stimuli). **D** ✦	*Sleep replenishes a client's energy and feelings of well-being.*
Implement measures to decrease excessive coughing and frequency of asthma attacks (e.g., protect client from exposure to irritants such as smoke, flowers, and powder; avoid extremely hot or cold foods/fluids). **D** ● ✦	*Altered respiratory function such as excessive coughing can lead to inadequate tissue oxygenation, which results in less efficient energy production and a reduced ability to tolerate activity. Improving respiratory status increases the amount of oxygen available for energy production.*
Discourage smoking and excessive intake of beverages high in caffeine such as coffee, tea, and colas.	*Excessive intake of nicotine and caffeine can increase cardiac workload and myocardial oxygen utilization, thereby decreasing oxygen availability.*

NDx = NANDA-I Diagnosis   **D** = Delegatable Action   ● = UAP   ✦ = LVN/LPN   ℮▶ = Go to ℮volve for animation

Continued...

THERAPEUTIC INTERVENTIONS	RATIONALE
Perform actions to improve respiratory status (e.g., place client in semi- to high-Fowler's position; instruct client to deep breathe or use incentive spirometry every 1 to 2 hours; maintain bed rest as ordered; and use oxygen as needed). **D** ✦	*Improvement of respiratory status is done to relieve dyspnea, decrease frequency of asthma attacks, and improve tissue oxygenation.*
Perform actions to maintain adequate nutritional status (e.g., increase activity as tolerated potentially improving appetite; encourage a rest period before meals to reduce fatigue; assist with oral hygiene before meals; maintain a clean environment and a relaxed, pleasant atmosphere). **D** ● ✦	*Adequate nutritional status is important in order to maintain ADL.*
Instruct a client to: • Report a change in the frequency and consistency of asthma attacks. • Report a decreased tolerance for activity. • Stop any activity that causes increased chest pain, increased shortness of breath, dizziness, or extreme fatigue or weakness.	*Changes in a client's activity tolerance should be reported immediately. Assessment of the change will allow for timely diagnosis of the cause and subsequent treatment.*
Dependent/Collaborative Actions	
Consult appropriate health care providers (e.g., respiratory therapist, physician, dietitian) if signs and symptoms of activity intolerance persist or worsen.	*Notifying the appropriate health care provider allows for modification of the treatment plan.*

DISCHARGE TEACHING/CONTINUED CARE

Nursing Diagnosis | # DEFICIENT KNOWLEDGE ɴᴅx; INEFFECTIVE HEALTH MAINTENANCE ɴᴅx; OR INEFFECTIVE SELF-HEALTH MANAGEMENT* ɴᴅx

Definition: Absence or deficiency of cognitive information related to specific topic (lack of specific information necessary for clients/significant others) to make informed choices regarding condition/treatment/lifestyle changes; inability to identify, manage, and/or seek out help to manage health pattern of regulating and integrating into daily living a therapeutic regimen for treatment of illness and the sequelae of illness that is unsatisfactory for meeting specific health goals

CLINICAL MANIFESTATIONS

Subjective	Objective
Verbalizes inability to manage illness; verbalizes inability to follow prescribed regimen	Increased frequency and intensity of asthma attacks

RISK FACTORS

• Cognitive deficit • Financial concerns • Smoking	• Inability to care for oneself • Difficulty in modifying personal habits and integrating treatments into lifestyle

NURSING ASSESSMENT	RATIONALE
Assess client readiness and ability to learn Assess meaning of illness to client	*Early recognition of client's readiness to learn and meaning of their illness allows for implementation of the appropriate teaching interventions.*

---

*The nurse should select the diagnostic label that is most appropriate for the client's discharge teaching.

NOC OUTCOMES

Knowledge: treatment regimen; knowledge: energy conservation; knowledge: treatment procedure(s); knowledge: health resources; knowledge: illness care; compliance behavior; health beliefs; perceived ability to perform: knowledge of treatment regimen

NIC INTERVENTIONS

Health system guidance; teaching: individual; teaching: disease process; teaching: prescribed activity/exercise; teaching: prescribed medication; self-modification assistance; values clarification; discharge planning; medication management; smoking cessation assistance

THERAPEUTIC INTERVENTIONS	RATIONALE

Desired Outcome: The client will identify ways to prevent or minimize respiratory problems.

Independent Actions
Instruct client in ways to maintain respiratory health:

- Maintain overall general good health (e.g., reduce stress, eat a well-balanced diet, obtain adequate rest).

- Stop smoking.

- Avoid exposure to respiratory irritants such as smoke, dust, aerosol sprays, paint fumes, and solvents; wear a mask or scarf over nose and mouth if exposure to high levels of these irritants is unavoidable.

- Remain indoors as much as possible when air pollution levels are high.
- Avoid extremes in hot and cold weather.

- Avoid prolonged close contact with persons who have respiratory infection.
- Receive immunizations against influenza and pneumococcal pneumonia.

Have client keep a log/diary of the frequency, duration, and intensity of asthma attacks, and morning peak flow rates.

Include significant others in explanations and teaching sessions and encourage their support.

Good general health supports the individual's ability to fight off infection.
The irritants in smoke and respiratory irritants increase mucus production, impair ciliary function, and can cause inflammation and damage to the bronchial and alveolar walls.

Air pollution in high levels is harmful to persons with existing lung disease.
Exposure to extreme hot and cold air may cause bronchoconstriction, allowing less air into and out of the lungs.
Increases a client's potential for a respiratory infection

Immunizations help to prevent further respiratory disease.

Changes in the incidence of asthma attacks should be reported to the client's health care provider because they may indicate a change in the disease process, effectiveness of medications, and/ or a concurrent illness.
Involvement of the client's significant others contribute to adherence to the treatment regimen.

THERAPEUTIC INTERVENTIONS	RATIONALE

Desired Outcome: The client will verbalize ways to maintain adherence to the medication regimen including rationale, food and drug interactions, side effects, methods of administration, and the importance of taking medications as prescribed.

Independent Actions
Educate the patient about the disease process and treatment of asthma:

- Explain asthma in terms the client can understand; stress that adherence to the treatment plan is necessary in order to prevent complications and reactivation of the disease.
- Explain that asthma can be treated, but only if the client adheres to the prescribed medication regimen.
- Provide written instructions about and encourage client to participate in the treatment plan.
- Provide client with written instructions about disease process, signs and symptoms to report, medication therapy, and follow-up appointments.

Understanding of the disease and its treatment plan provides patients with a sense of control, and they will be more likely to comply with the treatment regimen.

Written instructions allow the client to refer to them as needed. The instructions should include all information needed to understand disease processes and treatment.

Continued...

THERAPEUTIC INTERVENTIONS	RATIONALE
Explain the rationale for side effects of drugs, food and drug interactions, the importance of taking medications as prescribed, and drugs to manage side effects.	*Knowledge of medications and how they impact the system improves client adherence and helps enhance the client's understanding of the importance of adhering to the prescribed medication regimen. The client must be able to recognize alterations in functioning related to medication administration.*
Examples of asthma medications: • Corticosteroids • Mast cell stabilizers • Anticholinergics • IgE antagonists • Leukotriene modifiers • Beta$_2$-Adrenergic agonists • Methylxanthines	*Corticosteroids suppress inflammation and the normal immune process. Mast cell stabilizers decrease the frequency and intensity of allergic reactions. Anticholinergics provide adjunctive management of bronchospasms caused by asthma. IgE antagonists prevent the release of mediators of the allergic response. Leukotriene modifiers decrease the inflammatory process. Methylxanthines promote bronchodilation through relaxing the airways.*
Assist client to develop a method to promote adherence to the medication schedule. • Assist client to identify ways the medication regimen can be incorporated into the client's lifestyle.	*Knowledge of the medication regimen and the impact of these medications on the body, as well as how the medication regimen can be incorporated into the client's lifestyle, allows the client some mechanism of control of his/her disease and the ability to have an active part in treatment and care.*
Instruct client to take all medications as often as prescribed and avoid skipping doses or altering the prescribed dose; if a dose is missed, instruct client to take it as soon as remembered unless it is almost time for the next dose of the same medication.	*Consistent use of medication(s) is important in preventing asthma attacks.*
Teach the client how to use the different types of inhalers.	*Medication is not delivered to the lungs and remains in the oral pharynx when inhalers are used incorrectly, leading to infections in the oral pharynx.*
Reinforce the need to consult physician before discontinuing any medication or taking additional prescription and nonprescription medications.	*This is important to prevent exacerbations in asthma attacks.*
Provide information about and encourage utilization of community resources and social services that can assist client to comply with the medication regimen or to provide financial support if needed (e.g., local Department of Health and Human Services, local chapter of the American Lung Association, support groups).	*Provides for continuum of care and can help improve client adherence with the medication regimen and possibly financial assistance for medications.*

THERAPEUTIC INTERVENTIONS	RATIONALE
Desired Outcome: The client will state signs and symptoms to report to the health care provider.	
Independent Actions Instruct client to report the following to the health care provider: • Persistent or recurrent loss of appetite, nausea, weakness, fatigue, or weight loss • Fever, chills, continued or increased night sweats • Difficulty breathing, continued or increased cough, or chest pain • Unusual color, amount, and odor of vaginal secretions; white patches or ulcerated areas in mouth; stiff neck and headache; hoarseness; persistent sore throat; bone pain; swollen, red, painful joints; swollen lymph nodes • Signs and symptoms of adverse effects of medications	*These clinical manifestations indicate an infection or super infection and should be reported to the health care provider.*

THERAPEUTIC INTERVENTIONS	RATIONALE

Desired Outcome: The client will verbalize an understanding of a plan for adhering to recommended follow-up care including future appointments with health care provider and graded exercise program.

Independent Actions

Reinforce the importance of keeping appointments for follow-up tests (e.g., blood work, chest radiographs) and physical examinations to determine effectiveness of the medication regimen and assess for side effects.

Regular health care appointments are important to determine effectiveness of the medication regimen and assess for side effects.

ADDITIONAL NURSING DIAGNOSES

DISTURBED SLEEP PATTERN* NDx

Related to fear, anxiety, unfamiliar environment, excessive coughing, frequent assessments and treatments, side effects of medications (e.g., some bronchodilators, corticosteroids), and inability to assume usual sleep position associated with orthopnea

to meet self-care needs; and alterations in roles, lifestyle, and future plans

FEAR NDx AND ANXIETY NDx

Related to fear associated with difficulty breathing, fear of death during an asthma attack, potential changes in lifestyle

RISK FOR POWERLESSNESS NDx

Related to physical limitations; disease progression despite efforts to comply with treatment plan; dependence on others

CHRONIC OBSTRUCTIVE PULMONARY DISEASE

Chronic obstructive pulmonary disease (COPD) is a term used to describe a disease state characterized by the presence of airflow obstruction in the lungs. The airflow obstruction is chronic, usually progressive, and may be accompanied by airway hyperactivity. Other terms sometimes used to describe this condition are chronic obstructive lung disease (COLD) and chronic airflow limitation (CAL). Signs and symptoms usually include dyspnea, cough, and sputum production that worsen over time and during periodic exacerbations.

The two conditions that comprise COPD are chronic bronchitis and emphysema. Chronic bronchitis is characterized by a cough that persists at least 3 months of the year for 2 consecutive years and an excessive production of mucus in the bronchi due to inflammation of the bronchioles and hypertrophy and hyperplasia of the mucous glands. In contrast, emphysema is characterized by dyspnea and a mild cough. The impaired airflow that occurs with emphysema is related to loss of lung elasticity, narrowing of the terminal nonrespiratory bronchioles, and destructive changes in the walls of the alveolar and/or respiratory bronchioles. Both chronic bronchitis and emphysema are usually present in the person with COPD, although one of the two usually predominates.

Causative factors of COPD include chronic irritation of the lungs by cigarette smoke, exposure to air pollution and chemical irritants, and recurrent respiratory tract infections. In a small percentage of cases of emphysema, the destruction of lung tissue by proteolytic enzymes is a result of a genetic deficiency of alpha$_1$-antitrypsin.

This care plan focuses on care of the adult client with COPD who is hospitalized during an acute exacerbation. Much of the information is applicable to clients receiving follow-up care in an extended care facility or home setting.

OUTCOME/DISCHARGE CRITERIA

The client will:
1. Have improved respiratory function
2. Tolerate expected level of activity
3. Have no signs and symptoms of complications
4. Identify ways to prevent or minimize further respiratory problems
5. Verbalize ways to maintain an optimal nutritional status
6. Identify ways to conserve energy and/or reduce dyspnea and fatigue
7. Demonstrate proper chest physiotherapy and use of respiratory equipment
8. Verbalize an understanding of medications ordered including rationale, food and drug interactions, side effects, methods of administering, and importance of taking as prescribed
9. Identify precautions that should be adhered to when using oxygen
10. State signs and symptoms to report to the health care provider
11. Share feelings and thoughts about the effects of COPD on lifestyle and roles
12. Identify resources that can assist with financial needs, home management, and adjustment to changes resulting from COPD
13. Verbalize an understanding of and a plan for adhering to recommended follow-up care including future appointments with health care provider and graded exercise program.

NDx = NANDA-I Diagnosis   **D** = Delegatable Action   ● = UAP   ✦ = LVN/LPN   ⊜▶ = Go to ⊜volve for animation

Nursing Diagnosis IMPAIRED RESPIRATORY FUNCTION*

Definition: Inability of an individual to maintain adequate ventilation of the respiratory tract and perfusion of oxygen (O_2) and carbon dioxide (CO_2) between the lungs and vascular system to maintain adequate tissue oxygenation

Related to:

Ineffective breathing pattern NDx
Related to:
- Increased rate of respirations associated with fear and anxiety
- Decreased depth of respirations associated with weakness, fatigue, fear, anxiety, and presence of a flattened diaphragm (a result of prolonged hyperinflation of the lungs)

Ineffective airway clearance NDx
Related to:
- Narrowing of the airways associated with:
  - Excessive mucus production and inflammation and hyperplasia of the bronchial walls (especially with chronic bronchitis)
  - Destruction of the elastic fibers in the walls of the small airways (with emphysema)
- Stasis of secretions associated with:
  - Difficulty coughing up secretions resulting from fatigue, weakness, and presence of tenacious secretions if fluid intake is inadequate
  - Impaired ciliary function resulting from loss of ciliated epithelium (occurs with inflammation, destruction, and fibrosis of bronchial walls)
  - Decreased mobility

Impaired gas exchange NDx
Related to:
- Narrowing or obstruction of the small airways
- A decrease in effective lung surface (occurs as a result of collapse or destruction of alveolar walls)

CLINICAL MANIFESTATIONS

Subjective	Objective
Reports of confusion; disorientation; restlessness; irritability; somnolence; chest tightness	Rapid, shallow respirations; abnormal breath sounds; chronic cough; use of accessory muscles when breathing; increased anterior-posterior diameter; dyspnea; nasal flaring; central cyanosis (late sign); decreased expiratory and inspiratory pressure; decreased minute ventilation and vital capacity; significant decrease in oximetry results; abnormal arterial blood gas values; reduced activity tolerance

RISK FACTORS
- Smoking
- Obstruction of airways
- Excessive mucous production
- Impaired ciliary function
- Occupational dust and chemicals
- Alpha$_1$-Antitrypsin deficiency

DESIRED OUTCOMES

The client will maintain adequate respiratory function as evidenced by:
  a. Usual rate and depth of respiration
  b. Decreased dyspnea
  c. Usual or improved breath sounds
  d. Usual mental status
  e. Oximetry results within normal range for client
  f. Arterial blood gas values within normal range for client

NOC OUTCOMES

Respiratory status; airway patency; respiratory status: ventilation; respiratory status: gas exchange

NIC INTERVENTIONS

Respiratory monitoring; airway management; chest physiotherapy; cough enhancement; oxygen therapy; medication administration; ventilation assistance; cough enhancement; fear and anxiety reduction

---

*This diagnostic label includes the following nursing diagnoses: ineffective breathing pattern, ineffective airway clearance, and impaired gas exchange.

NURSING ASSESSMENT	RATIONALE
Assess for signs and symptoms of impaired respiratory function:	*Early recognition of signs and symptoms of ineffective breathing patterns allows for prompt intervention.*
• Rapid, shallow respirations	*Rapid, shallow respirations do not provide adequate ventilatory*
• Dyspnea, orthopnea	*support. Difficulty with breathing and the need to sit up to*
• Use of accessory muscles when breathing	*breathe, as well as use of accessory muscles, lead to client fatigue and further decline in respiratory status.*
• Abnormal breath sounds (e.g., diminished or absent, rhonchi, wheezes)	*Changes in the characteristics of breath sounds may be due to airway obstruction, mucus plugs, or retained secretions in larger airways.*
• Cough effectiveness	*Muscle fatigue/weakness may impair effective clearance of secretions.*
• Restlessness, irritability	*Restlessness, irritability, and change in mental status of level*
• Confusion, somnolence	*of consciousness indicate an oxygen deficiency and require immediate treatment.*
• Central cyanosis (a late sign)	*The bluish discoloration of the skin and mucous membranes occurs in the presence deoxygenated hemoglobin. This occurs when arterial oxygen saturation falls below 85% to 90%.*
Assess arterial blood gas and pulse oximetry values and report abnormal findings.	*Oximetry is a noninvasive method of measuring arterial oxygen saturation. The results assist in evaluating respiratory status. Decreasing PaO_2 and increasing CO_2 are indicators of respiratory problems.*

THERAPEUTIC INTERVENTIONS	RATIONALE

Independent Actions

Implement measures to improve respiratory status:	
• Reduce fear and anxiety.	*Prevent shallow and/or rapid breathing that can occur with fear*
• Maintain supportive environment.	*and anxiety.*
• Don't leave client during periods of acute respiratory distress.	*The client's anxiety may increase if left alone during periods of respiratory distress.*
• Open curtains and doors.	*Decreases client's feelings of being in an enclosed area, which can increase anxiety.*
• Place client in a semi-Fowler's position, and position overbed table so client can lean on it if desired. **D** ● ✦	*Positioning in semi-Fowler's position promotes optimal gas exchange by enabling chest expansion. Leaning on the overbed table decreases dyspnea through pressure on the gastric contents and diaphragmatic contraction.*
• Instruct client in and assist with diaphragmatic and pursed-lip breathing techniques.	*These techniques help clients slow their pace of breathing, which makes each breath more effective.*
Instruct client to deep breathe or use incentive spirometer every 1 to 2 hours. **D** ✦	*Forced deep breathing and use of incentive spirometry will increase expansion of the lungs and improve the client's ability to clear mucus from the lungs. The technique may also improve the amount of oxygen that is able to penetrate deep into the lungs.*
• Maintain client's fluid intake of at least 2500 mL/day unless contraindicated. **D** ✦	*Increased fluid intake promotes thinning of secretions and reduces dryness of the respiratory mucous membranes.*
• Perform suctioning if needed. **D** ✦	*Suctioning removes secretions from the large airways. It also stimulates coughing, which helps clear airways of mucus and foreign matter.*
• Instruct client to avoid intake of large meals, gas-forming foods (i.e., cauliflower, beans, cabbage, onions, etc.), and carbonated beverages.	*Gas-forming foods and carbonated beverages can cause abdominal bloating, which places pressure on the diaphragm and reduces lung expansion.*
• Discourage smoking.	*The irritants in smoke increase mucus production, impair ciliary function, and can cause inflammation and damage to the bronchial and alveolar walls; the carbon monoxide decreases oxygen availability.*
• Maintain activity restrictions and increase activity as allowed and tolerated. **D** ● ✦	*Conservation of energy through activity restrictions allows energy to be focused on breathing. Increasing activity as tolerated helps to mobilize secretions and promotes deeper breathing.*

NDx = NANDA-I Diagnosis   **D** = Delegatable Action   ● = UAP   ✦ = LVN/LPN   ⊖▶ = Go to ⊖volve for animation

Continued...

THERAPEUTIC INTERVENTIONS	RATIONALE

Dependent/Collaborative Actions

Implement measures to improve respiratory status:

- Assist with administration of mucolytics and diluent or hydrating agents via nebulizer if ordered. **D** ✦

- Avoid use of central nervous system (CNS) depressants. **D** ✦

- Administer and monitor oxygen as ordered. **D** ✦

- Administer the following medications if ordered:
- Bronchodilators
- Corticosteroids
- Antimicrobials
- *Alpha₁*-Proteinase inhibitor

Mucolytics and diluent or hydrating agents help to liquefy secretions for more effective removal.

CNS depressants further depress respiratory status, exacerbating the client's condition.

Oxygen should be administered at low doses. Question orders for high concentration, since many persons with COPD are depending on hypoxemia as a stimulus to breathe.

Bronchodilators relax smooth muscles of the airway, thus improving air exchange in the lungs. Corticosteroids decrease airway inflammation and thereby improve bronchial airflow. Antimicrobials may be given to prevent or treat pneumonia. Administration of alpha₁-proteinase inhibitor may be required if the cause of emphysema is a genetic deficiency of alpha₁-antitrypsin.

Consult appropriate health care providers (respiratory therapist and physician) if signs and symptoms of impaired respiratory function persist or worsen.

Notifying the appropriate health care professionals allows for a multidisciplinary approach to treatment.

Nursing Diagnosis   IMBALANCED NUTRITION: LESS THAN BODY REQUIREMENTS NDx

Definition: Inability of the individual to maintain adequate nutrition due to increased expenditure of energy to support the work of breathing

Related to:
- Decreased oral intake associated with:
  - Dyspnea, weakness, and fatigue
  - Nausea (can occur in response to noxious stimuli such as the sight of expectorated sputum and as a side effect of some medications)
  - Early satiety resulting from compression of the stomach by flattened diaphragm
- Increased metabolic needs associated with increased energy expenditure resulting from strenuous breathing efforts and persistent coughing

CLINICAL MANIFESTATIONS

Subjective	Objective
Report of painful oral mucous membrane	Weight loss; weight less than normal for client's age, height, and body frame; abnormal blood urea nitrogen (BUN) and low serum prealbumin levels; inflamed mucous membranes; pale conjunctiva; excessive hair loss; poor muscle tone

RISK FACTORS

- Lack of appetite
- Shortness of breath causing difficulty with eating
- Poor diet
- Lack of resources

DESIRED OUTCOMES

The client will maintain adequate nutrition status as evidenced by:
  a. Weight within normal range for client
  b. Normal BUN and serum prealbumin and albumin levels
  c. Usual strength and activity tolerance
  d. Healthy oral mucous membrane

NOC OUTCOMES	NIC INTERVENTIONS
Nutritional status	Nutritional monitoring; nutrition management; nutrition therapy; nausea management

NURSING ASSESSMENT	RATIONALE
Assess for and report signs and symptoms of malnutrition:	*Early recognition of signs and symptoms of malnutrition allows for prompt intervention.*
Weight significantly below a client's usual weight or less than normal for client's age, height, and body frame	*Inadequate nutritional intake may be exhibited by significant weight loss or a weight that is less than normal for a client's age, height, and body frame. If a significant amount of weight loss occurs in a short period of time, this may be an indication of another disease process occurring.*

- Abnormal BUN and low serum prealbumin and albumin levels
- Increased weakness and fatigue
- Sore, inflamed oral mucous membranes
- Pale conjunctiva

THERAPEUTIC INTERVENTIONS	RATIONALE

Independent Actions

Monitor percentage of meals and snacks client consumes. Report a pattern of inadequate intake. **D** ✦

Monitoring a client's intake helps to identify when a patient is at risk for inadequate nutrition.

Implement measures to maintain an adequate nutritional status:
- Perform actions to improve oral intake:
  - Implement measures to improve respiratory status.

    Interventions that relieve dyspnea allow the patient to eat a meal without interruption or need to rest.

  - Schedule treatments that assist in mobilizing mucus (e.g., aerosol treatments, postural drainage therapy) at least 1 hour before or after meals.

    Appropriate scheduling of treatments assists in decreasing nausea.

  - Increase activity as allowed and tolerated. **D** ✦

    Activity usually promotes a sense of well-being and can help improve an individual's appetite.

  - Encourage a rest period before meals. **D** ● ✦

    Rest before a meal helps to minimize fatigue during a meal.

  - Eliminate noxious sights and odors from the environment; provide client with an opaque, covered container for expectorated sputum. **D** ● ✦

    Noxious sites and odors can inhibit the feeding center in the hypothalamus. By eliminating them, the client's intake may improve.

  - Maintain a clean environment and a relaxed, pleasant atmosphere. **D** ● ✦
  - Provide oral hygiene before meals. **D** ● ✦

    Oral hygiene moistens the mouth, which makes it easier to chew and swallow; it also removes unpleasant tastes, which often improves the taste of foods and fluids.

  - Assist the client who is dyspneic in selecting foods that require little or no chewing.

    Because a person cannot swallow and breathe at the same time, relief of dyspnea increases the likelihood of maintaining a good oral intake. Foods that require little or no chewing are easier to eat and help to maintain a client's nutritional status.

  - Serve frequent, small meals rather than large ones if client is weak, fatigues easily, or has a poor appetite. **D** ✦

    Providing small rather than large meals can enable a client who is weak or fatigues easily to finish a meal. Also, a client who has a poor appetite is often more willing to attempt to eat smaller meals because they seem less overwhelming than larger ones. If smaller meals are served, the number of meals per day should be increased to help ensure adequate nutrition.

  - Place client in a high-Fowler's position for meals. **D** ● ✦

    Because a person cannot swallow and breathe at the same time, relief of dyspnea increases the likelihood of maintaining a good oral intake.

  - Allow adequate time for meals; reheat foods/fluids if necessary. **D** ● ✦

    Clients who feel rushed during meals tend to become anxious, lose their appetite, and stop eating. Appetite is also suppressed if foods/fluids normally served hot or warm become cold and do not appeal to the client.

NDx = NANDA-I Diagnosis   **D** = Delegatable Action   ● = UAP   ✦ = LVN/LPN   ⊖▶ = Go to ⊖volve for animation

Continued...

THERAPEUTIC INTERVENTIONS	RATIONALE
• Limit fluid intake with meals (unless the fluid has high nutritional value). **D** ✦	*When the stomach becomes distended, its volume receptors stimulate the satiety center in the hypothalamus and clients reduce their oral intake. Drinking liquids with meals distends the stomach and may cause satiety before an adequate amount of food is consumed.*
• Ensure that meals are well balanced and high in essential nutrients; offer dietary supplements if indicated.	*Clients must consume a diet that is well balanced and high in essential nutrients in order to meet their nutritional needs. Dietary supplements are often needed to help accomplish this.*

Dependent/Collaborative Actions

Implement measures to maintain an adequate nutritional status:

• Perform actions to improve oral intake:	
• Provide supplemental oxygen during meals. **D** ✦	*Supplemental oxygen therapy relieves dyspnea and the client's anxiety about and preoccupation with breathing efforts and increases the ability to focus on eating and drinking.*
• Obtain a dietary consult to assist the client in selecting foods/fluids that meet nutritional needs, are appealing, and adhere to personal and cultural preferences.	*Notifying the appropriate health care professionals allows for a multidisciplinary approach to treatment.*
• Administer vitamins and minerals if ordered. **D** ✦	*Administration of vitamins and minerals help to maintain nutritional status.*
Perform a calorie count if ordered. Report information to dietitian and physician.	*A calorie count provides information about the caloric and nutritional value of the foods/fluids the client consumes. The information obtained helps the dietitian and physician determine whether an alternative method of nutritional support is needed.*
Consult physician about an alternative method of providing nutrition (e.g., parenteral nutrition, tube feedings) if client does not consume enough food or fluids to meet nutritional needs.	*If the client's oral intake is inadequate, an alternative method of providing nutrients needs to be implemented.*

Nursing Diagnosis ACTIVITY INTOLERANCE NDx

Definition: Insufficient physiological or psychological energy to endure or complete required or desired daily activities

Related to:
• Tissue hypoxia associated with impaired gas exchange
• Inadequate nutrition status
• Difficulty resting and sleeping associated with dyspnea, excessive coughing, fear, anxiety, frequent assessment and treatments, and side effects of medication therapy (e.g., some bronchodilators, corticosteroids)
• Increased energy expenditure associated with strenuous breathing efforts and persistent coughing

CLINICAL MANIFESTATIONS

Subjective	Objective
Verbal report of fatigue or weakness	Abnormal heart rate or B/P response to activity; exertional discomfort or dyspnea; electrocardiographic changes reflecting dysrhythmias or ischemia; unable to speak with physical activity

RISK FACTORS
• Exertional dyspnea
• Dyspnea during rest and sleep
• Anxiety and fear
• Increased energy expenditure—coughing and breathing efforts

DESIRED OUTCOMES

The client will demonstrate an increased tolerance for activity as evidenced by:
  a. Verbalization of feeling less fatigued and weak
  b. Ability to perform activities of daily living without exertional dyspnea, chest pain, diaphoresis, dizziness, and significant changes in vital signs

NOC OUTCOMES

Activity tolerance; endurance; fatigue level; vital signs; self-care: activities of daily living; energy conservation

NIC INTERVENTIONS

Activity therapy; energy management; oxygen therapy; nutrition management; sleep enhancement; cardiac care; cardiac rehabilitation; teaching regarding prescribed activity

NURSING ASSESSMENT	**RATIONALE**
Assess for signs and symptoms of activity intolerance: • Statements of fatigue or weakness • Exertional dyspnea, chest pain, diaphoresis, or dizziness • Abnormal heart rate response to activity (e.g., increase in rate of 20 beats/min above resting rate, rate not returning to preactivity level within 3 minutes after stopping activity, change from regular to irregular rate) • Significant change (15-20 mm Hg) in B/P with activity	*Early recognition of signs and symptoms of activity intolerance allows for prompt intervention and treatment.*

THERAPEUTIC INTERVENTIONS	**RATIONALE**

Independent Actions

Implement measures to promote rest and/or conserve energy (e.g., maintain prescribed activity restrictions, minimize environmental activity and noise, provide uninterrupted rest periods, assist with care, keep supplies and personal articles within easy reach, limit the number of visitors, use shower chair when showering, sit to brush teeth or comb hair). **D** ● ✦	*Cells use oxygen and fat, protein, and carbohydrates to produce the energy needed for all body activities. Rest and activities that conserve energy result in a lower metabolic rate, which preserves nutrients and oxygen for necessary activities.*
Implement measures to promote sleep (e.g., elevated head of bed and support arms on pillows to facilitate breathing, discourage intake of fluids high in caffeine in the evening, and reduce environmental stimuli). **D** ✦	*Sleep replenishes a client's energy and feeling of well-being.*
Implement measures to decrease excessive coughing (e.g., protect client from exposure to irritants such as smoke, flowers, and powder; avoid extremely hot or cold foods/fluids). **D** ● ✦	*Altered respiratory function such as excessive coughing can lead to inadequate tissue oxygenation, which results in less efficient energy production and a reduced ability to tolerate activity. Improving respiratory status increases the amount of oxygen available for energy production.*
Discourage smoking and excessive intake of beverages high in caffeine such as coffee, tea, and colas.	*Excessive intake of nicotine and caffeine can increase cardiac workload and myocardial oxygen utilization, thereby decreasing oxygen availability.*
Perform actions to improve respiratory status (e.g., place client in semi- to high-Fowler's position; assist client to deep breathe or use incentive spirometry every 1 to 2 hours; maintain bed rest as ordered; and use oxygen as needed). **D** ● ✦	*Improvement of respiratory status through increased lung expansion.*
Perform actions to maintain adequate nutritional status (e.g., increase activity as tolerated, potentially improving appetite; encourage a rest period before meals to reduce fatigue; assist with oral hygiene before meals; maintain a clean environment and a relaxed pleasant atmosphere). **D** ✦	*Adequate nutritional status is important in order to maintain ADL.*
Increase client's activity gradually as allowed and tolerated. **D** ✦	*Gradual increase will slowly improve strength and ability in performance of activities.*
Instruct a client to: • Report a decreased tolerance for activity. • Stop any activity that causes increased chest pain, increased shortness of breath, dizziness, or extreme fatigue or weakness.	*Changes in a client's activity tolerance should be reported immediately. Assessment of the change will allow for timely diagnosis of the cause and subsequent treatment.*

Continued...

THERAPEUTIC INTERVENTIONS	RATIONALE
Dependent/Collaborative Actions Consult appropriate health care providers (e.g., respiratory therapist, physician, dietitian) if signs and symptoms of activity intolerance persist or worsen.	*Notifying the appropriate health care provider allows for modification of the treatment plan.*

Nursing Diagnosis RISK FOR INFECTION NDx (PNEUMONIA)

Definition: At increased risk for the lungs being invaded by pathogens

Related to:
* Stasis of secretions in the lungs (secretions provide a good medium for bacterial growth)
* Inhalation of pathogens (especially if client is using respiratory equipment or medication delivery devices that are not being cleaned adequately or routinely)

CLINICAL MANIFESTATIONS

Subjective	Objective
Verbalization of pleuritic pain	Increased respiratory rate; dyspnea; abnormal breath sounds (crackles, rales); productive cough with purulent green or rust-colored sputum; chills and diaphoresis; fever; elevated white blood cell (WBC) count; significant decrease in pulse oximetry values; worsening arterial blood gas values

RISK FACTORS
* Stasis of secretions
* Inhalation of pathogens
* Debilitated state
* Smoking

DESIRED OUTCOMES

The client will not develop pneumonia as evidenced by:
a. Usual breath sounds and percussion note over lungs
b. Absence of tachypnea
c. Cough productive of clear mucus only
d. Afebrile status
e. WBC count within normal range
f. Arterial blood gas values within normal range for client
g. Negative sputum culture
h. Ability to perform ADL without increased dyspnea, chest pain, diaphoresis, dizziness, and a significant change in vital signs

NOC OUTCOMES	NIC INTERVENTIONS
Infection severity; immune status	Infection protection; infection control; cough enhancement; airway management

NURSING ASSESSMENT	RATIONALE
Assess for and report signs and symptoms of pneumonia: • Abnormal breath sounds (e.g., crackles [rales], pleural friction rub, bronchial breath sounds, diminished or absent breath sounds) • Dull percussion note over affected lung area • Increase in respiratory rate • Cough productive of purulent, green, or rust-colored sputum • Chills and fever • Pleuritic pain • Elevated WBC count	*Early recognition of signs and symptoms of pneumonia allows for prompt intervention.*

NURSING ASSESSMENT	RATIONALE

- Significant decrease in oximetry results
- Worsening of arterial blood gas values
- Positive sputum culture results
- Chest radiograph results indicative of pneumonia

THERAPEUTIC INTERVENTIONS	RATIONALE

Independent Actions

Implement measures to prevent pneumonia:

- Perform actions to improve respiratory status (e.g., place client in semi- to high-Fowler's position; assist client to deep breathe or use incentive spirometer every 1 to 2 hours; improve activity tolerance; maintain fluid intake of at least 2500 mL/day unless contraindicated). **D** ✦

Positioning the client in semi- to high-Fowler's position promotes optimal gas exchange by enabling chest expansion. Forced deep breathing and use of incentive spirometry will increase expansion of the lungs and improve the client's ability to clear mucus from the lungs. Maintaining fluid intake will help to liquefy secretions for expectoration.

- Protect client from persons with respiratory tract infections. **D** ✦

The potential for illness is decreased through avoidance of persons with respiratory infections and crowds during the cold and flu season.

- Encourage and assist client to perform frequent oral hygiene. **D** ● ✦

Frequent oral hygiene helps to decrease the rate of infection through removal of pathogens and secretions that could be aspirated.

- Replace or cleanse equipment used for respiratory care as often as needed.

Equipment that is inadequately or incompletely cleaned after use harbors bacteria may lead to an respiratory infection.

- Instruct and assist client to rinse and clean medication delivery devices (e.g., dry powder inhaler, metered-dose inhaler, spacer) according to manufacturer's instructions.

Inhaled medication devices only deliver a certain percentage of the medication to the lungs. The rest of the medication is deposited in the oropharynx, which with some medications, increases the risk for infection, dysphonia, and/or candidiasis.

Dependent/Collaborative Actions

If signs and symptoms of pneumonia occur, administer antimicrobials as ordered. **D** ✦

Early administration of antibiotics at the first sign of infection can decrease the impact and duration of the infection.

Consult other health care providers at the first signs and symptoms of an infection.

Notifying the appropriate health care provider allows for modification of the treatment plan.

Collaborative Diagnosis ## RISK FOR RIGHT-SIDED HEART FAILURE

Definition: A condition where the right side of the heart is unable to pump blood efficiently

Related to:

- Increased cardiac workload associated with:
  - Pulmonary hypertension (can result from pulmonary vasoconstriction that occurs in response to hypoxia and the release of vasoactive substances)
  - Compensatory response to decreased pulmonary blood flow that results from compression of the pulmonary capillaries by hyperinflated alveoli (with emphysema) and loss of large portions of the pulmonary vascular bed (occurs in emphysema as a result of destruction of the alveolar walls)

CLINICAL MANIFESTATIONS

Subjective	Objective
Reports of weakness and fatigue	Tachypnea; tachycardia; dyspnea; restlessness; confusion; irritability; peripheral edema; decreased urine output; distended neck veins

Continued...

RISK FACTORS

- Hypertension
- Chronic respiratory disease
- Smoking
- Obesity

DESIRED OUTCOMES

The client will not develop right-sided heart failure as evidenced by:
   a. Pulse rate of 60 to 100 beats/min
   b. Usual mental status
   c. Usual strength and activity tolerance
   d. Adequate urine output
   e. Stable weight
   f. Absence of edema and distended neck veins

NURSING ASSESSMENT

Assess for and report signs and symptoms of right-sided heart failure:
- Further increase in pulse rate
- Restlessness, confusion
- Weakness and fatigue
- Decreased urine output
- Weight gain
- Dependent peripheral edema
- Distended neck veins
- Chest radiograph results showing cardiomegaly

RATIONALE

Early recognition of signs and symptoms of right-sided heart failure allows for prompt intervention.

THERAPEUTIC INTERVENTIONS

Dependent/Collaborative Actions

Implement measures to improve respiratory status (e.g., cough and deep breathe every 2-3 hours, ambulate as tolerated, maintain fluid restriction).

If signs and symptoms of right-sided heart failure occur
- Maintain oxygen therapy as ordered.

- Maintain client on strict bed rest in a semi-Fowler's to high-Fowler's position.

- Maintain fluid and sodium restrictions if ordered

- Administer medications that may reduce vascular congestion and/or cardiac workload (e.g., diuretics, cardiotonics, vasodilators).

RATIONALE

These interventions will reduce cardiac workload and the subsequent risk of right-sided heart failure by decreasing the pressure against which the heart must pump.

Supplemental O_2 helps to relieve dyspnea and improves gas exchange.

Placing the client on strict bed rest will help to conserve energy during periods of acute respiratory distress. Positioning the client in a semi- to high-Fowler's position promotes optimal gas exchange by enabling chest expansion.

Restricting a client's sodium and fluid intake will help reduce fluid volume overload.

Diuretics decrease fluid volume through inhibiting reabsorption of water, which decreases fluid volume.

Cardiotonics increase the contractile force of the heart, which increases cardiac output.

Vasodilators dilate the arterioles, which decreases B/P and decreases the work of the heart.

Collaborative Diagnosis   # RISK FOR RESPIRATORY FAILURE

Definition: Failure of the lungs to provide adequate oxygenation to the body

Related to:
- Severe ventilation/perfusion imbalance associated with end-stage COPD
- Acute exacerbation of COPD

CLINICAL MANIFESTATIONS

Subjective	Objective
Verbalization of increased fatigue and abdominal tenderness	Increased pulse rate >100 beats/min; confusion; restlessness; increased weakness; decreased urine output; dependent peripheral edema; hypoxemia; hypercapnia; weight gain; distended neck veins; enlarged liver; chest radiograph results demonstrating cardiomegaly

RISK FACTORS
- Pneumonia
- Pneumothorax
- Smoking
- Obesity

DESIRED OUTCOMES

The client will not experience respiratory failure as evidenced by:
  a. Usual skin color
  b. Usual mental status
  c. Partial pressure of oxygen in arterial blood (PaO_2) above 50 mm Hg and partial pressure of carbon dioxide in arterial blood ($PaCO_2$) below 50 mm Hg

NURSING ASSESSMENT

Assess for and report signs and symptoms of severe respiratory distress:
- Increased sternocleidomastoid and intercostal muscle retraction
- Cyanotic skin color
- Drowsiness, confusion
- PaO_2 of 50 mm Hg or less, $PaCO_2$ of 50 mm Hg or greater

RATIONALE

Early recognition of signs and symptoms of severe respiratory distress allows for prompt intervention.

THERAPEUTIC INTERVENTIONS

RATIONALE

Dependent/Collaborative Actions
Implement measures to prevent respiratory failure:
- Maintain client on strict bed rest in a semi- to high-Fowler's position **D** ● ✦

- Maintain oxygen therapy as ordered. **D** ✦

- Instruct client in and assist with diaphragmatic and pursed-lip breathing techniques. **D** ✦
- Instruct client to deep breathe or use incentive spirometer every 1 to 2 hours. **D** ✦

- Instruct client to avoid intake of large meals, gas-forming foods (i.e., cauliflower, beans, cabbage, onions, etc.), and carbonated beverages.
- Discourage smoking.

- Maintain activity restrictions and increase activity as allowed and tolerated. **D** ● ✦

- Maintain fluid and sodium restrictions as ordered.

- Administer diuretics and/or vasodilators ordered. **D** ✦

- Administer angiotensin-converting enzyme (ACE) inhibitors. **D** ✦

Placing the client on strict bed rest will help to conserve energy. Positioning in semi- to high Fowler's position promotes optimal gas exchange by enabling chest expansion.
Supplemental O_2 helps to relieve dyspnea and provides vasodilating effects that decrease pulmonary hypertension, thus decreasing the workload of the right side of the heart.
These techniques help clients slow their pace of breathing, which makes each breath more effective.
Forced deep breathing and use of incentive spirometry will increase expansion of the lungs and improve the client's ability to clear mucus from the lungs. The technique may also improve the amount of oxygen that is able to penetrate deep into the lungs.
Gas-forming foods and carbonated beverages can cause abdominal bloating, which places pressure on the diaphragm and reduces lung expansion.
The irritants in smoke increase mucus production, impair ciliary function, and can cause inflammation and damage to the bronchial and alveolar walls; the carbon monoxide decreases oxygen availability
Conservation of energy through activity restrictions allows energy to be focused on breathing. Increasing activity as tolerated helps to mobilize secretions and promotes deeper breathing.
Excess fluid volume is an isotonic retention of both sodium and water. Restricting sodium intake will result in less sodium and subsequently less water being reabsorbed by the kidneys, thus reducing cardiac workload.
Diuretics reduce excess fluid volume, reduce sodium retention, and decrease cardiac workload. Vasodilators augment diuretics in decreasing cardiac workload by reducing preload and afterload.
ACE inhibitors cause arterial and venous dilation and suppress aldosterone release. These actions decrease preload and afterload as well as decrease fluid volume through increased excretion of sodium and water. Long-term ACE inhibitor therapy has been shown to decrease the myocardial remodeling seen in heart failure.

Continued...

THERAPEUTIC INTERVENTIONS	RATIONALE
Administer beta-blockers (carvedilol). **D** ✦	*Beta-blockers decrease heart rate and B/P. The subsequent increase in cardiac output has been shown to slow the progression of heart failure and decrease the risk of death.*
If signs and symptoms of respiratory failure occur, assist with intubation and mechanical ventilatory support, and transfer to intensive care unit if indicated.	*Early recognition of signs and symptoms allows for early notification of appropriate members of the health care team and treatment.*

Nursing Diagnosis FEAR/ANXIETY NDx

Definition: Fear—Response to perceived threat (real or imagined) that is consciously recognized as a danger.
Anxiety—Vague uneasy feeling of discomfort or dread accompanied by an autonomic response (the source is often nonspecific or unknown to the individual); a feeling of apprehension caused by anticipation of danger

Related to:
- Exacerbation of symptoms (e.g., increased dyspnea, feeling of suffocation), need for hospitalization, and concern about prognosis
- Lack of understanding of the diagnosis, diagnostic tests, treatments, and prognosis
- Financial concerns about hospitalization and lifelong treatment
- Feeling of lack of control over the progression of COPD and its effects on lifestyle and roles

CLINICAL MANIFESTATIONS

Subjective	Objective
Verbalization of anxiety and fear	Unusual sleep patterns; relaxed facial expressions and body movements; stable vital signs; restlessness; shakiness; diaphoresis; self-focused behavior

RISK FACTORS
- Shortness of breath
- Feelings of suffocation
- Fear of dying

DESIRED OUTCOMES

The client will experience a reduction in fear and anxiety as evidenced by:
    a. Verbalization of feeling less anxious
    b. Usual sleep pattern
    c. Relaxed facial expression and body movements
    d. Stable vital signs
    e. Usual perceptual ability and interactions with others

NOC OUTCOMES

Anxiety level; fear level; anxiety self-control; fear self-control

NIC INTERVENTIONS

Anxiety reduction; calming technique; emotional support; presence; pain management

NURSING ASSESSMENT	RATIONALE
Assess client for signs and symptoms of fear and anxiety (e.g., verbalization of feeling anxious, insomnia, tenseness, shakiness, restlessness, diaphoresis, elevated B/P, tachycardia, self-focused behaviors).	*Moderate anxiety enhances the client's ability to solve problems. With severe anxiety or panic, the client is not able to follow directions and may become hyperactive and extremely agitated.*
Validate perceptions carefully, remembering that some behavior may result from hypoxia and/or hypercapnia.	*Assessment of the client's fear helps to determine whether the coping mechanisms are effective and which need to be strengthened.*

THERAPEUTIC INTERVENTIONS	RATIONALE

Independent Actions

Implement measures to reduce fear and anxiety:

- Orient client to hospital environment, equipment, and routines. **D** ● ✦

  Familiarity with the environment and usual routines reduces the client's anxiety about the unknown, provides a sense of security, and increases the client's sense of control, all of which help decrease anxiety.

- Introduce staff who will be participating in client's care. If possible, maintain consistency in staff assigned to client's care.

  Introduction to staff familiarizes clients with those individuals who will be working with them, which provides clients with a feeling of stability, which reduces the anxiety that typically occurs with change.

- Assure client that staff members are nearby; respond to call signal as soon as possible. **D** ● ✦

  Close contact and a prompt response to requests provide a sense of security and facilitate the development of trust, thus reducing the client's anxiety.

- Maintain a calm, supportive, confident manner when interacting with client; encourage verbalization of fear and anxiety.

  A sense of calmness and confidence conveys to the client that someone is in control of the situation, which helps reduce anxiety.

- Reinforce physician's explanations and clarify misconceptions the client has about the disease process, treatment plan, and possible recurrence; encourage questions.

  Factual information and an awareness of what to expect help decrease the anxiety that arises from uncertainty.

Implement measures to reduce respiratory distress if present:

- Elevate the head of the bed.

  Improvement of respiratory status helps relieve anxiety associated with the feeling of not being able to breathe.

- Encourage the client to breathe deeply and more slowly. **D** ● ✦

- Implement measures to reduce pain:

  Pain can create or increase anxiety because it is often perceived as a threat to well-being.

  - Instruct client in relaxation techniques and encourage participation in diversional activities once the period of acute pain and respiratory distress has subsided.

    Pain also causes sympathetic nervous system stimulation with subsequent feelings of tenseness and increased anxiety.

- When appropriate, assist the client to meet spiritual needs (e.g., arrange for a visit from the clergy).

  Spiritual support is a source of comfort and security for many people and can help reduce the client's fear and anxiety.

- Provide information based on current needs of client at a level that can be understood.

  Providing information that the client is not ready to process or cannot understand tends to increase anxiety.

  - Encourage the client to ask questions and to seek clarification of information provided.

    Making the client feel comfortable enough to ask questions or clarify information helps to reduce anxiety.

- Provide a calm, restful environment. **D** ● ✦

  A calm, restful environment facilitates relaxation and promotes a sense of security, which reduces fear and anxiety.

- Encourage significant others to project a caring, concerned attitude without obvious fear and anxiousness.

  Anxiety is easily transferable from one person to another. If significant others convey empathy, provide reassurance, and do not appear anxious, they can help reduce the client's fear and anxiety.

Dependent/Collaborative Actions

Implement measures to reduce fear and anxiety:

- Administer oxygen via nasal cannula rather than mask if possible. **D** ✦

  The use of a mask for some clients seems restrictive and suffocating. The use of a nasal cannula is more comfortable and less constraining. Improvement of respiratory status helps relieve anxiety associated with the feeling of not being able to breathe.

- Administer prescribed antianxiety agents if indicated. **D** ✦

  Decreases anxiety

Consult appropriate health care provider (e.g., psychiatric nurse clinician, physician) if above actions fail to control fear and anxiety.

Notifying the appropriate health care provider allows for modification of the treatment plan.

NDx = NANDA-I Diagnosis   **D** = Delegatable Action   ● = UAP   ✦ = LVN/LPN   ⊜▶ = Go to ⊜volve for animation

Nursing Diagnosis INEFFECTIVE SELF-HEALTH MANAGEMENT NDx

Definition: Pattern of regulating and integrating into daily living a therapeutic regimen for treatment of illness and the sequelae of illness that is unsatisfactory for meeting specific health goals

CLINICAL MANIFESTATIONS

Subjective	Objective
Verbalizes inability to manage illness; to follow prescribed regimen	Inaccurate follow through with instructions; inappropriate behaviors; experience of preventable complications of COPD; frequent exacerbation of illness

RISK FACTORS

- Cognitive impairment
- Insufficient resources
- Feeling of lack of control over disease progression
- Difficulty modifying personal habits (e.g., smoking) and integrating necessary treatments into lifestyle

DESIRED OUTCOMES

The client will demonstrate the probability of effective self-health management as evidenced by:
  a. Willingness to learn about and participate in treatments and care
  b. Statements reflecting ways to modify personal habits and integrate treatments into lifestyle
  c. Statements reflecting an understanding of the implications of not following the prescribed treatment plan

NOC OUTCOMES

Treatment behavior: illness or injury; compliance behavior; health beliefs; perceived ability to perform: knowledge of treatment regimen

NIC INTERVENTIONS

Self-modification assistance; values clarification; teaching: disease process; health system guidance; financial resource assistance; discharge planning; medication management; smoking cessation assistance

NURSING ASSESSMENT

Assess client's knowledge base related to the disease process. Assess for indications that the client may be unable to effectively manage the therapeutic regimen:
- Statements reflecting inability to manage care at home
- Failure to adhere to treatment plan (e.g., refusing to use proper breathing techniques, refusing medications)
- Statements reflecting a lack of understanding of factors that may cause further progression of COPD
- Statements reflecting an unwillingness or inability to modify personal habits and integrate necessary treatments into lifestyle
- Statements reflecting view that the COPD is incurable or that the situation is hopeless, and efforts to comply with the treatment plan are useless

RATIONALE

The client's knowledge base provides the basis for education. Early recognition of inability to understand disease process or self-care allows for change in teaching modality.

THERAPEUTIC INTERVENTIONS	RATIONALE

Independent Actions

Implement measures to promote effective therapeutic regimen management:

- Explain COPD in terms the client can understand; stress that COPD is a chronic condition, and adherence to the treatment program is necessary.

- Encourage questions and clarify misconceptions client has about COPD and its effects.

- Encourage client to participate in treatment plan (e.g., postural drainage therapy, breathing exercises).

- Consult occupational and/or physical therapist if indicated about a home evaluation to identify assistive devices and necessary environmental modifications.

- Assist client to develop a system for recording frequency of use of medications and respiratory treatments in order to avoid omission of those that should be used routinely and to avoid excessive use of those that should be used on an "as needed" basis (in times of respiratory distress, the client may tend to overuse medications because of fear, anxiety, and impaired cognition).

- Provide client with written instructions about chest physiotherapy, ways to prevent further respiratory problems, prescribed medications, signs and symptoms to report, where to obtain needed equipment and supplies, and future appointments with health care provider.

- Assist client to identify ways treatments can be incorporated into lifestyle; focus on modifications of lifestyle rather than complete change (e.g., statements reflecting plans for integrating treatments into lifestyle, active participation in treatment plan, changes in personal habits).

- Encourage client to discuss concerns regarding cost of hospitalization, medications, oxygen equipment, and follow-up care; obtain a social service consult to assist with financial planning and to obtain financial aid if indicated.

- Provide information about and encourage utilization of community resources that can assist the client to make necessary lifestyle changes (e.g., American Lung Association; pulmonary rehabilitation groups; counseling, vocational, and social services; smoking cessation programs).

- Include significant others in explanations and teaching sessions, and encourage their support; reinforce the need for the client to assume responsibility for managing as much of care as possible.

Dependent/Collaborative Actions

Consult appropriate health care provider about referrals to community health agencies if continued instruction, support, or supervision is needed.

The client should understand that COPD is a chronic illness, and adherence to the treatment program is necessary in order to delay and/or prevent complications; however, caution client that some complications may occur despite strict adherence to treatment plan.

Everyone does not understand the information as presented. Questioning allows for clarification and for clients to put the information within a context they understand.

Client involvement in care helps to reinforce the individual's understanding of lifestyle changes necessary to maintain health status.

Involvement of a variety of individuals on the health care team allows for a multifaceted plan of care and discharge planning that assists clients to be more independent in their living situation.

Adherence to the medication regimen is required to improve and/or maintain the client's health status. Working with the client to develop a system for monitoring the medication regimen improves the potential for adherence.

Written instructions provide the client with information as a reference to use as needed.

To improve the potential for adherence to the treatment/medication regimen, the client must be actively involved in how/when and what lifestyle modifications are implemented. An individual's chance of success is decreased if one has to make a total lifestyle change.

Financial concerns play a large part in an individual's ability to adhere to a treatment regimen. Involvement of social services may be required to obtain financial assistance needed by the patient.

Knowledge of community resources provides ongoing support and access to resources outside the acute care facility.

Involvement of significant others in client teaching improves adherence to discharge instructions and lifestyle changes.

Consult health care providers in the community for a continuum of care postdischarge.

DISCHARGE TEACHING/CONTINUED CARE

Nursing Diagnosis **DEFICIENT KNOWLEDGE NDx OR INEFFECTIVE HEALTH MAINTENANCE* NDx**

Definition: Absence or deficiency of cognitive information related to specific topic (lack of specific information necessary for clients/significant others to make informed choices regarding condition/treatment/lifestyle changes); inability to identify, manage, and/or seek help to manage health

CLINICAL MANIFESTATIONS

Subjective	Objective
Verbalization of the problem	Inaccurate follow through of instructions; inappropriate behaviors

RISK FACTORS
- Denial of disease process
- Cognitive deficiency
- Failure to take action to reduce risk factors

NOC OUTCOMES

Knowledge: treatment regimen; knowledge: energy conservation; knowledge: treatment procedure(s); knowledge: health resources; knowledge: illness care

NIC INTERVENTIONS

Health system guidance; teaching: individual; teaching: disease process; teaching: prescribed activity/exercise; teaching: prescribed medication

NURSING ASSESSMENT	**RATIONALE**
Assess client understanding of illness and treatment plan. Assess client's ability and readiness to learn. Assess client's understanding of teaching.	*Learning is more effective when client is motivated and understands the importance of what is to be learned.* *Readiness to learn changes based on situations and physical and emotional challenges.*

THERAPEUTIC INTERVENTIONS	**RATIONALE**

Desired Outcome: The client will identify ways to prevent or minimize further respiratory problems.

Independent Actions

Instruct client in ways to prevent or minimize further respiratory problems:

- Maintain overall general good health (e.g., reduce stress, eat a well-balanced diet, obtain adequate rest, adhere to prescribed graded exercise program).
- Stop smoking.

- Avoid exposure to respiratory irritants such as smoke, dust, some perfumes, aerosol sprays, paint fumes, and solvents; wear a mask or scarf over nose and mouth if exposure to high levels of irritants such as smoke, fumes, and dust is unavoidable.

There are a variety of ways a client can maintain general good health and support interventions focusing on the respiratory system.

The irritants in smoke increase mucus production, impair ciliary function, and can cause inflammation and damage to the bronchial and alveolar walls; the carbon monoxide decreases oxygen availability.

Exposure to respiratory irritants increases the risk of infection and impacts ciliary function.

---

*The nurse should select the diagnostic label that is most appropriate for the client's discharge teaching needs.

THERAPEUTIC INTERVENTIONS	RATIONALE
• Remain indoors when air pollution levels and/or pollen counts are high and/or outdoor temperatures are extremely hot or cold.	Air pollution in high levels is harmful to persons with existing lung disease. Exposure to extreme hot and cold air may cause bronchoconstriction, allowing less air into and out of the lungs.
• Avoid high altitudes; if air travel is required, consult physician about the need for supplemental oxygen.	The oxygen content at high altitudes is decreased, which may cause significant dyspnea if supplemental oxygen is not available.
• Adhere to chest physiotherapy (e.g., breathing exercises, postural drainage therapy) as ordered.	Chest physiotherapy is important to handle secretions and maintain positive respiratory status.
• Take medications such as bronchodilators and mucolytics as prescribed.	Adherence to medication regimen is important to maintain and improve respiratory status.
• Avoid contact with persons who have respiratory tract infections; avoid crowds and poorly ventilated areas; receive immunizations against influenza and pneumococcal pneumonia.	These actions decrease the client's risk of infection.
• Drink at least 10 glasses of liquid per day unless contraindicated.	Adequate fluid intake is necessary to liquefy secretions.
• Take antimicrobials as prescribed (some physicians instruct clients to begin antimicrobial therapy if sputum color becomes yellow or green).	Early treatment of infections may decrease the severity of the impact on the client with COPD.
• Clean medication administration devices (e.g., metered-dose inhaler, dry powder inhaler, spacer, table-top nebulizer), oxygen delivery devices (e.g., mask, nasal cannula), humidifier, and air filters as instructed by health care provider and manufacturer.	Equipment that is inadequately cleaned after use harbors bacteria, which may lead to an infection. Inhaled medication devices only deliver a certain percentage of the medication to the lungs. The rest of the medication is deposited in the oropharynx, which with some medications, increases the risk for infection, dysphonia, and/or candidiasis.

THERAPEUTIC INTERVENTIONS	RATIONALE

Desired Outcome: The client will verbalize ways to maintain an optimal nutritional status.

Independent Actions

Provide instructions regarding ways to maintain an optimal nutritional status:

• Rest before meals; do the majority of food preparation in advance rather than just before eating.	Preparing food in advance of eating and adequate rest before meals decrease fatigue that may occur when eating.
• Perform good oral hygiene before meals.	Good oral hygiene reduces unpleasant tastes in the mouth and moistens the mouth, making it easier to chew and swallow.
• Eat sitting down in a pleasant environment.	Eating in a pleasant environment helps to increase a client's appetite.
• Eat foods that require little or no chewing when energy is low and/or dyspnea is increased.	Because a person cannot swallow and breathe at the same time, relief of dyspnea increases the likelihood of maintaining a good oral intake. Foods that require little or no chewing will be easier to eat and help to maintain a client's nutritional status.
• Eat meals that are well balanced; drink nutritional supplements if needed to maintain an adequate caloric intake.	Clients must consume a diet that is well balanced and high in essential nutrients in order to meet their nutritional needs. Dietary supplements are often needed to help accomplish this.

Dependent/Collaborative Actions

Provide instructions regarding ways to maintain an optimal nutritional status:

• Use supplemental oxygen via nasal cannula during meals if needed.	Relief of dyspnea through the use of oxygen therapy decreases the client's anxiety about and preoccupation with breathing efforts and increases the ability to focus on eating and drinking.
• Take vitamins and minerals as prescribed.	Administration of vitamins and minerals help to maintain nutritional status.

Continued...

THERAPEUTIC INTERVENTIONS	RATIONALE

Desired Outcome: The client will identify ways to conserve energy and/or reduce dyspnea and fatigue.

Independent Actions

Instruct client in ways to conserve energy and/or reduce dyspnea and fatigue:

- Sit rather than stand during activities such as preparing food, rinsing dishes, ironing, showering, shaving, and talking on the phone.
- Have most frequently used food items, dishes, cleaning supplies, and clothing at waist level whenever possible rather than on high or low shelves.
- Pace yourself during any activity; stop, relax your muscles, and take a few deep breaths as often as needed.
- Simplify your life whenever possible; spread large projects over several days or weeks.
- Allow others to assist you with or actually do strenuous or lengthy tasks.
- Modify activities to avoid bending, reaching, and raising arms whenever possible (e.g., use long-handled assistive devices, simplify hair style so that it does not need to be blown dry or curled, sit with elbows resting on table while shaving).
- Do not try to carry on a conversation during activities that also require energy (e.g., walking, eating, cleaning, gardening).
- Use bronchodilators before activity as needed and prescribed.
- Use oxygen during activity as needed and prescribed; have portable oxygen system readily available.
- Use positions that minimize energy expenditure during sexual activity (e.g., side-lying).

Each of these actions is a method of conserving energy during a variety of activities.

THERAPEUTIC INTERVENTIONS	RATIONALE

Desired Outcome: The client will demonstrate proper chest physiotherapy and use of respiratory equipment.

Independent Actions

Reinforce instructions about proper breathing techniques (e.g., pursed-lip breathing, diaphragmatic breathing), postural drainage therapy (may be indicated if large amounts of mucus continue to be produced), and use of respiratory equipment (e.g., oxygen, incentive spirometer).

A variety of techniques and therapy are required for clients with COPD to maintain their health status.

Allow time for questions, clarification, and return demonstration.

Making the client feel comfortable enough to ask questions or clarify information and to provide a return demonstration will help improve adherence to treatment regimens.

THERAPEUTIC INTERVENTIONS	RATIONALE

Desired Outcome: The client will verbalize an understanding of medications ordered including rationale, food and drug interactions, side effects, methods of administration, and importance of taking as prescribed.

THERAPEUTIC INTERVENTIONS	RATIONALE

Independent Actions

Explain the rationale for, side effects of, and importance of taking medications prescribed.

A client's understanding of why medications are required, their side effects, and the importance of taking them as prescribed will promote adherence.

Inform client of pertinent food and drug interactions.

Clients need to understand what type of foods and other medications may impact their respiratory medications.

Have blood levels evaluated periodically, if indicated.

There are many medications where a blood level is required. The client needs to be aware of the importance of having these levels monitored to ensure appropriate dosing and to prevent toxic levels.

If client is discharged on medications via inhalation:
- Provide information about the proper use, cleaning, and replacement of the medication delivery devices (e.g., nebulizer, dry powder inhaler, metered-dose inhaler, spacer).

Equipment that is inadequately cleaned after use harbors bacteria, which may lead to an infection.

- Instruct to rinse mouth with water after using inhalers (removing remaining drug particles from the mouth helps reduce unpleasant tastes, dryness or irritation of the oral mucosa, and systemic absorption of the drug).

Inhaled medication devices only deliver a certain percentage of the medication to the lungs. The rest of the medication is deposited in the oropharynx. Rinsing the mouth after medication administration will remove remaining particles from the mouth.

- Instruct to observe for and report side effects such as persistent sore throat, increased cough, hoarseness, and/or white patches in mouth (could indicate candidiasis that can occur with corticosteroid use).

Some inhaled medications increase the risk for infection, dysphonia, and/or candidiasis.

- Instruct to use the prescribed bronchodilator before inhaling the corticosteroid and to wait 5 minutes between these two medications (this maximizes the effectiveness of the corticosteroid).

Separation of inhaled medications by 5 minutes is important in maximizing the effectiveness of the medications, particularly corticosteroids.

If client is discharged on a corticosteroid, instruct to:
- Take oral preparations with food to reduce gastric irritation.
- Expect that certain effects such as facial rounding, slight weight gain and swelling, increased appetite, and slight mood changes may occur.

The client should be taught the correct method of administration to decrease the incidence of side effects and adverse reactions.

- Report undesirable effects such as marked swelling in extremities, significant weight gain, extreme emotional and behavioral changes, extreme weakness, tarry stools, bloody or coffee-ground vomitus, frequent or persistent headaches, insomnia, lack of menses, and persistent gastric irritation.

Clients should be educated about the physical changes that can occur while taking corticosteroids, and the importance of notifying their health care professional for treatment and potential readjustment of medication dosage.

- Avoid contact with persons who have an infection.

Corticosteroids reduce the ability of the body to fight off infection; therefore, it is important for the client to avoid contact with persons who have an infection

- Follow recommendations about ways to reduce the risk for developing osteoporosis if long-term corticosteroid use is expected (e.g., take calcium and vitamin D supplements, stop smoking, do 30-60 minutes of weight-bearing exercise each day if able).

Long-term use of corticosteroids increases the client's risk of developing osteoporosis. It is important to provide the client with methods of decreasing this risk.

If client is discharged on a beta-adrenergic agonist (e.g., albuterol, metaproterenol, terbutaline, salmeterol), instruct to:
- Take oral preparations with meals to reduce gastric irritation.
- Expect that certain effects such as nervousness, restlessness, and slight tremor can occur.

Clients need to be educated on the form of administration, side effects, and adverse reactions. Clients must also be informed that if undesirable effects occur, to notify their health care provider.

- Report undesirable effects such as persistent or excessive nervousness, restlessness, tremors, headache, and gastric irritation; chest pain; vomiting; irregular heart beat; and wheezing.

Continued...

THERAPEUTIC INTERVENTIONS	RATIONALE
Instruct client to take regularly scheduled medications as often as prescribed and to avoid skipping doses, altering the prescribed dose, making up for missed doses, and discontinuing medication without permission of the health care provider.	*Many medications require a blood level to be obtained in order for an appropriate client response. The client must be made aware of what to do when doses are missed, generic medications are used if they were not used initially when the medication was prescribed, and the importance of not discontinuing the medication without the permission of the health care provider.*
Reinforce instructions about the frequency and dosage of medications prescribed on an "as needed" basis.	*The client should be educated on how to take medications that are prescribed to be used as needed. It should be emphasized that the client should not increase the frequency or dosage of these medications without permission from the health care provider.*
Instruct client to inform all health care providers of medications and herbal supplements being taken.	*Many clients have more than one physician and should be educated to inform all health care providers of all medications and herbal supplements being taken. This is important so that the health care provider is aware of all medications and herbal supplements taken by the client so if new medications are ordered, the health care provider can determine the impact of drug-to-drug interactions.*
Reinforce the need to consult physician before taking nonprescription medications.	*Many over-the-counter (OTC) medications can cause significant drug-to-drug interactions.*

THERAPEUTIC INTERVENTIONS	RATIONALE

Desired Outcome: The client will identify precautions that should be adhered to when using oxygen.

Independent Actions

Instruct client about precautions that should be adhered to when using oxygen: • Do not smoke. • Do not set oxygen flow rate at a level higher than prescribed by physician.	*A client using oxygen outside the health care facility should be educated on its use and safety issues. Oxygen is not a combustible gas by itself, but when exposed to an open flame or a spark, it can exacerbate a fire.*
• Do not allow the oxygen system to be within 10 feet of an open flame (e.g., gas stove, kerosene heater or lamp, fireplace, candle) or a source of sparks (e.g., electric razor, portable radio, wool blanket, hair dryer).	*Oxygen is highly flammable and should be placed at a safe distance from anything with an open flame. In the event of fire, the oxygen system should be shut off and removed from the area.*
• Post "No Smoking" signs in and around areas of oxygen use.	*Prevents accidental smoking around oxygen*
• Ensure that all electrical equipment in the area of the oxygen source is grounded.	*Decreases risk of oxygen-related fire*
• Always have a battery-operated oxygen delivery system readily available.	*A backup battery-operated system is necessary for power failures and when away from a hard wire power source.*
• Demonstrate to the client how to recognize when the oxygen supply is low, and how to get the oxygen source refilled or replaced.	*The client needs to be aware of how to assess the level of oxygen on hand and at what level to have it replenished to ensure it is available when it is required.*
• Instruct client to have the oxygen delivery system checked regularly by the supplier.	*This check helps to ensure it is working properly.*
• Always wear a medical alert identification bracelet or tag.	*Wearing a medical alert identification bracelet provides information important to ensure that the appropriate oxygen flow rate for diagnosis is administered in emergency situations and to the client's history of COPD.*
Instruct client on ways to prevent skin and mucous membrane irritation and breakdown resulting from the use of oxygen and/or oxygen delivery devices: • Assess areas of skin and mucous membranes that are in contact with the oxygen mask or nasal cannula (e.g., nares, bridge of nose, tops of ears) a few times each day for redness and irritation.	*A client who continuously uses oxygen should be taught methods to prevent skin and mucous membrane irritation. Oxygen is a dry gas and can cause dryness of the skin and mucous membranes that may lead to skin breakdown.*

THERAPEUTIC INTERVENTIONS	**RATIONALE**
• Pad areas of pressure and ensure that straps are not too tight.	*Pressure areas not padded and/or straps that are too tight may lead to skin breakdown.*
• Keep skin areas under straps and mask clean and dry.	*Helps to reduce dryness and cracking of the mucous membranes.*
• Refill oxygen humidification reservoir as needed, perform frequent oral hygiene, and apply water-based gel to nares and lips to reduce dryness of the mucous membranes.	

THERAPEUTIC INTERVENTIONS	**RATIONALE**

Desired Outcome: The client will state signs and symptoms to report to the health care provider.

Independent Actions

Instruct client to report:

• Changes in sputum characteristics (e.g., increase in volume or consistency, yellow or green color)	*A respiratory infection increases dyspnea and may precipitate respiratory failure.*
• Sputum that does not return to usual color after 3 days of antimicrobial therapy	*Instruct the client on signs and symptoms of an infection. When these appear, the client is to contact the health care provider immediately. Prompt treatment may prevent the infection from becoming severe and precipitating respiratory infection.*
• Cough that becomes worse	
• Increased fatigue, weakness, and shortness of breath	
• Increased need for medications and/or oxygen therapy	
• Elevated temperature	
• Drowsiness, confusion, new or increased irritability	*May indicate cardiac complications of COPD and require medical treatment.*
• Chest pain	
• Persistent weight loss or sudden weight gain	
• Swelling in ankles and/or feet	

THERAPEUTIC INTERVENTIONS	**RATIONALE**

Desired Outcome: The client will identify resources that can assist with financial needs, home management, and adjustment to changes resulting from COPD.

Independent Actions

Provide information regarding resources that can assist client and significant others with financial needs, home management, and adjustment to changes resulting from COPD (e.g., American Lung Association; respiratory equipment suppliers; pulmonary rehabilitation programs; counseling, vocational, and social services; Meals on Wheels; transportation services; home health agencies).	*COPD is a chronic illness and can significantly impact an individual's and family's financial status. Providing information specific to community resources is important to provide a continuum of care and may impact the client's health status.*
Initiate a referral to community and home health agencies if indicated.	*Provides for continuum of care postdischarge*

THERAPEUTIC INTERVENTIONS	**RATIONALE**

Desired Outcome: The client will verbalize an understanding of a plan for adhering to recommended follow-up care including future appointments with health care provider and graded exercise program.

Independent Actions

Implement measures to promote effective therapeutic regimen management (adhere to an appropriate diet and an exercise plan; stop smoking and maintain medication regimen).	*A chronic illness requires lifestyle changes. Client involvement in a comprehensive program of lifestyle changes (i.e., diet, exercise, stop smoking, etc.) has been shown to provide improved health status and slows the progression of the disease.*
Reinforce importance of lifelong follow-up care.	
Reinforce physician's instructions about a graded exercise program (e.g., walking for 20 minutes 3 times a week, stationary bicycling).	

ADDITIONAL NURSING DIAGNOSES

SELF-CARE DEFICIT NDx
Related to weakness, fatigue, and dyspnea

DISTURBED SLEEP PATTERN NDx
Related to fear, anxiety, unfamiliar environment, excessive coughing, frequent assessments and treatments, side effects of medications (e.g., some bronchodilators, corticosteroids), and inability to assume usual sleep position associated with orthopnea

DISTURBED BODY IMAGE NDx
Related to:
* Change in appearance (e.g., "barrel" chest, clubbing of fingers, retraction of tissues around the neck and shoulders)

* Dependence on others to meet self-care needs
* Possible alteration in sexual functioning (may result from dyspnea, weakness, fatigue, and persistent cough)
* Stigma associated with chronic illness
* Possible changes in lifestyle and roles

RISK FOR POWERLESSNESS NDx
Related to physical limitations; disease progression despite efforts to comply with treatment plan; dependence on others to meet self-care needs; and alterations in roles, lifestyle, and future plans.

MECHANICAL VENTILATION

Mechanical ventilation, intended for use as a temporary, life-saving therapy, is indicated for clients with acute respiratory failure who are unable to maintain normal gas exchange. Implemented using a variety of modes and techniques, methods of mechanical ventilation used in acute and long-term care settings are influenced by the type of underlying disease process and the need for an artificial airway.

Acute respiratory failure can be a result of either the failure to oxygenate, the failure to ventilate, or a combination of both. Two categories of respiratory failure influence the method of mechanical ventilation selected for ventilatory support. Type I, or hypoxemic respiratory failure, is defined as the inability to maintain a PaO_2 greater than 60 mm Hg with the client at rest and breathing room air. A variety of disease processes interfere with the normal exchange of oxygen and carbon dioxide across the alveolar membrane, leading to disturbances in diffusion. These processes include pulmonary fibrosis, pulmonary edema, acute respiratory distress syndrome (ARDS), and loss of functional lung tissue (pneumonectomy). Effective gas exchange is influenced by even distribution of gas (ventilation) and blood (perfusion) in all portions of the lung. Disturbances in the relationship between ventilation and perfusion also contribute to type I or hypoxemic respiratory failure and include pulmonary emboli, atelectasis, pneumonia, emphysema, and bronchitis, as well as ARDS. Type II failure, or the failure to ventilate, results from disease processes that interfere with a client's ability to effectively ventilate the waste products of respiration (CO_2). Characterized by a $PaCO_2$ greater than 60 mm Hg or a pH less than 7.35, type II respiratory failure, or hypercarbic respiratory failure, can occur as a result of disease processes that impair normal alveolar minute ventilation. These disease processes include COPD, restrictive pulmonary diseases (obesity, pneumothorax, diaphragmatic paralysis), neuromuscular defects (Guillain-Barré syndrome, myasthenia gravis, multiple sclerosis, muscular dystrophy, spinal cord injury), and chest trauma.

Invasive positive pressure ventilation is the most common method of mechanical ventilation used in the acute care setting. Invasive ventilation techniques require the use of an artificial airway (tracheostomy, endotracheal tube [ETT]). With this method of ventilation, the client's respiratory function is supported as positive pressure delivers the appropriate volume of air and concentration using the appropriate ventilator settings. The degree of mechanical support and the duration of therapy are determined by the client's underlying disease process and current state of health. As duration of mechanical support increases, the client is at increased risk for the development of complications associated with mechanical ventilation: tracheal damage, acid-base imbalances, aspiration pneumonia, nutritional imbalances, deep vein thrombosis (DVT), stress ulcers, immobility, and ventilator dependence.

To ensure the safe and effective care of a client requiring mechanical ventilation, a multidisciplinary approach is required. Collaboration among the physician provider, respiratory therapist, dietician, physical therapist, and nurse is essential in order to resolve the underlying disease process, prevent complications, and return the client to baseline pulmonary function. In addition, as with any artificial lifesaving or life-extending therapy, client and family choice must be respected if end-of-life issues arise.

This care plan focuses on the adult client hospitalized in an acute care setting with acute respiratory failure requiring support with mechanical ventilation.

OUTCOME/DISCHARGE CRITERIA

The client will:
1. Return to independent respiratory function
2. Tolerate an expected level of activity
3. Maintain a balanced nutritional state
4. Have no signs or symptoms of infection
5. Identify ways to maintain respiratory health
6. Verbalize an understanding of the treatment plan including prescribed medications, diet, and follow-up care
7. State signs and symptoms to report to health care provider

Nursing Diagnosis IMPAIRED RESPIRATORY FUNCTION* NDx

Definition: Inability of an individual to maintain adequate ventilation of the respiratory tract and perfusion of oxygen (O_2) and carbon dioxide (CO_2) between the lungs and vascular system to maintain adequate tissue oxygenation

Impaired spontaneous ventilation NDx
Related to:
- Metabolic factors, respiratory muscle fatigue

Ineffective breathing pattern NDx
Related to:
- Cognitive impairment, neuromuscular dysfunction, respiratory muscle fatigue, spinal cord injury, obesity, hyperventilation/hypoventilation

Ineffective airway clearance NDx
Related to:
- Presence of an artificial airway, retained secretions, secretions in the bronchi, excessive mucus, infection

Impaired gas exchange NDx
Related to:
- Alveolar-capillary membrane changes, ventilation-perfusion imbalance

CLINICAL MANIFESTATIONS

Subjective	Objective
Reports of fatigue; confusion; restlessness; somnolence; verbal report of shortness of breath	Dyspnea; orthopnea; use of accessory muscles; abnormal breath sounds; limited chest excursion; abnormal skin color; diaphoresis; decreased pulse oximetry values; abnormal arterial blood gas values

RISK FACTORS

- Apnea, or impending inability to breathe
- Acute respiratory failure
- Severe hypoxia
- Respiratory muscle fatigue

DESIRED OUTCOMES

The client will experience adequate respiratory function as evidenced by:
a. Normal rate and depth of breathing
b. Decrease or absence of dyspnea
c. Normal breath sounds
d. Usual mental status
e. Oximetry results within baseline range
f. Arterial blood gas values within baseline range

NOC OUTCOMES

Respiratory status: airway patency; respiratory status: gas exchange; respiratory status: ventilation; mechanical ventilation response: adult; vital signs

NIC INTERVENTIONS

Respiratory monitoring; ventilation assistance; airway management: artificial; mechanical ventilation management: invasive; acid-base management

NURSING ASSESSMENT	RATIONALE
Assess for and report signs and symptoms of impaired respiratory function: • Rapid, shallow, respirations • Dyspnea, orthopnea • Use of accessory muscles • Abnormal breath sounds • Limited chest excursion • Restlessness, irritability • Confusion • Somnolence	*Early recognition of signs and symptoms of impaired respiratory function allows for prompt intervention.*
Monitor arterial blood gas values/oximetry values. Monitor vital signs.	*Allows for evaluation of therapy effectiveness* *Allows for assessment of client tolerance to ventilator settings. Changes in vital signs can indicate a decline in respiratory function.*

*This diagnostic label includes the following nursing diagnoses: impaired spontaneous ventilation, ineffective breathing pattern, ineffective airway clearance, and impaired gas exchange.

NDx = NANDA-I Diagnosis   **D** = Delegatable Action   ● = UAP   ✦ = LVN/LPN   ⊖▶ = Go to ⊖volve for animation

Continued...

NURSING ASSESSMENT	RATIONALE
Assess proper functioning of equipment: • Ventilator connections • Artificial airway (presence of cuff leak)	*Any equipment malfunction can compromise safe and effective mechanical ventilation.*
Monitor chest radiograph results.	*Chest radiograph confirms proper position of ETT. Potential complications such as pneumothorax, right mainstem intubation, and infection can be assessed by assessing chest radiograph results.*

THERAPEUTIC INTERVENTIONS	RATIONALE

Independent Actions

Implement measures to ensure airway patency: • Maintain ETT or tracheostomy. • Secure with tape or other device. • Perform endotracheal suctioning as appropriate.	*Actions that ensure airway patency contribute to adequate oxygenation and acid-base balance. An artificial airway must be maintained in proper position to ensure ventilation of both lung fields. Suctioning should occur as needed to clear the large airways of accumulated secretions.*
• Maintain appropriate bag-valve device (Ambu bag).	*An appropriate bag-valve device (Ambu) must be at the bedside of a client receiving mechanical ventilation in the event of equipment failure.*
Reposition client every 1 to 2 hours. **D** ●	*Frequent repositioning helps to loosen and mobilize secretions.*
Position client in a semi- to high-Fowler's position. **D** ●	*A semi- to high-Fowler's position allows for maximal diaphragmatic excursion and lung expansion.*

Dependent/Collaborative Actions

Maintain appropriate ventilator settings: Oxygen concentration (fraction of inspired oxygen [FIO_2]) Tidal volume (V_t) Ventilator rate (f) Positive end-expiratory pressure (PEEP)	*Adjustment of ventilator settings is accomplished collaboratively between the physician provider and the respiratory therapist.* *Settings are adjusted to reduce the work of breathing and facilitate adequate ventilation and oxygenation. The nurse should always reassess the client's physiological response to ventilator changes through physical assessment and examination of arterial blood gas values.*
Implement measures to ensure airway patency: • Monitor cuff pressure of ETT/tracheostomy tube.	*Inflating the cuff with the minimal amount of air needed to prevent leakage of air around the cuff ensures delivery of adequate V_t and prevents aspiration of oral secretions.*
Implement measures to thin secretions and maintain adequate moisture of the respiratory mucous membranes: • Humidify inspired air. • Regulate fluid intake to optimize fluid balance.	*Adequate hydration and humidified inspired air help thin secretions, which facilitates the mobilization and expectoration of secretions. These actions also reduce dryness of the respiratory mucous membrane, which helps enhance mucociliary clearance.*
Maintain integrity of ventilator circuit: • Keep ventilator circuit free of excess moisture. • Respond to ventilator alarms. • Monitor ventilator connections.	*These actions help to maximize the effectiveness of mechanical ventilation, ensure a patent airway, and promote patient safety.*
Assist with the administration of mucolytics as ordered: • Acetylcysteine • Water, saline	*Mucolytics and diluent or hydrating agents are mucokinetic substances that reduce the viscosity of mucus, thus making it easier for the client to mobilize and clear secretions from the respiratory tract.*
Administer the following medications if ordered: • Bronchodilators • Corticosteroids • Leukotriene modifiers	*These medications increase the patency of the airways and enhance bronchial airflow. Bronchodilators produce bronchodilation by relaxing the bronchial smooth muscle. Corticosteroids and leukotriene modifiers reduce inflammation in the airways, which results in decreased bronchial hyperactivity and constriction, and decreased mucus production.*

THERAPEUTIC INTERVENTIONS	RATIONALE
Collaborate with physician to develop a sedation plan: • Administer sedatives as ordered* (e.g., propofol [Diprivan]). • Administer neuromuscular blocking agents as ordered: • Cisatracurium besylate (Nimbex)	*These strategies will help facilitate optimum ventilation and gas exchange, reducing ventilator asynchrony.*
Consult appropriate health care provider if signs and symptoms of impaired respiratory function persist or worsen.	*Notifying the appropriate health care provider allows for modification of the treatment plan.*

Nursing Diagnosis RISK FOR INJURY NDx

Definition: At risk for injury as a result of the interaction of environmental conditions; interacting with the individual's adaptive and defensive resources

Related to:
• **External factors** such as cognitive impairment resulting from neuromuscular blockade/sedation, use of restraints during mechanical ventilation, presence of an artificial airway, and malfunction of equipment
• **Internal factors** such as confusion

CLINICAL MANIFESTATIONS

Subjective	Objective
Not evident in an intubated client	Altered neurovascular function in restrained limbs; breakdown of oral mucosa around ETT; ventilator malfunction: increased blood pressure, use of respiratory accessory muscles; gasping breaths

RISK FACTORS	DESIRED OUTCOMES
• Restraint of limbs during mechanical ventilation • Equipment failure • Agitation/confusion	The client will remain free of injuries.

NOC OUTCOMES	NIC INTERVENTIONS
Risk control; risk detection; mobility	Environmental risk protection

NURSING ASSESSMENT	RATIONALE

Assess the client's environment for potential and actual risk:
• Assess client for confusion/agitation.
• Assess working status of mechanical ventilator.
• Assess for the presence of appropriate emergency equipment:
  • Ambu bag
  • Power source
	Early recognition of potential risk factors for injury allows for modification of client's environment.

Assess artificial airway for proper securing: • Note the position of the ETT at lip line. • Assess bilateral breath sounds for symmetry. • Assess artificial airway cuff volume.	*Identifies risk for accidental extubation or improper placement of the ETT into the right mainstem bronchus.*
Assess for presence of skin breakdown: • Assess condition of lips.	*Identifies potential skin breakdown. Allows for modification of the treatment plan.*

---

*Important note: A client should never be rendered paralyzed without adequate sedation.

NDx = NANDA-I Diagnosis   **D** = Delegatable Action   ● = UAP   ✦ = LVN/LPN   ⊝▶ = Go to ⊝volve for animation

Continued...

THERAPEUTIC INTERVENTIONS	RATIONALE

Independent Actions

Implement measures to reduce incidence of injury.

Reposition ETT from side to side every 24 hours.

Keep bag-valve device at bedside at all times:
- Ambu bag

Respond to all ventilator alarms:

High-pressure alarms (biting on the tube, presence of excessive secretions)

Low-pressure alarms (disconnection from ventilator circuit, cuff leak)

Reduces the risk of skin breakdown

Provides a source for manual ventilation in the event of equipment failure.

Alarm systems alert the nurse to possible machine malfunctions and should be responded to immediately to reduce the risk of inadequate ventilation or loss of airway.

Dependent/Collaborative Actions

Obtain a physician's order for the use of restraints.
- Apply soft bilateral wrist restraints.

Restraints are often a standard of care for client's who are receiving mechanical ventilation.

Circulation to affected extremities should be checked in accordance to safety standards to avoid complications associated with the use of restraints.

Notify the appropriate health care provider in the event of patient injury.

Notifying the appropriate health care provider allows for modification of the treatment plan.

Nursing Diagnosis   # IMBALANCED NUTRITION: LESS THAN BODY REQUIREMENTS NDx

Definition: Intake of nutrients insufficient to meet metabolic demands

Related to: Inability to absorb nutrients and ingest food

CLINICAL MANIFESTATIONS

Subjective	Objective
Not evident in an intubated client	Evidence of lack of food; poor muscle tone; hyperactive bowel sounds; decreased subcutaneous fat; weight loss; sore, inflamed buccal cavity; low serum albumin and total protein levels, iron deficiency; electrolyte imbalances

RISK FACTORS
- Inadequate nutritional therapy
- Increased caloric requirements
- Altered gastrointestinal motility

DESIRED OUTCOMES

The client will:
- a. Consume adequate nourishment
- b. Be free of signs of malnutrition
- c. Weigh within normal range for height and age

NOC OUTCOMES

Nutritional status

NIC INTERVENTIONS

Nutritional monitoring; nutritional management; nutritional therapy

NURSING ASSESSMENT	RATIONALE

Assess for and report signs and symptoms of malnutrition:
- Weight significantly below client's usual weight or below normal for client's age, height, and body frame
- Weakness and fatigue
- Sore, inflamed oral mucous membrane
- Pale conjunctiva

Early recognition of signs and symptoms of malnutrition allows for prompt intervention.

NURSING ASSESSMENT	RATIONALE
Assess for return of bowel function every 2 to 4 hours.	
Monitor serum albumin, prealbumin, total protein, ferritin, transferrin, hemoglobin, hematocrit, and serum electrolyte levels as indicated.	*Serum albumin levels less than 3.5 g/100 dL are considered a risk for poor nutritional status. Early recognition of abnormal lab values reflective of the client's overall nutritional state allows for prompt intervention.*

THERAPEUTIC INTERVENTIONS	RATIONALE
Dependent/Collaborative Actions	
Consult physician about an alternative method of providing nutrition: • Enteral nutrition • Parenteral nutrition	*Enteral feeding is the preferred method to meet the hypermetabolic nutritional needs of the ventilated client. If the client is unable to be fed enterally, nutritional support in the form of parenteral nutrition must be provided.*

Nursing Diagnosis **RISK FOR INFECTION NDx (VENTILATOR-ACQUIRED PNEUMONIA [VAP])**

Definition: At increased risk for being invaded by pathogenic organisms

Related to:
- Inadequate primary defenses
- Decrease in mucociliary action
- Stasis of pulmonary secretions
- Malnutrition
- Presence of invasive artificial airway
- Increased environmental exposure to pathogens

CLINICAL MANIFESTATIONS

Subjective *Not applicable*	Objective Increased temperature, B/P

RISK FACTORS
- Pooling of oropharyngeal secretions
- Immobility
- Malnutrition

DESIRED OUTCOMES

The client will remain free of infection as evidenced by:
  a. No increase in temperature
  b. Absence of purulent sputum
  c. Normal breath sounds
  d. Normal chest radiograph findings
  e. WBC and differential counts returning to normal or within normal limits

NOC OUTCOMES	NIC INTERVENTIONS
Immune status; infection severity	Infection protection; infection control

NURSING ASSESSMENT	RATIONALE
Assess for signs and symptoms of VAP: • Elevated temperature • Purulent sputum • Odorous sputum • Abnormal breath sounds (crackles, rhonchi)	*Early recognition of signs and symptoms of VAP allows for prompt intervention.*

Continued...

NURSING ASSESSMENT	RATIONALE
Assess WBC and differential cell counts for abnormalities.	*An increase in the WBC count above previous levels and/or a significant change in the differential may indicate the presence of an infection. Monitoring results allows for modification of treatment plan.*
Monitor chest radiograph results.	*The presence of pulmonary infiltrates on chest radiograph indicates the presence of pneumonia.*
Monitor results of sputum cultures.	*Monitoring results allows for modification of treatment plan.*

THERAPEUTIC INTERVENTIONS	RATIONALE

Independent Actions

Implement measures to reduce the risk for VAP:

- Elevate head of the bed a minimum of 30° to 45°.

  Head of the bed elevation reduces the risk of aspiration of gastric secretions.

- Use proper hand hygiene:
  - Frequent hand washing before and after suctioning
  - Wear gloves when in contact with the patient and change gloves between activities.

  Prevents the transmission of bacteria to the patient.

- Drain excess condensation in ventilator circuit.
- Suction oral cavity at least every 4 hours.

  Removes bacteria from the oropharynx and prevents aspiration of bacteria-laden secretions.

- Provide oral care.
- Maintain integrity of ETT/tracheostomy cuff.

Dependent/Collaborative Actions

Notify the appropriate health care provider if signs and symptoms of VAP develop.

Notifying the appropriate health care provider allows for modification of the treatment plan.

Obtain cultures as ordered.

Nursing Diagnosis | # ACTUAL/RISK FOR DYSFUNCTIONAL VENTILATORY WEANING RESPONSE NDx

Definition: Inability to adjust to lowered levels of mechanical ventilator support that interrupts and prolongs the weaning process

Related to:

- **Physiological factors:** ineffective airway clearance; sleep disturbance; inadequate nutrition; uncontrolled pain or discomfort
- **Psychological factors:** knowledge deficient of the weaning process; moderate amount of anxiety or fear; hopelessness; powerlessness; insufficient trust in health care team
- **Situational factors:** uncontrolled energy demands; inappropriate pacing of diminished ventilator support; inadequate social support; adverse environment; low nurse-to-client ratio; history of ventilator dependence greater than 4 days to 1 week; history of multiple unsuccessful weaning attempts

CLINICAL MANIFESTATIONS

Subjective	Objective
Expressed feelings of increased need for oxygen; queries about possible machine malfunction	Apprehension; agitation; baseline increase in respiratory rate (<5 breaths/minute); diaphoresis; adventitious breath sounds; asynchronized breathing with the ventilator; cyanosis; decreased level of consciousness; use of respiratory accessory muscles; gasping breaths; increase from baseline blood pressure; inability to cooperate; inability to respond to coaching

RISK FACTORS

- Prolonged mechanical ventilation
- Muscle weakness
- Activity intolerance
- Debilitated state

DESIRED OUTCOMES

The client will wean from mechanical ventilation as evidenced by:
   a. Arterial blood gas values within client's normal baseline
   b. Absence of dyspnea
   c. Absence of restlessness
   d. Ability to effectively clear secretions
   e. Tolerating and maintaining airway after extubation
   f. Vital signs within normal limits

NOC OUTCOMES

Anxiety self-control; mechanical ventilation weaning response: adult; respiratory status: gas exchange; respiratory status: ventilation; vital signs

NIC INTERVENTIONS

Mechanical ventilatory weaning; mechanical ventilation management: invasive

NURSING ASSESSMENT

Assess client's readiness for weaning:
- Resolution of underlying disease process
- Hemodynamic stability
- Absence of fever
- Normal state of consciousness
- Metabolic fluid balance
- Adequate nutritional status
- Adequate sleep

Assess client's psychological readiness to wean.
Assess client's tolerance of weaning process:
- Work of breathing
- Vital signs
- Pulse oximetry values
- Arterial blood gas values

Monitor hemoglobin (Hgb)/hematocrit (Hct); serum electrolyte levels; serum albumin/prealbumin levels; chest radiograph for improvements

RATIONALE

Early recognition of readiness to wean allows for prompt intervention.

THERAPEUTIC INTERVENTIONS

Independent Actions
Implement measures to facilitate the weaning process:
- Provide a safe, comfortable environment.
- Coordinate pain and sedation medications to minimize sedative effects.
- Schedule weaning periods for the time of the day when the client is most rested.
- Promote a normal sleep-wake cycle.
- Limit visitors to supportive persons.
- Coach client through periods of anxiety.
- Cluster care activities to promote successful weaning.
- Educate patient and family about the weaning process.

Evaluate patient tolerance of the weaning process.

Dependent/Collaborative Actions
Assist respiratory therapist in assessing readiness to wean by assessing:
- Minute ventilation
- Negative inspiratory force
- Vital capacity

RATIONALE

Comfort will facilitate the weaning process.
Fatigued respiratory muscles require 12 to 24 hours to recover.

Educating the client and family allows for the appropriate level of psychological support.
Allows for modification of the weaning plan

Assessment of the mechanics of weaning allows for determination of the client's ability to support normal ventilation.

NDx = NANDA-I Diagnosis   **D** = Delegatable Action   ● = UAP   ✦ = LVN/LPN   ⊖▶ = Go to ⊖volve for animation

Continued...

THERAPEUTIC INTERVENTIONS	RATIONALE
Use evidenced-based protocols for weaning.	*Protocol-driven weaning provides a standardized approach to the weaning process.*
Recommend a spontaneous breathing trial: • 30 to 120 minutes with PEEP/continuous positive airway pressure (CPAP) or t-piece	*Tolerance of a weaning trial helps to demonstrate readiness for extubation.*
Notify appropriate health care provider of signs and symptoms of dysfunctional weaning: • Respiration rate less than 8 or greater than 30 breaths/min • B/P changes greater than 20% of baseline • Heart rate changes greater than 20% of baseline • Pulse oximetry less than 90% • Decrease in spontaneous tidal volume • Labored respirations • Diaphoresis • Restlessness • Anxiety	*Notifying the appropriate health care provider allows for modification of the treatment plan.*

Collaborative Diagnosis   RISK FOR DECREASED CARDIAC OUTPUT NDx

Definition: Inability of the heart to maintain client's normal output

Related to: Altered hemodynamics related to increased intrathoracic pressure associated with positive pressure mechanical ventilation

CLINICAL MANIFESTATIONS

Subjective	Objective
Not evident in an intubated client	Hypotension; tachycardia; decreased level of consciousness

RISK FACTORS	DESIRED OUTCOMES

• Large tidal volumes
• PEEP
	The client will maintain normal cardiac output as evidenced by:
	   a. B/P within baseline range
	   b. Heart rate within baseline range
	   c. Measured cardiac output/index within normal range

NURSING ASSESSMENT	RATIONALE
Assess for and report signs and symptoms of decreased cardiac output. Monitor vital signs frequently. Measure cardiac output/index if ordered.	*Early recognition of signs and symptoms of decreased cardiac output allows for prompt intervention.*

THERAPEUTIC INTERVENTIONS	RATIONALE
Independent Actions Monitor client's response to ventilator changes: • Adding of PEEP	*PEEP increases intrathoracic pressure, which may further decrease venous return, compromising cardiac output.*

THERAPEUTIC INTERVENTIONS	RATIONALE
Dependent/Collaborative Actions	
Administer intravenous fluids as ordered.	*Helps to restore circulating volume, which helps to minimize cardiovascular effects*
Administer vasoactive infusions to restore normal cardiac output:	*Helps to maintain normal cardiac output*
• Inotropes	*Inotropes increase the force of cardiac contractions, which increases cardiac output.*
• Vasopressors	*Vasopressors should only be used if circulating volume has been restored.*
Notify physician provider if signs and symptoms of decreased cardiac output persist or worsen.	*Notifying the appropriate health care provider allows for modification of the treatment plan.*

Collaborative Diagnosis | RISK FOR BAROTRAUMA

Definition: Damage to the lungs

Related to:
• Increased lung inflation pressures
• Noncompliant lungs

CLINICAL MANIFESTATIONS

Subjective	Objective
Not evident in an intubated client	Pneumomediastinum on chest radiograph; pneumothorax on chest radiograph; subcutaneous emphysema in the neck area; high peak inspiratory pressures; absence of breath sounds on affected side

RISK FACTORS	DESIRED OUTCOMES
• Large tidal volumes • PEEP • Reduced lung compliance/stiff lungs	The client will maintain normal lung inflation as evidenced by: 　a. Normal chest radiograph results 　b. Normal or baseline peak inspiratory pressures 　c. Absence of subcutaneous emphysema 　d. Symmetrical breath sounds

NURSING ASSESSMENT	RATIONALE
Assess for and report signs and symptoms barotrauma: • Sudden occurrence of unexplained subcutaneous emphysema • Asymmetrical/absent breath sounds Monitor results of chest radiograph.	*Early recognition of signs and symptoms of barotrauma allows for prompt intervention.*

THERAPEUTIC INTERVENTIONS	RATIONALE
Dependent/Collaborative Actions Notify physician provider of signs/symptoms of barotrauma. Prepare for insertion of chest tube.	*Notifying the appropriate health care provider allows for modification of the treatment plan.*

Collaborative Diagnosis RISK FOR FLUID RETENTION/FLUID VOLUME OVERLOAD

Definition: Changes in the body that head to fluid imbalance

Related to:
- Ventilator humidification
- Stimulation of the renin-angiotensin-aldosterone mechanism leading to retention of sodium and water

CLINICAL MANIFESTATIONS

Subjective	Objective
Not evident in an intubated client	Increase in weight; anasarca; positive fluid balance; adventitious breath sounds; increase in B/P; decrease in urine output.

RISK FACTORS

- Decreased cardiac output
- Diminished renal perfusion
- Pressure changes within the thorax

DESIRED OUTCOMES

The client will maintain normal fluid volume status as evidenced by:
a. Weight within client's baseline range
b. Balanced intake and output
c. Vital signs within client's normal baseline
d. Normal breath sounds

NURSING ASSESSMENT	RATIONALE
Assess for and report signs and symptoms of fluid volume overload: • Abnormal breath sounds (crackles) • Increase in weight • Positive fluid balance • Increased B/P • Increased heart rate Monitor results of chest radiograph. Monitor vital signs/pulse oximetry values.	*Early recognition and reporting of signs and symptoms of fluid volume overload allow for prompt intervention.*

THERAPEUTIC INTERVENTIONS	RATIONALE
Dependent/Collaborative Actions Notify physician provider of signs/symptoms of fluid volume overload.	*Notifying the appropriate health care provider allows for modification of the treatment plan.*

Collaborative Diagnosis RISK FOR GASTROINTESTINAL BLEEDING

Definition: Bleeding within the gastrointestinal tract

Related to:
- Positive pressure ventilation
- Stress of critical illness/stress ulcers
- Atrophy of mucosal lining of stomach due to lack of enteral feeding

CLINICAL MANIFESTATIONS

Subjective	Objective
Not evident in an intubated client	Bleeding in stools; hematemesis

RISK FACTORS

- Stress of acute illness

DESIRED OUTCOMES

The client will not experience gastrointestinal bleeding.

NURSING ASSESSMENT	RATIONALE
Assess for and report signs and symptoms.	*Early recognition of signs and symptoms of gastrointestinal bleeding allows for prompt intervention.*

THERAPEUTIC INTERVENTIONS	RATIONALE
Dependent/Collaborative Actions	
Administer histamine (H₂) receptor blockers; proton pump inhibitors.	*Medications act to decrease gastric acidity and diminish the risk of stress ulcers.*
Administer enteral feedings as ordered.	*Stimulates the intestinal mucosa, preventing atrophy and disruption*
Notify physician provider if signs and symptoms persist or worsen.	*Notifying the appropriate health care provider allows for modification of the treatment plan.*

ADDITIONAL NURSING DIAGNOSES

FEAR/ANXIETY NDx
Related to the perceived need for mechanical ventilation; inability to communicate effectively; psychological ventilator dependence

RISK FOR ASPIRATION NDx
Related to presence of an artificial airway that bypasses normal upper airway defenses

IMPAIRED PHYSICAL MOBILITY NDx
Related to mechanical ventilation

IMPAIRED VERBAL COMMUNICATION NDx
Related to artificial airway and mechanical ventilation

IMPAIRED ORAL MUCOUS MEMBRANE NDx
Related to the presence of an artificial airway; bypass of normal physiological humidification process

POWERLESSNESS NDx
Related to illness-related regimen; lifestyle of helplessness

PNEUMONIA

Pneumonia or pneumonitis is an acute inflammation of lung tissue that can be caused by a variety of infectious agents, chemical irritants, or radiation therapy. Infectious organisms that cause pneumonia reach the lungs by inhalation, aspiration of nasopharyngeal or oropharyngeal contents, or by hematogenous spread of infection from another site in the body.

Pneumonia may be classified according to the causative organism (e.g., pneumococcal pneumonia, staphylococcal pneumonia, viral pneumonia), the area of involvement (e.g., lobar pneumonia), or the etiological factor (e.g., aspiration pneumonia, radiation pneumonitis). Pneumonia may also be classified as community-acquired pneumonia (CAP) or hospital-acquired pneumonia (HAP), the latter often referred to as nosocomial.

Most persons hospitalized with pneumonia have bacterial pneumonia. The onset of bacterial pneumonia is often abrupt and manifested by chills, fever, a cough productive of purulent or blood-tinged sputum, and pleuritic chest pain (in some cases). Elderly persons, who often have impaired immune mechanisms, may present with a change in mental status and a recent history of weakness, fatigue, and a decline in appetite rather than the symptoms of typical pneumonia.

This care plan focuses on the adult client hospitalized with bacterial pneumonia. Much of the information is applicable to clients receiving follow-up care in an extended care facility or home setting.

OUTCOME/DISCHARGE CRITERIA

The client will:
1. Have improved respiratory function
2. Tolerate expected level of activity
3. Have no signs and symptoms of complications
4. State signs and symptoms to report to the health care provider
5. Verbalize an understanding of and a plan for adhering to recommended follow-up care including future appointments with health care provider, medications prescribed, and activity limitations

Nursing Diagnosis   IMPAIRED RESPIRATORY FUNCTION*

Definition: Inability of an individual to maintain adequate ventilation of the respiratory tract and perfusion of oxygen and carbon dioxide between the lungs and vascular system to maintain adequate tissue oxygenation

Ineffective breathing pattern NDx

Related to:

- Decreased depth of respirations associated with:
  - Weakness, fatigue, and reluctance to breathe deeply because of chest pain
  - Decreased lung compliance (distensibility) if pleural effusion is present
- Increased rate of respirations associated with:
  - Compensation for hypoxia that results from impaired gas exchange
  - The increase in metabolic rate that occurs with an infectious process

Ineffective airway clearance NDx

Related to:

- Tracheobronchial inflammation and increased production of mucus associated with the infectious process
- Stasis of secretions associated with decreased activity, poor cough effort resulting from fatigue and chest pain, impaired ciliary function (results from increased viscosity and volume of mucus that occurs with the infectious process

Impaired gas exchange NDx

Related to:

- A decrease in effective lung surface associated with the accumulation of mucus and consolidation of lung tissue

CLINICAL MANIFESTATIONS

Subjective	Objective
Report of shortness of breath and chest tightness	Tachypnea; pharyngitis; dullness on percussion over consolidated areas; abnormal breath sounds; productive cough; fever; irritability; confusion; disorientation; restlessness; somnolence; use of accessory muscles when breathing; pink, rusty, purulent, green, yellow, or white sputum; significant decrease in oximetry results; abnormal arterial blood gas values; abnormal chest radiograph results; declining results in pulmonary function tests; reduced activity tolerance; asymmetrical chest excursion

RISK FACTORS

- Smoking
- Outdoor/indoor pollutants
- Exposure to second-hand cigarette smoke
- Allergies
- Low birth weight
- Periodontal disease
- Individuals older than 60 years
- White male

DESIRED OUTCOMES

The client will maintain adequate respiratory function as evidenced by:

  a. Normal rate and depth of respirations
  b. Decreased dyspnea
  c. Usual or improved breath sounds
  d. Symmetrical chest excursion
  e. Usual mental status
  f. Oximetry results within normal range for client
  g. Arterial blood gas values within normal range for client

NOC OUTCOMES

Respiratory status: airway patency; respiratory status: ventilation; respiratory status: gas exchange

NIC INTERVENTIONS

Respiratory monitoring; airway management; tube care: chest; cough enhancement; oxygen therapy; ventilation assistance; anxiety reduction

---

*This diagnostic label includes the following nursing diagnoses: ineffective breathing pattern, ineffective airway clearance, and impaired gas exchange.

NURSING ASSESSMENT	RATIONALE
Assess for signs and symptoms of impaired respiratory function:	*Early recognition of signs and symptoms of ineffective breathing patterns allows for prompt intervention.*
• Dyspnea, orthopnea	
• Use of accessory muscles when breathing	
• Abnormal breath sounds (e.g., diminished, bronchial, crackles, wheezes)	*Changes in the characteristics of breath sounds may be due to airway obstruction, mucous plugs, or retained secretions in larger airways.*
• Asymmetrical or limited chest excursion	
• Cough (usually a productive cough of rust-colored, purulent, or blood-tinged sputum)	
• Restlessness, irritability	*Restlessness, irritability, and changes in mental status or level of consciousness indicate an oxygen deficiency and require immediate treatment.*
• Confusion, somnolence	
• Central cyanosis (a late sign)	
• Significant decrease in oximetry results	*Oximetry is a noninvasive method of measuring arterial oxygen saturation. The results assist in evaluating respiratory status.*
• Abnormal arterial blood gas values	*Decreasing PaO_2 and increasing $PaCO_2$ are indicators of respiratory problems.*
• Changes in vital signs	*Increased work of breathing or hypoxia may cause tachycardia and/or hypertension.*
Assess arterial blood gas values, oximetry values, and chest radiograph results. Report abnormal findings.	*Changes in infiltrates noted in the lungs require prompt treatment.*

THERAPEUTIC INTERVENTIONS	RATIONALE

Independent Actions

Implement measures to improve respiratory status:

• Place client in a semi-Fowler's position and position overbed table so client can lean on it if desired. **D** ● ✦	*Positioning in semi-Fowler's position promotes optimal gas exchange by enabling chest expansion. Leaning on the overbed table decreases dyspnea through pressure on the gastric contents and diaphragmatic contraction.*
• Instruct client to breathe slowly if hyperventilating.	*Slowing the pace of breathing makes each breath more effective.*
• If client must remain flat in bed, assist with position change at least every 2 hours. **D** ✦ ●	*Prevents consolidation of secretions*
• Assist client to deep breathe or use incentive spirometer every 1 to 2 hours. **D** ✦	*Forced deep breathing and use of incentive spirometry will increase expansion of the lungs and improve the client's ability to clear mucus from the lungs. The technique may also improve the amount of oxygen that is able to penetrate deep into the lungs.*
• Maintain client fluid intake of at least 2500 mL/day unless contraindicated. **D** ✦	*Increased fluid intake promotes thinning of secretions and reduces dryness of the respiratory mucous membranes.*
• Instruct client to avoid intake of large meals, gas-forming foods (i.e., cauliflower, beans, cabbage, onions, etc.), and carbonated beverages.	*Gas-forming foods and carbonated beverages can cause abdominal bloating, which places pressure on the diaphragm and reduces lung expansion.*
• Discourage smoking.	*The irritants in smoke increase mucus production, impair ciliary function, and can cause inflammation and damage to the bronchial and alveolar walls; the carbon monoxide decreases oxygen availability.*
• Maintain activity restrictions and increase activity as allowed and tolerated. **D** ● ✦	*Conservation of energy through activity restrictions allows energy to be focused on breathing. Increasing activity as tolerated helps to mobilize secretions and promotes deeper breathing.*

Dependent/Collaborative Actions

Implement measures to improve respiratory status:

• Assist with or perform postural drainage therapy if ordered.	*Prevents consolidation of secretions*
• Perform suctioning if ordered. **D** ✦	*Removes secretions from the large airways. It also stimulates coughing, which helps clear airways of mucus and foreign matter.*
• Humidify inspired air as ordered. **D** ✦	*Liquefies secretions, improving client's ability to eliminate them through expectoration*
• Assist with administration of mucolytics and diluent or hydrating agents via nebulizer if ordered. **D** ✦	*Mucolytics and diluent or hydrating agents help to liquefy secretions for more effective removal.*

NDx = NANDA-I Diagnosis   **D** = Delegatable Action   ● = UAP   ✦ = LVN/LPN   ⊝▶ = Go to ⊝volve for animation

Continued...

THERAPEUTIC INTERVENTIONS	RATIONALE
• Avoid use of central nervous system (CNS) depressants.	*CNS depressants further depress respiratory status, exacerbating the client's condition.*
• Administer and monitor oxygen as ordered. **D** ✦	*Provides supplemental oxygen if required by client*
• Administer bronchodilators, antimicrobials, expectorants. **D** ✦	*Bronchodilators relax smooth muscles of the airway, thus improving air exchange in the lungs. Antimicrobials may be given to prevent or treat pneumonia. Expectorants help client to remove secretions from the lungs.*
Consult appropriate health care providers—(respiratory therapist and physician) if signs and symptoms of impaired respiratory function persist or worsen.	*Notifying the appropriate health care professionals allows for a multidisciplinary approach to treatment.*

Nursing Diagnosis RISK FOR DEFICIENT FLUID VOLUME NDx

Definition: At risk for experiencing vascular, cellular, or intracellular dehydration

Related to: Decreased oral intake and excessive fluid loss (occurs with profuse diaphoresis and hyperventilation if present)

CLINICAL MANIFESTATIONS

Subjective	Objective
Report of thirst	Decreased B/P; decreased pulse pressure; decreased pulse volume; decreased skin turgor; decreased urine output; dry skin; elevated Hct; increased temperature; increased pulse rate; weakness

RISK FACTORS

- Active fluid volume loss
- Failure of regulatory mechanisms
- Decreased fluid volume intake
- Increased insensible loss of fluid

DESIRED OUTCOMES

The client will not experience a deficient fluid volume as evidenced by:
  a. Normal skin turgor
  b. Moist mucous membrane
  c. Stable weight
  d. B/P and pulse rate within normal range for client and stable with position change
  e. Capillary refill time less than 2 to 3 seconds
  f. Usual mental status
  g. BUN and Hct within normal range
  h. Balanced intake and output
  i. Urine specific gravity within normal range

NOC OUTCOMES

Fluid balance; hydration; kidney function; vital signs

NIC INTERVENTIONS

Fluid management; fluid monitoring; fluid resuscitation; hypovolemia management; intravenous therapy

NURSING ASSESSMENT	RATIONALE
Assess for signs and symptoms of deficient fluid volume: • Decreased skin turgor • Dry mucous membranes, thirst • Weight loss of 2% or greater over a short period • Postural hypotension and/or low B/P • Weak, rapid pulse • Capillary refill time greater than 2 to 3 seconds • Neck veins flat when client is supine • Change in mental status • Elevated BUN and Hct • Decreased urine output with increased specific gravity (reflects an actual rather than potential fluid volume deficit)	*Early recognition of signs and symptoms of deficient fluid volume allows for prompt intervention.*

THERAPEUTIC INTERVENTIONS	RATIONALE
Independent Actions	
Implement measures to reduce nausea and vomiting if present:	*Nausea often causes the client to have decreased fluid volume intake. Persistent vomiting results in excessive loss of fluid.*
• Instruct client to ingest food/fluid slowly.	
• Eliminate noxious sights and odors. **D ● ✦**	
Implement measures to control diarrhea if present:	*Persistent or severe diarrhea results in excessive loss of gastrointestinal fluid.*
• Discourage intake of spicy foods and foods high in fiber or lactose.	
Implement measures to reduce fever if present:	*Fever may be accompanied by diaphoresis, which can result in excessive loss of fluid.*
• Sponge bath client with tepid water. **D ● ✦**	
• Remove excessive clothing or bedcovers. **D ● ✦**	
Carefully measure drainage:	*Accurate intake/output records must be maintained to ensure fluid loss is replaced appropriately.*
• Nasogastric **D ✦**	
• Wound **D ✦**	
• Urine **D ✦**	
Dependent/Collaborative Actions	
Maintain a fluid intake of at least 2500 mL/day unless contraindicated. **D ✦**	*Adequate fluid intake needs to be provided in order to ensure adequate hydration.*
Implement measures to reduce nausea and vomiting if present:	*Nausea often causes the client to have decreased fluid volume intake. Persistent vomiting results in excessive loss of fluid.*
• Administer antiemetics as ordered. **D ✦**	
Implement measures to control diarrhea if present:	*Persistent or severe diarrhea results in excessive loss of gastrointestinal fluid.*
• Administer antidiarrheal agents as ordered. **D ✦**	
Implement measures to reduce fever if present:	*Fever may be accompanied by diaphoresis, which can result in excessive loss of fluid.*
• Administer antipyretics as ordered. **D ✦**	
Administer and maintain intravenous replacement fluids as ordered.	*Replacing fluid volume that is lost helps prevent/treat deficient fluid volume.*
Consult physician if signs and symptoms of deficient fluid volume persist or worsen.	*Notifying the physician allows for modification of the treatment plan.*

Nursing Diagnosis ## IMBALANCED NUTRITION: LESS THAN BODY REQUIREMENTS NDx

Definition: Intake of nutrients insufficient to meet metabolic needs

Related to: Increased expenditure of energy to support the work of breathing

CLINICAL MANIFESTATIONS

Subjective	Objective
Complaints of sore oral mucous membrane; complaints of altered taste sensations	Weight loss; weight less than normal for client's age, height, and body frame; abnormal BUN and low serum prealbumin and albumin levels; inflamed mucous membranes; pale conjunctiva; dyspnea on exertion

RISK FACTORS

- Smoking
- Aerosol treatments
- Productive cough
- Dyspnea
- Excessive coughing

DESIRED OUTCOMES

The client will maintain adequate nutrition status as evidenced by:
  a. Weight within normal range for client
  b. Normal BUN and serum prealbumin and albumin levels
  c. Usual strength and activity tolerance
  d. Healthy oral mucous membrane

NDx = NANDA-I Diagnosis   **D** = Delegatable Action   ● = UAP   ✦ = LVN/LPN   ⊖▶ = Go to Evolve for animation

Continued...

NOC OUTCOMES	NIC INTERVENTIONS
Nutritional status	Nutritional monitoring; nutrition management; nutrition therapy

NURSING ASSESSMENT	RATIONALE
Assess for and report signs and symptoms of malnutrition: • Weight significantly below client's usual weight or less than normal for client's age, height, and body frame • Abnormal BUN and low serum prealbumin and albumin levels • Increased weakness and fatigue • Sore, inflamed oral mucous membrane • Pale conjunctiva	*Early recognition of signs and symptoms of malnutrition allows for prompt intervention.*

THERAPEUTIC INTERVENTIONS	RATIONALE

Independent Actions

Monitor percentage of meals and snacks client consumes. Report inadequate intake. **D** ● ✦

Monitoring a client's intake helps to identify when a patient is at risk for inadequate nutrition and allows for prompt intervention.

Implement measures to maintain an adequate nutritional status:
* Schedule treatments that assist in mobilizing mucus (e.g., aerosol treatments, postural drainage therapy) at least 1 hour before or after meals. **D** ✦

The foul odor and taste of sputum and some aerosols are likely to decrease appetite. Appropriate scheduling of treatments also assists in decreasing nausea.

* Increase activity as tolerated. **D** ● ✦

Activity usually promotes a sense of well-being and can help improve an individual's appetite.

* Encourage a rest period before meals.

Rest before a meal helps to minimize the fatigue that may occur when eating.

* Eliminate noxious sights and odors from the environment; provide client with an opaque, covered container for expectorated sputum. **D** ● ✦

Noxious sights and odors can decrease one's appetite. By eliminating them, the patient's intake may improve.

* Maintain a clean environment and a relaxed, pleasant atmosphere. **D** ● ✦

A clean environment and a relaxed atmosphere may increase intake.

* Provide oral hygiene before meals. **D** ● ✦

Oral hygiene moistens the mouth, which makes it easier to chew and swallow. It also removes unpleasant tastes, which often improves the taste of foods/fluids.

* Assist the client who is quite dyspneic in selecting foods that require little or no chewing.

Dyspnea decreases the ability of an individual to eat complete meals.

* Serve frequent, small meals rather than large ones if the client is weak, fatigues easily, or has a poor appetite. **D** ● ✦

Small, frequent meals decrease fatigue and help to maintain an individual's nutritional status.

* Limit fluid intake with meals unless the fluid has high nutritional value. **D** ✦

Decreasing fluid intake during meals helps to reduce early satiety and subsequent decreased food intake.

* Allow for adequate time for meals. **D** ● ✦

Clients who feel rushed during meals tend to become anxious, lose their appetite, and stop eating.

* Ensure that meals are well balanced and high in essential nutrients.

A diet that is well balanced and high in essential nutrients meets the client's nutritional needs.

Dependent/Collaborative Actions

Implement measures to maintain an adequate nutritional status:
* Place client in a high-Fowler's position for meals and provide supplemental oxygen therapy during meals if indicated. **D** ✦

Supplemental oxygen helps to relieve dyspnea.

* Obtain a dietary consult to assist client in selecting foods/fluids that meet nutritional needs, are appealing, and adhere to personal and cultural preferences.

Notifying the appropriate health care professionals allows for a multifaceted approach to treatment.

THERAPEUTIC INTERVENTIONS	RATIONALE
• Perform a calorie count if ordered and report information to dietitian and physician.	*A calorie count provides information about the caloric and nutritional value of the foods/fluids consumed. The information helps the dietitian and physician determine whether an alternative method of nutritional support is needed.*
• Administer vitamins and minerals if ordered. **D** ✦	*Administration of vitamins and minerals helps to partially maintain nutritional status if dietary intake is not adequate.*
Consult a physician about an alternative method of providing nutrition (e.g., parenteral nutrition, tube feedings) if client does not consume enough food or fluids to meet nutritional needs.	*If a client is unable to eat, collaboration with the physician is required to determine alternative methods of maintaining nutritional status.*

Nursing Diagnosis ACUTE PAIN NDx (CHEST)

Definition: Unpleasant sensory and emotional experience arising from actual or potential tissue damage or described in terms of such damage (International Association for the Study of Pain); sudden or slow onset of any intensity from mild to severe with an anticipated or predictable end and a duration of <6 months

Related to:
• Extension of the inflammatory/infection process to the pleura
• Muscle strain associated with excessive coughing

CLINICAL MANIFESTATIONS

Subjective	Objective
Verbalization of pain in chest with breathing and coughing	Increased blood pressure; increased heart rate; changes in respiratory rate; diaphoresis

RISK FACTORS	DESIRED OUTCOMES

• Excessive coughing
• Increased sputum production
• Smoking and exposure to second-hand smoke
	The client will experience diminished chest pain as evidenced by:
	   a. Verbalization of a decrease in or absence of pain
	   b. Relaxed facial expression and body positioning
	   c. increased participation in activities

NOC OUTCOMES	NIC INTERVENTIONS
Comfort level; pain control	Pain management; environmental management; analgesic administration

NURSING ASSESSMENT	RATIONALE
Assess for signs and symptoms of pain (e.g., verbalization of pain, grimacing, reluctance to move, guarding of affected side of chest).	*Early recognition of signs and symptoms of pain allows for prompt intervention and improved pain control.*
Assess client's perception of the severity of pain using a pain intensity rating scale.	*An awareness of the severity of pain being experienced helps determine the most appropriate interventions for pain management. Use of a pain intensity scale gives the nurse a clearer understanding of the pain being experienced and promotes consistency when communicating with others about the client's pain experience.*
Assess the client's pain pattern (e.g., location, quality, onset, duration, precipitating factors, aggravating factors, alleviating factors).	*Knowledge of the client's pain pattern assists in the identification of effective pain management interventions.*

NDx = NANDA-I Diagnosis   **D** = Delegatable Action   ● = UAP   ✦ = LVN/LPN   ⊝▶ = Go to ⊝volve for animation

Continued...

NURSING ASSESSMENT	RATIONALE
Ask the client to describe previous pain experiences and methods used to manage pain effectively.	*Many variables affect a client's response to pain (e.g., age, sex, coping style, previous experience with pain, culture, cause of pain). Knowledge of the client's usual response to pain and methods previously used to manage pain effectively enables the nurse to evaluate the client's pain more accurately and facilitates the identification of effective strategies for pain management.*

THERAPEUTIC INTERVENTIONS	RATIONALE

Independent Actions

Implement measures to reduce fear and anxiety (e.g., assure client that chest pain is common with pneumonia and should subside with treatment of the pneumonia; assure the client that the need for pain relief is understood). **D ✦**	*Fear and anxiety can decrease the client's threshold and tolerance for pain and thereby heighten the perception of pain. In addition, pain management methods are not as effective if the client is tense and unable to relax.*
Implement measures to promote rest (e.g., minimize environmental activity and noise). **D ● ✦**	*Fatigue can decrease the client's threshold and tolerance for pain and thereby heighten the perception of pain. A client who is well rested often experiences decreased pain and increased effectiveness of pain management measures.*
Instruct and assist the client to splint the chest with hands or pillows when deep breathing, coughing, or changing position. **D ✦**	*Splinting the chest with deep breathing, coughing, or changing position reduces pain and promotes a more effective cough.*

Dependent/Collaborative Actions

Administer analgesics before activities and procedures that can cause pain and before pain becomes severe. **D ✦**	*The administration of analgesics before a pain-producing event helps minimize the pain that may be experienced during a procedure.*
Consult appropriate health care provider (e.g., physician, pharmacist, pain management specialist) if above measures fail to provide adequate pain relief	*Notifying the appropriate health care provider allows for modification of the treatment plan.*

Nursing Diagnosis   **HYPERTHERMIA** NDx

Definition: Body temperature elevated above normal

Related to: Stimulation of the thermoregulatory center in the hypothalamus by endogenous pyrogens that are related to an infectious process

CLINICAL MANIFESTATIONS

Subjective	Objective
Verbalization of chills	Increased temperature; elevated heart rate; diaphoresis; elevated respiratory rate; flushed skin; skin warm to touch

RISK FACTORS

- Infection
- Smoking
- Smog
- Inadequate primary defenses
- Dehydration

DESIRED OUTCOMES

The client will experience resolution of hyperthermia as evidenced by:
   a. Skin usual temperature and color
   b. Pulse rate between 60 and 100 beats/min
   c. Respiratory rate 12 to 20 breaths/min
   d. Normal body temperature

NOC OUTCOMES

Thermoregulation

NIC INTERVENTIONS

Fever treatment

NURSING ASSESSMENT	RATIONALE
Assess for signs and symptoms of hyperthermia (e.g., warm, flushed skin; tachycardia; tachypnea; elevated temperature; chills; and excessive diaphoresis).	*Early recognition of signs and symptoms of a fever allows for prompt intervention.*

THERAPEUTIC INTERVENTIONS	RATIONALE

Independent Actions

Perform actions to resolve the infectious process:

- Assist client to cough and deep breathe frequently. **D** ● ✦

Deep breathing and coughing will help to remove secretions.

- Minimize environmental noise and activity. **D** ● ✦

These actions promote rest and help to conserve energy.

- Organize nursing care to allow for periods of uninterrupted rest. **D** ● ✦

- Provide adequate caloric and protein intake.

Adequate nutrition is needed to support functioning of the immune system.

Implement measures to reduce elevated temperature

Administer tepid sponge bath and/or apply cold cloths to groin and axillae. **D** ● ✦

These interventions will work to decrease the client's temperature.

Use a room fan to provide cool circulating air. **D** ● ✦

Dependent/Collaborative Actions

Implement measure to reduce elevated temperature.

Helps to decrease elevated temperature

Apply a cooling blanket if ordered. **D** ● ✦

Administer antipyretics and antimicrobials if ordered. **D** ✦

Antipyretics will help to reduce elevated temperature. Appropriately prescribed anti-infectives can effectively treat the client's infection.

Consult physician if temperature remains elevated.

Notify the physician if a client's temperature does not respond to treatment.

Nursing Diagnosis ## ACTIVITY INTOLERANCE NDx

Definition: Insufficient physiological or psychological energy to endure or complete required or desired daily activity

Related to:

- Tissue hypoxia associated with impaired gas exchange
- Difficulty resting and sleeping associated with excessive coughing, dyspnea, discomfort, unfamiliar environment, anxiety, and frequent assessments and treatments
- Inadequate nutritional status
- Increased energy expenditure associated with persistent coughing and the increased metabolic rate that is present in an infectious process

CLINICAL MANIFESTATIONS

Subjective	Objective
Verbal report of fatigue or weakness	Abnormal heart rate or B/P response to activity; exertional discomfort or dyspnea; electrocardiographic changes reflecting dysrhythmias or ischemia; unable to speak with physical activity

RISK FACTORS

- Bedrest or immobility
- Generalized weakness
- Sedentary lifestyle
- Imbalance between oxygen supply and demand

DESIRED OUTCOMES

The client will demonstrate an increased tolerance for activity as evidenced by:

a. Verbalization of feeling less fatigued and weak

b. Ability to perform ADL without dizziness, increased dyspnea, chest pain, diaphoresis, and a significant change in vital signs

---

NDx = NANDA-I Diagnosis   **D** = Delegatable Action   ● = UAP   ✦ = LVN/LPN   ⊖▶ = Go to ⊖volve for animation

Continued...

NOC OUTCOMES	NIC INTERVENTIONS
Energy conservation; rest; activity tolerance	Energy management; oxygen therapy; sleep enhancement; nutrition management; infection control

NURSING ASSESSMENT	RATIONALE
Assess for signs and symptoms of activity intolerance: • Statements of fatigue or weakness • Exertional dyspnea, chest pain, diaphoresis, or dizziness • Abnormal heart rate response to activity (e.g., increase in rate of 20 beats/min above resting rate, rate not returning to preactivity level within 3 minutes after stopping activity, change from regular to irregular rate) • Significant change (15-20 mm Hg) in B/P with activity	*Early recognition of signs and symptoms of activity intolerance allows for prompt intervention.*

THERAPEUTIC INTERVENTIONS	RATIONALE

Independent Actions

Implement measures to promote rest and/or conserve energy (e.g., maintain prescribed activity restrictions, minimize environmental activity and noise, provide uninterrupted rest periods, assist with care, keep supplies and personal articles within easy reach, limit the number of visitors, use shower chair when showering, sit to brush teeth or comb hair). **D** ● ✦

Rest and activities that conserve energy result in a lower metabolic rate, which preserves nutrients and oxygen for necessary activities.

Implement measures to promote sleep (e.g., elevated head of bed and support arms on pillows to facilitate breathing, maintain oxygen therapy during sleep, discourage intake of fluids high in caffeine in the evening, reduce environmental stimuli). **D** ✦

Sleep replenishes a client's energy and feeling of well-being.

Implement measures to decrease excessive coughing (e.g., protect client from exposure to irritants such as smoke, flowers, and powder; avoid extremely hot or cold foods/fluids). **D** ● ✦

Excessive coughing can lead to inadequate tissue oxygenation, which results in less efficient energy production and a reduced ability to tolerate activity. Improving respiratory status increases the amount of oxygen available for energy production.

Discourage smoking and excessive intake of beverages high in caffeine such as coffee, tea, and colas. **D** ✦

Excessive intake of nicotine and caffeine can increase cardiac workload and myocardial oxygen utilization, thereby decreasing oxygen availability.

Perform actions to improve respiratory status (e.g., place client in semi- to high-Fowler's position; assist client to deep breathe or use incentive spirometry every 1 to 2 hours; maintain bed rest as ordered; and use oxygen as needed). **D** ✦

Improvement of respiratory status is done to relieve dyspnea and improve tissue oxygenation.

Perform actions to maintain adequate nutritional status (e.g., increase activity as tolerated potentially improving appetite; encourage a rest period before meals to reduce fatigue; assist with oral hygiene before meals; maintain a clean environment and a relaxed, pleasant atmosphere). **D** ● ✦

Adequate nutritional status is important in order to maintain ADL.

Increase client's activity gradually as allowed and tolerated. **D** ● ✦

A gradual increase in activity will slowly improve strength and ability in performance of activities.

Instruct a client to:
• Report a decreased tolerance for activity.
• Stop any activity that causes increased chest pain, increased shortness of breath, dizziness, or extreme fatigue or weakness.

Changes in a client's activity tolerance should be reported immediately.

Assessment of the change will allow for timely diagnosis of the cause and subsequent treatment.

Dependent/Collaborative Actions

Consult appropriate health care providers (e.g., respiratory therapist, physician, dietitian) if signs and symptoms of activity intolerance persist or worsen.

Notifying the appropriate health care provider allows for modification of the treatment plan.

Nursing Diagnosis | # RISK FOR INFECTION: EXTRAPULMONARY (E.G., BACTEREMIA, PERICARDITIS, ENDOCARDITIS, MENINGITIS, SEPTIC ARTHRITIS) AND/OR SUPERINFECTION (E.G., CANDIDIASIS) NDx

Definition: At increased risk for being invaded by pathogenic organisms

Related to:
- Spread of infecting organisms into the blood and to other sites associated with inadequate host defenses and resistance to antimicrobial agents
- Interruption in the balance of usual endogenous microbial flora associated with the administration of antimicrobial agents

CLINICAL MANIFESTATIONS

Subjective	Objective
Verbalization of chest pain, joint pain, fatigue, stiff neck, headache	Abnormal vital signs; unusual drainage from a body cavity; abnormal WBC and differential counts; white patches and/or ulcerations in the mouth; yeast infections

RISK FACTORS
- Smoking
- Hospitalization
- Exposure to infectious agents
- Overuse of antimicrobial agents

DESIRED OUTCOMES

The client will not develop an extrapulmonary infection or a superinfection as evidenced by:
  a. Gradual return of vital signs to the client's normal range
  b. Usual mental status
  c. Absence of a pericardial friction rub, precordial pain, and a pathological murmur
  d. Absence of joint pain and swelling
  e. Absence of unusual drainage from any body cavity
  f. Absence of white patches and ulcerations in the mouth
  g. Absence of stiff neck and headache
  h. WBC and differential counts returning toward normal range for the client

NOC OUTCOMES

Immune status; infection severity

NIC INTERVENTIONS

Infection protection; infection control

NURSING ASSESSMENT	RATIONALE

Assess for and report signs and symptoms of an extrapulmonary infection or a superinfection:
- Increase in temperature and pulse rate above previous levels
- Change in mental status
- Pericardial friction rub, precordial pain, or development of a pathological murmur
- Swollen, red, painful joints
- Unusual color, amount, and odor of vaginal drainage (fungal infections are common superinfections with antimicrobial therapy); perineal itching; white patches or ulcerated areas in the mouth
- Stiff neck, headache, increase in WBC count above previous levels and/or significant change in differential

Early recognition of signs and symptoms of an extrapulmonary or superinfection allows for prompt intervention.

Continued...

THERAPEUTIC INTERVENTIONS	RATIONALE

Independent Actions

Implement measures to prevent an extrapulmonary infection and/or a superinfection:

- Use good hand hygiene and encourage client to do the same. **D** ● ✦

  Good hand hygiene removes transient flora, which reduces the risk of transmission of pathogens. Use of products such as an antibacterial soap, a chlorhexidine solution, or an alcohol-based handrub agent can actually inhibit the growth of or kill microorganisms, which further reduces infection risks.

- Maintain sterile technique during all invasive procedures (e.g., urinary catheterizations, venous and arterial punctures, injections). **D** ✦

  Use of sterile technique reduces the possibility of introducing pathogens into the body.

- Change peripheral intravenous line sites according to hospital policy.

  Peripheral intravenous line sites are changed routinely to reduce persistent irritation of one area of a vein wall and the resultant colonization of microorganisms at that site.

- Protect client from others with infection. **D** ● ✦

  Protecting the client from others with infections reduces the client's risk of exposure to pathogens.

- Anchor catheters/tubings (e.g., urinary, intravenous) securely. **D** ✦

  Trauma to the tissues and the risk for introduction of pathogens associated with in-and-out movement of the tubing are reduced.

- Change equipment, tubings, and solutions used for treatments such as intravenous infusions and respiratory care according to hospital policy.

  The longer equipment, tubings, and solutions are in use, the greater the chance of colonization of microorganisms, which can then be introduced into the body.

- Maintain a closed system for drains (e.g., urinary catheter) and intravenous infusions whenever possible. **D** ✦

  Each time a drainage or infusion system is opened, pathogens from the environment have an opportunity to enter the body. Maintaining a closed system decreases this risk, which reduces the possibility of infection.

- Instruct and assist client to perform good perineal care routinely and after each bowel movement. **D** ✦

  Routine cleansing of the perineal area reduces the risk of colonization of organisms and subsequent perineal, urinary tract, and/or vaginal infection.

- Reinforce importance of frequent oral hygiene. **D** ✦

  Frequent oral hygiene helps to prevent infection by removing most of the food, debris, and many of the microorganisms that are present in the mouth. It also helps maintain the integrity of the oral mucous membranes, which provides a physical and chemical barrier to pathogens.

Dependent/Collaborative Actions

If signs and symptoms of an extrapulmonary infection or a superinfection occur:

- Prepare client for and/or assist with diagnostic tests (e.g., lumbar puncture, cultures, joint aspiration) if planned.
- Implement appropriate comfort measures for symptoms experienced.

  An extrapulmonary and/or a superinfection should be addressed immediately. Preparation of the client for procedures that may be involved in the diagnostic process is important to alleviate associated fears and anxiety.

- Administer antimicrobials as ordered.

  Antimicrobials should be administered as soon as a culture and sensitivity has been obtained.

Collaborative Diagnosis **RISK FOR PLEURAL EFFUSION**

Definition: An abnormal accumulation of fluid in the pleural cavity

Related to: Pulmonary infection; increased permeability of capillary beds

CLINICAL MANIFESTATIONS

Subjective	Objective
Verbalization of chest pain (pleural); dyspnea	Dull percussion note and diminished or absent breath sounds; chest radiograph showing pleural effusion; respiratory rate greater than 20 breaths/min; fever; night sweats; cough; weight loss

RISK FACTORS
* Pulmonary infection
* Increased permeability of capillary beds

DESIRED OUTCOMES

The client will not develop pleural effusion as evidenced by:
   a. No increase in dyspnea
   b. Symmetrical chest excursion
   c. Improved breath sounds and percussion note throughout lung fields

NURSING ASSESSMENT

Assess for and report signs and symptoms of pleural effusion (e.g., dyspnea, chest pain, decreased chest excursion on affected side, dull percussion note, decreased or absent breath sounds over the affected area, chest radiograph showing pleural effusion)

RATIONALE

Early recognition of signs and symptoms of pleural effusion allows for prompt intervention.

THERAPEUTIC INTERVENTIONS

Dependent/Collaborative Actions
Implement measures to resolve the infectious process:

* Encourage coughing and deep breathing.
* Administer antimicrobials as ordered.

If signs and symptoms of pleural effusion occur:
* Continue with actions to improve respiratory status (e.g., increase activity tolerance; instruct client in and assist with diaphragmatic and pursed-lip breathing techniques; instruct client to deep breathe or use incentive spirometer every 1 to 2 hours; encourage coughing and deep breathing; place client in high semi-Fowler's position).
* Prepare client for a thoracentesis if planned.

RATIONALE

Resolution of an infectious process reduces the risk for development of pleural effusion and/or atelectasis.
Helps to expand lungs and mobilize secretions
Treats infection

Maintenance/improvement of the client's respiratory status and removal of secretions decrease the potential of infection or the occurrence of a pleural effusion.

Removal of fluid from the lungs will help to improve the client's ability to maintain adequate gas exchange.

Collaborative Diagnosis   # RISK FOR ATELECTASIS

Definition: Collapse of lung tissue caused by hypoventilated alveoli

Related to: Shallow respirations; stasis of secretion

CLINICAL MANIFESTATIONS

Subjective	Objective
Report of dyspnea	Decreased breath sounds and/or crackles; cough; sputum production; low-grade fever; heart rate greater than 60 to 100 beats/min; increased respiratory rate above 20 breaths/min/effort Chest radiograph, ultrasound, or computed tomography results showing patchy infiltrates

RISK FACTORS
* Ineffective cough effort
* Immobility
* Smoking

DESIRED OUTCOMES

The client will not develop atelectasis as evidenced by:
   a. Clear, audible breath sounds
   b. Resonant percussion note over lungs
   c. Unlabored respirations at 12 to 20 breaths/min
   d. Pulse rate within normal range for client
   e. Afebrile status

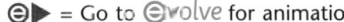

NDx = NANDA-I Diagnosis   **D** = Delegatable Action   ● = UAP   ◆ = LVN/LPN   ⊝▶ = Go to ⊝volve for animation

Continued...

NURSING ASSESSMENT	RATIONALE
Assess for and report signs and symptoms of atelectasis: • Diminished or absent breath sounds • Dull percussion note over affected area • Increased respiratory rate • Dyspnea • Tachycardia • Elevated temperature	*Early recognition of signs and symptoms of atelectasis allows for implementation of the appropriate interventions.*
Monitor pulse oximetry results as indicated.	*Pulse oximetry is an indirect measure of arterial oxygen saturation. Monitoring pulse oximetry (SaO_2) allows for early detection of hypoxia and implementation of the appropriate interventions.*
Monitor chest radiograph results.	*Chest radiograph provides radiographic confirmation of atelectasis.*

THERAPEUTIC INTERVENTIONS	RATIONALE

Dependent/Collaborative Actions
Implement measures to prevent atelectasis:
• Perform actions to improve breathing pattern:
  • Encourage client to deep breathe.
  • Incentive spirometry
• Perform actions to promote effective airway clearance.
  • Turn, cough, and deep breathe.
	Lack of movement places a client at risk for atelectasis. Changing positions frequently, coughing, and deep breathing help to expand the lungs, enhancing alveolar expansion.

Administer antibiotics as ordered.	*Helps to mobilize secretions* *Treats infection*
If signs and symptoms of atelectasis occur: • Increase frequency of position change, coughing or "huffing," deep breathing, and use of incentive spirometer.	*Improves lung expansion and mobilization of secretions*
Consult physician if signs and symptoms of atelectasis persist or worsen.	*Allows for prompt alterations in interventions*

DISCHARGE TEACHING: CONTINUED CARE

Nursing Diagnosis DEFICIENT KNOWLEDGE NDx, INEFFECTIVE HEALTH MAINTENANCE NDx, OR INEFFECTIVE SELF-HEALTH MANAGEMENT* NDx

Definition: Absence or deficiency of cognitive information related to specific topic (lack of specific information necessary for clients/significant others) to make informed choices regarding condition/treatment/lifestyle changes; inability to identify, manage, and/or seek out help to maintain health; pattern of regulating and integrating into daily living a therapeutic regimen for treatment of illness and the sequelae of illness that is unsatisfactory for meeting specific health goals

CLINICAL MANIFESTATIONS

Subjective	Objective
Verbalization of the problem	Inaccurate follow through of instructions; inappropriate behaviors

RISK FACTORS
• Denial of disease process
• Cognitive deficiency
• Failure to take action to reduce risk factors

---

*The nurse should select the diagnostic label that is most appropriate for the client's discharge teaching needs.

NOC OUTCOMES	NIC INTERVENTIONS
Knowledge: disease process; knowledge: treatment regimen; knowledge: infection control	Health system guidance; teaching: individual; teaching: disease process; teaching: prescribed medications

NURSING ASSESSMENT	RATIONALE
Assess client's ability and readiness to learn. Assess the client's understanding of teaching.	*Learning is more effective when the client is motivated and understands the importance of what is to be learned. Readiness to learn changes based on situations, physical and emotional challenges.*

THERAPEUTIC INTERVENTIONS	RATIONALE

Desired Outcome: The client will identify ways to maintain respiratory health.

Independent Actions
Instruct client in ways to maintain respiratory health:

- Consume a well-balanced diet.

  A well-balanced diet is important for the proper functioning of the immune system.
- Drink at least 10 glasses of liquid per day unless contraindicated.

  Adequate fluid intake is necessary to liquefy secretions.
- Maintain a balanced program of rest and exercise.

  Rest and exercise are important to maintain psychological and physical well-being.
- Avoid crowds during flu and cold season.
- Avoid contact with persons who have respiratory infections.

  The potential for illness is decreased through avoidance of persons with respiratory infections and of crowds during the cold and flu season.
- Consult physician about vaccinations available if at high risk for recurrent pneumonia.

  Immunizations augment the client's immune system in fighting off infection.
- Continue coughing and deep breathing exercises for at least a few weeks after discharge and during any period of decreased physical activity or respiratory infection.

  Deep breathing and coughing will help to remove secretions.
- Maintain good oral hygiene.

  Good oral hygiene reduces the number of organisms in the oropharynx.
- Avoid excessive alcohol intake and stop smoking to prevent depression of pulmonary antimicrobial defenses.

  Avoidance of alcohol and smoking prevents depression of the pulmonary antimicrobial defenses.
- Avoid exposure to respiratory irritants (e.g., smoke and other environmental pollutants).

  Respiratory irritation caused by smoke and other environmental pollutants can cause changes in respiratory status in susceptible persons.

THERAPEUTIC INTERVENTIONS	RATIONALE

Desired Outcome: The client will state signs and symptoms to report to the health care provider.

Independent Actions
Instruct client to report the following signs and symptoms:

- Persistent or recurrent temperature elevation
- Chills
- Difficulty breathing
- Restlessness, irritability, drowsiness, or confusion
- Persistent or increased chest pain
- Persistent weight loss
- Persistent fatigue
- Persistent cough
- Unusual color, amount, and odor of vaginal secretions; white patches or ulcerated areas in the mouth; stiff neck and headache; or swollen, red, painful joints.

The patient's understanding of the signs and symptoms associated with infection, superinfection, extension of infection to another site, pleural effusion, and atelectasis is important for prompt identification, reporting, and treatment.

Reinforce the importance of keeping follow-up appointments with health care provider.

A follow-up appointment with the health care provider is important to monitor continued recovery.

NDx = NANDA-I Diagnosis   **D** = Delegatable Action   ● = UAP   ✦ = LVN/LPN   ⊖▶ = Go to ⊖volve for animation

Continued...

THERAPEUTIC INTERVENTIONS	RATIONALE

Desired Outcome: The client will verbalize an understanding of a plan for adhering to recommended follow-up care including future appointment with health care provider, medications prescribed, and activity limitations.

Independent Actions

Explain the rationale for, side effects of, and importance of taking medications prescribed (e.g., antimicrobials). Inform client of pertinent food and drug interactions.

An informed client is more likely to adhere to medication regimens.

Implement measures to improve client compliance:
- Include significant others in all discharge teaching sessions if possible.
- Encourage questions and allow time for reinforcement and clarification of information provided.

Involvement of significant others in patient teaching improves adherence to discharge instructions.

Everyone does not understand information as presented, so set aside time for questions to allow for clarification of information.

Provide written instructions regarding scheduled appointments with health care provider, medications prescribed, fluid requirements, respiratory care, and signs and symptoms to report.

Written instructions allow the client to refer to instructions as needed.

ADDITIONAL NURSING DIAGNOSES

NAUSEA NDx
Related to stimulation of the vomiting center associated with noxious stimuli (e.g., foul taste of sputum and some aerosol treatments, sight of sputum)

DISTURBED SLEEP PATTERN NDx
Related to unfamiliar environment, discomfort, excessive coughing, anxiety, inability to assume usual sleep position

because of dyspnea, and frequent assessments and treatments

FEAR/ANXIETY NDx
Related to severity of symptoms (e.g., cough, chest pain, shortness of breath) and need for hospitalization, unfamiliar environment, and separation from significant others

PNEUMOTHORAX

Pneumothorax occurs when air accumulates in the pleural space and causes complete or partial collapse of a lung. Clinical manifestations vary with the degree of lung collapse but usually include sudden onset of unilateral sharp chest pain, tachypnea, dyspnea, anxiety, agitation, absent or diminished breath sounds, and tachycardia. When the pneumothorax is symptomatic and involves greater than 15% of the lung tissue, it is usually treated with placement of a chest tube into the intrapleural space. The tube is then connected to suction through a closed water-seal drainage system or, less frequently, to a flutter (Heimlich) valve to evacuate the intrapleural air, reestablish negative intrapleural pressure, and reexpand the lung. After lung reexpansion, obliteration of the pleural space may be necessary in some situations to minimize the risk of a recurrent pneumothorax. Methods for accomplishing this include chemical or mechanical pleurodesis, partial pleurectomy, or pleural stapling.

A pneumothorax can be classified in a variety of ways (e.g., open, closed, iatrogenic, spontaneous [primary, secondary], traumatic [penetrating, blunt]). An open pneumothorax occurs when air enters the pleural space through an opening in the chest wall. This opening can result from a penetrating injury (e.g., gunshot wound, stab wound), surgery involving the chest or diaphragm, or a complication of a diagnostic or therapeutic procedure (e.g., thoracentesis, lung biopsy, insertion of a pacemaker, subclavian venipuncture).

A closed pneumothorax occurs when air enters the pleural space without evidence of an external wound. The most common type of closed pneumothorax occurs in the absence of obvious respiratory disease and is often referred to as a primary spontaneous pneumothorax. Persons at greatest risk for this are men who are tall, 20 to 40 years of age, smokers, and have a family history of spontaneous pneumothorax. Other causes of a closed pneumothorax include damage to lung tissue as a result of a complication of pulmonary disease (e.g., COPD, cystic fibrosis, lung cancer, tuberculosis), mechanical ventilation, a fractured rib, and migration of a subclavian catheter or pacemaker lead.

This care plan focuses on the adult client hospitalized for diagnosis and treatment of a pneumothorax.

OUTCOME/DISCHARGE CRITERIA

The client will:
1. Experience reexpansion of affected lung
2. Have adequate respiratory function

3. Identify safety measures related to care of chest tube insertion site and flutter valve (if present)
4. Identify ways to reduce the risk of another pneumothorax
5. State signs and symptoms to report to the health care provider

6. Verbalize an understanding of and a plan for adhering to recommended follow-up care including future appointments with health care provider and activity restrictions.

Nursing Diagnosis INEFFECTIVE BREATHING PATTERN NDx

Definition: Inspiration and/or expiration that does not provide adequate ventilation

Related to:
• Increased rate of respirations associated with fear and anxiety
• Decreased rate of respirations associated with the depressant effect of some medications (e.g., narcotic [opioid] analgesics)
• Decreased depth of respirations associated with:
  • Reluctance to breathe deeply resulting from chest pain and fear of dislodging chest tube or experiencing another pneumothorax
  • Complete or partial collapse of the lung
  • Anxiety and the depressant effect of some medications (e.g., narcotic [opioid] analgesics)

CLINICAL MANIFESTATIONS

Subjective	Objective
Verbalization of pain, anxiety, fear/agitation, shortness of breath	Tachypnea; dyspnea; hypotension; impaired chest wall expansion; cough and/or hemoptysis; diaphoresis; diminished breath sounds; tachycardia; use of accessory muscles when breathing; significant decrease in oximetry results; abnormal arterial blood gas values; chest radiograph—collapsed lung

RISK FACTORS
• Fear
• Anxiety
• Pain

DESIRED OUTCOMES

The client will experience an effective breathing pattern as evidenced by:
  a. Normal rate and depth of respirations
  b. Decreased dyspnea
  c. Symmetrical chest excursion

NOC OUTCOMES

Respiratory status: ventilation

NIC INTERVENTIONS

Respiratory monitoring; ventilation assistance; anxiety management; pain management

NURSING ASSESSMENT

Assess for signs and symptoms of an ineffective breathing pattern (e.g., shallow respirations, tachypnea, dyspnea, asymmetrical chest excursion, use of accessory muscles when breathing).

RATIONALE

Early recognition of signs and symptoms of infective breathing patterns allows for prompt intervention.

THERAPEUTIC INTERVENTIONS

Independent Actions
Implement measures to improve breathing pattern:
• Perform actions to reduce chest pain (e.g., orient client to the hospital environment, equipment; maintain a calm, supportive, environment; instruct and assist client to splint chest when coughing or deep breathing). **D** ● ✦

RATIONALE

Reduction of chest pain increases the client's willingness to move and breathe more deeply.

NDx = NANDA-I Diagnosis   **D** = Delegatable Action   ● = UAP   ✦ = LVN/LPN   ⊖▶ = Go to ⊖volve for animation

Continued...

THERAPEUTIC INTERVENTIONS	RATIONALE
• Perform actions to reduce fear and anxiety (e.g., assure client that staff members are nearby; respond to call signal as soon as possible; provide calm, restful environment; instruct in relaxation techniques; encourage family to project a supportive attitude without obvious anxiousness). **D** ✦	*Reduction of fear and anxiety assists in preventing the shallow and/or rapid breathing associated with these emotions.*
• Place the client in semi- to high-Fowler's position unless contraindicated; position with pillows to prevent slumping. **D** ● ✦	*Positioning the client in semi- to high-Fowler's position promotes optimal gas exchange by enabling chest expansion.* *Positioning with pillows prevents slumping.*
• Instruct client to deep breathe or use incentive spirometer every 1 to 2 hours. **D** ✦	*Forced deep breathing and use of incentive spirometry will increase expansion of the lungs and improve the client's ability to clear mucus from the lungs. The technique may also increase the amount of oxygen that is able to penetrate deep into the lungs.*
• Assure the client that deep breathing and turning should not dislodge the chest tube or increase the risk of another pneumothorax.	*This assurance will decrease the client's anxiety and fear associated with the chest tube and the original pneumothorax.*
• Instruct the client to breathe slowly, if hyperventilating.	*Hyperventilation is an ineffective breathing pattern that can eventually lead to respiratory alkalosis. Clients can often slow their breathing rate if they concentrate on doing so.*
• Increase activity as allowed and tolerated. **D** ● ✦	*During activity, especially ambulation, the client usually takes deeper breaths, thus increasing lung expansion.*

Dependent/Collaborative Actions

Implement measures to improve breathing pattern:

• Medicate with analgesics as needed. **D** ✦	*Pain relief increases client's willingness to take deep breaths and improve lung expansion.*
• Administer central nervous system depressants judiciously; hold medications and consult physician if respiratory rate is less than 12 breaths/min. **D** ✦	*Central nervous system depressants cause depression of the respiratory center in the brainstem, which can result in a decreased rate and depth of respiration.*
Consult appropriate health care provider (e.g., respiratory therapist, physician) if ineffective breathing pattern continues.	*Notifying the appropriate health care provider allows for modifications of treatment.*

Nursing Diagnosis   # IMPAIRED GAS EXCHANGE NDx

Definition: Deficit in oxygenation and/or carbon dioxide elimination at the alveolar-capillary membrane

Related to: Loss of effective lung surface, associated with partial or complete lung collapse

CLINICAL MANIFESTATIONS

Subjective	Objective
Verbalization of restlessness, irritability, confusion, and somnolence	Tachypnea; dyspnea; significant decrease in oximetry results; decreased PaO_2 and/or increased $PaCO_2$; chest radiograph—presence of air or blood in the pleural space on the affected side and any mediastinal shift; abnormal arterial blood gases-oxygen saturation less than 90%; hypoxemia; hypercarbia; decreased hemoglobin and hematocrit associated with blood loss in a hemothorax; hypoxemia; hypocarbia; nasal flaring; tachycardia

RISK FACTORS
- Decreased lung expansion
- Pain
- Muscle fatigue
- Obesity

DESIRED OUTCOMES

The client will experience adequate O_2/CO_2 exchange as evidenced by:
    a. Usual mental status
    b. Unlabored respirations of 12 to 20 breaths/min
    c. Oximetry results within normal range
    d. Arterial blood gas values within normal range

NOC OUTCOMES

Respiratory status: gas exchange

NIC INTERVENTIONS

Respiratory monitoring; oxygen therapy; chest tube care; acid-base management

NURSING ASSESSMENT	RATIONALE
Assess for and report signs and symptoms of impaired gas exchange: • Restlessness, irritability • Confusion, somnolence • Tachypnea, dyspnea • Significant decrease in oximetry results • Decreased PaO_2 and/or increased $PaCO_2$	*Early recognition of signs and symptoms of ineffective gas exchange allows for prompt intervention.*

THERAPEUTIC INTERVENTIONS	RATIONALE
Independent Actions Implement measures to improve gas exchange: • Perform actions to promote lung reexpansion:	
• Prepare client for and assist with insertion of chest tube (the tube is then connected to a drainage system [with or without suction] or, less commonly, to a flutter valve).	*Provide client with information related to the procedure to decrease the experience of fear and anxiety.*
• After chest tube insertion, implement measures to maintain patency and integrity of chest drainage system:	*These actions help to ensure maintenance of the chest tube drainage system and facilitate drainage.*
• Maintain fluid level in water seal and suction chambers as ordered.	*Fluid level determines the level of suction in a closed drainage system.*
• Maintain occlusive dressing over chest tube insertion site.	*Maintains a seal around the chest tube insertion site, preventing air leaks and loss of negative pressure*
• Tape all connections securely.	*Supports maintenance of a closed system and reduces the risk of air leaks*
• Tape the tubing to the chest wall close to insertion site.	*Taping the tubing to the chest wall close to the insertion site reduces the risk of inadvertent removal of the tube.*
• Position tubing to avoid kinks; coil excess tubing on the bed rather than allowing it to hang down below the collection device. **D** ✦	*Excess tubing hanging over the bed in a dependent loop allows drainage to collect in the loop and could occlude the drainage system. Kinked tubing blocks drainage and may promote fluid or blood accumulation in the pleural cavity.*
• Keep drainage collection device below level of client's chest at all times.	*The system must be lower than the level of the client's chest to promote chest tube drainage.*
• Maintain suction as ordered; ensure that the air vent is open on the drainage collection device if the system is to water seal only; if a flutter valve is present, ensure that there is no fluid in the valve and that the distal end is open).	*These actions facilitate the escape of air from the pleural space.*
• Avoid stripping or clamping a chest tube.	*Stripping a chest tube may cause high negative pressure in the pleural space and can potentially damage the lung tissue. Clamping a chest tube can block air from escaping the pleural space, which may lead to a tension pneumothorax.*

Continued...

THERAPEUTIC INTERVENTIONS	RATIONALE
• Keep a petrolatum gauze dressing at the bedside.	*This dressing is applied to the insertion site if the chest tube becomes dislodged. This will maintain an airtight seal, preventing a recurrence of a pneumothorax.*
• Keep a bottle of sterile water at the bedside.	*If the chest tube becomes disconnected, submerging it in a bottle of sterile water will provide a temporary closed drainage system.*
• Perform actions to improve breathing patterns (e.g., place client in semi- to high-Fowler's position to improve air exchange; instruct client to deep breathe or use incentive spirometer every 1 to 2 hours).	*Positioning the client in semi- to high-Fowler's position promotes optimal gas exchange by enabling chest expansion.* *Forced deep breathing and use of incentive spirometry will increase expansion of the lungs and improve the client's ability to clear mucus from the lungs. The technique may also increase the amount of oxygen that is able to penetrate deep into the lungs.*
• Discourage smoking.	*Smoking impairs gas exchange because it (1) reduces effective airway clearance by increasing mucus production and impairing ciliary function; (2) decreases oxygen availability (hemoglobin binds with the carbon monoxide in smoke rather than with oxygen); (3) causes damage to the bronchial and alveolar walls; and (4) causes vasoconstriction and subsequently reduces pulmonary blood flow.*

Dependent/Collaborative Actions

Implement measures to improve gas exchange:

• Maintain activity restrictions as ordered; increase activity gradually as allowed and tolerated. **D** ● ✦	*Conservation of energy through activity restrictions allows energy to be focused on breathing. Increasing activity as tolerated helps mobilize excretions and promotes deeper breathing and lung expansion.*
• Maintain oxygen therapy as ordered. **D** ✦	*Supplemental oxygen helps to relieve dyspnea.*
Consult appropriate health care provider (e.g., respiratory therapist, physician) if signs and symptoms of impaired gas exchange persist or worsen.	*Notifying the appropriate health care professionals allows for a prompt and multifaceted approach to treatment.*

Nursing Diagnosis **ACUTE PAIN** NDx **(CHEST)**

Definition: Unpleasant sensory and emotional experience arising from actual or potential tissue damage or described in terms of such damage; may be sudden or slow onset of any intensity from mild to severe with an anticipated or predictable end and a duration of <6 months.

Related to: Irritation of the parietal pleura and associated with:
• Stretching of the pleura resulting from air in the pleural space
• Tissue irritation associated with insertion and presence of a chest tube

CLINICAL MANIFESTATIONS

Subjective	Objective
Verbalization of chest pain with breathing and coughing	Grimacing; rubbing chest; reluctance to move; shallow respirations; restlessness; increased B/P; tachycardia

RISK FACTORS

• Excessive coughing
• Increased sputum production
• Chest tubes

DESIRED OUTCOMES

The client will experience diminished chest pain as evidenced by:
   a. Verbalization of a decrease in or absence of pain
   b. Relaxed facial expression and body positioning
   c. Improve breathing pattern
   d. Increased participation in activities
   e. Stable vital signs

NOC OUTCOMES	NIC INTERVENTIONS
Pain control; comfort level	Pain management; environmental management; analgesic administration

NURSING ASSESSMENT	RATIONALE
Assess for signs and symptoms of chest pain (e.g., verbalization of pain, grimacing, rubbing chest, guarding of affected side of chest, reluctance to move, shallow respirations, restlessness, increased B/P, tachycardia).	*Early recognition of signs and symptoms of pain allows for prompt intervention and improved pain control.*
Assess client's perception of the severity of pain using a pain intensity rating scale.	*An awareness of the severity of pain being experienced helps determine the most appropriate interventions for pain management. Use of a pain intensity rating scale gives the nurse a clearer understanding of the pain being experienced and promotes consistency when communicating with others about the client's pain experience.*
Assess the client's pain pattern (e.g., location, quality, onset, duration, precipitating factors, aggravating factors, alleviating factors).	*Knowledge of the client's pain pattern assists in the identification of effective pain management interventions.*
Ask the client to describe previous pain experiences and methods used to manage pain effectively.	*Many variables affect a client's response to pain (e.g., age, sex, coping style, previous experience with pain, culture, cause of pain). Knowledge of the client's usual response to pain and methods previously used to manage pain effectively enables the nurse to evaluate the client's pain more accurately and facilitates the identification of effective strategies for pain management.*

THERAPEUTIC INTERVENTIONS	RATIONALE

Independent Actions

Implement measures to reduce fear and anxiety (e.g., assure client that chest pain is common with pneumothorax and should subside with treatment; assure client that the need for pain relief is understood).	*Fear and anxiety can decrease the client's threshold and tolerance for pain and thereby heighten the perception of pain. In addition, pain management methods are not as effective if the client is tense and unable to relax.*
Implement measures to promote rest (e.g., minimize environmental activity and noise). **D** ● ✦	*Fatigue can decrease the client's threshold and tolerance for pain and thereby heighten the perception of pain. A client who is well rested often experiences decreased pain and increased effectiveness of pain management measures.*
Perform actions to facilitate the escape of air from the pleural space (e.g., maintain suction as ordered; ensure the air vent is open on the drainage collective device if system is to water seal only; if flutter valve is present, ensure that there is not fluid in the valve and that the distal end is open).	*These actions promote the removal of air from the pleural space and work to expand lung tissue.*
Instruct and assist the client to splint the chest with hands or pillows when deep breathing, coughing, or changing position.	*Splinting the chest with deep breathing, coughing, or changing position reduces pain and promotes a more effective cough.*
Provide or assist with nonpharmacological methods for pain relief (e.g., position change; progressive relaxation exercises; restful environment; diversional activities such as watching television, reading, or conversing).	*Nonpharmacological pain management includes a variety of interventions. It is believed that most of these are effective because they stimulate closure of the gating mechanism in the spinal cord and subsequently block the transmission of pain impulses. In addition, some interventions are thought to stimulate the release of endogenous analgesics (e.g., endorphins) that inhibit the transmission of pain impulses and/or alter the client's perception of pain. Many of the nonpharmacological interventions also help decrease pain by promoting relaxation.*
Securely anchor the chest tube.	*Limiting movement of the chest tube prevents resulting tissue irritation from the chest tube.*

Continued...

THERAPEUTIC INTERVENTIONS	RATIONALE
Collaborative/Dependent Interventions Administer analgesics before activities and procedures that can cause pain and before pain becomes severe; and as ordered. **D** ✦	*The administration of analgesics before a pain-producing event helps minimize the pain that will be experienced. When given prior to a procedure, analgesics improve the client's ability to tolerate activities.*
Consult appropriate health care provider (e.g., pharmacist, pain management specialist, physician) if the above measures fail to provide adequate pain relief.	*Notifying the appropriate health care professionals allows for a prompt and multifaceted approach to treatment.*

Collaborative Diagnosis — RISK FOR TENSION PNEUMOTHORAX WITH MEDIASTINAL SHIFT

Definition: Rapid accumulation of air in the pleural space causing severely high intrapleural pressures with resultant increased tension on the heart and great vessels; related to a significant increase in intrapleural pressure associated with inability of air to leave pleural space during expiration (can occur as a result of chest tube or flutter valve malfunction)

Related to: High intrapleural pressures, chest tube malfunction

CLINICAL MANIFESTATIONS

Subjective	Objective
Reports of pain; fear; anxiety	Lack of fluctuations in water seal chamber; dyspnea; subcutaneous emphysema; expanding area of absent breath sounds with hyperresonant percussion note; heart rate irregular and greater than 100 beats/min; low B/P; neck vein distention; hypoxemia ($PaO_2 <$ 80 mm Hg); hypercarbia ($PaCO_2 > 45$ mm Hg); respiratory acidosis (pH < 7.35); chest radiograph— expanding size of the pneumothorax and mediastinal shift

RISK FACTORS

- Ineffective lung expansion
- Immobility
- Stasis of secretions

DESIRED OUTCOMES

The client will not develop tension pneumothorax with mediastinal shift as evidenced by:
  a. No sudden increase in dyspnea
  b. Vital signs within normal range for client
  c. Usual mental status
  d. Absence of neck vein distention
  e. Trachea in midline position
  f. Usual skin color
  g. Arterial blood gas values returning toward normal

NURSING ASSESSMENT	RATIONALE
Assess for and immediately report signs and symptoms of: • Malfunction of chest drainage system (e.g., respiratory distress, lack of fluctuation in the water seal chamber without evidence of lung reexpansion, excessive bubbling in water seal chamber, significant increase in subcutaneous emphysema) • Malfunction of the flutter valve if present (e.g., respiratory distress, abrupt cessation of air flow from the distal end of the valve during exhalation)	*Early recognition of signs and symptoms of a malfunction in the chest tube drainage system allows for prompt intervention and decreases the potential prevention of an extension of the pneumothorax.*

NURSING ASSESSMENT	RATIONALE

- Extended pneumothorax (e.g., extended area of absent breath sounds with hyperresonant percussion note, increased dyspnea, chest radiograph showing an increase in size of pneumothorax)
- Tension pneumothorax (e.g., severe dyspnea, rapid and/or irregular heart rate, hypotension, restlessness, agitation, confusion, neck vein distention, shift in trachea from midline, arterial blood gas values that have worsened, chest radiograph showing a mediastinal shift).

THERAPEUTIC INTERVENTIONS	RATIONALE

Dependent/Collaborative Actions

Implement measures to promote lung reexpansion (e.g., maintain proper functioning of the closed chest drainage system).

Proper functioning of a closed chest drainage system reduces the risk of tension pneumothorax with mediastinal shift.

If signs and symptoms of tension pneumothorax with mediastinal shift occur:
- Maintain client on bed rest in a semi- to high-Fowler's position.
- Maintain oxygen therapy as ordered.

Positioning the client in semi- to high-Fowler's position promotes optimal gas exchange by enabling chest expansion.
Supplemental oxygen helps to relieve dyspnea and improves gas exchange.

- Assist with clearing existing chest tube or flutter valve, insertion of new tube, and/or needle aspiration of air from the pleural space.

By clearing existing chest tube/flutter valve, inserting a new tube, and/or performing needle aspiration, intrapleural pressure is reduced and lung expansion is promoted.

Nursing Diagnosis **FEAR/ANXIETY** NDx

Definition: Fear—Response to perceived threat that is consciously recognized as a danger.

Anxiety—Vague uneasy feeling of discomfort or dread accompanied by an autonomic response (the source is often nonspecific or unknown to the individual); a feeling of apprehension caused by anticipation of danger. It is an alerting signal that warns of impending danger and enables the individual to take measures to deal with the threat.

Related to:
- Exacerbation of symptoms (e.g., increased dyspnea, feeling of suffocation), need for hospitalization, and concern about prognosis
- Lack of understanding of the diagnosis, diagnostic tests, treatments, and prognosis
- Financial concerns about hospitalization

CLINICAL MANIFESTATIONS

Subjective	Objective
Verbalization of anxiety; usual perceptual ability and interactions with others	Unusual sleep patterns; unstable vital signs; restlessness; shakiness; diaphoresis; self-focused behavior

RISK FACTORS
- Pain
- Fear of unknown
- Fear of environment

DESIRED OUTCOMES

The client will experience a reduction in fear and anxiety as evidenced by:
    a. Verbalization of feeling less anxious
    b. Usual sleep pattern
    c. Relaxed facial expression and body movements
    d. Stable vital signs
    e. Usual perceptual ability and interactions with others

Continued...

NOC OUTCOMES	NIC INTERVENTIONS
Anxiety level; fear level; anxiety self-control; fear self-control	Anxiety reduction; calming technique; emotional support; presence; pain management

NURSING ASSESSMENT	RATIONALE
Assess client for signs and symptoms of fear and anxiety (e.g., verbalization of feeling anxious, insomnia, tenseness, shakiness, restlessness, diaphoresis, elevated B/P, tachycardia, self-focused behaviors).	*Moderate anxiety enhances the client's ability to solve problems. With severe anxiety or panic, the client is not able to follow directions and may become hyperactive and extremely agitated.*
Validate perceptions carefully, remembering that some behavior may result from hypoxia and/or hypercapnia.	*Assessment of the client's fear helps to determine whether the coping mechanisms are effective and which need to be strengthened.*

THERAPEUTIC INTERVENTIONS	RATIONALE

Independent Actions

Implement measures to reduce fear and anxiety:

- Orient client to hospital environment, equipment, and routines. **D** ● ✦

  Familiarity with the environment and usual routines reduces the client's anxiety about the unknown, provides a sense of security, and increases the client's sense of control, all of which help decrease anxiety.

- Introduce staff who will be participating in the client's care. If possible, maintain consistency in staff assigned to client's care.

  Introduction to staff familiarizes clients with those individuals who will be working with them, which provides clients with a feeling of stability, which reduces the anxiety that typically occurs with change.

- Assure client that staff members are nearby; respond to call signal as soon as possible. **D** ● ✦

  Close contact and a prompt response to requests provide a sense of security and facilitate the development of trust, thus reducing the client's anxiety.

- Maintain a calm, supportive, confident manner when interacting with client; encourage verbalization of fear and anxiety. **D** ● ✦

  A sense of calmness and confidence conveys to the client that someone is in control of the situation, which helps reduce anxiety.

- Reinforce physician's explanations and clarify misconceptions the client has about the pneumothorax, treatment plan, and possible recurrence; encourage questions.

  Factual information and an awareness of what to expect help decrease the anxiety that arises from uncertainty.

- Implement measures to reduce respiratory distress if present:
  - Elevate the head of the bed.
  - Encourage the client to breathe deeply and more slowly. **D** ● ✦

  Improvement of respiratory status helps relieve the anxiety associated with the feeling of not being able to breathe.

- Implement measures to reduce pain:
  - Instruct client in relaxation techniques and encourage participation in diversional activities once the period of acute pain and respiratory distress has subsided.

  Pain can create or increase anxiety because it is often perceived as a threat to well-being.

  Pain also causes sympathetic nervous system stimulation with subsequent feelings of tenseness and increased anxiety.

- When appropriate, assist the client to meet spiritual needs (e.g., arrange for a visit from the clergy).

  Spiritual support is a source of comfort and security for many people and can help reduce the client's fear and anxiety.

- Provide information based on current needs of client at a level that can be understood.

  Providing information that the client is not ready to process or cannot understand tends to increase anxiety.

  - Encourage the client to ask questions and to seek clarification of information provided.

  Making the client feel comfortable enough to ask questions or clarify information helps to reduce anxiety.

- Provide a calm, restful environment. **D** ● ✦

  A calm, restful environment facilitates relaxation and promotes a sense of security, which reduces fear and anxiety.

- Encourage significant others to project a caring, concerned attitude without obvious fear and anxiousness. **D** ✦

  Anxiety is easily transferable from one person to another. If significant others convey empathy, provide reassurance, and do not appear anxious, they can help reduce the client's fear and anxiety.

THERAPEUTIC INTERVENTIONS	RATIONALE

Dependent/Collaborative Actions
Implement measures to reduce fear and anxiety:

- Administer oxygen via nasal cannula rather than mask if possible. **D** ✦

  The use of a mask for some clients seems restrictive and suffocating. The use of a nasal cannula is more comfortable and less constraining. Improvement of respiratory status helps relieve anxiety associated with the feeling of not being able to breathe.

- Administer prescribed antianxiety agents if indicated. **D** ✦

  Reduces client's fear and anxiety

Consult appropriate health care provider (e.g., psychiatric nurse clinician, physician) if above actions fail to control fear and anxiety.

Notifying the appropriate health care provider allows for modification of the treatment plan.

DISCHARGE TEACHING/CONTINUED CARE

Nursing Diagnosis

DEFICIENT KNOWLEDGE NDx, INEFFECTIVE HEALTH MAINTENANCE NDx, OR INEFFECTIVE SELF-HEALTH MANAGEMENT* NDx

Definition: Absence or deficiency of cognitive information related to specific topic (lack of specific information necessary for clients/significant others) to make informed choices regarding condition/treatment/lifestyle changes; inability to identify, manage, and/or seek out help to maintain health; pattern of regulating and integrating into daily living a therapeutic regimen for treatment of illness and the sequelae of illness that is unsatisfactory for meeting specific health goals

CLINICAL MANIFESTATIONS

Subjective	Objective
Verbalization of the problem	Inaccurate follow through of instructions; inappropriate behaviors

RISK FACTORS

- Denial of disease process
- Fear and anxiety that blocks ability to understand

NOC OUTCOMES	NIC INTERVENTIONS
Knowledge: treatment regimen; knowledge: health promotion	Health system guidance; teaching: individual; teaching: procedure/treatment

NURSING ASSESSMENT	RATIONALE
Assess client's readiness and ability to learn.	*Early recognition of readiness to learn and meaning of illness to client allows for implementation of the appropriate teaching interventions.*

THERAPEUTIC INTERVENTIONS	RATIONALE

Desired Outcome: The client will identify safety measures related to care of chest tube insertion site and flutter valve (if present).

---

*The nurse should select the diagnostic label that is most appropriate for the individual client's teaching needs.

NDx = NANDA-I Diagnosis   **D** = Delegatable Action   ● = UAP   ✦ = LVN/LPN   ⊕▶ = Go to ⊕volve for animation

Continued...

THERAPEUTIC INTERVENTIONS	RATIONALE

Independent Actions

If the chest tube is removed before discharge, explain the importance of keeping a dressing over the insertion site until instructed by physician to remove it.

The occlusive dressing over the insertion site maintains a seal to the area where the chest tube was removed, preventing potential air leaks and loss of negative pressure during healing. Removal of this by someone other than a physician may cause a recurrence of the pneumothorax.

If client is discharged with a flutter valve in place, reinforce the following safety measures:
* Maintain an occlusive dressing around the insertion site.

The occlusive dressing around the insertion site prevents potential air leaks and loss of negative pressure.

* Ensure that the connection between the chest tube and flutter valve is taped securely and anchored to the chest wall using tape.

Supports maintenance of a closed system and reduces the risk of air leaks. Anchoring tubing to the chest wall close to the insertion site reduces the risk of inadvertent removal of the tube.

* Maintain patency of the flutter valve (e.g., avoid occluding the distal end of the flutter valve, contact physician if fluid collects in the valve, avoid activities such as swimming and bathing [the valve should not be submerged in water]).

A decrease in patency of the flutter valve causes a loss of negative pressure and may cause a recurrence of the pneumothorax.

Allow time for questions and clarification of information provided.

Everyone does not understand information as presented, so set aside time for questions to allow for clarification of information.

THERAPEUTIC INTERVENTIONS	RATIONALE

Desired Outcome: The client will identify ways to reduce the risk of another pneumothorax.

Independent Actions

Caution client to avoid activities that involve experiencing marked changes in atmospheric pressure (e.g., scuba diving, flying in an unpressurized aircraft, mountain climbing).

Changes in atmospheric pressure may cause a recurrence in an individual recovering from a pneumothorax.

Encourage client to stop smoking.

Smoking impairs gas exchange because it (1) reduces effective airway clearance by increasing mucus production and impairing ciliary function; (2) decreases oxygen availability (hemoglobin binds with the carbon monoxide in smoke rather than with oxygen); (3) causes damage to the bronchial and alveolar walls; and (4) causes vasoconstriction and subsequently reduces pulmonary blood flow.

Instruct client to continue treatment of any underlying lung disease (e.g., COPD, tuberculosis)

Treatment of underlying lung disease helps to prevent recurrence of a pneumothorax.

THERAPEUTIC INTERVENTIONS	RATIONALE

Desired Outcome: The client will state signs and symptoms to report to the health care provider.

Independent Actions

Instruct client to report the following signs and symptoms:
* Difficulty breathing
* Chest pain
* Elevated temperature
* Chills
* Increased redness and warmth at chest tube insertion site
* Purulent drainage from chest tube insertion site or flutter valve

Recognition of signs and symptoms of infection leads to early treatment of respiratory infections.

THERAPEUTIC INTERVENTIONS	RATIONALE

Desired Outcome: The client will verbalize an understanding of and a plan for adhering to recommended follow-up care including future appointments with health care provider and activity restrictions.

Independent Actions

Reinforce importance of keeping follow-up appointments with health care provider.

A follow-up appointment with the health care provider is important to monitor continued recovery.

Instruct client to avoid excessive physical exertion and lifting objects over 10 lb until permitted by physician.

Lifting an object over 10 lb and physical exertion may place the client at risk for recurrence of a pneumothorax.

Reinforce physician's explanation about the possibility of another pneumothorax.

Clients need to be aware that they are at risk for a recurrence of a pneumothorax.

Assist client to develop a plan for obtaining emergency assistance if pneumothorax recurs.

An informed client is more likely to adhere to medication regimens.

Encourage client to continue with deep breathing exercises and use of incentive spirometer for the length of time recommended by physician.

Forced deep breathing and use of incentive spirometry will increase expansion of the lungs and improve the client's ability to clear mucus from the lungs. The technique may also improve the amount of oxygen that is able to penetrate deep into the lungs.

Implement measures to improve client compliance:

- Include significant others in teaching sessions if possible.

Involvement of significant others in patient teaching improves adherence to discharge instructions.

- Encourage questions and allow time for reinforcement and clarification of information provided.

Information is presented with time for questions to allow for clarification of information.

- Provide written instructions about precautions related to chest tube insertion site and flutter valve (if present), signs and symptoms to report, future appointments with health care provider, and activity restrictions.

Written instructions allow the client to refer to instructions as needed.

ADDITIONAL NURSING DIAGNOSES

NAUSEA NDx
Related to stimulation of the vomiting center associated with noxious stimuli (e.g., foul taste of sputum and some aerosol treatments, sight of sputum) because of dyspnea, and frequent assessments and treatments.

DISTURBED SLEEP PATTERN NDx
Related to unfamiliar environment, discomfort, excessive coughing, anxiety, inability to assume usual sleep position

FEAR/ANXIETY NDx
Related to severity of symptoms (e.g., cough, chest pain, shortness of breath) and need for hospitalization, unfamiliar environment, and separation from significant others

PULMONARY EMBOLISM

Pulmonary embolism is the partial or complete obstruction of one of the pulmonary arterial vessels by an embolus. The most common source of the embolus is a thrombus that originates in a deep vein of the lower extremities. The embolus can also originate in the right side of the heart; the upper extremities; and vessels that have sustained endothelial injury caused by factors such as trauma, surgery, or the presence of an indwelling central venous catheter. Nonthrombotic sources of pulmonary embolism include air, fat, amniotic fluid, tumor cells, and foreign material (e.g., broken intravenous catheter, talc [often used to "cut" drugs injected by intravenous drug abusers]).

The clinical manifestations of pulmonary embolism are varied and nonspecific. The extensiveness of the signs and symptoms depends on the size and number of emboli, size of the vessel that is occluded, extent of vessel occlusion, and presence of preexisting cardiac or pulmonary disease. The classic signs and symptoms of a moderate-size pulmonary embolism are sudden onset of dyspnea, tachypnea, tachycardia, and a feeling of apprehension or impending doom. The person may also experience chest pain, cough, and low-grade fever.

Medical treatment varies depending on the source of the embolus and its effect on cardiopulmonary function. When the source is a thrombus, treatment usually consists of bed rest and initiation of intravenous anticoagulant therapy. A thrombolytic agent might be administered if the thromboembolus is occluding a large vessel, cardiopulmonary status is

NDx = NANDA-I Diagnosis   **D** = Delegatable Action   ● = UAP   ✦ = LVN/LPN   ⊝▶ = Go to ⊝volve for animation

Continued...

severely compromised, or both. Anticoagulant therapy (subcutaneous and/or oral) often continues for 3 to 6 months after discharge. If thrombolytic agents and anticoagulant therapy are contraindicated or unsuccessful or the source of the embolus is nonthrombotic, surgical removal of the embolus may be indicated.

This care plan focuses on the adult client hospitalized for treatment of a pulmonary embolism resulting from a deep vein thrombus. Much of the information is also applicable to clients receiving follow-up care at home.

OUTCOME/DISCHARGE CRITERIA

The client will:
1. Have adequate respiratory function
2. Have no signs and symptoms of complications

3. Identify ways to reduce the risk of recurrent thrombus formation and pulmonary embolism
4. Verbalize an understanding of medications ordered including rationale, food and drug interactions, side effects, schedule for taking, and importance of taking as prescribed
5. Demonstrate the ability to correctly draw up and administer heparin subcutaneously if prescribed
6. Identify ways to prevent bleeding associated with anticoagulant therapy
7. State signs and symptoms to report to the health care provider
8. Verbalize an understanding of and a plan for adhering to recommended follow-up care including future appointments with health care provider and activity level.

Nursing Diagnosis | INEFFECTIVE BREATHING PATTERN NDx

Definition: Inspiration and/or expiration that does not provide adequate ventilation

Related to:
- Increased rate of respirations associated with fear, anxiety, and stimulant effects of hypoxia
- Decreased rate of respirations associated with the depressant effect of some medications (e.g., narcotic [opioid] analgesics)
- Decreased depth of respirations associated with:
  - Fear, anxiety, and reluctance to breathe deeply because of chest pain if present
  - Depressant effect of some medications (e.g., narcotic [opioid] analgesics)
  - Decreased mobility

CLINICAL MANIFESTATIONS

Subjective	Objective
Verbalization of restlessness, anxiety, nausea, chest pain, shortness of breath	Dyspnea; tachypnea; tachycardia; hypotension; impaired chest wall expansion; cough and/or hemoptysis; transient pleural rub; jugular vein distention; diaphoresis; cyanosis; abnormal breath sounds—crackles; S_1 and S_4 gallop rhythms; transient pleural friction rub; fever; use of accessory muscles when breathing; significant decrease in oximetry results; abnormal arterial blood gas values; chest radiograph—normal or elevated hemidiaphragm; after 24 hours—small infiltrates

RISK FACTORS
- Deep vein thrombosis (DVT)
- Pain
- Muscle fatigue
- Obesity
- Immobility

NOC OUTCOMES

Respiratory status; ventilation

DESIRED OUTCOMES

The client will experience an effective breathing pattern as evidenced by:
  a. Normal rate and depth of respirations
  b. Absence of dyspnea

NIC INTERVENTIONS

Respiratory monitoring; ventilation assistance; anxiety management; pain management

NURSING ASSESSMENT	RATIONALE
Assess for signs and symptoms of an ineffective breathing pattern: • Rapid, shallow respirations • Restlessness • Significant decrease in oximetry results • Abnormal arterial blood gas values Assess for significant abnormalities in chest radiograph reports.	*Early recognition of signs and symptoms of ineffective breathing patterns allows for prompt intervention.*

THERAPEUTIC INTERVENTIONS	RATIONALE

Independent Actions

Implement measures to improve breathing pattern:
- Perform actions to reduce chest pain:
  - Splint chest with pillow or hands when deep breathing, coughing, and changing position. **D** ● ✦

  - Provide or assist with nonpharmacological methods for pain relief (e.g., relaxation techniques, restful environment, diversional activities).

- Perform actions to reduce fear and anxiety:
  - Remain with client during periods of respiratory distress.
  - Provide a calm, restful environment. **D** ● ✦

- Elevate the head of the bed.
- Encourage the client to breathe deeply and more slowly. **D** ● ✦
- Perform actions to improve gas exchange:
  - Place client in a semi- to high-Fowler's position unless contraindicated. **D** ● ✦
  - Position with pillows. **D** ● ✦
- Instruct client to breathe slowly; if hyperventilating, instruct client to deep breathe or use incentive spirometer every 1 to 2 hours.
- Increase activity when allowed. **D** ● ✦

Splinting the chest with deep breathing, coughing, or changing position reduces pain and promotes a more effective respiratory effort.

Relaxation and diversional activities help to alleviate pain, fear, and anxiety. Pain causes sympathetic nervous system stimulation with subsequent feelings of tenseness and increased anxiety, and can increase respiratory distress.

Reduction in fear and anxiety prevents the shallow and/or rapid breathing that can occur with fear and anxiety.

A calm, restful environment facilitates relaxation and promotes a sense of security, and reduces the rapid breathing associated with fear and anxiety.

Provides for improved expansion of the lungs

Helps calm the client while improving ventilation

Placing the client in a semi- to high-Fowler's position promotes optimal gas exchange by enabling chest expansion.

Positioning with pillows helps to prevent slumping.

Deep breathing and use of incentive spirometry help to reduce dyspnea and improve tissue oxygenation.

Conservation of energy through activity restrictions allows energy to be focused on breathing. Increasing activity as tolerated helps mobilize excretions and promotes deeper breathing and lung expansion.

Dependent/Collaborative Actions

Implement measures to improve breathing pattern:
- Perform actions to reduce chest pain:
  - Administer analgesics as needed.
- Administer central nervous system depressants judiciously; hold medication and consult physician if respiratory rate is less than 12 breaths/min.

Consult appropriate health care provider (e.g., respiratory therapist, physician) if ineffective breathing pattern persists or worsens.

Pain relief increases client's willingness to take deep breaths and improves lung expansion.

Central nervous system depressants cause depression of the respiratory center in the brainstem, which can result in a decreased rate and depth of respiration.

Notifying the appropriate health care professionals allows for a prompt and multidisciplinary approach to treatment.

Nursing Diagnosis   **IMPAIRED GAS EXCHANGE** NDx

Definition: Deficit in oxygenation and/or carbon dioxide elimination at the alveolar-capillary membrane

Related to:
- Decreased pulmonary perfusion associated with obstruction of pulmonary arterial blood flow by the embolus and vasoconstriction resulting from the release of vasoactive substances (e.g., serotonin, endothelin, some prostaglandins)
- Decreased bronchial airflow associated with bronchoconstriction resulting from:
  - The release of substances such as serotonin and some prostaglandins
  - A compensatory response to an increase in the amount of dead space in the underperfused lung area (the compensatory bronchoconstriction also affects airways in perfused lung areas)
- Loss of effective lung surface associated with atelectasis if it occurs

CLINICAL MANIFESTATIONS

Subjective	Objective
Reports of restlessness; confusion; irritability; somnolence; shortness of breath	Tachypnea; dyspnea; diaphoresis; hypotension; decreased chest wall expansion; use of accessory muscles when breathing; significant decrease in oximetry results; abnormal arterial blood gas values; hypoxemia; hypocarbia; nasal flaring; tachycardia

RISK FACTORS
- DVT
- Pain
- Muscle fatigue
- Obesity
- Decreased lung expansion

DESIRED OUTCOMES

The client will experience adequate O_2/CO_2 exchange as evidenced by:
  a. Usual mental status
  b. Unlabored respirations at 12 to 20 breaths/min
  c. Oximetry results within normal range
  d. Arterial blood gas values within normal range

NOC OUTCOMES

Respiratory status: gas exchange

NIC INTERVENTIONS

Respiratory monitoring; oxygen therapy; airway management; ventilation assistance; acid-base management

NURSING ASSESSMENT	RATIONALE
Assess for and report signs and symptoms of impaired gas exchange: • Restlessness, irritability • Confusion, somnolence • Tachypnea, dyspnea • Abnormal arterial blood gas values • Significant decrease in oximetry results • Decreased PaO_2 and/or increased $PaCO_2$	*Early recognition of signs and symptoms of impaired gas exchange allows for prompt intervention.*

THERAPEUTIC INTERVENTIONS	RATIONALE

Independent Actions
Implement measures to improve gas exchange:

• Maintain client on bed rest; increase activity gradually as allowed and tolerated. **D** ● ✦	*Placing the client on strict bed rest will help to conserve energy during periods of acute respiratory distress. Increasing activity gradually will improve strength and ability to perform activities.*
• Discourage smoking.	*The carbon monoxide in smoke decreases oxygen availability, and the nicotine can cause vasoconstriction and further reduce pulmonary blood flow.*

THERAPEUTIC INTERVENTIONS	RATIONALE
Dependent/Collaborative Actions Implement measures to improve gas exchange:	
• Maintain oxygen therapy as ordered. **D** ✦	*Supplemental oxygen helps to relieve dyspnea and improves gas exchange.*
• Administer anticoagulants (e.g., continuous intravenous heparin, low-molecular-weight heparin, warfarin) as ordered.	*Anticoagulants will prevent blood clotting, which will help to improve pulmonary blood flow.*
• Prepare client for the following if planned:	
• Injection of a thrombolytic agent (e.g., streptokinase, urokinase, alteplase)	*Thrombolytics convert plasminogen to plasmin, which then degrades the fibrin in clots. The loss of the fibrin results in the lysis of a clot.*
• Embolectomy	*An embolectomy is the surgical removal of a blood clot. The patient should be educated about the procedure and postoperative care.*
Consult appropriate health care provider (e.g., respiratory therapist, physician) if signs and symptoms of impaired gas exchange persist or worsen.	*Notifying the appropriate health care provider allows for a multifaceted treatment plan.*

Nursing Diagnosis ACUTE PAIN NDx (CHEST)

Definition: Unpleasant sensory and emotional experience arising from actual or potential tissue damage or described in terms of such damage; may be sudden or slow onset of any intensity from mild to severe with an anticipated or predictable end and a duration of <6 months.

Related to:
- Decreased pulmonary tissue perfusion associated with obstructed pulmonary blood flow
- Inflammation of the parietal pleura associated with tissue damage if infarction occurs

CLINICAL MANIFESTATIONS

Subjective	Objective
Verbalization of chest pain with breathing and coughing	Grimacing; rubbing chest; reluctance to move; shallow respiration; tachycardia; increased B/P

RISK FACTORS
- DVT
- Excessive coughing
- Increased sputum production

DESIRED OUTCOMES
The client will experience diminished chest pain as evidenced by:
  a. Verbalization of a decrease in or absence of pain
  b. Relaxed facial expression and body positioning
  c. Increased participation in activities when allowed
  d. Pulse and B/P within normal range for client

NOC OUTCOMES
Pain control; pain level

NIC INTERVENTIONS
Analgesic administration; pain management; environmental management: comfort; analgesic administration

NURSING ASSESSMENT	RATIONALE
Assess for signs and symptoms of pain (e.g., verbalization of pain, grimacing, reluctance to move, rubbing chest, guarding of affected side of chest, shallow respirations, increased B/P, tachycardia).	*Early recognition of signs and symptoms of pain allows for prompt intervention and improved pain control.*

NDx = NANDA-I Diagnosis   **D** = Delegatable Action   ● = UAP   ✦ = LVN/LPN   ⊜▶ = Go to ⊜volve for animation

Continued...

NURSING ASSESSMENT	RATIONALE
Assess client's perception of the severity of pain using a pain intensity rating scale.	*An awareness of the severity of pain being experienced helps determine the most appropriate interventions for pain management. Use of a pain intensity scale gives the nurse a clearer understanding of the pain being experienced and promotes consistency when communicating with others about the client's pain experience.*
Assess the client's pain pattern (e.g., location, quality, onset, duration, precipitating factors, aggravating factors, alleviating factors).	*Knowledge of the client's pain pattern assists in the identification of effective pain management interventions.*
Ask the client to describe previous pain experiences and methods used to manage pain effectively.	*Many variables affect a client's response to pain (e.g., age, sex, coping style, previous experience with pain, culture, cause of pain). Knowledge of the client's usual response to pain and methods previously used to manage pain effectively enables the nurse to evaluate the client's pain more accurately and facilitates the identification of effective strategies for pain management.*

THERAPEUTIC INTERVENTIONS	RATIONALE

Independent Actions

Implement measures to reduce fear and anxiety (e.g., assure client that chest pain is common with embolism and should subside with treatment; assure the client that the need for pain relief is understood).	*Fear and anxiety can decrease the client's threshold and tolerance for pain and thereby heighten the perception of pain. In addition, pain management methods are not as effective if the client is tense and unable to relax.*
Implement measures to improve gas exchange:	
• Maintain client on bed rest and increase activity gradually as allowed and tolerated. **D** ● ✦	*Placing the client on strict bed rest will help to conserve energy during periods of acute respiratory distress. Increasing activity gradually will improve strength and ability to perform activities.*
• Place client in a semi- to high-Fowler's position unless contraindicated. **D** ● ✦	*Positioning the client in semi- to high-Fowler's position promotes optimal gas exchange by enabling chest expansion.*
• Position with pillows. **D** ● ✦	*Positioning with pillows helps to prevent slumping.*
• Instruct and assist the client to splint the chest with hands or pillows when deep breathing, coughing, or changing position. **D** ● ✦	*Splinting the chest with deep breathing, coughing, or changing position reduces pain and promotes a more effective cough.*
• Instruct client to breathe slowly if hyperventilating.	
• Instruct client to deep breathe or use incentive spirometer every 1 to 2 hours. **D** ✦	*Deep breathing and use of incentive spirometry helps to expand the lungs and improve oxygenation.*
• Provide or assist with nonpharmacological methods for pain relief (e.g., relaxation techniques, restful environment, diversional activities).	*Relaxation and diversional activities help to alleviate pain, fear, and anxiety, which in turn will decrease dyspnea.*
• Implement measures to promote rest (e.g., minimize environmental activity and noise). **D** ● ✦	*A calm, restful environment facilitates relaxation and promotes a sense of security, and reduces rapid breathing associated with fear and anxiety.*

Dependent/Collaborative Actions

Implement measures to improve gas exchange:	
• Maintain oxygen therapy as ordered. **D** ✦	*Supplemental oxygen helps to relieve dyspnea and improves gas exchange.*
Administer analgesics before activities and procedures that can cause pain and before pain becomes severe. **D** ✦	*The administration of analgesics before a pain-producing event helps minimize the pain that will be experienced. Analgesics are also more effective if given before a procedure and will improve the client's ability to tolerate the procedure.*
Consult appropriate health care provider (e.g., physician, pharmacist, pain management specialist) if above measures fail to provide adequate pain relief.	*Notifying the appropriate health care provider allows for a multifaceted treatment plan.*

Collaborative Diagnoses # RISK FOR RIGHT-SIDED HEART FAILURE

Definition: A condition where the right side of the heart is unable to pump blood efficiently

Related to:
Increased cardiac workload associated with:
- Pulmonary hypertension (can result from pulmonary vasoconstriction that occurs in response to hypoxia and the release of vasoactive substances)
- Compensatory response to decreased pulmonary blood flow that results from obstruction of multiple and/or large pulmonary vessels

CLINICAL MANIFESTATIONS

Subjective	Objective
Reports of weakness and fatigue	Tachypnea; tachycardia; dyspnea; restlessness; confusion; irritability; peripheral edema; decreased urine output; distended neck veins

RISK FACTORS
- Smoking
- Chronic respiratory disease
- Obesity
- Hypertension

DESIRED OUTCOMES

The client will not develop right-sided heart failure as evidenced by:
   a. Pulse rate of 60 to 100 beats/min
   b. Usual mental status
   c. Usual strength and activity tolerance
   d. Adequate urine output
   e. Stable weight
   f. Absence of edema and distended neck veins

NURSING ASSESSMENT	RATIONALE
Assess for and report signs and symptoms of right-sided heart failure: • Further increase in pulse rate • Restlessness, confusion • Weakness and fatigue • Decreased urine output • Weight gain • Dependent peripheral edema • Distended neck veins • Chest radiograph results showing cardiomegaly	*Early recognition of signs and symptoms of right-sided heart failure allows for prompt intervention.*

THERAPEUTIC INTERVENTIONS	RATIONALE

Dependent/Collaborative Actions
Implement measures to improve pulmonary blood flow:
 	
• Administer anticoagulants (e.g., continuous intravenous heparin, low-molecular-weight heparin, warfarin (as ordered).
• Prepare client for the following if planned:
  • Injection of a thrombolytic agent (e.g., streptokinase, urokinase, alteplase)
 	
  • Embolectomy
	These interventions will reduce cardiac workload and the subsequent risk of right-sided heart failure by decreasing the pressure against which the heart must pump.
	Anticoagulants will prevent blood clotting which will help to improve pulmonary blood flow and decrease the potential of an extension or recurrence of a pulmonary embolism.
	
	Thrombolytics convert plasminogen to plasmin, which then degrades the fibrin in clots. The loss of the fibrin results in the lysis of a clot.
	An embolectomy is the surgical removal of a blood clot. The patient should be educated about the procedure and postoperative care.

Continued...

THERAPEUTIC INTERVENTIONS	RATIONALE
If signs and symptoms of right-sided heart failure occur	
• Maintain oxygen therapy as ordered.	*Supplemental oxygen helps to relieve dyspnea and improves gas exchange.*
• Maintain client on strict bed rest in a semi- to high-Fowler's position	*Placing the client on strict bed rest will help to conserve energy during periods of acute respiratory distress. Positioning the client in a semi- to high-Fowler's position promotes optimal gas exchange by enabling chest expansion.*
• Maintain fluid and sodium restrictions if ordered.	*Restricting a client's sodium and fluid will help reduce fluid volume overload.*
• Administer medications that may reduce vascular congestion and/or cardiac workload (e.g., diuretics, cardiotonics, vasodilators)	*Diuretics decrease fluid volume through inhibiting reabsorption of water, which decreases fluid volume.*
	Cardiotonics increase the contractile force of the heart, which increases cardiac output.
	Vasodilators dilate the arterioles, which decreases B/P and decreases the work of the heart.

Collaborative Diagnosis RISK FOR EXTENDED OR RECURRENT PULMONARY EMBOLISM

Definition: A sudden blockage of the pulmonary artery or one or more branches that usually occurs from a blood clot that formed in the legs

Related to: Inadequate response to therapy

CLINICAL MANIFESTATIONS

Subjective	Objective
Reports of shortness of breath, persistent chest pain	Dyspnea; tachycardia; cough with blood-streaked sputum; declining oximetry O_2 levels; pleural rub; cyanosis

RISK FACTORS
- Sedentary lifestyle
- Smoking
- Obesity
- Dehydration

DESIRED OUTCOMES

The client will not experience an extension or recurrence of a pulmonary embolism as evidenced by:
 a. Absence of or diminishing chest pain
 b. Absence of or decrease in dyspnea
 c. Pulse rate 60 to 100 beats/min
 d. Arterial blood gas values returning to normal

NURSING ASSESSMENT	RATIONALE
Assess for and report signs and symptoms of extended or recurrent pulmonary embolism (e.g., development of persistent or increased chest pain, dyspnea, apprehension, tachypnea, tachycardia, declining PaO_2).	*Early recognition of signs and symptoms of pulmonary embolism allows for prompt treatment.*

THERAPEUTIC INTERVENTIONS	RATIONALE
Dependent/Collaborative Actions	
Implement measures to prevent recurrence of a pulmonary embolism:	
• Encourage and assist client to perform active foot and leg exercises every 1 to 2 hours while awake. **D** ● ✦	*Exercise of the legs and feet while on bedrest helps to maintain return of blood flow from the lower extremities to the heart.*
• Instruct client to avoid positions that compromise blood flow (e.g., pillows under knees, crossing legs, sitting for long periods).	*These positions (i.e., placing pillows under knees, crossing legs) compromise blood flow and increase the potential for a thrombus.*

THERAPEUTIC INTERVENTIONS	RATIONALE
• Elevate foot of bed for 20-minute intervals several times a shift unless contraindicated. **D** ● ✦	*This action increases return of blood flow from the lower extremities to the heart.*
• Maintain a minimum fluid intake of 2500 mL/day unless contraindicated to prevent increased blood viscosity.	*Maintaining a minimum fluid intake of 2500 mL/day prevents increased blood viscosity and the potential for a thrombus.*
• Consult physician about an order for antiembolism stockings or an intermittent pneumatic compression device.	*Antiembolic stockings and/or an intermittent pneumatic compression device will maintain blood flow from the lower extremities to the heart and decrease the incidence of a thrombus.*
Perform actions to prevent dislodgment of thrombus:	
• Maintain client on strict bed rest in a semi- to high-Fowler's position. **D** ● ✦	*Immobility in a patient who has a blood clot will help to prevent the clot from dislodging and moving in the circulatory system.*
If signs and symptoms of extended or recurrent pulmonary embolism occur:	
• Maintain oxygen therapy as ordered. **D** ✦	*Supplemental oxygen helps to relieve dyspnea and improves gas exchange.*
• Prepare client for diagnostic tests (e.g., ventilation-perfusion lung scan, arterial blood gases, d-dimer level, pulmonary angiography) if indicated.	*Before any diagnostic exam or surgical procedure, explain the procedure to the client and family. An explanation decreases fear and anxiety.*
• Prepare client for surgical interventions (e.g., embolectomy) if planned.	
• Assess for and report signs and symptoms of pulmonary infarction (e.g., hemoptysis, fever, increased WBC count).	*Recognition of signs and symptoms of a pulmonary infarction allows for prompt treatment, which may decrease the impact of the infarction.*
• Implement measures to improve breathing pattern and gas exchange (e.g., encourage coughing and deep breathing, use incentive spirometry every 1 to 2 hours, place client in semi- to high-Fowler's position).	*These actions improve lung expansion and gas exchange to further reduce the risk of atelectasis.*

Collaborative Diagnosis **RISK FOR ATELECTASIS**

Definition: Collapse of lung tissue caused by hypoventilated alveoli

Related to:
• Shallow respirations
• Stasis of secretions in alveoli and bronchioles
• Decreased surfactant production (results from inadequate deep breathing and changes in regional blood flow in the lungs)

CLINICAL MANIFESTATIONS

Subjective	Objective
Verbal reports of difficulty breathing	Diminished or absent breath sounds; dull percussion over affected area; increased respiratory rate; dyspnea; tachycardia; elevated temperature

RISK FACTORS
• Immobility
• Ineffective airway clearance
• Smoking
• Obesity

DESIRED OUTCOMES

The client will not develop atelectasis as evidenced by:
a. Clear, audible breath sounds
b. Resonant percussion note over lungs
c. Unlabored respirations at 12 to 20 breaths/min
d. Pulse rate within normal range for client
e. Afebrile status

NURSING ASSESSMENT	RATIONALE
Assess for and report signs and symptoms of atelectasis: • Diminished or absent breath sounds • Dull percussion note over affected area • Increased respiratory rate • Dyspnea • Tachycardia • Elevated temperature	*Early recognition of signs and symptoms of atelectasis allows for implementation of the appropriate interventions.*

 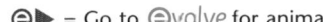

Continued...

NURSING ASSESSMENT	RATIONALE
Monitor pulse oximetry results as indicated.	*Pulse oximetry is an indirect measure of arterial oxygen saturation. Monitoring pulse oximetry (SaO₂) allows for early detection of hypoxia and implementation of the appropriate interventions.*
Monitor chest radiograph results.	*Chest radiograph provides radiographic confirmation of atelectasis.*

THERAPEUTIC INTERVENTIONS	RATIONALE

Independent Actions

Implement measures to prevent atelectasis: **D** ✦	*Improves client ability to expand lung tissue and improve oxygenation and clearance of mucous.*
• Perform actions to improve breathing pattern:	
• Encourage client to deep breathe.	
• Incentive spirometry	
• Perform actions to promote effective airway clearance.	
• Turn, cough, and deep breathe.	
If signs and symptoms of atelectasis occur:	*Lack of movement places a client at risk for atelectasis. Changing positions frequently, coughing, and deep breathing help to expand the lungs, enhancing alveolar expansion.*
• Increase frequency of position change, coughing or "huffing," deep breathing, and use of incentive spirometer.	
Consult physician if signs and symptoms of atelectasis persist or worsen.	*Notifying the appropriate health care provider will allow for modification of the treatment plan.*

Collaborative Diagnosis   # RISK FOR UNUSUAL BLEEDING

Definition: Bleeding related to therapeutic regimen

Related to: Excessive use of thrombolytics and anticoagulants

CLINICAL MANIFESTATIONS

Subjective	**Objective**
Not applicable	Petechiae; bruises easily; prolonged bleeding from puncture sites; unusual joint pain; hypotension; tachycardia; decreases in Hgb and Hct

RISK FACTORS	DESIRED OUTCOMES

• Smoking
• Multiple IV insertions
	The client will not experience unusual bleeding as evidenced by:
	   a. Skin and mucous membranes free of petechiae, purpura, ecchymoses, and active bleeding
	   b. Absence of unusual joint pain
	   c. No increase in abdominal girth
	   d. Absence of frank and occult blood in stool, urine, and vomitus
	   e. Usual menstrual flow
	   f. Vital signs within normal range for client
	   g. Stable Hct and Hgb

NURSING ASSESSMENT	RATIONALE
Assess client for and report signs and symptoms of unusual bleeding: • Petechiae, purpura, ecchymoses • Gingival bleeding • Prolonged bleeding from puncture sites • Epistaxis, hemoptysis • Unusual joint pain • Increase in abdominal girth	*Early recognition of signs and symptoms of unusual bleeding, which may occur as part of the infarction process and from medications (i.e., thrombolytics and anticoagulants) during treatment of a thrombus or pulmonary embolism, allows for implementation of the appropriate interventions.*

NURSING ASSESSMENT	RATIONALE

- Frank or occult blood in stool, urine, or vomitus
- Menorrhagia
- Restlessness, confusion
- Decreasing B/P and increased pulse rate
- Decrease in Hct and Hgb levels

THERAPEUTIC INTERVENTIONS	RATIONALE

Dependent/Collaborative Actions

Monitor platelet count and coagulation test results (e.g., prothrombin time or international normalized ratio [INR], activated partial thromboplastin time). Report a low platelet count and coagulation test results that exceed the therapeutic range.

Monitoring effectiveness and dosage requirements of heparin and warfarin is done via prothrombin time/INR/activated partial thromboplastin time. Platelet counts should be monitored every 2 to 3 days because these medications may cause mild thrombocytopenia.

If platelet count is low, coagulation test results are abnormal, or Hct and Hgb levels decrease, test all stools, urine, and vomitus for occult blood. Report positive results.

Increased bleeding may occur when a patient is receiving anticoagulant therapy. Reporting any signs of bleeding, including a positive result for occult blood, allows for timely treatment and changes in medication dosage as needed.

Implement measures to prevent bleeding:
- Avoid giving injections whenever possible; consult physician about prescribing an alternative route for medications ordered to be given intramuscularly or subcutaneously.

It is important to prevent bleeding while the patient is receiving anticoagulants. Injections may cause increased bleeding and oozing from the injection sites.

  - When giving injections or performing venous or arterial punctures, use the smallest gauge needle possible and apply gentle, prolonged pressure to the site after the needle is removed. **D** ✦

Use of the smallest needle possible and application of gentle, prolonged pressure at the puncture site will help to prevent excessive bleeding.

- Caution client to avoid activities that increase the risk for trauma (e.g., shaving with a straight-edge razor, using stiff bristle toothbrush or dental floss).

These activities increase the risk of trauma and associated bleeding.

- Whenever possible, avoid intubations (e.g., nasogastric) and procedures that can cause injury to the rectal mucosa (e.g., taking temperature rectally, inserting a rectal suppository, administering an enema).

Procedures that may cause injury to the mucous membranes may cause excessive bleeding. If the client must undergo one of these procedures, the nurse must monitor the client closely for bleeding.

- Perform actions to reduce the risk for falls (e.g., keep bed in low position with side rails up when client is in bed, avoid unnecessary clutter in room, instruct client to wear slippers/shoes with nonslip soles when ambulating). **D** ● ✦

Falls are another way that a client who is receiving anticoagulants may experience increased bleeding. Mechanisms should be put in place to decrease the risk of falls.

- Pad side rails if client is confused or restless.
- Instruct client to avoid blowing nose forcefully or straining to have a bowel movement; consult physician about an order for a decongestant and/or laxative if indicated.

Forcefully blowing one's nose or straining with a bowel movement should be avoided during anticoagulant therapy because these actions may increase bleeding.

If bleeding occurs and does not subside spontaneously:
- Apply firm, prolonged pressure to bleeding areas if possible.

Pressure at the site helps to promote clotting.

- If epistaxis occurs, place client in a high-Fowler's position and apply pressure and ice pack to nasal area.

Placing the client in high-Fowler's and applying pressure and ice to the nasal area helps to promote clotting.

- Maintain oxygen therapy as ordered. **D** ✦

Oxygen therapy will assist in maintaining oxygen saturation if bleeding occurs.

- Administer protamine sulfate (antidote for heparin), vitamin K (e.g., phytonadione), and/or whole blood or blood products (e.g., fresh frozen plasma, platelets) as ordered.

Administration of the antidotes for heparin and warfarin will reverse the effects of these medications and decrease bleeding.

Nursing Diagnosis	**FEAR/ANXIETY** NDx

Definition: Fear—Response to perceived threat that is consciously recognized as a danger

Anxiety—Vague, uneasy feeling of discomfort or dread accompanied by an autonomic response (the source often nonspecific or unknown to the individual); a feeling of apprehension caused by anticipation of danger. It is an alerting signal that warns of impending danger and enables the individual to take measures to deal with a threat

Related to:
- Exacerbation of symptoms (e.g., increased dyspnea, feeling of suffocation)
- Lack of understanding of the diagnosis, diagnostic tests, treatments, and prognosis
- Unfamiliar environment
- Possibility of recurrent embolism; threat of death

CLINICAL MANIFESTATIONS

Subjective	Objective
Verbalization of fear and/or anxiety	Unusual sleep patterns; unstable vital signs; restlessness; shakiness; diaphoresis; self-focused behavior

RISK FACTORS
- Fear of the unknown
- Fear of death
- Pain
- Unknown environment
- Fear of recurrence of embolism

DESIRED OUTCOMES

The client will experience a reduction in fear and anxiety as evidenced by:
  a. Verbalization of feeling less anxious
  b. Usual sleep pattern
  c. Relaxed facial expression and body movements
  d. Stable vital signs
  e. Usual perceptual ability and interactions with others

NOC OUTCOMES

Anxiety level; fear level; anxiety self-control; fear self-control

NIC INTERVENTIONS

Anxiety reduction; calming technique; emotional support; presence; pain management

NURSING ASSESSMENT	RATIONALE

Assess client for signs and symptoms of fear and anxiety (e.g., verbalization of feeling anxious, insomnia, tenseness, shakiness, restlessness, diaphoresis, elevated B/P, tachycardia, self-focused behaviors).

Moderate anxiety enhances the client's ability to solve problems. With severe anxiety or panic, the client is not able to follow directions and may become hyperactive and extremely agitated.

Validate perceptions carefully, remembering that some behavior may result from hypoxia and/or hypercapnia.

Assessment of the client's fear helps to determine whether the coping mechanisms are effective and which need to be strengthened.

THERAPEUTIC INTERVENTIONS	RATIONALE

Independent Actions
Implement measures to reduce fear and anxiety:
- Orient client to hospital environment, equipment, and routines. **D** ● ✦

Familiarity with the environment and usual routines reduces the client's anxiety about the unknown, provides a sense of security, and increases the client's sense of control, all of which help decrease anxiety.

- Introduce staff who will be participating in the client's care. If possible, maintain consistency in staff assigned to client's care.

Introduction to staff familiarizes clients with those individuals who will be working with them, which provides clients with a feeling of stability, which reduces the anxiety that typically occurs with change.

- Assure client that staff members are nearby; respond to call signal as soon as possible. **D** ● ✦

Close contact and a prompt response to requests provide a sense of security and facilitate the development of trust, thus reducing the client's anxiety.

THERAPEUTIC INTERVENTIONS	RATIONALE
• Maintain a calm, supportive, confident manner when interacting with client; encourage verbalization of fear and anxiety. **D** ● ✦	*A sense of calmness and confidence conveys to the client that someone is in control of the situation, which helps reduce anxiety.*
• Reinforce physician's explanations and clarify misconceptions the client has about the pulmonary embolus, treatment plan, and possible recurrence; encourage questions.	*Factual information and an awareness of what to expect help decrease the anxiety that arises from uncertainty.*
• Implement measures to reduce respiratory distress if present: • Elevate the head of the bed. • Encourage the client to breathe deeply and more slowly. **D** ● ✦	*Improvement of respiratory status helps relieve anxiety associated with the feeling of not being able to breathe.*
• Implement measures to reduce pain: • Instruct client in relaxation techniques and encourage participation in diversional activities once the period of acute pain and respiratory distress has subsided	*Pain can create or increase anxiety because it is often perceived as a threat to well-being.* *Pain also causes sympathetic nervous system stimulation with subsequent feelings of tenseness and increased anxiety.*
• When appropriate, assist the client to meet spiritual needs (e.g., arrange for a visit from the clergy).	*Spiritual support is a source of comfort and security for many people and can help reduce the client's fear and anxiety.*
• Provide information based on current needs of the client at a level that can be understood. • Encourage the client to ask questions and to seek clarification of information provided.	*Providing information that the client is not ready to process or cannot understand tends to increase anxiety.* *Making the client feel comfortable enough to ask questions or clarify information helps to reduce anxiety.*
• Provide a calm, restful environment. **D** ● ✦	*A calm, restful environment facilitates relaxation and promotes a sense of security, which reduces fear and anxiety.*
• Encourage significant others to project a caring, concerned attitude without obvious fear and anxiousness.	*Anxiety is easily transferable from one person to another. If significant others convey empathy, provide reassurance, and do not appear anxious, they can help reduce the client's fear and anxiety.*

Dependent/Collaborative Actions

Implement measures to reduce fear and anxiety:	
• Administer oxygen via nasal cannula rather than mask if possible. **D** ✦	*The use of a mask for some clients seems restrictive and suffocating. The use of a nasal cannula is more comfortable and less constraining. Improvement of respiratory status helps relieve anxiety associated with the feeling of not being able to breathe.*
• Administer prescribed antianxiety agents if indicated. **D** ✦	*Decreasing anxiety may improve respiratory status.*
Consult appropriate health care provider (e.g., psychiatric nurse clinician, physician) if above actions fail to control fear and anxiety.	*Notifying the appropriate health care provider allows for modification of the treatment plan.*

DISCHARGE TEACHING/CONTINUED CARE

Nursing Diagnosis

DEFICIENT KNOWLEDGE NDx, INEFFECTIVE HEALTH MAINTENANCE NDx, OR INEFFECTIVE SELF-HEALTH MANAGEMENT* NDx

Definition: Absence or deficiency of cognitive information related to specific topic (lack of specific information necessary for clients/significant others) to make informed choices regarding condition/treatment/lifestyle changes; inability to identify, manage, and/or seek out help to maintain health; pattern of regulating and integrating into daily living a therapeutic regimen for treatment of illness and the sequelae of illness that is unsatisfactory for meeting specific health goals

*The nurse should select the diagnostic label that is most appropriate for the individual client's teaching needs.

NDx = NANDA-I Diagnosis **D** = Delegatable Action ● = UAP ✦ = LVN/LFN ⊜▶ = Go to ⊜volve for animation

Continued...

CLINICAL MANIFESTATIONS

Subjective	Objective
Verbalization of the problem	Inaccurate follow through of instructions; inappropriate behaviors

RISK FACTORS
- Denial of disease process
- Fear and anxiety that blocks ability to understand

NOC OUTCOMES	NIC INTERVENTIONS
Knowledge: disease process; knowledge: treatment regimen	Health system guidance; teaching: individual; teaching: prescribed medication; teaching: prescribed activity/exercise; teaching: psychomotor skill

NURSING ASSESSMENT	RATIONALE
Assess client readiness to learn Assess meaning of illness to client	*Early recognition of readiness to learn and meaning of illness to client allows for appropriate teaching interventions.*

THERAPEUTIC INTERVENTIONS	RATIONALE

Desired Outcome: The client will identify ways to reduce the risk of recurrent thrombus formation and pulmonary embolism.

Independent Actions

Provide the following instructions on ways to promote venous blood flow and reduce the risk of thrombus recurrence:

- Avoid wearing constrictive clothing (e.g., garters, girdles, narrow-banded knee-high hose). — *Wearing constrictive clothing decreases blood flow from the lower extremities, increasing the risk of a thrombus.*
- Avoid sitting and standing in one position for long periods. — *Decreases the ability of veins to prevent stasis of blood.*
- Avoid crossing legs and lying or sitting with pillows under knees. — *Decreases blood flow and increases the risk of developing a thrombus.*
- Wear graduated compression stockings or support hose during the day. — *Compression stockings and support hose prevent venous dilation and increase blood flow to the heart.*
- Engage in regular aerobic exercise (e.g., swimming, walking, cycling) — *Each of these activities stimulates venous blood return to the heart, decreasing the incidence of a thrombus.*
- Elevate legs periodically, especially when sitting.
- Dorsiflex feet regularly.
- Maintain recommended weight for age, height, and body frame. — *Overweight individuals are at a higher risk for development of a thrombus because of increased endothelial fibrinolytic dysfunction and an increased risk for atherothrombotic events.*

- Inform client that smoking and the use of estrogen or oral contraceptives can increase the risk for recurrent thrombus formation. — *Smoking and the use of estrogens or oral contraceptives have been associated with thrombus formation and pulmonary embolism.*
- Instruct client to avoid trauma to or massage of any area of suspected thrombus formation in order to decrease the risk of pulmonary embolism. — *Trauma or massage to an area of suspected thrombus may dislodge the thrombus into the vascular system and place the patient at risk for a pulmonary embolism.*
- Provide information regarding exercise programs and support groups that can assist the client to stop smoking and/or lose weight. — *Providing information on community resources provides a continuum of care.*

THERAPEUTIC INTERVENTIONS	RATIONALE

Desired Outcome: The client will verbalize an understanding of medications ordered including rationale, food and drug interactions, side effects, schedule for taking, and importance of taking as prescribed.

THERAPEUTIC INTERVENTIONS	RATIONALE
Independent Actions Explain the rationale for, side effects of, and importance of taking medications prescribed.	*Understanding of the impact of medications improves adherence.*
If client is discharged on warfarin (e.g., Coumadin), instruct to:	
• Keep scheduled appointments for periodic blood studies to monitor coagulation time.	*Appropriate dosing of warfarin is based on monitoring of lab values (INR) and bleeding time. If these values are not monitored, the client's dosage may become too high, increasing the risk of bleeding, or too low, increasing the risk of thrombus.*
• Take medication at the same time each day, do not stop taking medication abruptly, and do not attempt to make up for missed doses.	*Appropriate medication administration is important to obtain the most beneficial effects.*
• Avoid regular and/or excessive intake of alcohol (may alter responsiveness to warfarin).	*Alcohol intake beyond 1 to 2 drinks per day decreases the effects of warfarin; in clients with liver disease, alcohol will increase the effects of warfarin.*
• Avoid significantly increasing or decreasing consumption of foods high in vitamin K (e.g., green leafy vegetables).	*Increasing the amount of foods high in vitamin K will antagonize warfarin's anticoagulant effects.*
• Report prolonged or excessive bleeding from skin, nose, or mouth; red, rust-colored, or smoky urine; bloody or tarry stools; blood in vomitus or sputum; prolonged or excessive menses; excessive bruising; severe or persistent headache; or sudden abdominal or back pain.	*Increased incidence of bleeding must be reported to the client's health care provider for appropriate intervention.*
• Inform physician immediately if pregnancy is suspected or if breast-feeding (warfarin crosses the placental barrier and enters the breast milk).	*Warfarin is contraindicated in pregnancy because it crosses the placenta and is found in breast milk.*
• Wear a medical alert identification bracelet or tag identifying self as being on anticoagulant therapy.	*This allows health care providers to be aware of health conditions and prescribed medications if the client is unable to provide this information.*
• Inform physician of any other medications being taken because there are some that affect the anticoagulant activity of warfarin (e.g., nonsteroidal anti-inflammatory drugs [NSAIDs], various antimicrobials, phenytoin).	*There are some medications that affect the anticoagulant activity of warfarin (e.g., NSAIDs, various antimicrobials, phenytoin).*
• Notify health care provider immediately of any sudden changes in the skin, such as bruised, darkened, or painful areas.	*Warfarin can cause necrosis of the skin.*
• Instruct client to inform all health care providers of medications and herbal supplements being taken.	*Health care providers must be aware of all medications and herbal supplements taken because they can interact with prescribed medications.*

THERAPEUTIC INTERVENTIONS	RATIONALE
Desired Outcome: The client will demonstrate the ability to correctly draw up and administer heparin subcutaneously if prescribed.	
Independent Actions If client is to be discharged on subcutaneous heparin, provide instructions about subcutaneous injection technique.	*The client should be instructed on the proper method of medication administration.*
Allow time for questions, practice, and return demonstration.	*Allowing for questioning, practice, and return demonstration of proper medication administration helps clients feel confident that they can perform this once they are at home.*

THERAPEUTIC INTERVENTIONS	RATIONALE
Desired Outcome: The client will identify ways to prevent bleeding associated with anticoagulant therapy.	

Continued...

THERAPEUTIC INTERVENTIONS	RATIONALE

Independent Actions

Instruct client about ways to minimize the risk of bleeding while receiving anticoagulant therapy:

- Use an electric rather than straight-edge razor.
- Floss and brush teeth; use waxed floss and a soft bristle toothbrush.
- Avoid putting sharp objects (e.g., toothpicks) in mouth.
- Do not walk barefoot.
- Cut nails carefully.
- Avoid situations that could result in injury (e.g., contact sports).
- Do not blow nose forcefully.
- Avoid straining to have a bowel movement.

All of these mechanisms will help to minimize the risk of bleeding.

Instruct client to control any bleeding by applying firm, prolonged pressure to the area if possible.

Application of firm, prolonged pressure will promote clotting.

THERAPEUTIC INTERVENTIONS	RATIONALE

Desired Outcome: The client will state signs and symptoms to report to the health care provider.

Independent Actions

Stress the importance of reporting the following:

- Tenderness, swelling, or pain in extremity
- Sudden chest pain
- New or increased shortness of breath
- Extreme anxiousness or restlessness
- Cough productive of blood-tinged sputum
- Unusual bleeding
- Fever

These symptoms are indicative of an embolism or increased bleeding from the use of anticoagulants. Immediate reporting allows for prompt treatment.

THERAPEUTIC INTERVENTIONS	RATIONALE

Desired Outcome: The client will verbalize an understanding of and a plan for adhering to recommended follow-up care including future appointments with health care provider and activity level.

Independent Actions

Reinforce the importance of keeping follow-up appointments with health care provider.

Follow-up appointments are important to monitor the client's recovery and medication regimen.

Reinforce the physician's instructions regarding activity limitations.

Clients may not fully understand the instructions regarding activity limitations, as they are feeling better and may increase activities prematurely.

Implement measures to improve client compliance:

- Include significant others in teaching sessions if possible.

Involvement of significant others in patient teaching improves adherence to discharge instructions.

- Encourage questions and allow time for reinforcement and clarification of information provided.

Everyone does not understand information as presented, so set aside time for questions to allow for clarification of information.

- Provide written instructions regarding future appointments with health care provider, medications prescribed, activity restrictions, signs and symptoms to report, and future laboratory studies.

Written instructions allow the client to refer to instructions as needed.

THORACIC SURGERY

Thoracic surgery is a term used to refer to surgical procedures that involve entry into the thoracic cavity to gain access to the lungs, heart, aorta, or esophagus. Types of thoracic surgery performed to treat pulmonary disorders include pneumonectomy, lobectomy, segmental resection, and wedge resection. The surgery may be performed to repair lung damage resulting from trauma and to remove benign or malignant tumors; areas of bronchiectasis, fungal infection, or tuberculosis; abscesses; blebs; and bullae. Although some thoracic surgery can be accomplished using an intercostally inserted endoscope, an open thoracic approach is needed to treat conditions requiring surgery deep in the lung, extensive removal of lung tissue, or both.

This care plan focuses on the adult client hospitalized for thoracic surgery to remove a portion or all of a lung. Much of the information is applicable to clients receiving follow-up care in an extended care facility or home setting.

3. Have surgical pain controlled
4. Have no signs and symptoms of postoperative complications
5. Identify ways to promote optimal respiratory health
6. Demonstrate the ability to perform prescribed arm and shoulder exercises
7. State signs and symptoms to report to the health care provider
8. Identify community resources that can assist with home management and adjustment to the diagnosis, effects of surgery, and subsequent treatment if planned
9. Verbalize an understanding of and a plan for adhering to recommended follow-up care including future appointments with health care provider, medications prescribed, activity level, pain management, wound care, and subsequent treatment of the underlying disorder.

OUTCOME/DISCHARGE CRITERIA

The client will:
1. Have optimal respiratory function
2. Have evidence of normal healing of surgical wound

PREOPERATIVE USE IN CONJUNCTION WITH THE PREOPERATIVE CARE PLAN

Nursing Diagnosis FEAR AND ANXIETY NDx

Definition: Fear—Response to perceived threat (real or imagined) that is consciously recognized as a danger
Anxiety—Vague uneasy feeling of discomfort or dread accompanied by an autonomic response (the source often nonspecific or unknown to the individual); a feeling of apprehension caused by anticipation of danger. It is an alerting signal that warns of impending danger and enables the individual to take measures to deal with the threat

Related to:
- Lack of understanding of the diagnosis, surgical procedure, and postoperative management
- Unfamiliar environment and financial concerns
- Anticipated loss of control associated with effects of anesthesia
- Potential embarrassment or loss of dignity associated with body exposure
- Anticipated pain and/or difficulty breathing
- Possible changes in usual lifestyle (e.g., activity limitations, cessation of smoking)

CLINICAL MANIFESTATIONS

Subjective	Objective
Verbalization of fear and/or anxiety	Unusual sleep patterns; unstable vital signs; restlessness; shakiness; diaphoresis; self-focused behavior

Continued...

RISK FACTORS

- Fear of the unknown
- Fear of lifestyle changes
- Fear of pain after surgery
- Fear of death
- Fear of disfigurement

DESIRED OUTCOMES

The client will experience a reduction in fear and anxiety.

NOC OUTCOMES

Anxiety level; fear level; anxiety self-control; fear self-control

NIC INTERVENTIONS

Anxiety reduction; calming technique; emotional support; presence; pain management

NURSING ASSESSMENT

Assess client for signs and symptoms of fear and anxiety (e.g., verbalization of feeling anxious, insomnia, tenseness, shakiness, restlessness, diaphoresis, elevated B/P, tachycardia, self-focused behaviors).

Validate perceptions carefully, remembering that some behavior may result from hypoxia and/or hypercapnia.

RATIONALE

Moderate anxiety enhances the client's ability to solve problems. With severe anxiety or panic, the client is not able to follow directions and may become hyperactive and extremely agitated.

Assessment of the client's fear helps to determine whether the coping mechanisms are effective and which need to be strengthened.

THERAPEUTIC INTERVENTIONS

RATIONALE

Independent Actions

Implement measures to reduce fear and anxiety:

- Preoperatively, orient client to hospital environment, equipment, and routines.

Familiarity with the environment and usual routines reduces the client's anxiety about the unknown, provides a sense of security, and increases the client's sense of control, all of which help decrease anxiety.

- Introduce staff who will be participating in the client's care. If possible, maintain consistency in staff assigned to client's care.

Introduction to staff familiarizes clients with those individuals who will be working with them, which provides clients with a feeling of stability, which reduces the anxiety that typically occurs with change.

- Assure client that staff members are nearby; respond to call signal as soon as possible. **D** ✦

Close contact and a prompt response to requests provide a sense of security and facilitate the development of trust, thus reducing the client's anxiety.

- Maintain a calm, supportive, confident manner when interacting with client; encourage verbalization of fear and anxiety. **D** ✦

A sense of calmness and confidence conveys to the client that someone is in control of the situation, which helps reduce anxiety.

- Reinforce physician's explanations and anticipated effect of loss of lung tissue on activity tolerance; if appropriate, reassure client that the remaining lung tissue should be able to provide adequate respiratory function.

Factual information and an awareness of what to expect help decrease the anxiety that arises from uncertainty and concerns about the client's future life.

- Provide instructions about the purpose of the chest drainage system that will be present after removal of the portion of the lung (chest tubes are rarely inserted if a pneumonectomy is performed).

Information about what to expect after surgery may help decrease fears and anxieties perioperatively.

- Assure client that supplemental oxygen will be given after surgery, if needed.

Knowledge that oxygen will be available if needed may help to relieve anxiety associated with the feeling of not being able to breathe.

- Implement measures to reduce respiratory distress if present:
  - Elevate the head of the bed.
  - Encourage the client to breathe deeply and more slowly.

Improvement of respiratory status helps relieve anxiety associated with the feeling of not being able to breathe.

THERAPEUTIC INTERVENTIONS	RATIONALE
• Implement measures to reduce pain: • Instruct client in relaxation techniques and encourage participation in diversional activities once the period of acute pain and respiratory distress has subsided. • When appropriate, assist the client to meet spiritual needs (e.g., arrange for a visit from the clergy). • Provide information based on current needs of client at a level that can be understood. • Encourage the client to ask questions and to seek clarification of information provided. • Provide a calm, restful environment. **D** ● ✦ • Encourage significant others to project a caring, concerned attitude without obvious fear and anxiousness.	*Pain can create or increase anxiety because it is often perceived as a threat to well-being.* *Pain also causes sympathetic nervous system stimulation with subsequent feelings of tenseness and increased anxiety.* *Spiritual support is a source of comfort and security for many people and can help reduce the client's fear and anxiety.* *Providing information that the client is not ready to process or cannot understand tends to increase anxiety.* *Making the client feel comfortable enough to ask questions or clarify information helps to reduce anxiety.* *A calm, restful environment facilitates relaxation and promotes a sense of security, which reduces fear and anxiety.* *Anxiety is easily transferable from one person to another. If significant others convey empathy, provide reassurance, and do not appear anxious, they can help reduce the client's fear and anxiety.*

Dependent/Collaborative Actions

Implement measures to reduce fear and anxiety:

• Administer oxygen via nasal cannula rather than mask if possible. **D** ✦ • Administer prescribed antianxiety agents if indicated. **D** ● ✦ Consult appropriate health care provider if above actions fail to control fear and anxiety.	*The use of a mask for some clients seems restrictive and suffocating. The use of a nasal cannula is more comfortable and less constraining. Improvement of respiratory status helps relieve anxiety associated with the feeling of not being able to breathe.* *Notifying the appropriate health care provider allows for modification of the treatment plan.*

POSTOPERATIVE

Nursing Diagnosis ## IMPAIRED RESPIRATORY FUNCTION*

Definition: Inability of an individual to maintain adequate ventilation of the respiratory tract and perfusion of O_2 and CO_2 between the lungs and vascular system to maintain adequate tissue oxygenation

Ineffective breathing pattern NDx
Related to:
• Increased rate of respirations associated with fear and anxiety
• Decreased rate of respirations associated with the depressant effect of anesthesia and some medications (e.g., narcotic [opioid] analgesics, some antiemetics)
• Decreased depth of respirations associated with:
  • Reluctance to breathe deeply resulting from incisional pain and fear of dislodging chest tube(s) if in place
  • Weakness, fatigue, fear, and anxiety
  • Depressant effect of anesthesia and some medications (e.g., narcotic [opioid] analgesics, some antiemetics)
  • Limited chest expansion resulting from positioning and elevation of the diaphragm (can occur if abdominal distention is present or if the phrenic nerve was injured during surgery)

Ineffective airway clearance NDx
Related to:
• Occlusion of the pharynx in the immediate postoperative period associated with relaxation of the tongue resulting from the effect of anesthesia and some medications (e.g., narcotic [opioid] analgesics)

---

*This diagnostic label includes the following nursing diagnoses: ineffective breathing pattern, ineffective airway clearance, and impaired gas exchange.

NDx = NANDA-I Diagnosis   **D** = Delegatable Action   ● = UAP   ✦ = LVN/LPN   ⊜▶ = Go to ⊜volve for animation

Continued...

- Stasis of secretions associated with:
  - Decreased activity
  - Depressed ciliary function resulting from effects of anesthesia
  - Difficulty coughing up secretions resulting from the depressant effect of anesthesia and some medications (e.g., narcotic [opioid] analgesics, some antiemetics), pain, weakness, fatigue, and presence of tenacious secretions (can occur as a result of deficient fluid volume)
- Increased secretions associated with irritation of the respiratory tract (can result from inhalation anesthetics, endotracheal intubation, and surgically induced lung tissue injury and inflammation)

Impaired gas exchange NDx
Related to:
A decrease in alveolar surface area and pulmonary vasculature associated with the extensive removal of lung tissues

CLINICAL MANIFESTATIONS

Subjective	Objective
Report of pain; anxiety; fear/agitation; restlessness; irritability; confusion	Tachypnea; orthopnea; dyspnea; diminished breath sounds; tachycardia; productive cough; significant decrease in oximetry values; abnormal arterial blood gas values; chest radiograph changes

RISK FACTORS

- Increased secretions
- Postoperative incision pain
- Anxiety
- Analgesics
- Potential immobility
- Anesthesia

DESIRED OUTCOMES

The client will experience adequate respiratory function as evidenced by:
  a. Normal rate and depth of respirations
  b. Absence of dyspnea
  c. Normal breath sounds over remaining lung tissue
  d. Usual mental status
  e. Usual skin color
  f. Oximetry results within normal range
  g. Arterial blood gas values within normal range

NURSING ASSESSMENT	RATIONALE
Assess for signs and symptoms of impaired respiratory function:	*Early recognition of signs and symptoms of infective breathing patterns allows for prompt intervention.*
- Rapid, shallow respirations	
- Dyspnea, orthopnea	*Changes in the characteristics of breath sounds may be due to airway obstruction, mucous plugs, or retained secretions in larger airways.*
- Use of accessory muscles when breathing	*Muscle fatigue/weakness may impair effective clearance of secretions.*
- Abnormal breath sounds (e.g., diminished or absent over remaining lung tissue)	
- Development of or increase in cough	
- Restlessness, irritability	*Restlessness, irritability, and changes in mental status or level of consciousness indicate an oxygen deficiency and require immediate treatment.*
- Confusion, somnolence	
- Significant decrease in oximetry results	*Oximetry is a noninvasive method of measuring arterial oxygen saturation. The results assist in evaluating respiratory status.*
- Abnormal arterial blood gas values	*Decreasing PaO_2 and increasing $PaCO_2$ are indicators of respiratory problems.*
- Changes in vital signs	*Increased work of breathing or hypoxia may cause tachycardia and/or hypertension.*
- Significant abnormalities in chest radiograph reports	*Changes in infiltrates noted in the lungs require prompt treatment.*

THERAPEUTIC INTERVENTIONS	RATIONALE

Independent Actions

Implement measures to maintain adequate respiratory function:

- Perform actions to reduce chest pain (e.g., orient client to the hospital environment, equipment; maintain a calm, supportive environment; instruct and assist client to splint chest when coughing or deep breathing). **D** ✦

  Reduction chest pain increases the client's willingness to move and breathe more deeply.

- Perform actions to reduce fear and anxiety (e.g., assure client that staff members are nearby; respond to call signal as soon as possible; provide calm, restful environment; instruct in relaxation techniques; encourage family to project a supportive attitude without obvious anxiousness). **D** ✦

  Reduction of fear and anxiety assists in preventing the shallow and/or rapid breathing associated with these emotions.

- Perform actions to reduce the accumulation of gas and fluid in the gastrointestinal (GI) tract (e.g., ambulate as early as possible, progress to solid foods slowly).

  This helps to decrease the pressure on the diaphragm, allowing the individual to have greater lung expansion.

- Position client as ordered (e.g., usually on back or operative side after pneumonectomy, on back or either side after removal of a portion of the lung).

  Proper positioning after surgery allows for full expansion of the remaining lung tissue.

- When positioning clients on their side, use a 30° to 45° "tip" position (rather than complete lateral positioning).

  This position helps to minimize lateral compression of lung tissue.

- Instruct client to deep breathe or use incentive spirometer every 1 to 2 hours. **D** ● ✦

  Forced deep breathing and use of incentive spirometry will increase expansion of the lungs and improve the client's ability to clear mucus from the remaining lung tissue. The technique may also improve the amount of oxygen that is able to penetrate deep into the lungs.

- Assure the client that deep breathing and turning should not dislodge the chest tube.

  This assurance will decrease the client's anxiety and fear associated with the chest tube.

- Maintain activity restrictions as ordered; increase activity gradually as allowed and tolerated. **D** ● ✦

  During activity, especially ambulation, the client usually takes deeper breaths, thus increasing expansion of remaining lung tissue.

Dependent/Collaborative Actions

Implement measures to maintain adequate respiratory function:

- Administer bronchodilators (e.g., methylxanthines, sympathomimetics) if ordered.

  These medications will dilate the bronchioles, improve the volume of air reaching the lungs, and improve arterial blood gas values.

- Administer pain medications as ordered.

  Reduction of chest pain increases the client's willingness to move and breathe more deeply.

- Maintain oxygen therapy as ordered. **D** ✦

  Improves oxygenation of body tissues

Consult appropriate health care provider (e.g., respiratory therapist, physician) if signs and symptoms of impaired respiratory function persist or worsen.

Notifying the appropriate health care provider allows for modifications of treatment.

Nursing Diagnosis ## ACUTE PAIN NDx (CHEST)

Definition: Unpleasant sensory and emotional experience arising from actual or potential tissue damage or described in terms of such damage (International Association for the Study of Pain); may be sudden or slow onset of any intensity from mild to severe with an anticipated or predictable end and a duration of <6 months

Related to:
- Tissue trauma, reflex muscle spasm, and disruption of intercostal nerves associated with the surgery
- Irritation of the parietal pleura associated with surgical trauma and stretching of the pleura (occurs if there is an accumulation of blood or air in the pleural space)
- Tissue irritation associated with the presence of chest tubes
- Stress on surgical area associated with deep breathing

Continued...

CLINICAL MANIFESTATIONS

Subjective	Objective
Verbalization of pain in chest with breathing and coughing and pain around the chest tube insertion site	Increased B/P; tachycardia; shallow respirations; grimacing with movement

RISK FACTORS

- Frequent coughing
- Suture line pain
- Chest tubes
- Anxiety

DESIRED OUTCOMES

The client will experience diminished chest pain as evidenced by:
- a. Verbalization of a decrease in or absence of pain
- b. Relaxed facial expression and body positioning
- c. Increased participation in activities
- d. Stable vital signs

NOC OUTCOMES

Pain control; comfort level

NIC INTERVENTIONS

Pain management; analgesic administration; environmental management: comfort

NURSING ASSESSMENT	RATIONALE
Assess for signs and symptoms of pain (e.g., verbalization of pain, grimacing, reluctance to move, guarding of affected side of chest, shallow respirations, increased B/P, tachycardia).	*Early recognition of signs and symptoms of pain allows for prompt intervention and improved pain control.*
Assess client's perception of the severity of pain using a pain intensity rating scale.	*An awareness of the severity of pain being experienced helps determine the most appropriate interventions for pain management. Use of a pain intensity scale gives the nurse a clearer understanding of the pain being experienced and promotes consistency when communicating with others about the client's pain experience.*
Assess the client's pain pattern (e.g., location, quality, onset, duration, precipitating factors, aggravating factors, alleviating factors).	*Knowledge of the client's pain pattern assists in the identification of effective pain management interventions.*
Ask the client to describe previous pain experiences and methods used to manage pain effectively.	*Many variables affect a client's response to pain (e.g., age, sex, coping style, previous experience with pain, culture, cause of pain). Knowledge of the client's usual response to pain and methods previously used to manage pain effectively enables the nurse to evaluate the client's pain more accurately and facilitates the identification of effective strategies for pain management.*

THERAPEUTIC INTERVENTIONS	RATIONALE
Independent Actions	
Implement measures to reduce fear and anxiety (e.g., assure client that chest pain is expected postoperatively, and assure the client that the need for pain relief is understood).	*Fear and anxiety can decrease the client's threshold and tolerance for pain and thereby heighten the perception of pain. In addition, pain management methods are not as effective if the client is tense and unable to relax.*
Perform actions to promote rest (e.g., minimize environmental activity and noise). **D** ● ✦	*A restful environment reduces fatigue and subsequently increases the client's threshold and tolerance for pain.*
Provide or assist with nonpharmacologic methods for pain relief (e.g., relaxation techniques, restful environment, watching television, reading).	*Relaxation and diversional activities help to alleviate pain, fear, and anxiety, which may increase tolerance for pain.*
Instruct and assist client to support chest incision with a pillow or hands when turning, coughing, and deep breathing. **D** ● ✦	*Supporting the chest incision with a pillow or hands when turning, coughing, and deep breathing supports the incision and makes the activity less painful.*
Securely anchor chest tubes.	*Anchoring of chest tubes decreases irritation from the movement of the tubes.*

THERAPEUTIC INTERVENTIONS	RATIONALE

Dependent/Collaborative Actions

Administer analgesics before activities and procedures that can cause pain and before pain becomes severe. **D** ✦

The administration of analgesics before a pain-producing event helps minimize the pain that will be experienced. Analgesics given before procedures will improve the client's ability to tolerate the procedures before the pain becomes severe.

Encourage client to use the patient-controlled analgesia device as instructed.

Patient-controlled analgesia allows the client to control pain medication administration. Clients using patient-controlled analgesia have been shown to use less medication and ambulate more quickly after surgery than patients receiving nurse-controlled analgesia.

Maintain integrity of analgesia delivery system (epidural, intravenous, subcutaneous, transdermal).

Consult appropriate health care provider (e.g., physician, pharmacist, pain management specialist) if above measures fail to provide adequate pain relief.

Notifying the appropriate health care provider allows for a multifaceted treatment plan.

Collaborative Diagnosis **RISK FOR INEFFECTIVE LUNG EXPANSION**

Definition: Inability to expand the lung to provide adequate oxygenation to the body

Extended pneumothorax

Related to:

An increase in intrapleural pressure associated with accumulation of air in pleural space (can occur if the chest drainage system malfunctions and/or air leaks into the pleural space through the incision)

Hemothorax

Related to:

Intraoperative or postoperative bleeding and/or malfunction of the chest drainage system

Mediastinal shift

Related to:

- A significant increase in intrapleural pressure on the operative side after a lobectomy associated with an accumulation of fluid and air in the pleural space
- Excessive negative pressure on the operative side after pneumonectomy associated with inadequate serous fluid accumulation in the empty thoracic space (the position of the mediastinum is maintained by accumulation of serous fluid in the empty thoracic space)

CLINICAL MANIFESTATIONS

Subjective	Objective
Verbalization of shortness of breath	Absent breath sounds; hyperresonant percussion with pneumothorax; dull percussion with hemothorax; rapid, shallow, and/or labored respirations; restlessness; agitation; confusion; arterial blood gas values that have worsened; chest radiograph results showing a lung collapse; further decrease in Hct and Hgb

RISK FACTORS

- Surgery
- Smoking
- Pain
- Anesthetics

DESIRED OUTCOMES

The client will experience normal lung reexpansion as evidence by:

    a. Audible breath sounds and resonant percussion note over remaining lung tissue by third or fourth postoperative day

    b. Unlabored respirations at 12 to 20 breaths/min

    c. Arterial blood gas values within normal range

    d. Absence of or no sudden increase in dyspnea

    e. Vital signs within normal limits

    f. Usual mental status

    g. Trachea in midline position

    h. Absence of neck vein distention

    i. Chest radiograph showing lung reexpansion

Continued...

NURSING ASSESSMENT	RATIONALE
Assess for and immediately report signs and symptoms of: • Malfunction of chest drainage system (e.g., respiratory distress, lack of fluctuation in water seal chamber without evidence of lung reexpansion, excessive bubbling in water seal chamber, significant increase in subcutaneous emphysema) • Extended pneumothorax (e.g., extended area of absent breath sounds with hyperresonant percussion note; rapid, shallow, and/or labored respirations; restlessness; agitation; confusion; arterial blood gas values that have worsened; chest radiograph results showing delayed lung reexpansion or further lung collapse). • Mediastinal shift (e.g., severe dyspnea, rapid and/or irregular pulse rate, hypotension, restlessness, agitation, confusion, shift in trachea from midline, neck vein distention, arterial blood gas values that have worsened, chest radiograph results showing a deviation of trachea from midline)	*Early recognition of signs and symptoms of respiratory problems after thoracic surgery allows for prompt intervention.*

THERAPEUTIC INTERVENTIONS	RATIONALE
Independent Actions Implement measures to promote lung reexpansion and prevent further lung collapse: • Perform actions to maintain patency and integrity of chest drainage system:	
• Maintain fluid levels in the water seal and suction chambers as ordered.	*Maintains negative pressure within the lungs.*
• Maintain occlusive dressing over chest tube insertion site.	*Maintains negative pressure seal.*
• Tape all connections securely.	*Prevents tubing from being disconnected and maintains a closed drainage system.*
• Tape the tubing to the chest wall close to insertion site.	*Reduces the risk of inadvertent removal of the chest tube.*
• Position tubing to promote optimum drainage (e.g., coil excess tubing on bed rather than allowing it to hang down below the collection device, keep tubing free of kinks). **D** ✦	*Promotes drainage.*
• Drain fluid that accumulates in tubing into the collection chamber.	*Maintains patency of the drainage system.*
• Avoid stripping of chest tubes. If ordered, milk tubing using a hand over hand method while moving along the drainage tube.	*Chest tube stripping increases high negative pressures in the pleural space and may damage lung tissues.*
• Keep drainage collection device below level of client's chest at all times. **D** ✦	*Prevents backflow of drainage into the lungs.*
• Perform actions to facilitate the escape of air from the pleural space (e.g., maintain suction as ordered, ensure that the air vent is open on the drainage collection device if system is to water seal only).	*Improves lung expansion and removal of secretions.*
• Perform actions to improve breathing pattern and facilitate airway clearance (e.g., encourage client to cough and deep breathe every 1 to 2 hours; use incentive spirometry every 2 hours; ambulate as ordered and as tolerated). **D** ✦	
Dependent/Collaborative Actions If signs and symptoms of further lung collapse or a hemothorax or mediastinal shift occur: • Maintain client on bed rest in a semi- to high-Fowler's position.	*Improves client's ability to expand the lungs.*

THERAPEUTIC INTERVENTIONS	RATIONALE
• Maintain oxygen therapy as ordered. **D** ✦	*Helps to maintain tissue oxygenation.*
• Assess for and immediately report signs and symptoms of tension pneumothorax (e.g., severe dyspnea, increased restlessness and agitation, rapid and/or irregular pulse rate, hypotension, neck vein distention, shift in trachea from midline).	*Emergency treatment is required to prevent further respiratory difficulty.*
• Assist with clearing of existing chest tube and/or insertion of a new tube.	*Reestablishes a closed drainage system.*
• Assist with autotransfusion of blood from chest tube and/or administer blood products and/or volume expanders if ordered.	*Addresses decreased Hct and Hgb.*
• Assist with clearing of existing chest tubes, thoracentesis, or insertion of chest tube if not already present.	*Prevents drainage from accumulating in the lungs.*
• Prepare client for surgical intervention to ligate bleeding vessels if indicated.	*Decreases anxiety.*

Collaborative Diagnosis RISK FOR CARDIAC DYSRHYTHMIAS

Definition: A disturbance of the heart's normal rhythm. Dysrhythmias can range from missed or rapid beats to serious disturbances that impair the pumping ability of the heart

Related to: Altered nodal function and myocardial conductivity associated primarily with myocardial hypoxia (may result from impaired gas exchange and diminished myocardial blood flow that can occur with hypovolemia and sympathetic nervous system–medicated vasoconstriction in the immediate postoperative period)

CLINICAL MANIFESTATIONS

Subjective	Objective
Verbal reports of palpitations or "skipped beats"	Irregular apical pulse; heart rate less than 60 or greater than 100 beats/min; apical-radial pulse deficit; syncope; palpitations; abnormal rate, rhythm, or configuration on electrocardiogram (ECG)

RISK FACTORS
• Electrolyte imbalance
• Activity intolerance
• Myocardial hypoxia
• Hypovolemia

DESIRED OUTCOMES

The client will maintain normal sinus rhythm as evidenced by:
  a. Regular apical pulse rate at 50 to 100 beats/min
  b. Equal apical and radial pulse rates
  c. Absence of syncope and palpitations
  d. ECG showing normal sinus rhythm

NURSING ASSESSMENT	RATIONALE
Assess for and report signs and symptoms of cardiac dysrhythmias (e.g., irregular apical pulse; pulse rate less than 60 and greater than 100 beats/min; apical-radial pulse deficit; syncope; palpitations; abnormal rate, rhythm, or configurations on ECG).	*Early recognition of signs and symptoms of cardiac dysrhythmias after thoracic surgery allows for prompt intervention.*

Continued...

THERAPEUTIC INTERVENTIONS	RATIONALE

Independent Actions

Implement measures to prevent cardiac dysrhythmias:

- Reduce pain, fear, and anxiety (e.g., assure client need for pain relief is understood, and plan methods for achieving pain control with client; orient client to environment, equipment, and routines; maintain a calm, supportive environment; encourage/instruct client in use of relaxation techniques; allow client to discuss anxiety and fears). **D** ✦

Pain, anxiety, and fear cause stimulation of the sympathetic nervous system, which increases the heart rate and causes vasoconstriction, both of which increase cardiac workload and decrease oxygen availability to the myocardium.

Dependent/Collaborative Actions

If cardiac dysrhythmias occur:

- Administer antidysrhythmics (e.g., digoxin) as ordered.
- Restrict client's activity based on client's tolerance and severity of the dysrhythmia.
- Maintain oxygen therapy as ordered.

- Assess cardiovascular status frequently and report signs and symptoms of inadequate tissue perfusion (e.g., decrease in B/P, cool skin, cyanosis, diminished peripheral pulses, urine output less than 30 mL/h, restlessness and agitation, increased shortness of breath).

Prevention of dysrhythmias.
Reduces client's potential for injury.

Provides supplemental oxygenation, which may decrease dysrhythmias.
Provides for prompt treatment of dysrhythmias.
Indications of decreased cardiac output.

Collaborative Diagnosis ## RISK FOR ACUTE PULMONARY EDEMA

Definition: Accumalation of fluid in the lungs that leads to impaired O_2/CO_2 exchange

Related to:
- Increased pulmonary capillary permeability associated with hypoxia
- Increased hydrostatic pressure in the remaining pulmonary vessels associated with reduced size of the pulmonary vascular bed and decreased effectiveness of lymphatic drainage resulting from extensive removal of pulmonary tissue (especially if pneumonectomy was performed)

CLINICAL MANIFESTATIONS

Subjective	Objective
Verbal reports of shortness of breath and difficulty breathing	Adventitious breath sounds (e.g., rales), productive cough (e.g. blood tinged, frothy sputum; increased work of breathing, increased respiratory rate; decreased oxygen saturation; diaphoresis; dyspnea; tachypnea; auscultated; wheezes; decreasing pulse oximetry; abnormal arterial blood gases

RISK FACTORS

- Increased pulmonary hydrostatic pressure
- Decreased effectiveness of the lymph drainage
- Smoking

DESIRED OUTCOMES

The client will not develop pulmonary edema as evidenced by:
  a. Unlabored respirations at 12 to 20 breaths/min
  b. Clear breath sounds and resonant percussion note over nonoperated lung tissue
  c. Absence of productive, persistent cough
  d. Usual skin color
  e. Oximetry results within normal range
  f. Arterial blood gas values within normal range

NURSING ASSESSMENT	RATIONALE
Pulmonary edema (e.g., severe dyspnea, tachycardia, development of or increase in crackles [rales] or wheezes, dull percussion note over remaining lung tissue, persistent cough productive of frothy and/or blood-tinged sputum, cyanosis, significant decrease in oximetry results, decrease in PaO_2 and/or increase in $PaCO_2$, chest radiograph results showing pulmonary edema).	*Early recognition of signs and symptoms of pulmonary edema allows for prompt intervention.*

THERAPEUTIC INTERVENTIONS	RATIONALE

Independent Actions

Implement measures to maintain adequate respiratory function (e.g., encourage use of incentive spirometry every 2 to 3 hours; ambulate as tolerated; provide supplemental oxygen as needed; maintain patency of chest tube).	*Improves lung expansion and mobilization of secretions.*

Dependent/Collaborative Actions

If signs and symptoms of pulmonary edema occur, administer bronchodilators and agents to reduce pulmonary vascular congestion (e.g., diuretics and morphine sulfate).	*Improves bronchial airflow and decreases pulmonary congestion.*

Collaborative Diagnosis   RISK FOR BRONCHOPLEURAL FISTULA

Definition: A fistula between the lungs and the pleural space

Related to: Inadequate bronchial closure and healing after a partial or complete resection of the lungs (most often associated with preoperative radiation to the lungs and/or residual cancer of the bronchial stump)

CLINICAL MANIFESTATIONS

Subjective	Objective
Verbalization of pain; verbal reports of shortness of breath, difficulty breathing	Hyperthermia; cough with purulent sputum; continuous bubbling of chest drainage system; increasing subcutaneous emphysema around neck and incision; elevated WBC count; chest radiograph with presence of bronchopleural fistula

RISK FACTORS

- Surgery
- Radiation

DESIRED OUTCOMES

The client will experience resolution of a bronchopleural fistula if it occurs as evidenced by:
- a. Afebrile status
- b. Absence of cough
- c. Absence of continuous bubbling in water seal chamber of chest drainage system
- d. Unlabored respirations at 12 to 20 breaths/min
- e. WBC and differential counts returning toward normal

NURSING ASSESSMENT	RATIONALE
Assess for and report signs and symptoms of bronchopleural fistula (e.g., fever, cough, purulent sputum, continuous bubbling in water seal chamber of chest drainage system, increasing subcutaneous emphysema around incision and neck, respiratory distress, persistent elevation of WBC count and significant change in differential, chest radiograph results showing presence of bronchopleural fistula).	*Early recognition of the signs and symptoms of bronchopleural fistula allows for prompt intervention.*

NDx = NANDA-I Diagnosis   **D** = Delegatable Action   ● = UAP   ✦ = LVN/LPN   ⊖▶ = Go to ⊖volve for animation

Continued...

THERAPEUTIC INTERVENTIONS	RATIONALE

Independent Actions

If signs and symptoms of a bronchial fistula occur:

- Turn client to operative side unless contraindicated.
- Have tracheostomy tray readily available.

- Prepare client for chest tube insertion, thoracentesis, and surgical repair of bronchial stump if planned.

Reduces risk for aspiration of pleural fluid.
Severe subcutaneous emphysema in the neck can compress trachea and obstruct the airway.
Decreases client anxiety.

Collaborative Diagnosis **RESTRICTED ARM AND SHOULDER MOVEMENT**

Definition: Decreased movement of the upper limbs

Related to: Decreased activity of the arm and shoulder on the operative side associated with weakness, fatigue, pain, and adhesion formation between incised muscles

CLINICAL MANIFESTATIONS

Subjective	Objective
Verbalization of difficulty/inability in moving arm and shoulder, pain with movement	Limited range of motion of arm and shoulder

RISK FACTORS

- Limited movement
- Fatigue
- Pain
- Weakness

DESIRED OUTCOMES

The client will maintain normal arm and shoulder function as evidenced by ability to move arm and shoulder on operative side through usual range of motion.

NURSING ASSESSMENT	RATIONALE
Assess for and report signs and symptoms of restricted arm and shoulder movement on operative side (e.g., inability to move arm and shoulder through usual range of motion, inability to use arm in ADL).	*Early recognition of signs and symptoms of reduced arm and shoulder movement allows for prompt intervention.*

THERAPEUTIC INTERVENTIONS	RATIONALE

Dependent/Collaborative Actions

Implement measures to prevent restriction of arm and shoulder movement on operative side:

- Instruct client in and assist with arm and shoulder exercises ordered (usually passive range of motion is started the evening of surgery, and active range of motion exercises are started by the second postoperative day).
- Perform actions to reduce pain (e.g., administer analgesics). **D ✦**
- Encourage client to use arm on operative side to perform self-care activities. **D ● ✦**
- Place frequently used articles and bed stand on operative side. **D ● ✦**
- Anchor pull rope at foot of bed. **D ● ✦**

Early intervention and movement of the arms and shoulders are important in preventing restricted movement.

Reduction of pain will increase client's ability and willingness to move arm and shoulder.
Use of the arm on the operative side by the client helps to maintain movement.
Place articles on the operative side of the bed so that client will be more likely to use that arm.

DISCHARGE TEACHING/CONTINUED CARE

| Nursing Diagnosis | **DEFICIENT KNOWLEDGE, NDx INEFFECTIVE HEALTH MAINTENANCE NDx, OR INEFFECTIVE SELF-HEALTH MANAGEMENT* NDx** |

Definition: Absence or deficiency of cognitive information related to specific topic (lack of specific information necessary for clients/significant others) to make informed choices regarding condition/treatment/lifestyle changes; inability to identify, manage, and/or seek out help to maintain health; pattern of regulating and integrating into daily living a therapeutic regimen for treatment of illness and the sequelae of illness that is unsatisfactory for meeting specific health goals

CLINICAL MANIFESTATIONS

Subjective	Objective
Verbalization of the problem	Inaccurate follow through of instructions; inappropriate behaviors

RISK FACTORS

- Denial of disease process
- Cognitive deficiency
- Failure to take action to reduce risk factors

NOC OUTCOMES

Knowledge: health promotion; knowledge: health resources; knowledge: treatment regimen

NIC INTERVENTIONS

Health system guidance; teaching: individual; teaching: prescribed activity/exercise; teaching: disease process

NURSING ASSESSMENT	RATIONALE
Assess client readiness to learn Assess meaning of illness to client	*Early recognition of readiness to learn and meaning of illness to client allows for appropriate teaching interventions.*

THERAPEUTIC INTERVENTIONS	RATIONALE

Desired Outcome: The client will identify ways to promote optimal respiratory health.

Independent Actions
Instruct client in ways to promote optimal respiratory health:

- Maintain overall general good health (e.g., reduce stress, eat a well-balanced diet, obtain adequate rest, obtain adequate exercise).

  Maintenance of good general health helps to fight off respiratory infections and maintain adequate respiratory status.

- Stop smoking.
- Avoid exposure to respiratory irritants such as smoke, dust, aerosol sprays, paint fumes, and solvents.

  The irritants in smoke and other respiratory irritants increase mucus production, impair ciliary function, and can cause inflammation and damage to the bronchial and alveolar walls; the carbon monoxide decreases oxygen availability.

- Remain indoors as much as possible when air pollution levels are high.

  High levels of air pollution are lung irritants and impair ciliary function.

- Wear a mask or scarf over nose and mouth if exposure to high levels of irritants such as smoke, fumes, and dust is unavoidable.

  Wearing a mask or scarf decreases the level of exposure to irritants in the air.

- Take medications as prescribed to treat any underlying respiratory disease such as chronic obstructive pulmonary disease, cancer of the lung, or tuberculosis.

  Helps to maintain adequate lung functioning and oxygenation of body tissues.

- Decrease the risk of respiratory tract infections:

  Each of these actions helps to decrease the incidence of infections and maintain good lung health.

  - Avoid contact with persons who have respiratory tract infections.
  - Avoid crowds and poorly ventilated areas.

*The nurse should select the diagnosis that is most appropriate for the client's teaching needs.

NDx = NANDA-I Diagnosis   **D** = Delegatable Action   ● = UAP   ✦ = LVN/LPN   ⊖▶ = Go to ⊖volve for animation

Continued...

THERAPEUTIC INTERVENTIONS	RATIONALE
• Drink at least 10 glasses of liquid/day unless contraindicated.	*Maintains adequate circulatory volume.*
• Receive immunizations against influenza and pneumococcal pneumonia.	*Improves client's resistance to influenza and pneumococcal pneumonia.*

Desired Outcome: The client will demonstrate the ability to perform prescribed arm and shoulder exercises

Instruct client regarding the importance of exercising the arm and shoulder on the operative side. Emphasize that the exercises should be performed at least 5 times per day for several weeks.	*Exercise of the arm and shoulder on the operative side prevents restriction of arm and shoulder movement.*
Demonstrate appropriate arm and shoulder exercises (e.g., shoulder shrugs, arm circles).	*The client's ability to perform the exercises should be evaluated before leaving the health care facility.*
Allow time for questions, clarification, and return demonstration.	*Everyone does not understand information as presented; allowing time for questioning helps clients assimilate the information in terms they can understand. Return demonstration allows the nurse to verify client's ability to perform exercises.*

Desired Outcome: The client will state signs and symptoms to report to the health care provider

Instruct the client to report these signs and symptoms:	*Clients need to be aware of the signs and symptoms that should be reported to their health care provider to allow for prompt treatment of complications.*
• Increased discomfort in or decreased ability to move arm and shoulder on operative side	
• Increased shortness of breath	
• Persistent cough	
• Persistent low-grade fever	
• Difficulty breathing	
• Chest pain	
• Increasing weakness or inability to tolerate prescribed activity level	
• Separation of wound edges	
• Increased redness, warmth, pain, or swelling around the wound	
• Unusual or excessive drainage from any wound site	

Desired Outcome: The client will identify community resources that can assist with home management and adjustment to the diagnosis, effects of surgery, and subsequent treatment if planned

Provide information about community resources that can assist the client and significant others with home management and adjustment to the diagnosis, effects of surgery, and subsequent treatment if planned (e.g., American Lung Association, American Cancer Society, smoking cessation program, Meals on Wheels, counselors, support groups, home health agencies).	*Information on how to access community resources and information related to home management is important to maintain client's recovery.*

Desired Outcome: The client will verbalize an understanding of and a plan for adhering to recommended follow-up care including future appointments with health care provider, medications prescribed, activity level, pain management, wound care, and subsequent treatment of the underlying disorder

Reinforce physician's instructions about activity level:	*Reinforcement of instructions and providing written instructions for the client provide a reference for questions once the client is home.*
• Gauge activity according to tolerance and ensure adequate rest periods.	
• Stop any activity that causes excessive fatigue, dyspnea, or chest pain.	
• Avoid lifting heavy objects and doing strenuous upper body exercises until complete healing of chest muscles has occurred (usually 3 to 6 months).	

THERAPEUTIC INTERVENTIONS	RATIONALE
Inform client that numbness and discomfort in the operative area can persist for several weeks but are usually temporary.	*The client should be aware of when numbness and discomfort in the operative area will resolve, so they won't become anxious if pain and numbness persist.*
Clarify plans for subsequent treatment of underlying disorder (e.g., chemotherapy, radiation therapy) if appropriate.	*Client should be aware that the surgery may not completely remove the necessity of treatment of the underlying condition.*

TUBERCULOSIS

Tuberculosis (TB) is an infectious disease caused by *Mycobacterium tuberculosis*, a gram-positive, acid-fast bacillus. It is spread by airborne droplets released when a person with active TB disease coughs, sneezes, or speaks. These droplets can cause infection in others if contact with the infected person is close and repeated or prolonged. The inhaled tubercle bacilli implant themselves in the lung, multiply, and can spread to other areas of the body through the lymphatic channels (lymphatic dissemination) and blood (hematogenous dissemination).

Most people who are infected with tubercle bacilli do not develop an active form of TB. Those who do are usually part of high-risk populations that include persons who are immunosuppressed, persons in continued close contact with people with active untreated TB, and those who have been exposed to virulent strains of multidrug-resistant tuberculosis (MDR-TB). In addition, TB that has previously been inactive (latent, dormant) in a person with an effective immune system can become active if that person experiences situations that suppress the immune response (e.g., chemotherapy treatment, long-term corticosteroid use, malnutrition, human immunodeficiency virus [HIV] infection, advanced age).

Signs and symptoms of active TB can include fatigue, anorexia, weight loss, night sweats, fever (usually low grade), cough (usually progresses from a dry cough to one that is productive of mucopurulent or blood-tinged sputum), dyspnea, and/or pleuritic pain (in some cases).

A person with suspected active TB is placed on precautions to prevent airborne transmission of the tubercle bacilli and started on a regimen of multiple antitubercular/antimicrobial medications while awaiting results of sputum cultures. If the diagnosis is confirmed, a major health care focus becomes one of promoting compliance with the lengthy (usually 6-18 months), multiple-drug treatment regimen.

This care plan focuses on the adult client hospitalized with signs and symptoms of active pulmonary tuberculosis. Much of the information presented here is applicable to clients receiving follow-up care in an extended care facility or home setting.

OUTCOME/DISCHARGE CRITERIA

The client will:
1. Have an adequate respiratory status
2. Tolerate expected level of activity
3. Have no signs and symptoms of complications
4. Identify ways to maintain respiratory health
5. Identify ways to prevent the spread of TB to others
6. Verbalize an understanding of medications ordered including rationale, food and drug interactions, side effects, and importance of taking as prescribed
7. State signs and symptoms to report to the health care provider
8. Verbalize an understanding of and a plan for adhering to recommended follow-up care including future appointments with health care provider.

Nursing Diagnosis **IMPAIRED RESPIRATORY FUNCTION***

Definition: Inability of an individual to maintain adequate ventilation of the respiratory tract and perfusion of O_2 and CO_2 between the lungs and vascular system to maintain adequate oxygenation

Ineffective breathing pattern NDx
Related to:
- Decreased depth of respirations associated with weakness, fatigue, and reluctance to breathe deeply if chest pain is present
- Increased rate of respirations associated with the increase in metabolic rate that occurs with an infectious process

Ineffective airway clearance NDx
Related to:
- Tracheobronchial inflammation
- Increase in secretions associated with the infectious process and the necrosis and subsequent liquefaction of tubercle nodules (the nodules, or caseations, are lesions that consist of tubercle bacilli surrounded by a fibrous capsule)

*This diagnostic label includes the following nursing diagnoses: ineffective breathing pattern, ineffective airway clearance, and impaired gas exchange.

NDx = NANDA-I Diagnosis   **D** = Delegatable Action   ● = UAP   ✦ = LVN/LPN   ⊜▶ = Go to ⊜volve for animation

Continued...

- Stasis of secretions associated with decreased activity; poor cough effort resulting from weakness, fatigue, and chest pain (if present); and impaired ciliary function (results from the increased viscosity and volume of mucus that occurs with the infectious process)

Impaired gas exchange NDx
Related to:
- A decrease in effective lung surface associated with the accumulation of secretions
- Destruction of normal lung tissue that occurs with the presence of the tubercle nodules

CLINICAL MANIFESTATIONS

Subjective	Objective
Verbalization of fatigue, pleuritic pain, confusion, restlessness, and somnolence	Dyspnea; orthopnea; use of accessory muscles; fever (usually low grade); cough—progressive from a dry cough to one that is productive of mucopurulent or blood-tinged sputum; decreased expiratory and inspiratory pressures; abnormal breath sounds; limited chest excursion; significantly decreased oximetry results; abnormal arterial blood gas values; sputum positive for acid-fast stain; chest radiograph—nodular calcification, enlargement of hilar lymph nodes, parenchymal infiltrate, pleural effusion, and cavitation

RISK FACTORS
- Exposure to someone who has TB
- Increased secretions
- Smoking and exposure to second-hand smoke
- Ineffective medication regimen

DESIRED OUTCOMES
The client will experience adequate respiratory function as evidenced by:
  a. Normal rate and depth of respirations
  b. Absence of dyspnea
  c. Normal breath sounds over remaining lung tissue
  d. Usual mental status
  e. Usual skin color
  f. Oximetry results within normal range
  g. Arterial blood gas values within normal range

NURSING ASSESSMENT

Assess for and report signs and symptoms of impaired respiratory function:
- Rapid, shallow respirations
- Dyspnea, orthopnea
- Use of accessory muscles when breathing
- Abnormal breath sounds (e.g., diminished, crackles [rales], rhonchi)
- Cough (usually a productive cough of mucopurulent or blood-tinged sputum)
- Limited chest excursion
- Restlessness, irritability
- Confusion, somnolence

Assess arterial blood gas values, oximetry values, and chest radiograph results. Report abnormal findings.

RATIONALE

Early recognition of signs and symptoms of impaired respiratory function allows for prompt intervention.

THERAPEUTIC INTERVENTIONS

Independent Actions
Implement measures to improve respiratory status:
- Perform actions to reduce chest pain if present (e.g., splint chest with pillow when coughing and deep breathing).

D ✦

RATIONALE

These actions increase the client's willingness to move, cough, and deep breathe.

THERAPEUTIC INTERVENTIONS	RATIONALE
• Place client in a semi- to high-Fowler's position unless contraindicated; position with pillows. **D** ● ✦	*Positioning in semi- to high-Fowler's position promotes optimal gas exchange by enabling chest expansion. Positioning with pillows prevents slumping.*
• If client must remain flat in bed, assist with position change at least every 2 hours. **D** ● ✦	*Changing positions every 2 hours helps to mobilize secretions for expectoration.*
• Instruct client to deep breathe or use inspiratory exercises every 1 to 2 hours. **D** ● ✦	*Forced deep breathing and use of incentive spirometry will increase expansion of the lungs and improve the client's ability to clear mucus from the lungs. The technique may also improve the amount of oxygen that is able to penetrate deep into the lungs.*
• Perform actions to promote removal of pulmonary secretions:	*Coughing or "huffing" every 1 to 2 hours will help to remove secretions.*
• Assist client to cough or "huff" every 1 to 2 hours. **D** ● ✦	
• Implement measures to thin tenacious secretions and reduce dryness of the respiratory mucous membrane:	*Increasing fluid intake will help liquefy secretions.*
Maintain a fluid intake of at least 2500 mL/day unless contraindicated. **D** ● ✦	
• Increase activity as allowed and tolerated. **D** ● ✦	*Conservation of energy through activity restrictions allows energy to be focused on breathing. Increasing activity as tolerated helps to mobilize secretions and promotes deeper breathing.*
• Discourage smoking.	*Irritants in smoke increase mucus production, impair ciliary function, and can cause inflammation and damage to the bronchial and alveolar walls; the carbon monoxide decreases oxygen availability.*

Dependent/Collaborative Actions

Implement measures to improve respiratory status:
- Assist with positive airway pressure techniques (e.g., continuous positive airway pressure [CPAP], bilevel positive airway pressure [BiPAP], flutter/positive expiratory pressure [PEP] device) if ordered.

  Improves volume of air that is breathed into the lungs.
- Maintain oxygen as ordered. **D** ✦ *Supplemental oxygen helps to relieve dyspnea.*
- Humidify air as ordered. **D** ✦ *Humidity will help to liquefy secretions.*
- Administer central nervous system (CNS) depressants judiciously; hold medication and consult physician if respiratory rate is less than 12 breaths/min. **D** ✦ *CNS depressants may significantly decrease respiratory rate, leading to respiratory acidosis and hypoxemia.*
- Administer the following medications as ordered:
  - Bronchodilators (e.g., methylxanthines, sympathomimetic [adrenergic] agents). *Bronchodilators open bronchioles and allow for improved ventilation of the lungs.*
  - Antitubercular/antimicrobial agents *Antitubercular agents impact the active infection.*

Consult appropriate health care provider (e.g., respiratory therapist, physician) if signs and symptoms of impaired respiratory function persist or worsen. *Notifying the appropriate health care professionals allows for a prompt and multifaceted approach to treatment.*

Nursing Diagnosis # IMBALANCED NUTRITION: LESS THAN BODY REQUIREMENTS NDx

Definition: Intake of nutrients insufficient to meet metabolic needs

Related to:
- Decreased oral intake associated with dyspnea, weakness, fatigue, excessive coughing, and the foul order and taste of sputum and some aerosol treatments
- Nausea (can occur in response to noxious stimuli such as the sight of expectorated sputum and as a side effect of some medications)
- Increased nutritional needs associated with the increase in metabolic rate that occurs with an infectious process

Continued...

CLINICAL MANIFESTATIONS

Subjective	Objective
Verbalization of sore buccal membranes; report of altered taste sensation	Weight loss; weight less than normal for client's age, height, and body frame; abnormal BUN and low serum prealbumin and albumin levels; inflamed mucous membranes; pale conjunctiva; poor muscle tone; excessive hair loss

RISK FACTORS

- Shortness of breath
- Lack of appetite
- Inappropriate diet
- Nausea
- Respiratory treatments
- Productive cough

DESIRED OUTCOMES

The client will maintain adequate nutrition status as evidenced by:
  a. Weight within normal range for clients
  b. Normal BUN and serum prealbumin and albumin levels
  c. Usual strength and activity tolerance
  d. Healthy oral mucous membrane

NOC OUTCOMES

Nutritional status

NIC INTERVENTIONS

Nutritional monitoring; nutrition management; nutrition therapy

NURSING ASSESSMENT

Assess for and report signs and symptoms of malnutrition:
- Weight significantly below client's usual weight or less than normal for client's age, height, and body frame
- Abnormal BUN and low serum prealbumin and albumin levels
- Increased weakness and fatigue
- Sore, inflamed oral mucous membrane
- Pale conjunctiva
- Sore buccal membranes
- Excessive hair loss
- Poor muscle tone

RATIONALE

Early recognition of signs and symptoms of malnutrition allows for prompt intervention.

THERAPEUTIC INTERVENTIONS

Independent Actions

Monitor percentage of meals and snacks client consumes. Report inadequate intake. **D** ✦

Implement measures to maintain an adequate nutritional status:
- Schedule treatments that assist in mobilizing mucus (e.g. aerosol treatments, postural drainage therapy) at least 1 hour before or after meals.
- Increase activity as tolerated. **D** ● ✦

- Encourage a rest period before meals. **D** ● ✦

- Eliminate noxious sights and odors from the environment; provide client with an opaque, covered container for expectorated sputum. **D** ● ✦
- Maintain a clean environment and a relaxed, pleasant atmosphere. **D** ● ✦
- Provide oral hygiene before meals. **D** ● ✦

RATIONALE

Monitoring a client's intake helps to identify when a patient is at risk for inadequate nutrition and allows for prompt intervention

The foul odor and taste of sputum and some aerosols are likely to decrease appetite. Appropriate scheduling of treatments also assists in decreasing nausea.

Activity usually promotes a sense of well-being and can help improve an individual's appetite.

Rest before a meal helps to minimize fatigue that may occur when eating.

Noxious sights and odors can decrease one's appetite. By eliminating them, the patient's intake may improve.

A clean environment and a relaxed atmosphere may increase intake.

Oral hygiene moistens the mouth, which makes it easier to chew and swallow. It also removes unpleasant tastes, which often improves the taste of foods/fluids.

THERAPEUTIC INTERVENTIONS	RATIONALE
• Assist the client who is quite dyspneic in selecting foods that require little or no chewing.	*Dyspnea decreases the ability of an individual to eat complete meals.*
• Serve frequent, small meals rather than large ones if the client is weak, fatigues easily, or has a poor appetite. **D** ● ✦	*Small, frequent meals decrease fatigue and help to maintain an individual's nutritional status.*
• Place client in a high-Fowler's position for meals. **D** ✦	*The high-Fowler's position improves lung expansion and helps to relieve dyspnea.*
• Limit fluid intake with meals unless the fluid has high nutritional value. **D** ● ✦	*Decreasing fluid intake during meals helps to reduce early satiety and subsequent decreased food intake.*
• Allow for adequate time for meals. **D** ● ✦	*Clients who feel rushed during meals tend to become anxious, lose their appetite, and stop eating.*
• Ensure that meals are well balanced and high in essential nutrients.	*A diet that is well balanced and high in essential nutrients meets the client's nutritional needs.*

Dependent/Collaborative Actions

Implement measures to maintain an adequate nutritional status:

• Administer dietary supplements as needed. **D** ✦	*If dietary intake does not provide the recommended daily allowances of vitamins and minerals, supplements may be necessary.*
	Dietary supplements are often needed to accomplish appropriate nutritional status.
• Administer supplemental oxygen while eating. **D** ✦	*Maintains appropriate oxygenation while client is eating, which may improve intake*
• Obtain a dietary consult to assist client in selecting foods/fluids that meet nutritional needs, are appealing, and adhere to personal and cultural preferences.	
• Perform a calorie count if ordered and report information to dietitian and physician.	*A calorie count provides information about the caloric and nutritional value of the foods/fluids consumed. The information helps the dietitian and physician determine whether an alternative method of nutritional support is needed.*
Consult a physician about an alternative method of providing nutrition (e.g., parenteral nutrition, tube feedings) if client does not consume enough food or fluids to meet nutritional needs.	*If a client is unable to eat, collaboration with the physician is required to determine alternative methods of maintaining nutritional status.*

Nursing Diagnosis ## ACTIVITY INTOLERANCE NDx

Definition: Insufficient physiological or psychological energy to endure or complete required or desired daily activities

Related to:
• Tissue hypoxia associated with impaired gas exchange
• Difficulty resting and sleeping associated with frequent coughing, dyspnea, and frequent assessments and treatment
• Inadequate nutritional status
• Increased energy expenditure associated with persistent coughing and the increased metabolic rate that is present in an infectious process

CLINICAL MANIFESTATIONS

Subjective	Objective
Verbal report of fatigue, weakness, and/or dizziness	Abnormal heart rate or B/P response to activity; exertional discomfort or dyspnea; electrocardiographic changes reflecting dysrhythmias or ischemia; unable to speak during physical activity

---

NDx = NANDA-I Diagnosis **D** = Delegatable Action ● = UAP ✦ = LVN/LPN   ⊜▶ = Go to ⊜volve for animation

Continued...

RISK FACTORS

- Generalized weakness
- Imbalance between oxygen supply/demand
- Debilitated condition
- Immobility
- Sedentary lifestyle

DESIRED OUTCOMES

The client will demonstrate an increased tolerance for activity as evidenced by:
  a. Verbalization of feeling less fatigued and weak
  b. Ability to perform ADL without exertional dyspnea, chest pain, diaphoresis, dizziness, and significant changes in vital signs

NOC OUTCOMES

Activity tolerance, endurance: fatigue level; vital signs; energy conservation; symptom severity

NIC INTERVENTIONS

Activity therapy; energy management; oxygen therapy; nutrition management; sleep enhancement; cardiac care; cardiac rehabilitation; teaching regarding prescribed activity

NURSING ASSESSMENT

Assess for signs and symptoms of activity intolerance:
- Statements of fatigue or weakness
- Exertional dyspnea, chest pain, diaphoresis, or dizziness
- Abnormal heart rate response to activity (e.g., increase in rate of 20 beats/min above resting rate, rate not returning to preactivity level within 3 minutes after stopping activity, change from regular to irregular rate)
- Significant change (15-20 mm Hg) in B/P with activity

RATIONALE

Early recognition of signs and symptoms of activity intolerance allows for prompt intervention.

THERAPEUTIC INTERVENTIONS

RATIONALE

Independent Actions

Implement measures to improve activity tolerance:
- Conserve energy.
- Maintain prescribed activity restrictions.
- Minimize environmental activity and noise.
- Provide uninterrupted rest periods.
- Assist with care.
- Keep supplies and personal articles within easy reach.
- Limit the number of visitors.
- Assist client in energy-saving techniques (e.g., using a shower chair when showering, sitting to brush teeth or comb hair).
- Implement measures to promote sleep (e.g., maintain a quiet, restful environment; discourage client from napping during the day, participating in group care activities to allow for periods of rest).
- Increase client's activity gradually as allowed and tolerated. **D** ● ✦
- Discourage smoking and excessive intake of beverages high in caffeine such as coffee, tea, and colas.

- Implement measures to improve respiratory status (e.g., encourage use of incentive spirometer; elevate head of bed; assist with turning, coughing, and deep breathing) if ineffective breathing pattern, ineffective airway clearance, or impaired gas exchange is contributing to client's activity intolerance. **D** ✦

Instruct client to report a decreased tolerance for activity and to stop any activity that causes chest pain, shortness of breath, dizziness, or extreme fatigue or weakness.

Cells use oxygen and fat, protein, and carbohydrates to produce the energy needed for all body activities. Rest and activities that conserve energy result in a lower metabolic rate, which preserves nutrients and oxygen for necessary activities.

Progressive increase in activity helps strengthen the myocardium, which enhances cardiac output and improves activity tolerance.
Both nicotine and excessive caffeine intake can increase cardiac workload and myocardial oxygen utilization, thereby decreasing the amount of oxygen necessary for energy production.
Improving respiratory status increases the amount of oxygen available for energy production. It also eases the work of breathing, which reduces energy expenditure.

These symptoms indicate that insufficient oxygen is reaching the tissues and that activity has been increased beyond a therapeutic level.

THERAPEUTIC INTERVENTIONS	RATIONALE

Dependent/Collaborative Actions

Implement measures to improve activity tolerance:

- Implement measures to increase cardiac output (e.g., administer positive inotropic agents, vasodilators, or antidysrhythmics as ordered; elevate the head of the bed) if decreased cardiac output is contributing to the client's activity intolerance.

  Sufficient cardiac output is necessary to maintain an adequate blood flow and oxygen supply to the tissues. Adequate tissue oxygenation promotes more efficient energy production, which subsequently improves client's activity tolerance.

- Implement measures to reduce fever if present (e.g., administer tepid sponge bath, administer antipyretics as ordered). **D** ✦

  An elevated temperature increases the metabolic rate with subsequent depletion of available energy and a decrease in the ability to tolerate activity.

- Maintain oxygen therapy as ordered. **D** ✦

  Supplemental oxygen helps to alleviate hypoxia and restore the more efficient aerobic metabolism, thereby improving energy levels and activity tolerance.

- Implement measures to maintain an adequate nutritional status (e.g., provide a diet high in essential nutrients, provide dietary supplements as indicated, administer vitamins and minerals as ordered).

  Metabolism is the process by which nutrients are transformed into energy. If nutrition is inadequate, energy production is decreased, which subsequently reduces one's ability to tolerate activity.

- Implement measures to treat anemia if present (e.g., administer prescribed iron, folic acid, and/or vitamin B_{12}; administer packed red blood cells as ordered).

  Anemia reduces the blood's oxygen-carrying capacity. Resolution of anemia increases oxygen availability to the cells, which increases the efficiency of energy production and subsequently improves activity tolerance.

Consult physician if signs and symptoms of activity intolerance persist.

Notifying the physician allows for modification of the treatment plan.

Nursing Diagnosis

RISK FOR INFECTION: NDx EXTRAPULMONARY (E.G., PERICARDIAL, LARYNGEAL, SKELETAL, JOINT, RENAL, BRAIN, ADRENAL, LYMPHATIC) AND/OR SUPERINFECTION (E.G., CANDIDIASIS)

Definition: At increased risk for being invaded by pathogenic organisms

Related to:

- Spread of the tubercle bacilli into the lymph nodes (lymphatic dissemination) and blood (hematogenous dissemination)
- Decreased resistance to infection associated with inadequate nutritional status and/or presence of other disease (e.g., HIV infection, chronic obstructive pulmonary disease) and side effects of the treatment of those diseases
- Interruption in the balance of usual endogenous microbial flora associated with the administration of antitubercular/antimicrobial agents

CLINICAL MANIFESTATIONS

Subjective	Objective
Reports of precordial pain; bone pain; painful joints; headache	Increase in temperature; increased pulse rate; pericardial friction rub and/or precordial pain; swollen lymph nodes; swollen, reddened joints; unusual color, amount, and odor of vaginal drainage; perineal itching; white patches or ulcerated areas in the mouth; increased weakness or fatigue; hoarseness, sore throat; increase in WBC count above previous levels and/or significant change in differential

Continued...

RISK FACTORS

- Inadequate primary defenses
- Inadequate secondary defenses (decreased hemoglobin level, leukopenia, suppressed inflammatory response)
- Inadequate acquired immunity
- Malnutrition
- Ineffective pharmaceutical agents
- Insufficient knowledge to avoid exposure to pathogens

DESIRED OUTCOMES

The client will not develop extrapulmonary infection or superinfection as evidenced by:
  a. No increase in temperature
  b. Pulse rate within client's normal range
  c. Absence of a pericardial friction rub and precordial pain
  d. Absence of heat, pain, redness, swelling, and unusual drainage in any area
  e. Absence of white patches and ulcerations in mouth
  f. No reports of increased weakness and fatigue
  g. Normal voice quality
  h. Absence of headache
  i. WBC and differential counts returning toward normal

NOC OUTCOMES

Immune status; infection severity

NIC INTERVENTIONS

Infection protection; infection control

NURSING ASSESSMENT	RATIONALE
Assess for and report signs and symptoms of extrapulmonary infection or superinfection: • Further increase in temperature • Increased pulse rate • Pericardial friction rub and/or precordial pain • Bone pain • Swollen, red, painful joints • Swollen lymph nodes • Unusual color, amount, and odor of vaginal drainage; perineal itching • White patches or ulcerated areas in the mouth • Increased weakness or fatigue • Hoarseness, sore throat • Headache • Increase in WBC count above previous levels and/or significant change in differential	*Early recognition of signs and symptoms of infection allows for prompt treatment.* *Fungal infections are common superinfections with antimicrobial therapy.*

THERAPEUTIC INTERVENTIONS	RATIONALE
Independent Actions Implement measures to reduce the risk for extrapulmonary infection and/or superinfection:	
• Use good hand hygiene and encourage client to do the same. **D ● ✦**	*Good hand washing prevents spread of infection.*
• Perform actions to maintain an adequate nutritional status (provide frequent meals, provide oral hygiene before meals, decrease fluid intake with meals).	*Adequate nutritional status is important to prevent infections.*
• Maintain sterile technique during all invasive procedures (e.g., venous and arterial punctures, injections, urinary catheterization).	*Sterile technique during invasive procedures is important to prevent exposure to infectious agents.*
• Change peripheral intravenous line sites, and change equipment, tubing, and solutions used for treatments such as intravenous infusions and respiratory care according to hospital policy.	*Changing intravenous line sites, equipment, tubings, etc., helps to prevent infection.*
Protect client from others with an infection. **D ● ✦**	*Exposure to others with infection increases the client's risk.*
• Anchor catheters/tubings (e.g., urinary, intravenous) securely.	*Securing catheters/tubing reduces trauma to the tissues and the risk for introduction of pathogens associated with the in-and-out movement of the tubing.*

THERAPEUTIC INTERVENTIONS	RATIONALE
• Maintain a closed system for drains (e.g., urinary catheter) and intravenous infusions whenever possible.	*Closed drainage systems prevent the introduction of infectious agents into the system.*
• Assist client to perform good perineal care routinely and after each bowel movement. **D** ● ✦	*Good perineal care and hygiene prevent skin breakdown and exposure to potential infectious agents.*
• Reinforce importance of frequent oral hygiene. **D** ✦	*Good oral hygiene prevents accumuluation of infectious agents.*

Dependent/Collaborative Actions

If signs and symptoms of an extrapulmonary infection or superinfection occur:

• Prepare client for and/or assist with diagnostic tests (e.g., blood, vaginal, pleural fluid, and urine cultures; lumbar puncture; aspiration of joint fluid; bone marrow aspiration).	*If an infection occurs, a culture and sensitivity of the infected area allow for prescription of appropriate antibiotics.*
• Administer additional or alternative antitubercular/antimicrobial medications as ordered.	*Antitubercular and antimicrobial agents help to resolve the infectious process.*

Collaborative Diagnosis ## RISK FOR PLEURAL EFFUSION

Definition: An abnormal accumulation of fluid in the pleural cavity

Related to: An increase in capillary permeability of the pulmonary and pleural vessels associated with the inflammatory response to the presence of tubercle bacilli in the lung and pleural space

CLINICAL MANIFESTATIONS

Subjective	Objective
Report of dyspnea; verbalization of chest pain (pleural)	Dull percussion note and diminished or absent breath sounds; chest radiograph showing pleural effusion; respiratory rate greater than 20 breaths/min; fever; night sweats; cough; weight loss

RISK FACTORS	DESIRED OUTCOMES

• Pulmonary infection
• Increased permeability of capillary beds
	The client will not develop pleural effusion as evidenced by:
	  a. No increase in dyspnea
	  b. Symmetrical chest excursion
	  c. Improved breath sounds and percussion note throughout lung fields

NURSING ASSESSMENT	RATIONALE
Assess for and report signs and symptoms of pleural effusion (e.g., dyspnea, chest pain, decreased chest excursion on affected side, dull percussion note, decreased or absent breath sounds over the affected area, chest radiograph showing pleural effusion)	*Early recognition of signs and symptoms of pleural effusion allows for prompt intervention.*

THERAPEUTIC INTERVENTIONS	RATIONALE
Dependent/Collaborative Actions Implement measures to resolve the infectious process: • Encourage coughing and deep breathing. • Administer antimicrobials as ordered.	*Resolution of an infectious process reduces the risk for development of pleural effusion and/or atelectasis.* *Treats infection.*

Continued...

THERAPEUTIC INTERVENTIONS	RATIONALE
If signs and symptoms of pleural effusion occur: • Continue with actions to improve respiratory status (e.g., increase activity tolerance; instruct client in and assist with diaphragmatic and pursed-lip breathing techniques; instruct client to deep breathe or use incentive spirometer every 1 to 2 hours; encourage coughing and deep breathing; place client in semi- to high-Fowler's position). • Prepare client for a thoracentesis if planned.	*Maintenance/improvement of the client's respiratory status and removal of secretions decrease the potential of infection or the occurrence of a pleural effusion.* *Removal of fluid from the lungs will help to improve the client's ability to maintain adequate gas exchange.*

Collaborative Diagnosis | RISK FOR PNEUMOTHORAX

Definition: Accumulation of air in the pleural space that causes complete or partial collapse of a lung

Related to: Accumulation of air in the pleural space associated with formation of a bronchopleural fistula or rupture of a subpleural bleb

CLINICAL MANIFESTATIONS

Subjective	Objective
Verbalization of shortness of breath	Absent breath sounds; hyperresonant percussion; rapid, shallow, and/or labored respirations; restlessness; agitation; confusion; arterial blood gas values that have worsened; chest radiograph results showing a lung collapse

RISK FACTORS

• Rupture of a subpleural bleb
• Bronchopleural fistula

DESIRED OUTCOMES

The client will experience normal lung reexpansion if pneumothorax occurs as evidenced by:
  a. Audible breath sounds and resonant percussion note by the third or fourth postoperative day
  b. Unlabored respirations at 12 to 20 breaths/min
  c. Arterial blood gas values returning toward normal
  d. Chest radiograph showing lung reexpansion

NURSING ASSESSMENT	RATIONALE
Assess for and immediately report signs and symptoms of pneumothorax (e.g., absent breath sounds with hyperresonant percussion note over involved area; rapid, shallow, and/or labored respirations; tachycardia; sudden onset of chest pain; restlessness; agitation; confusion; significant decrease in oximetry results; abnormal arterial blood gas values; chest radiograph results showing lung collapse).	*Early recognition of the signs and symptoms of pneumothorax allows for prompt intervention.*

THERAPEUTIC INTERVENTIONS	RATIONALE
Dependent/Collaborative Actions If signs and symptoms of lung collapse occur: • Maintain client on bed rest in a semi- to high-Fowler's position. • Maintain oxygen therapy as ordered.	*Improves client's ability to expand the lungs.* *Helps to maintain tissue oxygenation.*

THERAPEUTIC INTERVENTIONS	RATIONALE
• Assess for and immediately report signs and symptoms of tension pneumothorax (e.g., severe dyspnea, increased restlessness and agitation, rapid and/or irregular pulse rate, hypotension, neck vein distention, shift in trachea from midline).	*Emergency treatment is required to prevent further respiratory difficulty.*
• Assist with clearing of existing chest tube and/or insertion of a new tube.	*Reestablishes a closed drainage system.*

Collaborative Diagnosis **RISK FOR ATELECTASIS**

Definition: Collapse of lung tissue caused by hypoventilated alveoli

Related to:
• Consolidation of lung tissue
• Proliferation of the infection
• Stasis of secretions

CLINICAL MANIFESTATIONS

Subjective	Objective
Report of dyspnea	Decreased breath sounds and/or crackles; cough; sputum production; low-grade fever; heart rate greater than 60 to 100 beats/min; increased respiratory rate >20 breaths/min/increased work of breathing; chest radiograph, ultrasound, or computed tomography results showing patchy infiltrates

RISK FACTORS	DESIRED OUTCOMES
• Ineffective treatment regimen • Smoking • Immobility	The client will not develop atelectasis as evidenced by: a. Clear, audible breath sounds b. Resonant percussion note over lungs c. Unlabored respirations at 12 to 20 breaths/min d. Pulse rate within normal range for client e. Afebrile status

NURSING ASSESSMENT	RATIONALE
Assess for and report signs and symptoms of atelectasis: • Diminished or absent breath sounds • Dull percussion note over affected area • Increased respiratory rate • Dyspnea • Tachycardia • Elevated temperature	*Early recognition of signs and symptoms of atelectasis allows for implementation of the appropriate interventions.*
Monitor pulse oximetry results as indicated.	*Pulse oximetry is an indirect measure of oxygen saturation. Monitoring pulse oximetry (SaO$_2$) allows for early detection of hypoxia and implementation of the appropriate interventions.*
Monitor chest radiograph results.	*Chest radiograph provides radiographic confirmation of atelectasis.*

Continued...

THERAPEUTIC INTERVENTIONS	RATIONALE

Dependent/Collaborative Actions

Implement measures to prevent atelectasis:

- Perform actions to improve breathing pattern:
  - Encourage client to deep breathe
  - Use of incentive spirometry
- Perform actions to promote effective airway clearance:
  - Turn, cough, and deep breathe.

Administer antibiotics as ordered.

If signs and symptoms of atelectasis occur:

- Increase frequency of position change, coughing or "huffing," deep breathing, and use of incentive spirometer.

Consult physician if signs and symptoms of atelectasis persist or worsen.

Lack of movement places a client at risk for atelectasis. Changing positions frequently, coughing, and deep breathing help to expand the lungs, enhancing alveolar expansion.

Treats infection.
Improves lung expansion and mobilization of secretions.

Allows for prompt alterations in interventions.

PATIENT AND DISCHARGE TEACHING/CONTINUED CARE

Nursing Diagnosis **DEFICIENT KNOWLEDGE, NDx INEFFECTIVE HEALTH MAINTENANCE NDx, OR INEFFECTIVE SELF-HEALTH MANAGEMENT* NDx**

Definition: Absence or deficiency of cognitive information related to specific topic (lack of specific information necessary for clients/significant others) to make informed choices regarding condition/treatment/lifestyle changes); inability to identify, manage, and/or seek out help to maintain health; pattern of regulating and integrating into daily living a therapeutic regimen for treatment of illness and the sequelae of illness that is unsatisfactory for meeting specific health goals

CLINICAL MANIFESTATIONS

Subjective	Objective
Verbalization of the problem	Inaccurate follow through of instructions; inappropriate behaviors

RISK FACTORS

- Denial of disease process
- Cognitive deficiency
- Failure to take action to reduce risk factors

NOC OUTCOMES

Knowledge: medication; knowledge: health promotion; knowledge: disease process; knowledge: infection control; treatment behavior: illness or injury; compliance behavior; health beliefs: perceived resources; health beliefs: perceived ability to perform; health beliefs: perceived control

NIC INTERVENTIONS

Health system guidance; teaching: individual; teaching: disease process; teaching: prescribed medication management; communicable disease management; self-modification assistance; values clarification; teaching: disease process; support system enhancement

---

*The nurse should select the diagnostic label that is most appropriate for the client's discharge teaching.

NURSING ASSESSMENT	RATIONALE
Assess client readiness and ability to learn Assess meaning of illness to client	*Early recognition of readiness to learn and meaning of illness to client allows for implementation of the appropriate teaching interventions.*

THERAPEUTIC INTERVENTIONS	RATIONALE

Desired Outcome: The client will identify ways to maintain respiratory health and ways to prevent spread of TB to others.

Dependent/Collaborative Actions

Instruct client in ways to maintain respiratory health:

• Maintain overall general good health (e.g., reduce stress, eat a well-balanced diet, obtain adequate rest).	*Good general health supports the individual's ability to fight off infection.*
• Stop smoking.	*The irritants in smoke and respiratory irritants increase mucus production, impair ciliary function, and can cause inflammation and damage to the bronchial and alveolar walls; the carbon monoxide decreases oxygen availability*
• Avoid exposure to respiratory irritants such as smoke, dust, aerosol sprays, paint fumes, and solvents; wear a mask or scarf over nose and mouth if exposure to high levels of these irritants is unavoidable.	
• Remain indoors as much as possible when air pollution levels are high.	*Air pollution in high levels is harmful to persons with existing lung disease.* *Exposure to extreme hot and cold air may cause bronchoconstriction, allowing less air into and out of the lungs and decreasing oxygen/CO$_2$ exchange.*
• Avoid prolonged close contact with persons who have active TB or any other respiratory infection.	*Leads to increased potential for an infection and the spread of TB*
• Avoid crowds and poorly ventilated areas.	
• Drink at least 10 glasses of liquid per day unless contraindicated.	*Increased fluid intake is necessary with many of the medications used in the treatment of TB to maintain adequate hydration. Increased fluid intake is important to thin or liquefy secretions making them easier to expectorate.*
• Receive immunizations against influenza and pneumococcal pneumonia.	*Immunizations help to prevent further respiratory disease.*

Educate the patient on the disease process and treatment of TB:

• Explain TB in terms the client can understand; stress that TB is an infectious disease and that adherence to the treatment plan is necessary in order to prevent transmission to others, complications, and reactivation of the disease.	*Understanding of the disease and its treatment plan provides the patient with a sense of control and makes it more likely that the patient will be adherent to the treatment regimen.*
• Explain that active TB can be treated successfully but only if the client adheres to the prescribed multiple drug therapy.	*The client must understand that TB can be successfully treated only with a multiple drug regimen.*
• Provide written instructions about and encourage the client to participate in the treatment plan (e.g., protecting others from the infection, adhering to medication regimen, participating in respiratory care treatments).	*Written instructions allow the client to refer to them as needed. The instructions should include all information needed to understand disease processes and treatment.*
• Provide client with written instructions about disease transmission, signs and symptoms to report, medication therapy, and follow-up appointments.	

Educate the patient on ways to prevent the spread of TB to others:

• Cover nose and mouth with a tissue when coughing, sneezing, and laughing.	*These actions are important to prevent the spread of TB. TB is an airborne bacteria and is spread through close contact with someone who is infected.*
• Refrain from spitting or do so into a tissue.	

Continued...

THERAPEUTIC INTERVENTIONS	RATIONALE
• Practice good hand hygiene (e.g., wash hands using an antimicrobial soap, use an alcohol-base hand rub), especially after placing hands over mouth or nose and handling soiled tissues.	*Appropriate hand washing and care of soiled tissues helps prevent spread of infection.*
• Dispose of soiled tissues properly (e.g., place in paper or plastic bag, flush down toilet).	
• Avoid close contact with people who are at high risk for infection (e.g., those who are very young or elderly, those with HIV infection); wear a mask if close contact is unavoidable.	*Individuals who are at high risk for infection are at high risk for contracting TB.*
• Adhere strictly to the prescribed medication regimen for the treatment of TB.	*Medications require an adequate blood level to be effective.*
• Inform clients that they will continue to be infectious until 3 consecutive sputum cultures show absence of the tubercle bacilli (this usually occurs after a couple of weeks of taking the antitubercular/antimicrobial agents) and that in order to not become infectious again, they must continue with the medication regimen for the prescribed length of time (usually 6-18 months).	*Clients need to know that they will be infectious for an extended period even though they continue taking medications. The longer the medication regimen, the greater the incidence of nonadherence.*

THERAPEUTIC INTERVENTIONS	RATIONALE

Desired Outcome: The client will verbalize an understanding of medications ordered including rationale, food and drug interactions, side effects, and importance of taking as prescribed.

Dependent/Collaborative Actions

Explain the rationale for, side effects of, and importance of taking medications prescribed, as well as food and drug interactions, and drugs to manage side effects.	*Knowledge of the medication regimen and the impact of these medications on the body, as well as how the medication regimen can be incorporated into the client's lifestyle, allows the client some mechanism of control of his/her disease and the ability to have an active part in treatment and care.*
Examples of TB drugs: isoniazid, rifampin, ethambutol, pyrazinamide, and streptomycin	*Treatment failures often result from clients not taking their medications correctly or prematurely stopping their medications.*
Assist client to identify ways the medication regimen can be incorporated into the client's lifestyle.	*Clients must understand that they increase their chance of developing a "drug-resistant" strain of TB if the medications are not taken as prescribed.*
Assist client to develop a method to promote adherence to the medication schedule (e.g., filling a pill box or empty egg carton with the medications that need to be taken that day/week, setting a timer or alarm as a reminder of when to take medications, using a checklist to document when each medication is due and taken).	
Remind client of the consequences of not adhering to the multiple drug regimen.	*Nonadherence to the multiple drug regimen may cause spread of TB from lungs to other parts of the body, development of a strain of TB that will be very difficult to treat, and transmission of TB to others.*
Reinforce the need to consult a physician before discontinuing any medication or taking additional prescription and nonprescription medications.	*There may be drug-drug interactions that occur when taking TB prescriptions. A physician should approve of any medications taken to alleviate potential negative effects.*
Instruct client to take all medications as often as prescribed and avoid skipping doses or altering the prescribed dose; if a dose is missed, instruct client to take it as soon as remembered unless it is almost time for the next dose of the same medication.	*Proper treatment occurs when medications are taken as prescribed. If the clients are unable to take medications as prescribed, it may prolong treatment time and lead to exacerbation of the disease.*
Instruct client to consult health care provider if considering becoming pregnant, if pregnancy occurs, and if breast-feeding.	*Some of the medications used to treat TB are contraindicated in pregnancy and if breast-feeding.*

THERAPEUTIC INTERVENTIONS	RATIONALE

Desired Outcome: The client will state signs and symptoms to report to the health care provider.

Dependent/Collaborative Actions

Instruct client to report the following:

- Persistent or recurrent loss of appetite, nausea, weakness, fatigue, or weight loss
- Fever, chills, continued or increased night sweats
- Difficulty breathing, continued or increased cough, or chest pain
- Unusual color, amount, and odor of vaginal secretions; white patches or ulcerated areas in mouth
- Stiff neck and headache
- Hoarseness; persistent sore throat
- Bone pain; swollen, red, painful joints
- Swollen lymph nodes

These signs and symptoms may indicate a superinfection or spread of infection to another site, ineffectiveness of medications, inadequate nutrition, and/or adverse effects of medication regimen.

THERAPEUTIC INTERVENTIONS	RATIONALE

Desired Outcome: The client will verbalize an understanding of and a plan for adhering to recommended follow-up care including future appointments with health care provider.

Dependent/Collaborative Actions

Reinforce the importance of keeping appointments for follow-up tests (e.g., blood work, hearing tests, sputum cultures, chest radiographs) and physical examinations to determine the effectiveness of the medication regimen and assess for side effects such as liver and kidney damage.

Provide information about and encourage utilization of community resources and social services that can assist the client to comply with the medication regimen or to provide financial support if needed (e.g., home health agencies, local Department of Health and Human Services, directly observed therapy [DOT] programs, local chapter of the American Lung Association, support groups).

Include significant others in explanations and teaching sessions and encourage their support.

Monitoring of TB is critical in maintaining client's health and the effectiveness of the medication regimen.

Provide for continuum of care and can help client's adherence with the medication regimen and possibly financial assistance for medications.

Involvement of the client's significant others contribute to treatment regimen adherence and may help with medication administration if needed.

ADDITIONAL NURSING DIAGNOSES

FEAR/ANXIETY NDx
Related to unfamiliar environment, separation from significant others, financial concerns, and fear of transmitting disease to others

RISK FOR DEFICIENT FLUID VOLUME NDx
Related to decreased oral fluid intake and excessive fluid loss (can occur with night sweats and profuse diaphoresis)

ACUTE PAIN: CHEST NDx
Related to extension of the inflammatory/infectious process to the pleura and muscle strain (can result from excessive coughing)

DISTURBED SLEEP PATTERN NDx
Related to an unfamiliar environment, night sweats, persistent coughing, anxiety, and frequent assessments and treatments

See Bibliography at the back of the book.

The Client with Alterations in Cardiovascular Function

ABDOMINAL AORTIC ANEURYSM

An abdominal aortic aneurysm is an abnormal dilation of the wall of the abdominal aorta. The aneurysm usually develops in the segment of the vessel that is between the renal arteries and the iliac branches of the aorta. The most common cause of an abdominal aortic aneurysm is atherosclerosis. The plaque that forms on the wall of the artery causes degenerative changes in the medial layer of the vessel. These changes lead to loss of elasticity, weakening, and eventual dilation of the affected segment. Some other causes of abdominal aortic aneurysm include inflammation (arteritis), trauma, infection, congenital abnormalities of the vessel, and connective tissue disorders that cause vessel wall weakness.

Most abdominal aortic aneurysms are asymptomatic and are discovered during a routine physical examination (signs include palpation of a pulsatile mass in the abdomen and/or auscultation of a bruit over the abdominal aorta) or during a review of x-ray results of the abdomen or lower spine. The presence of symptoms such as mild to severe abdominal, lumbar, or flank pain and/or lower extremity arterial insufficiency is usually indicative of a large aneurysm that is exerting pressure on surrounding tissues or an aneurysm that is leaking.

Surgical repair of an aneurysm is usually performed if the aneurysm is growing rapidly and/or reaches a size of 5 to 6 cm or larger, or if the client experiences symptoms. The procedure often involves the use of a synthetic graft, which is inserted to replace or support the weakened vessel.

This care plan focuses on the adult client hospitalized for surgical repair of an abdominal aortic aneurysm. Much of the postoperative information is applicable to clients receiving follow-up care in an extended care facility or home setting.

OUTCOME DISCHARGE CRITERIA

The client will:
1. Tolerate prescribed diet
2. Tolerate expected level of activity
3. Have surgical pain controlled
4. Have clear, audible breath sounds throughout lungs
5. Have evidence of normal healing of surgical wounds
6. Have no signs and symptoms of postoperative complications
7. Identify ways to prevent or slow the progression of atherosclerosis
8. State signs and symptoms to report to the health care provider
9. Verbalize an understanding of and a plan for adhering to recommended follow-up care including future appointments with health care provider, medications prescribed, activity level, and wound care.

PREOPERATIVE: USE IN CONJUNCTION WITH THE STANDARDIZED PREOPERATIVE CARE PLAN

Related Preoperative Nursing/Collaborative Diagnoses — ANXIETY NDx/FEAR NDx

Definition: Response to a perceived threat that is recognized as danger; vague, uneasy feeling of discomfort or dread

Related to:
- Unfamiliar environment and separation from significant others
- Lack of understanding of diagnostic tests, surgical procedure, and postoperative care
- Anticipated loss of control associated with effects of anesthesia risk of disease if blood transfusions are necessary
- Anticipated postoperative discomfort and potential change in sexual functioning
- Possibility of death

POTENTIAL COMPLICATIONS OF ABDOMINAL AORTIC ANEURYSM: HYPOVOLEMIC SHOCK

Related to excessive blood loss if the aneurysm ruptures

Postoperative Nursing/Collaborative Diagnosis*

Nursing/Collaborative Diagnosis | **RISK FOR IMBALANCED FLUID** NDx **AND RISK FOR ELECTROLYTE IMBALANCE** NDx

Definition: At risk for a decrease, increase, or rapid shift from one to the other of intravascular, interstitial, and/or intracellular fluid; at risk for a change in serum electrolyte levels

Related to:
- **Third-spacing of fluid** related to:
  - Increased capillary permeability in surgical area associated with the inflammation that occurs after extensive dissection of tissue during major abdominal surgery
  - Increased vascular hydrostatic pressure associated with excess fluid volume if present
  - Hypoalbuminemia associated with the escape of proteins from the vascular space into the peritoneum (a result of increased capillary permeability in the surgical area)
- **Excess fluid volume** NDx related to:
  - Vigorous fluid replacement
  - Fluid retention associated with increased secretion of antidiuretic hormone (ADH; output of ADH is stimulated by trauma, pain, and anesthetic agents) and/or renal insufficiency (can occur if there is inadequate blood flow to the kidneys during or after surgery)
  - Reabsorption of third-space fluid (occurs about the third postoperative day)
- **Deficient fluid volume** NDx related to restricted oral fluid intake before, during, and after surgery; blood loss; and loss of fluid associated with nasogastric tube drainage
- **Hypokalemia, hypochloremia, and metabolic alkalosis** related to loss of electrolytes and hydrochloric acid associated with nasogastric tube drainage

CLINICAL MANIFESTATIONS

Subjective	Objective
Excessive fluid volume: Not applicable	Excessive fluid volume: Weight gain of 2% or greater in a short period; elevated B/P (B/P may not be elevated if cardiac output is poor or fluid has shifted out of the vascular space); presence of an S_3 heart sound; intake greater than output; change in mental status; crackles (rales) dyspnea, orthopnea; edema, distended neck veins; elevated CVP (use internal jugular vein pulsation method to estimate CVP if monitoring device is not present)
Deficient fluid volume: Verbal report of thirst	Deficient fluid volume: Hypotension; tachycardia; decreased urine output; tenting skin turgor; dry mucous membranes; thick, tenacious pulmonary secretions
Hypokalemia: Complaints of muscular weakness, leg cramps; paresthesia; palpitations	Hypokalemia: Decreased or absent deep tendon reflexes; anorexia; nausea; vomiting; rhabdomyolysis; orthostatic hypotension; ventricular arrhythmias; cardiac arrest
Hypochloremia: Complaints of muscle cramps, weakness, and/or twitching; irritability	Hypochloremia: Tetany; hyperactive deep tendon reflexes; arrhythmias; seizures, coma
Metabolic alkalosis: Complaints of muscle cramps, weakness, and/or twitching; irritability; complaints of numbness and tingling of fingers, nose, and/or mouth	Metabolic alkalosis: Apathy; confusion; slow, shallow respirations; hyperactive reflexes; seizures; stupor; anorexia; nausea; vomiting

---

*Use in conjunction with the Standardized Postoperative Care Plan.

NDx = NANDA-I Diagnosis   **D** = Delegatable Action   ● = UAP   ✦ = LVN/LPN   ⊝▶ = Go to ⊝volve for animation

Continued...

RISK FACTORS

- Aneurysm rupture resulting in hypovolemic shock
- Excessive volume replacement during resuscitation
- Excessive electrolyte loss through nasogastric drainage

DESIRED OUTCOMES

The client will experience resolution of third-spacing as evidenced by:
   a. Absence of ascites
   b. B/P and pulse rate within normal range for client and stable with position changes

The client will not experience excess fluid volume as evidenced by:
   a. Stable B/P
   b. Absence of an S_3 heart sound
   c. Balanced intake and output
   d. Normal breath sounds

The client will not experience deficient fluid volume, hypokalemia, hypochloremia, or metabolic acidosis as evidenced by:
   a. B/P and pulse rate within normal range for client and stable with position change
   b. Balanced intake and output within 48 hours after surgery
   c. Absence of cardiac dysrhythmias, muscle weakness, paresthesias, twitching, spasms, and dizziness
   d. Blood urea nitrogen (BUN), serum electrolytes, and arterial blood gas values within normal range

NOC OUTCOMES

Fluid balance; fluid overload severity; electrolyte and acid/base balance

NIC INTERVENTIONS

Fluid monitoring; fluid management; electrolyte management: hypokalemia; fluid/electrolyte management; acid-base monitoring; acid-base management: metabolic alkalosis

NURSING ASSESSMENT	RATIONALE
Assess for and report signs and symptoms of third-spacing: • Ascites (e.g., increase in abdominal girth, dull percussion note over abdomen with finding of shifting dullness) • Evidence of vascular depletion (e.g., postural hypotension; weak, rapid pulse).	*Early recognition of signs and symptoms of third-spacing allows for prompt intervention.*
Monitor serum albumin levels. Report below-normal levels.	*Low serum albumin levels result in fluid shifting out of vascular space because albumin normally maintains plasma colloid osmotic pressure.*
Monitor serum electrolyte values. Report abnormal values.	*Early recognition of signs of electrolyte imbalances allows for prompt intervention.*
Assess quantity of nasogastric tube drainage.	*Excessive nasogastric tube drainage can lead to hypokalemia, hypochloremia, and metabolic alkalosis.*

THERAPEUTIC INTERVENTIONS	RATIONALE
Dependent/Collaborative Actions Implement measures to prevent further third-spacing of fluid/fluid volume overload: • Administer fluid replacement judiciously. • Maintain fluid restrictions as ordered.	*Actions help to reduce the risk of fluid volume overload.*
• If client is receiving intravenous fluids that contain sizeable amounts of sodium (0.9% sodium chloride [NaCl] or lactated Ringer's), consult the physician about a change in solution or a decrease in the rate of infusion.	*Actions help to reduce the risk of third-spacing and electrolyte imbalances.*
• Administer albumin infusions if ordered.	*Administration of albumin helps to increase colloid osmotic pressure, promoting mobilization of fluid back into the vascular space.*

THERAPEUTIC INTERVENTIONS	RATIONALE
• Administer diuretics if ordered. **D** ✦	*Diuretics help to increase excretion of water.* *Diuretics should only be administered if signs and symptoms of fluid volume overload are evident.*
Implement measures to prevent or treat deficient fluid volume, hypokalemia, hypochloremia, and metabolic alkalosis:	
• Administer fluid and electrolytes as ordered.	
• Carefully measure all drainage (e.g., wound, nasogastric) and administer fluid replacement as ordered. **D** ✦	
Consult physician if signs and symptoms of third-spacing, fluid volume deficit, fluid volume overload, or electrolyte imbalances persist or worsen.	*Consulting the appropriate health care provider allows for modification of the treatment plan.*

Collaborative Diagnosis ## RISK FOR HYPOVOLEMIC SHOCK

Definition: A type of low blood flow shock that occurs when there is a loss of intravascular fluid volume. Loss of fluid volume may be absolute, resulting from fluid lost from hemorrhage, diuresis, or gastrointestinal losses

Related to: Hypovolemia associated with blood loss during surgery, third-space fluid shift, and hemorrhage (can occur as a result of inadequate wound closure and/or stress on and subsequent leakage or rupture of anastomotic sites)

CLINICAL MANIFESTATIONS

Subjective	Objective
Verbalizations of anxiety; confusion; agitation	Tachypnea; decreased urine output; pallor; cool, clammy skin

RISK FACTOR
• Aneurysm rupture

DESIRED OUTCOMES

The client will not develop hypovolemic shock as evidenced by:
  a. Usual mental status
  b. Stable vital signs
  c. Skin warm and usual color
  d. Palpable peripheral pulses
  e. Urine output at least 30 mL/h

NURSING ASSESSMENT	RATIONALE
Assess for and report signs and symptoms of leakage at anastomotic sites:	*Early recognition of signs and symptoms of hypovolemic shock allows for prompt intervention.*
• New or expanding hematoma at incision site and/or ecchymosis of flank or perineal area	
• Increased abdominal girth (can also occur with third-spacing)	
• New or increased reports of lumbar, flank, abdominal, pelvic, or groin pain	
• Increasing feeling of abdominal and/or gastric fullness unrelated to oral intake	
• Diminishing or absent peripheral pulses	
• Decreased motor or sensory function in lower extremities	
• Decreasing B/P, increasing pulse rate	

NDx = NANDA-I Diagnosis   **D** = Delegatable Action   ● = UAP   ✦ = LVN/LPN   ⊝▶ = Go to ⊝volve for animation

Continued...

NURSING ASSESSMENT	RATIONALE
Assess for and report signs and symptoms of hypovolemic shock: • Restlessness, agitation, changes in mental status • Significant decrease in B/P • Postural hypotension • Rapid, weak pulse • Rapid respirations • Cool skin • Pallor, cyanosis • Diminished or absent peripheral pulses • Urine output less than 30 mL/h	
Monitor red blood cell (RBC) count, hematocrit (Hct), and hemoglobin (Hgb) values for abnormal trends.	*While decreasing values may be indicative of hemorrhage, lab value trends should be evaluated in light of overall fluid status because fluid volume overload may dilute actual Hgb values.*

THERAPEUTIC INTERVENTIONS	RATIONALE
Dependent/Collaborative Actions	

Implement measures to prevent hypovolemic shock:
• Perform actions to prevent or treat hypovolemia:
  • If bleeding occurs, apply firm pressure to area if possible.
  • Administer blood and/or volume expanders (colloids/crystalloids) as ordered.
  • Provide maximum fluid intake allowed.	

• Perform actions to reduce stress on and separation of anastomotic sites: **D** ✦
  • Instruct client to avoid positions that compromise peripheral blood flow (use of knee gatch, crossing legs).
  • Instruct client to avoid activities that create a Valsalva response (e.g., straining to have a bowel movement, holding breath while moving up in bed).
  • Instruct client to avoid vigorous coughing.
	Stress on anastomotic sites increases the risk for disruption of suture lines, which may lead to hemorrhage and/or hypovolemic shock due to blood loss.

• Implement measures to reduce the accumulation of gas and fluid in the gastrointestinal tract (e.g., insert nasogastric tube).	*Interstitial fluid accumulation in the gastrointestinal tract along with excessive gas accumulation can result in excessive stress on anastomotic sites, increasing the risk of disruption of suture lines and subsequent hemorrhage.*
• Administer fluid replacement therapy judiciously. • Maintain fluid restrictions if ordered.	*Interstitial fluid accumulation in the gastrointestinal tract can lead to excessive stress on anastomotic sites, increasing the risk of disruption of suture lines and subsequent hemorrhage.*
• Administer antihypertensives if ordered. **D** ✦	*Elevated B/P must be reduced to a level that does not stress vascular anastomotic sites. Medications must be administered to keep a client's B/P within an acceptable range, especially within the immediate postoperative period.*
If signs and symptoms of hypovolemic shock occur: • Place client flat in bed unless contraindicated. • Monitor vital signs frequently. • Administer oxygen as ordered.	
Prepare client for surgery if signs and symptoms of hypovolemic shock occur, persist, or worsen.	*Surgical exploration will aid in identifying and controlling suspected sources of hemorrhage.*

Collaborative Diagnosis # RISK FOR LOWER EXTREMITY ARTERIAL EMBOLIZATION

Definition: A sudden disruption in the arterial blood supply to an extremity

Related to: Dislodgment of necrotic debris or clot from surgical site

CLINICAL MANIFESTATIONS

Subjective	Objective
Verbal reports of sudden, severe pain in affected limb; numbness in affected limb *Six P's of acute arterial ischemia: pain, pallor, pulselessness; paresthesia; paralysis; poikilothermia*	Diminished or absent pulses in affected limb; pale, cool, mottled extremity

RISK FACTOR

- Virchow's triad: venous stasis, hypercoagulability of blood, endothelial damage at surgical site

DESIRED OUTCOMES

The client will not experience lower extremity arterial embolization as evidenced by:
  a. No reports of pain or diminished sensation in lower extremities
  b. Palpable peripheral pulses
  c. Usual temperature and color of extremities

NURSING ASSESSMENT

Assess for and report signs and symptoms of lower extremity arterial embolization:
- Sudden, severe onset of pain in extremity
- Diminishing or absent peripheral pulses (pulses may be absent for a few hours after surgery as a result of vasospasm)
- Cool, pale, or mottled extremities

RATIONALE

Early recognition of signs and symptoms of arterial embolization allows for prompt intervention.

THERAPEUTIC INTERVENTIONS

Dependent/Collaborative Actions
Implement measures to reduce risk of embolization: **D** ✦
- Limit client's activity as ordered.
- Instruct client to avoid activities that create a Valsalva response.

If signs and symptoms of lower extremity arterial embolization occur:
- Maintain client on bed rest. **D** ✦
- Prepare client for the following if planned:
  - Diagnostic studies (e.g., Doppler ultrasound, arteriography)
  - Embolectomy

RATIONALE

In order to prevent dislodgment of existing thrombi.

To restore blood flow, an embolus should be removed as soon as possible after identification/location of the obstruction.

Collaborative Diagnosis # RISK FOR CARDIAC DYSRHYTHMIAS

Definition: Abnormal cardiac rhythms

Related to: Altered nodal function and myocardial conductivity associated with:
- Myocardial hypoxia resulting from:
  - Altered respiratory function
  - Diminished myocardial blood flow that can result from preexisting coronary artery disease, hypotension (can occur as a result of hypovolemia, vasodilation associated with rapid warming, and effects of some medications), and sympathetic nervous system–mediated vasoconstriction that results from pain, stress, and hypothermia.
  - Myocardial damage if a perioperative myocardial infarction has occurred
  - Hypokalemia if present

NDx = NANDA-I Diagnosis   **D** = Delegatable Action   ● = UAP   ✦ = LVN/LPN   ⊖▶ = Go to ⊖*volve* for animation

Continued...

CLINICAL MANIFESTATIONS

Subjective	Objective
Verbalization of syncope; palpitations NOTE: *Signs and symptoms are dependent upon how the client is tolerating the dysrhythmia.*	Irregular apical pulse; pulse rate less than 60 or greater than 100 beats/min; electrocardiogram (ECG) tracing abnormalities

RISK FACTORS

- Stress associated with general anesthesia
- Preexisting cardiovascular disease
- Electrolyte imbalances

DESIRED OUTCOMES

The client will maintain normal sinus rhythm as evidenced by:
  a. Regular apical pulse at 60 to 100 beats/min
  b. Equal apical and radial pulse rates
  c. Absence of syncope and palpitations
  d. ECG reading showing normal sinus rhythm

NURSING ASSESSMENT

Assess for and report signs and symptoms of cardiac dysrhythmias:
- Irregular apical pulse
- Pulse rate less than 60 or greater than 100 beats/min
- Apical-radial pulse deficit
- Syncope
- Palpitations
- Abnormal rate, rhythm, or configurations on ECG

Monitor continuous ECG if indicated.
Monitor serum electrolyte results for abnormalities.

RATIONALE

Early recognition of signs and symptoms of cardiac dysrhythmia allows for prompt intervention.

THERAPEUTIC INTERVENTIONS

Dependent/Collaborative Actions
Implement measures to prevent cardiac dysrhythmias (e.g., place client in semi- to high-Fowler's position):
- Perform actions to maintain an adequate respiratory status.
- Perform actions to decrease stimulation of the sympathetic nervous system:
  - Implement measures to reduce pain and anxiety.
  - Implement measures to keep client from getting cold.
- Perform actions to prevent or treat hypokalemia:
  - Prevent nausea and vomiting.
  - Administer fluid and electrolyte replacements as ordered.
- Perform actions to prevent or treat hypotension:
  - Consult physician before giving negative inotropic agents, diuretics, and vasodilating agents if systolic B/P is below 90 to 100 mm Hg.
  - Perform actions to prevent hypovolemic shock.
  - Administer narcotic (opioid) analgesics judiciously, being alert to the synergistic effect of the narcotic ordered and the anesthetic that was used during surgery.
  - Gradually bring client's body temperature to normal if hypothermic.
  - Administer sympathomimetics (e.g., dopamine) if ordered.

RATIONALE

Actions help to maintain adequate myocardial tissue oxygenation. Sympathetic stimulation increases the heart rate and causes vasoconstriction, both of which increase cardiac workload and decrease oxygen availability to the myocardium.

Electrolyte imbalances, particularly hypokalemia and hypocalcemia, can contribute to cardiac dysrhythmias.

Actions help to ensure adequate vascular volume, tissue perfusion, and delivery of oxygen to the myocardial tissue.

Rapid warming results in vasodilation, which may reduce B/P and tissue perfusion.

Sympathomimetics mimic the action of the sympathetic nervous system, causing vasoconstriction, which elevates B/P.

THERAPEUTIC INTERVENTIONS	RATIONALE
If cardiac dysrhythmias occur: • Administer antidysrhythmics as ordered. • Restrict client's activity based on his/her tolerance and severity of the dysrhythmia. • Maintain oxygen therapy as ordered. • Assess cardiovascular status frequently and report signs and symptoms of inadequate tissue perfusion (e.g., decrease in B/P, cool skin, cyanosis, diminished peripheral pulses, urine output less than 30 mL/h, restlessness and agitation, shortness of breath). • Have emergency cart readily available for cardioversion, defibrillation, or cardiopulmonary resuscitation.	*Cardiac dysrhythmias may deteriorate and become life-threatening. Life-threatening dysrhythmias or those that render the client unstable are treated with electrical therapy.*

Collaborative Diagnosis RISK FOR ISCHEMIC COLITIS

Definition: Inflammation of the colon resulting from impaired blood flow

Related to: Diminished blood supply to the colon associated with ligation of the inferior mesenteric artery during surgery, hypovolemia, and/or embolization

CLINICAL MANIFESTATIONS

Subjective	Objective
Verbalization of nausea; abdominal pain	Low-grade fever; diarrhea; vomiting; bright red, bloody stools

RISK FACTORS
• Hypovolemic shock/low perfusion states
• Thromboembolism

DESIRED OUTCOMES
The client will not develop ischemic colitis as evidenced by:
a. Absence of blood in stools
b. Absence of diarrhea
c. Absence of or decrease in abdominal pain
d. Soft, nontender abdomen

NURSING ASSESSMENT	RATIONALE
Assess for and report signs and symptoms of ischemic colitis: • Blood in stools • Diarrhea • Reports of new or increasing abdominal pain • Distended abdomen	*Early recognition of signs and symptoms of ischemic colitis allows for prompt intervention.*

THERAPEUTIC INTERVENTIONS	RATIONALE
Dependent/Collaborative Actions Implement measures to prevent hypovolemic shock and embolization: • To prevent hypovolemic shock if bleeding occurs, apply firm, prolonged pressure; maintain adequate fluid replacement as ordered. • For embolization, maintain adequate fluid intake; prevent peripheral pooling of blood; administer anticoagulants.	*Actions help to maintain adequate blood supply to the colon.*

Continued...

THERAPEUTIC INTERVENTIONS	RATIONALE

If signs and symptoms of ischemic colitis occur:
• Administer antimicrobials if ordered.
• Prepare client for the following if planned:
  • Colonoscopy
  • Colon resection (usually performed if client has extensive tissue necrosis or gangrenous patches)
  • Embolectomy
	Invasive interventions may be necessary to remove areas of necrosis and/or restore circulation to the intestines.

Collaborative Diagnosis   # IMPAIRED RENAL FUNCTION

Definition: Impaired ability to excrete metabolic waste products and water leading to functional disturbances of all body systems

Related to: Insufficient blood flow to the kidneys associated with hypovolemia and prolonged aortic clamp time

CLINICAL MANIFESTATIONS

Subjective	Objective
Not applicable	Oliguria; fixed urine specific gravity at 1.010 or less; elevated BUN/creatinine levels; decreased glomerular filtration rate (GFR); decreased creatinine clearance

RISK FACTORS
• Hypovolemic shock/low perfusion states
• Thromboembolism

DESIRED OUTCOMES

The client will maintain adequate renal function as evidenced by:
   a. Urine output at least 30 mL/h
   b. BUN and serum creatinine levels and creatinine clearance within normal range

NURSING ASSESSMENT	RATIONALE
Assess for and report signs and symptoms of impaired renal function: • Urine output less than 30 mL/h • Urine specific gravity fixed at or less than 1.010 • Elevated BUN and serum creatinine levels • Decreased creatinine clearance	*Early recognition of signs and symptoms of impaired renal function allows for prompt intervention.*

THERAPEUTIC INTERVENTIONS	RATIONALE
Dependent/Collaborative Actions Implement measures to prevent hypovolemic shock (e.g., administer fluid boluses).	*Actions help to maintain adequate renal blood flow.*
If signs and symptoms of impaired renal function occur, assess for and report signs of acute renal failure: • Oliguria or anuria; weight gain; edema • Elevated B/P; lethargy and confusion • Increasing BUN and serum creatinine, phosphorus, and potassium levels	*Identification of signs and symptoms of developing acute renal failure allows for modification of the treatment plan.*

DISCHARGE TEACHING/CONTINUED CARE

Nursing Diagnosis # DEFICIENT KNOWLEDGE NDx; INEFFECTIVE HEALTH MAINTENANCE NDx; OR INEFFECTIVE SELF-HEALTH MANAGEMENT* NDx

Definition: Absence or deficiency of cognitive information related to specific topic; (lack of specific information necessary for clients/significant others to make informed choices regarding condition/treatment/lifestyle changes); inability to identify, manage, and/or seek out help to manage health; pattern of regulating and integrating into daily living a program for treatment of illness and the sequelae of illness that is unsatisfactory for meeting specific health goals

CLINICAL MANIFESTATIONS

Subjective	**Objective**
Verbalization of the problem	Inaccurate follow through of instructions; inappropriate behaviors

RISK FACTORS
- Denial of disease process
- Cognitive deficiency
- Failure to take action to reduce risk factors

NOC OUTCOMES	NIC INTERVENTIONS
Knowledge: treatment regimen; knowledge: cardiac disease management	Health system guidance; teaching: individual; teaching: disease process; teaching: prescribed diet

NURSING ASSESSMENT	**RATIONALE**
Assess client's readiness and ability to learn. Assess meaning of illness to client.	*Early recognition of readiness to learn and meaning of illness to client allows for implementation of the appropriate teaching interventions.*

THERAPEUTIC INTERVENTIONS	**RATIONALE**

Desired Outcome: The client will identify ways to prevent or slow the progression of atherosclerosis.

Independent Actions
Inform the client that certain modifiable factors such as elevated serum lipid levels, a sedentary lifestyle, smoking, and hypertension have been shown to increase the risk of atherosclerosis.

Assist client to identify changes in lifestyle that could reduce the risk for atherosclerosis:
- Dietary modifications
- Smoking cessation
- Physical exercise on a regular basis

Provide instructions on ways the client can reduce intake of saturated fat and cholesterol:
- Reduce intake of meat fat (e.g., trim visible fat off meat; replace fatty meats such as fatty cuts of steak, hamburger, and processed meats with leaner products).
- Reduce intake of milk fat (e.g., avoid dairy products containing more than 1% fat).

After vascular surgery, clients should be educated as to health promotion activities that slow the progression of atherosclerosis.
Clients should be encouraged to control B/P, increase physical activity, stop smoking, and maintain normal body weight and serum lipid levels.
Appropriate modifications of diet, exercise, and smoking cessation can modify the progression of coronary artery disease.

Decreasing intake of saturated fat and cholesterol and increasing complex carbohydrates can reduce the risk of coronary artery disease by lowering LDL cholesterol.

---

*The nurse should select the diagnosis that is most appropriate for the client's discharge teaching needs.

NDx = NANDA-I Diagnosis   **D** = Delegatable Action   ● = UAP   ✦ = LVN/LFN   ⊖▶ = Go to ⊖volve for animation

Continued...

THERAPEUTIC INTERVENTIONS	RATIONALE
• Reduce intake of *trans* fats (e.g., avoid stick margarine and shortening and foods such as commercial baked goods that are prepared with these products).	
• Use vegetable oil rather than coconut or palm oil in cooking and food preparation.	
• Use cooking methods such as steaming, baking, broiling, poaching, microwaving, and grilling rather than frying.	
• Restrict intake of eggs (recommendations about the number of whole eggs allowed per week vary depending on the client's lipid levels).	
Instruct client to take lipid-lowering agents (e.g., HMG-CoA [3-hydroxy-3-methylglutaryl-coenzyme A] reductase inhibitors ["statins"], ezetimibe, gemfibrozil, niacin) as prescribed.	*Lipid-lowering agents inhibit the synthesis of cholesterol in the liver. The result of this inhibition is an increase in hepatic LDL receptors. This results in the liver being able to remove more LDLs from the blood.*

THERAPEUTIC INTERVENTIONS	RATIONALE

Desired Outcome: The client will state signs and symptoms to report to the health care provider.

Independent Actions

Instruct client to report these additional signs and symptoms:	*Additional signs and symptoms indicate internal bleeding. Prompt treatment for the client exhibiting signs and symptoms of internal bleeding from graft site reduces the risk of life-threatening complications.*
• Sudden or gradual increase in lower back, flank, groin, or abdominal pain	
• Chest pain	
• Coolness, pallor, or blueness of lower extremities	
• Increased weakness and fatigue	
• Decreased urine output	
• Bloody or persistent diarrhea	
• Increased bruising of incision site, flank area, or perineum	
• Impotence	

THERAPEUTIC INTERVENTIONS	RATIONALE

Desired Outcome: The client will verbalize an understanding of and a plan for adhering to recommended follow-up care including future appointments with health care provider, medications prescribed, activity level, and wound care.

Independent Actions

Reinforce the physician's instructions regarding:	*The nurse should reinforce the need to follow-up with the physician/surgeon provider as instructed to ensure adherence to all aspects of the treatment plan.*
• Importance of scheduling adequate rest periods	
• Ways to prevent constipation and subsequent straining to have a bowel movement (e.g., drink at least 10 glasses of liquid per day unless contraindicated, increase intake of foods high in fiber, take stool softeners if necessary)	
• The need to avoid sexual intercourse, isometric exercise/activity (e.g., lifting objects over 10 lb, pushing heavy objects), and strenuous exercise for specified length of time (usually 4-12 weeks depending on the activity)	
• The need to take prophylactic antimicrobials before any dental work or invasive procedure (some physicians recommend this for the first 6-12 months after surgical placement of a synthetic graft)	

ADDITIONAL NURSING DIAGNOSIS

SEXUAL DYSFUNCTION
Related to:
- Decreased libido associated with operative site discomfort and fear of surgical site bleeding
- Impotence associated with prolonged reduction in blood flow in the mesenteric or internal iliac arteries (can occur as a result of prolonged aortic clamp time during surgery, persistent hypovolemia, embolization, or graft occlusion) and/or nerve damage (can occur during surgery)

RELATED CARE PLANS

Standardized Preoperative Care Plan
Standardized Postoperative Care Plan

ANGINA PECTORIS

Angina pectoris is transient chest pain or discomfort that is caused by an imbalance between myocardial oxygen supply and demand. The discomfort typically occurs in the retrosternal area; may or may not radiate; and is described as a tight, heavy, squeezing, burning, or choking sensation. The most common cause of angina pectoris is decreased coronary blood supply due to atherosclerosis of a major coronary artery. The atherosclerosis causes narrowing of the vessel lumen and an inability of the vessel to dilate and supply sufficient blood to the myocardium at times when myocardial oxygen needs are increased. Other conditions that can compromise coronary blood flow (e.g., spasm and/or thrombosis of a coronary artery, hypovolemia) and conditions that reduce oxygen availability and/or increase myocardial workload and oxygen demands (e.g., anemia, smoking, exercise, heavy meals, increased altitude, exposure to cold, stress) may precipitate or increase the frequency of angina attacks by widening the gap between oxygen needs and availability.

The two major types of angina pectoris are stable (classic exertional) angina and unstable angina. Stable angina, the most common type, is usually precipitated by physical exertion or emotional stress, lasts 3 to 5 minutes, and is relieved by rest and nitroglycerin. Unstable angina is characterized by an increasing frequency and/or severity of attacks that occur with less provocation or at rest. It is considered to be an acute coronary syndrome, which is associated with thrombus formation in a coronary artery. Persons with unstable angina are usually hospitalized and treated with heparin and antiplatelet agents while decisions regarding medical versus surgical treatment are made. A third type of angina is Prinzmetal's variant angina. It is less common than stable or unstable angina and is caused by severe focal spasm of a coronary artery.

This care plan focuses on the adult client hospitalized during an episode of chest pain/discomfort suspected to be unstable angina.

OUTCOME DISCHARGE CRITERIA

The client will:
1. Perform activities of daily living and ambulate without angina
2. Have angina controlled by oral medication
3. Have no signs and symptoms of complications
4. Verbalize a basic understanding of angina pectoris
5. Identify factors that may precipitate angina attacks and ways to control these factors
6. Identify modifiable cardiovascular risk factors and ways to alter these factors
7. Verbalize an understanding of the rationale for and components of a diet designed to lower serum cholesterol and triglyceride levels
8. Demonstrate accuracy in counting pulse
9. Verbalize an understanding of medications ordered including rationale, food and drug interactions, side effects, schedule for taking, and importance of taking as prescribed
10. State signs and symptoms to report to the health care provider
11. Identify community resources that can assist in making necessary lifestyle changes and adjusting to the effects of angina pectoris
12. Verbalize an understanding of and a plan for adhering to recommended follow-up care including future appointments with health care provider.

Nursing Diagnosis ## ACTUAL/RISK FOR DECREASED CARDIAC OUTPUT NDx

Definition: Risk for or actual inadequate volume of blood being pumped by the heart per minute to meet the metabolic demands of the body

Related to: Mechanical and/or electrical dysfunction of the heart associated with severe or prolonged myocardial ischemia

Continued...

CLINICAL MANIFESTATIONS

Subjective	Objective
Verbalization of palpitations; fatigue; shortness of breath/dyspnea; orthopnea; anxiety	Dysrhythmias; ECG changes; altered preload (jugular venous distention [JVD], edema, weight gain, increased central venous pressure [CVP], murmurs); altered afterload (cold, clammy skin; cyanosis; prolonged capillary refill time; decreased peripheral pulses); altered contractility (crackles, cough, decreased cardiac output); restlessness

RISK FACTORS

- Altered heart rate
- Altered heart rhythm
- Altered stroke volume

DESIRED OUTCOMES

The client will maintain adequate cardiac output as evidenced by:
 a. B/P within client's normal range
 b. Apical pulse regular and between 60 and 100 beats/min
 c. Absence of S_3, S_4 heart sounds (gallop)
 d. Absence of fatigue and weakness
 e. Unlabored respirations at 12 to 20 breaths/min
 f. Clear, audible breath sounds
 g. Usual mental status
 h. Absence of dizziness and syncope
 i. Palpable peripheral pulses
 j. Capillary refill time less than 2 to 3 seconds
 k. Urine output of at least 30 mL/h
 l. Absence of edema and JVD

NOC OUTCOMES

Circulation status; cardiac pump effectiveness; tissue perfusion: cardiac; tissue perfusion: peripheral

NIC INTERVENTIONS

Cardiac care: acute; hemodynamic regulation; cardiac precautions; cardiac care: rehabilitative

NURSING ASSESSMENT	RATIONALE
Assess for and report signs and symptoms of decreased cardiac output: • Variations in B/P • Tachycardia • Presence of extra heart sounds (gallop) • Fatigue and weakness • Dyspnea, tachypnea • Crackles (rales) • Restlessness, change in mental status • Dizziness, syncope • Diminished or absent peripheral pulses • Cool extremities • Capillary refill time greater than 2 to 3 seconds • Oliguria • Edema • JVD	*Early recognition of signs and symptoms of decreased cardiac output allows for prompt intervention.*
Monitor and report abnormal chest radiograph, arterial blood gas, or pulse oximetry values.	*Diagnostic tests may demonstrate vascular congestion (pulmonary edema) indicative of decreased cardiac output. Arterial blood gas/pulse oximetry values may indicate hypoxia as cardiac output decreases and pulmonary congestion worsens.*
Monitor and report abnormal ECG readings.	*May demonstrate findings associated with ischemia such as dysrhythmias, ST-segment depression/elevation, or inverted T waves.*
Monitor and report elevated cardiac enzymes (creatine kinase–MB [CK-MB]; troponin).	*Elevated values may indicate myocardial ischemia/damage. Extensive damage may further decrease cardiac output.*

THERAPEUTIC INTERVENTIONS	RATIONALE

Independent Actions

Implement measures to improve cardiac output:

- Maintain a calm, quiet environment, limit the number of visitors, and maintain activity restrictions. **D** ✦

Instruct client to avoid activities that create a Valsalva response:

- Straining to have a bowel movement
- Holding breath while moving up in bed

Discourage excessive intake of beverages high in caffeine such as coffee, tea, and colas.

Discourage smoking.

Actions promote emotional and physical rest and help to reduce cardiac workload.

Excessive straining can increase cardiac workload.

Caffeine is a myocardial stimulant and can increase myocardial oxygen consumption.

Nicotine has a cardiostimulatory effect and causes vasoconstriction; the carbon monoxide in smoke reduces oxygen availability.

Dependent/Collaborative Actions

Maintain oxygen therapy as ordered. **D** ✦

Administer the following medications if ordered:

- Nitrates

- Beta-adrenergic blockers

- Calcium channel blockers

- Anticoagulants

Prepare client for percutaneous coronary intervention if planned:

- Balloon angioplasty
- Atherectomy
- Intracoronary stenting
- Coronary artery bypass grafting (CABG)

Increase activity as allowed and tolerated. **D** ✦

Oxygen helps to improve oxygenation and reduce damage to the myocardium.

Medications act to improve blood flow to the coronary arteries helping to maintain adequate cardiac output.

Nitrates dilate the coronary and peripheral (primarily venous) blood vessels, thereby improving myocardial blood flow and reducing cardiac workload and myocardial oxygen consumption.

Beta blockers reduce myocardial oxygen requirements by decreasing the heart rate and force of myocardial contractility.

Calcium channel blockers dilate the coronary arteries and also reduce cardiac workload by dilating peripheral vessels.

Anticoagulants prevent obstruction of the coronary arteries by thrombosis.

Nursing Diagnosis ## ACUTE PAIN NDx (RADIATING OR NONRADIATING CHEST PAIN/DISCOMFORT)

Definition: Unpleasant sensory and emotional experience arising from actual or potential tissue damage

Related to: Decreased myocardial oxygenation (an insufficient oxygen supply forces the myocardium to convert to anaerobic metabolism; the end products of anaerobic metabolism act as irritants to myocardial neural receptors)

CLINICAL MANIFESTATIONS

Subjective	Objective
Verbal report of chest discomfort or pain over the sternal border, radiating to the neck, jaw, left arm; indigestion	ECG changes (ST-segment depression/elevation); dysrhythmias

RISK FACTORS

- Arteriosclerosis
- Increased oxygen demand
- Decreased oxygen supply
- Hypertension

DESIRED OUTCOMES

The client will experience relief of chest pain/discomfort as evidenced by:
   a. Verbalization of the same
   b. Relaxed facial expression and body positioning
   c. Increased participation in activities
   d. Stable vital signs

NDx = NANDA-I Diagnosis **D** = Delegatable Action ● = UAP ✦ = LVN/LFN ⊖▶ = Go to ⊖volve for animation

Continued...

NOC OUTCOMES	NIC INTERVENTIONS
Comfort level; pain control	Pain management; analgesic administration

NURSING ASSESSMENT	RATIONALE
Assess for signs and symptoms of pain/discomfort: • Verbalization of pain • Grimacing • Rubbing neck, jaw, or arm • Reluctance to move • Clutching chest • Restlessness • Diaphoresis • Increased B/P • Tachycardia Assess client's perception of the severity of the pain/discomfort using an intensity rating scale. Assess the client's pattern of pain/discomfort (location, quality, onset, duration, precipitating factors, aggravating factors, alleviating factors).	*Early recognition and reporting of signs and symptoms of ischemic chest pain allow for prompt intervention.*
Monitor and report abnormal ECG readings.	*May demonstrate findings associated with ischemia such as dysrhythmias, ST-segment depression/elevation, or inverted T waves.*
Monitor and report elevated cardiac enzymes (CK-MB; troponin).	*Elevated values may indicate myocardial ischemia.*

THERAPEUTIC INTERVENTIONS	RATIONALE
Independent Actions Provide or assist with nonpharmacological measures for relief of discomfort: **D** ✦ • Position change • Relaxation techniques • Restful environment	*Activities that promote rest help to reduce myocardial oxygen consumption.*
Dependent/Collaborative Actions Administer nitroglycerin as ordered. Maintain oxygen therapy as ordered. **D** ✦	*Nitrates dilate the coronary and peripheral (primarily venous) blood vessels, thereby improving myocardial blood flow and reducing cardiac workload and myocardial oxygen consumption.*
Administer a narcotic (opioid) analgesic (e.g., morphine sulfate) as ordered if pain/discomfort is unrelieved by rest and nitroglycerin within 15 to 20 minutes (narcotic analgesics are usually administered intravenously).	*Narcotic analgesics help to alleviate pain and anxiety, lower B/P, and decrease myocardial oxygen consumption.*
Consult physician if pain/discomfort persists or worsens. Prepare client for percutaneous coronary intervention if planned: • Balloon angioplasty • Atherectomy • Intracoronary stenting • CABG	*Consulting the appropriate health care provider allows for modification of the treatment plan.*

Collaborative Diagnosis   **RISK FOR CARDIAC DYSRHYTHMIAS**

Definition: A disturbance of the heart's normal rhythm. Dysrhythmias can range in severity from missed or rapid beats to serious disturbances that impair the pumping ability of the heart

⊖▶ Related to: Myocardial irritability associated with myocardial hypoxia

CLINICAL MANIFESTATIONS

Subjective	Objective
Verbal report of palpitations or skipped beats; syncope	ECG rate or rhythm abnormalities

RISK FACTORS

- Myocardial ischemia
- Electrolyte disturbances
- Coronary artery disease

DESIRED OUTCOMES

The client will maintain normal sinus rhythm as evidenced by:
- a. Regular apical pulse at 60 to 100 beats/min
- b. Equal apical and radial pulse rates
- c. Absence of syncope and palpitations
- d. ECG showing normal sinus rhythm

NURSING ASSESSMENT

Assess for and report signs and symptoms of cardiac dysrhythmias:
- Irregular apical pulse
- Pulse rate less than 60 or greater than 100 beats/min
- Apical-radial pulse deficit
- Syncope
- Palpitations
- Abnormal rate, rhythm, or configurations on ECG

Assess cardiovascular status frequently and report signs and symptoms of inadequate cardiac output.

Assess ECG tracing.

RATIONALE

Early recognition of signs and symptoms of dysrhythmias allows for prompt intervention.

THERAPEUTIC INTERVENTIONS

RATIONALE

Independent Actions

Restrict client's activity based on his/her tolerance and severity of the dysrhythmia. **D** ✦

Have emergency cart readily available for cardioversion, defibrillation, or cardiopulmonary resuscitation.

Dependent/Collaborative Actions

Maintain oxygen therapy as ordered. **D** ✦

Implement measures to help maintain an adequate cardiac output:
- Antidysrhythmics
- Add the following categories of medications: Nitrates, beta-adrenergic blocking agents; calcium channel blockers, anticoagulants

Decreases myocardial workload.

Many dysrhythmias can be lethal and may only respond to electrical therapy.

Oxygen helps to improve oxygenation and reduce myocardial ischemia.

Classes of medications are administered in order to improve myocardial blood flow and oxygenation, reducing the risk for dysrhythmias. Antidysrhythmics help to reduce myocardial irritability.

Collaborative Diagnosis # RISK FOR MYOCARDIAL INFARCTION

Definition: Irreversible myocardial damage

Related to: Persistent ischemia or complete occlusion of a coronary artery

CLINICAL MANIFESTATIONS

Subjective	Objective
Verbal report of sudden, severe, chest pain; nausea	Q-wave tracing on ECG; diaphoresis; variations in B/P; increased heart rate; abnormal or extra heart sounds; pericardial friction rub; increased CK-MB level; elevated tropin level

---

NDx = NANDA-I Diagnosis   **D** = Delegatable Action   ● = UAP   ✦ = LVN/LPN   ⊖▶ = Go to ⊖volve for animation

Continued...

RISK FACTORS

- Coronary artery disease
- Hypertension
- Hyperlipidemia
- Smoking
- Diabetes

DESIRED OUTCOMES

The client will not experience a myocardial infarction as evidenced by:
  a. Resolution of chest pain within 15 to 20 minutes
  b. Stable vital signs
  c. Cardiac enzyme levels within normal range
  d. Absence of ST-segment depression or elevation, T-wave inversion, and abnormal Q waves on ECG

NURSING ASSESSMENT	RATIONALE
Assess for and report signs and symptoms of a myocardial infarction: • Chest pain that lasts longer than 20 minutes • Increase in pulse rate • Significant change in B/P • Labored respirations Assess for elevation of cardiac enzymes: • CK-MB • Troponin Assess ECG tracing for abnormalities: • ST-segment depression or elevation • T-wave inversion • Abnormal Q waves on ECG	*Early recognition of signs and symptoms of a myocardial infarction allows for prompt intervention.*

THERAPEUTIC INTERVENTIONS	RATIONALE
Independent Actions Maintain client on strict bed rest in a semi- to high-Fowler's position. **D** ✦	*Reduces myocardial oxygen consumption.*
Dependent/Collaborative Actions Maintain oxygen therapy as ordered. **D** ✦	*Oxygen helps to improve oxygenation and reduce myocardial ischemia.*
Administer the following medications if ordered: • Morphine sulfate	*Reduces pain and anxiety and decreases cardiac workload.*
• Nitrates	*Improve myocardial blood flow and reduce myocardial oxygen requirements.*
Beta-adrenergic blockers	*Reduce myocardial oxygen requirements by decreasing heart rate and force of myocardial contraction.*
Prepare client for the following procedures that may be performed: • Injection of a thrombolytic agent (e.g., streptokinase, alteplase [tissue-type plasminogen activator; tPA], anistreplase [APSAC, Eminase], reteplase, tenecteplase [TNK-tPA]) • Percutaneous coronary intervention • Insertion of an intra-aortic balloon pump (IABP)	*Procedures may be performed to improve myocardial blood flow.*

DISCHARGE TEACHING/CONTINUED CARE

Nursing Diagnosis ## DEFICIENT KNOWLEDGE NDx; INEFFECTIVE FAMILY THERAPEUTIC REGIMEN MANAGEMENT NDx; OR INEFFECTIVE SELF-HEALTH MANAGEMENT NDx*

Definition: Absence or deficiency of cognitive information related to specific topic (lack of specific information necessary for clients/significant others to make informed choices regarding condition/treatment/lifestyle changes); pattern of regulating and integrating into daily living a program for treatment of illness and the sequelae of illness that is unsatisfactory for meeting specific health goals; inability to identify, manage, and/or seek out help to manage health

CLINICAL MANIFESTATIONS

Subjective	Objective
Verbalization of unfamiliarity with information resources; collateral report of exaggerated behaviors	Inaccurate follow through of instructions; inaccurate performance of a test; lack of recall

RISK FACTORS
- Denial of disease process
- Cognitive deficiency
- Failure to take action to reduce risk factors

NOC OUTCOMES	NIC INTERVENTIONS
Knowledge: treatment regimen; knowledge: cardiac disease management	Teaching: individual; teaching: disease process; teaching: prescribed activity/exercise; teaching: prescribed medication; health system guidance

NURSING ASSESSMENT	RATIONALE
Assess client's readiness and ability to learn. Assess meaning of illness to client.	*Early recognition of readiness to learn and meaning of illness to client allows for implementation of the appropriate teaching interventions.*

THERAPEUTIC INTERVENTIONS	RATIONALE

Desired Outcome: The client will verbalize a basic understanding of angina pectoris.

Independent Actions
Explain angina pectoris in terms that client can understand:
- Use teaching aids (e.g., pamphlets, diagrams) whenever possible.

Clients vary in physical and cognitive ability to learn. When educating clients, nurses need to determine their ability to read and understand written materials. If literacy barriers are present, alternative educational materials should be provided.

THERAPEUTIC INTERVENTIONS	RATIONALE

Desired Outcome: The client will identify factors that may precipitate an angina attack and ways to control these factors.

Independent Actions
Provide the following instructions regarding ways to reduce risk of precipitating an angina attack:
- Take nitroglycerin before strenuous activity or sexual intercourse and during times of high emotional stress.
- Gradually increase activity by engaging in a regular aerobic exercise program (e.g., walking, biking, swimming).

Clients with diagnosed cardiovascular disease should be educated to learn what may precipitate angina and ways to decrease the risk for angina. In addition, clients should be taught to recognize that changes in their individual pattern of angina may indicate advancing disease, and if changes occur, prompt treatment should occur.

*The nurse should select the diagnostic label that is most appropriate for the client's discharge teaching needs.

NDx = NANDA-I Diagnosis   **D** = Delegatable Action   ● = UAP   ✦ = LVN/LPN   ⊖▶ = Go to ⊖volve for animation

Continued...

THERAPEUTIC INTERVENTIONS	RATIONALE
• Avoid strenuous exercise and activities that involve pushing or lifting heavy objects (e.g., weightlifting).	
• Avoid exercising for at least an hour after eating, and exercise with caution at higher altitude and when the environmental temperature is extremely hot or cold.	
• Avoid tobacco use before exercise.	
• Rest between activities.	
• Stop any activity that causes shortness of breath, palpitations, dizziness, or extreme fatigue or weakness.	*Activities eliciting these reponses may lead to angina and should be discontinued.*
• Begin a cardiovascular fitness program if recommended by physician.	*Physical activity, if recommended, should be regular, rhythmic, and repetitive.*
• Adhere to the following precautions regarding sexual activity:	*Resumption of sexual activity should be based on the physiological status of the patient.*
• Avoid intercourse for at least 1 to 2 hours after a heavy meal or alcohol consumption and when fatigued or stressed.	
• Engage in sexual activity in a familiar environment and in a position that minimizes exertion (e.g., side-lying, partner on top).	
• Recognize that a new sexual relationship can be started but may result in greater energy expenditure initially.	
• Avoid hot or cold showers just before and after intercourse.	

THERAPEUTIC INTERVENTIONS	RATIONALE

Desired Outcome: The client will identify modifiable cardiovascular risk factors and ways to alter these factors.

Independent Actions

Inform client that certain modifiable factors such as elevated serum lipid levels, a sedentary lifestyle, hypertension, and smoking have been shown to increase the risk for coronary artery disease.	*A person with modifiable risk factors should be encouraged to make lifestyle changes to reduce the risk for coronary artery disease (CAD). For the motivated client, knowing how to reduce the risk may be all the information that is needed.*
Assist client to identify changes in lifestyle that can help to eliminate or reduce the above risk factors and help to manage angina:	
• Dietary modification	
• Physical exercise on a regular basis	
• Moderation of alcohol intake	
• Smoking cessation	
Encourage client to limit daily alcohol consumption. Current recommendations:	*Daily alcohol intake exceeding 1 oz of ethanol may contribute to the development of hypertension and some forms of heart disease.*
• No more than 2 drinks per day for men	
• No more than 1 drink per day for women and lighter-weight persons.	
(A "drink" is considered to be ½ oz of ethanol [e.g., 1½ oz of 80-proof whiskey, 12 oz of beer, 5 oz of wine].)	

THERAPEUTIC INTERVENTIONS	RATIONALE

Desired Outcome: The client will verbalize an understanding of the rationale for and components of a diet designed to lower serum cholesterol and triglyceride levels.

Independent Actions

Explain the rationale for a diet low in saturated fat and cholesterol.	*Fat intake should be approximately 30% of calories with most coming from monosaturated fats found in nuts and oils such as olive oil or canola oil.*

THERAPEUTIC INTERVENTIONS	RATIONALE
Provide instructions on ways the client can reduce intake of saturated fat and cholesterol:	*Dietary modifications that reduce LDLs help reduce the risk of CAD.*

- Reduce intake of meat fat (e.g., trim visible fat off meat; replace fatty meats such as fatty cuts of steak, hamburger, and processed meats with leaner products).
- Reduce intake of milk fat (e.g., avoid dairy products containing more than 1% fat).
- Reduce intake of *trans* fats (e.g., avoid stick margarine and shortening and foods such as commercial baked goods that are prepared with these products).
- Use vegetable oil rather than coconut or palm oil in cooking and food preparation.
- Use cooking methods such as steaming, baking, broiling, poaching, microwaving, and grilling rather than frying.
- Restrict intake of eggs (recommendations about the number of whole eggs allowed per week vary depending on the client's lipid levels).

Encourage client to increase intake of omega-3 fatty acids (e.g., flaxseed, cold water ocean fish such as salmon and halibut) to help lower triglyceride levels and increase high-density lipoprotein (HDL) levels.	*Omega-3 fatty acids have been shown to reduce the risk for CAD if consumed regularly.*

THERAPEUTIC INTERVENTIONS	RATIONALE

Desired Outcome: The client will demonstrate accuracy in counting pulse.

Independent Actions

Teach clients how to count their pulse, being alert to the regularity of the rhythm. Allow time for return demonstration and accuracy check.	*Educating clients to their baseline rhythm allows for early detection of irregularities warranting immediate attention from a health care provider. Early detection may reduce the incidence of sudden death.*

THERAPEUTIC INTERVENTIONS	RATIONALE

Desired Outcome: The client will verbalize an understanding of medications ordered including rationale, food and drug interactions, side effects, schedule for taking, and importance of taking as prescribed.

Independent Actions

Explain the rationale for, side effects of, and importance of taking the medications prescribed. Inform client of pertinent food and drug interactions.	*Taking medications as prescribed ensures that therapeutic drug levels will be maintained.* *Clients should be instructed not to discontinue taking medications if they feel better. Clients without financial resources should be assisted in accessing appropriate resources to obtain needed medications (e.g., pharmacy assistance programs).*

- Nitrates
- Nitroglycerin skin patches
- Beta-adrenergic blockers
- Calcium channel blockers
- Lipid-lowering agents

Instruct client to consult physician before taking other prescription and nonprescription medications.	*Drug-drug interactions may render medications inactive or result in life-threatening side effects.*
Instruct client to inform all health care providers of medications being taken.	*Continuity of health care information is critical to reduce the incidence of prescribing medications with potential adverse drug-drug interactions.*

THERAPEUTIC INTERVENTIONS	RATIONALE

Desired Outcome: The client will state signs and symptoms to report to the health care provider.

Continued...

THERAPEUTIC INTERVENTIONS	RATIONALE

Independent Actions

Stress the importance of reporting the following signs and symptoms:
- Chest, arm, neck, or jaw discomfort unrelieved by rest and/ or nitroglycerin taken every 5 minutes for 15 minutes
- Shortness of breath
- Irregular pulse or a resting pulse less than 56 or greater than 100 beats/min (the rate the client should report may vary depending on the medications prescribed, the client's baseline pulse rate, and physician's preference)
- Fainting spells
- Diminished activity tolerance
- Swelling of feet or ankles
- Increase in severity or frequency of angina attacks

Early identification of signs and symptoms of advancing coronary disease allows for prompt intervention by the appropriate health care provider.

THERAPEUTIC INTERVENTIONS	RATIONALE

Desired Outcome: The client will identify community resources that can assist in making necessary lifestyle changes and adjusting to the effects of angina pectoris.

Independent Actions

Provide information about community resources that can assist client in making lifestyle changes and adjusting to effects of angina pectoris (e.g., weight loss, smoking cessation, and stress management programs; American Heart Association; counseling services).

Cardiac disease can significantly impact an individual's and family's socioeconomic status. Providing information specific to community resources is important to provide a necessary continuum of care and may impact the client's health status preventing future hospitalizations.

THERAPEUTIC INTERVENTIONS	RATIONALE

Desired Outcome: The client will verbalize an understanding of and a plan for adhering to recommended follow-up care including future appointments with health care provider.

Independent Actions

Reinforce the importance of keeping follow-up appointments with health care provider.

Implement measures to improve client compliance:
- Include significant others in teaching sessions if possible.

- Encourage questions and allow time for reinforcement and clarification of information provided.
- Provide written instructions regarding future appointments with health care provider, dietary modifications, activity level, medications prescribed, and signs and symptoms to report.

Regular health care appointments are important to determine the effectiveness of the prescribed treatment plan.

Involvement of significant others in patient teaching improves adherence to discharge instructions.

Everyone does not understand information as presented, so set aside time for questions to allow for clarification of information.

Written instructions allow the client to refer to instructions as needed.

ADDITIONAL NURSING DIAGNOSES

FEAR/ANXIETY NDx
Related to:
- Discomfort during angina attack and threat of recurrent attacks

- Lack of understanding of diagnostic tests, diagnosis, and treatment plan
- Unfamiliar environment
- Effect of angina pectoris on future lifestyle and roles

CARDIAC DYSRHYTHMIAS

Cardiac dysrhythmias are disturbances in the normal heart rate or rhythm that are caused by a disorder in the initiation and/or conduction of intrinsic electrical impulses. Dysrhythmias can be classified according to the site of impulse formation and the site or degree of conduction block. Supraventricular dysrhythmias (e.g., sinus dysrhythmia, sinus tachycardia, sinus bradycardia, premature atrial contractions, atrial flutter, atrial fibrillation, junctional rhythm) originate above the ventricle. Ventricular rhythms (e.g., premature ventricular contractions, idioventricular rhythm, ventricular tachycardia, Torsades de pointes, ventricular fibrillation) originate in the ventricle. Impulse conduction defects (e.g., first-degree atrioventricular [AV] block, second-degree AV block, third-degree AV block, bundle branch block) result from a delay or block in the transmission of impulses. Causes of dysrhythmias include myocardial ischemia, cardiomyopathy, valvular heart disease, hypoxemia, electrolyte and acid-base imbalances, thyroid dysfunction, certain medications, infection, anemia, excessive caffeine or alcohol intake, smoking, pain, and emotional distress.

Dysrhythmias vary in severity and their effect on cardiac function. They can be benign and require no treatment or be life-threatening. The etiological factors and the clinical significance of the dysrhythmia determine the therapeutic management. Drug therapy is often successful at controlling a dysrhythmia. Other treatment options, depending on the type and severity of the dysrhythmia, include electrical cardioversion, a pacemaker, an implantable cardioverter-defibrillator (ICD), radiofrequency catheter ablation, surgery (e.g., elimination of offending area of myocardium by surgical excision, cryosurgery, or laser; maze procedure), and cardiopulmonary resuscitation and defibrillation.

This care plan focuses on the adult client needing acute management of a dysrhythmia in a medical setting.

OUTCOME DISCHARGE CRITERIA

The client will:
1. Have fewer or no dysrhythmias
2. Have adequate cardiac output and tissue perfusion
3. Tolerate expected level of activity
4. Have no signs and symptoms of complications
5. Verbalize a basic understanding of cardiac dysrhythmias
6. Demonstrate accuracy in counting pulse
7. Verbalize an understanding of medications ordered including rationale, food and drug interactions, side effects, schedule for taking, and importance of taking as prescribed
8. Verbalize an understanding of ways to avoid precipitating or exacerbating dysrhythmias
9. State signs and symptoms to report to the health care provider
10. Verbalize an understanding of and a plan for adhering to recommended follow-up care including activity restrictions and future appointments with health care provider.

Nursing Diagnosis ## RISK FOR DECREASED CARDIAC OUTPUT NDx

Definition: Risk for inadequate volume of blood being pumped by the heart per minute to meet the metabolic demands of the body

Related to:
• A slow heart rate (if client has a bradydysrhythmia)
• Decreased ventricular filling and emptying associated with a rapid and/or irregular heart rate

CLINICAL MANIFESTATIONS

Subjective	Objective
Complaints of fatigue; dyspnea; anxiety; palpitations	Restlessness; tachycardia; bradycardia; arrhythmias, EKG changes; increased central venous pressure; increased pulmonary artery wedge pressure; cool, clammy skin; dyspnea; orthopnea; decreased peripheral pulses; prolonged capillary refill; variations in blood pressure readings; S_3, S_4 heart sounds

Continued...

RISK FACTORS

- Altered heart rate
- Altered heart rhythm
- Altered stroke volume

DESIRED OUTCOMES

The client will maintain adequate cardiac output as evidenced by:

- a. B/P within normal range for client
- b. Apical pulse between 60 and 100 beats/min and more regular
- c. Absence of extra heart sounds (S_3, S_4 gallop)
- d. No reports of fatigue and weakness
- e. Unlabored respirations at 12 to 20 breaths/min
- f. Clear, audible breath sounds
- g. Usual mental status

NOC OUTCOMES

Cardiac pump effectiveness; circulation status

NIC INTERVENTIONS

Cardiac care; cardiac precautions; dysrhythmia management

NURSING ASSESSMENT

Assess for and report signs and symptoms of dysrhythmias:

- ECG showing rate less than 60 or greater than 100 beats/min, an irregular rhythm, or missed or ectopic beats
- Palpitations
- Dizziness or syncope
- Apical-radial pulse deficit

Assess for and report signs and symptoms of decreased cardiac output:

- Variations in B/P (may be increased because of compensatory vasoconstriction; may be decreased when compensatory mechanisms and pump fail)
- Presence of gallop rhythm
- Fatigue and weakness
- Dyspnea, orthopnea, tachypnea
- Crackles (rales)
- Restlessness, change in mental status
- Dizziness, syncope
- Diminished or absent peripheral pulses
- Cool extremities
- Pallor or cyanosis of skin
- Capillary refill time greater than 2 to 3 seconds
- Oliguria
- Edema
- Jugular venous distention

Monitor pulse oximetry and chest radiograph results.

Monitor serum electrolytes.

RATIONALE

Early recognition of signs and symptoms of decreased cardiac output allows for prompt intervention.

Cardiac dysrhythmias alter the normal pumping action of the heart. Rhythms that are too fast or too slow have the potential to alter/decrease cardiac output.

Chest radiograph report along with pulse oximetry values can help to identify heart failure that may accompany some cardiac dysrhythmias.

Serum potassium (K^+) and magnesium (Mg^+) abnormalities can contribute to dysrhythmias.

THERAPEUTIC INTERVENTIONS

Independent Actions

Perform actions to reduce cardiac workload: **D** ✦

- Place client in a semi- to high-Fowler's position.
- Instruct client to avoid activities such as straining to have a bowel movement and holding breath while moving up in bed.
- Implement measures to promote rest and conserve energy.

RATIONALE

The Valsalva maneuver not only increases cardiac workload but can also slow the heart rate.

THERAPEUTIC INTERVENTIONS	RATIONALE
• Discourage smoking.	*Nicotine has a cardiostimulatory effect and causes vasoconstriction; the carbon monoxide in smoke reduces oxygen availability, which not only increases cardiac workload but contributes to myocardial irritability.*
• Discourage excessive intake of beverages high in caffeine such as coffee, tea, and colas.	*Caffeine is a myocardial stimulant and can increase myocardial irritability.*

Dependent/Collaborative Actions

Perform actions to reduce cardiac workload:

• Maintain oxygen therapy as ordered. **D** ✦	*Supplemental oxygen supports myocardial tissue oxygenation.*
Implement measures to maintain an adequate cardiac output:	*Medications that control heart rate and dysrhythmias help to sustain adequate cardiac output.*
• Administer antidysrhythmic agents.	
• Administer anticholinergic agents.	*Defibrillation is the most effective method of terminating lethal dysrhythmias or certain dysrhythmias unresponsive to drug therapy.*
• Assist with vagal maneuvers.	
• Assist with cardioversion or defibrillation if performed.	

• Administer electrolyte replacement therapy to keep values within normal range:
  • K^+
  • Mg^+	

• Prepare client for an electrophysiological study (EPS) if planned.	*EPS studies help to determine the cause and treatment options for the dysrhythmias.*

• Prepare client for the following procedures if planned:
  • Insertion of a pacemaker or ICD
  • Radiofrequency catheter ablation
  • Surgery (e.g., maze procedure, endocardial resection, "corridor" procedure)	

Nursing Diagnosis ## RISK FOR ACTIVITY INTOLERANCE NDx

Definition: At risk for experiencing insufficient physiological or psychological energy to endure or complete required or desired daily activities

Related to:
• Tissue hypoxia if cardiac output is decreased
• Difficulty resting and sleeping associated with frequent assessments and treatments, fear, and anxiety

CLINICAL MANIFESTATIONS

Subjective	Objective
Verbal reports of exertional discomfort; fatigue; weakness	Abnormal blood pressure response to activity (e.g., excessive rise in blood pressure–systolic >180 or diastolic >110 mm Hg; excessive hypotension—drop in systolic blood pressure of 10 mm Hg from baseline blood pressure); abnormal heart rate response to activity (e.g., inappropriate bradycardia—drop in heart rate >10 beats per minute; increased heart rate >100 beats per minute); EKG changes reflecting arrhythmias or ischemia

RISK FACTORS
• Presence of respiratory problems
• Presence of circulatory problems
• Inexperience with activity

DESIRED OUTCOMES

The client will not experience activity intolerance as evidenced by:
  a. No reports of fatigue or weakness
  b. Ability to perform activities of daily living without exertional dyspnea, chest pain, diaphoresis, dizziness, and a significant change in vital signs

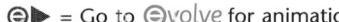

NDx = NANDA-I Diagnosis   **D** = Delegatable Action   ● = UAP   ✦ = LVN/LPN   ⊖▶ = Go to ⊖volve for animation

Continued...

NOC OUTCOMES	NIC INTERVENTIONS
Activity tolerance; rest; energy conservation; self-care: activities of daily living	Energy management; oxygen therapy; sleep enhancement; cardiac care

NURSING ASSESSMENT	RATIONALE
Assess for and report signs and symptoms of activity intolerance: • Statements of fatigue or weakness • Exertional dyspnea, chest pain, diaphoresis, or dizziness • Abnormal heart rate response to activity • Increase in rate of 20 beats/min above resting rate • Rate not returning to preactivity level within 3 minutes after stopping activity • Change from regular to irregular rate • Significant change (15-20 mm Hg) in B/P with activity	*Early recognition of signs and symptoms of activity intolerance allows for prompt intervention.*

THERAPEUTIC INTERVENTIONS	RATIONALE

Independent Actions

Implement measures to prevent activity intolerance: **D** ● ✦   *Actions help to promote rest and/or conserve energy.*
- Maintain activity restrictions as ordered.
- Minimize environmental activity and noise.
- Organize nursing care to allow for periods of uninterrupted rest.
- Limit the number of visitors and their length of stay.
- Assist client with self-care activities as needed.
- Keep supplies and personal articles within easy reach.
- Instruct client in energy-saving techniques (e.g., using shower chair when showering, sitting to brush teeth or comb hair).
- Implement measures to reduce fear and anxiety (e.g., provide instruction before interaction with client).
- Implement measures to promote sleep (e.g., maintain quiet environment).

Instruct client to:
- Report a decreased tolerance for activity.
- Stop any activity that causes chest pain, shortness of breath, dizziness, or extreme fatigue or weakness.

Dependent/Collaborative Actions

Perform actions to maintain an adequate cardiac output:
- Administer antidysrhythmic agents.   *Medications that control heart rate and dysrhythmias help to*
- Administer anticholinergic agents.   *sustain adequate cardiac output.*
- Assist with vagal maneuvers.
- Assist with cardioversion or defibrillation if performed.   *Defibrillation is the most effective method of terminating lethal dysrhythmias or certain dysrhythmias unresponsive to drug therapy.*

- Maintain oxygen therapy as ordered. **D** ✦   *Supplemental oxygen helps to alleviate hypoxia and restore more efficient aerobic metabolism, thereby improving energy levels and activity tolerance.*

- Increase client's activity gradually as allowed and tolerated. **D** ✦

Consult appropriate health care provider (e.g., cardiac rehabilitation therapist, physician) if signs and symptoms of activity intolerance develop and persist or worsen.   *Consulting the appropriate health care provider allows for modification of the treatment plan.*

Nursing Diagnosis **RISK FOR FALLS** NDx

Definition: Increased susceptibility to falling that may cause physical harm

Related to:
- Lightheadedness, dizziness, or syncope associated with inadequate cerebral blood flow resulting from decreased cardiac output and the hypotensive effect of some antidysrhythmic agents
- Weakness and fatigue that can occur with decreased cardiac output

CLINICAL MANIFESTATIONS

Subjective	Objective
Verbal reports of difficulty with gait; sleeplessness	Anemia; arthritis; decreased lower extremity strength; faintness when turning or extending neck; foot problems; hearing difficulties; impaired balance; impaired physical mobility; neuropathy; orthostatic hypotension; proprioceptive deficits; visual difficulties

RISK FACTORS
- Diminished mental status
- Faintness
- Anemia

DESIRED OUTCOME

The client will not experience falls.

NOC OUTCOMES

Falls occurrence; fall prevention behavior

NIC INTERVENTIONS

Fall prevention

NURSING ASSESSMENT	**RATIONALE**
Assess client for risk for falls using an approved scale: • Morris Falls Scale	*Early recognition of a client's risk for falls allows for prompt intervention.*

THERAPEUTIC INTERVENTIONS	**RATIONALE**

Independent Actions

Encourage client to request assistance whenever needed; have call signal within easy reach. **D** ● ✦

Accompany client during ambulation. **D** ● ✦

Provide ambulatory aids (e.g., walker) if client is weak or unsteady on feet.

Instruct and assist client to rise and change positions slowly.

Perform actions to increase strength and help prevent activity intolerance (e.g., assist client with self care activities).

Make sure that shower has a nonslip bottom surface and that shower chair, secure bath mat, grab bars, and adequate lighting are present. **D** ● ✦

Include client and significant others in planning and implementing measures to prevent falls.

If client falls, initiate first aid measures if appropriate and notify physician.

Arranging environment within reach of the client allows access to the appropriate assistance.

In order to reduce lightheadedness and dizziness associated with postural hypotension.

Dependent/Collaborative Actions

Perform actions to maintain adequate cerebral blood flow:
- Implement measures to maintain an adequate cardiac output:
  - Administer ordered medications.
- Consult physician before giving diuretics and medications with a negative inotropic or vasodilatory effect if client is hypotensive.

Maintaining adequate cerebral blood flow helps to decrease the risk of a syncopal episode, which may increase the risk for falls.

NDx = NANDA-I Diagnosis   **D** = Delegatable Action   ● = UAP   ✦ = LVN/LPN   ⊖▶ = Go to ⊖volve for animation

Collaborative Diagnosis | RISK FOR SYSTEMIC ARTERIAL EMBOLISM

Definition: Embolism is the obstruction of a vessel by an embolus—a bolus of matter circulating in the bloodstream. An embolus travels in the bloodstream until it reaches a vessel through which it cannot fit

Related to:

- Formation of thrombi in the heart associated with stasis of blood in the heart resulting from ineffective contractions (particularly a risk for clients in atrial fibrillation)
- Dislodgment of existing thrombi from the heart associated with a sudden restoration of coordinated mechanical contractions (a concern after cardioversion)

CLINICAL MANIFESTATIONS

Subjective	Objective
NOTE: *Subjective/objective clinical manifestations are dependent upon the vessel occluded by the embolus.*	The degree and extent of clinical manifestations depend on the size and location of the obstruction.

RISK FACTORS

- Immobilization
- History of DVT
- Malignancy
- Surgery within last 3 months
- Obesity
- Smoking

DESIRED OUTCOMES

The client will not experience systemic arterial embolization as evidenced by:
a. Absence of new or unusual pain in extremities
b. Usual temperature and color of extremities
c. Palpable and equal peripheral pulses
d. Usual mental status
e. Usual sensory and motor function
f. Absence of sudden chest pain and dyspnea

NURSING ASSESSMENT	RATIONALE
Assess for and report signs and symptoms of:	*Early recognition and reporting of signs and symptoms of systemic arterial emboli allow for prompt intervention.*
• **Arterial embolus** in an extremity (e.g., diminished or absent peripheral pulses; pallor, coolness, numbness, and/or pain in extremity)	
• **Cerebral embolism** (e.g., decreased level of consciousness, alteration in usual sensory and motor function)	
• **Pulmonary embolism** (e.g., sudden chest pain, dyspnea, restlessness or apprehension, significant decrease in arterial oxygen saturation [SaO_2])	

THERAPEUTIC INTERVENTIONS	RATIONALE
Independent Actions	
If signs and symptoms of an arterial embolus in an extremity occur:	
• Maintain client on bed rest with affected extremity in a level or slightly dependent position.	*Elevation of the extremity helps to improve arterial blood flow.*
If signs and symptoms of cerebral embolism occur:	
• Maintain client on bed rest (head of bed should be flat if systolic B/P is less than 90 mm Hg); keep head and neck in neutral, midline position.	*Actions focus on maintaining cerebral perfusion and reducing cerebral edema by facilitating venous drainage from the head.*
If signs and symptoms of pulmonary embolism occur:	
• Maintain client on bed rest in a semi- to high-Fowler's position.	*Positioning helps to facilitate optimum lung expansion/ventilation.*

THERAPEUTIC INTERVENTIONS	RATIONALE

Dependent/Collaborative Actions

If signs and symptoms of an arterial embolus in an extremity occur:

- Prepare client for the following if planned:
  - Injection of a thrombolytic agent (e.g., streptokinase)
  - Embolectomy
- Prepare client for diagnostic studies (e.g., Doppler or duplex ultrasound, arteriography) if planned.

If signs and symptoms of cerebral embolism occur:

- Maintain oxygen therapy as ordered.

If signs and symptoms of pulmonary embolism occur:

- Maintain oxygen therapy as ordered.
- Prepare client for diagnostic tests (e.g., arterial blood gases, D-dimer level, ventilation-perfusion lung scan, pulmonary angiography).
- Prepare client for the following if planned:
  - Injection of a thrombolytic agent (e.g., streptokinase, urokinase, alteplase [tPA])
- Vena caval interruption (e.g., insertion of an intracaval filtering device) to prevent further pulmonary emboli
- Embolectomy

Perform actions to prevent dysrhythmias.

Administer anticoagulants if ordered.

Actions aid in restoring blood flow to the affected extremity.

Prevention of dysrhythmias such as atrial fibrillation helps to reduce the risk of thrombus formation.

Controlling dysrhythmias and administering anticoagulants help to reduce the risk of thrombus formation in the heart and the subsequent risk for arterial embolization.

Collaborative Diagnosis ## RISK FOR HEART FAILURE

Definition: Impaired cardiac pumping

Related to: The decreased cardiac output that can occur with a rapid, irregular, or slow heart rate

CLINICAL MANIFESTATIONS

Subjective	Objective
Reports of fatigue; dyspnea; chest pain	Tachycardia; edema; nocturia; cool, clammy skin; diminished/absent hair growth in lower extremities; weight gain; abnormal breath sounds; frothy pink sputum

RISK FACTORS

- Hypertension
- Coronary artery disease (CAD)
- Diabetes
- Obesity

DESIRED OUTCOMES

The client will not develop heart failure as evidenced by:
a. Absence of an S_3 heart sound
b. Usual mental status
c. Clear, audible breath sounds
d. Absence of dyspnea, orthopnea, and a cough
e. No reports of increased fatigue and weakness
f. Palpable peripheral pulses
g. Urine output at least 30 mL/h
h. Stable weight
i. Absence of edema and distended neck veins

Continued...

NURSING ASSESSMENT	RATIONALE
Assess for and report signs and symptoms of heart failure: • Presence of an S$_3$ heart sound • Restlessness, agitation, confusion, or other change in mental status • Crackles (rales) • Dyspnea, orthopnea • Dry, hacking cough or cough productive of frothy or blood-tinged sputum • Development of or increased weakness and fatigue • Diminished or absent peripheral pulses • Decreased urine output during the day, nocturia • Weight gain • Edema • Distended neck veins Monitor results of chest radiograph for pulmonary vascular congestion, pleural effusion, or pulmonary edema.	*Early recognition and reporting of signs and symptoms of heart failure allow for prompt intervention.*

THERAPEUTIC INTERVENTIONS	RATIONALE
Dependent/Collaborative Actions Perform actions to maintain an adequate cardiac output: • Administer antidysrhythmic agents. • Administer anticholinergic agents. • Assist with vagal maneuvers. • Assist with cardioversion or defibrillation if performed.	*Medications that control heart rate and dysrhythmias help to sustain adequate cardiac output.* *Defibrillation is the most effective method of terminating lethal dysrhythmias or certain dysrhythmias unresponsive to drug therapy.*

If signs and symptoms of heart failure occur:
• Maintain oxygen therapy as ordered.
• Administer the following medications if ordered:
  • Positive inotropic agents (e.g., dopamine, dobutamine, digoxin)
  • Diuretics, vasodilators (e.g., nitroglycerin), and/or angiotensin-converting enzyme (ACE) inhibitors (e.g., captopril, ramipril)
  • Morphine sulfate
	
	Positive inotropes help to increase myocardial contractility.
	
	Medications act to decrease cardiac workload.
	
	Used most often in clients with pulmonary edema, morphine helps reduce preload and anxiety.

Collaborative Diagnosis RISK FOR SUDDEN CARDIAC DEATH

Definition: Death from a cardiac cause, most often from ventricular dysrhythmias—specifically, ventricular tachycardia or ventricular fibrillation

Related to: A lack of effective electrical and mechanical activity in the heart

CLINICAL MANIFESTATIONS

Subjective	Objective
Not applicable	Unresponsiveness; apnea; pulseless; absence of B/P; ECG tracing abnormalities (pulseless ventricular tachycardia, pulseless electrical activity, ventricular fibrillation, asystole)

RISK FACTORS

- Ventricular dysrhythmia
- Ventricular tachycardia
- Ventricular fibrillation

DESIRED OUTCOMES

The client will not experience sudden cardiac death as evidenced by:
  a. Stable vital signs
  b. Palpable peripheral pulses
  c. Usual mental status
  d. No evidence of cardiac arrest (flat line/asystole) or ventricular defibrillation on ECG

NURSING ASSESSMENT

Assess for and report signs and symptoms of sudden cardiac death:
- Pulselessness (ECG may continue to show electrical activity, which is referred to as pulseless electrical activity)
- Very low or no B/P
- Unresponsiveness
- ECG showing long pauses, flat line, or ventricular fibrillation

RATIONALE

Early recognition and reporting of signs and symptoms of sudden cardiac death allow for prompt intervention.

THERAPEUTIC INTERVENTIONS

Independent Actions
If signs and symptoms of sudden cardiac death occur, initiate cardiopulmonary resuscitation (CPR) and call a "code."

Dependent/Collaborative Actions
Implement measures to treat cardiac dysrhythmias.

RATIONALE

In the event lethal dysrhythmias occur, initiate advanced cardiac life support (ACLS) promptly.

Treatment with antidysrhythmics may reduce the risk for sudden cardiac death.

DISCHARGE TEACHING/CONTINUED CARE

Nursing Diagnosis | # DEFICIENT KNOWLEDGE NDx; INEFFECTIVE HEALTH MAINTENANCE NDx; OR INEFFECTIVE SELF-HEALTH MANAGEMENT NDx*

Definition: Absence or deficiency of cognitive information related to specific topic (lack of specific information necessary for clients/significant others to make informed choices regarding condition/treatment/lifestyle changes); inability to identify, manage, and/or seek out help to manage health; pattern of regulating and integrating into daily living a program for treatment of illness and the sequelae of illness that is unsatisfactory for meeting specific health goals

CLINICAL MANIFESTATIONS

Subjective	Objective
Exaggerated behaviors; unfamiliarity with information resources	Inaccurate follow through of instructions; inaccurate performance of a test; lack of recall

RISK FACTORS

- Denial of disease process
- Cognitive deficiency
- Failure to take action to reduce risk factors

NOC OUTCOMES

Knowledge: treatment regimen; knowledge: medication regimen

NIC NTERVENTIONS

Teaching: individual; teaching: disease process; teaching: prescribed medications; health system guidance

*The nurse should select the diagnostic label that is most appropriate for the client's discharge teaching needs.

 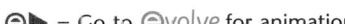

Continued...

NURSING ASSESSMENT	RATIONALE
Assess client's readiness and ability to learn. Assess meaning of illness to client.	*Early recognition of readiness to learn and meaning of illness to client allows for implementation of the appropriate teaching interventions.*

THERAPEUTIC INTERVENTIONS	RATIONALE

Desired Outcome: The client will verbalize a basic understanding of cardiac dysrhythmias.

Independent Actions

Explain cardiac dysrhythmias in terms the client can understand. Use appropriate teaching aids (e.g., pictures, videotapes).	*Clients vary in their physical and cognitive ability to learn. When educating clients, nurses need to determine their ability to read and understand written materials. If literacy barriers are present, alternative educational materials should be provided.*

THERAPEUTIC INTERVENTIONS	RATIONALE

Desired Outcome: The client will demonstrate accuracy in counting pulse.

Independent Actions

Teach clients how to count their pulse, being alert to the regularity of the rhythm. Allow time for return demonstration and accuracy check.	*Educating clients to their baseline rhythm allows for early detection of irregularities warranting immediate attention from a health care provider. Early detection may reduce the incidence of sudden death.*

THERAPEUTIC INTERVENTIONS	RATIONALE

Desired Outcome: The client will verbalize an understanding of medications ordered including rationale, food and drug interactions, side effects, schedule for taking, and importance of taking as prescribed.

Independent Actions

Explain the rationale for and importance of taking the medications prescribed.

Provide client with written instructions that include a schedule of times to take medications, the side effects to be alert for, and pertinent food and drug interactions.

Caution client to avoid driving and other hazardous activities if experiencing dizziness or lightheadedness.

Instruct client to:
- Limit intake of alcoholic beverages because of the B/P-lowering effects of alcohol and many antidysrhythmic agents
- Change from a lying to sitting or standing position slowly if dizziness or lightheadedness is a problem.
- Avoid skipping doses, trying to make up for missed doses, altering the prescribed dose, and discontinuing medication without first discussing it with health care provider.
- Check pulse before taking medication if medication prescribed is known to slow pulse, and consult health care provider if pulse is unusually slow.
- Wear or carry medical identification specifying the name of the medication being taken.
- Consult physician before taking other prescription and nonprescription medications.
- Inform all health care providers of medications being taken.

Taking medications as prescribed ensures that therapeutic drug levels will be maintained.

Clients should be instructed not to discontinue taking medications if they feel better. Clients without financial resources should be assisted in accessing appropriate resources to obtain needed medications (e.g., pharmacy assistance programs).

Drug-drug interactions may render medications inactive or result in life-threatening side effects.

Continuity of health care information is critical to reduce the incidence of prescribing medications with potential adverse drug-drug interactions.

THERAPEUTIC INTERVENTIONS	RATIONALE

Desired Outcome: The client will verbalize an understanding of ways to avoid precipitating or exacerbating dysrhythmias.

Independent Actions

Provide client with the following information about ways to reduce the risk for precipitating or exacerbating dysrhythmias:
- If client has a bradydysrhythmia, instruct to avoid activities that stimulate the vagus nerve (e.g., putting pressure on carotid artery or on eyes, bearing down or straining during a bowel movement, performing activities that involve using arms over head for a prolonged time).
- If client has a tachydysrhythmia, instruct to:
  - Avoid activities that have a cardiostimulatory effect (e.g., drinking caffeinated beverages, smoking).
  - Avoid stressful situations whenever possible and develop and use stress management techniques (stress has a cardiostimulatory effect).
  - Eat foods high in potassium (e.g., bananas, cantaloupe, potatoes, raisins, avocados) and take prescribed potassium supplement if taking a potassium-depleting diuretic.

Clients with diagnosed cardiac dysrhythmias should be educated as to what may precipitate angina and ways to decrease the risk for angina. In addition, clients should be taught to recognize that changes in their baseline heart rhythm may indicate serious changes that require prompt treatment.

THERAPEUTIC INTERVENTIONS	RATIONALE

Desired Outcome: The client will state signs and symptoms to report to the health care provider.

Independent Actions

Instruct the client to report:
- Any significant change in the rate or rhythm of pulse, particularly a rate of less than 50 or greater than 100 beats/min and increased irregularity
- Significant weight gain or swelling of feet or ankles
- Shortness of breath or a persistent cough
- Unusual weakness or fatigue
- Persistent lightheadedness or dizziness or any fainting episodes
- Increased awareness of being able to feel the heart beating (palpitations)
- Chest, arm, neck, jaw, or back discomfort

Early identification of signs and symptoms of a cardiac dysrhythmia allows for prompt intervention.

RISK FACTORS
- Myocardial infarction
- Heart failure
- Cardiomyopathy
- Electrolyte balance
- Acid-base imbalance

THERAPEUTIC INTERVENTIONS	RATIONALE

Desired Outcome: The client will verbalize an understanding of and a plan for adhering to recommended follow-up care including activity restrictions and future appointments with health care provider.

Continued...

THERAPEUTIC INTERVENTIONS	RATIONALE

Independent Actions

Reinforce the importance of keeping follow-up appointments with health care provider.

Reinforce instructions from the cardiac rehabilitation therapist and physician about activity level.

Implement measures to improve client compliance:

* Include significant others in teaching sessions if possible.

* Encourage questions and allow time for reinforcement and clarification of information provided.

* Provide written instructions on future appointments with health care provider, activity progression, medications prescribed, and signs and symptoms to report.

Regular health care appointments are important to determine effectiveness of the prescribed treatment plan.

Involvement of significant others in patient teaching improves adherence to discharge instructions.

Everyone does not understand information as presented, so set aside time for questions to allow for clarification of information.

Written instructions allow the client to refer to instructions as needed.

ADDITIONAL NURSING DIAGNOSIS

FEAR/ANXIETY

Related to:

* Symptoms being experienced as a result of the dysrhythmias (e.g., palpitations, dizziness, shortness of breath)
* Possibility of sudden death
* Possible changes in lifestyle and roles
* Unfamiliar environment and separation from significant others

* Lack of understanding of diagnostic tests, diagnosis, and treatment modalities
* Financial concerns about the cost of hospitalization, life-long medication therapy, and/or invasive treatment modalities (e.g., insertion of a pacemaker or implantable cardioverter-defibrillator)

CAROTID ENDARTERECTOMY

Carotid endarterectomy is the surgical removal of atherosclerotic plaque from the intima of the carotid artery. The most common site of plaque formation in the carotid artery is the bifurcation. Access to this extracranial area is gained through an incision along the anterior sternocleidomastoid muscle. Surgery is performed to improve carotid artery blood flow and to reduce the risk of cerebral embolization and stroke.

This care plan focuses on the adult client hospitalized for a carotid endarterectomy. Much of the postoperative information is applicable to clients receiving follow-up care in an extended care facility or home setting.

OUTCOME/DISCHARGE CRITERIA

The client will:

1. Have adequate cerebral blood flow
2. Have surgical pain controlled
3. Have evidence of normal wound healing
4. Identify ways to prevent or slow the progression of atherosclerosis
5. Identify ways to manage signs and symptoms resulting from cranial nerve damage if it has occurred
6. State signs and symptoms to report to the health care provider
7. Verbalize an understanding of and a plan for adhering to recommended follow-up care including future appointments with health care provider, medications prescribed, activity level, and wound care.

NURSING/COLLABORATIVE DIAGNOSIS: PREOPERATIVE

Use in conjunction with the Standardized Preoperative Care Plan.

| Nursing Diagnosis | **RISK FOR INEFFECTIVE CEREBRAL TISSUE PERFUSION** NDx |

Definition: Decrease in oxygen resulting in failure to nourish tissues at the capillary level

Related to:
- Partial or complete occlusion of the carotid artery by atherosclerotic plaque and/or a thrombus
- A cerebral embolus associated with dislodgment of atherosclerotic plaque or a thrombus from the carotid artery

CLINICAL MANIFESTATIONS

Subjective	Objective
Reports of behavioral changes; changes in motor response	Altered mental status; changes in pupillary reactions; difficulty swallowing; extremity weakness; paralysis; speech abnormalities

RISK FACTORS
- Arterial fibrillation
- Carotid stenosis
- Hypertension
- Hypercholesterolemia
- Embolism

DESIRED OUTCOMES

The client will maintain adequate cerebral tissue perfusion as evidenced by:
a. Mentally alert and oriented
b. Absence of dizziness, visual disturbances, and speech impairments
c. Normal motor and sensory function

NOC OUTCOMES

Tissue perfusion: cerebral; neurological status; cognition

NIC INTERVENTIONS

Cerebral perfusion promotion; neurological monitoring

NURSING ASSESSMENT	RATIONALE
Assess for and report signs and symptoms of carotid artery occlusion and/or cerebral embolization: - Agitation - Lethargy - Confusion - Dizziness - Diplopia - Ipsilateral blindness - Homonymous hemianopsia - Slurred speech - Expressive aphasia - Paresthesias - Hemiparesis - Hemiplegia	*Early recognition and reporting of signs and symptoms of ineffective cerebral tissue perfusion allow for prompt intervention.*

THERAPEUTIC INTERVENTIONS	RATIONALE

Independent Actions
Implement measures to maintain adequate cerebral tissue perfusion:
- Caution client to avoid activities that create a Valsalva response.
  - Straining to have a bowel movement
  - Holding breath while moving up in bed
Perform actions to prevent hypertension in order to reduce the risk of cerebral embolism:
- Implement measures to reduce stress (e.g., explain procedures, maintain calm environment).
	Actions help to prevent dislodgment of existing thrombi.

Continued...

THERAPEUTIC INTERVENTIONS	RATIONALE
If signs and symptoms of decreased cerebral tissue perfusion persist or worsen: • Provide emotional support to client and significant others; be aware that the development of signs and symptoms usually necessitates postponement or cancellation of planned surgery.	

Dependent/Collaborative Actions
Implement measures to maintain adequate cerebral tissue perfusion:
• Administer anticoagulants if ordered:
  • Heparin
  • Warfarin
  • Antiplatelet agents
	Anticoagulants act to prevent new or extended thrombus formation and further occlusion of the carotid artery. NOTE: These medications might be discontinued before surgery to reduce the risk of intraoperative and postoperative hemorrhage.

Perform actions to prevent hypertension in order to reduce the risk of cerebral embolism: • Administer antihypertensives as ordered.	*These medications are sometimes discontinued before surgery to reduce the risk of a critical drop in B/P during and immediately after surgery.*
If signs and symptoms of decreased cerebral tissue perfusion persist or worsen: • Administer anticoagulants if ordered. • Maintain client on bed rest with head of bed flat unless contraindicated. • Notify the appropriate health care provider.	*Notification of the appropriate health care provider allows for modification of the treatment plan.*

Postoperative

Use in conjunction with the Standardized Postoperative Care Plan.

Collaborative Diagnosis # RISK FOR CEREBRAL ISCHEMIA

Definition: Decrease in blood supply to the brain caused by constriction or obstruction of blood vessels

Related to:
• Prolonged carotid artery clamp time during surgery and/or vasospasm associated with clamping and manipulation of cerebral vessels
• Compression of carotid vessels associated with inflammation, edema, and/or development of a hematoma in the operative area
• Hypotension associated with:
  • Hypovolemia resulting from intraoperative and/or postoperative blood loss
  • Stimulation of the carotid sinus baroreceptors resulting from surgical manipulation and/or improved blood flow in the carotid artery after surgery
• Increased cerebral vascular dilation and pressure associated with inability of the autoregulatory system to adjust to increased blood flow in cerebral vessels distal to the surgical site (this hyperperfusion syndrome can occur in the initial postoperative period in clients who have had a high-grade, long-term carotid artery blockage that has resulted in chronic cerebral vessel dilation)
• Embolization during or after surgery and/or formation of a thrombus at surgical site

CLINICAL MANIFESTATIONS

Subjective	Objective
Verbal reports of dizziness	Agitation; lethargy; confusion; visual disturbances (e.g., blurred or dimmed vision, diplopia, ipsilateral blindness, homonymous hemianopsia); speech impairments (e.g., slurred speech, expressive aphasia); paresthesias, paresis, paralysis

RISK FACTORS
- Arteriosclerosis
- Hypertension

DESIRED OUTCOMES

The client will maintain adequate cerebral blood flow as evidenced by:
a. Mentally alert and oriented
b. Absence of dizziness, visual disturbances, and speech impairments
c. Normal sensory and motor function

NURSING ASSESSMENT	RATIONALE
Assess for and report signs and symptoms of: • Cerebral ischemia • Excessive operative site bleeding • New or expanding hematoma • Continued bright red bleeding from incision or wound drain • Hypovolemic shock Assess RBC count, Hct and Hgb levels for abnormalities.	*Early recognition and reporting of signs and symptoms of cerebral ischemia allow for prompt intervention.*

THERAPEUTIC INTERVENTIONS	RATIONALE

Dependent/Collaborative Actions

Implement measures to prevent cerebral ischemia:
- Perform actions to prevent or treat hypovolemic shock.
- Perform actions to reduce pressure on carotid vessels:
  - Implement measures to reduce operative site inflammation and/or edema:
- Keep head of bed elevated 30 degrees unless contraindicated.
- Apply cooling pad or ice pack to incisional area as ordered.
- Administer corticosteroids if ordered.
- Maintain patency of wound drain (e.g., keep tubing free of kinks, empty collection device as often as necessary) if present.
- Instruct client to support head and neck with hands during position changes and to avoid turning head abruptly or hyperextending neck.
- Caution client to avoid activities that create a Valsalva response (e.g., straining to have a bowel movement, holding breath while moving up in bed)
- Administer the following medications if ordered:
  - Antihypertensives
  - Sympathomimetics

Interventions that focus on maintaining adequate cerebral blood flow and vessel patency help to prevent cerebral ischemia.

Corticosteriods help reduce operative site inflammation and/or edema reducing pressure on carotid vessels.

Action helps to reduce stress on the suture line and prevent subsequent bleeding and hematoma formation.

Action helps to prevent dislodgment of existing thrombi and reduce stress on and subsequent bleeding from the suture line.

Medications help to maintain B/P within a safe range, preventing either hypotension, which can reduce cerebral blood flow, or hypertension, which can stress and disrupt the operative vessel leading to hemorrhage.

Collaborative Diagnosis **RISK FOR RESPIRATORY DISTRESS**

Definition: Inability of a client to get enough oxygen to support respiration; can result from upper airway obstruction or lung disease

Related to: Airway obstruction associated with tracheal compression (can occur as a result of inflammation, edema, and/or hematoma formation in the surgical area)

CLINICAL MANIFESTATIONS

Subjective	Objective
Verbal reports of difficulty getting "air" or breathing	Agitation; restlessness; rapid/labored respirations; stridor; sternocleidomastoid muscle retraction

Continued...

RISK FACTOR

• Surgical manipulation in close proximity to airway

DESIRED OUTCOMES

The client will not experience respiratory distress as evidenced by:
  a. Usual mental status
  b. Unlabored respirations at 12 to 20 breaths/min
  c. Absence of stridor and sternocleidomastoid muscle retraction
  d. Oximetry results within normal range
  e. Arterial blood gas values within normal range

NURSING ASSESSMENT

Assess for and report:
• Increased edema or expanding hematoma in surgical area
• Deviation of trachea from midline
• New or increased difficulty swallowing
• Signs and symptoms of respiratory distress:
  • Restlessness
  • Agitation
  • Rapid and/or labored respirations
  • Stridor
  • Sternocleidomastoid muscle retraction
Monitor arterial blood gas values and pulse oximetry values for abnormalities.

RATIONALE

Early recognition of signs and symptoms of respiratory distress allows for prompt intervention.

THERAPEUTIC INTERVENTIONS

Dependent/Collaborative Actions
Have tracheostomy and suction equipment readily available.

Implement measures to prevent compression of the trachea:
• Perform actions to prevent inflammation, edema, and hematoma formation in the operative area (e.g., maintnain head and neck in alignment, place client in semi- to high-fowlers, apply ice to operative area as ordered).
• Perform actions to prevent excessive pressure:
  • Caution client to avoid activities that create a Valsalva response (e.g., straining to have a bowel movement, holding breath while moving up in bed)
  • Administer antihypertensives if ordered.
If signs and symptoms of respiratory distress occur:
• Place client in a high-Fowler's position unless contraindicated.
• Loosen neck dressing if it appears tight.
• Administer oxygen as ordered.
• Assist with intubation or tracheostomy if performed.
• Prepare client for evacuation of hematoma or surgical repair of the bleeding vessel if planned.

RATIONALE

An emergency tracheostomy may be necessary if a client's airway becomes compromised.
Compression of the trachea can result in respiratory distress. During the postoperative period, frequent assessment of the position of the trachea (midline, shifted to the left or right) is critical.

Interventions and medications help to prevent excessive pressure in the operative vessel and subsequent bleeding and hematoma formation.

Identification of signs and symptoms of respiratory distress allows for modification of the treatment plan and initiation of emergency measures if indicated.

Collaborative Diagnosis   **RISK FOR CRANIAL NERVE DAMAGE (FACIAL, HYPOGLOSSAL, GLOSSOPHARYNGEAL, VAGUS, AND/OR ACCESSORY NERVES)**

Definition: Damage to cranial nerve(s)

Related to: Surgical trauma and/or compression of the nerves (can occur as a result of inflammation, edema, and/or hematoma formation)

CLINICAL MANIFESTATIONS

Subjective	Objective
Facial: Verbal reports of altered taste sensations	**Facial:** Difficulty raising eyebrows, closing eyes tightly, pursing lips, and/or smiling.
Hypoglossal: Not applicable	**Hypoglossal:** Inability to protrude tongue or move tongue side to side
Glossopharyngeal/vagus: Not applicable	**Glossopharyngeal/vagus:** Absence of gag reflex; difficulty in swallowing
Accessory nerves: Not applicable	**Accessory nerves:** Inability to shrug shoulders against resistance.

RISK FACTOR

- Surgical retraction

DESIRED OUTCOMES

The client will experience beginning resolution of cranial nerve damage if it occurs as evidenced by:
  a. Gradual return of facial symmetry and usual taste sensation
  b. Increased ability to chew and swallow
  c. Improved speech
  d. Return of usual shoulder movements

NURSING ASSESSMENT

Assess for and report signs and symptoms of the following:
- Facial nerve damage (e.g., facial ptosis on affected side, impaired sense of taste)
- Vagus and glossopharyngeal nerve damage (e.g., loss of gag reflex, difficulty swallowing, hoarseness, inability to speak clearly)
- Hypoglossal nerve damage (e.g., tongue biting when chewing, tongue deviation toward affected side, difficulty swallowing and speaking).
- Accessory nerve damage (e.g., unilateral shoulder sag, difficulty raising shoulder against resistance)

RATIONALE

Early recognition and reporting of signs and symptoms of nerve damage allow for prompt intervention.

THERAPEUTIC INTERVENTIONS

Dependent/Collaborative Actions
Implement measures to prevent compression of the cranial nerves at the operative site:
- Keep head of bed elevated 30 degrees unless contraindicated.
- Apply ice pack to incisional area.
- Maintain patency of wound drain.
- Avoid Valsalva maneuvers. **D** ✦
If signs and symptoms of cranial nerve damage occur:
- If the facial, hypoglossal, vagus, and/or glossopharyngeal nerves are affected:
  - Withhold oral foods/fluids until gag reflex returns and client is better able to chew and swallow; provide parenteral nutrition or tube feeding if indicated.
  - When oral intake is allowed and tolerated:
    - Implement measures to improve client's ability to chew and/or swallow:
      - Place client in high-Fowler's position for meals and snacks.
      - Assist client to select foods that require little or no chewing and are easily swallowed (e.g., custard, eggs, canned fruits, mashed potatoes).

RATIONALE

These actions decrease edema at the surgical site.

Actions help to reduce the risk of aspiration.

Continued...

THERAPEUTIC INTERVENTIONS	RATIONALE
• Avoid serving foods that are sticky (e.g., peanut butter, soft bread, honey).	
• Serve thick rather than thin fluids or add a thickening agent (e.g., "Thick-It," gelatin, baby cereal) to thin fluids.	
• Instruct client to add extra sweeteners or seasonings to foods/fluids if desired.	*Action helps to compensate for impaired sense of taste.*
• Implement measures to facilitate communication (e.g., maintain quiet environment; provide pad and pencil, Magic Slate, or word cards; listen carefully when client speaks).	
• Consult speech pathologist about additional ways to facilitate swallowing and communication.	
• If the accessory nerve is affected, instruct client in and assist with exercises (e.g., range of motion of affected shoulder, wall climbing with fingers, shoulder shrugs).	*Exercises help to prevent atrophy of trapezius and sternocleidomastoid muscles.*
• Provide emotional support to client and significant others; assure them that the nerve damage is usually not permanent, but caution them that the symptoms may take months to resolve.	

DISCHARGE TEACHING/CONTINUED CARE

Nursing Diagnosis ## DEFICIENT KNOWLEDGE NDx; INEFFECTIVE HEALTH MAINTENANCE NDx; OR INEFFECTIVE SELF-HEALTH MANAGEMENT NDx*

Definition: Absence or deficiency of cognitive information related to specific topic (lack of specific information necessary for clients/significant others to make informed choices regarding condition/treatment/lifestyle changes); inability to identify, manage, and/or seek out help to manage health; pattern of regulating and integrating into daily living a program for treatment of illness and the sequelae of illness that is unsatisfactory for meeting specific health goals

CLINICAL MANIFESTATIONS

Subjective	Objective
Verbalization of unfamiliarity with information resources	Inaccurate follow-through of instructions

RISK FACTORS
• Denial of disease process
• Cognitive deficiency
• Failure to take action to reduce risk factors

NOC OUTCOMES	NIC INTERVENTIONS
Knowledge: treatment regimen; knowledge: cardiac disease management	Health system guidance; teaching: disease process; teaching: individual; teaching: prescribed diet

NURSING ASSESSMENT	RATIONALE
Assess client's readiness and ability to learn. Assess meaning of illness to client.	*Early recognition of readiness to learn and meaning of illness to client allows for implementation of the appropriate teaching interventions.*

*The nurse should select the diagnostic label that is most appropriate for the client's discharge teaching needs.

THERAPEUTIC INTERVENTIONS	RATIONALE

Desired Outcome: The client will identify ways to prevent or slow the progression of atherosclerosis.

Independent Actions

Inform the client that certain modifiable factors such as elevated serum lipid levels, a sedentary lifestyle, cigarette smoking, and hypertension have been shown to increase the risk of atherosclerosis.

Assist client to identify changes in lifestyle that could reduce the risk for atherosclerosis (e.g., smoking cessation, dietary modifications, physical exercise on a regular basis).

Provide instructions on ways the client can reduce intake of saturated fat and cholesterol:

- Reduce intake of meat fat (e.g., trim visible fat off meat; replace fatty meats such as fatty cuts of steak, hamburger, and processed meats with leaner products).
- Reduce intake of milk fat (e.g., avoid dairy products containing more than 1% fat).
- Reduce intake of *trans* fats (e.g., avoid stick margarine and shortening and foods such as commercial baked goods that are prepared with these products).
- Use vegetable oil rather than coconut or palm oil in cooking and food preparation.
- Use cooking methods such as steaming, baking, broiling, poaching, microwaving, and grilling rather than frying.
- Restrict intake of eggs (recommendations about the number of whole eggs allowed per week vary depending on the client's lipid levels).

Instruct client to take lipid-lowering agents (e.g., HMG-CoA reductase inhibitors ["statins"], ezetimibe, gemfibrozil, niacin) and antiplatelet agents (e.g., low-dose aspirin) as prescribed.

A person with modifiable risk factors should be encouraged to make lifestyle changes to reduce the risk for atherosclerosis in order to prevent progression of the disease.

THERAPEUTIC INTERVENTIONS	RATIONALE

Desired Outcome: The client will identify ways to manage signs and symptoms resulting from cranial nerve damage if it has occurred.

Independent Actions

If signs and symptoms of hypoglossal, facial, vagus, and/or glossopharyngeal nerve damage are present:

- Reinforce techniques to improve swallowing and speaking.
- Assist client in identifying foods that are nutritious and easy to chew and swallow; obtain a dietary consult if needed.
- Instruct client to increase the amount of sweeteners and seasonings usually used and/or to try different seasonings in foods and beverages if sense of taste is altered.

If signs and symptoms of accessory nerve damage are present, reinforce exercises that should be performed to maintain shoulder muscle tone and prevent contractures.

Educating the client as to normal nerve function allows for early detection of irregularities warranting immediate attention from a health care provider. Early detection may reduce the incidence of permanent nerve damage.

THERAPEUTIC INTERVENTIONS	RATIONALE

Desired Outcome: The client will state signs and symptoms to report to the health care provider.

Continued...

THERAPEUTIC INTERVENTIONS	RATIONALE

Independent Actions

Instruct client to also report any of the following signs and symptoms to the health care provider:

- Increased swelling or purple discoloration at wound site
- New or increased difficulty chewing, swallowing, or speaking
- Any loss of or change in vision
- Dizziness
- Numbness, tingling, or weakness of arms or legs
- Increasing irritability
- Lethargy, confusion
- Failure of signs and symptoms of cranial nerve damage to resolve as expected; remind client that it can take months for reversible signs and symptoms to resolve.

Early identification of signs and symptoms of complications associated with surgery allows for prompt intervention.

THERAPEUTIC INTERVENTIONS	RATIONALE

Desired Outcome: The client will verbalize an understanding of and a plan for adhering to recommended follow-up care including future appointments with health care provider, medications prescribed, activity level, and wound care.

Independent Actions

Reinforce the physician's instructions regarding:

- Ways to prevent constipation and subsequent straining to have a bowel movement (e.g., drink at least 10 glasses of liquid per day unless contraindicated, increase intake of foods high in fiber, take stool softeners if necessary)
- The need to avoid isometric exercise/activity (e.g., lifting objects over 10 lb, pushing heavy objects) and strenuous exercise for specified length of time (usually 4-12 weeks depending on the activity)

Actions help to prevent increasing straining, which may lead to wound or vascular graft dehiscence.

RELATED CARE PLANS

Standardized Preoperative Care Plan
Standardized Postoperative Care Plan

DEEP VEIN THROMBOSIS

Venous thrombosis occurs when a thrombus forms in a superficial or deep vein. This condition is often called thrombophlebitis because of the associated inflammation in the involved vessel wall. The predisposing factors for venous thrombus formation are venous stasis, damage to the endothelium of the vein wall, and/or hypercoagulability. Conditions/factors associated with a high risk for venous thrombosis include surgery (especially orthopedic and abdominal surgery), immobility, advanced age, heart failure, certain malignancies, fractures or other injuries of the pelvis or lower extremities, varicose veins, pregnancy, obesity, estrogen and oral contraceptive use, sepsis, venous cannulation, administration of vessel irritants (e.g., hypertonic solutions, chemotherapeutic agents, high-dose antibiotics), history of deep vein thrombosis, and inherited coagulation abnormalities.

Deep vein thrombosis usually develops in a lower extremity; however, the incidence of subclavian venous thrombosis is rising because of the increased use of central venous catheters. Clinical manifestations of deep vein thrombosis are often not distinctive and, in many cases, the client is asymptomatic. Signs and symptoms that may be present include pain, tenderness, swelling, unusual warmth, and/or positive Homans' sign in the involved extremity. The greatest danger associated with deep vein thrombosis is that the clot, or parts of it, will detach and cause embolic occlusion of a pulmonary vessel.

Persons with deep vein thrombosis are usually treated medically rather than surgically unless there is massive occlusion of a vessel and anticoagulation and thrombolytic therapy are contraindicated. With the increasing use of thrombolytic therapy, thrombectomies and embolectomies are rarely performed. Medical treatment varies depending on the location of the thrombus, the person's risk for bleeding and history of previous thrombus, and whether a coagulation abnormality exists. Anticoagulant therapy is not universally used to treat calf vein thrombosis because the incidence of pulmonary embolism is low if there is no proximal vein involvement. However, there is a risk of extension of calf vein thrombi into a proximal venous segment if untreated, and because of this risk, many persons with calf vein thrombosis are treated with anticoagulants. There is also some variation in the anticoagulant regimen in relation to the time that oral anticoagulants are initiated and the route and type of heparin ordered (e.g., continuous intravenous heparin, intermittent intravenous heparin, adjusted-dose subcutaneous heparin, low-molecular-weight heparin).

This care plan focuses on the adult client hospitalized for treatment of deep vein thrombosis in a lower extremity. The information is also applicable to clients receiving follow-up care at home.

OUTCOME DISCHARGE CRITERIA

The client will:
1. Have adequate tissue perfusion in affected extremity
2. Have no evidence of tissue irritation or breakdown
3. Have no signs and symptoms of complications
4. Identify ways to promote venous blood flow and reduce the risk of chronic venous insufficiency and recurrent thrombus formation
5. Verbalize an understanding of medications ordered including rationale, food and drug interactions, side effects, schedule for taking, and importance of taking as prescribed
6. Demonstrate the ability to correctly draw up and administer heparin subcutaneously if prescribed
7. Identify precautions necessary to prevent bleeding associated with anticoagulant therapy
8. State signs and symptoms to report to the health care provider
9. Verbalize an understanding of and a plan for adhering to recommended follow-up care including future appointments with health care provider and activity level.

Nursing Diagnosis INEFFECTIVE TISSUE PERFUSION: PERIPHERAL NDx

Definition: Decrease in oxygen resulting in failure to nourish tissues at the capillary level

Related to:
- Obstructed venous blood flow in affected extremity associated with the presence of a thrombus and inflammation of the vessel
- Venous stasis associated with decreased mobility

CLINICAL MANIFESTATIONS

Subjective	Objective
Verbalization of tenderness/pressure over involved vein; extremity pain	Edema; brawny hemosideric skin discoloration; dependent blue or purple skin color; positive Homans' sign; slow healing of lesions; skin temperature changes; altered sensations; weak or absent pulses

RISK FACTOR

- Virchow's triad: venous stasis, endothelial damage due to trauma or inflammation, blood hypercoagulability

DESIRED OUTCOME

The client will have improved venous blood flow in the affected extremity as evidenced by diminished pain, tenderness, swelling, and distention of superficial blood vessels in extremity.

NOC OUTCOMES

Tissue perfusion: peripheral

NIC INTERVENTIONS

Embolus care: peripheral; circulatory care: venous insufficiency; lower extremity monitoring

Continued...

NURSING ASSESSMENT	RATIONALE
Assess for signs and symptoms of impaired venous blood flow in the affected extremity: • Pain or tenderness in extremity • Increase in circumference of extremity • Distention of superficial blood vessels in extremity	*Early recognition of signs and symptoms of altered peripheral tissue perfusion allows for prompt intervention.*
Assess activated clotting time (ACT), activated partial thromboplastin time (aPTT), bleeding time, Hgb level, Hct, international normalized ratio (INR), platelet count, and D-dimer for abnormalities.	*Alterations in lab values may indicate risk factors for the formation of deep vein thrombosis (DVT). D-dimer elevation is suggestive of DVT.*

THERAPEUTIC INTERVENTIONS	RATIONALE
Independent Actions Elevate affected extremity 10 degrees to 20 degrees above the level of the heart. **D** ✦	*Actions help to reduce venous stasis.*
Maintain the client on bed rest.	*Bed rest until the thrombus is considered stable helps to reduce the risk of dislodgment.*
Discourage positions that compromise blood flow (e.g., pillows under knees, crossing legs, sitting or standing for long periods). **D** ✦	
Dependent/Collaborative Actions Perform actions to treat the thrombosis: • Administer medications as ordered.	*Administration of identified medications helps to improve venous blood flow.*
• Indirect thrombin inhibitors	*Indirect thrombin inhibitors are divided into two classes: unfractionated heparin, which acts upon both intrinsic and extrinsic pathways, and low-molecular-weight heparin (LMWH), which acts as an antithrombin.*
• Direct thrombin inhibitors	*Direct thrombin inhibitors bind with thrombin, inhibiting its function.*
• Factor Xa inhibitors	*Factor Xa inhibitors inhibit factor Xa directly or indirectly.*
• Anticoagulants	*Anticoagulants act by inhibiting clotting factors.*
• Vitamin K antagonists	*Vitamin K antagonists inhibit vitamin K–dependent clotting factors II, VII, IX, and X.*
• Prepare client for intravenous injection of a thrombolytic agent or catheter-directed fibrinolysis.	
Maintain a minimum fluid intake of 2500 mL (unless contraindicated). **D** ✦	*Ensuring adequate fluid intake helps to prevent increased blood viscosity.*
Apply antiembolism stockings or intermittent compression devices if ordered. **D** ● ✦	*Actions help to reduce venous stasis.*
Consult physician if signs and symptoms of impaired venous blood flow in affected extremity persist or worsen.	*Notification of the appropriate health care provider allows for modification of the treatment plan. Clients may require surgical intervention to remove an embolus (embolectomy) or prevent a pulmonary embolus (vena caval interruption device—Greenfield filter).*

Nursing Diagnosis ACUTE PAIN NDx (AFFECTED EXTREMITY)

Definition: An unpleasant sensory and emotional experience arising from actual or potential tissue damage

Related to:
• Decreased tissue perfusion and swelling associated with obstructed venous blood flow
• Inflammation of vein

CLINICAL MANIFESTATIONS

Subjective	**Objective**
Verbal report of pain in the affected extremity	Diaphoresis, B/P and heart rate changes; increased respiratory rate

RISK FACTORS

- Arteriosclerosis
- Venous stasis
- Immobility

DESIRED OUTCOMES

The client will experience diminished pain in the affected extremity as evidenced by:
  a. Verbalization of a decrease in pain
  b. Relaxed facial expression and body positioning
  c. Increased participation in activities when allowed

NOC OUTCOMES

Comfort level; pain control

NIC INTERVENTIONS

Pain management; analgesic administration; heat/cold application

NURSING ASSESSMENT	**RATIONALE**
Assess for signs and symptoms of pain (e.g., verbalization of pain, grimacing, rubbing affected area, restlessness, reluctance to move). Assess client's perception of the severity of pain using a pain intensity rating scale. Assess client's pain pattern (e.g., location, quality, onset, duration, precipitating factors, aggravating factors, alleviating factors).	*Early recognition of signs and symptoms of pain allows for prompt intervention.*

THERAPEUTIC INTERVENTIONS	**RATIONALE**

Dependent/Collaborative Actions
Implement measures to reduce pain:
- Perform actions to protect the affected extremity from trauma, pressure, or excessive movement: **D** ✦
  - Avoid jarring the bed.
  - Use a bed cradle or footboard.   *Bed cradles help to relieve pressure from bed linens.*
  - Support extremity during position changes.
  - Maintain activity restrictions as ordered.
  - Instruct client to move affected extremity slowly and cautiously.
- Provide or assist with nonpharmacological methods for pain relief: **D** ● ✦
  - Position change
  - Relaxation techniques
  - Restful environment
  - Diversional activities
- Instruct client and significant others that the painful extremity should not be rubbed to relieve pain.   *Rubbing the affected extremity could dislodge the thrombus, resulting in a thromboembolism.*

Independent Actions
Implement measures to reduce pain:
- Administer analgesics and anti-inflammatory agents if ordered. **D** ✦
- Consult physician if above measures fail to provide adequate pain relief.   *Notification of the appropriate health care provider allows for modification of the treatment plan.*

Nursing Diagnosis: RISK FOR IMPAIRED TISSUE INTEGRITY NDx

Definition: At risk for skin being adversely altered

Related to:

* Accumulation of waste products and decreased oxygen and nutrient supply to the skin and subcutaneous tissue associated with prolonged pressure on tissues as a result of decreased mobility
* Damage to the skin and/or subcutaneous tissue associated with friction or shearing that can occur with movement while on bed rest
* Increased skin fragility in affected extremity associated with insufficient blood flow and edema

CLINICAL MANIFESTATIONS

Subjective	Objective
Verbal report of pain or altered sensation at site of tissue impairment	Color changes; redness; swelling; warmth of skin areas demonstrating impairment

RISK FACTORS

* Altered circulation
* Impaired mobility
* Mechanical factors: shear

DESIRED OUTCOMES

The client will maintain tissue integrity as evidenced by:
  a. Absence of redness and irritation
  b. No skin breakdown

NOC OUTCOMES

Tissue integrity: skin and mucous membranes

NIC INTERVENTIONS

Skin surveillance; pressure management; pressure ulcer prevention

NURSING ASSESSMENT

Inspect the skin (especially bony prominences, dependent areas, and affected extremity) for pallor, redness, and breakdown.

RATIONALE

Early recognition of impaired skin integrity allows for prompt intervention.

THERAPEUTIC INTERVENTIONS

RATIONALE

Dependent/Collaborative Actions
Implement measures to prevent tissue breakdown: **D** ●

* Assist client with turning every 2 hours.
* Use pressure-relieving devices to position client properly:
  * Pillows, gel or foam cushions
* Keep client's skin dry.
* Keep bed linens dry and wrinkle free.

Implement measures to prevent tissue breakdown in involved extremity:

* Perform actions to protect affected extremity from trauma and/or excessive pressure: **D** ✦
  * Use a bed cradle or footboard to relieve pressure from bed linens.
  * Keep heel off bed by elevating extremity on foam block or pillows or using heel protector.
  * Instruct and assist client to move affected extremity cautiously.
  * Remove antiembolism stockings for 30 to 60 minutes at least twice daily.
  * Use caution when applying heat to extremity.

Prolonged pressure on the skin obstructs capillary blood flow.

Excessive moisture on the skin softens epidermal cells and makes them less resistant to damage.

THERAPEUTIC INTERVENTIONS	RATIONALE

Dependent/Collaborative Actions

If tissue breakdown occurs:
- Notify appropriate health care provider (e.g., wound care specialist, physician).
- Perform care of involved areas as ordered or per standard hospital procedure.

Notification of the appropriate health care provider allows for modification of the treatment plan.

Collaborative Diagnosis ## RISK FOR PULMONARY EMBOLISM

Definition: Occlusion of a portion of the pulmonary vascular bed by an embolus, which can be a thrombus (blood clot)

Related to: Dislodgment of thrombus

CLINICAL MANIFESTATIONS

Subjective	Objective
Verbal reports of chest or pleural pain	Pleural friction rub; pleural effusion; tachycardia; tachypnea; dyspnea; unexplained anxiety

RISK FACTOR
- Virchow's triad: venous stasis, endothelial trauma or inflammation, blood hypercoagulability

DESIRED OUTCOMES

The client will not experience a pulmonary embolism as evidenced by:
a. Absence of sudden chest pain
b. Unlabored respirations at 12 to 20 breaths/min
c. Pulse rate 60 to 100 beats/min
d. Arterial blood gas values within normal range

NURSING ASSESSMENT	RATIONALE

Assess for and report signs and symptoms of a pulmonary embolism:
- Sudden chest pain
- Dyspnea
- Tachypnea
- Tachycardia
- Apprehension

Assess pulse oximetry and arterial blood gas values for abnormalities.

Assess vital signs for signs of shock associated with massive pulmonary embolism.

Early recognition of signs and symptoms of a pulmonary embolism allows for prompt intervention.

Clinical stability of the client is dependent upon the degree of obstruction associated with the embolism (e.g., massive occlusion, embolus with infarction, embolus without infarction, or chronic/recurrent pulmonary embolism).

THERAPEUTIC INTERVENTIONS	RATIONALE

Dependent/Collaborative Actions

Implement measures to prevent a pulmonary embolism: **D** ✦
- Maintain client on bed rest as ordered.
- Do not exercise or check for Homans' sign in affected extremity during acute phase of deep vein thrombosis.
- Never massage affected extremity, and caution client not to allow significant others to massage extremity.

Actions help to prevent dislodgment of thrombus.

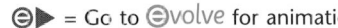

NDx = NANDA-I Diagnosis   **D** = Delegatable Action   ● = UAP   ✦ = LVN/LPN   ⊖▶ = Go to ⊖*volve* for animation

Continued...

THERAPEUTIC INTERVENTIONS	RATIONALE
• Caution client to avoid activities that create a Valsalva response (e.g., straining to have a bowel movement, blowing nose forcefully, holding breath while moving up in bed)	
• Administer anticoagulants as ordered. **D** ✦	*While anticoagulants will not dissolve clots, they will prevent development of new thrombi.*
• Prepare client for a vena caval interruption (e.g., insertion of an intracaval filtering device) if planned.	*These devices allow for filtration of clots without interruption of blood flow, reducing the risk of an embolus.*
If signs and symptoms of a pulmonary embolism occur:	
• Maintain client on bed rest in a semi- to high-Fowler's position.	*Semi- to high-Fowler's position facilitates adequate lung expansion.*
• Maintain oxygen therapy as ordered.	
• Prepare client for diagnostic tests (e.g., arterial blood gases, D-dimer level, ventilation-perfusion lung scan, pulmonary angiography).	
• Administer anticoagulants as ordered.	*Anticoagulants (e.g., heparin) prevent the formation of new clots, while thrombolytic agents dissolve pulmonary embolism.*
• Prepare client for the following if planned:	
• Injection of a thrombolytic agent (e.g., streptokinase, urokinase, tissue plasminogen activator [tPA])	
• Vena caval interruption (e.g., insertion of an intracaval filtering device)	*Vena caval interruption techniques assist in preventing further pulmonary embolization.*
• Embolectomy	*Primary indication for surgery is to prevent the recurrence of a pulmonary embolism.*

Collaborative Diagnosis | RISK FOR BLEEDING

Definition: Loss of blood from the circulatory system

Related to: Prolonged coagulation time associated with anticoagulant therapy and possible heparin-induced thrombocytopenia

CLINICAL MANIFESTATIONS

Subjective	Objective
Verbal reports of bleeding	Petechiae, purpura, ecchymoses; gingival bleeding; prolonged bleeding from puncture sites; epistaxis, hemoptysis; unusual joint pain; increase in abdominal girth; frank or occult blood in stool, urine, or vomitus; menorrhagia; restlessness, confusion; decreasing B/P and increased pulse rate; decrease in Hct and Hgb levels

RISK FACTORS

- Anticoagulant therapy
- Prolonged clotting times
- Heparin-induced thrombocytopenia

DESIRED OUTCOMES

The client will not experience unusual bleeding as evidenced by:
  a. Skin and mucous membranes free of petechiae, purpura, ecchymoses, and active bleeding
  b. Absence of unusual joint pain
  c. No increase in abdominal girth
  d. Absence of frank and occult blood in stool, urine, and vomitus
  e. Usual menstrual flow
  f. Vital signs within normal range for client
  g. Stable Hct and Hgb

NURSING ASSESSMENT	RATIONALE
Assess client for and report signs and symptoms of unusual bleeding:	*Early recognition of signs and symptoms of bleeding allows for prompt intervention.*

Assess client for and report signs and symptoms of unusual bleeding:
- Petechiae, purpura, ecchymoses
- Gingival bleeding
- Prolonged bleeding from puncture sites
- Epistaxis, hemoptysis
- Unusual joint pain
- Increase in abdominal girth
- Frank or occult blood in stool, urine, or vomitus
- Menorrhagia
- Restlessness, confusion
- Decreasing B/P and increased pulse rate
- Decrease in Hct and Hgb levels

Monitor Hct, platelet count, and coagulation test results (prothrombin time [PT], international normalized ratio [INR], activated partial thromboplastin time [aPTT], partial thromboplastin time [PTT]), and report abnormal values.

Assess stool, urine, and vomitus for blood.

Monitor and assess vital signs.

Early recognition of signs and symptoms of bleeding allows for prompt intervention.

THERAPEUTIC INTERVENTIONS	RATIONALE

Dependent/Collaborative Actions

Implement measures to prevent bleeding:
- Avoid giving injections whenever possible; consult physician for alternative routes.
- When giving injections or performing venous or arterial punctures, use the smallest gauge needle possible and apply gentle, prolonged pressure to the site after the needle is removed. **D** ▶
- Caution client to avoid activities that increase the risk for trauma (e.g., shaving with a straight-edge razor, using a stiff bristle toothbrush or dental floss).
- Pad side rails if client is confused or restless.
- Whenever possible, avoid intubations (e.g., nasogastric) and procedures that can cause injury to rectal mucosa (e.g., inserting a rectal suppository or tube, administering an enema).
- Perform actions to reduce the risk for falls (e.g., keep bed in low position with side rails up when client is in bed, avoid unnecessary clutter in room, instruct client to wear shoes with nonslip soles when ambulating). **D** ✦
- Instruct client to avoid blowing nose forcefully or straining to have a bowel movement; consult physician about an order for a decongestant and/or laxative if indicated.

Nursing activities should be adjusted to reduce the risk of bleeding while a client is undergoing anticoagulation therapy.

If bleeding occurs and does not subside spontaneously:
- Apply firm, prolonged pressure to bleeding areas if possible.
- If epistaxis occurs, place client in a high-Fowler's position and apply pressure and ice pack to nasal area.
- Maintain oxygen therapy as ordered.
- Administer protamine sulfate (antidote for heparin), vitamin K (e.g., phytonadione), and/or whole blood or blood products (e.g., fresh frozen plasma, platelets) as ordered.

If bleeding occurs, efforts must be directed at controlling active bleeding, replacing blood products as needed, and reversing anticoagulant therapy effects.

DISCHARGE TEACHING/CONTINUED CARE

Nursing Diagnosis ## DEFICIENT KNOWLEDGE NDx; INEFFECTIVE HEALTH MAINTENANCE NDx; OR INEFFECTIVE SELF-HEALTH MANAGEMENT NDx*

Definition: Absence or deficiency of cognitive information related to specific topic (lack of specific information necessary for clients/significant others to make informed choices regarding condition/treatment/lifestyle changes); inability to identify, manage, and/or seek out help to manage health; pattern of regulating and integrating into daily living a program for treatment of illness and the sequelae of illness that is unsatisfactory for meeting specific health goals

NOC OUTCOMES	NIC INTERVENTIONS
Knowledge: disease process; knowledge: treatment regimen	Health system guidance; teaching: individual; teaching: prescribed medication; teaching: prescribed activity/exercise

CLINICAL MANIFESTATIONS

Subjective	Objective
Verbalization of unfamiliarity with information	Inaccurate follow-through of instructions

RISK FACTORS
- Denial of disease process
- Cognitive deficiency
- Failure to take action to reduce risk factors

NURSING ASSESSMENT	RATIONALE
Assess client's readiness and ability to learn. Assess meaning of illness to client.	*Early recognition of readiness to learn and meaning of illness to client allows for implementation of the appropriate teaching interventions.*

THERAPEUTIC INTERVENTIONS	RATIONALE

Desired Outcome: The client will identify ways to promote venous blood flow and reduce the risk of chronic venous insufficiency and recurrent thrombus formation.

Independent Actions
Educate the client regarding interventions to reduce the risk of deep vein thrombosis:
- Avoid wearing constrictive clothing (e.g., garters, girdles, narrow-banded knee-high hose).
- Avoid sitting and standing in one position for long periods.
- Wear graduated compression stockings or support hose during the day.
- Avoid crossing legs and lying or sitting with pillows under knees.
- Engage in regular aerobic exercise (e.g., swimming, walking, bicycling).
- Elevate legs periodically, especially when sitting.
- Dorsiflex feet regularly.
- Maintain an ideal body weight for age, height, and body frame.

Inform client that smoking and the use of estrogen or oral contraceptives can increase the risk for recurrent thrombus formation.

Clients identified as at risk for the development of deep vein thrombosis should be educated as to what may precipitate embolic events. In addition, clients should be taught to recognize that vascular changes may indicate serious problems that require prompt treatment.

*The nurse should select the diagnostic label most appropriate for the client's discharge teaching needs.

THERAPEUTIC INTERVENTIONS	RATIONALE

Desired Outcome: The client will verbalize an understanding of medications ordered including rationale, food and drug interactions, side effects, schedule for taking, and importance of taking as prescribed.

Independent Actions

Educate the client regarding prescribed medications including rationale, food and drug interactions, side effects, dosing schedule, and importance of taking medications as prescribed.
- Coumadin
- Heparin

Taking medications as prescribed ensures that therapeutic drug levels will be maintained and adverse reactions avoided.
Clients should be instructed not to discontinue taking medications if they feel better. Clients without financial resources should be assisted in accessing appropriate resources to obtain needed medications (e.g., pharmacy assistance programs).

THERAPEUTIC INTERVENTIONS	RATIONALE

Desired Outcome: The client will demonstrate the ability to correctly draw up and administer heparin subcutaneously if prescribed.

Independent Actions

Provide instructions on subcutaneous injection techniques as needed.
Assess understanding through return demonstration.

Return demonstration of skill allows the nurse to evaluate client's understanding and implement additional education if necessary.

THERAPEUTIC INTERVENTIONS	RATIONALE

Desired Outcome: The client will identify precautions necessary to prevent bleeding associated with anticoagulant therapy.

Independent Actions

Instruct client about ways to minimize risk of bleeding:
- Use an electric rather than straight-edge razor.
- Floss and brush teeth gently; use waxed floss and a soft bristle toothbrush.
- Avoid putting sharp objects (e.g., toothpicks) in mouth.
- Do not walk barefoot.
- Cut nails carefully.
- Avoid situations that could result in injury (e.g., contact sports).
- Avoid blowing nose forcefully.
- Avoid straining to have a bowel movement.

Instruct client to control any bleeding by applying firm, prolonged pressure to the area if possible.

Actions that reduce the risk of bleeding prevent the development of complications.

THERAPEUTIC INTERVENTIONS	RATIONALE

Desired Outcome: The client will state signs and symptoms to report to the health care provider.

Independent Actions

Instruct the client to report the following signs and symptoms to the appropriate health care provider:
- Recurrent tenderness, pain, distention of superficial veins, or swelling in extremity
- Sudden chest pain accompanied by shortness of breath
- Unusual bleeding

Early identification of signs and symptoms of bleeding associated with drug therapy or the development of deep vein thrombosis allows for prompt intervention by the appropriate health care provider.

NDx = NANDA-I Diagnosis   **D** = Delegatable Action   ● = UAP   ✦ = LVN/LPN   ⊖▶ = Go to ⊖volve for animation

Continued...

THERAPEUTIC INTERVENTIONS	RATIONALE
• Discoloration or itching of affected extremity (indicative of stasis dermatitis associated with chronic venous insufficiency)	
• Skin breakdown on affected extremity	
Reinforce importance of keeping follow-up appointments with health care provider.	*Regular health care appointments are important to determine effectiveness of the prescribed treatment plan.*
Reinforce physician's instructions regarding activity limitations.	
Implement measures to improve client compliance:	
• Include significant others in teaching sessions if possible.	*Involvement of significant others in patient teaching improves adherence to discharge instructions.*
• Encourage questions and allow time for reinforcement and clarification of information provided.	*Everyone does not understand information as presented, so set aside time for questions to allow for clarification of information.*
• Provide written instructions regarding future appointments with health care provider, medications prescribed, activity restrictions, signs and symptoms to report, and future laboratory studies.	*Written instructions allow the client to refer to instructions as needed.*

FEMOROPOPLITEAL BYPASS

Lower extremity arterial bypass is performed to treat peripheral artery insufficiency that has not responded well to conservative management. The impaired blood flow can occur as a result of acute conditions (e.g., trauma, embolization), but most often is caused by atherosclerotic changes in the vessels. The femoropopliteal arterial segment is the most common site of occlusion in persons with lower extremity arterial disease. Surgical intervention is usually indicated when the client experiences signs and symptoms of severe occlusion (e.g., intermittent claudication that has become disabling, foot pain that is present at rest, presence of lower extremity ischemic ulcers) and/or when more conservative invasive treatment measures such as balloon angioplasty, laser angioplasty, stent placement, or percutaneous atherectomy have been unsuccessful.

Surgical treatment of the diseased femoropopliteal arterial segment can be accomplished by endarterectomy or removal of the segment and replacement with a synthetic graft, but the most commonly performed procedure is to bypass the segment using a synthetic or an autogenous vein graft. The saphenous vein is the preferred autogenous graft for femoropopliteal bypass because it is thick walled and has an adequate lumen diameter. Before grafting the saphenous vein proximal and distal to the occluded arterial segment, reversal of the vein or division of its valve cusps is done to allow unimpeded arterial blood flow.

This care plan focuses on the adult client with atherosclerotic occlusion of the femoropopliteal arterial segment who is hospitalized for a femoropopliteal bypass. Much of the postoperative information is applicable to clients receiving follow-up care in an extended care facility or home setting.

OUTCOME/DISCHARGE CRITERIA

The client will:
1. Have adequate circulation in the operative extremity
2. Have surgical pain controlled
3. Tolerate expected level of activity
4. Have evidence of normal wound healing
5. Have no signs and symptoms of postoperative complications
6. Identify ways to prevent or slow the progression of atherosclerosis
7. Identify ways to promote blood flow in the operative extremity
8. State signs and symptoms to report to the health care provider
9. Verbalize an understanding of and a plan for adhering to recommended follow-up care including future appointments with health care provider, medications prescribed, activity level, and wound care.

PREOPERATIVE: USE IN CONJUNCTION WITH THE STANDARDIZED PREOPERATIVE CARE PLAN

Nursing Diagnosis ## INEFFECTIVE TISSUE PERFUSION: PERIPHERAL NDx

Definition: Decrease in oxygen resulting from failure to nourish tissues at the capillary level

Related to: Diminished blood flow in the affected lower extremity associated with:
- Atherosclerotic changes in the femoral and popliteal arteries
- Thrombus formation in the affected vessel

CLINICAL MANIFESTATIONS

Subjective	Objective
Verbal reports of altered sensation to the affected extremity; intermittent claudication; slow healing of lesions	Altered skin characteristics (hair, moisture) or nails; cold extremities; diminished arterial pulses; pale skin upon leg elevation; pallor; shiny, waxy skin; weak or absent pulses

RISK FACTOR
- Virchow's triad: venous stasis, endothelial trauma (surgery), blood hypercoagulability

DESIRED OUTCOMES

The client will not experience further reduction in arterial blood flow in the affected lower extremity as evidenced by:
  a. No increase in lower extremity pain
  b. No further decrease in peripheral pulses
  c. No increase in capillary refill time
  d. Usual temperature and color of extremity

NOC OUTCOMES

Tissue perfusion: peripheral

NIC INTERVENTIONS

Circulatory care: arterial insufficiency; circulatory care: venous insufficiency; lower extremity monitoring

NURSING ASSESSMENT	**RATIONALE**
Assess for and report signs and symptoms of a further reduction in arterial blood flow in the affected lower extremity: • Intermittent claudication occurring with increased intensity and/or with less activity than previously • Development of or increase in intensity of rest pain (the foot and toe pain that occurs when the client is in a horizontal position results from decreased blood flow to the skin and subcutaneous tissue; because it occurs in the absence of lower extremity muscle activity, it reflects a severe reduction in the femoropopliteal arterial blood flow) • Diminishing peripheral pulses • Increase in usual capillary refill time • Increased coolness and numbness of foot and lower leg • Increased pallor or blanching of foot and lower leg when extremity is elevated • More rapid appearance of rubor or cyanosis in foot and lower leg when extremity is in a dependent position	*Early recognition of signs and symptoms of altered peripheral tissue perfusion allows for prompt intervention.*

Continued...

THERAPEUTIC INTERVENTIONS	RATIONALE
Independent Actions	
Implement measures to prevent further reduction in and/or improve blood flow in the affected lower extremity: **D** ✦	
• Discourage positions that compromise blood flow in lower extremities (e.g., crossing legs, pillows under knees, use of knee gatch, elevating legs when in bed, sitting for long periods).	*Prevents pooling of blood in the extremities.*
• Perform actions to prevent vasoconstriction:	*Reduces vascular response to the neuroendocrine stimulation.*
• Implement measures to reduce stress (e.g., maintain a calm environment, control pain, explain preoperative and postoperative care).	
• Discourage smoking.	*Stimulates release of norepinephrine.*
• Implement measures to keep client from getting cold (e.g., maintain a comfortable room temperature; provide adequate clothing, warm socks, and blankets).	
• Encourage short walks unless contraindicated.	*Promotes venous return.*
Dependent/Collaborative Actions	
Administer the following medications if ordered:	*Hemorrheologic agents help to improve the flow of blood to the ischemic area. Anticoagulants help to prevent or treat thrombi.*
• A hemorrheologic agent	
• Anticoagulants	
Consult physician if signs and symptoms of further reduction in lower extremity tissue perfusion occur.	*Notification of the appropriate health care provider allows for modification of the treatment plan.*

Nursing Diagnosis   # ACUTE/CHRONIC PAIN NDx (INTERMITTENT CLAUDICATION AND REST PAIN)

Definitions:

Acute pain—Unpleasant sensory and emotional experience arising from actual or potential tissue damage with a duration of less than 6 months

Chronic pain—Unpleasant sensory and emotional experience arising from actual or potential tissue damage without an anticipated end and a duration of greater than 6 months; can be associated with a chronic pathological process or recurs at intervals for months or years

Related to: Diminished arterial blood flow in the affected lower extremity (ischemia results in the release of anaerobic metabolites that irritate the nerve endings of the affected lower extremity)

CLINICAL MANIFESTATIONS

Subjective	Objective
Client's self report of pain; helplessness; anxiety	Expressions of pain are variable; diaphoresis, B/P and pulse changes

RISK FACTORS	DESIRED OUTCOMES
• Immobility	The client will experience diminished lower extremity pain as evidenced by:
• Blood hypercoagulability	a. Verbalization of same
• Peripheral vascular disease	b. Relaxed facial expression and body positioning

NOC OUTCOMES	NIC INTERVENTIONS
Comfort level; pain control	Pain management

NURSING ASSESSMENT	RATIONALE
Assess for and report signs and symptoms of pain in the affected lower extremity: • Intermittent claudication (e.g., verbalization of pain, aching, and/or cramping [usually in the calf muscle] during ambulation) • Rest pain (e.g., awakening at night with reports of severe burning or aching in foot or toes) • Grimacing, restlessness, reluctance to move, and/or rubbing leg or foot Assess client's perception of the severity of pain using a pain intensity rating scale. Assess the client's pain pattern (e.g., location, quality, onset, duration, precipitating factors, aggravating factors, alleviating factors).	*Early recognition of signs and symptoms of acute/chronic pain allows for prompt intervention.*

THERAPEUTIC INTERVENTIONS	RATIONALE
Independent Actions Implement measures to reduce pain in the affected extremity: **D** ✦ • Perform actions to prevent further reduction in and/or improve blood flow in the affected lower extremity: • Discourage positions that compromise blood flow in lower extremities (e.g., crossing legs, pillows under knees, use of knee gatch, elevating legs when in bed, sitting for long periods).	*Improves blood flow from the lower extremities.*
• Perform actions to reduce fear and anxiety about the pain experience (e.g., assure client that the need for pain relief is understood, plan methods for achieving pain control with client).	*Fear and anxiety can decrease the client's threshold and tolerance for pain and thereby heighten the perception of pain.*

• Perform actions to reduce the number of episodes of intermittent claudication:
  • Encourage client to stop activity minutes before symptoms are usually experienced (intermittent claudication is predictable, and clients are often aware of how far or how long they can ambulate before the discomfort begins or intensifies).
  • Maintain client on bed rest if experiencing severe intermittent claudication.
	Limiting activity decreases muscle contractions in and subsequent ischemia of the affected lower extremity.

• If client is experiencing rest pain in the affected extremity, perform actions to facilitate gravity flow of arterial blood to the ischemic area: **D** ✦
  • Allow client to sleep in a recliner with legs in a dependent position or, if in bed, to hang affected lower leg over the side of bed.
  • Instruct client to avoid horizontal positioning and elevation of affected extremity for prolonged periods.
• Provide lightweight blankets or a foot cradle if external pressure aggravates lower extremity pain.
• Provide or assist with nonpharmacological measures for relief of pain (e.g., relaxation techniques; position change; diversional activities such as conversing, watching television, or reading). **D** ✦	

Dependent/Collaborative Actions Implement measures to reduce pain in the affected extremity: • Administer analgesics (if ordered). **D** ✦ Consult physician if above measures fail to provide adequate pain relief.	*Notification of the appropriate health care provider allows for modification of the treatment plan.*

NDx = NANDA-I Diagnosis   **D** = Delegatable Action   ● = UAP   ✦ = LVN/LPN   ⊖▶ = Go to ⊖volve for animation

POSTOPERATIVE: USE IN CONJUNCTION WITH THE STANDARDIZED POSTOPERATIVE CARE PLAN

Nursing Diagnosis   INEFFECTIVE TISSUE PERFUSION: PERIPHERAL NDx

Definition: Decrease in oxygen resulting from failure to nourish tissues at the capillary level

Related to: Diminished blood flow in the operative extremity associated with:
- Inflammation of the femoral and popliteal arteries at the sites of graft anastomoses
- Pressure on vessels in the operative extremity resulting from edema that can occur as a result of decreased venous return and dissection of tissue around perivascular lymphatics
- Venous stasis resulting from decreased mobility and decreased venous return if the saphenous vein was used for the bypass graft (can result in impaired venous return until collateral venous circulation improves)
- Graft occlusion
- Hypovolemia resulting from blood loss during surgery and decreased fluid intake

CLINICAL MANIFESTATIONS

Subjective	Objective
Verbal reports of pain unrelieved by analgesics; numbness	Diminished or absent pulses; diminished or absent Doppler flow; coolness/cyanosis of foot; increased edema in operative extremity; capillary refill time greater than 2 to 3 seconds

RISK FACTOR
- Virchow's triad: venous stasis, endothelial trauma (surgery), blood hypercoagulability

DESIRED OUTCOMES

The client will maintain adequate tissue perfusion in the operative extremity as evidenced by:
  a. Resolution of leg and foot pain
  b. Palpable peripheral pulses
  c. Adequate Doppler flow readings in operative extremity
  d. Absence of coolness, numbness, and cyanosis in foot and lower leg
  e. Resolution of edema in operative extremity
  f. Capillary refill time less than 2 to 3 seconds

NOC OUTCOMES

Tissue perfusion: peripheral

NIC INTERVENTIONS

Circulatory care: arterial insufficiency; circulatory care: venous insufficiency; lower extremity monitoring

NURSING ASSESSMENT

Assess for and report signs and symptoms of ineffective tissue perfusion in operative extremity:
- Pain unrelieved by prescribed analgesics
- Diminished or absent pulses (the pulses may be difficult to palpate for 4 to 12 hours after surgery because of vasospasm that can occur in the operative extremity)
- Diminished or absent Doppler flow readings over operative extremity
- Coolness, numbness, or cyanosis of foot and lower leg
- Increase in edema in the operative extremity
- Capillary refill time greater than 2 to 3 seconds

RATIONALE

Early recognition and reporting of signs and symptoms of ineffective peripheral tissue perfusion allow for prompt intervention.

THERAPEUTIC INTERVENTIONS	RATIONALE

Independent Actions

Implement measures to promote adequate tissue perfusion in operative extremity: **D** ✦

- Avoid 90 degrees flexion of the hip as much as possible (e.g., place client in high-Fowler's position for meals only, limit length of time that client is in straight-back chair, provide recliner for client's use when sitting up).

  Extensive flexing of the hip can reduce perfusion to the operative limb.

- Limit length of time that operative leg is in dependent position (e.g., allow client to sit up for meals only; encourage short, frequent walks rather than long walks).

  Sitting for an extended period with legs in a dependent position may increase peripheral edema, stressing suture line.

- Instruct client to keep knee in a neutral or slightly flexed position.
- Perform actions to prevent graft occlusion.
- If lower extremity edema is present, elevate foot of bed 15 degrees as ordered.

  Elevation of the edematous operative extremity helps to promote venous return without compromising arterial flow.

- Place a bed cradle over lower extremities.

  Bed cradles help to minimize pressure from bed linens.

- Instruct client to perform active foot and leg exercises every 1 to 2 hours while awake.
- Perform actions to prevent vasoconstriction:

  Vasoconstriction narrows vessel lumens, which results in diminished blood flow through affected vessels.

  - Implement measures to reduce stress (e.g., control pain, maintain a calm environment, explain postoperative care).

    Stress stimulates the sympathetic nervous system, which results in vasoconstriction.

  - Discourage smoking.

    Nicotine increases catecholamine output, which subsequently causes vasoconstriction.

  - Implement measures to keep client from getting cold (e.g., maintain a comfortable room temperature; provide adequate clothing, warm socks, and blankets).

    When the body is cold, peripheral vasoconstriction occurs in an attempt to conserve heat.

Dependent/Collaborative Actions

Implement measures to promote adequate tissue perfusion in operative extremity:

- Maintain a minimum fluid intake of 2500 mL/day unless contraindicated; if oral intake is inadequate or contraindicated, maintain intravenous fluid therapy as ordered.

  Intravenous fluids and/or blood help maintain vascular volume, which is essential for adequate tissue perfusion.

- Administer blood and blood products as ordered.

Consult physician if signs and symptoms of diminished tissue perfusion in the operative extremity persist or worsen.

  Notification of the appropriate health care provider allows for modification of the treatment plan.

Collaborative Diagnosis | # RISK FOR GRAFT OCCLUSION

Definition: Obstruction of blood flow to the vascular graft

Related to: Thrombus formation, kink in graft, inadequate vessel lumen diameter at sites of anastomoses, or dislodgment of surgical site debris

CLINICAL MANIFESTATIONS

Subjective	Objective
Verbal reports of sudden, severe pain in affected extremity	Diminished or absent pulses; capillary refill time greater than 2 to 3 seconds; cyanosis; coolness or diminished sensation in foot

Continued...

RISK FACTORS

- Blood hypercoagulability
- Immobility

DESIRED OUTCOMES

The client will maintain a patent graft in the operative extremity as evidenced by:
  a. No reports of sudden, severe toe or foot pain
  b. Palpable peripheral pulses
  c. Capillary refill time less than 2 to 3 seconds
  d. Absence of cyanosis, coolness, and diminishing sensation in the foot

NURSING ASSESSMENT

Assess for and report signs and symptoms of graft occlusion in the operative extremity:
- Sudden, severe pain in toes or foot
- Diminishing or absent peripheral pulses
- Capillary refill time greater than 2 to 3 seconds
- Cyanosis, coolness, or diminished sensation in the foot

RATIONALE

Early recognition of signs and symptoms of acute graft occlusion allows for prompt intervention.

THERAPEUTIC INTERVENTIONS

Dependent/Collaborative Actions

Instruct client to avoid prolonged flexion of the knee on the operative extremity (e.g., limit sitting as ordered, do not place pillows under knees when in bed).

Implement measures to promote adequate tissue perfusion in operative extremity: **D** ✦
- Avoid 90 degrees flexion of the hip.
- Elevate the affected extremity if edematous.
- Perform actions to prevent vasoconstriction.
- Administer anticoagulants if ordered.

If signs and symptoms of graft occlusion occur:
- Maintain client on bed rest with operative leg in a level or slightly dependent position.
- Administer anticoagulants as ordered.
- Prepare client for surgical intervention (e.g., removal of debris or thrombus, straightening of graft, widening of lumen at site[s] of anastomosis) if planned.

RATIONALE

Actions help to prevent kinking of the graft and subsequent graft occlusion.

Actions help to reduce the risk of thrombus formation.

Prevents pooling of blood in lower extremities as well as dependent edema, which may stress suture lines.

Action helps to improve arterial blood flow.

Collaborative Diagnosis   RISK FOR COMPARTMENT SYNDROME

Definition: Elevated intracompartmental pressure within a confined myofascial compartment compromises the neurovascular function of tissues within that space

Related to: Severe edema of the operative extremity (an infrequent but serious complication that can occur as a result of surgical site inflammation, reperfusion of the ischemic muscles, or dissection of tissue around the perivascular lymphatics)

CLINICAL MANIFESTATIONS

Subjective	Objective
Verbal reports of increasing leg pain; new onset or increasing numbness of affected extremity; difficulty moving foot	Diminished or absent peripheral pulses; cyanotic, cool leg

RISK FACTORS

- Acute arterial occlusion
- Prolonged ischemia to tissues

DESIRED OUTCOMES

The client will not experience compartment syndrome in the operative extremity as evidenced by:
   a. No complaints of increasing leg pain
   b. No statements of new or increasing numbness and tingling in foot or leg, or tightness and tenseness of thigh or calf muscle
   c. Ability to move leg and foot
   d. No decrease in or absence of peripheral pulses
   e. Absence of cyanosis and coldness of leg and foot

NURSING ASSESSMENT

Assess for and report signs and symptoms of compartment syndrome in the operative extremity:
- Sudden, severe pain in toes or foot
- Diminishing or absent peripheral pulses
- Capillary refill time greater than 2 to 3 seconds
- Cyanosis, coolness, or diminished sensation in the foot

Assess for and report reddish-brown discoloration of urine.

RATIONALE

Early recognition of signs and symptoms of compartment syndrome allows for prompt intervention.

Assessment finding of reddish-brown urine discoloration could indicate myoglobinuria resulting from the release of myoglobin from the damaged muscle cells. If an excessive amount of myoglobin is released, it can get trapped in the renal tubules and cause renal failure.

THERAPEUTIC INTERVENTIONS

Dependent/Collaborative Actions

Limit length of time that operative leg is in a dependent position (e.g., limit sitting and walking as ordered).

Elevate operative extremity 15 degrees if ordered.

Administer osmotic diuretics if ordered.

If signs and symptoms of compartment syndrome occur:
- Maintain client on bed rest.
- Prepare client for a fasciotomy if planned.

RATIONALE

Measures help to prevent an increase in edema in operative leg in order to reduce the risk of development of compartment syndrome.

Surgical decompression (fasciotomy) may be necessary to decompress soft tissue and improve circulation.

Collaborative Diagnosis **RISK FOR SAPHENOUS NERVE DAMAGE**

Definition: Damage to the saphenous nerve

Related to:
- Inadvertent or unavoidable dissection of the nerve during surgery
- Trauma to the nerve during surgery

CLINICAL MANIFESTATIONS

Subjective	Objective
Verbal reports of numbness and tingling in affected extremity; heightened sensitivity to affected extremity	Not applicable

RISK FACTOR

- Vascular surgery

DESIRED OUTCOME

The client will have resolution of or adapt to operative extremity saphenous nerve damage if it has occurred.

NDx = NANDA-I Diagnosis   **D** = Delegatable Action   ● = UAP   ✦ = LVN/LPN   ⊖▶ = Go to ⊖volve for animation

Continued...

NURSING ASSESSMENT	RATIONALE
Assess for and report signs and symptoms of saphenous nerve damage: • Numbness, tingling • Hypersensitivity of the operative extremity	*Early recognition of signs and symptoms of saphenous nerve damage allows for prompt intervention.*

THERAPEUTIC INTERVENTIONS	RATIONALE

Dependent/Collaborative Actions
If signs and symptoms of saphenous nerve damage are present:
• Adhere to and instruct client in the following safety precautions:
  • Wear shoes or slippers whenever out of bed.
  • Do not apply heat or cold to the affected extremity.
  • Test temperature of bath water before use.
  • Protect operative extremity from trauma.
• Reinforce information from physician regarding permanence of numbness, tingling, or hypersensitivity.
 	
• Consult physician if signs and symptoms increase in severity.
	
	Nerve damage eliminates ability to sense temperature changes which can lead to tissue damage.
	These symptoms are permanent if the nerve was severed during surgery; if the nerve was just traumatized, the symptoms are temporary and expected to resolve within 1 year.
	Notification of the appropriate health care provider allows for modification of the treatment plan.

DISCHARGE TEACHING/CONTINUED CARE

Nursing Diagnosis | # DEFICIENT KNOWLEDGE NDx; INEFFECTIVE FAMILY THERAPEUTIC REGIMEN MANAGEMENT NDx; OR INEFFECTIVE SELF-HEALTH MANAGEMENT NDx*

Definition: Absence or deficiency of cognitive information related to specific topic (lack of specific information necessary for clients/significant others to make informed choices regarding condition/treatment/lifestyle changes); pattern of regulating and integrating into daily living and family processes a program for treatment of illness and the sequelae of illness that is unsatisfactory for meeting specific health goals

CLINICAL MANIFESTATIONS

Subjective	Objective
Verbalization of unfamiliarity with information	Inaccurate follow-through of instructions

NOC OUTCOMES	NIC INTERVENTIONS
Knowledge: treatment regimen; knowledge: cardiac disease management	Health system guidance; teaching: individual; teaching: disease process; teaching: prescribed diet; teaching: prescribed activity/exercise

RISK FACTORS
• Denial of disease process
• Cognitive deficiency
• Failure to take action to reduce risk factors

NURSING ASSESSMENT	RATIONALE
Assess client's readiness and ability to learn. Assess meaning of illness to client.	*Early recognition of readiness to learn and meaning of illness to client allows for implementation of the appropriate teaching interventions.*

*The nurse should select the diagnostic label that is most appropriate for the client's discharge teaching needs.

THERAPEUTIC INTERVENTIONS	RATIONALE

Desired Outcome: The client will identify ways to prevent or slow the progression of atherosclerosis.

Independent Actions

Inform the client that certain modifiable factors such as elevated serum lipid levels, a sedentary lifestyle, smoking, and hypertension have been shown to increase the risk of atherosclerosis.

After vascular surgery, clients should be educated as to health promotion activities that slow the progression of atherosclerosis.

Assist client to identify changes in lifestyle that could reduce the risk for atherosclerosis (e.g., smoking cessation, dietary modifications, physical exercise on a regular basis).

Making these changes will decrease the incidence of hypertension and improve circulatory status to the lower extremities.

Provide instructions on ways the client can reduce intake of saturated fat and cholesterol:

Dietary modifications that reduce saturated fat and cholesterol intake may slow the progression of arteriosclerosis.

- Reduce intake of meat fat (e.g., trim visible fat off meat; replace fatty meats such as fatty cuts of steak, hamburger, and processed meats with leaner products).
- Reduce intake of milk fat (e.g., avoid dairy products containing more than 1% fat).
- Reduce intake of *trans* fats (e.g., avoid stick margarine and shortening and foods such as commercial baked goods that are prepared with these products).
- Use vegetable oil rather than coconut or palm oil in cooking and food preparation.
- Use cooking methods such as steaming, baking, broiling, poaching, microwaving, and grilling rather than frying.
- Restrict intake of eggs (recommendations about the number of whole eggs allowed per week vary depending on the client's lipid levels).

Instruct client to take lipid-lowering agents as prescribed.

Lipid-lowering agents help to keep cholesterol within normal limits, reducing the risk of atherosclerosis.

THERAPEUTIC INTERVENTIONS	RATIONALE

Desired Outcome: The client will identify ways to promote blood flow in the operative extremity.

Independent Actions

Provide the following instructions about ways to promote blood flow in the operative extremity:

Actions reduce the risk of compression of vessels, which may compromise blood flow.

- Avoid wearing constrictive clothing (e.g., garters, girdles, narrow-banded knee-high stockings).
- Avoid positions that compromise blood flow (e.g., pillows under knees, crossing legs, sitting or standing for prolonged periods).
- Do active foot and leg exercises for 5 minutes every hour while awake.

Dorsiflexion/plantar extension exercises help to stimulate blood flow to the extremities.

- Maintain a regular exercise program (walking and swimming are recommended).
- Stop smoking.
- Drink at least 10 glasses of liquid per day unless contraindicated.

Proper hydration thins circulating blood volume, allowing for optimum flow through vessels.

THERAPEUTIC INTERVENTIONS	RATIONALE

Desired Outcome: The client will state signs and symptoms to report to the health care provider.

NDx = NANDA-I Diagnosis   **D** = Delegatable Action   ● = UAP   ✦ = LVN/LPN   ⊖▶ = Go to ⊖volve for animation

Continued...

THERAPEUTIC INTERVENTIONS	RATIONALE

Independent Actions

Instruct client to report these additional signs and symptoms:

- Sudden or gradual increase in operative leg or foot pain
- Increased swelling or purple discoloration at incision sites
- Pallor, coldness, or bluish color of the operative extremity
- Diminishing or sudden absence of peripheral pulses (client may be instructed to monitor his/her peripheral pulses)
- Significant increase in swelling of operative extremity (edema is expected to resolve gradually within the first 2 to 8 weeks after surgery)
- Difficulty moving foot on operative side
- Increasing numbness and/or tingling sensation of operative lower leg or foot
- Any area of persistent skin irritation or breakdown of foot on operative side

Early identification of signs and symptoms of bleeding associated with drug therapy or the development of arterial or venous thrombosis allows for prompt intervention by the appropriate health care provider.

THERAPEUTIC INTERVENTIONS	RATIONALE

Desired Outcome: The client will verbalize an understanding of and a plan for adhering to recommended follow-up care including future appointments with health care provider, medications prescribed, activity level, and wound care.

Independent Actions

Reinforce the physician's instructions regarding:

- Importance of scheduling adequate rest periods
- Need to avoid sitting or standing for long periods
- Need to take prophylactic antimicrobials before any dental work or invasive procedure (some physicians recommend this for the first 6 to 12 months after surgical placement of a synthetic graft)

Promotes healing.
Decreases pooling of blood in the lower extremities.
Prevents infection.

RELATED CARE PLANS

Standardized Preoperative Care Plan
Standardized Postoperative Care Plan

HEART FAILURE

Heart failure is a syndrome in which the heart is unable to pump an adequate supply of blood to meet the body's metabolic needs. To compensate for decreased cardiac output, there is an increase in sympathetic nervous system activity and stimulation of renin-angiotensin-aldosterone output and antidiuretic hormone (ADH) release. These neurohormonal compensatory mechanisms temporarily aid in maintaining an adequate cardiac output but are thought to contribute to cardiac remodeling (changes in the structure of the ventricle [e.g., dilation, hypertrophy]). The increase in fluid volume that results from increased aldosterone and ADH causes elevated pressure in the cardiac chambers, which stimulates the release of natriuretic peptides (atrial natriuretic factor [ANF] and brain natriuretic peptide [BNP]). These hormones coun-

teract the effects of the increased levels of norepinephrine, renin, angiotensin II, and aldosterone and promote sodium and water excretion and vasodilation. Chronic distention of the heart chambers eventually exhausts stores of these natriuretic hormones and the effects of norepinephrine, renin, aldosterone, and ADH prevail, leading to heart failure.

Numerous conditions can lead to heart failure including coronary artery disease, myocardial infarction, cardiomyopathy, cardiac valve malfunction, hypertension, congenital heart defects, and systemic conditions that increase the metabolic rate (e.g., thyrotoxicosis, infection) or cause prolonged or severe hypoxia. Heart failure can be classified in a number of ways. It is often classified as left-sided or right-sided, backward or forward, and/or systolic or diastolic failure. A functional classification system based on the relationship between symptoms and the amount of activity needed to provoke the symptoms was developed by the New York Heart Association and is commonly used by many practitioners. In this system, which has 4 levels or classes, a person is said to have Class I heart failure if no symptoms are experienced with ordinary physical activity and Class IV failure when symptoms occur with any physical activity and possibly at rest.

Signs and symptoms of heart failure are dependent on which side of the heart is failing as well as whether there is forward or backward failure. Symptoms of forward failure are caused by low cardiac output. Symptoms of backward failure are associated with the ventricle failing to empty completely, which results in blood flow backup. In left-sided failure, there is reduced emptying of the left ventricle, which results in decreased systemic tissue perfusion as well as blood flow backup in the left atrium and pulmonary vasculature. Pulmonary vascular congestion leads to pulmonary edema with symptoms such as tachypnea, dyspnea, cough, and abnormal breath sounds. In right-sided failure, the effect of reduced function and emptying of the right ventricle is decreased pulmonary blood flow and backup of blood in the right atrium. This results in systemic venous congestion, which is manifested by peripheral edema and signs of major organ enlargement and dysfunction. Initially only one side of the heart may fail (more commonly the left side), but as failure progresses, both sides are usually affected.

The focus of treatment is to improve performance of the failing heart. Diuretic therapy and an angiotensin-converting enzyme (ACE) inhibitor remain the cornerstone of treatment. A positive inotropic agent is often added to ameliorate symptoms. Recent studies have shown that the addition of a beta-adrenergic blocking agent and spironolactone also improve the clinical status of many persons with chronic heart failure. It is thought that ACE inhibitors, beta blockers, and spironolactone interfere with the compensatory neurohormonal activity that occurs with heart failure and alter the course of cardiac remodeling, subsequently slowing disease progression. The pharmacological treatment of heart failure varies somewhat depending on whether the client has systolic failure (an impaired inotropic state characterized by inadequate ventricular emptying) or diastolic failure (impaired filling of the ventricle). Positive inotropic agents are contraindicated for treatment of diastolic failure.

As long as the body's compensatory mechanisms and/or treatment measures are able to maintain cardiac output that is sufficient to prevent or relieve symptoms, a state of compensated heart failure exists. If the myocardium is severely damaged and intrinsic compensatory mechanisms and treatment measures fail to maintain adequate cardiac output and tissue perfusion, a state of decompensated heart failure exists. When this state persists and is no longer responsive to medical treatment, it is termed intractable or refractory heart failure.

This care plan focuses on the adult client hospitalized for management of heart failure. Much of the information is applicable to clients receiving follow-up care in an extended care facility or home setting.

OUTCOME/DISCHARGE CRITERIA

The client will:
1. Have vital signs within a safe range and evidence of adequate peripheral circulation
2. Tolerate expected level of activity without undue fatigue or dyspnea
3. Have achieved dry weight and have minimal or no edema
4. Have clear, audible breath sounds throughout lungs
5. Have oxygen saturation within normal limits for client's age
6. Identify modifiable cardiovascular risk factors and ways to alter these factors
7. Verbalize an understanding of the rationale for and components of a diet low in sodium
8. Demonstrate accuracy in counting pulse
9. Verbalize an understanding of medications ordered including rationale, food and drug interactions, side effects, schedule for taking, and importance of taking as prescribed
10. State signs and symptoms to report to the health care provider
11. Identify community resources that can assist with home management and adjustment to changes resulting from heart failure
12. Share feelings and concerns about changes in body functioning and usual roles and lifestyle
13. Verbalize an understanding of and a plan for adhering to recommended follow-up care including future appointments with health care provider and activity limitations.

USE IN CONJUNCTION WITH THE CARE PLAN ON IMMOBILITY

Nursing Diagnosis **DECREASED CARDIAC OUTPUT** NDx

Definition: Inadequate volume of blood pumped by the heart per minute to meet metabolic demands of the body

Related to:
* Alterations in preload, afterload, and myocardial contractility associated with the cardiac condition causing the heart failure (e.g., ischemia of the myocardium, valve malfunction, cardiomyopathy)
* The effects of sympathetic nervous system and renin-angiotensin-aldosterone stimulation that occur in response to decreased cardiac output
* Structural changes in the heart (e.g., dilation, hypertrophy) that occur with prolonged activation of neurohormonal adaptive responses

NDx = NANDA-I Diagnosis   **D** = Delegatable Action   ● = UAP   ✦ = LVN/LPN   ⊖▶ = Go to ⊖volve for animation

Continued...
CLINICAL MANIFESTATIONS

Subjective	Objective
Fatigue; weakness; dyspnea; orthopnea; dizziness	Variations in B/P; tachycardia; pulsus alternans; S_3 heart sounds; tachypnea; dry, hacking cough; productive cough with pink, frothy sputum; abnormal breath sounds (e.g., crackles/rales, wheezes); syncope; diminished or absent pulses; cool extremities; capillary refill time greater than 3 seconds; decreased urine output; nocturia; edema; jugular venous distention; elevated serum levels of BNP and ANF; increased central venous pressure (CVP); chest radiograph evidence of pulmonary vascular congestion or pulmonary edema

DESIRED OUTCOMES

The client will have improved cardiac output as evidenced by:
a. B/P within normal range for client
b. Apical pulse between 60 and 100 beats/min and regular
c. Resolution of gallop rhythm
d. Verbalization of feeling less fatigued and weak
e. Unlabored respirations at 12 to 20 breaths/min
f. Improved breath sounds
g. Usual mental status
h. Absence of dizziness and syncope
i. Palpable peripheral pulses
j. Skin warm and usual color
k. Capillary refill time less than 2 to 3 seconds
l. Urine output at least 30 mL/h
m. Decrease in edema and jugular vein distention
n. CVP within normal range

NOC OUTCOMES

Cardiac pump effectiveness; circulation status; tissue perfusion: peripheral

NIC INTERVENTIONS

Cardiac care: acute; invasive hemodynamic monitoring; hemodynamic regulation; cardiac precautions; dysrhythmia management; hypervolemia management; cardiac care: rehabilitative

NURSING ASSESSMENT

Assess for signs and symptoms of heart failure and decreased cardiac output:
- Dyspnea, orthopnea
- Variations in B/P
- Tachycardia
- Pulsus alternans
- S_3 heart sounds
- Tachypnea
- Dry, hacking cough
- Productive cough with pink, frothy sputum
- Abnormal breath sounds (e.g., crackles/rales, wheezes)
- Syncope
- Diminished or absent pulses
- Cool extremities
- Capillary refill time greater than 3 seconds
- Decreased urine output
- Nocturia
- Edema
- Jugular venous distention

Assess chest radiograph for abnormalities (e.g., pulmonary vascular congestion or pulmonary edema).
Assess serum levels of ANF and BNP for abnormalities.

RATIONALE

Early recognition of signs and symptoms of heart failure and decreased cardiac output allows for prompt intervention.

THERAPEUTIC INTERVENTIONS	RATIONALE

Independent Actions
Implement measures to improve cardiac output:
• Perform actions to reduce cardiac workload:
  • Place client in a semi- to high-Fowler's position. **D** ● ✦
  • Instruct client to avoid activities that create a Valsalva response (e.g., straining to have a bowel movement, holding breath while moving up in bed).
  • Implement measures to promote emotional and physical rest:
    • Maintain a calm, quiet environment.
    • Limit the number of visitors.
    • Maintain activity restrictions. **D** ● ✦
	Measures that impact preload, afterload, and contractility help to improve cardiac performance, resulting in increased cardiac output.

• Implement measures to improve respiratory status.
  • Position in semi- to high-Fowler's position
  • Administer supplemental oxygen
	Actions help improve alveolar gas exchange and promote adequate tissue oxygenation to the heart, improving performance.

• Discourage smoking. **D** ✦	*Nicotine has a cardiostimulatory effect and causes vasoconstriction; the carbon monoxide in smoke reduces oxygen availability.*
• Provide small meals rather than large ones. **D** ✦	*Large meals can increase cardiac workload because they require a greater increase in blood supply to gastrointestinal tract for digestion.*
• Discourage excessive intake of beverages high in caffeine such as coffee, tea, and colas. **D** ✦ • Increase activity gradually as allowed and tolerated. **D** ● ✦	*Caffeine is a myocardial stimulant and can increase myocardial oxygen consumption.*
Dependent/Collaborative Actions Implement measures to improve cardiac output: • Perform actions to reduce cardiac workload: • Implement measures to reduce excess fluid volume. • Administer diuretics (e.g., Lasix) • Administer the following medications if ordered:	*Decreasing circulating fluid volume reduces preload, reducing the workload of the heart.* *In addition, reducing excess fluid volume helps to decrease pulmonary vascular congestion.*
• Diuretics	*Reduce sodium and water retention and subsequently reduce cardiac workload.*
• ACE inhibitors	*Reduce vascular resistance and subsequently decrease cardiac workload; they also alter the course of cardiac remodeling and slow disease progression.*
• Positive inotropic agents	*To improve myocardial contractility*
• Beta-adrenergic blocking agents	*To blunt the effects of sympathetic nervous system stimulation on the heart and kidney*
• B-type natriuretic peptide (nesiritide)	*To promote diuresis and vasodilation*
• Vasodilators	*To reduce cardiac workload*
Consult physician if signs and symptoms of decreased cardiac output persist or worsen.	*Consulting the appropriate health care provider allows for modification of the treatment plan.*

Nursing Diagnosis **IMPAIRED RESPIRATORY FUNCTION***

Definition: Inspiration and/or expiration that does not provide adequate ventilation; inability to clear secretions or obstructions from the respiratory tract to maintain a clear airway

Ineffective breathing pattern NDx related to:
• Increased rate of respirations associated with fear and anxiety
• Decreased depth of respirations associated with:
  • Weakness, fatigue, and decreased mobility
  • Decreased lung compliance (distensibility) as a result of pleural effusion or accumulation of fluid in the pulmonary interstitium
  • Pressure on the diaphragm if ascites is present

---

*This diagnostic label includes the following nursing diagnoses: ineffective breathing pattern, ineffective airway clearance, and impaired gas exchange.

NDx = NANDA-I Diagnosis   **D** = Delegatable Action   ● = UAP   ✦ = LVN/LPN   ⊖▶ = Go to ⊖volve for animation

Continued...

Ineffective airway clearance NDx related to:
- Increased airway resistance associated with edema of the bronchial mucosa and pressure on the airways resulting from engorgement of the pulmonary vessels
- Stasis of secretions associated with decreased mobility and poor cough effort

Impaired gas exchange NDx related to:
- Impaired diffusion of gases associated with accumulation of fluid in the pulmonary interstitium and alveoli
- Decreased pulmonary tissue perfusion associated with decreased cardiac output

CLINICAL MANIFESTATIONS

Subjective	Objective
Reports of dyspnea; orthopnea; restlessness; irritability	Rapid, shallow, slow, or irregular respirations; use of accessory muscles when breathing; adventitious breath sounds (e.g., crackles [rales], wheezes); diminished or absent breath sounds; dry, hacking cough or cough productive of frothy or blood-tinged sputum; limited chest excursion; confusion, somnolence; central cyanosis (a late sign); significant decrease in oximetry results; abnormal arterial blood gas values; abnormal chest radiograph results

RISK FACTORS
- Fluid volume overload
- Structural valve defects
- Myocardial infarction

DESIRED OUTCOMES

The client will experience adequate respiratory function as evidenced by:
  a. Normal rate, rhythm, and depth of respirations
  b. Decreased dyspnea
  c. Usual or improved breath sounds
  d. Symmetrical chest excursion
  e. Usual mental status
  f. Oximetry results within normal range
  g. Arterial blood gas values within normal range

NOC OUTCOMES

Respiratory status: ventilation; respiratory status: airway patency; respiratory status: gas exchange

NIC INTERVENTIONS

Respiratory monitoring; airway management; chest physiotherapy; cough enhancement; ventilation assistance; oxygen therapy; anxiety reduction

NURSING ASSESSMENT	RATIONALE
Assess for signs and symptoms of impaired respiratory function: • Dyspnea, orthopnea • Restlessness, irritability • Rapid, shallow, slow, or irregular respirations • Use of accessory muscles when breathing • Adventitious breath sounds (e.g., crackles [rales], wheezes) • Diminished or absent breath sounds • Dry, hacking cough or cough productive of frothy or blood-tinged sputum • Limited chest excursion • Confusion, somnolence • Central cyanosis (a late sign) Assess results of chest radiograph, pulse oximetry, and arterial blood gases for abnormalities.	*Early recognition of signs and symptoms of impaired respiratory dysfunction allows for prompt intervention.*

THERAPEUTIC INTERVENTIONS	RATIONALE

Independent Actions
Implement measures to improve respiratory status:

- Perform actions to reduce fear and anxiety:
  - Maintain a calm, supportive, confident manner when interacting with the client.
- Instruct client to breathe slowly if hyperventilating.
- Place client in a semi- to high-Fowler's position unless contraindicated; position overbed table so client can lean forward on it if desired. **D** ● ✦
- Instruct client to change position and deep breathe or use incentive spirometer every 1 to 2 hours.
- Perform actions to increase strength and activity tolerance.
- Perform actions to promote removal of pulmonary secretions:
  - Instruct and assist client to cough or "huff" every 1 to 2 hours.
  - Humidify inspired air as ordered. **D** ✦
- Instruct client to avoid intake of gas-forming foods (e.g., beans, cauliflower, cabbage, onions), carbonated beverages, and large meals.
- Discourage smoking.

- Maintain activity restrictions; increase activity gradually as allowed and tolerated. **D** ● ✦

Dependent/Collaborative Actions
Implement measures to improve respiratory status:
- Perform actions to improve cardiac output:
  - Administer positive inotropic agents.

- Maintain oxygen therapy as ordered.
- Assist with positive airway pressure techniques (e.g., continuous positive airway pressure [CPAP], bilevel positive airway pressure [BiPAP], flutter/positive expiratory pressure [PEP] device) if ordered.
- Administer central nervous system depressants judiciously; hold medication and consult physician if respiratory rate is less than 12 breaths/min.
- Administer the following medications if ordered:
  - Diuretics **D** ✦
  - Theophylline **D** ✦
  - Morphine sulfate

- Assist with thoracentesis/paracentesis if performed.
- Consult appropriate health care provider (e.g., physician, respiratory therapist) if signs and symptoms of impaired respiratory function persist or worsen.

To improve pulmonary tissue perfusion and reduce fluid accumulation in the lungs.
Decreases respiratory rate and anxiety.

Improves lung expansion and decreases stasis of secretions.

Increasing strength and activity help with mobilization and removal of secretions.

To keep secretions thin.
In order to prevent gastric distention and an increase in pressure on the diaphragm.

The irritants in smoke increase mucus production, impair ciliary function, and can cause damage to the bronchial and alveolar walls; the carbon monoxide in smoke decreases oxygen availability.
Improves strength.

Positive inotropic agents increase cardiac output by improving myocardial contractility.
Improves tissue oxygenation.
Positive airway pressure techniques help to improve oxygenation by keeping terminal airways and alveoli open. The more alveoli that remain open, the better the gas exchange.

Diuretics help to decrease pulmonary vascular congestion.
Theophylline helps to dilate the bronchioles.
Morphine has a vasodilatory action that helps to reduce myocardial workload; morphine also reduces apprehension associated with dyspnea.
Removes excess fluid to allow increased lung expansion.
Allows for multidisciplinary client care.

Collaborative Diagnosis **RISK FOR IMBALANCED FLUID NDx AND RISK FOR ELECTROLYTE IMBALANCE NDx**

Definition: At risk for a decrease, increase, or rapid shift from one to the other of intravascular, interstitial, and/or intracellular fluid; at risk for a change in serum electrolyte levels

NDx = NANDA-I Diagnosis   **D** = Delegatable Action   ● = UAP   ✦ = LVN/LPN   ⊖▶ = Go to ⊖volve for animation

Continued...
Related to:

- **Excess fluid volume NDx** related to:
  - Retention of sodium and water associated with a decreased glomerular filtration rate (GFR) and activation of the renin-angiotensin-aldosterone mechanism (both are a result of the reduced renal blood flow that occurs with decreased cardiac output)
  - Decreased excretion of water associated with increased ADH output (a compensatory response to decreased cardiac output)
- **Third-spacing of fluid** related to:
  - Increased intravascular pressure associated with excess fluid volume
  - Low plasma colloid osmotic pressure if serum albumin is decreased as a result of malnutrition or impaired liver function (occurs with hepatic venous congestion)
- **Hyponatremia** related to:
  - Hemodilution associated with excess fluid volume
  - Sodium loss associated with diuretic therapy and increased release of natriuretic peptide hormones

CLINICAL MANIFESTATIONS

Subjective	Objective
Fluid overload: Reports of dyspnea; orthopnea	**Fluid overload:** Weight gain of 2% or greater in a short period; elevated B/P (B/P may not be elevated if cardiac output is poor or fluid has shifted out of the vascular space); presence of an S_3 heart sound; intake greater than output; change in mental status; crackles (rales); low Hct (may be normal or even increased if fluid has shifted out of the vascular space); edema; distended neck veins; elevated CVP (use internal jugular vein pulsation method to estimate CVP if monitoring device not present)
Third-spacing: Reports of increased dyspnea	**Third-spacing:** Ascites; diminished or absent breath sounds; evidence of vascular depletion (e.g., postural hypotension; weak, rapid pulse; decreased urine output)
Hyponatremia: Reports of nausea; weakness	**Hyponatremia:** Vomiting; abdominal cramps; confusion; seizures; low serum sodium level

DESIRED OUTCOMES

The client will experience resolution of fluid imbalance as evidenced by:
a. Decline in weight toward client's normal
b. B/P and pulse within normal range for client and stable with position change
c. Resolution of S_3 heart sound
d. Balanced intake and output
e. Usual mental status
f. Improved breath sounds
g. Hct returning toward normal range
h. Decreased dyspnea and orthopnea
i. Decrease in edema and ascites
j. Resolution of neck vein distention
k. CVP within normal range

The client will maintain a safe serum sodium level as evidenced by:
a. Usual mental status
b. Usual muscle strength
c. Absence of seizure activity
d. Serum sodium level within normal range

NOC OUTCOMES

Fluid balance; fluid overload severity; electrolyte and acid-base balance

NIC INTERVENTIONS

Fluid monitoring; fluid/electrolyte management; electrolyte management: hyponatremia; hypervolemia management

NURSING ASSESSMENT	RATIONALE
Assess for signs and symptoms of fluid and electrolyte imbalance:	*Early recognition of signs and symptoms of fluid and electrolyte imbalance allows for prompt intervention.*

Assess for signs and symptoms of fluid and electrolyte imbalance:
- Fluid overload
  - Dyspnea, orthopnea
  - Weight gain of 2% or greater in a short period
  - Elevated B/P (B/P may not be elevated if cardiac output is poor or fluid has shifted out of the vascular space)
  - Presence of an S_3 heart sound
  - Intake greater than output
  - Change in mental status
  - Crackles (rales),
  - Low Hct (may be normal or even increased if fluid has shifted out of the vascular space)
  - Edema
  - Distended neck veins
  - Elevated CVP (use internal jugular vein pulsation method to estimate CVP if monitoring device not present)
- Third-spacing
  - Increased dyspnea
  - Ascites
  - Diminished or absent breath sounds
  - Evidence of vascular depletion (e.g., postural hypotension; weak, rapid pulse; decreased urine output)
- Hyponatremia
  - Nausea, weakness
  - Vomiting
  - Abdominal cramps
  - Confusion
  - Seizures
  - Low serum sodium level

Monitor chest x-ray results for indications of pulmonary vascular congestion, pleural effusion, or pulmonary edema.

Monitor serum albumin levels for abnormalities.

Low serum albumin levels result in fluid shifting out of the vascular space because albumin normally maintains plasma colloid osmotic pressure.

THERAPEUTIC INTERVENTIONS	RATIONALE

Dependent/Collaborative Actions

Implement measures to restore fluid balance:
- Perform actions to reduce excess fluid volume:
  - Restrict sodium intake as ordered.
  - Maintain fluid restrictions if ordered.
  - Implement measures to improve cardiac output.
  - If client is receiving numerous and/or large-volume intravenous medications, consult pharmacist about ways to prevent excessive fluid administration (e.g., stop primary infusion during administration of intravenous medications, dilute medications in the minimum amount of solution).
  - Administer diuretics as ordered.
- Perform actions to prevent further third-spacing and promote mobilization of fluid back into the vascular space:
  - Administer albumin infusions if ordered.

  - Assist with thoracentesis or paracentesis if performed

All actions help to reduce circulating fluid volume, helping to decrease preload and reduce the workload of the heart. Decreasing circulating fluid volume and implementing measures to optimize cardiac output help to restore circulation and improve oxygenation and tissue perfusion to the vital organs.

Diuretics help increase excretion of water.

Increasing colloid osmotic pressure with the infusion of protein-based fluids pulls accumulated third-spaced fluid back into the vascular space, reducing edema.

Remove excess fluid from the pleural space or peritoneal cavity.

Continued...

THERAPEUTIC INTERVENTIONS	RATIONALE
Implement measures to treat hyponatremia: • Maintain fluid restrictions if ordered. • Administer intravenous saline solution if ordered (if client's hyponatremia is thought to be due to "salt wasting," treatment includes administration of saline and discontinuation of diuretics). • Consult physician about a decrease in or discontinuation of diuretics and temporary discontinuation of dietary sodium restriction if sodium level is significantly reduced. Consult physician if signs and symptoms of imbalanced fluid and/or hyponatremia persist or worsen.	*For hyponatremia induced by water excess, fluid restrictions are implemented to treat the problem.* *If hyponatremia is severe and associated with neurological symptoms, 3% saline may be administered to restore sodium levels while the body is returning to a normal fluid balance.* *Diuretic therapy causes loss of sodium.* *Consulting the appropriate health care provider allows for modification of the treatment plan.*

Collaborative Diagnosis   RISK FOR RENAL INSUFFICIENCY

Definition: A deficiency in the kidney's ability to clear waste products; a sign of inadequate glomerular filtration

Related to: A prolonged or severe decrease in renal blood flow associated with low cardiac output, volume depletion (may result from third-spacing, increased output of natriuretic hormones, and/or excessive diuretic use), and vasodilator-induced hypotension

CLINICAL MANIFESTATIONS

Subjective	Objective
Not applicable	Urine output less than 30 mL/h; urine specific gravity fixed at or less than 1.010; elevated BUN and serum creatinine levels; decreased creatinine clearance

RISK FACTORS
• Decreased cardiac output
• Volume depletion

DESIRED OUTCOMES

The client will maintain adequate renal function as evidenced by:
   a. Urine output at least 30 mL/h
   b. BUN, serum creatinine, and creatinine clearance values within normal range

NURSING ASSESSMENT	RATIONALE
Assess for and report signs and symptoms of impaired renal function: • Subjective • Objective Monitor serum electrolyte, BUN/creatinine results for abnormalities.	*Early recognition and reporting of signs and symptoms of renal insufficiency allow for prompt intervention.*

THERAPEUTIC INTERVENTIONS	RATIONALE
Dependent/Collaborative Actions Implement measures to maintain adequate renal blood flow: • Perform actions to improve cardiac output. • Perform actions to reduce third-spacing. • Ensure a minimum fluid intake of 1000 mL/day unless ordered otherwise. • Consult physician before giving vasodilators and diuretics if client is hypotensive.	*Prerenal causes of renal insufficiency/renal failure include such factors as decreased cardiac output and hypovolemia, which can reduce blood flow to the kidneys, decreasing the glomerular perfusion and filtration.*

THERAPEUTIC INTERVENTIONS	RATIONALE
If signs and symptoms of impaired renal function occur: • Consult physician about possible need to reduce the digitalis dosage. • Consult physician about lowering the dose of or discontinuing angiotensin-converting enzyme (ACE) inhibitors and diuretics if BUN and serum creatinine levels continue to rise significantly. • Assess for and report signs of acute renal failure (e.g., oliguria or anuria; further weight gain; increasing edema; increased B/P; lethargy and confusion; increasing BUN and serum creatinine, phosphorus, and potassium levels). • Prepare client for dialysis if indicated.	*Digitalis is excreted by the kidney and will quickly reach toxic levels when renal function is impaired.* *ACE inhibitors and many diuretics should be used cautiously in persons with impaired renal function because they can have an adverse effect on renal function.*

Collaborative Diagnosis RISK FOR CARDIAC DYSRHYTHMIAS

Definition: Irregularities of the heart rate or rhythm

Related to:
• Impaired nodal function and/or altered myocardial conductivity associated with:
  • Hypoxia
  • Sympathetic nervous system stimulation (a compensatory response to low cardiac output)
  • Structural changes in the myocardium (e.g., dilation, hypertrophy)
  • Imbalanced electrolytes (particularly the magnesium and potassium depletion that can result from diuretic therapy)

CLINICAL MANIFESTATIONS

Subjective	Objective
Verbal reports of lightheadedness/dizziness	Irregular apical pulse; pulse rate below 60 or above 100 beats/min; apical-radial pulse deficit; syncope; palpitations; abnormal rate, rhythm, or configurations on ECG

RISK FACTORS
• Diuretic administration
• Myocardial infarction

DESIRED OUTCOMES

The client will maintain normal sinus rhythm as evidenced by:
  a. Regular apical pulse at 60 to 100 beats/min
  b. Equal apical and radial pulse rates
  c. Absence of syncope and palpitations
  d. ECG reading showing normal sinus rhythm

NURSING ASSESSMENT	RATIONALE
Assess for and report signs and symptoms of cardiac dysrhythmias: • Subjective • Objective Monitor ECG for abnormalities. Monitor serum electrolyte levels for abnormalities.	*Early recognition of signs and symptoms of cardiac dysrhythmias allows for prompt intervention.*

THERAPEUTIC INTERVENTIONS	RATIONALE
Dependent/Collaborative Actions Implement measures to prevent cardiac dysrhythmias: • Perform actions to improve cardiac output.	*Adequate cardiac output helps to promote adequate myocardial tissue perfusion and oxygenation. Myocardial ischemia can lead to dysrhythmias.*

NDx = NANDA-I Diagnosis   D = Delegatable Action   ● = UAP   ✦ = LVN/LPN   ☺▶ = Go to ☺volve for animation

Continued...

THERAPEUTIC INTERVENTIONS	RATIONALE
• Perform actions to improve respiratory status.	*Optimum respiratory function helps to improve tissue oxygenation, reducing the potential for myocardial ischemia.*
• Consult physician regarding an order for a potassium (K^+) or magnesium (Mg^+) replacement if serum levels of either are below normal.	K^+ *and* Mg^+ *abnormalities can cause cardiac dysrhythmias.*
If cardiac dysrhythmias occur:	
• Initiate cardiac monitoring if not already being done.	
• Administer antidysrhythmics if ordered.	
• Restrict client's activity based on client's tolerance and severity of the dysrhythmia.	*Decreases stress on the heart.*
• Maintain oxygen therapy as ordered.	*Increases tissue oxygenation.*
• Assess cardiovascular status frequently and report signs and symptoms of a further decline in cardiac output and tissue perfusion.	
• Prepare client for catheter ablation or insertion of a pacemaker or implantable cardioverter-defibrillator (ICD) if planned.	*Decreases fear and anxiety.*
• Have emergency cart readily available for cardioversion, defibrillation, or cardiopulmonary resuscitation.	

Collaborative Diagnosis RISK FOR ACUTE PULMONARY EDEMA

Definition: Excess water in the lungs, usually a result of heart failure

Related to: Accumulation of fluid in the lungs associated with increased hydrostatic pressure in the pulmonary vessels as a result of blood flow backup in the left ventricle

CLINICAL MANIFESTATIONS

Subjective	**Objective**
Sudden development of or increased dyspnea or orthopnea	Increased crackles (rales) or wheezes; disorientation; increased restlessness and anxiousness; cough productive of frothy or blood-tinged sputum; significant decrease in oximetry results; worsening arterial blood gas results; chest radiograph showing pulmonary edema

RISK FACTORS

- Acute myocardial infarction
- Decreased cardiac output
- High afterload

DESIRED OUTCOMES

The client will not develop acute pulmonary edema as evidenced by:
  a. Decreased dyspnea
  b. Usual or improved breath sounds
  c. Usual mental status
  d. Arterial blood gas values within normal range

NURSING ASSESSMENT	RATIONALE
Assess for and report signs and symptoms of acute pulmonary edema: • Subjective • Objective Monitor pulse oximetry and arterial blood gas values and chest radiograph results for abnormalities.	*Early recognition of signs and symptoms of acute pulmonary edema allows for prompt intervention.*

THERAPEUTIC INTERVENTIONS	RATIONALE
Dependent/Collaborative Actions Implement measures to improve cardiac output.	*Improving cardiac output results in a decrease in pulmonary vascular congestion as the left side of the heart improves performance.*
If signs and symptoms of pulmonary edema occur: • Place client in a high-Fowler's position unless contraindicated. • Maintain oxygen therapy as ordered. • Administer the following medications if ordered: • Diuretics • Theophylline • Morphine sulfate	*Interventions for acute pulmonary edema focus on the immediate improvement of oxygenation and relief of pulmonary vascular congestion by improving cardiac output and diuresis to reduce fluid accumulation in the lungs.* *Morphine sulfate is very beneficial in acute pulmonary edema because it helps to reduce anxiety and decrease pulmonary vascular congestion (increases venous capacitance, which lowers venous return to the heart).*
• Vasodilators	*Vasodilators help to reduce afterload and improve left ventricular emptying, which reduces pulmonary blood flow backup.*

Collaborative Diagnosis **RISK FOR THROMBOEMBOLISM**

Definition: A clot attached to a vessel wall that detaches and circulates within the blood

Related to:
• Venous stasis in the periphery associated with decreased cardiac output and decreased mobility
• Stasis of blood in the heart associated with decreased ventricular emptying (risk increases if dysrhythmias are present)

CLINICAL MANIFESTATIONS

Subjective	Objective
Reports of deep vein thrombus: Pain, tenderness	Deep vein thrombus: Swelling, unusual warmth, and/or positive Homans' sign in extremity
Reports of arterial thrombus: Numbness and/or pain in extremity	Arterial thrombus: Diminished or absent peripheral pulses; pallor, coolness,
Cerebral ischemia: Not applicable	Cerebral ischemia: Decreased level of consciousness; alteration in usual sensory and motor function
Reports of pulmonary embolism: Sudden onset of chest pain; increased dyspnea	Pulmonary embolism: Increased restlessness and apprehension; significant decrease in arterial oxygen saturation (Sao_2)

RISK FACTORS
• Venous stasis
• Atrial fibrillation
• Mural thrombus

DESIRED OUTCOMES

The client will not develop a thromboembolism as evidenced by:
a. Absence of pain, tenderness, swelling, and numbness in extremities
b. Usual temperature and color of extremities
c. Palpable and equal peripheral pulses
d. Usual mental status
e. Usual sensory and motor function
f. Absence of sudden chest pain and increased dyspnea

Continued...

NURSING ASSESSMENT	RATIONALE
Assess for and report signs and symptoms of deep vein thrombus, arterial embolus in an extremity, cerebral ischemia, or pulmonary embolism: • Pain/tenderness in extremity • Chest pain • Shortness of breath • Altered mental status • Diminished/absent pulses	*Early recognition of signs and symptoms of thromboembolism allows for prompt intervention.*

THERAPEUTIC INTERVENTIONS	RATIONALE

Dependent/Collaborative Actions
Implement additional measures to prevent the development of thromboemboli:
• Perform actions to improve cardiac output.
• Perform actions to treat cardiac dysrhythmias if present.
• Administer anticoagulants or antiplatelet agents if ordered.
If signs and symptoms of an arterial embolus in an extremity occur:
• Maintain client on bed rest with affected extremity in a level or slightly dependent position.
• Prepare client for the following if planned:
  • Diagnostic studies (e.g., Doppler or duplex ultrasound, arteriography)
  • Injection of a thrombolytic agent
  • Embolectomy
• Administer anticoagulants as ordered.
If signs and symptoms of cerebral ischemia occur:
• Maintain client on bed rest; keep head and neck in neutral, midline position.
• Administer anticoagulants as ordered.
	Adequate cardiac output ensures that blood flow continues to the extremities without pooling. Dysrhythmias, especially atrial fibrillation, allow blood to pool in the atria, leading to clot formation. Anticoagulant therapy is used to prevent clot formation.
	
	Improves arterial blood flow.
	
	Decreases fear and anxiety.
	
	Actions help to reduce intracranial pressure that accompanies cerebral ischemia.

Collaborative Diagnosis   # RISK FOR CARDIOGENIC SHOCK

Definition: Decreased cardiac output and evidence of tissue hypoxia in the presence of adequate intravascular volume

Related to: Inability of heart, intrinsic compensatory mechanisms, and treatments to maintain adequate tissue perfusion to vital organs

CLINICAL MANIFESTATIONS

Subjective	Objective
Verbal reports of increased restlessness, lethargy, or confusion	Systolic B/P below 80 mm Hg; rapid, weak pulse; diminished or absent peripheral pulses; increased coolness and duskiness or cyanosis of skin; urine output less than 30 mL/h

RISK FACTORS
• Acute myocardial infarction
• Cardiomyopathy

DESIRED OUTCOMES

The client will not develop cardiogenic shock as evidenced by:
  a. Stable or improved mental status
  b. Systolic B/P greater than 80 mm Hg
  c. Palpable peripheral pulses
  d. Stable or improved skin temperature and color
  e. Urine output at least 30 mL/h

NURSING ASSESSMENT	RATIONALE
Assess for and immediately report signs and symptoms of cardiogenic shock: • Confusion • Hypertension • Rapid, weak pulse • Diminished/absent pulse • Urine output <30 mL/h	*Early recognition of signs and symptoms of cardiogenic shock allows for prompt intervention.*

THERAPEUTIC INTERVENTIONS	RATIONALE

Dependent/Collaborative Actions
Implement measures to prevent cardiogenic shock:
• Perform actions to improve cardiac output.
• Perform actions to treat cardiac dysrhythmias if present.
If signs and symptoms of cardiogenic shock occur:
• Maintain oxygen therapy as ordered.
• Administer the following medications if ordered:
  • Sympathomimetics
 	
  • Vasodilators
 	
• Assist with intubation and insertion of hemodynamic monitoring device (e.g., Swan-Ganz catheter) and intra-aortic balloon pump (IABP) if indicated.
	Treating dysrhythmias and restoring a stable cardiac rhythm improves filling time of the ventricles, enhancing cardiac output.
	
	Increases tissue oxygenation.
	
	Sympathomimetics increase cardiac output and maintain arterial pressure.
	If the client's B/P is not too low, vasodilators can be used to decrease afterload, reducing cardiac workload.
	Cardiogenic shock unresponsive to drug therapy requires more invasive intervention to obtain numeric values that guide treatment or to assist the heart if function continues to deteriorate.

Nursing Diagnosis

DEFICIENT KNOWLEDGE NDx; INEFFECTIVE FAMILY THERAPEUTIC REGIMEN MANAGEMENT NDx; OR INEFFECTIVE SELF-HEALTH MANAGEMENT NDx*

Definition: Absence or deficiency of cognitive information related to specific topic (lack of specific information necessary for clients/significant others to make informed choices regarding condition/treatment/lifestyle changes); inability to identify, manage, and/or seek out help to manage health; pattern of regulating and integrating into daily living a program for treatment of illness and the sequelae of illness that is unsatisfactory for meeting specific health goals

CLINICAL MANIFESTATIONS

Subjective	**Objective**
Verbalization of unfamiliarity with information	Inability to follow through with instructions

RISK FACTORS
• Denial of disease process
• Cognitive deficiency
• Failure to take action to reduce risk factors

NOC OUTCOMES	NIC INTERVENTIONS
Knowledge: treatment regimen; knowledge: cardiac disease management; knowledge: disease process; knowledge: medication regimen	Health system guidance; teaching: individual; teaching: disease process; teaching: prescribed diet; teaching: prescribed medication; teaching: prescribed activity/exercise

NURSING ASSESSMENT	RATIONALE
Assess client's readiness and ability to learn. Assess meaning of illness to client.	*Early recognition of readiness to learn and meaning of illness to client allows for implementation of the appropriate teaching interventions.*

*The nurse should select the nursing diagnostic label that is most appropriate for the client's discharge teaching needs.

NDx = NANDA-I Diagnosis   **D** = Delegatable Action   ● = UAP   ✦ = LVN/LPN   ⊝▶ = Go to ⊝volve for animation

Continued...

THERAPEUTIC INTERVENTIONS	RATIONALE

Desired Outcome: The client will identify modifiable cardiovascular risk factors and ways to alter these factors.

Independent Actions

Inform client that certain modifiable factors such as elevated serum lipid levels, excessive alcohol intake, a sedentary lifestyle, hypertension, and smoking have been shown to increase the risk for coronary artery disease and certain forms of heart disease.

Assist client to identify changes in lifestyle that can help the client manage the above risk factors (e.g., dietary modification, physical exercise on a regular basis, moderation of alcohol intake, smoking cessation).

Encourage client to limit daily alcohol consumption. Current recommendations are no more than 2 drinks per day for men and no more than 1 drink per day for women and lighter-weight persons. A "drink" is considered to be ½ oz of ethanol (e.g., 1½ oz of 80-proof whiskey, 12 oz of beer, 5 oz of wine).

Thorough education is a critical component of the care of a client with heart failure. The client must have a thorough understanding of the importance of adhering to diet, medication, activity/ exercise, and nutritional recommendations to prevent an exacerbation and control the disease.

Improves client's ability to maintain or improve state of health.

Daily alcohol intake exceeding 1 oz of ethanol may contribute to the development of hypertension and some forms of heart disease.

THERAPEUTIC INTERVENTIONS	RATIONALE

Desired Outcome: The client will verbalize an understanding of the rationale for and components of a diet low in sodium.

Independent Actions

Explain the rationale for a diet low in sodium.

Provide the following information about decreasing sodium intake:

- Read labels on foods/fluids and calculate sodium content of items; avoid those products that tend to have a high sodium content (e.g., canned soups and vegetables, tomato juice, commercial baked goods, commercially prepared frozen or canned entrees and sauces).
- Do not add salt when cooking foods or to prepared foods; use low-sodium herbs and spices if desired.
- Avoid cured and smoked foods.
- Avoid salty snack foods (e.g., crackers, nuts, pretzels, potato chips).
- Avoid commercially prepared fast foods.
- Avoid routine use of over-the-counter medications with a high sodium content (e.g., Alka-Seltzer, some antacids).

Obtain a dietary consult to assist client in planning meals that will meet prescribed dietary modifications.

The edema associated with chronic heart failure is often treated with a reduction in dietary sodium. The degree of sodium restriction depends on the severity of heart failure and the effectiveness of diuretic therapy.

THERAPEUTIC INTERVENTIONS	RATIONALE

Desired Outcome: The client will demonstrate accuracy in counting pulse.

Independent Actions

Teach clients how to count their pulse, being alert to the regularity of the rhythm.

Allow time for return demonstration and accuracy check.

Educating clients to their baseline heart rate allows for early detection of irregularities that warrant immediate attention from a health care provider. Early detection may reduce the incidence of exacerbation of heart failure.

THERAPEUTIC INTERVENTIONS	RATIONALE

Desired Outcome: The client will verbalize an understanding of medications ordered including rationale, food and drug interactions, side effects, schedule for taking, and importance of taking as prescribed.

Independent Actions

Explain the rationale for, side effects of, and importance of taking the medications prescribed. Inform client of pertinent food and drug interactions.

- Digitalis preparations

  Digitalis is a positive inotrope that improves cardiac contractility, increasing cardiac output.

- Diuretics

  Diuretics help to mobilize edematous fluid, reducing pulmonary venous pressure and preload.

- ACE inhibitors

  ACE inhibitors block the effects of angiotensin-converting enzyme, which facilitates the conversion of angiotensin I to angiotensin II, a potent vasoconstrictor.

- Beta-adrenergic blockers

  Beta blockers reduce the effects of the sympathetic nervous system on the failing heart by slowing the heart rate.

Instruct client to take medications on a regular basis and avoid skipping doses, altering prescribed dose, making up for missed doses, and discontinuing medication without permission of health care provider.

Taking medications as prescribed ensures that therapeutic drug levels will be maintained.

Instruct client to consult physician before taking other prescription and nonprescription medications.

Instruct client to inform all health care providers of medications being taken.

Clients should be instructed not to discontinue taking medications if they feel better. Clients without financial resources should be assisted in accessing appropriate resources to obtain needed medications (e.g., pharmacy assistance programs).

THERAPEUTIC INTERVENTIONS	RATIONALE

Desired Outcome: The client will state signs and symptoms to report to the health care provider.

Independent Actions

Instruct client to report:

- Weight gain of more than 2 lb in a day or 4 lb in a week
- Increased swelling of ankles, feet, or abdomen
- Persistent cough
- Increasing shortness of breath
- Chest discomfort/pain
- Increased weakness and fatigue
- Frequent nighttime urination
- Signs and symptoms of digitalis toxicity
- Side effects of diuretic therapy

Reporting signs and symptoms of heart failure to the appropriate provider allows for modification of the treatment plan and possibly can prevent a client's readmission to the hospital.

THERAPEUTIC INTERVENTIONS	RATIONALE

Desired Outcome: The client will identify community resources that can assist with home management and adjustment to changes resulting from heart failure.

Independent Actions

Provide information regarding community resources that can assist with home management and adjustment to changes resulting from heart failure (e.g., Meals on Wheels, home health agencies, transportation services, American Heart Association, counseling services).

Heart failure can significantly impact an individual's and family's socioeconomic status. Providing information specific to community resources is important to provide a necessary continuum of care and may impact the client's health status, preventing future hospitalizations.

Continued...

THERAPEUTIC INTERVENTIONS	RATIONALE

Desired Outcome: Verbalize an understanding of and a plan for adhering to recommended follow-up care including future appointments with health care provider and activity limitations.

Independent Actions

Reinforce the importance of keeping follow-up appointments with health care provider.

Regular health care appointments are important to determine effectiveness of the prescribed treatment plan.

Provide the following instructions regarding activity:
- Increase activity gradually and only as tolerated.
- Stop any activity that causes chest pain, dizziness, or a significant increase in shortness of breath or fatigue.
- Plan and adhere to rest periods during the day.
- Adhere to physician's recommendations about activities that should be avoided.
- Notify physician if activity tolerance declines.
- Reduce dyspnea and fatigue during sexual activity by:
  - Avoiding sexual activity when unusually fatigued
  - Waiting 1 to 2 hours after a heavy meal or alcohol intake before engaging in sexual activity
  - Identifying and using positions that minimize energy expenditure
  - Using portable oxygen during sexual activities

Implement measures to improve client adherence:
- Include significant others in teaching sessions if possible.

Involvement of significant others in patient teaching improves adherence to discharge instructions.

- Encourage questions and allow time for reinforcement and clarification of information provided.

Everyone does not understand information as presented, so set aside time for questions to allow for clarification of information.

- Provide written instructions regarding scheduled appointments with health care provider, medications prescribed, dietary sodium restrictions, and signs and symptoms to report.

Written instructions allow the client to refer to instructions as needed.

- Ensure client has the necessary financial or social support resources to meet the conditions of the treatment plan.

ADDITIONAL NURSING DIAGNOSES

RISK FOR FALLS NDx
Related to:
- Weakness
- Dizziness and syncope associated with inadequate cerebral blood flow resulting from decreased cardiac output and the hypotensive effect of some medications (e.g., ACE inhibitors, diuretics)
- Getting up without assistance as a result of restlessness, agitation, forgetfulness, and confusion (can result from cerebral hypoxia and imbalanced fluid and electrolytes)

DISTURBED SLEEP PATTERN NDx
Related to: Unfamiliar environment, frequent assessments and treatments, decreased physical activity, fear, anxiety, and inability to assume usual sleep position associated with orthopnea

ACTIVITY INTOLERANCE NDx
Related to:
- Tissue hypoxia associated with impaired alveolar gas exchange and decreased cardiac output
- Inadequate nutritional status
- Difficulty resting and sleeping associated with dyspnea, frequent assessments and treatments, fear, and anxiety

RISK FOR IMPAIRED TISSUE INTEGRITY NDx
Related to:
- Damage to the skin and/or subcutaneous tissue associated with prolonged pressure on the tissues, friction, and/or shearing if mobility is decreased
- Increased fragility of the skin associated with edema, poor tissue perfusion, and inadequate nutritional status

IMBALANCED NUTRITION: LESS THAN BODY REQUIREMENTS NDx
Related to:
- Decreased oral intake associated with:
  - Anorexia and nausea (result from venous congestion in the gastrointestinal tract and can occur if digitalis levels exceed a therapeutic level)
  - Weakness, fatigue, dyspnea, and dislike of prescribed diet
- Elevated metabolic rate associated with the increased oxygen needs of the heart and the increased work of breathing
- Impaired absorption of nutrients associated with poor tissue perfusion

FEAR/ANXIETY NDx
Related to:
- Exacerbation of symptoms and need for hospitalization
- Lack of understanding of diagnostic tests, the diagnosis, and treatments
- Cost of hospitalization and lifelong treatment
- Possibility of early disability and death

NAUSEA NDx
Related to: Stimulation of the vomiting center associated with:
- Stimulation of the visceral afferent pathways resulting from vascular congestion in the heart and gastrointestinal tract
- Stimulation of the cerebral cortex resulting from stress
- Stimulation of the chemoreceptor trigger zone by certain medications (e.g., digitalis preparations)

DISTURBED THOUGHT PROCESSES NDx
Related to:
- Cerebral hypoxia associated with impaired alveolar gas exchange and inadequate cerebral tissue perfusion (a result of decreased cardiac output)
- Imbalanced fluid and electrolytes

INEFFECTIVE COPING NDx
Related to: Fear, anxiety, possible need to alter lifestyle, and knowledge that condition is chronic and will require lifelong medical supervision and medication therapy

HEART SURGERY: CORONARY ARTERY BYPASS GRAFTING OR VALVE REPLACEMENT

Heart surgery is performed for a variety of reasons including myocardial revascularization, valve repair or replacement, repair of congenital or acquired structural abnormalities, placement of a mechanical assist device, and heart transplantation. Two common heart surgeries are coronary artery bypass grafting (CABG), which is done to treat severe coronary artery disease, and heart valve replacement. CABG involves removing a segment of a vein (e.g., saphenous, cephalic) or an artery (e.g., internal mammary, radial, gastroepiploic) to create an anastomosis between the aorta or other major artery and a point on the coronary artery distal to the obstruction. Heart valve replacement involves replacing the stenotic or regurgitant valve with a mechanical prosthesis or a biological (tissue) valve (porcine or bovine valve, human valve).

Heart surgery is usually performed through a median sternotomy. Cardiopulmonary bypass (CPB; extracorporeal circulation) is maintained during surgery by a machine that diverts the blood from the heart and lungs, oxygenates the blood and removes carbon dioxide, maintains the desired body temperature, filters the blood, and then recirculates the blood into the arterial system. Systemic hypothermia (provided by the CPB machine) can reduce tissue oxygen requirements to 50% of normal, which affords the major organs additional protection from ischemic injury. Cold cardioplegia (infusion of a cold alkaline solution containing potassium into the coronary circulation) is used to precipitate cardiac arrest and provide additional protection to the myocardium during surgery. An isotonic crystalloid solution is used to prime the bypass machine. This dilutes the client's blood, which improves blood flow and reduces the risk of microemboli formation. Before closing the chest, pacing electrodes are usually placed on the epicardial surface of the heart and brought out through the chest wall to be used for temporary pacing if needed. A chest tube is placed in the mediastinum to drain blood, and if needed, one is also placed in the pleural space to promote lung reexpansion.

In addition to the traditional sternotomy approach performed on CPB, heart surgery may be performed "off pump" (referred to as off pump coronary bypass [OPCAB]) or using a minimally invasive approach (e.g., small incision in left sternal border, a series of holes or "ports" using video-assisted equipment). Minimally invasive procedures such as a MIDCAB (minimally invasive direct coronary artery bypass) can be performed without CPB or with a less invasive, catheter-based system of CPB. Several techniques are used to stabilize the operative area during a beating heart procedure (stabilizer device to "still" certain areas of the heart while the rest keeps beating, drugs that decrease the heart rate or cause transient asystole). Because "off pump" and minimally invasive approaches reduce the risk for some of the major complications (e.g., mediastinitis, emboli associated with cross-clamping the aorta) and shorten hospitalization and rehabilitation time they promise to become more common.

This care plan focuses on the adult client hospitalized for either CABG or valve replacement surgery. Much of the postoperative information is applicable to clients receiving follow-up care in an extended care facility or home setting.

NDx = NANDA-I Diagnosis   **D** = Delegatable Action   ● = UAP   ✦ = LVN/LPN   ⊝▶ = Go to ⊝volve for animation

Continued...

OUTCOME/DISCHARGE CRITERIA

The client will:
1. Have adequate cardiac output and tissue perfusion
2. Have clear, audible breath sounds throughout lungs
3. Have evidence of normal healing of surgical wound(s)
4. Have oxygen saturation within normal limits for client's age
5. Tolerate expected level of activity
6. Have surgical pain controlled
7. Have no signs and symptoms of complications
8. Identify modifiable cardiovascular risk factors and ways to alter these factors
9. Verbalize an understanding of the rationale for and components of a diet restricted in sodium, saturated fat, and cholesterol
10. Verbalize an understanding of activity restrictions and the rate of activity progression
11. Verbalize an understanding of medications ordered including rationale, food and drug interactions, side effects, schedule for taking, and importance of taking as prescribed
12. State signs and symptoms to report to the health care provider
13. Identify community resources that can assist with cardiac rehabilitation and adjustment to having had heart surgery
14. Verbalize an understanding of and a plan for adhering to recommended follow-up care including future appointments with health care provider, wound care, and pain management.

PREOPERATIVE: USE IN CONJUNCTION WITH THE STANDARDIZED PREOPERATIVE CARE PLAN

Related Preoperative Nursing/Collaborative Diagnoses FEAR NDx/ANXIETY NDx

Definition: Response to a perceived threat that is recognized as danger; vague, uneasy feeling of discomfort on dread

Related to:
- Unfamiliar environment and separation from significant others
- Lack of understanding of diagnostic tests, preoperative procedures/preparation, planned surgery, and postoperative course
- Anticipated loss of control associated with effects of anesthesia
- Financial concerns associated with surgery and hospitalization
- Anticipated postoperative discomfort and alterations in lifestyle and roles
- Risk of disease if blood transfusions are necessary
- Potential embarrassment or loss of dignity associated with body exposure
- Possibility of death

POSTOPERATIVE: USE IN CONJUNCTION WITH THE STANDARDIZED POSTOPERATIVE CARE PLAN

Nursing Diagnosis DECREASED CARDIAC OUTPUT NDx

Definition: Inadequate volume of blood pumped by the heart per minute to meet metabolic demands of the body

Related to:
- Preexisting compromise in cardiac function
- Trauma to the heart during surgery
- Increased afterload associated with:
  - Vasoconstriction resulting from hypothermia and an increase in catecholamine output and plasma renin levels (these increases occur with CPB and the effect of stressors [e.g., pain, anxiety])
  - Fluid overload
- Decreased preload associated with:
  - Hypovolemia (can result from blood loss, fluid shifting from the intravascular to interstitial space, loss of fluid from nasogastric tube, decreased fluid intake, and excessive diuresis)
- Hypotension (can occur if body is warmed rapidly after surgery and as a result of the effect of anesthesia and certain medications [e.g., narcotic analgesics, beta-adrenergic blockers, vasodilators])
- Effects of anesthesia, hypothermia, hypoxemia, and acid-base and/or electrolyte imbalances on contractility and conductivity of the heart

CLINICAL MANIFESTATIONS

Subjective	Objective
Reports of fatigue and weakness	Low B/P; resting pulse rate greater than 100 beats/min; postural hypotension; cool, pale, or cyanotic skin; capillary refill time greater than 2 to 3 seconds; diminished or absent peripheral pulses; urine output less than 30 mL/h; low central venous pressure (CVP); crackles (rales); presence of gallop rhythm; dyspnea, tachypnea; restlessness, change in mental status; edema; jugular venous distention (JVD); chest radiograph results showing pulmonary vascular congestion, pulmonary edema, or pleural effusion; abnormal arterial blood gas values; significant decrease in oximetry results; dysrhythmias

DESIRED OUTCOMES

The client will maintain adequate cardiac output as evidenced by:
  a. B/P within range of 100/60 to 130/80 mm Hg
  b. Apical pulse regular and between 60 and 100 beats/min
  c. Absence of or no increase in intensity of gallop rhythm
  d. Increased strength and activity tolerance
  e. Unlabored respirations at 12 to 20 breaths/min
  f. Absence of adventitious breath sounds
  g. Usual mental status
  h. Absence of dizziness and syncope
  i. Palpable peripheral pulses
  j. Skin warm and usual color
  k. Capillary refill time less than 2 to 3 seconds
  l. Urine output at least 30 mL/h
  m. Absence of edema and JVD

NOC OUTCOMES

Cardiac pump effectiveness; circulation status; tissue perfusion: peripheral; tissue perfusion: cardiac

NIC INTERVENTIONS

Cardiac care: acute; invasive hemodynamic monitoring; hemodynamic regulation; cardiac precautions; dysrhythmia management; cardiac care: rehabilitative

NURSING ASSESSMENT

Assess for and report signs and symptoms of decreased cardiac output:
- Hypotension
- Cool, pale, cyanotic skin
- Diminished/absent pulses
- Urine output <30 mL/h
- Jugulovenous distention
- Tachypnea
- Dyspnea

Monitor ECG for dysrhythmias.
Monitor chest radiograph, pulse oximetry, and arterial blood gas values for abnormalities.

RATIONALE

Early recognition of signs and symptoms of decreased cardiac output allows for prompt intervention.

THERAPEUTIC INTERVENTIONS

RATIONALE

Independent Actions

Implement measures to maintain an adequate cardiac output:
- Perform actions to prevent or treat hypotension:
  - Avoid rapid rewarming; gradually bring client's body temperature to normal if client is hypothermic.

Vasodilation occurs with warming. Warming measures should be gradual to prevent hypotension.

Continued...

THERAPEUTIC INTERVENTIONS	RATIONALE

• Perform actions to reduce cardiac workload:
  • Place client in a semi- to high-Fowler's position **D** ● ✦
  • Instruct client to avoid activities that create a Valsalva response (e.g., straining to have a bowel movement, holding breath while moving up in bed).
  • Implement measures to promote rest (e.g., maintain activity restrictions, limit the number of visitors, reduce anxiety).
  • Discourage smoking.
 	
  • Discourage excessive intake of beverages high in caffeine such as coffee, tea, and colas.
	Nicotine has a cardiostimulatory effect and causes vasoconstriction; the carbon monoxide in smoke reduces oxygen availability. Caffeine is a myocardial stimulant and can increase myocardial oxygen consumption.

Dependent/Collaborative Actions

Administer prescribed pain medications.
Implement measures to maintain an adequate cardiac output:
• Perform actions to prevent or treat hypovolemia:
  • Administer blood and/or colloid or crystalloid solutions as ordered.
  • Maintain a minimum fluid intake of 1000 mL/day unless ordered otherwise.
  • Implement measures to prevent and control bleeding.
• Perform actions to prevent or treat hypotension:
  • Consult physician before giving negative inotropic agents, diuretics, and vasodilating agents if client is hypotensive.
  • Administer narcotic (opioid) analgesics judiciously; in the immediate postoperative period, be alert to the synergistic effect of the narcotic ordered and the anesthetic that was used during surgery.
  • Administer sympathomimetics if ordered.
 	
• Administer positive inotropic agents (e.g., dopamine, dobutamine, digitalis preparations) if ordered.
• Perform actions to prevent or treat cardiac dysrhythmias.
• Administer antidysrhythmic medications.
• Replace K+, Mg+ electrolytes.
• Perform actions to reduce cardiac workload:
  • Perform actions to prevent or treat hypertension:
    • Implement measures to gradually rewarm client (e.g., increased room temperature, radiant heat lamp, warm blankets) if client is hypothermic.
    • Implement measures to reduce stress (e.g., initiate pain relief measures, reduce fear and anxiety).
    • Administer vasodilators if ordered.
  • Implement measures to maintain adequate respiratory function.
  • Implement measures to prevent or treat excess fluid volume:
    • Administer diuretics.
    • Limit excess fluid intake.
  • Increase activity gradually as allowed and tolerated.
Consult physician if signs and symptoms of decreased cardiac output persist or worsen.
	Actions help to maintain or restore circulating blood volume. An adequate circulating blood volume is necessary to achieve the optimum preload necessary for effective cardiac output.
	
	Opioids promote vasodilation.
	
	Sympathomimetics may be administered as a temporary measure to improve B/P if adequate circulating fluid volume has been restored.
	Positive inotropic agents increase myocardial contractility, improving cardiac output.
	Cardiac dysrhythmias can alter ventricular filling time and significantly reduce cardiac output.
	
	Actions help to prevent vasoconstriction associated with hypothermia and also prevent shivering, which elevates the metabolic rate and increases cardiac workload.
	
	Reduces vasoconstriction.
	
	Promotes adequate tissue oxygenation.
	
	Consulting the appropriate health care provider allows for modification of the treatment plan.

Nursing Diagnosis **RISK FOR IMPAIRED RESPIRATORY FUNCTION***

Definition: Inspiration and/or expiration that does not provide adequate ventilation; inability to clear secretions or obstructions from the respiratory tract to maintain a clear airway

Related to:
Ineffective breathing pattern NDx related to:
- Increased rate of respirations associated with fear and anxiety
- Decreased rate of respirations associated with the depressant effect of anesthesia and some medications (e.g., narcotic [opioid] analgesics)
- Decreased depth of respirations associated with:
  - Weakness, fatigue, and decreased mobility
  - Depressant effect of anesthesia and some medications (e.g., narcotic [opioid] analgesics)
  - Reluctance to breathe deeply because of chest incision and fear of dislodging chest tube
  - Hemiparesis of the diaphragm if the phrenic nerve was injured
  - Decreased lung compliance (distensibility) if pleural effusion is present

Ineffective airway clearance NDx related to:
- Stasis of secretions associated with decreased activity, depressed ciliary function resulting from the effect of anesthesia, and a weak cough effort
- Increased secretions associated with irritation of the respiratory tract (can result from inhalation anesthetics and endotracheal intubation)

Impaired gas exchange NDx related to ventilation/perfusion imbalances associated with:
- Atelectasis resulting from:
  - Deflation of the alveoli while on the CPB machine
  - Decreased surfactant production/function (occurs because of lack of alveolar expansion and decreased pulmonary blood flow during CPB and as a result of a systemic inflammatory response to the bypass machine)
  - Postoperative hypoventilation or ineffective clearance of secretions
  - Accumulation of fluid in the pulmonary interstitium and alveoli (can occur as a result of excess fluid volume)
  - Decreased pulmonary blood flow resulting from decreased cardiac output

CLINICAL MANIFESTATIONS

Subjective	Objective
Reports of restlessness; irritability	Rapid, shallow, or slow respirations; dyspnea, orthopnea; use of accessory muscles when breathing; adventitious breath sounds (e.g., crackles [rales], rhonchi); diminished or absent breath sounds; asymmetrical chest excursion; cough; confusion, somnolence; abnormal arterial blood gas values; significant decrease in oximetry results; abnormal chest radiograph results

RISK FACTORS
- Immobility
- Atelectasis
- Ineffective clearance of secretions

DESIRED OUTCOMES

The client will experience adequate respiratory function as evidenced by:
  a. Normal rate and depth of respirations
  b. Absence of dyspnea
  c. Normal breath sounds by third to fourth postoperative day
  d. Symmetrical chest excursion
  e. Usual mental status
  f. Oximetry results within normal range
  g. Arterial blood gas values within normal range

---

*This diagnostic label includes the following nursing diagnoses: ineffective breathing pattern, ineffective airway clearance, and impaired gas exchange.

NDx = NANDA-I Diagnosis   **D** = Delegatable Action   ● = UAP   ✦ = LVN/LPN   ⊖▶ = Go to ⊖volve for animation

Continued...

NOC OUTCOMES	NIC INTERVENTIONS
Respiratory status: ventilation; respiratory status: airway patency; respiratory status: gas exchange	Respiratory monitoring; airway management; chest physiotherapy; cough enhancement; ventilation assistance; oxygen therapy; anxiety reduction

NURSING ASSESSMENT	RATIONALE
Assess for and report signs and symptoms of impaired respiratory function: • Rapid, shallow, or slow respirations • Dyspnea, orthopnea • Use of accessory muscles when breathing • Adventitious breath sounds (e.g., crackles [rales], rhonchi) • Diminished or absent breath sounds • Asymmetrical chest excursion • Cough • Confusion, somnolence Monitor pulse oximetry and arterial blood gas values, and chest radiograph results for abnormalities.	*Early recognition of signs and symptoms of impaired respiratory function allows for prompt intervention.*

THERAPEUTIC INTERVENTIONS	RATIONALE

Independent Actions

Implement measures to maintain adequate respiratory function:

• Perform actions to decrease fear and anxiety (e.g., explain procedures, interact with client in a confident manner, initiate pain relief measures).	*Actions that decrease fear and anxiety help to prevent the shallow and/or rapid breathing that can occur with fear and anxiety.*
• Place client in a semi- to high-Fowler's position unless contraindicated.	*Improves lung expansion.*
• If client must remain flat in bed, assist with position change at least every 2 hours.	*Actions help to mobilize secretions and prevent alveolar collapse associated with immobility.*
• Instruct and assist client to cough and deep breathe or use incentive spirometer every 1 to 2 hours; assure client that chest tube is sutured in place and that these activities should not dislodge the tube.	*Improves lung expansion and prevents stasis of secretions.*
• Instruct client to avoid intake of gas-forming foods (e.g., beans, cauliflower, cabbage, onions), carbonated beverages, and large meals.	*Helps to prevent gastric distention and subsequent pressure on the diaphragm.*
• Discourage smoking.	*The irritants in smoke increase mucus production, impair ciliary function, and can cause damage to the bronchial and alveolar walls; the carbon monoxide in smoke decreases oxygen availability.*

Dependent/Collaborative Actions

Implement measures to maintain adequate respiratory function:

• Monitor mechanical ventilation carefully to ensure that ventilatory rate and pressures are correct.	*The nurse collaborates with the respiratory therapist to ensure that mechanical ventilation is delivered therapeutically without adverse outcomes.*
• Perform actions to decrease pain and increase strength and activity (e.g., administer analgesics before activities that can cause pain).	*Providing adequate pain relief helps to increase client's willingness and ability to move, cough, deep breathe, and use incentive spirometer.*
• Perform actions to maintain an adequate cardiac output.	*Adequate cardiac output ensures pulmonary blood flow, facilitating gas exchange.*
• Administer blood and blood products as ordered.	
• Perform actions to prevent or treat excess fluid volume and third-spacing (e.g., administer diuretics as ordered).	*Actions help to reduce the risk for pleural effusion and pulmonary edema.*
• Maintain an adequate fluid intake and humidify inspired air if ordered.	*Actions help to thin tenacious secretions and reduce dryness of the respiratory mucous membrane.*
• Maintain oxygen therapy as ordered.	*Maintains tissue oxygenation.*
• Maintain activity restrictions as ordered; increase activity gradually as allowed and tolerated.	

THERAPEUTIC INTERVENTIONS	RATIONALE
• Administer central nervous system depressants judiciously; hold medication and consult physician if respiratory rate is less than 12 breaths/min.	*Prevents decreased tissue oxygenation.*
Consult appropriate health care provider (e.g., respiratory therapist, physician) if signs and symptoms of impaired respiratory function persist or worsen.	*Consulting the appropriate health care provider allows for modification of the treatment plan.*

Nursing/Collaborative Diagnosis

RISK FOR IMBALANCED FLUID NDx AND RISK FOR ELECTROLYTE IMBALANCE NDx

Definition: At risk for a decrease, increase, or rapid shift from one to the other of intravascular, interstitial, and/or intracellular fluid; at risk for a change in serum electrolyte levels

Related to:

Excess fluid volume NDx related to:

• Vigorous fluid therapy during and immediately after surgery (the CPB machine is primed with a large amount of crystalloid solution to decrease blood viscosity and the risk for embolic complications, decrease hemolysis of cells, and help maintain adequate circulation throughout the body)
• Increased production of antidiuretic hormone (ADH; output of ADH is stimulated by trauma, pain, and anesthetic agents)
• Reshifting of fluid from the interstitial space back into the intravascular space approximately 3 days after surgery
• Decreased glomerular filtration rate and activation of the renin-angiotensin-aldosterone mechanism (a result of nonpulsatile renal perfusion while on the bypass machine and the decreased renal blood flow that can occur with decreased cardiac output)
• Presence of preexisting heart failure

Third-spacing of fluid related to increased capillary permeability (a result of the systemic inflammatory response that occurs with CPB) and the subsequent low plasma colloid osmotic pressure associated with decreased plasma proteins

Deficient fluid volume NDx related to:

• Restricted oral intake before, during, and after surgery
• Blood loss during surgery and via chest tube after surgery
• Loss of fluid associated with nasogastric tube drainage and excessive diuresis
• Third-spacing of intravascular fluid

Hypokalemia, hypochloremia, and/or metabolic alkalosis related to loss of electrolytes and hydrochloric acid associated with nasogastric tube drainage (diuretic therapy and the hemodilution created by priming the bypass machine with large amounts of fluid also contribute to the imbalanced electrolytes)

CLINICAL MANIFESTATIONS

Subjective	Objective
Excess fluid volume: Not applicable	**Excess fluid volume:** Weight gain of 2% or greater in a short period; elevated B/P (B/P may not be elevated if cardiac output is poor or fluid has shifted out of the vascular space); presence of an S_3 heart sound; intake greater than output; change in mental status; crackles (rales); dyspnea, orthopnea; edema, distended neck veins; elevated CVP (use internal jugular vein pulsation method to estimate CVP if monitoring device is not present)
Third-spacing: Not applicable	**Third-spacing:** Ascites; increased dyspnea and diminished or absent breath sounds; evidence of vascular depletion (e.g., postural hypotension; weak, rapid pulse; decreased urine output)
Deficient fluid volume: Reports of thirst	**Deficient fluid volume:** Hypotension; tachycardia; decreased urine output; tenting skin turgor; dry mucous membranes; thick, tenacious pulmonary secretions

---

NDx = NANDA-I Diagnosis   **D** = Delegatable Action   ● = UAP   ◆ = LVN/LPN   ⊖▶ = Go to ⊖volve for animation

Continued...

DESIRED OUTCOMES

The client will experience resolution of excess fluid volume and third-spacing as evidenced by:
  a. Decline in weight toward client's normal
  b. B/P and pulse within normal range for client and stable with position change
  c. Resolution of S$_3$ heart sound
  d. Balanced intake and output
  e. Usual mental status
  f. Improved breath sounds
  g. Decreased dyspnea and orthopnea
  h. Decrease in edema and ascites
  i. Resolution of neck vein distention
  j. CVP within normal range

The client will not experience deficient fluid volume, hypokalemia, hypochloremia, or metabolic alkalosis.

NOC OUTCOMES	NIC INTERVENTIONS
Fluid balance; fluid overload severity; electrolyte and acid-base balance	Fluid monitoring; electrolyte monitoring; acid-base monitoring; fluid management; electrolyte management: hypokalemia; acid-base management: metabolic alkalosis

NURSING ASSESSMENT	RATIONALE
Assess for and report signs and symptoms of excess fluid volume and third-spacing.	*Early recognition of signs and symptoms of excess fluid volume and third-spacing allows for prompt intervention.*
Monitor chest radiograph for abnormal findings: • Pulmonary vascular congestion • Pleural effusion • Pulmonary edema	
Monitor serum albumin levels for abnormal values.	*Low serum albumin levels result in fluid shifting out of the vascular space because albumin normally maintains plasma colloid osmotic pressure.*
Monitor postoperative drains (mediastinal tubes/chest tubes) for amount and consistency of drainage.	*Excessive postoperative drainage can lead to deficient circulating fluid volume.*

THERAPEUTIC INTERVENTIONS	RATIONALE

Dependent/Collaborative Actions
Implement measures to restore fluid balance:
• Perform actions to reduce excess fluid volume:
  • Perform actions to maintain adequate renal blood flow.

Adequate renal blood flow helps to maintain normal glomerular filtration with subsequent fluid removal.

  • Maintain adequate blood pressure within client's baseline normal values.
  • Administer diuretics if ordered.

Decreases fluid volume excess.

  • Maintain fluid and sodium restrictions as ordered (2500 mL fluid and 3-4 g sodium restrictions are common).

High sodium levels cause fluid retention.

• Perform actions to prevent further third-spacing and promote mobilization of fluid back into the vascular space:
  • Administer albumin infusions if ordered.

Albumin helps to increase colloid osmotic pressure, pulling fluid back into the vascular space and helping to reduce third-spacing.

• Administer the following if ordered to treat deficient fluid volume and hypokalemia:
  • Blood and/or colloid or crystalloid solutions

Colloid solutions may be used rather than crystalloid solutions because they help maintain colloid osmotic pressure and subsequently reduce shifting of fluid from the intravascular to the interstitial space.

  • Potassium supplements

Keeping the serum potassium at 4.0 to 4.5 mEq/L reduces the risk for dysrhythmias.

Consult physician if signs and symptoms of excess fluid volume and third-spacing persist or worsen.

Allows for prompt alterations in interventions.

Nursing Diagnosis	**RISK FOR INFECTION** NDx

Definition: At increased risk for being invaded by pathogenic organisms

Related to:
- **Pneumonia** related to:
  - Stasis of pulmonary secretions associated with decreased activity
  - Depressed ciliary function resulting from the effect of anesthesia
  - A poor cough effort resulting from weakness, surgical site pain, and fear of dislodging chest tube
- **Wound infection and mediastinitis** related to:
  - Wound contamination associated with introduction of pathogens during or after surgery
  - Decreased resistance to infection associated with factors such as inadequate nutritional status and diminished tissue perfusion to wound area (an increased risk if client is elderly or has diabetes or if on CPB a prolonged time or cardiac output is low for a prolonged time)

CLINICAL MANIFESTATIONS

Subjective	Objective
Verbal reports of increased pain at wound site	Increased temperature; redness; warmth, discharge in close proximity to wound; thick, malodorous pulmonary secretions

DESIRED OUTCOMES

The client will not develop pneumonia.	The client will remain free of wound infection and mediastinitis.

NOC OUTCOMES	NIC NTERVENTIONS
Immune status; infection severity; wound healing: primary intention	Infection protection; infection control; cough enhancement; airway management; incision site care

NURSING ASSESSMENT	RATIONALE
Assess for and report signs and symptoms of sternal wound infection and mediastinitis: • Fever persisting beyond the fourth postoperative day • Grating sound and/or movement of sternum when client moves or coughs Monitor chest radiograph results for abnormalities.	*Early recognition of signs and symptoms of pneumonia or sternal wound infection/mediastinitis allows for prompt intervention. Signs and symptoms of sternal infection and mediastinitis are often not manifested until the second week after surgery.*

THERAPEUTIC INTERVENTIONS	RATIONALE

Independent Actions
Implement additional measures to reduce the risk for pneumonia:
• Perform actions to maintain adequate respiratory function:
  • Encourage cough and deep breathing.
  • Increase activity as tolerated.
• Have client splint chest incision with a pillow when turning, coughing, and deep breathing.
	Improves lung expansion and decreases stasis of secretions.
	
	Splinting the incision helps increase client's willingness to move, cough, and deep breathe.

Dependent/Collaborative Actions If signs and symptoms of a sternal wound infection and mediastinitis occur: • Administer antimicrobial agents as ordered. • Prepare client for surgical debridement, drainage, and anti-biotic irrigation of wound if planned.	*Treats infection.* *Decreases fear and anxiety.*

Collaborative Diagnosis RISK FOR MYOCARDIAL INFARCTION

Definition: Necrosis of the myocardium due to interruption in blood flow for an extended period

Related to: An increased myocardial oxygen demand and/or insufficient coronary blood flow (can result from coronary artery spasm, hypotension, or thrombosis or embolism of a native coronary vessel or bypass grafts)

CLINICAL MANIFESTATIONS

Subjective	Objective
Reports of sudden severe, persistent chest pain	Change in vital signs; increase in cardiac enzyme levels; new and persistent ST-segment depression or elevation, T-wave inversion, and/or abnormal Q waves on ECG; abnormal extra heart sounds

RISK FACTORS

* Extended low perfusion states
* Vasospasm
* Thrombus

DESIRED OUTCOMES

The client will not experience an MI as evidenced by:
  a. No episodes of sudden and persistent chest pain
  b. Stable vital signs
  c. Cardiac enzyme levels declining toward normal range
  d. Absence of pathological Q wave, ST-segment depression or elevation, and T-wave inversion on ECG

NURSING ASSESSMENT

Assess for and report signs and symptoms of a myocardial infarction:
* Change in vital signs
* Increase in cardiac enzyme levels
* New and persistent ST-segment depression or elevation, T-wave inversion, and/or abnormal Q waves on ECG
* Abnormal extra heart sounds
* Sudden severe, persistent chest pain

RATIONALE

Early recognition of signs and symptoms of a myocardial infarction allows for prompt intervention.

THERAPEUTIC INTERVENTIONS

RATIONALE

Dependent/Collaborative Actions
Implement measures to maintain adequate cardiac output.

If signs and symptoms of a myocardial infarction occur:
* Initiate cardiac monitoring if not currently being done.
* Maintain client on bed rest in a semi- to high-Fowler's position.
* Maintain oxygen therapy as ordered.
* Administer the following medications if ordered:
  * Morphine sulfate

  * Nitrates

  * Beta-adrenergic blocking agents

Adequate cardiac output helps to improve myocardial blood supply and reduce the risk of myocardial infarction.

Improves ability to detect changes quickly.
Promotes lung expansion.

Maintains tissue oxygenation.

Morphine helps reduce pain and anxiety and decrease cardiac workload.
Nitrates help to improve coronary blood flow and reduce myocardial oxygen requirements.
Beta blockers help to reduce myocardial oxygen requirements by decreasing heart rate and the force of myocardial contractility.

| Collaborative Diagnosis | **RISK FOR CARDIAC DYSRHYTHMIAS** |

Definition: Disturbance of the heart rhythm

Related to: Impaired nodal function and/or altered myocardial conductivity associated with trauma to the heart during surgery, hypothermia, hypoxia, sympathetic stimulation (can result from anxiety, volume depletion, and pain), or electrolyte and acid-base imbalances

CLINICAL MANIFESTATIONS

Subjective	Objective
Verbal report of palpitations; lightheadedness	Irregular apical pulse; pulse rate below 60 or above 100 beats/min; apical-radial pulse deficit; syncope; palpitations; abnormal rate, rhythm, or configurations on ECG

RISK FACTORS

- Electrolyte imbalances
- Myocardial ischemia

DESIRED OUTCOMES

The client will maintain normal sinus rhythm as evidenced by:
   a. Regular apical pulse at 60 to 100 beats/min
   b. Equal apical and radial pulse rates
   c. Absence of syncope and palpitations
   d. ECG showing normal sinus rhythm

NURSING ASSESSMENT

Assess for and report signs and symptoms of cardiac dysrhythmias:
- Irregular apical
- Pulse rate <60 or >100 beats/min
- Palpitations

Monitor ECG, levels of serum cardiac enzymes/troponin for abnormalities.

RATIONALE

Early recognition of signs and symptoms of excess of cardiac dysrhythmias allows for prompt intervention.

THERAPEUTIC INTERVENTIONS

RATIONALE

Dependent/Collaborative Actions

Implement measures to prevent cardiac dysrhythmias:
- Perform actions to maintain adequate cardiac output and myocardial blood flow.
- Maintain oxygen therapy as ordered.
- Monitor serum electrolyte levels; consult physician about administration of a potassium or magnesium supplement if serum levels of either are low.
- Perform actions to maintain adequate respiratory function.

- Administer prophylactic antidysrhythmic agents if ordered.

If cardiac dysrhythmias occur:
- Initiate cardiac monitoring if not still being done.
- Administer antidysrhythmics if ordered.
- Maintain temporary pacemaker function as ordered.
- Restrict client's activity based on client's tolerance and severity of the dysrhythmia.
- Maintain oxygen therapy as ordered.

Optimum respiratory function helps to improve tissue oxygenation and prevent respiratory acidosis or alkalosis (myocardial conductivity is altered by hypoxia and acid-base imbalance).

Continued...

THERAPEUTIC INTERVENTIONS	RATIONALE
• Assess cardiovascular status frequently and report signs and symptoms of inadequate tissue perfusion (e.g., decrease in B/P, cool skin, cyanosis, diminished peripheral pulses, urine output less than 30 mL/h, restlessness and agitation, shortness of breath).	
• Have emergency cart readily available for cardioversion, defibrillation, or cardiopulmonary resuscitation.	

Collaborative Diagnosis ## RISK FOR HEART FAILURE

Definition: Cardiac dysfunction that results in inadequate perfusion of tissues with vital blood-borne nutrients

Related to: Preexisting myocardial dilation or hypertrophy and decreased cardiac output postoperatively associated with damage to and further stress on the heart

CLINICAL MANIFESTATIONS

Subjective	Objective
Report of restlessness; anxiousness; increased weakness/ fatigue	Increased pulse rate; S_3 heart sounds; confusion; change in mental status; crackles; dyspnea; orthopnea; dry, hacking cough; diminished or absent pulses; decreased urine output; weight gain; distended neck veins; increased CVP; chest radiograph results showing pulmonary congestion

RISK FACTORS
• Myocardial infarction
• Decreased cardiac output

DESIRED OUTCOMES

The client will not develop heart failure as evidenced by:
  a. Pulse rate 60 to 100 beats/min
  b. Absence of an S_3 heart sound
  c. Usual mental status
  d. Absence of adventitious breath sounds
  e. Absence of dyspnea, orthopnea, and cough
  f. Palpable peripheral pulses
  g. No increase in fatigue and weakness
  h. Urine output at least 30 mL/h
  i. Stable weight
  j. Absence of edema and distended neck veins
  k. CVP within normal limits

NURSING ASSESSMENT	RATIONALE
Assess for signs and symptoms of heart failure: • Increased pulse rate • S_3 heart sounds • Confusion • Crackles • Dyspnea • Distended neck veins • Restlessness	*Early recognition of signs and symptoms of heart failure allows for prompt intervention.*

THERAPEUTIC INTERVENTIONS	RATIONALE
Dependent/Collaborative Actions Implement measures to prevent heart failure: • Perform actions to maintain adequate cardiac output (e.g., administer intravenous fluids and positive inotropic medications as ordered). • Perform actions to prevent and treat cardiac dysrhythmias (e.g., administer antiarrhythmic agents as ordered).	*Dysrhythmias contribute to the development of heart failure.*

THERAPEUTIC INTERVENTIONS	RATIONALE

If signs and symptoms of heart failure occur:
* Maintain oxygen therapy as ordered. — *Maintains tissue oxygenation.*
* Administer the following medications if ordered:
  * Positive inotropic agents — *Inotropes help to increase myocardial contractility.*
  * Diuretics, ACE inhibitors, and/or vasodilators — *To decrease cardiac workload.*
  * Morphine sulfate — *Morphine helps to reduce preload and anxiety.*

Collaborative Diagnosis | RISK FOR CARDIAC TAMPONADE

Definition: Pericardial effusion that creates sufficient pressure to cause cardiac compression

Related to: Accumulation of fluid (usually blood) in the pericardial sac and/or mediastinum associated with excessive bleeding and/or obstructed drainage of the mediastinal tube

CLINICAL MANIFESTATIONS

Subjective	Objective
Not applicable	Sudden decrease in chest tube drainage; chest radiograph report of widening mediastinum; decreased B/P; narrowed pulse pressure; pulsus paradoxus; distant muffled heart sounds

RISK FACTORS
* Cardiac surgery
* Obstructed postsurgical draining

DESIRED OUTCOMES

The client will not experience cardiac tamponade as evidenced by:
  a. Stable vital signs
  b. Audible heart sounds
  c. Absence of jugular venous distention
  d. Absence of pulsus paradoxus
  e. CVP within normal limits

NURSING ASSESSMENT	RATIONALE

Assess for and report signs and symptoms of cardiac tamponade: — *Early recognition of signs and symptoms of cardiac tamponade allows for prompt intervention.*
* Decreased blood pressure
* Pulsus paradoxus
* Muffled heart sounds

THERAPEUTIC INTERVENTIONS	RATIONALE

Dependent/Collaborative Actions

Implement measures to reduce the risk of cardiac tamponade
* Perform actions to maintain patency and integrity of chest drainage system. — *Prevents pressure buildup on the heart.*
* If chest tube becomes obstructed, assist with clearing of existing tube and/or insertion of a new tube. — *Maintains patency.*
* When removing the pacemaker catheter(s), do it carefully. — *Avoid trauma to the surrounding vessels and subsequent bleeding.*

If signs and symptoms of cardiac tamponade occur:
* Prepare client for echocardiography. — *Decreases fear and anxiety.*
* Administer intravenous fluids and/or vasopressors if ordered. — *Maintains mean arterial pressure.*
* Prepare client for surgical drainage of pericardial fluid. — *Decreases fear and anxiety.*

Collaborative Diagnosis RISK FOR BLEEDING

Definition: Loss of blood from the circulatory system

Related to:
- Impaired platelet function associated with mechanical damage to the platelets by the bypass machine and possible heparin-induced thrombocytopenia
- Incomplete neutralization of the heparin used during surgery to prevent thrombus formation in the bypass machine
- Decreased release and function of clotting factors associated with systemic hypothermia during surgery
- Anticoagulant therapy (relevant primarily for clients who have had valve replacement and are taking warfarin)
- Inadequate surgical hemostasis or disruption of suture lines associated with hypertension if it occurs

CLINICAL MANIFESTATIONS

Subjective	Objective
Reports of unusual joint pain	Excessive amount of bloody drainage from chest tube; continuous oozing of blood from incisions; prolonged bleeding from puncture sites; gingival bleeding; petechiae, purpura, ecchymoses; epistaxis, hemoptysis; increase in abdominal girth; frank or occult blood in stool, urine, or vomitus; menorrhagia; restlessness, confusion; significant drop in B/P accompanied by an increased pulse rate; decrease in Hct and Hgb levels

DESIRED OUTCOMES

The client will not experience unusual bleeding as evidenced by:
  a. Gradual decrease in amount of bloody drainage from chest tube
  b. Skin and mucous membranes free of active bleeding, petechiae, purpura, and ecchymoses
  c. Absence of unusual joint pain
  d. No increase in abdominal girth
  e. Absence of frank and occult blood in stool, urine, and vomitus
  f. Usual menstrual flow
  g. Usual mental status
  h. Vital signs within normal range for client
  i. Stable or improved Hct and Hgb levels

NURSING ASSESSMENT	RATIONALE
Assess for and report signs and symptoms of unusual bleeding: • Excessive amounts of bleeding from chest tubes • Decreased B/P • Increased heart rate Monitor platelet count and coagulation tests for abnormal results or results that exceed the therapeutic range for clients receiving anticoagulant therapy.	*Early recognition of signs and symptoms of unusual bleeding allows for prompt intervention.*

THERAPEUTIC INTERVENTIONS	RATIONALE
Dependent/Collaborative Actions Test all stools, urine, and vomitus for occult blood if platelet count and coagulation tests are abnormal.	*Early detection of abnormal bleeding.*
Implement measures to prevent bleeding: • When giving injections or performing venous and arterial punctures, use the smallest gauge needle possible and apply gentle, prolonged pressure to the site after the needle is removed.	*In order to maintain systolic B/P at a level less than 140 mm Hg and subsequently decrease the risk for disruption of suture lines.*
• Perform actions to prevent and treat hypertension.	
• Caution client to avoid activities that increase the risk for trauma (e.g., shaving with a straight-edge razor, using stiff bristle toothbrush or dental floss).	*Prevents injury.*
• Pad side rails if client is confused or restless.	

THERAPEUTIC INTERVENTIONS	RATIONALE
• Perform actions to reduce the risk for falls (e.g., keep bed in low position with side rails up when client is in bed, avoid unnecessary clutter in room, instruct client to wear shoes/slippers with nonslip soles when ambulating).	
• Instruct client to avoid blowing nose forcefully or straining to have a bowel movement; consult physician regarding order for a decongestant and/or laxative if indicated.	
• Administer the following if ordered:	*Promotes blood clotting.*
• Vitamin K	*Vitamin K counteracts the effect of warfarin therapy.*
• Protamine sulfate	*Protamine sulfate further neutralizes the heparin used to prime the bypass machine.*
If bleeding occurs and does not subside spontaneously:	
• Apply firm, prolonged pressure to bleeding area(s) if possible.	
• Maintain oxygen therapy as ordered.	
• Autotransfuse blood from the chest drainage device if ordered.	
• Administer the following if ordered:	*Promotes blood clotting.*
• Vitamin K or protamine sulfate	
• Whole blood or packed red blood cells	
• Blood products	
• Prepare client for return to surgery.	*Decreases fear and anxiety.*

| Collaborative Diagnosis | # RISK FOR THROMBOEMBOLISM |

Definition: A clot attached to a vessel wall that detaches and circulates within the blood

Related to:
- Trauma to the blood vessels associated with bypass grafting, cannulation for CPB, and cross-clamping of the aorta
- Thrombi formation at the prosthetic valve site (with valve replacement surgeries)
- Formation of microemboli associated with incomplete emptying of cardiac chambers if atrial fibrillation or heart failure occurs
- Venous stasis associated with diminished cardiac output and decreased activity
- Hypercoagulability associated with activation of the coagulation cascade during CPB (the body does not recognize the non-endothelial surfaces of the bypass machine and initiates the inflammatory and coagulation cascades in response to what it perceives as a foreign substance)

CLINICAL MANIFESTATIONS

Subjective	Objective
Deep vein thrombus: Reports of pain, tenderness	Deep vein thrombus: Swelling, unusual warmth, and/or positive Homans' sign in extremity
Arterial thrombus: Reports of numbness and/or pain in extremity	Arterial thrombus: Diminished or absent peripheral pulses; pallor, coolness
Cerebral ischemia: Not applicable	Cerebral ischemia: Decreased level of consciousness; alteration in usual sensory and motor function
Pulmonary embolism: Reports of sudden onset of chest pain; increased dyspnea	Pulmonary embolism: Increased restlessness and apprehension; significant decrease in arterial oxygen saturation (SaO_2)

Continued...

RISK FACTOR

- Virchow's triad: venous stasis, endothelial trauma (surgery), blood hypercoagulability

DESIRED OUTCOMES

The client will not develop a thromboembolism as evidenced by:
  a. Absence of pain, tenderness, swelling, and numbness in extremities
  b. Usual temperature and color of extremities
  c. Palpable and equal peripheral pulses
  d. Usual mental status
  e. Usual sensory and motor function
  f. Absence of sudden chest pain and dyspnea

NURSING ASSESSMENT	**RATIONALE**
Assess for and report signs and symptoms of deep vein thrombus, arterial embolus in an extremity, cerebral ischemia, or pulmonary embolism. • Swelling, warmth, redness in extremity • Diminished or absent pulses • Altered level of consciousness • Restlessness • Apprehension	*Early recognition of signs and symptoms of thromboembolism allows prompt intervention.*

THERAPEUTIC INTERVENTIONS	**RATIONALE**

Dependent/Collaborative Actions
Implement measures to prevent thrombi and microemboli formation in the heart:
• Perform actions to prevent stasis of blood in the heart:
  • Implement measures to prevent and treat cardiac dysrhythmias.
  • Implement measures to maintain an adequate cardiac output.
	With atrial fibrillation and the resultant decrease in cardiac output due to ineffective atrial contractions, thrombi may form in the atria as a result of blood stasis.

• Administer anticoagulants if ordered.	*Decreases potential for blood clotting.*
If signs and symptoms of an arterial embolus occur: • Maintain client on strict bed rest with affected extremity in a level or slightly dependent position.	*Improves arterial blood flow.*
• Prepare client for diagnostic studies (e.g., Doppler or duplex ultrasound, arteriography).	*Decreases fear and anxiety.*
• Administer anticoagulants if ordered. • Prepare client for surgical intervention (e.g., embolectomy, revascularization) if planned.	*Decreases potential for clotting.* *Improves blood flow by removing thrombus.*

Collaborative Diagnosis **RISK FOR NEUROLOGICAL DYSFUNCTION**

Definition: Decreased level of consciousness and client's normal cognitive, sensory, and motor function

Related to:
- Inadequate cerebral blood flow associated with:
  - Decreased systemic arterial pressure while on CPB
  - An embolus (can result from dislodgment of atherosclerotic plaque during cross-clamping of the aorta and cannulation for bypass, dislodgment of debris from calcified valve, incomplete filtration of air by bypass machine, or cardiac thrombus formation on prosthetic valve or as a result of dysrhythmias)
  - Hypotension or low cardiac output postoperatively
- Cerebral edema initiated by a systemic inflammatory response to the CPB machine
- Possible poor cerebral protection during CPB from inadequate temperature regulation (hypothermia must be adequate to help protect the central nervous system)

CLINICAL MANIFESTATIONS

Subjective	Objective
Reports of visual disturbances; swallowing difficulties; paresthesias	Slurred speech, expressive or receptive aphasia; decreased level of consciousness, delirium, hallucinations, confusion; impaired memory, lack of ability to concentrate, difficulty problem-solving; weakness of extremity, facial droop, ptosis, paralysis Decline in client's normal sensory and motor function

RISK FACTORS

- Thromboembolism
- Altered cerebral perfusion during bypass

DESIRED OUTCOMES

The client will maintain usual neurological function as evidenced by:
- a. Absence of visual disturbances, swallowing difficulties, and speech impairments
- b. Mentally alert and oriented
- c. Usual memory and problem-solving abilities
- d. Normal sensory and motor function

NURSING ASSESSMENT

Assess for and report signs and symptoms of neurological dysfunction:
- Slurred speech
- Expressive/receptor dysphagia
- Decreased level of consciousness
- Weakness of extremity
- Facial droop
- Ptosis
- Swallowing difficulties

RATIONALE

Early recognition of signs and symptoms of neurological dysfunction allows prompt intervention.

THERAPEUTIC INTERVENTIONS

Dependent/Collaborative Actions

Implement measures to promote adequate cerebral blood flow and reduce the risk for neurological dysfunction:
- Keep head of bed flat until B/P is stabilized at a satisfactory level (at least 90 mm Hg systolic).
- Keep head and neck in neutral, midline position.
- Perform actions to maintain adequate cardiac output (e.g., administer positive inotropic medications as ordered).
- Perform actions to prevent thrombi and microemboli formation in the heart.
- Perform actions to reduce the risk for increased intracranial pressure (ICP):
  - Limit activities that can increase ICP (e.g., excessive suctioning, instruct client to avoid excessive coughing and straining to have a bowel movement).
  - Implement measures to maintain adequate respiratory function and gas exchange.

If signs and symptoms of neurological dysfunction occur:
- Maintain client on bed rest until physician evaluates symptoms.
- Maintain oxygen therapy as ordered.
- Administer anticoagulants if ordered.

RATIONALE

Improves blood flow to the central nervous system.

To prevent dilation of the cerebral vessels associated with hypoxia and hypercapnia.

Maintains tissue oxygenation.
Decreases potential for thrombi.

NDx = NANDA-I Diagnosis   **D** = Delegatable Action   ● = LAP   ✦ = LVN/LPN   ⊖▶ = Go to ⊖volve for animation

RISK FOR IMPAIRED RENAL FUNCTION

Definition: Renal insufficiency refers to a decline in renal function to about 25% of normal

Related to: Deposit of hemolyzed red blood cell products in renal tubules or inadequate renal blood flow associated with CPB, low cardiac output, hypotension, an embolus, or effect of vasopressor drugs (risk is increased if client is elderly or has preexisting renal disease)

CLINICAL MANIFESTATIONS

Subjective	Objective
Reports of confusion	Urine output less than 30 mL/h; urine specific gravity fixed at or less than 1.010; elevated BUN and serum creatinine levels; decreased creatinine clearance

RISK FACTORS

- Decreased cardiac output
- Thromboembolism

DESIRED OUTCOMES

The client will maintain adequate renal function as evidenced by:
  a. Urine output at least 30 mL/h
  b. BUN, serum creatinine, and creatinine clearance values within normal range

NURSING ASSESSMENT	RATIONALE
Assess for and report signs and symptoms of impaired renal function: • Urine output >30 mL/h • Elevsted BUN, creatinine values Monitor serum creatinine levels for abnormalities.	*Early recognition of signs and symptoms of impaired renal function allows prompt intervention.*

THERAPEUTIC INTERVENTIONS	RATIONALE
Dependent/Collaborative Actions Implement measures to maintain adequate renal blood flow: • Maintain a minimum fluid intake of 1000 mL/day unless ordered otherwise. • Perform actions to maintain adequate cardiac output. • Perform actions to prevent thrombi and microemboli formation in the heart. If signs and symptoms of impaired renal function occur: • Administer diuretics. • Consult physician about discontinuing any potentially nephrotoxic medications. • Assess for and report signs of acute renal failure (e.g., oliguria or anuria; weight gain; edema; elevated B/P; lethargy and confusion; increasing BUN and serum creatinine, phosphorus, and potassium levels). • Prepare client for dialysis if indicated.	 *Maintains adequate fluid volume.* *To reduce the risk for occlusion of the renal artery by an embolus.* *To increase urine output and subsequently reduce further accumulation of hemolyzed red blood cell products in the renal tubules.* *Potentially improves renal functioning.* *Allows for prompt alteration in interventions.* *Decreases fear and anxiety.*

RISK FOR PNEUMOTHORAX

Definition: Presence of air or gas in the pleural space caused by rupture of the visceral pleural or the parietal pleura and chest wall

Related to: The accumulation of air in the pleural space if the pleura was opened during surgery

CLINICAL MANIFESTATIONS

Subjective	Objective
Reports of sudden pleural pain; verbalization of shortness of breath	Tachypnea; dyspnea; absent or decreased breath sounds; hyperresonance to percussion on affected side; chest radiograph abnormalities; abnormal arterial blood gas values

RISK FACTORS

- Surgical procedures within the chest cavity
- Invasive line placement in great vessels (e.g., subclavian)

DESIRED OUTCOMES

The client will experience normal lung re-expansion as evidenced by:
   a. Audible breath sounds and a resonant percussion note over lungs by third to fourth postoperative day
   b. Unlabored respirations at 12 to 20 breaths/min
   c. Arterial blood gas values returning toward normal
   d. Chest radiograph showing lung reexpansion

NURSING ASSESSMENT

Assess for and immediately report signs and symptoms of pneumothorax:
- Subjective
- Objective

Assess for malfunction of chest drainage system:
- Respiratory distress
- Excessive bubbling in water seal chamber
- Significant increase in subcutaneous emphysema

Monitor chest radiograph results.

RATIONALE

Early recognition of signs and symptoms of a pneumothorax allows prompt intervention.

THERAPEUTIC INTERVENTIONS

Dependent/Collaborative Actions

Perform actions to maintain patency and integrity of chest drainage system:
- Maintain fluid level in the water seal and suction chambers as ordered.
- Maintain occlusive dressing over chest tube insertion site.
- Tape all connections securely.
- Tape the tubing to the chest wall close to insertion site.
- Position tubing to promote optimum drainage (e.g., coil excess tubing on bed rather than allowing it to hang down below the collection device, keep tubing free of kinks).
- Drain any fluid that accumulates in tubing into the collection chamber and milk tube gently if indicated to dislodge clots.
- Keep drainage collection device below level of client's chest at all times.

Perform actions to facilitate the escape of air from the pleural space (e.g., maintain suction as ordered, ensure that the air vent is open on the drainage collection device if system is to water seal only).

Perform actions to maintain adequate respiratory function:
- Encourage use of incentive spirometer every 2 hours.
- Increase activity as tolerated.

If signs and symptoms of further lung collapse occur:
- Maintain client on bed rest in a semi- to high-Fowler's position.
- Maintain oxygen therapy as ordered.

RATIONALE

Measures help to promote lung reexpansion and prevent further lung collapse.
Maintains negative pressure.
To reduce the risk of inadvertent removal of the tube.

Dislodges clots.

Prevents backflow and stasis of drainage.

Promotes full lung expansion.

Promotes lung expansion and prevents stasis of secretions.

Improves ability for lung expansion.

Maintains tissue oxygenation.

NDx = NANDA-I Diagnosis   **D** = Delegatable Action   ● = UAP   ✦ = LVN/LPN   ⊝▶ = Go to ⊝volve for animation

Continued...

THERAPEUTIC INTERVENTIONS	RATIONALE
• Assess for and immediately report signs and symptoms of tension pneumothorax (e.g., severe dyspnea, increased restlessness and agitation, rapid and/or irregular pulse rate, hypotension, neck vein distention, shift in trachea from midline).	*Allows for prompt alterations in interventions.*
• Assist with clearing of existing chest tube and/or insertion of a new tube.	

Nursing Diagnosis

DEFICIENT KNOWLEDGE NDx; INEFFECTIVE FAMILY THERAPEUTIC REGIMEN MANAGEMENT NDx; OR INEFFECTIVE SELF-HEALTH MANAGEMENT NDx*

Definition: Absence or deficiency of cognitive information related to specific topic (lack of specific information necessary for clients/significant others to make informed choices regarding condition/treatment/lifestyle changes); pattern of regulating and integrating into daily living a program for treatment of illness and the sequelae of illness that is unsatisfactory for meeting specific health goals; inability to identify, manage, and/or seek out help to manage health

CLINICAL MANIFESTATIONS

Subjective	**Objective**
Verbalization of unfamiliarity with information	Inability to follow instructions

RISK FACTORS
• Denial of disease process
• Cognitive deficiency
• Failure to take action to reduce risk factors

NOC OUTCOMES	NIC INTERVENTIONS
Knowledge: treatment regimen; knowledge: cardiac disease management; knowledge: disease process	Health system guidance; teaching: individual; teaching: disease process; teaching: prescribed diet; teaching: prescribed medication; teaching: prescribed activity/exercise

NURSING ASSESSMENT	RATIONALE
Assess client's readiness and ability to learn.	*Early recognition of readiness to learn and meaning of illness to client allows for implementation of the appropriate teaching interventions.*
Assess meaning of illness to client.	

THERAPEUTIC INTERVENTIONS	RATIONALE

Desired Outcome: The client will identify modifiable cardiovascular risk factors and ways to alter these factors.

Independent Actions

Inform client that certain modifiable factors such as elevated serum lipid levels, a sedentary lifestyle, hypertension, excessive alcohol intake, and smoking have been shown to increase the risk for coronary artery disease and certain forms of heart disease.	*Thorough education is a critical component of the care of a client after open heart surgery. Continued lifestyle modifications consistent with recommendations for clients with cardiovascular disease are necessary to maintain patency of vessel grafts. The client must have a thorough understanding of the importance of adhering to diet, medication, activity/exercise, and nutritional recommendations to prevent an exacerbation and control the disease.*

---

*The nurse should select the nursing diagnostic label that is most appropriate for the client's discharge teaching needs.

THERAPEUTIC INTERVENTIONS	RATIONALE

Assist clients to identify changes in lifestyle that can help them to eliminate or reduce the above risk factors (e.g., dietary modification, physical exercise on a regular basis, moderation of alcohol intake, smoking cessation).

Encourage client to limit daily alcohol consumption. Current recommendations are no more than 2 drinks per day for men and no more than 1 drink per day for women and lighter-weight persons. A "drink" is considered to be ½ oz of ethanol (e.g., 1½ oz of 80-proof whiskey, 12 oz of beer, 5 oz of wine).

Daily alcohol intake exceeding 1 oz of ethanol may contribute to the development of hypertension and some forms of heart disease.

THERAPEUTIC INTERVENTIONS	RATIONALE

Desired Outcome: The client will verbalize an understanding of the rationale for and components of a diet restricted in sodium, saturated fat, and cholesterol.

Independent Actions

Explain the rationale for a diet restricting sodium, saturated fat, and cholesterol intake.

Provide the following information about decreasing sodium intake:
- Read labels on foods/fluids and calculate sodium content of items; avoid those products that tend to have a high sodium content (e.g., canned soups and vegetables, tomato juice, commercial baked goods, commercially prepared frozen or canned entrees and sauces).
- Do not add salt when cooking foods or to prepared foods; use low-sodium herbs and spices if desired.
- Avoid cured and smoked foods.
- Avoid salty snack foods (e.g., crackers, nuts, pretzels, potato chips).
- Avoid commercially prepared fast foods.
- Avoid routine use of over-the-counter medications with a high sodium content (e.g., Alka-Seltzer, some antacids).

Provide instructions on ways the client can reduce intake of saturated fat and cholesterol:
- Reduce intake of meat fat (e.g., trim visible fat off meat; replace fatty meats such as fatty cuts of steak, hamburger, and processed meats with leaner products).
- Reduce intake of milk fat (e.g., avoid dairy products containing more than 1% fat).
- Reduce intake of *trans* fats (e.g., avoid stick margarine and shortening and foods such as commercial baked goods that are prepared with these products).
- Use vegetable oil rather than coconut or palm oil in cooking and food preparation.
- Use cooking methods such as steaming, baking, broiling, poaching, microwaving, and grilling rather than frying.
- Restrict intake of eggs (recommendations about the number of whole eggs allowed per week vary depending on the client's lipid levels).

Obtain a dietary consult to assist client in planning meals that will meet the prescribed restrictions of sodium, saturated fat, and cholesterol.

Current daily dietary sodium intake is less than 2400 mg. Excessive sodium intake causes water to be retained, resulting in increased circulating fluid volume, increased cardiac workload, and hypertension.

Understanding of disease limitations improves client adherence to treatment regimen.

The risk of coronary artery disease (CAD) is associated with a serum cholesterol level of more than 200 mg/dL or a fasting triglyceride level of more than 150 mg/dL. Elevated serum lipid levels are one of the most firmly established risk factors for CAD.

Continued...

THERAPEUTIC INTERVENTIONS	RATIONALE

Desired Outcome: The client will verbalize an understanding of activity restrictions and the rate of activity progression.

Independent Actions

Reinforce physician's instructions regarding activity. Instruct client to:

- Gradually rebuild activity level by adhering to a planned exercise program (often begins with walking and light household activities).
- Take frequent rest periods for 4 to 6 weeks after surgery.
- Avoid lifting heavy objects in order to allow incision to heal and prevent a sudden increase in cardiac workload.
- Avoid driving a car and riding a bicycle, motorcycle, lawn mower, tractor, or a horse for 4 to 6 weeks; if minimally invasive surgery was performed, these activities will probably be allowed much sooner.
- Check with physician or cardiac rehabilitation therapist before resuming sexual activity (usually permitted 3 to 4 weeks after surgery once able to walk 2 blocks or climb 2 flights of stairs without shortness of breath).
- Stop any activity that causes chest pain, shortness of breath, palpitations, dizziness, or extreme fatigue or weakness.
- Participate in a cardiac rehabilitation program if recommended by physician.

While the benefits of physical activity are an integral part of cardiac rehabilitation, the level of activity should be increased gradually. Physical activity guidelines after acute coronary syndromes focus on frequency, intensity, type, and time of activity.

THERAPEUTIC INTERVENTIONS	RATIONALE

Desired Outcome: The client will verbalize an understanding of medications ordered including rationale, food and drug interactions, side effects, schedule for taking, and importance of taking as prescribed.

Independent Actions

Explain the rationale for, side effects of, and importance of taking medications prescribed. Inform client of pertinent food and drug interactions.
- Warfarin (Coumadin)

Instruct client to inform physician before taking other prescription and nonprescription medications.
Instruct client to inform all health care providers of medications being taken.

Taking medications as prescribed ensures that therapeutic drug levels will be maintained. Clients should be instructed not to discontinue taking medications if they feel better. Clients without financial resources should be assisted in accessing appropriate resources to obtain needed medications (e.g., pharmacy assistance programs).

THERAPEUTIC INTERVENTIONS	RATIONALE

Desired Outcome: The client will state signs and symptoms to report to the health care provider.

Independent Actions

Instruct client to report these additional signs and symptoms:

- Chest pain that seems unrelated to incisional discomfort
- Development of or increased shortness of breath
- Dizziness, fainting
- Increased fatigue and weakness

Reporting concerning signs and symptoms to the appropriate provider allows for modification of the treatment plan.
May indicate a pulmonary embolism.
May indicate decreased cardiac output.

THERAPEUTIC INTERVENTIONS	RATIONALE
• Weight gain of more than 2 lb in a day or 4 lb in a week	*May indicate decreased renal function.*
• Swelling of feet or ankles	
• Persistent cough, especially if productive of yellow, green, rust-colored, or frothy sputum	*May indicate infection or pulmonary embolism.*
• Significant change in pulse rate or rhythm (check with physician about client's need to monitor pulse at home)	*May indicate decreased cardiac output.*
• Persistent low-grade fever or temperature above 101° F (38.3° C) for more than 1 day	*May indicate dehydration and/or infection.*
• Depression or problems with concentration or memory that last more than 6 weeks	*A common feature after bypass surgery, but it should be resolved by 6 weeks.*
• A fever in combination with chest pain and malaise occurring 1 week to 1 month after surgery	*May be indicative of postpericardiotomy syndrome and require treatment with anti-inflammatory agents.*

THERAPEUTIC INTERVENTIONS	RATIONALE

Desired Outcome: The client will identify community resources that can assist with cardiac rehabilitation and adjustment to having had heart surgery.

Independent Actions

Provide information about community resources that can assist client with cardiac rehabilitation and adjustment to having had heart surgery (e.g., American Heart Association, Mended Hearts Club, counseling services).

Cardiac disease can significantly impact an individual's and family's socioeconomic status. Providing information specific to community resources is important to provide a necessary continuum of care and may impact the client's health status, preventing future hospitalizations.

THERAPEUTIC INTERVENTIONS	RATIONALE

Desired Outcome: The client will verbalize an understanding of and a plan for adhering to recommended follow-up care including future appointments with health care provider, wound care, and pain management.

Independent Actions

Provide the client with routine postoperative instructions and measures to improve adherence.

If valve replacement surgery was done, instruct the client to:
• Not have dental work for 6 months.
• Inform health care providers of valve surgery so prophylactic antimicrobials may be started before any dental work, invasive diagnostic procedures, or surgery.
• Perform good oral hygiene in order to reduce the risk for infective endocarditis.

Regular health care appointments are important to determine effectiveness of the prescribed treatment plan.
Actions are important to prevent the development of endocarditis.

ADDITIONAL NURSING DIAGNOSES

ACTIVITY INTOLERANCE NDx
Related to:
• Tissue hypoxia associated with decreased cardiac output, impaired alveolar gas exchange, and anemia (results from hemodilution, blood loss, and red cell hemolysis [red cells are traumatized by the CPB machine])

• Difficulty resting and sleeping associated with frequent assessments and treatments, discomfort, fear, and anxiety

RELATED CARE PLANS

Standardized Preoperative Care Plan
Standardized Postoperative Care Plan

HYPERTENSION

Hypertension is defined by the Joint National Committee on Prevention, Detection, Evaluation, and Treatment of High Blood Pressure as a systolic blood pressure (SBP) of 140 mm Hg or greater, a diastolic blood pressure (DBP) of 90 mm Hg or greater, or taking antihypertensive medication. Isolated systolic hypertension (ISH) is present when the SBP is greater than 140 mm Hg and the DBP is less than 90 mm Hg. The classification of hypertension is based on the level of the blood pressure. The current classification system includes a category designated as prehypertension (SBP of 120-139 mm Hg or DBP of 80-89 mm Hg) and divides hypertension into two stages.

Stage 1 hypertension is an average SBP of 140 to 159 mm Hg or a DBP of 90 to 99 mm Hg. Stage 2 hypertension is a SBP of greater than 160 mm Hg or a DBP greater than 100 mm Hg. In addition to classifying the stages of hypertension on the basis of average blood pressure readings, the clinician usually also specifies the presence or absence of target organ disease and the additional risk factors for cardiovascular disease that are present. Hypertensive crisis, urgency, or emergency are terms used to describe a situation in which the pressure elevation poses an immediate threat to the client's life.

The two major types of hypertension are essential (primary or idiopathic) hypertension and secondary hypertension. Essential hypertension, which constitutes approximately 95% of the cases, has an unknown etiology. Secondary hypertension has identifiable causes, which include renal parenchymal or vascular disease, Cushing's syndrome, certain neurological disorders, pheochromocytoma, primary aldosteronism, coarctation of the aorta, and use of certain drugs (e.g., adrenal steroids, oral contraceptives, nonsteroidal antiinflammatories, cyclooxygenase-2 inhibitors, sympathomimetics such as decongestants and anorexiants, amphetamines, cocaine).

The pathological hallmark of hypertension is an increase in systemic vascular resistance. In order to sustain adequate tissue perfusion when vascular resistance is increased, the heart must pump harder. A prolonged increase in cardiac workload eventually leads to ventricular hypertrophy and heart failure. The prolonged increase in vascular pressure causes widespread pathological changes in the blood vessels. The end result of all the changes in the cardiovascular system is a decreased blood supply to the tissues, with target organ damage occurring most often in the eyes, kidneys, brain, and heart. This target organ damage is often what causes the initial symptoms in the person with hypertension.

Initial treatment of hypertension may be nonpharmacologic and consists of lifestyle modifications such as weight reduction, regular aerobic exercise, and moderation of dietary sodium and alcohol intake. If these measures do not achieve the desired control of blood pressure, pharmacological therapy is initiated. A diuretic alone or in combination with an angiotensin-converting enzyme inhibitor, an angiotensin II receptor antagonist, a calcium-channel blocking agent, or a beta-adrenergic blocking agent is considered appropriate for initial pharmacological therapy. If the person's blood pressure is inadequately controlled by the initial drug, a second drug from another class is added or another drug is substituted until the desired control of blood pressure is achieved with a minimum of side effects.

This care plan focuses on the adult client hospitalized with severe hypertension that is either newly diagnosed or uncontrolled.

OUTCOME/DISCHARGE CRITERIA

The client will:
1. Have B/P within a safe range
2. Have evidence of adequate tissue perfusion
3. Have no signs and symptoms of complications
4. Verbalize a basic understanding of hypertension and its effects on the body
5. Identify modifiable risk factors for hypertension and ways to alter these factors
6. Verbalize an understanding of medications ordered including rationale, food and drug interactions, side effects, schedule for taking, and importance of taking as prescribed
7. Verbalize an understanding of the rationale for and components of the recommended diet
8. State signs and symptoms to report to the health care provider
9. Identify community resources that can assist in making lifestyle changes necessary for effective control of hypertension.
10. Verbalize an understanding of and a plan for adhering to recommended follow-up care including future appointments with health care provider.

Nursing Diagnosis   INEFFECTIVE TISSUE PERFUSION NDx

Definition: Decrease in oxygen resulting in failure to nourish tissues at the capillary level

Related to:
- Increased peripheral vascular resistance
- Atherogenic changes in the blood vessels associated with the effects of prolonged or excessive elevation of B/P
- Possible decrease in cardiac output associated with the increased cardiac workload and eventual myocardial hypertrophy that result from elevated B/P
- Excessive lowering of B/P by antihypertensive medications

CLINICAL MANIFESTATIONS

Subjective	Objective
Not applicable	Altered mental status, restlessness, confusion, cold extremities, diminished pulses, pallor in extremities, absent bowel sounds, abdominal pain, anemia, elevated BUN

RISK FACTORS

- Peripheral vascular disease
- Atherosclerosis
- Decreased hemoglobin
- Interruption of blood flow

DESIRED OUTCOMES

The client will maintain adequate tissue perfusion as evidenced by:
  a. B/P declining toward normal range for client
  b. Usual mental status
  c. Extremities warm with absence of pallor and cyanosis
  d. Palpable peripheral pulses
  e. Capillary refill time less than 2 to 3 seconds
  f. Absence of exercise-induced pain
  g. Urine output at least 30 mL/h

NOC OUTCOMES

Circulation status; tissue perfusion: cerebral

NIC INTERVENTIONS

Vital signs monitoring; hemodynamic regulation; cerebral perfusion promotion

NURSING ASSESSMENT	RATIONALE

Assess for and report the following:
• Further increase in B/P, failure of B/P to decline in response to antihypertensive agents, or rapid or excessive decline in B/P.
• Signs and symptoms of diminished tissue perfusion:
  • Restlessness
  • Confusion
  • Cool extremities
  • Pallor or cyanosis of extremities
  • Diminished or absent peripheral pulses
  • Low capillary refill
  • Angina
  • Increasing BUN and serum creatinine levels
  • Oliguria
Assess and monitor B/P.
	Early recognition of signs and symptoms of ineffective tissue perfusion allows for prompt intervention.

THERAPEUTIC INTERVENTIONS	RATIONALE
Independent Actions Implement measures to reduce anxiety (e.g., provide a calm, restful environment). Implement measures to relieve headache (e.g., minimize environmental stimulation). Implement measures to promote rest: **D** ● ✦ • Maintain a calm environment. • Limit the number of visitors. • Maintain activity restrictions.	*Identified independent nursing actions help to reduce sympathetic nervous system stimulation, which could increase B/P and heart rate.*
Discourage excessive intake of beverages high in caffeine such as coffee, tea, and colas. **D** ✦	*Caffeine has a vasoconstrictive effect.* *Vasoconstriction reduces the size/diameter of arterial vessel walls, increasing systemic vascular resistance or afterload. As a result of an increase in afterload, B/P must be increased to maintain adequate tissue perfusion.*
Discourage smoking.	*Nicotine causes vasoconstriction, which elevates B/P by increasing afterload/systemic vascular resistance.*

NDx = NANDA-I Diagnosis   **D** = Delegatable Action   ● = LAP   ✦ = LVN/LPN   ⊖▶ = Go to ⊖volve for animation

Continued...

THERAPEUTIC INTERVENTIONS	RATIONALE
Maintain dietary sodium restrictions as ordered. **D** ✦	*Restricting sodium intake helps to reduce fluid retention, which can increase preload and B/P.*
Dependent/Collaborative Actions	
Administer the following medications if ordered: **D** ✦ • Adrenergic inhibiting agents • Centrally acting adrenergic inhibitors • Alpha-adrenergic blockers • Peripheral adrenergic inhibitors • Beta-adrenergic blockers Combined alpha-adrenergic and beta-adrenergic blockers • Vasodilators for immediate reduction in B/P • Angiotensin-converting enzyme inhibitors • Calcium-channel blocking agents • Angiotensin II receptor antagonists • Diuretics	*Medications are administered to reduce B/P in order to improve tissue perfusion.* *Persistent, untreated hypertension leads to myocardial hypertrophy and possibly heart failure.*
Consult physician: • Before administering antihypertensive medications if client has an excessive or rapid drop in B/P • If signs and symptoms of diminished tissue perfusion persist or worsen.	*A rapid drop in B/P of more than 20% to 25% in a person with severe hypertension can reduce perfusion to vital organs.* *Notification of the appropriate health care provider allows for modification of the treatment plan.*

Nursing Diagnosis ACUTE PAIN NDx (HEADACHE)

Definition: Unpleasant sensory and emotional experience arising from actual or potential tissue damage

Related to: Distention of the cerebral blood vessels associated with increased vascular pressure

CLINICAL MANIFESTATIONS

Subjective	Objective
Verbal reports of pain such as "pressure," "squeezing tightness" in the skull, face, or both	Increased B/P; increased heart rate

RISK FACTORS	DESIRED OUTCOMES
• Increased B/P • Increased cerebral blood flow	The client will obtain relief of headache as evidenced by: a. Verbalization of same b. Relaxed facial expression and body positioning c. Increased participation in activities

NOC OUTCOMES	NIC INTERVENTIONS
Comfort level; pain control	Pain management; environmental management: comfort; analgesic administration

NURSING ASSESSMENT	RATIONALE
Assess for signs and symptoms of headache: • Statements of same • Restlessness • Irritability • Grimacing • Rubbing head • Avoidance of bright lights and noises • Reluctance to move	*Early recognition of signs and symptoms of acute headache pain allows for prompt intervention.*

NURSING ASSESSMENT	RATIONALE
Assess client's perception of the severity of the headache using a pain intensity rating scale.	
Assess the client's pain pattern (e.g., location, quality, onset, duration, precipitating factors, aggravating factors, alleviating factors).	

THERAPEUTIC INTERVENTIONS	RATIONALE
Independent Actions	
Perform actions to reduce fear and anxiety about the pain experience.	*Fear and anxiety can stimulate the sympathetic nervous system, causing an increase in B/P and heart rate.*
	Decreasing fear and anxiety helps to promote relaxation and increase the client's threshold and tolerance for pain.
Provide a quiet environment. **D** ● ✦	*Patients with migraine-type headaches can benefit from a dimly lit environment.*
Avoid jarring bed or startling client to minimize risk of sudden movements. **D** ● ✦	
Provide or assist with nonpharmacological measures for headache relief: **D** ✦	
• Cool cloth to forehead	
• Back and neck massage	
• Elevation of head	
• Relaxation exercises	
• Diversional activities	
Dependent/Collaborative Actions	
Perform actions to reduce B/P:	*Elevated B/P, if extreme, can cause headaches in some individuals.*
• Administer ordered antihypertensive medications. **D** ✦	
Administer analgesics as ordered and before headache becomes severe. **D** ✦	
Consult appropriate health care provider (e.g., pharmacist, physician) if above measures fail to relieve headache.	*Notification of the appropriate health care provider allows for modification of the treatment plan.*

Collaborative Diagnosis | # RISK FOR CEREBROVASCULAR ACCIDENT/HYPERTENSIVE ENCEPHALOPATHY

Definition: Death of brain cells due to ischemia (lack of blood flow) to a part of the brain, or hemorrhage into the brain

Related to:

Cerebrovascular accident related to cerebral thrombosis, embolism, or hemorrhage associated with injury to the arterial walls resulting from atherosclerosis and/or a prolonged increase in pressure in the cerebral vessels

Hypertensive encephalopathy related to cerebral edema associated with hyperperfusion of the brain (excessive cerebral blood flow results from decompensation of the cerebral blood flow autoregulatory mechanism in response to markedly elevated B/P)

CLINICAL MANIFESTATIONS

Subjective	Objective
Verbal reports of difficulty swallowing	Speech difficulty, impaired mobility, decreased level of consciousness, facial droop, ptosis

---

NDx = NANDA-I Diagnosis **D** = Delegatable Action ● = UAP ✦ = LVN/LPN ⊜▶ = Go to ⊜volve for animation

Continued...

RISK FACTORS
- Hypertension
- Cerebrovascular disease
- Smoking
- Obesity
- Metabolic syndrome

DESIRED OUTCOMES

The client will not experience a cerebrovascular accident or hypertensive encephalopathy as evidenced by:
 a. Absence of dizziness, syncope, visual disturbances, and speech impairments
 b. Absence or resolution of headache
 c. Absence of vomiting
 d. Mentally alert and oriented
 e. Pupils equal and normally reactive to light
 f. Normal sensory and motor function

NURSING ASSESSMENT

Assess for signs and symptoms of cerebrovascular accident/hypertensive encephalopathy:
- Dizziness, syncope
- Visual disturbances (e.g., diplopia, blurred vision, loss of vision)
- Slurred speech, aphasia
- Persistent or increasing headache
- Vomiting
- Decreased level of consciousness
- Unequal pupils or a sluggish or absent pupillary reaction to light
- Paresthesias, facial droop, ptosis, weakness of extremity, paralysis
- Seizures

RATIONALE

Early recognition of signs and symptoms of cerebrovascular accident and/or hypertensive encephalopathy allows for prompt intervention.

THERAPEUTIC INTERVENTIONS

Dependent/Collaborative Actions
Perform actions to reduce B/P:
- Administer medications as ordered. **D** ✦

Instruct client to avoid activities that create a Valsalva response (e.g., straining to have a bowel movement, holding breath while moving up in bed).

Keep head of bed elevated at least 30 degrees and encourage client to keep head and neck in neutral, midline position. **D** ✦ ●

If signs and symptoms of a cerebrovascular accident or hypertensive encephalopathy occur:
- Administer antihypertensive agents if ordered:
  - Vasodilators
- Maintain client on bed rest.
- Initiate appropriate safety measures (e.g., side rails up, seizure precautions).
- Administer osmotic diuretics and corticosteroids if ordered.

RATIONALE

Collectively, all collaborative actions help to reduce the risk of a cerebrovascular accident and hypertensive encephalopathy.
Actions help to prevent a sudden increase in intracranial pressure and dislodgment of an existing thrombus.

Actions help to promote adequate venous return from the cerebral vessels.

Provides for rapid B/P reduction.
Medications help to reduce intracranial pressure.

Collaborative Diagnosis **RISK FOR ANGINA AND/OR MYOCARDIAL INFARCTION**

Definition: Angina is the clinical manifestation of myocardial ischemia caused by the imbalance between myocardial oxygen supply and demand. Myocardial infarction is irreversible myocardial damage

Related to:
- Insufficient myocardial blood flow associated with coronary artery disease (a sequela of inadequately controlled hypertension)
- Myocardial oxygen demands exceeding the oxygen supply (a result of the increased cardiac workload that occurs with increased vascular resistance)

CLINICAL MANIFESTATIONS

Subjective	Objective
Verbal reports of chest pain; sensation of heaviness/pressure; nausea	Diaphoresis; variations in vital signs; dysrhythmias; ECG changes

RISK FACTORS

- Coronary artery disease
- Obesity
- Smoking
- Hypertension
- Metabolic syndrome

DESIRED OUTCOMES

The client will not experience episodes of myocardial ischemia as evidenced by:
  a. Absence of chest pain
  b. Unlabored respirations at 12 to 20 breaths/min
  c. Cardiac enzyme levels within normal range
  d. Absence of ST-segment depression or elevation, T-wave inversion, and abnormal Q waves on ECG

NURSING ASSESSMENT

Assess for signs and symptoms of myocardial ischemia:
- Chest pain/discomfort
- Dyspnea

Monitor ECG for abnormalities.

RATIONALE

Early recognition of signs and symptoms of angina and/or myocardial infarction allows for prompt intervention.

THERAPEUTIC INTERVENTIONS

RATIONALE

Dependent/Collaborative Actions

Instruct client to avoid activities that create a Valsalva response (e.g., straining to have a bowel movement, holding breath while moving up in bed).

Decreases intrathoracic pressure.

Increase activity gradually as allowed and tolerated.

If signs and symptoms of myocardial ischemia occur:
- Consult physician about an order for cardiac enzyme levels and ECG; report significant elevation of cardiac enzymes and ST-segment depression or elevation, T-wave inversion, and/or abnormal Q waves on ECG.

Notification of the appropriate health care provider allows for modification of the treatment plan.

- Maintain client on strict bed rest in a semi- to high-Fowler's position.

Improves lung expansion and tissue oxygenation.

- Maintain oxygen therapy as ordered.

Maintains tissue oxygenation.

- Administer the following medications if ordered:
  - Nitrates

Nitrates work to improve coronary blood flow and reduce myocardial oxygen requirements.

  - Morphine

Morphine works to reduce pain and anxiety and decrease cardiac workload.

  - Beta blockers

Beta blockers work to reduce myocardial oxygen requirements by decreasing heart rate and the force of myocardial contractility.

Collaborative Diagnosis # RISK FOR IMPAIRED RENAL FUNCTION

Definition: Renal insufficiency refers to a decline in renal function to about 25% of normal

Related to: Vascular changes in the kidneys associated with effects of prolonged or severe hypertension

CLINICAL MANIFESTATIONS

Subjective	Objective
Complaints of shortness of breath	Oliguria; fluid and electrolyte imbalances; weight gain; elevated B/P; crackles/rales

---

Continued...

RISK FACTORS

- Myocardial infarction
- Hypertension
- Arteriosclerosis

DESIRED OUTCOMES

The client will maintain adequate renal function as evidenced by:
  a. Urine output at least 30 mL/h
  b. Absence of proteinuria
  c. BUN, serum creatinine, and creatinine clearance values within normal range

NURSING ASSESSMENT

Assess for signs and symptoms of impaired renal function:
- Nocturia
- Urine output less than 30 mL/h
- Urine specific gravity fixed at or less than 1.010
- Proteinuria

Assess BUN/serum creatinine levels for abnormalities.

RATIONALE

Early recognition of signs and symptoms of impaired renal function allows for prompt intervention.

THERAPEUTIC INTERVENTIONS

Dependent/Collaborative Actions

Perform actions to reduce B/P:
- Administer antihypertensive agents.
- Maintain an adequate fluid intake to reduce risk of dehydration.
  - Encourage oral fluid intake.
  - Administer intravenous fluids as ordered.

If signs and symptoms of impaired renal function occur:
- Consult physician about lowering the dose of or discontinuing angiotensin-converting enzyme (ACE) inhibitors if BUN and serum creatinine levels continue to rise significantly.
- Prepare client for dialysis if indicated.

RATIONALE

Collaborative actions help to improve renal blood flow.

ACE inhibitors should be used cautiously in persons with impaired renal function because they can have an adverse effect on renal function.

Decreases fear and anxiety.

Collaborative Diagnosis   # RISK FOR HEART FAILURE

Definition: Cardiac dysfunction that results in inadequate perfusion of tissues with vital blood-borne nutrients

Related to: The prolonged increase in cardiac workload associated with increased systemic vascular resistance

CLINICAL MANIFESTATIONS

Subjective	Objective
Left-sided heart failure: Complaints of shortness of breath	Left-sided heart failure: Dyspnea; orthopnea; frothy sputum; decreased urine output; edema; hypotension/hypertension; S₃ gallop Right-sided heart failure: Hepatosplenomegaly; peripheral edema; jugular venous distention

RISK FACTORS

- Hypertension
- Obesity
- Smoking
- Coronary artery disease

DESIRED OUTCOMES

The client did not develop heart failure as evidenced by:
  a. Pulse rate 60 to 100 beats/min
  b. Absence of an S₃ heart sound
  c. Usual mental status
  d. Clear, audible breath sounds
  e. Absence of dyspnea, orthopnea, and cough
  f. Increased strength and activity tolerance
  g. Palpable peripheral pulses
  h. Urine output at least 30 mL/h
  i. Stable weight
  j. Absence of edema and distended neck veins

NURSING ASSESSMENT	RATIONALE
Assess for signs and symptoms of heart failure: • Tachycardia • Presence of an S₃ heart sound • Restlessness, agitation, confusion, or other change in mental status • Crackles (rales) • Dyspnea, orthopnea • Dry, hacking cough or cough productive of frothy or blood-tinged sputum • Development of or increased weakness and fatigue • Diminished or absent peripheral pulses • Decreased urine output during the day, nocturia • Weight gain • Edema • Distended neck veins Monitor results of chest radiograph for abnormalities.	*Early recognition of signs and symptoms of heart failure allows for prompt intervention.*

THERAPEUTIC INTERVENTIONS	RATIONALE

Dependent/Collaborative Actions
Implement measures to reduce B/P:
• Reduce noxious stimuli.
• Decrease anxiety.
• Administer antihypertensive agents.
If signs and symptoms of heart failure occur:
• Maintain oxygen therapy as ordered.
• Administer the following medications if ordered:
  • Positive inotropic agents
  • Diuretics, vasodilators
  • Morphine sulfate
	Reducing B/P helps to reduce cardiac workload and prevent heart failure.
	
	Positive inotropes increase myocardial contractility.
	Diuretics and vasodilators act to reduce myocardial workload.
	Morphine helps to reduce anxiety.

Collaborative Diagnosis RISK FOR AORTIC DISSECTION

Definition: A tear in the wall of the aorta that allows blood to flow between the layers of the wall of the aorta, forcing the layers apart

Related to: Weakening and degeneration of the aortic media associated with a severe or prolonged increase in pressure in the aorta

CLINICAL MANIFESTATIONS

Subjective	Objective
Verbal report of tearing, stabbing, or shearing-type pain that is severe with sudden onset	Widening of the mediastinum; hemodynamic instability; lack of peripheral pulses

RISK FACTOR
• Hypertension

DESIRED OUTCOMES

The client will not experience dissection of the aorta as evidenced by:
  a. Absence of sudden, severe chest pain
  b. Palpable peripheral pulses with no change in pulse pattern
  c. Usual sensory and motor function
  d. Usual mental status
  e. Stable vital signs
  f. Skin warm and usual color

 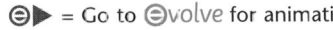

Continued...

NURSING ASSESSMENT	RATIONALE
Assess for signs and symptoms of aortic dissection: • Sudden, severe chest pain that may radiate to back • Abnormal pulse pattern in extremities • Sudden lack of pulse in an extremity Assess for signs and symptoms of hypovolemic shock: • Restlessness • Agitation • Significant decrease in B/P • Rapid, weak pulse • Cool skin • Pallor • Diminished or absent pulses	*Early recognition of signs and symptoms of aortic dissection allows for prompt intervention.*

THERAPEUTIC INTERVENTIONS	RATIONALE
Dependent/Collaborative Actions Perform actions to reduce B/P: • Administer antihypertensives. • Alleviate pain. • Alleviate anxiety.	*Actions help to prevent aortic dissection.*
Instruct client to avoid activities that create a Valsalva response (e.g., straining to have a bowel movement, holding breath while moving up in bed).	*Increases intrathoracic pressure.*
If signs and symptoms of aortic dissection occur: • Maintain client on strict bed rest. • Monitor vital signs frequently. • Administer oxygen as ordered. • Prepare client for diagnostic studies (e.g., transesophageal echocardiogram, computed tomography) if planned. • Administer antihypertensive agents. • Prepare client for surgery if planned.	*Helps to maintain B/P.* *Maintains tissue oxygenation.* *Decreases fear and anxiety.* *Decreases B/P.* *Decreases fear and anxiety.*

Nursing Diagnosis INEFFECTIVE FAMILY THERAPEUTIC REGIMEN MANAGEMENT NDx

Definition: Pattern of regulating and integrating into family processes a program for treatment of illness and the sequelae of illness that is unsatisfactory for meeting specific health needs

Related to:
• Lack of understanding of the implications of not following the prescribed treatment plan
• Difficulty modifying personal habits (e.g., alcohol intake, dietary preferences)
• Undesirable side effects of some antihypertensive agents
• Insufficient financial resources

CLINICAL MANIFESTATIONS

Subjective	Objective
Verbalized difficulty with regulating one or more prescribed regimens for treatment and illness; verbalized that did not take action to include treatment regimen in daily routines	Acceleration of illness symptoms; choice of daily living ineffective for meeting goals of a treatment program

RISK FACTORS

- Complex therapeutic regimen
- Excessive demands

DESIRED OUTCOMES

The client will demonstrate the probability of effective management of the therapeutic regimen as evidenced by:

a. Willingness to learn about and participate in treatments and care

b. Statements reflecting ways to modify personal habits

c. Statements reflecting an understanding of the implications of not following the prescribed treatment plan

NOC OUTCOMES

Compliance behavior; treatment behavior: illness or injury; knowledge: treatment regimen; health beliefs: perceived resources; knowledge: cardiac disease management; health beliefs: perceived ability to perform

NIC INTERVENTIONS

Self-modification assistance; medication management; values clarification; exercise promotion; smoking cessation assistance; teaching: prescribed diet; weight reduction assistance; financial resource assistance

NURSING ASSESSMENT

Assess for indications that the client may be unable to effectively manage the therapeutic regimen:

- Statements reflecting inability to manage care at home
- Failure to adhere to treatment plan (e.g., not adhering to dietary modifications, refusing medications)
- Statements reflecting a lack of understanding of factors that may cause progression of hypertension
- Statements reflecting an unwillingness or inability to modify personal habits
- Statements reflecting view that hypertension will reverse itself or that the situation is hopeless and efforts to comply with the therapeutic regimen are useless
- Statements reflecting that the side effects of medications are too uncomfortable and that the client feels better when not taking medication
- Statements reflecting that medications are too expensive

RATIONALE

Identification of indications of the inability to effectively manage a therapeutic regimen allows for implementation of the appropriate support/interventions.

THERAPEUTIC INTERVENTIONS

Independent Actions

Implement measures to promote effective management of the therapeutic regimen:

- Explain hypertension in terms the client can understand; stress that hypertension is a chronic condition and that adherence to the treatment plan is necessary in order to delay and/or prevent complications.
- Encourage questions and clarify misconceptions client has about hypertension and its effects, and the side effects of medications.
- Provide instructions on and encourage client to participate in the treatment plan (e.g., calculating sodium intake, monitoring B/P); determine areas of misunderstanding and reinforce teaching as necessary.
- Provide client with written instructions about dietary modifications, signs and symptoms to report, medication therapy, B/P monitoring, and exercise regimen.
- Assist client to identify ways medication regimen, exercise, and dietary modifications can be incorporated into lifestyle; focus on modifications of lifestyle rather than complete change.

RATIONALE

To promote effective management of a therapeutic regimen, the nurse must ensure that the client understands expectations. In addition, the nurse must ensure that the client has the appropriate resources to adhere to the treatment plan (e.g., financial, social support).

Continued...

THERAPEUTIC INTERVENTIONS	RATIONALE

- Assist client to identify a reward system for self that will assist him/her to effect necessary change(s).
- Initiate and reinforce discharge teaching.
- Provide information about and encourage utilization of community resources that can assist client to make necessary lifestyle changes (e.g., cardiovascular fitness, weight loss, and smoking cessation programs; stress management classes).
- Encourage client to discuss concerns about the cost of medications and visits with health care provider; obtain a social service consult to assist with financial planning and to obtain financial aid if indicated.
- Encourage client to attend follow-up educational classes
- Reinforce behaviors suggesting future compliance with the therapeutic regimen (e.g., statements reflecting plan for adhering to treatment plan, statements reflecting an understanding of hypertension and its long-term effects).
- Include significant others in explanations and teaching sessions and encourage their support; reinforce the need for client to assume responsibility for managing as much of care as possible.

Dependent/Collaborative Actions

Consult appropriate health care provider (e.g., social worker, physician) regarding referrals to community health agencies if continued instruction or support is needed.	*Consulting the appropriate health care provider allows for modification of discharge teaching/continued care.*

Nursing Diagnosis	**DEFICIENT KNOWLEDGE NDx OR INEFFECTIVE HEALTH MAINTENANCE NDx***

Definition: Absence or deficiency of cognitive information related to specific topic (lack of specific information necessary for clients/significant others to make informed choices regarding condition/treatment/lifestyle changes); inability to identify, manage, and/or seek out help to manage health

CLINICAL MANIFESTATIONS

Subjective	Objective
Verbalization of unfamiliarity with information	Inability to accurately follow instructions

NOC OUTCOMES	NIC INTERVENTIONS
Knowledge: treatment regimen; knowledge: cardiac disease management	Health system guidance; teaching: individual; teaching: prescribed diet; teaching: prescribed medication

NURSING ASSESSMENT	RATIONALE
Assess client's readiness and ability to learn.	*Early recognition of readiness to learn and meaning of illness to client allows for implementation of the appropriate teaching interventions.*
Assess meaning of illness to client.	

THERAPEUTIC INTERVENTIONS	RATIONALE

Desired Outcome: The client will verbalize a basic understanding of hypertension and its effects on the body.

---

*The nurse should select the nursing diagnostic label that is most appropriate for the client's discharge teaching needs.

THERAPEUTIC INTERVENTIONS	RATIONALE

Independent Actions

Explain hypertension and its effects in terms client can understand. Use available teaching aids (e.g., pamphlets, videotapes).

Inform client that hypertension is often asymptomatic and that absence of symptoms is not a reliable indication that B/P is within a safe range.

Educating clients in terms they understand regarding their underlying disease process can facilitate understanding as to the importance of adhering to a treatment plan.

THERAPEUTIC INTERVENTIONS	RATIONALE

Desired Outcome: The client will identify modifiable risk factors for hypertension and ways to alter these factors.

Independent Actions

Inform client that certain modifiable factors such as elevated serum lipid levels, excessive alcohol intake, a sedentary lifestyle, smoking, and excess body weight have been shown to increase the risk for cardiovascular disease and hypertension.

Assist client to identify changes in lifestyle that can help the client to manage hypertension (e.g., dietary modification, physical exercise on a regular basis, smoking cessation, moderation of alcohol intake, weight loss if overweight).

Encourage client to limit daily alcohol consumption (daily alcohol intake exceeding 1 oz of ethanol may contribute to the development of hypertension).

Instruct client to participate in a regular aerobic exercise program (e.g., walking, swimming) and avoid isometric exercise (e.g., weight training). Caution client to consult physician before beginning an exercise program.

Thorough education is a critical component of the care of a client with hypertension. The client must have a thorough understanding of the importance of adhering to diet, medication, activity/exercise, and nutritional recommendations to prevent an exacerbation and control the disease.

Current recommendations are no more than 2 drinks per day for men and no more than 1 drink per day for women and lighter-weight persons. A "drink" is considered to be ½ oz of ethanol (e.g., 1½ oz of 80-proof whiskey, 12 oz of beer, 5 oz of wine). Decreases weight and improves cardiovascular stamina.

THERAPEUTIC INTERVENTIONS	RATIONALE

Desired Outcome: The client will verbalize an understanding of medications ordered including rationale, food and drug interactions, side effects, schedule for taking, and importance of taking as prescribed.

Independent Actions

Explain the rationale for, side effects of, and importance of taking medications prescribed. Inform client of pertinent food and drug interactions.
- Diuretics
- Beta-adrenergic blockers
- Angiotensin-converting enzyme (ACE) inhibitors

Taking medications as prescribed ensures that therapeutic drug levels will be maintained.

Clients should be instructed not to discontinue taking medications if they feel better. Clients without financial resources should be assisted in accessing appropriate resources to obtain needed medications (e.g., pharmacy assistance programs).

THERAPEUTIC INTERVENTIONS	RATIONALE

Desired Outcome: The client will verbalize an understanding of the rationale for and components of the recommended diet.

Independent Actions

Explain the rationale for the recommended dietary modifications:
- Reduced sodium intake
- Reduced intake of saturated fat and cholesterol
- Include the recommended daily allowances of potassium, calcium, and magnesium in diet.

Reducing sodium intake to a recommended 2.4 g/day can help control hypertension by reducing the fluid retention associated with increased intake.

NDx = NANDA-I Diagnosis **D** = Delegatable Action ● = UAP ✦ = LVN/LPN ⊖▶ = Go to ⊖volve for animation

Continued...

THERAPEUTIC INTERVENTIONS	RATIONALE

Desired Outcome: The client will state signs and symptoms to report to the health care provider.

Independent Actions
Instruct the client to report:
- Persistent headache or headache present upon awakening
- Sudden and continued increase in B/P (if B/P is monitored at home)
- Chest pain
- Shortness of breath
- Significant weight gain or swelling of feet or ankles
- Changes in vision
- Frequent or uncontrollable nosebleeds
- Persistent dizziness, lightheadedness, or fainting
- Persistent side effects experienced from use of antihypertensive medications (e.g., impotence; dry mouth; depression; persistent dry cough; swelling of the tongue, face, or neck)
- Side effects of diuretic therapy

Reporting signs and symptoms indicative of hypertension to the appropriate provider allows for modification of the treatment plan and may prevent complications.

THERAPEUTIC INTERVENTIONS	RATIONALE

Desired Outcome: The client will identify community resources that can assist in making lifestyle changes necessary for effective control of hypertension.

Independent Actions
Provide information regarding community resources and support groups that can assist client in making lifestyle changes that are necessary for effective control of hypertension (e.g., cardiovascular fitness, weight loss, and smoking cessation programs; stress management classes).

Hypertension can significantly impact an individual's and family's socioeconomic status. Providing information specific to community resources is important to provide a necessary continuum of care and may impact the client's health status, preventing future hospitalizations.

THERAPEUTIC INTERVENTIONS	RATIONALE

Desired Outcome: The client will verbalize an understanding of and a plan for adhering to recommended follow-up care including future appointments with health care provider.

Independent Actions
Reinforce the importance of keeping follow-up appointments with health care provider and continuing lifelong medical supervision.

Regular health care appointments are important to determine effectiveness of the prescribed treatment plan.

RELATED NURSING DIAGNOSES

FEAR/ANXIETY NDx
Related to:
- Necessity for urgent treatment
- Possibility of severe disability or sudden death
- Unfamiliar environment
- Persistent or severe headache
- Lack of understanding of diagnostic tests, diagnosis, and treatment plan

IMPLANTABLE CARDIAC DEVICES

Pacemakers and implantable cardioverter-defibrillators (ICDs) are small battery-powered devices that monitor the heart rate and deliver electrical impulses to the heart to help correct dysrhythmias. Both pacemakers and ICDs consist of a pulse generator (contains the battery and electronic circuitry) and electrode catheters (leads). Both devices can be implanted during a minor surgical procedure under local anesthesia. The leads are inserted into the heart transvenously via the subclavian, jugular, or cephalic vein. The leads are then tunneled under the skin and attached to the pulse generator that is implanted in a subcutaneous pocket created in the subclavicular area or, less commonly, in the abdomen. A combined pacemaker and cardioverter-defibrillator is also available.

A pacemaker is used to stimulate the heart electrically when the heart fails to initiate or conduct intrinsic electrical impulses at a rate that is sufficient to maintain adequate perfusion. Pacemaker insertion is indicated for treatment of symptomatic bradydysrhythmias (e.g., sinus bradycardia, second- and third-degree heart block, sick sinus syndrome) and on some occasions, for treatment of tachydysrhythmias that have been unresponsive to other forms of therapy.

Pacemakers are either temporary or permanent. Temporary pacemakers are used to regulate the heart rate in emergency or short-term situations. In most instances, temporary pacing is done using external transcutaneous pacing electrodes or using temporary pacemaker electrodes that have been placed on the epicardium during thoracic surgery (e.g., heart surgery). Temporary pacemakers are attached to and regulated by an external power source. Permanent pacemakers are used for long-term management of certain dysrhythmias. There are a number of permanent pacemakers available. Their functional capabilities are described by a three- or five-letter code that specifies the chamber being paced, the chamber being sensed, mode of response, programmability/rate responsiveness, and antitachycardia functions.

Most pacemakers used now are dual-chambered pacemakers with leads in both the atrium and ventricle. Dual-chamber pacing allows for the physiological timing between atrial systole and ventricular systole to be maintained, which improves cardiac output. Present-day pacemakers can also be programmed externally, and most operate in a synchronous mode (a chamber of the heart is triggered to fire or is inhibited by the intrinsic activity of the heart) or a rate-responsive mode. The most frequently used rate-responsive systems have an activity sensor in the pulse generator that detects movement and then appropriately increases or decreases the pacing rate.

ICDs are used to treat life-threatening dysrhythmias. They are indicated for persons who have survived one or more incidents of sudden cardiac death, persons with recurrent ventricular tachycardia or ventricular fibrillation, and for persons with demonstrated risk factors for sudden cardiac death. The sensing lead of an ICD monitors the heart's electrical activity and if the heart rate exceeds the generator's programmed rate, the generator delivers a burst of antitachycardia pacing (ATP) to override the heart's pacemaker. If after a programmed number of ATP therapies the rate continues to exceed the desired rate, the ICD device then delivers low-energy and high-energy cardioversion shocks. If ventricular fibrillation is present, defibrillation shocks are delivered.

This care plan focuses on the adult client with a symptomatic dysrhythmia hospitalized for implantation of either a cardioverter-defibrillator or permanent pacemaker.

OUTCOME/DISCHARGE CRITERIA

The client will:
1. Have adequate cardiac output
2. Have no signs and symptoms of postoperative complications
3. Verbalize a basic understanding of the rationale for and function of an ICD/pacemaker
4. Demonstrate knowledge of how to monitor ICD function
5. Verbalize an understanding of appropriate actions to take if the ICD delivers a shock
6. Verbalize an understanding of recommended activity restrictions
7. Identify appropriate safety precautions associated with having an ICD/pacemaker
8. State signs and symptoms to report to the health care provider
9. Verbalize an understanding of and a plan for adhering to recommended follow-up care including future appointments with health care provider, medications prescribed, and wound care.

Nursing/Collaborative Diagnosis **PREOPERATIVE**

USE IN CONJUNCTION WITH THE STANDARDIZED PREOPERATIVE CARE PLAN.

Nursing Diagnosis **RISK FOR/ACTUAL DECREASED CARDIAC OUTPUT** NDx

Definition: Inadequate volume of blood pumped by the heart per minute to meet metabolic demands of the body

Related to:
- A slow heart rate (if client has a bradydysrhythmia)
- Decreased diastolic filling time associated with a rapid and/or irregular heart rate (if client has a tachydysrhythmia)

NDx = NANDA-I Diagnosis   **D** = Delegatable Action   ● = UAP   ✦ = LVN/LPN   ⊜▶ = Go to ⊖volve for animation

Continued...

- Decreased diastolic filling time and ineffective ventricular contractions if client has sustained ventricular tachycardia or ventricular fibrillation
- Related factors will depend upon the type of device implanted and underlying dysrhythmias.

CLINICAL MANIFESTATIONS

Subjective	Objective
Verbal reports of anxiety; fatigue; weakness; dizziness; syncope; exertional dyspnea	Change in mental status; B/P less than 90 mm Hg systolic or below normal for patient; irregular or absent pulses; diminished peripheral pulses; tachypnea; cool, pale skin; cool extremities; increased capillary refill time

RISK FACTOR

- Cardiac dysrhythmias

DESIRED OUTCOMES

The client will maintain an adequate cardiac output as evidenced by:
   a. Systolic B/P of at least 90 mm Hg
   b. Palpable peripheral pulses
   c. No increase in number or duration of dizziness or syncopal episodes
   d. Baseline mental status
   e. Absence of cyanosis
   f. Urine output at least 30 mL/h

NOC OUTCOMES

Circulation status; cardiac pump effectiveness

NIC INTERVENTIONS

Cardiac care; cardiac precautions; dysrhythmia management; tissue perfusion: cardiac

NURSING ASSESSMENT	RATIONALE
Assess client upon admission for baseline data regarding status of cardiac output.	
Assess for and report signs and symptoms of decreased cardiac output:	*Early recognition and reporting of signs and symptoms of decreased cardiac output allow for prompt intervention.*
• Change in mental status	
• B/P less than 90 mm Hg systolic or below normal for patient	
• Irregular or absent pulses	
• Diminished peripheral pulses	
• Tachypnea	
• Cool, pale skin	
• Cool extremities	
• Increased capillary refill time	
• Verbal reports of anxiety, fatigue, weakness, dizziness, syncope, exertional dyspnea	
Assess for and report ECG rhythm abnormalities that may alter cardiac output:	
• Bradydysrhythmias	
• Tachydysrhythmias	
• Ventricular tachycardia/fibrillation	

THERAPEUTIC INTERVENTIONS	RATIONALE

Independent Actions

Implement measures to maintain an adequate cardiac output before surgery:
- Perform actions to reduce cardiac workload:
  - Place client in a semi- to high-Fowler's position unless systolic B/P is less than 90 mm Hg (then head of bed should be flat).

THERAPEUTIC INTERVENTIONS	RATIONALE
• Implement measures to promote rest (e.g., reduce fear and anxiety, maintain activity restrictions, limit the number of visitors).	
• Discourage smoking.	*Nicotine has a cardiostimulatory effect and causes vasoconstriction; the carbon monoxide in smoke reduces oxygen availability.*
• Instruct client to avoid activities that create a Valsalva response (e.g., straining to have a bowel movement, holding breath while moving up in bed)	*Valsalva maneuvers can increase vagal stimulation, resulting in slowing of the heart rate. In addition, Valsalva maneuvers can also lead to a sudden increase in cardiac workload.*
• Notify physician if serum potassium level is abnormal.	*Abnormal potassium levels affect myocardial conductivity.*

Dependent/Collaborative Actions

Implement measures to maintain an adequate cardiac output before surgery:

• Perform actions to reduce cardiac workload:	
• Maintain oxygen therapy as ordered.	
• Administer the following medications if ordered:	
• Antidysrhythmics	
• Anticholinergics	*Anticholinergic drugs increase the heart rate by blocking the action of the vagal nerve in patients with symptomatic bradycardia.*
• Consult physician before giving prescribed digitalis preparations if client has heart block or ventricular dysrhythmias.	*Digitalis preparations can increase ventricular irritability.* *Prevents further compromise of cardiac output by decreasing heart rate.*
• Prepare for and assist with cardioversion or defibrillation if performed.	*Decreases fear and anxiety.*
• Maintain temporary pacing if ordered.	*Maintains cardiac output.*

NURSING/COLLABORATIVE DIAGNOSIS: POSTOPERATIVE

USE IN CONJUNCTION WITH THE STANDARDIZED POSTOPERATIVE CARE PLAN.

Collaborative Diagnoses
RISK FOR PACEMAKER/IMPLANTABLE CARDIOVERTER-DEFIBRILLATOR (ICD) MALFUNCTION

Definition: Failure of the implanted device to maintain cardiac output

Related to: Improper placement or dislodgment of the leads, break in or faulty attachment of the leads, or pulse generator malfunction

CLINICAL MANIFESTATIONS

Subjective	Objective
Client reports receiving multiple shocks without ECG evidence of tachydysrhythmia; dizziness; lightheadedness	ECG showing rapid and/or irregular rate without accompanying antitachycardia pacing; presence of sustained ventricular tachycardia or fibrillation on ECG; absence of pacer spikes when heart rate falls below the programmed pacing rate; pacer spikes present with normal P waves and QRS complexes; absence of P wave or QRS complex after a pacer spike; presence of ectopic beats; apical pulse less than programmed pacing rate; significant decrease in B/P; syncope; dyspnea

Continued...
DESIRED OUTCOMES

The client will experience normal cardioverter-defibrillator function as evidenced by:
  a. Absence of sustained ventricular dysrhythmias on ECG
  b. Client reports of receiving internal shocks when ventricular tachycardia or fibrillation is evident on the ECG

The client will experience normal pacemaker function as evidenced by:
  a. Regular pulse at a rate equal to or greater than the programmed pacing rate
  b. Stable B/P
  c. Absence of dizziness, syncope, and dyspnea
  d. ECG showing pacer spikes before the P wave and/or QRS complex when the pulse rate falls below the programmed pacing rate

NURSING ASSESSMENT	RATIONALE
Assess for and report signs and symptoms of cardioverter-defibrillator/pacemaker malfunction: • Multiple shocks without ECG evidence of tachydysrhythmia; dizziness; lightheadedness; significant decrease in BP; syncope; dyspnea • ECG with regular/irregular pulse rate without pacing spikes • Symptoms will depend upon type of implantable device. Ascertain the type of ICD/pacemaker the client has and how it is programmed (including the rate at which pacing should occur if a combination pacemaker cardioverter-defibrillator was implanted). Have information available about problem-solving techniques and activation and deactivation of the specific device.	*Early recognition and reporting of signs and symptoms of device malfunction allow for prompt intervention.*

THERAPEUTIC INTERVENTIONS	RATIONALE
Independent Actions Implement measures to reduce the risk for breakage and dislodgment of the ICD leads in order to prevent ICD malfunction: • Maintain activity restrictions as ordered. • Instruct client to limit movement of the arm and shoulder on the side that the ICD was inserted for the first 48 hours after surgery. If signs and symptoms of pacemaker malfunction occurs: • Turn the client to either side.	*Limiting movements during the first 48 hours after surgery allows for leads to embed in the myocardium.* *In the event of a pacemaker malfunction, such as failure to capture, turning the client to the left side may help facilitate placement of the lead(s) against the myocardium.*

Dependent/Collaborative Actions
If signs and symptoms of ICD malfunction occur:
• If the device is activated and ventricular fibrillation or pulseless ventricular tachycardia occurs:
  • Notify the physician.
  • Proceed with external defibrillation (the defibrillation paddles should be positioned at least 3-4 inches away from the pulse generator).
  • Administer antidysrhythmics.
• If the device is activated and delivering inappropriate shocks:
  • Notify the physician.
If signs and symptoms of pacemaker malfunction occur:
• Follow manufacturer's suggestions for problem solving:
  • Have a pacemaker magnet available.
  • If client has a temporary pacemaker, adjust sensitivity and/or output (MA) within prescribed limits until capture occurs.
• Prepare client for chest radiograph to check placement of leads.
• Prepare client for surgical repair or replacement of pulse generator if indicated.
	Allows for prompt intervention and prevention of a deleterious outcome.
	
	The physician or other trained personnel may need to deactivate the device.
	
	Increasing the sensitivity or output (MA) may help improve pacer capture of the myocardial wall, producing ventricular or atrial contraction.
	Decreases fear and anxiety.

Collaborative Diagnoses **RISK FOR CARDIAC TAMPONADE**

Definition: Rapid collection of blood in the pericardial sac that compresses the myocardium, preventing the heart from pumping effectively

Related to: Perforation of the atria or ventricle by the pacemaker leads

CLINICAL MANIFESTATIONS

Subjective	Objective
Pericardial pain; sense of fullness in chest	Pericardial friction rub; significant decrease in B/P; narrowed pulse pressure; pulsus paradoxus; distant or muffled heart sounds; jugular venous distention

RISK FACTOR
• Lead malposition

DESIRED OUTCOMES

The client will not experience cardiac tamponade as evidenced by:
a. Stable vital signs
b. Audible heart sounds
c. Absence of jugular venous distention

NURSING ASSESSMENT

Assess for and report signs and symptoms of cardiac perforation/cardiac tamponade:
• Decrease in B/P
• Pulsus paradoxus
• Narrow pulse pressure
• Muffled heart sounds
Assess chest radiograph results/echocardiogram results for abnormalities.

RATIONALE

Early recognition and reporting of signs and symptoms of cardiac tamponade allow for prompt intervention.

THERAPEUTIC INTERVENTIONS

Independent Actions
Implement measures to prevent dislodgment of the pacemaker/ICD leads:
• Maintain activity restrictions as ordered.
• Instruct client to limit movement of the arm and shoulder on the side that the ICD was inserted for the first 48 hours after surgery.

Dependent/Collaborative Actions
If signs and symptoms of cardiac perforation or tamponade occur:
• Prepare client for chest radiograph and echocardiogram.
• Prepare client for repositioning or replacement of the lead(s), repair of perforation, and/or pericardiocentesis if planned.

RATIONALE

Actions reduce the risk for perforation of the heart wall.

Collaborative Diagnoses **RISK FOR PNEUMOTHORAX**

Definition: Air in the pleural space with resulting collapse of the lung

Related to: Accumulation of air in the pleural space associated with accidental puncture of the pleura during subclavian insertion of the cardioverter-defibrillator leads

Continued...

CLINICAL MANIFESTATIONS

Subjective	Objective
Report of sudden onset of chest pain	Absent breath sounds with hyperresonant percussion note over involved area; rapid, shallow, and/or labored respirations; tachycardia; restlessness; confusion; significant decrease in oximetry results; abnormal arterial blood gas values; chest radiograph results showing lung collapse

RISK FACTOR

- Surgical implantation in close proximity to lung

DESIRED OUTCOMES

The client will have resolution of pneumothorax if it occurs as evidenced by:
- a. Audible breath sounds and a resonant percussion note over lungs
- b. Normal respiratory rate and pattern
- c. Usual mental status
- d. Arterial blood gas values returning to normal range

NURSING ASSESSMENT	RATIONALE
Assess for and immediately report signs and symptoms of pneumothorax: • Absent breath sounds • Dyspnea • Tachycardia • Restlessness • Confusion	*Early recognition and reporting of signs and symptoms of a pneumothorax allow for prompt intervention.*
Assess for and immediately report signs and symptoms of tension pneumothorax with mediastinal shift: • Severe dyspnea • Increased restlessness and agitation • Rapid and/or irregular heart rate • Hypotension • Neck vein distention • Shift in trachea from midline	*A tension pneumothorax is a rapid accumulation of air in the pleural space that can result from a pneumothorax.* *Compression of the great vessels can result in altered cardiac output. This complication is a medical emergency.*

THERAPEUTIC INTERVENTIONS	RATIONALE
Independent Actions If signs and symptoms of pneumothorax occur: • Maintain client on bed rest in a semi- to high-Fowler's position	*Promotes lung expansion.*
Dependent/Collaborative Actions If signs and symptoms of pneumothorax occur: • Maintain oxygen therapy as ordered. • Prepare client for insertion of chest tube if indicated.	*Maintains tissue oxygenation.* *A chest tube will evacuate accumulated air from the pleural space and reexpand the lung.*

Collaborative Diagnoses   **RISK FOR UNDESIRED STIMULATION OF THE HEART AND/ OR CERTAIN NERVES AND MUSCLES**

Definition: Adverse stimulation of the hear and nerves which may cause dysrhythmias, pain, or breathing problems

Related to: The presence of a foreign body in the heart and the emission of electrical impulses from the pacemaker lead(s) to nearby muscles and nerves such as the diaphragm, intercostals muscles, and phrenic nerve

CLINICAL MANIFESTATIONS

Subjective	Objective
Verbal reports of abdominal or chest wall twitching	Ventricular ectopic beats on ECG; hiccups

RISK FACTOR

- Malposition of leads

DESIRED OUTCOMES

The client will have resolution of ventricular irritability and undesired nerve and muscle stimulation as evidenced by:
  a. Absence of ventricular ectopic beats
  b. Absence of hiccups
  c. Absence of abdominal and intercostal muscle twitching

NURSING ASSESSMENT	RATIONALE
Assess for and report signs and symptoms of ventricular irritability and undesired nerve or muscle stimulation.	*Early recognition and reporting of signs and symptoms of ventricular irritability and undesired nerve or muscle stimulation allow for prompt intervention.*

THERAPEUTIC INTERVENTIONS	RATIONALE

Dependent/Collaborative Actions
If signs and symptoms persist:
• Consult physician.
• Turn client to left side.
• Prepare client for the following procedures if planned:
  • Chest x-ray to determine placement of lead(s)
  • Repositioning of the lead(s)
	Turning the client to the left side may help facilitate placement of the lead(s) against the myocardium.

DISCHARGE TEACHING/CONTINUED CARE

Nursing Diagnosis | # DEFICIENT KNOWLEDGE NDx; INEFFECTIVE FAMILY THERAPEUTIC REGIMEN MANAGEMENT NDx; OR INEFFECTIVE SELF-HEALTH MANAGEMENT NDx*

Definition: Absence or deficiency of cognitive information related to specific topic (lack of specific information necessary for clients/significant others to make informed choices regarding condition/treatment/lifestyle changes); pattern of regulating and integrating into daily living a program for treatment of illness and the sequelae of illness that is unsatisfactory for meeting specific health goals; inability to identify, manage, and/or seek out help to manage health

CLINICAL MANIFESTATIONS

Subjective	Objective
Verbalization of unfamiliarity with information	Inability to accurately follow instructions

RISK FACTORS

- Denial of disease process
- Cognitive deficiency
- Failure to take action to reduce risk factors

NOC OUTCOMES	NIC INTERVENTIONS
Knowledge: treatment regimen	Teaching: individual; teaching: prescribed activity/exercise

*The nurse should select the diagnosis that is most appropriate for the client's discharge teaching needs.

NDx = NANDA-I Diagnosis   **D** = Delegatable Action   ● = UAP   ✦ = LVN/LPN   ⊖▶ = Go to ⊖volve for animation

Continued...

NURSING ASSESSMENT	RATIONALE
Assess client's readiness and ability to learn.	*Early recognition of readiness to learn and meaning of illness to client allows for implementation of the appropriate teaching interventions.*
Assess meaning of treatment plan with client.	

THERAPEUTIC INTERVENTIONS	RATIONALE

Desired Outcome: The client will verbalize a basic understanding of the rationale for and function of an ICD/pacemaker.

Independent Actions	
Reinforce preoperative teaching regarding the rationale for and basic function of an ICD/pacemaker.	*Ensuring client's understanding preoperatively helps to reinforce necessity of the treatment plan and allows for additional client concerns to be addressed.*

THERAPEUTIC INTERVENTIONS	RATIONALE

Desired Outcome: The client will demonstrate knowledge of how to monitor ICD/pacemaker function.

Independent Actions

Inform the client with a combined pacemaker/cardioverter-defibrillator device of the pacemaker's programmed pacing rate and, if appropriate, provide instructions about how to take pulse and monitor both the rate and regularity. (Many physicians prefer that their clients not monitor their own pulse because of the confusion between paced beats and spontaneous beats.)

Proper education enables the client to monitor for possible device malfunction and seek out the appropriate health care provider if concerning signs and symptoms develop.

Instruct client with an ICD to monitor for and report the following:

- Signs of a heart rhythm disturbance such as dizziness, fainting, shortness of breath, unexplained fatigue, or feeling that heart is fluttering

May indicate malfunction of the ICD.

Instruct the client with a pacemaker to have pulse generator function checked regularly per physician's instructions or if experiencing symptoms such as dizziness, fainting, unexplained fatigue, or shortness of breath. Inform the client that monitoring may be done at the physician's office or by telephone monitoring device.

Decreases potential for malfunction and allows for alterations in settings as indicated.

THERAPEUTIC INTERVENTIONS	RATIONALE

Desired Outcome: The client will identify appropriate safety precautions associated with having an ICD/pacemaker.

Independent Actions

Instruct client to adhere to the following safety precautions:

- Inform all health care providers about the device (certain medical equipment such as a magnetic resonance imaging [MRI] machine, radiation therapy machine, and electrocautery equipment may actually damage the pulse generator and/or interfere with normal function of these devices).
- Avoid close proximity with strong magnets (e.g., MRI machine, large industrial magnets), high voltage electrical equipment (e.g., arc welder, running car engine), and large electromagnetic fields (e.g., radio and television transmitters).

Safety precautions are necessary to maintain proper functioning of device at all times.

THERAPEUTIC INTERVENTIONS	RATIONALE
• Move away from any electrical device if dizziness or light-headedness occurs. • If planning to travel, obtain name of a physician and/or pacemaker/ICD clinic at point(s) of destination. • Alert airport personnel to device (it may set off the security alarm). • Always wear a medical alert bracelet or tag and carry an identification card that includes the name of the manufacturer, model number, mode of operation, and insertion date of the device. • Clients with ICDs should adhere to restrictions on driving; typically, clients are not allowed to drive until they have had a 6-month discharge-free period (this is a law in some states for persons with ICDs).	

THERAPEUTIC INTERVENTIONS	RATIONALE

Desired Outcome: The client will verbalize an understanding of appropriate actions to take if the ICD delivers a shock.

Independent Actions

• Instruct client to call an ambulance or emergency rescue service and then to lie down if the ICD delivers a shock. • Instruct family members to call the client's physician and the ambulance or emergency rescue service if the client's ICD delivers a shock while they are present. Instruct them to get cardiopulmonary resuscitation (CPR) training and to initiate CPR if the client is having symptoms such as an irregular and rapid pulse along with dizziness, shortness of breath, chest pain, sweatiness, or loss of consciousness and the device fails to fire after 30 seconds or if the device fires unsuccessfully four to seven times.	*Delivery of a shock indicates a potentially life-threatening dysrhythmia has occurred. The appropriate health care provider should be notified for possible alteration of the treatment plan or hospitalization for further evaluation and stabilization of client's condition.*

THERAPEUTIC INTERVENTIONS	RATIONALE

Desired Outcome: The client will verbalize an understanding of recommended activity restrictions.

Independent Actions

Provide the following instructions about activity restrictions after ICD/pacemaker insertion:

• Limit movement of the arm and shoulder on the operative side for the first 48 hours after surgery. • Limit activities that put undue stress on the incision site (e.g., using arms over head, bowling, racquetball, tennis, lifting over 25 lb) until cleared by physician (usual time is 1-2 months). • Avoid letting anything rub on or hit the device. • Do not rub or "play with" the device under the skin. • Avoid immersing the device insertion site in water for at least 3 days after surgery. • Avoid activities that can cause blunt trauma to the pulse generator (e.g., contact sports, firing a rifle with the butt end of the gun against affected shoulder).	*Activity restrictions serve to ensure that the service wires embed in the appropriate position in the myocardium to achieve maximum device function. Additional restrictions serve to prevent the formation of a wound hematoma, wound infection, or device damage.*

Continued...

THERAPEUTIC INTERVENTIONS	RATIONALE

Desired Outcome: The client will state signs and symptoms to report to the health care provider.

Independent Actions

Instruct client to report these additional signs and symptoms to health care provider:

- Increased irregularity of pulse (if self-monitoring is being done) or episodes of feeling that heart is fluttering
- Unexplained fatigue
- Lightheadedness, dizziness, fainting
- Shortness of breath
- Redness, swelling, drainage, or increased soreness at implant site
- Unexplained fever
- Swelling of arm on the side of the device

Reporting signs and symptoms of device malfunction to the appropriate provider allows for modification of the treatment plan and may prevent life-threatening complications.

May indicate infection.

May indicate venous thrombosis associated with insertion/presence of leads in vein.

THERAPEUTIC INTERVENTIONS	RATIONALE

Desired Outcome: The client will verbalize an understanding of and a plan for adhering to recommended follow-up care including future appointments with health care provider, medications prescribed, and wound care.

Independent Actions

Remind client of the importance of keeping scheduled appointments with pacemaker/ICD clinic and for chest radiograph verification of lead placement.

Allow adequate time for questions and clarification of information provided.

Regular health care appointments are important to determine effectiveness of the prescribed treatment plan.

ADDITIONAL NURSING DIAGNOSES

FEAR/ANXIETY NDx
Related to unfamiliar environment, lack of understanding of surgical procedure, anticipated postoperative discomfort, possibility of ICD/ pacemaker malfunction, and possible changes in lifestyle as a result of having an ICD/pacemaker

RELATED CARE PLANS

Standardized Preoperative Care Plan
Standardized Postoperative Care Plan

MYOCARDIAL INFARCTION

A myocardial infarction (MI) is an acute coronary syndrome resulting from prolonged ischemia of the heart muscle and occurs when blood flow to an area of the myocardium is insufficient to meet the myocardial oxygen requirements. Sustained ischemia causes tissue necrosis and irreversible cellular damage, which results in disturbances in mechanical, biochemical, and electrical function in the necrotic or infarcted area. The degree of altered function depends on the area of the heart involved and the size of the infarct.

MIs may be classified in a number of ways. A transmural MI involves the full thickness of the myocardium. A significant Q wave develops with a transmural infarction, so this may be referred to as a Q-wave MI. A subendocardial infarction only involves a partial thickness of the myocardium and is often classified as a non–Q-wave MI because a pathological Q wave does not develop. MIs may also be classified as an ST-elevation MI or a non–ST-elevation MI (NSTEMI). In addition to these classification systems, many practitioners also describe an MI by the area of the heart that has been damaged (e.g., anterior MI, lateral MI, inferior MI).

Most MIs are caused by rupture of atherosclerotic plaque in a coronary artery, which leads to the release of substances that activate platelet aggregation and clotting factors and cause local vasoconstriction. Other less common causes include severe, persistent spasm of a coronary artery; severe or prolonged hypotension; a rapid ventricular rate; and cocaine use.

The classic symptom of an MI is intense retrosternal chest pain/discomfort. It is often described as a tight, heavy, squeezing, or crushing sensation or "heartburn"; may radiate to the left arm, neck, jaw, or back; lasts longer than 20 minutes; and is unrelieved by nitroglycerin and rest. However, 15% to 25% of infarctions go unrecognized because clients have only mild or no chest discomfort. Other signs and symptoms may include shortness of breath, diaphoresis, dizziness, weakness, pallor, nausea, and vomiting.

The extent of myocardial damage can be limited by early (within 4-6 hours of the onset of symptoms) restoration of coronary blood flow. This can be accomplished by injection of a thrombolytic agent to dissolve the clot obstructing the coronary artery or by a coronary angioplasty. In addition to early restoration of coronary blood flow, treatment with an antiplatelet agent, a beta blocker, an angiotensin-converting enzyme (ACE) inhibitor, and an HMG-CoA (3-hydroxy-3-methylglutaryl-coenzyme A) reductase inhibitor has been found to significantly reduce mortality after an MI. The prognosis for a client who has had an MI is largely influenced by size and location of the infarct, concurrent cardiovascular status, and promptness and effectiveness of treatment.

This care plan focuses on the adult client hospitalized during an episode of intense chest pain for definitive diagnosis and management of a myocardial infarction.

3. Verbalize a basic understanding of an MI
4. Demonstrate accuracy in counting pulse
5. Identify modifiable cardiovascular risk factors and ways to alter these factors
6. Verbalize an understanding of the rationale for and components of a diet designed to lower serum cholesterol and triglyceride levels
7. Verbalize an understanding of medications ordered including rationale, food and drug interactions, side effects, schedule for taking, and importance of taking as prescribed
8. Verbalize an understanding of activity restrictions and the rate at which activity can be progressed
9. State signs and symptoms to report to the health care provider
10. Identify community resources that can assist with cardiac rehabilitation and adjustment to the effects of an MI
11. Share feelings and concerns about changes in body functioning and usual roles and lifestyle
12. Verbalize an understanding of and a plan for adhering to recommended follow-up care including future appointments with health care provider.

OUTCOME/DISCHARGE CRITERIA

The client will:
1. Have adequate cardiac output and tissue perfusion
2. Tolerate prescribed activity without a significant change in vital signs, chest pain, dyspnea, dizziness, or extreme fatigue or weakness

Nursing Diagnosis ## RISK FOR DECREASED CARDIAC OUTPUT NDx

Definition: Risk for inadequate volume of blood pumped by the heart per minute to meet metabolic demands of the body

Related to: Possible decreased contractility and altered conductivity of the heart associated with the myocardial damage that has occurred with infarction

CLINICAL MANIFESTATIONS

Subjective	Objective
Verbal reports of anxiety; fatigue; weakness; dizziness; syncope; exertional dyspnea	Change in mental status; B/P less than 90 mm Hg systolic or below normal for patient; irregular or absent pulses; diminished peripheral pulses; tachypnea; cool, pale skin; cool extremities; increased capillary refill time

DESIRED OUTCOMES

The client will have adequate cardiac output as evidenced by:
a. B/P within normal range for client
b. Apical pulse between 60 and 100 beats/min and regular
c. Resolution of gallop rhythm(s)
d. No reports of fatigue and weakness
e. Unlabored respirations at 12 to 20 breaths/min
f. Clear, audible breath sounds

g. Usual mental status
h. Absence of dizziness and syncope
i. Palpable peripheral pulses
j. Skin warm and usual color
k. Capillary refill time less than 2 to 3 seconds
l. Urine output at least 30 mL/h
m. Absence of edema and jugular venous distention (JVD)

NDx = NANDA-I Diagnosis   **D** = Delegatable Action   ● = UAP   ✦ = LVN/LPN   ⊖▶ = Go to ⊖volve for animation

Continued...

NOC OUTCOMES	NIC INTERVENTIONS
Cardiac pump effectiveness; circulation status; tissue perfusion: peripheral; tissue perfusion: cardiac	Cardiac care: acute; hemodynamic regulation; cardiac precautions; dysrhythmia management; cardiac care: rehabilitative

NURSING ASSESSMENT	RATIONALE

Assess for signs and symptoms of decreased cardiac output:
* Variations in B/P (may be increased because of pain or compensatory vasoconstriction; may be decreased when compensatory mechanisms and pump fail)
* Tachycardia
* Presence of gallop rhythm(s)/S_4 heart sound
* Fatigue and weakness
* Dyspnea, orthopnea, tachypnea
* Crackles (rales)
* Restlessness, anxiousness, confusion, or other change in mental status
* Dizziness, syncope
* Diminished or absent peripheral pulses
* Cool extremities
* Pallor or cyanosis of skin
* Capillary refill time greater than 2 to 3 seconds
* Oliguria
* Edema
* JVD
* Chest radiograph results showing pulmonary vascular congestion, pulmonary edema, or pleural effusion
* Abnormal arterial blood gas values
* Significant decrease in oximetry results

Assess for diagnostic findings indicative of an MI:
* Elevated serum creatine kinase (CK)-MB level
* Elevated serum troponin level
* Elevated serum lactate dehydrogenase (LDH) level with an LDH_1 level that is higher than the LDH_2 (a reliable indicator of an acute MI)
* ECG showing ST-segment elevation or depression, inversion of T waves, and/or presence of abnormal Q waves (there may be no Q waves if client has had a subendocardial infarction)

Early recognition and reporting of signs and symptoms of an MI allow for prompt intervention.

THERAPEUTIC INTERVENTIONS	RATIONALE

Independent Actions

Perform actions to reduce cardiac workload:
* Place client in a semi- to high-Fowler's position. **D** ●

* Instruct client to avoid activities that create a Valsalva response (e.g., straining to have a bowel movement, holding breath while moving up in bed).
* Implement measures to promote rest and conserve energy. **D** ● ✦
* Discourage smoking.

* Provide small meals rather than large ones.

* Discourage excessive intake of beverages high in caffeine such as coffee, tea, and colas.
* Restrict sodium intake if ordered.

Elevation of client's upper body reduces cardiac workload by decreasing venous return from the periphery and subsequently reducing preload.

When a client exhales after the Valsalva maneuver, the intrathoracic pressure falls, causing a sudden increase in venous return and a subsequent increase in preload and cardiac workload.

Physical rest reduces cardiac workload by lowering the body's energy requirements and subsequent need for oxygen.

Nicotine has a cardiostimulatory effect and causes vasoconstriction; the carbon monoxide in smoke reduces oxygen availability.

Large meals require a greater increase in blood supply to the gastrointestinal tract for digestion.

Caffeine is a myocardial stimulant and can increase myocardial oxygen consumption.

Restricting sodium helps to prevent fluid retention.

THERAPEUTIC INTERVENTIONS	RATIONALE
• Increase activity gradually as allowed and tolerated.	*A gradual increase in activity prevents a sudden increase in cardiac workload.*

Dependent/Collaborative Actions

Implement measures to maintain an adequate cardiac output

• Prepare client for procedures that may be performed to improve coronary blood flow:
  • Injection of a thrombolytic agent
  • Percutaneous coronary intervention
  • Insertion of an intra-aortic balloon pump (IABP)
	Decreases fear and anxiety.

• Maintain oxygen therapy as ordered. **D** ✦ • Administer the following medications if ordered:	*When tissue oxygenation is adequate, the heart does not need to work as hard to supply oxygen to the tissues; thus more oxygen is available for myocardial use.*
• Nitrates	*Nitrates decrease cardiac workload and myocardial oxygen demands by relaxing peripheral veins and, to a lesser extent, arterioles.*
• Beta-adrenergic blocking agents	*Beta-adrenergic blockers reduce cardiac workload by blocking sympathetic nervous system stimulation of beta receptors in the heart.*
• ACE inhibitors	*ACE inhibitors/angiotensin II receptor antagonists block the vasoconstrictor effect of angiotensin II, which causes a decrease in aldosterone output.*
• Antidysrhythmics	*Antidysrhythmics improve cardiac output by correcting automaticity and/or conduction abnormalities in the heart.*
• Anticoagulants	*Anticoagulants help to restore/improve coronary blood flow.*
Consult physician if signs and symptoms of decreased cardiac output persist or worsen.	*Notifying the physician allows for modification of the treatment plan.*

Nursing Diagnosis

ACUTE PAIN NDx (CHEST PAIN/DISCOMFORT THAT MAY RADIATE TO ARM, NECK, JAW, OR BACK)

Definition: Unpleasant sensory and/or emotional experience arising from actual on potential tissue damage

Related to: Myocardial ischemia (a decreased oxygen supply forces the myocardium to convert to anaerobic metabolism; the end products of anaerobic metabolism act as irritants to myocardial neural receptors)

CLINICAL MANIFESTATIONS

Subjective	Objective
Verbal reports of pain	Grimacing; rubbing neck, jaw, or arm; reluctance to move; clutching chest; restlessness; diaphoresis; increased B/P and/or tachycardia

RISK FACTORS

• Coronary artery disease
• Increase in oxygen demand

DESIRED OUTCOMES

The client will experience relief of chest pain/discomfort as evidenced by:
 a. Verbalization of same
 b. Relaxed facial expression and body positioning
 c. Increased participation in activities
 d. Stable vital signs

NOC OUTCOMES

Comfort level; pain control

NIC INTERVENTIONS

Pain management; analgesic administration; oxygen therapy

NDx = NANDA-I Diagnosis   **D** = Delegatable Action   ● = UAP   ✦ = LVN/LPN   ⊖▶ = Go to ⊖volve for animation

Continued...

NURSING ASSESSMENT	RATIONALE
Assess signs and symptoms of chest pain/discomfort: • Verbalization of pain • Grimacing • Rubbing neck, jaw, or arm • Reluctance to move • Clutching chest • Restlessness • Diaphoresis • Increased B/P • Tachycardia Assess client's perception of the severity of the pain/discomfort using an intensity rating scale. Assess the client's pattern of pain/discomfort (e.g., location, quality, onset, duration, precipitating factors, aggravating factors, alleviating factors).	*Early recognition and reporting of signs and symptoms of chest pain allow for prompt intervention.*

THERAPEUTIC INTERVENTIONS	RATIONALE
Independent Actions Implement measures to relieve pain/discomfort: • Maintain client on bed rest in a semi- to high-Fowler's position. **D** ● ✦ • Provide or assist with nonpharmacological measures for pain relief (e.g., relaxation techniques, restful environment). **D** ✦	*Best rest helps to reduce myocardial oxygen demands by reducing cardiac workload.* *Nonpharmacological interventions are effective because they stimulate closure of the gating mechanism in the spinal cord and subsequently block the transmission of pain impulses.*

Dependent/Collaborative Actions
Implement measures to relieve pain/discomfort:
• Administer the following medications if ordered:
  • Intravenous narcotic (opioid) analgesics
  • Nitrates
	Intravenous rather than an intramuscular route should be used because intramuscular injections are poorly absorbed if tissue perfusion is decreased; intramuscular injections also elevate some serum enzyme levels, which may interfere with assessment of myocardial damage.

• Maintain oxygen therapy as ordered. **D** ✦ Implement measures to maintain an adequate cardiac output: Prepare client for procedures that may be performed to improve coronary blood flow: • Injection of a thrombolytic agent • Percutaneous coronary intervention • Insertion of an IABP Consult physician if pain/discomfort persists or worsens.	*Oxygen therapy helps to increase the myocardial oxygen supply.* *Decreases fear and anxiety.* *Notifying the physician allows for modification of the treatment plan.*

Nursing Diagnosis RISK FOR ACTIVITY INTOLERANCE NDx

Definition: At risk for experiencing insufficient physiological or psychological energy to endure or complete required or desired daily activities

Related to:
• Tissue hypoxia if cardiac output is decreased
• Difficulty resting and sleeping associated with discomfort, frequent assessments and treatments, fear, and anxiety

CLINICAL MANIFESTATIONS

Subjective	Objective
Verbal report of fatigue or weakness	Abnormal heart rate or B/P response to activity; exertional discomfort or dyspnea; ECG changes reflecting ischemia

RISK FACTORS

- Increased oxygen demand
- Immobility
- Generalized weakness

DESIRED OUTCOMES

The client will not experience activity intolerance as evidenced by:
a. No reports of fatigue or weakness
b. Ability to perform activities of daily living without exertional dyspnea, chest pain, diaphoresis, dizziness, and a significant change in vital signs

NOC OUTCOMES

Activity tolerance; energy conservation; self-care: activities of daily living

NIC INTERVENTIONS

Energy management; oxygen therapy; cardiac care: rehabilitative; sleep enhancement

NURSING ASSESSMENT

Assess for signs and symptoms of activity intolerance:
- Statements of fatigue or weakness
- Exertional dyspnea, chest pain, diaphoresis, or dizziness
- Abnormal heart rate response to activity (e.g., increase in rate of 20 beats/min above resting rate, rate not returning to preactivity level within 3 minutes after stopping activity, change from regular to irregular rate)
- Significant change (15-20 mm Hg) in B/P with activity

RATIONALE

Early recognition and reporting of signs and symptoms of activity intolerance allow for prompt intervention.

THERAPEUTIC INTERVENTIONS

Independent Actions

Implement measures to prevent activity intolerance:
- Perform actions to promote rest and/or conserve energy:
  - Maintain activity restrictions as ordered.
  - Minimize environmental activity and noise. **D** ✦
  - Organize nursing care to allow for periods of uninterrupted rest.
  - Limit the number of visitors and their length of stay.
  - Assist client with self-care activities as needed. **D** ●
  - Keep supplies and personal articles within easy reach.
  - Instruct client in energy-saving techniques (e.g., using shower chair when showering, sitting to brush teeth or comb hair).
  - Implement measures to reduce fear and anxiety.
  - Implement measures to promote sleep:
    - Encourage relaxing diversional activities in the evening.
    - Allow client to continue usual sleep practices unless contraindicated.
    - Reduce environmental distractions.
  - Implement nonpharmacological measures to relieve pain/discomfort. **D** ✦

Instruct client to:
- Report a decreased tolerance for activity.
- Stop any activity that causes chest pain, shortness of breath, dizziness, or extreme fatigue or weakness.

Dependent/Collaborative Actions

Implement measures to prevent activity intolerance:
- Perform actions to promote rest and/or conserve energy:
  - Implement measures to promote sleep:
    - Administer prescribed sedative-hypnotics.
    - Administer prescribed analgesics.

RATIONALE

Cells use oxygen and fat, protein, and carbohydrates to produce the energy needed for all body activities. Rest and activities that conserve energy result in a lower metabolic rate, which preserves nutrients and oxygen for necessary activities.

Continued...

THERAPEUTIC INTERVENTIONS	RATIONALE
• Perform actions to maintain an adequate cardiac output if decreased cardiac output is contributing to client's activity intolerance.	*Sufficient cardiac output is necessary to maintain an adequate blood flow and oxygen supply to the tissues. Adequate tissue oxygenation promotes more efficient energy production, which subsequently improves the client's activity tolerance.*
• Maintain oxygen therapy as ordered.	*Maintains tissue oxygenation.*
• Increase client's activity gradually as allowed and tolerated.	*Improves cardiac stamina.*
Consult appropriate health care provider (e.g., cardiac rehabilitation therapist, physician) if signs and symptoms of activity intolerance persist or worsen.	*Notifying the physician allows for modification of the treatment plan.*

Collaborative Diagnosis   RISK FOR CARDIAC DYSRHYTHMIAS

Definition: Disturbance of heart rhythm

CLINICAL MANIFESTATIONS

Subjective	Objective
Verbal report of palpitations; lightheadedness	Irregular apical pulse; pulse rate below 60 or above 100 beats/min; apical-radial pulse deficit; syncope; palpitations; abnormal rate, rhythm, or configurations on ECG

RISK FACTORS

- Electrolyte abnormalities
- Drug toxicities
- Myocardial ischemia

DESIRED OUTCOMES

The client will maintain normal sinus rhythm as evidenced by:
  a. Regular apical pulse at 60 to 100 beats/min
  b. Equal apical and radial pulse rates
  c. Absence of syncope and palpitations
  d. ECG showing normal sinus rhythm

NURSING ASSESSMENT	RATIONALE
Assess frequently for and report signs and symptoms of cardiac dysrhythmias: • Irregular apical pulse • Syncope • Palpitations	*Early recognition of dysrhythmias allows for prompt intervention.*

THERAPEUTIC INTERVENTIONS	RATIONALE
Independent Actions If cardiac dysrhythmias occur: • Initiate cardiac monitoring if not currently being done.	*Monitoring should be implemented in order to identify dysrhythmias that could cause further deterioration of the client's condition.*
• Restrict client's activity based on client's tolerance and severity of the dysrhythmia.	*Rest reduces the workload of the injured heart.*
Dependent/Collaborative Actions Implement measures to maintain an adequate cardiac output.	*Adequate cardiac output promotes adequate myocardial tissue perfusion and oxygenation and reduces the risk of cardiac dysrhythmias.*
If cardiac dysrhythmias occur: • Administer antidysrhythmics if ordered. • Maintain oxygen therapy as ordered.	*The most common complication after an MI is dysrhythmias due to the irritability of the heart muscle. Dysrhythmias are not usually treated unless they are life-threatening.*

THERAPEUTIC INTERVENTIONS	RATIONALE

- Prepare client for the following if planned:
  - Cardioversion
  - Insertion of a pacemaker or implantable cardioverter-defibrillator (ICD)
  - Catheter ablation of irritable site
- Have emergency cart readily available for defibrillation or cardiopulmonary resuscitation.

Collaborative Diagnosis | **RISK FOR HEART FAILURE**

Definition: Cardiac dysfunction due to impaired cardiac pumping that results in inadequate perfusion of tissues; may be classified primarily as left-sided or right-sided failure and may present either acutely after an MI or chronically

Related to: Cardiac dysfunction which decreases cardiac output due to impaired electrical conduction, tissue damage, and/or infection

CLINICAL MANIFESTATIONS

Subjective	Objective
Verbal reports of shortness of breath; increased anxiety; increased weakness; increased fatigue	Cyanosis; pallor; cool, clammy skin; severe dyspnea; tachycardia; S_3 heart sound; crackles; pink, frothy sputum; weight gain; edema; distended neck veins; decreased urine output; chest radiograph demonstrating vascular congestion

RISK FACTORS
- Acute MI
- Dysrhythmias
- Pulmonary emboli
- Hypertensive crisis
- Ruptured papillary muscle
- Myocarditis

DESIRED OUTCOMES

The client will not develop heart failure as evidenced by:
a. Pulse rate 60 to 100 beats/min
b. Absence of an S_3 heart sound
c. Usual mental status
d. Clear, audible breath sounds
e. Absence of or no increase in dyspnea and orthopnea
f. Absence of cough
g. Palpable peripheral pulses
h. No reports of increased fatigue and weakness
i. Urine output at least 30 mL/h
j. Stable weight
k. Absence of edema and distended neck veins

NURSING ASSESSMENT	RATIONALE

Assess for and report signs and symptoms of heart failure:
- Cyanosis
- Pallor
- Dyspnea
- Tachycardia
- S_3 heart sounds
- Crackles
- Decreased urine output

Monitor chest radiograph results for vascular congestion and arterial blood gas/pulse oximetry values for abnormalities.

Early recognition of signs and symptoms of heart failure allows for prompt intervention.

THERAPEUTIC INTERVENTIONS	RATIONALE

Independent Actions
Implement measures to prevent heart failure:
- Perform actions to maintain an adequate cardiac output.

Ensuring adequate cardiac output prevents the accumulation of fluid/blood in the pulmonary and vascular system.

NDx = NANDA-I Diagnosis **D** = Delegatable Action ● = UAP ✦ = LVN/LPN ⊖▶ = Go to ⊖volve for animation

Continued...

THERAPEUTIC INTERVENTIONS	RATIONALE

Dependent/Collaborative Actions
Implement measures to prevent heart failure:
• Perform actions to treat cardiac dysrhythmias if present
If signs and symptoms of heart failure occur:
• Maintain oxygen therapy as ordered.
• Administer the following medications if ordered:
   • Positive inotropic agents
 	
   • B-type natriuretic peptide (nesiritide)
   • Vasodilators
 	
   • ACE inhibitors
 	
   • Diuretics
 	
   • Morphine sulfate
	Dysrhythmias can contribute to the development of heart failure by altering normal filling time or filling volume.
	
	Inotropic agents improve cardiac output by increasing myocardial contractility.
	Nesiritide promotes diuresis and vasodilation.
	Vasodilators help to decrease preload and afterload, reducing the workload of the heart.
	ACE inhibitors help to decrease cardiac workload and reduce ventricular remodeling.
	Diuretics help to decrease intravascular volume, decreasing venous return, thereby reducing preload and helping to decrease pulmonary vascular congestion.
	Morphine helps to reduce anxiety, reduce preload through secondary vasodilation, and decrease the cardiovascular effects of the fight or flight response that can occur with anxiety.

Collaborative Diagnosis   RISK FOR THROMBOEMBOLISM

Definition: A clot attached to a vessel/cardiac chamber wall that becomes dislodged, circulating within the blood. After an acute MI, a thromboembolism may result from debris and clots that collect inside dilated aneurismal sacs in the ventricle or from infarcted endocardium

Related to:
• Venous stasis in the periphery associated with decreased cardiac output and decreased mobility
• Stasis of blood in the heart associated with decreased ventricular emptying (risk increases if dysrhythmias are present)

CLINICAL MANIFESTATIONS*

Subjective	Objective
Verbal reports of pain; apprehension; anxiety	Deep vein: Tenderness; swelling; positive Homans' sign; increased warmth Arterial: Diminished or absent peripheral pulses; pallor, coolness, numbness, and/or pain in extremity Cerebral: Decreased level of consciousness; alteration in usual sensory and motor function Pulmonary: Sudden onset of chest pain, dyspnea, increased restlessness, and significant decrease in arterial oxygen saturation (Sao_2)

RISK FACTORS
• Immobility
• Ventricular aneurysms
• Myocardial infarctions
• Hypercoagulability

DESIRED OUTCOMES

The client will not develop a thromboembolism as evidenced by:
  a. Absence of pain, tenderness, swelling, and numbness in extremities
  b. Usual temperature and color of extremities
  c. Palpable and equal peripheral pulses
  d. Usual mental status
  e. Usual sensory and motor function
  f. Absence of sudden chest pain and dyspnea

NURSING ASSESSMENT	RATIONALE
Assess for and report signs and symptoms of deep vein, arterial, cerebral, or pulmonary thromboembolism:	*Early recognition of signs and symptoms of thromboembolism allows for prompt intervention.*

*Clinical manifestations vary depending upon the location of the embolus and may occur in the veins and arteries located in the legs, brain, and pulmonary system.

NURSING ASSESSMENT	RATIONALE
Monitor results of echocardiogram and report findings of a cardiac thrombus.	

THERAPEUTIC INTERVENTIONS	RATIONALE

Independent Actions

If signs and symptoms of an arterial embolus in an extremity occur:

- Maintain client on bed rest with affected extremity in a level or slightly dependent position.

Positioning helps to improve arterial blood flow.

If signs and symptoms of cerebral ischemia occur:

- Maintain client on bed rest; keep head and neck in neutral, midline position.

Positioning helps to facilitate venous drainage of the head, reducing the risk of increased intracranial pressure (ICP).

Dependent/Collaborative Actions

Implement measures to prevent the development of thromboemboli:

- Perform actions to reduce the risk of thrombus formation in the heart:

The goal of dependent nursing actions is to prevent the formation of a thrombus by maintaining adequate blood flow and preventing venous stasis, reducing hypercoagulability of the blood, and limiting damage to the vessel linings.

  - Implement measures to maintain an adequate cardiac output.
  - Prepare client for procedures to improve coronary blood flow (e.g., PCTA, insertion of IABP—intraaortic balloon pump).

Procedures will help improve coronary blood flow and improve cardiac output.

  - Implement measures to treat dysrhythmias if present.
  - Administer antiarrythmic medications.

Reduces the risk of dysrhythmias that allow pooling of blood in the heart (e.g., atrial fibrillation).

  - Administer anticoagulants and antiplatelet agents if ordered.

If signs and symptoms of an arterial embolus in an extremity occur:

- Prepare client for diagnostic studies.
  - Doppler or duplex ultrasound
  - Arteriography
- Prepare client for the following if planned:

Procedures act to restore blood flow to affected vessel.

  - Injection of a thrombolytic agent
  - Embolectomy
- Administer anticoagulants as ordered.

Collaborative Diagnosis

RISK FOR RUPTURE OF A PORTION OF THE HEART (E.G., VENTRICULAR FREE WALL, INTERVENTRICULAR SEPTUM, PAPILLARY MUSCLE)

Definition: Tearing of cardiac tissues within the heart

Related to: Weakening of cardiac tissue from ischemia and/or necrosis

CLINICAL MANIFESTATIONS*

Subjective	Objective
Not applicable	Papillary muscle rupture: Holosystolic murmur; dyspnea; evidence of papillary muscle rupture on echocardiography or cardiac catheterization Ventricular septal defect: Holosystolic murmur; parasternal thrill; finding of septal defect on echocardiography or cardiac catheterization Cardiac tamponade: Significant decrease in B/P; narrowed pulse pressure; pulsus paradoxus; distant or muffled heart sounds; jugular venous distention; increased central venous pressure

---

*Clinical manifestations will vary depending upon which structures are affected.

NDx = NANDA-I Diagnosis   **D** = Delegatable Action   ● = UAP   ✦ = LVN/LPN   ⊖▶ = Go to ⊖volve for animation

Continued...

RISK FACTOR

- MI or damage

DESIRED OUTCOME

The client will not experience rupture of any portion of the heart as evidenced by absence of signs of acute heart failure and/or cardiogenic shock.

NURSING ASSESSMENT	RATIONALE
Assess for any report signs and symptoms of papillary muscle rupture, ventricular septal defect, and cardiac tamponade: • Holosystolic murmurs • Dyspned Assess for and immediately report signs and symptoms of acute heart failure and/or cardiogenic shock: • Increased restlessness/confusion • Systolic B/P less than 80 mm Hg • Rapid, weak pulse • Diminished or absent pulses • Increase coolness and duskiness of skin • Urine output less than 30 mL/h	*Early recognition of signs and symptoms of rupture of heart structures allows for prompt intervention.*

THERAPEUTIC INTERVENTIONS	RATIONALE
Independent Actions Implement measures to reduce cardiac workload and increase activity as allowed. Add the following actions: • Place client in semi-Fowler's position. • Instruct client to avoid activities that create a Valsalva response (e.g., straining). • Discourage smoking. If signs and symptoms of rupture of a portion of the heart occur: • Maintain client on bed rest.	*Reducing cardiac workload helps to reduce risk of rupture of the papillary muscle and ventricular free wall or septum.* *The client may become hemodynamically unstable and therefore should be maintained on bed rest.*

Dependent/Collaborative Actions
If signs and symptoms of rupture of a portion of the heart occur:
• Assist with pericardiocentesis if performed.
• Assist with measures to treat heart failure or cardiogenic shock.
• Prepare client for surgical intervention if planned:
  • Valve replacement
  • Repair of ventricular septal defect
	
	Cardiac tamponade is treated with pericardiocentesis.
	
	Decreases fear and anxiety.

Collaborative Diagnosis   RISK FOR PERICARDITIS

Definition: Inflammation of the pericardium

Related to:
- Exposure to pathogens
- Death of tissue

CLINICAL MANIFESTATIONS

Subjective	Objective
Verbal reports of precordial pain that frequently radiates to shoulder, neck, back, and arm; is intensified during deep inspiration, movement, and coughing; and usually is relieved by sitting up and leaning forward	Pericardial friction rub; persistent temperature elevation; further increase in white blood cell (WBC) count and sedimentation rate

RISK FACTORS
- MI
- Myocardial necrosis
- Infection

DESIRED OUTCOMES

The client will experience resolution of pericarditis if it develops as evidenced by:
  a. Fewer reports of precordial pain
  b. Absence of pericardial friction rub
  c. Temperature declining toward normal
  d. WBC count and sedimentation rate declining toward normal range

NURSING ASSESSMENT

Assess for and report signs and symptoms of pericarditis:
- Pericardial friction rub
- Elevated temperature
- Precordial pain

Monitor erythrocyte sedimentation rate, WBC and differential cell counts for abnormalities.

RATIONALE

Early recognition of signs and symptoms of pericarditis allows for prompt intervention.

THERAPEUTIC INTERVENTIONS

Independent Actions

If signs and symptoms of pericarditis occur:
- Allay client's anxiety.
- Assist client to assume position of comfort.

Dependent/Collaborative Actions

If signs and symptoms of pericarditis occur:
- Administer anti-inflammatory agents if ordered.

RATIONALE

The client may believe that symptoms indicate recurrent MI.
Pericarditic pain is best relieved with the patient sitting or leaning forward.

Pain and inflammation associated with pericarditis are usually treated with anti-inflammatory agents.

Collaborative Diagnosis # RISK FOR INFARCTION EXTENSION OR RECURRENCE

Definition: Expansion of tissue death from the MI and/or secondary MI

Related to: Inadequate treatment of original MI

CLINICAL MANIFESTATIONS

Subjective	Objective
Verbal reports of chest pain	Changes in vital signs; increase in cardiac enzyme levels; increase in ECG abnormalities (ST-segment elevation/Q waves)

RISK FACTOR
- Previous MI

DESIRED OUTCOMES

The client will not experience infarct extension or recurrence as evidenced by:
  a. No further episodes of persistent chest pain
  b. Stable vital signs
  c. Cardiac enzyme levels declining toward normal range
  d. Improved ECG readings

NURSING ASSESSMENT

Assess for and report signs and symptoms of infarct extension or recurrence (e.g., changes in vital signs; increase in cardiac enzyme levels; ECG changes [ST-segment elevation/Q waves]).

RATIONALE

Early recognition of signs and symptoms of reinfarction allows for prompt intervention.

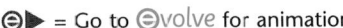

NDx = NANDA-I Diagnosis **D** = Delegatable Action ● = UAP ✦ = LVN/LPN ⊖▶ = Go to ⊖volve for animation

Continued...

THERAPEUTIC INTERVENTIONS	RATIONALE
Dependent/Collaborative Actions If client experiences signs and symptoms of infarct extension or recurrence: • Administer medications ordered: • Medications such as nitrates, ACE inhibitors, beta-blocking agents, aspirin, and heparin, act to optimize cardiac performance and reduce the risk of reinfarction. • Prepare the client for coronary angiogram, thrombolytic therapy, or revascularization procedure (e.g., percutaneous transluminal coronary angioplasty [PTCA], coronary artery bypass grafting [CABG]) if planned.	*The goal of dependent nursing actions is to reduce the workload of the heart, optimize function, and improve perfusion to the myocardium.* *Decreases fear and anxiety.*

Collaborative Diagnosis RISK FOR CARDIOGENIC SHOCK

Definition: Decreased cardiac output and evidence of tissue hypoxia in the presence of adequate intravascular volume

Related to:
• Inability of the heart to effectively provide perfusion to the tissues
• Cardiac tissue ischemia and/or necrosis

CLINICAL MANIFESTATIONS

Subjective	Objective
Reports of lethargy; restlessness	Systolic B/P below 80 mm Hg; rapid, weak pulse; diminished or absent peripheral pulses; increased coolness and duskiness or cyanosis of skin; urine output less than 30 mL/h

RISK FACTORS
• Myocardial ischemia
• MI
• Heart failure
• Pericardial infections

DESIRED OUTCOMES

The client will not develop cardiogenic shock as evidenced by:
  a. Stable or improved mental status
  b. Systolic B/P greater than 80 mm Hg
  c. Palpable peripheral pulses
  d. Stable or improved skin temperature and color
  e. Urine output at least 30 mL/h

NURSING ASSESSMENT	RATIONALE
Assess for and report signs and symptoms of cardiogenic shock: • Systolic B/P <80 mm Hg • Weak pulse • Diminished peripheral pulses • Cyanosis of skin • Urine output <30 mL/h	*Early recognition of signs and symptoms of cardiogenic shock allows for prompt intervention.*

THERAPEUTIC INTERVENTIONS	RATIONALE
Dependent/Collaborative Actions Implement measures to prevent cardiogenic shock: • Perform actions to maintain an adequate cardiac output (e.g., administer inotropic agents). • Perform actions to treat cardiac dysrhythmias if present (e.g., administer antiarrhythmics).	*Cardiogenic shock that is unresponsive to therapy has a high mortality rate.* *Medications geared toward optimizing cardiac performance and improving cardiac output are necessary. Cardiac assist devices support the failing heart when medication therapy is ineffective.*

THERAPEUTIC INTERVENTIONS	RATIONALE

- Perform actions to treat heart failure if it occurs.
- Perform actions to treat rupture of any portion of the heart if it occurs.

If signs and symptoms of cardiogenic shock occur:
- Maintain oxygen therapy as ordered.
- Adminster medications:
  - Positive inotropic agents   *Inotropic agents act to increase myocardial contractility and improve heart failure.*
- Administer the following if ordered:
  - Sympathomimetics
  - Vasodilators
  - Intravenous fluids
- Assist with intubation and insertion of hemodynamic monitoring devices and/or cardiac assist devices:
  - Swan Ganz
  - Intra-aortic balloon pump

DISCHARGE TEACHING/CONTINUED CARE

Nursing Diagnosis   ## DEFICIENT KNOWLEDGE NDx OR INEFFECTIVE SELF-HEALTH MANAGEMENT NDx*

Definition: Absence or deficiency of cognitive information related to specific topic (lack of specific information necessary for clients/significant others to make informed choices regarding condition/treatment/lifestyle changes); pattern of regulating and integrating into daily living a therapeutic regimen for treatment of illness and its sequelae that is unsatisfactory for meeting specific health goals

CLINICAL MANIFESTATIONS

Subjective	Objective
Verbalization of unfamiliarity with information	Inability to follow through with instructions

RISK FACTORS
- Denial of disease process
- Cognitive deficiency
- Failure to take action to reduce risk factors

NOC OUTCOMES	NIC INTERVENTIONS
Knowledge: treatment regimen; knowledge: disease process; knowledge: cardiac disease management	Health system guidance; teaching: individual; teaching: disease process; teaching: prescribed activity/exercise; teaching: prescribed medication

NURSING ASSESSMENT	RATIONALE
Assess client's readiness and ability to learn.	*Early recognition of readiness to learn and meaning of illness to client allows for implementation of the appropriate teaching interventions.*
Assess meaning of illness to client.	

THERAPEUTIC INTERVENTIONS	RATIONALE

Desired Outcome: The client will verbalize a basic understanding of an MI.

---

*The nurse should select the nursing diagnostic label that is most appropriate for the client's discharge teaching needs.

NDx = NANDA-I Diagnosis   **D** = Delegatable Action   ● = UAP   ✦ = LVN/LPN   ☺▶ = Go to ☺volve for animation

Continued...

THERAPEUTIC INTERVENTIONS	RATIONALE
Independent Actions Explain an MI in terms the client can understand. Use appropriate teaching aids (e.g., pictures, videotapes, heart models). Inform client that it takes approximately 6 to 8 weeks for the heart to heal after an MI.	*Clients vary in physical and cognitive ability to learn. When educating clients, nurses need to determine a client's ability to read and understand written materials. If literacy barriers are present, alternative educational materials should be provided. Better understanding of the clinical problem may enhance adherence.*

THERAPEUTIC INTERVENTIONS	RATIONALE
Desired Outcome: The client will demonstrate accuracy in counting pulse. **Independent Actions** Teach client how to count his/her pulse, being alert to the regularity of the rhythm. Allow time for return demonstration and accuracy check.	*Educating clients to assess their baseline pulse allows for early detection of irregularities warranting immediate attention from a health care provider. Early detection may reduce the incidence of sudden death.*

THERAPEUTIC INTERVENTIONS	RATIONALE
Desired Outcome: The client will identify modifiable cardiovascular risk factors and ways to alter these factors. **Independent Actions** Inform client that certain modifiable factors such as elevated serum lipid levels, a sedentary lifestyle, hypertension, and smoking have been shown to increase the risk for coronary artery disease.	*Thorough education is a critical component of the care of a client after an MI. Continued lifestyle modifications consistent with recommendations for clients with cardiovascular disease are necessary to prevent coronary reocclusion. The client must have a thorough understanding of the importance of adhering to diet, medication, activity/exercise, and nutritional recommendations to prevent an exacerbation and control the disease.*
Assist client to identify changes in lifestyle that can help the client to eliminate or reduce the above risk factors and to help prevent a recurrent MI (e.g., dietary modification, physical exercise on regular basis, moderation of alcohol intake, smoking cessation). Encourage client to limit daily alcohol consumption. Daily alcohol intake exceeding 1 oz of ethanol may contribute to the development of hypertension and some forms of heart disease.	*Current recommendations are no more than 2 drinks per day for men and no more than 1 drink per day for women and lighter-weight persons. A "drink" is considered to be ½ oz of ethanol (e.g., 1½ oz of 80-proof whiskey, 12 oz of beer, 5 oz of wine).*

THERAPEUTIC INTERVENTIONS	RATIONALE
Desired Outcome: The client will verbalize an understanding of the rationale for and components of a diet designed to lower serum cholesterol and triglyceride levels. **Independent Actions** Provide instructions on ways the client can reduce intake of saturated fat and cholesterol: • Reduce intake of meat fat (e.g., trim visible fat off meat; replace fatty meats such as fatty cuts of steak, hamburger, and processed meats with leaner products). • Reduce intake of milk fat (e.g., avoid dairy products containing more than 1% fat). • Reduce intake of *trans* fats (e.g., avoid stick margarine and shortening and foods such as commercial baked goods that are prepared with these products).	*The risk of coronary artery disease (CAD) is associated with a serum cholesterol level of more than 200 mg/dL or a fasting triglyceride level of more than 150 mg/dL. Elevated serum lipid levels are one of the most firmly established risk factors for CAD.*

THERAPEUTIC INTERVENTIONS	RATIONALE

- Use vegetable oil rather than coconut or palm oil in cooking and food preparation.
- Use cooking methods such as steaming, baking, broiling, poaching, microwaving, and grilling rather than frying.
- Restrict intake of eggs (recommendations about the number of whole eggs allowed per week vary depending on the client's lipid levels).
- Encourage client to increase intake of omega-3 fatty acids (e.g., flaxseed, cold water ocean fish such as salmon and halibut) to help lower triglyceride levels and increase high-density lipoprotein (HDL) levels.

THERAPEUTIC INTERVENTIONS	RATIONALE

Desired Outcome: The client will verbalize an understanding of medications ordered including rationale, food and drug interactions, side effects, schedule for taking, and importance of taking as prescribed.

Independent Actions

Explain the rationale for, side effects of, and importance of taking the medications prescribed. Inform client of pertinent food and drug interactions.

Taking medications as prescribed ensures that therapeutic drug levels will be maintained. Clients should be instructed not to discontinue taking medications if they feel better. Clients without financial resources should be assisted in accessing appropriate resources to obtain needed medications (e.g., pharmacy assistance programs).

Educate the client on the proper administration, dosing regimen, side effects, precautions, and storage of the following medications if ordered:
- Nitrates/nitrate patches/nitrate paste
- Beta-adrenergic blockers
- ACE inhibitors
- Lipid-lowering agents

Instruct the client to notify physician provider before taking other prescription medications and to inform all health care providers of medications being taken.

THERAPEUTIC INTERVENTIONS	RATIONALE

Desired Outcome: The client will state signs and symptoms to report to the health care provider.

Independent Actions

Instruct the client to report:
- Chest, arm, neck, jaw, or back discomfort unrelieved by nitroglycerin
- Shortness of breath
- Significant weight gain or swelling of feet or ankles
- Irregular pulse or a significant unexpected change in the pulse rate
- Persistent impotence or decreased libido (can be a side effect of certain medications or result from anxiety, depression, or fatigue)
- Inability to tolerate prescribed activity
- Increase in severity or frequency of episodes of angina

Reporting concerning signs and symptoms to the appropriate provider allows for modification of the treatment plan.

Continued...

THERAPEUTIC INTERVENTIONS	RATIONALE

Desired Outcome: The client will verbalize an understanding of activity restrictions and the rate at which activity can be progressed.

Independent Actions

Reinforce physician's instructions about activity. Instruct client to:

- Gradually increase activity by adhering to a regular aerobic exercise program (often begins with walking).
- Take frequent rest periods for about 4 to 8 weeks after discharge.
- Avoid physical conditioning programs such as jogging and aerobic dancing until advised by physician.
- Avoid strenuous exercise and activities that involve pushing or lifting heavy objects (e.g., weightlifting).
- Avoid exercising for at least an hour after eating and when the environmental temperature is extremely hot or cold.
- Avoid tobacco use before exercise.
- Stop any activity that causes chest pain, shortness of breath, palpitations, dizziness, or extreme fatigue or weakness.
- Begin a cardiovascular fitness program if recommended by physician.

Reinforce instructions regarding sexual activity:

- Sexual activity with usual partner can be resumed after the prescribed length of time (many physicians consider a client ready to resume sexual activity when the client is able to climb two flights of stairs briskly without dyspnea or angina).
- Assume a comfortable and unstrenuous position for intercourse (e.g., side-lying, partner on top).
- A new sexual relationship can be started but may result in greater energy expenditure until it becomes a more familiar or usual experience.
- Take nitroglycerin before sexual activity if angina occurs with sexual activity.
- Avoid intercourse for at least 1 to 2 hours after a heavy meal or alcohol consumption.
- Avoid sexual activity when fatigued or stressed.
- Avoid hot or cold showers just before and after intercourse.

While the benefits of physical activity are an integral part of cardiac rehabilitation, the level of activity should be increased gradually. Physical activity guidelines after acute coronary syndromes focus on frequency, intensity, type, and time of activity.

THERAPEUTIC INTERVENTIONS	RATIONALE

Desired Outcome: The client will identify community resources that can assist with cardiac rehabilitation and adjustment to the effects of an MI.

Independent Actions

Provide information on community resources and support groups that can assist client with cardiac rehabilitation and adjustment to the effects of an MI (e.g., American Heart Association, "coronary clubs," counseling services).

Cardiac disease can significantly impact an individual's and family's socioeconomic status. Providing information specific to community resources is important to provide a necessary continuum of care and may impact the client's health status, preventing future hospitalizations.

THERAPEUTIC INTERVENTIONS	**RATIONALE**

Desired Outcome: The client will verbalize an understanding of and a plan for adhering to recommended follow-up care including future appointments with health care provider.

Independent Actions

Reinforce the importance of keeping follow-up appointments with health care provider and for exercise stress testing and laboratory studies to monitor serum lipid levels.

Implement measures to improve client adherence:

Regular health care appointments are important to determine effectiveness of the prescribed treatment plan.

- Include significant others in teaching sessions if possible.

Involvement of significant others in patient teaching improves adherence to discharge instructions.

- Encourage questions and allow time for reinforcement and clarification of information provided.
- Provide written instructions on future appointments with health care provider, dietary modifications, activity progression, medications prescribed, and signs and symptoms to report.
- Obtain social service consult as needed to help client obtain financial assistance.

Everyone does not understand information as presented, so set aside time for questions to allow for clarification of information.

Written instructions allow the client to refer to instructions as needed.

ADDITIONAL NURSING DIAGNOSES

DISTURBED SLEEP PATTERN NDx
Related to:
- Symptoms being experienced with the MI (e.g., chest discomfort, shortness of breath)
- Frequent assessments and treatments
- Fear and anxiety

FEAR/ANXIETY NDx
Related to:
- Symptoms being experienced with the MI (e.g., chest discomfort, arm pain, and/or shortness of breath)

- Possible future disability, change in roles and lifestyle, and/or death associated with severe damage to the heart
- Unfamiliar environment and separation from significant others
- Lack of understanding of diagnostic tests, diagnosis, and treatment
- Financial concerns about the cost of hospitalization and future treatment

GRIEVING NDx
Related to:
- Loss of normal function of the heart
- Possible changes in lifestyle, occupation, and roles
- Uncertainty of prognosis

See Bibliography at the back of the book.

6 The Client with Alterations in Neurological Function

ALZHEIMER'S DISEASE/DEMENTIA

Alzheimer's disease is a slowly progressive disease that is characterized by stages of declining memory, cognitive and behavioral functioning. Approximately 5 million Americans have been diagnosed with Alzheimer's disease, with a predicted increase to 7.7 million by 2031 It is the most common form of dementia and affects more women than men (possibly because women live longer), and the risk for and incidence of this disease is slightly higher in African Americans and Hispanics than in other populations.

Although the cause of Alzheimer's disease is unknown, several uncontrollable risk factors are associated with the development of the disease, including age, family history/genetics, and gender. Age is one of the most important factors in the development of Alzheimer's disease. The chance of developing Alzheimer's doubles every 5 years in individuals older than 65 years. By the time an individual reaches the age of 85, there is a 50% chance that they will develop the disease. It can, however, rarely affect individuals younger than the age of 40.

The second risk factor is family and genetics. An individual who has a first-degree relative—a sister, brother, or parent—with Alzheimer's is at a greater risk for developing the disease. The risk increases even more if more than one family member has the illness. The gene identified that carries the risk of Alzheimer's disease is apolipoprotein E-e4 (APOE-e4). This form of APOE gene is one of three in the body and is responsible for the development of proteins in the blood that carry cholesterol The presence of APOE-e4 increases the risk of developing the disease however, the presence of this gene does not mean development of the disease is certain. Individuals who inherit a copy of the APOE-e4 gene are simply at increased risk for developing Alzheimer's. If the individual inherits two copies of the gene (one from each parent), he or she has an even greater risk of developing the disease; however, again inheriting the APOE-e4 gene is not a guarantee that the individual will develop Alzheimer's disease.

The last uncontrollable risk factor is gender. Women are at a higher risk of developing the disease because they usually live longer than men. Other potential risk factors are serious head injury, high blood pressure, poorly controlled diabetes, high cholesterol, obesity, and overall poor health during the aging process. A higher incidence of obesity, diabetes, and high cholesterol also increases a woman's likelihood of developing Alzheimer's.

Alzheimer's disease is a chronic, progressive disease that affects the brain structures. Changes that occur in the brain are the development of neurofibrillary tangles, amyloid or neurotic plaques, and the loss of connection between neurons. The plaques develop initially in the areas of the brain responsible for memory and cognitive functioning. Over time the plaques develop in the cerebral cortex in the areas that control language and reasoning.

The onset of Alzheimer's disease usually occurs between 50 and 60 years of age, but may affect people as early as age 40. In the early stage of Alzheimer's disease, the individual may appear healthy, but experiences forgetfulness, short-term memory loss, mild impairment in judgment, and difficulty in deciphering or calculating numbers. Loss of initiative and interest, decreased ability to make judgment, and geographic disorientation are also experienced. These clinical manifestations develop over time; the initial memory deterioration is so subtle that it may not be noticed. The timeframe for the early stage is 2 to 4 years.

In the middle or moderate stage, the clinical manifestations of the disease become more pronounced. The client may experience inability to recognize close family or friends, impairment of cognitive functions, disorientation to person, place, and time, agitation, confusion, possible paranoia hallucinations, and delusions. Affected individuals may wander away from their regular environment and become lost; they may experience mood swings and exhibit aggressive behaviors. The individual's lack of concern about personal hygiene and appearance also become more noticeable.

In the final stage, clients are unable to interact with or respond to their environment. They become bedridden and are totally dependent upon others for activities of daily living. They are unable to carry on a conversation and have no recognition of self or others. This stage lasts until the individual dies, which usually occurs about 14 years after diagnosis.

There is no cure for Alzheimer's disease. Treatment focuses on retaining memory, cognitive and physical functioning, and slowing the progression of the disease. Drug therapy consists of four medications that have been approved by the United States Food and Drug Administration: donepezil, rivastigmine, galantamine, and memantine. These medications regulate the neurotransmitters that transmit information from neuron to neuron. They are thought to help maintain cognitive and memory functioning and may control some of the behavioral symptoms. Other medications may be used to control the symptoms of insomnia, agitation, depression, and anxiety.

This care plan focuses on the adult client with Alzheimer's disease who has been hospitalized. However, much of the information is also applicable to clients with dementia who are receiving follow-up care in an extended care facility or home setting.

OUTCOME/DISCHARGE CRITERIA

The client will:
1. Maintain cognitive functioning as long as possible
2. Have a decline in number of wandering incidents
3. Have minimal episodes of aggressive behavior
4. Avoid behaviors that may harm self or others
5. Participate in activities of daily living
6. Engage in appropriate social interaction with others
7. Engage in a regular exercise program

Nursing Diagnosis ## RISK FOR VIOLENCE: SELF-DIRECTED OR OTHER-DIRECTED NDx

Definition: At risk for behaviors in which an individual demonstrates that he or she can be physically, emotionally, and/or sexually harmful to self and/or others

Related to: Cognitive changes in the client

CLINICAL MANIFESTATIONS

Subjective	Objective
Verbalization of being anxious	Altered perception of reality; frequently expresses anger or frustration; changes in sleep and rest patterns; changes in coping skills; becoming increasingly more aggressive; mood swings

RISK FACTORS

- Impaired cognitive function
- Inability to appropriately handle frustration
- Impaired assessment of the environment

DESIRED OUTCOMES

The client will not experience violence to self and/or others as evidenced by:
  a. No personal injury or injury to others
  b. No demonstration of aggressive behavior
  c. No verbal outburst
  d. No violation of others personal space

NOC OUTCOMES

Aggression control; cognitive ability; mood equilibrium; risk control

NIC INTERVENTIONS

Mood enhancement; environment management; violence prevention; behavior modification

NURSING ASSESSMENT

Assess for changes in cognitive capabilities that may lead to the development of violent actions:
- Decreased decision-making ability
- Decreased attention span
- Decreased ability to concentrate
- Impaired judgment
- Short-term memory impairment
- Decreased ability to communicate
- Inability to solve problems

Use an instrument to assess cognitive status such as the Folstein's Mini-Mental State Examination—assesses:
- Orientation
- Registration

RATIONALE

Changes in individuals with early Alzheimer's are often subtle. Early recognition allows for early intervention and prevention of violence.

Use of this or other instruments to assess cognitive status provides a baseline for evaluation and changes associated with Alzheimer's and other dementias.

Continued...

NURSING ASSESSMENT	RATIONALE
• Attention and calculation • Recall • Speech-language Monitor events that precipitate aggressive behaviors.	*Helps in developing a plan of action to decrease aggressive behaviors*

THERAPEUTIC INTERVENTIONS	RATIONALE
Independent Actions Involve client's cognitive functioning as much as possible. Have client engage in activities that require decision-making.	*Engagement in decision making helps maintain client's cognitive functioning.*
Implement measures to decrease stressful situations and overstimulation: • Place client in private room. • Provide as much autonomy as possible: • Choice of diet • Choice of clothing • Choice of activities	*These actions prevent overstimulation and allow client some control over his/her environment.*
• Provide verbal feedback specific to behavior in a non-threatening manner. • Ask questions about behavior.	*Behavior-specific feedback helps diffuse a situation in which client may be frustrated with limitations on behavior.* *Asking questions may identify what precipitated the inappropriate behavior.*
• Allow client increased personal space.	*Providing increased personal space helps decreases environmental stimuli and client's inappropriate behaviors*
• Speak slowly in a calm and soothing manner. Make comments as precise as possible. Repeat frequently if needed.	*Speaking clearly and precisely helps limit misunderstandings. Client may have some short-term memory loss; frequent repetition may be necessary.*
Implement actions to decrease client's potential to wander: • Provide supervision if patient wanders or expresses a need to go somewhere else, away from the current environment. **D ● ✦**	*Provides safety while allowing client to have need for a change of environment met*
• Provide activities that involve action to distract the client (e.g., folding clothes, take client for a walk, play a simple board game, set table for a meal).	*These actions meet the client's needs for activity and may help increase self-esteem in that the client can accomplish simple activities and they also decrease the client's tendency to wander.*
• Have client wear a sensory device/medic alert to assist in finding client who is known to wander.	*Sensory device/medic alert improves ability to locate client if the client becomes lost.*
• Develop a plan of action with the caregiver in case the client becomes lost.	*Development of an action plan helps locate the client.*
Implement actions to decrease or diffuse experiences of anger and/or exhibits aggressive behavior: • Speak calmly and clearly to the client. Allow verbalization, but do not try to discuss the client's anger. • Use distraction .	*The client is unable to reflect on his/her behavior or learn to control it.* *The client may have impaired short-term memory and distraction may calm aggressive behavior.*
• If able, leave the room and return in a few minutes.	*The client with short-term memory loss may forget what was causing his/her frustration while the other person is out of the room.*
Dependent/Collaborative Actions Use soft restraints if there is a threat of injury to the client or caregiver.	*Allows the client to be angry without causing harm to self and others*
Administer medications that reduce aggressive behavior.	*Medications may help diffuse the situation.*

Nursing Diagnosis | # SELF-CARE DEFICIT: DRESSING, BATHING, FEEDING, AND TOILETING NDx

Definition: Impaired ability to perform or complete bathing/hygiene/grooming/feeding activities for oneself

Related to:
- Inability to make decisions
- Loss of cognitive understanding
- Altered thought processes
- Difficulty in processing information

CLINICAL MANIFESTATIONS

Subjective	Objective
N/A	Inability to determine what to wear; inability to feed self; inability to run bath water or clean self after micturition or defecation

RISK FACTORS
- Impaired memory
- Confusion
- Impaired judgment

DESIRED OUTCOMES

The client will be able to perform activities of daily living as evidenced by:
  a. Ability to appropriately dress and groom self with no or minimal assistance
  b. Ability to feed self with no or minimal assistance
  c. Ability to care for personal hygiene with no or minimal assistance

NOC OUTCOMES

Self-care: bathing, grooming, eating, personal hygiene

NIC INTERVENTIONS

Self-care assistance: bathing, grooming, feeding, personal hygiene

NURSING ASSESSMENT	RATIONALE
Assess client's current self-care habits.	*Provides a baseline of client's ability and where interventions should be implemented*
Assess client's cognitive and physical ability to perform self-care habits.	*When a client's cognitive abilities are impaired, the client is unable to determine self-care needs.*

THERAPEUTIC INTERVENTIONS	RATIONALE

Independent Actions
Implement measures to involve client in activities of daily living: **D** ● ✦

• Allow client time for dressing and bathing in a quiet environment.	*Allowing a client time for ADLS in a quite environment decreases client's stress and frustration.*
• Follow a consistent routine for bathing, dressing, and grooming.	*Routines may prevent confusion, require less decision-making, and may decrease client's frustration.*
• Assist as needed in bathing and perineal care.	*Appropriate bathing and perineal care helps prevent skin breakdown.*
• Limit clothing choices by putting together complete outfits that are easy to put on and to take off.	*Limiting choices decreases frustration if clothing is easy to put on and remove.*
• Lay out or give client clothing in the order in which it will be put on. Start with the bottom half and then top half.	*When helping a client dress, this establishes a routine and simplifies the dressing process.*
• Encourage client independence when dressing; provide assistance as needed.	*Preserves client's independence as long as possible*
• Assist client in selecting foods that will provide appropriate nutrients. Allow client to choose foods he/she likes.	*Client self selection of food helps maintain client's nutritional status and decreases frustration if client receives foods he/she likes*

NDx = NANDA-I Diagnosis   **D** = Delegatable Action   ● = UAP   ✦ = LVN/LPN   ⊜▶ = Go to ⊜volve for animation

Continued...

THERAPEUTIC INTERVENTIONS	RATIONALE
• If assisting client, serve only two foods at a time.	*Keeping food selections to a minimum decreases frustration because client may not be able to decide which food to eat first.*
• Place food in a bowl rather than on a plate, or offer finger foods if client has impaired coordination.	*A bowl is easier for the client to eat from and helps maintain client's independence and decreases frustrations in trying to feed self.*

Nursing Diagnosis CHRONIC CONFUSION NDx

Definition: Irreversible, long-standing, and/or progressive deterioration of intellect and personality characterized by decreased ability to interpret environmental stimuli; decreased capacity for intellectual thought processes; manifested by disturbances of memory, orientation, or behavior

Related to: Degeneration of the CNS and cognitive functioning

CLINICAL MANIFESTATIONS

Subjective	Objective
N/A	Inaccurate interpretation of environment and time; memory loss; altered mood states (e.g., lability, hostility, irritability, inappropriate affect); inability to make decisions or problem solve; changes in attention span; disorientation; inappropriate social behavior; progressive cognitive impairment

RISK FACTORS

• Physiologic changes from progression of Alzheimer's disease

DESIRED OUTCOMES

The client will:
  a. Remain calm and display minimal aggressive behaviors
  b. Have limited disorientation to person, place, and time

NOC OUTCOMES

Cognition; distorted thought; self-control; safety behavior; information processing

NIC INTERVENTIONS

Dementia management; environmental management; behavioral management

NURSING ASSESSMENT	RATIONALE
Assess for episodes of disorientation to person, place, and time, episodes of inappropriate behavior, impaired decision-making ability, impaired memory and judgment, delusions, impaired attention span.	*Early recognition of signs and symptoms of confusion allows for prompt intervention.*

THERAPEUTIC INTERVENTIONS	RATIONALE
Independent Actions Implement measures to maintain client orientation to person, place, and time: • Maintain a structured environment with routine activities, while continuing to monitor the client.	*A predictable environment helps client maintain a sense of security.*
• Orient to person, place, and time frequently. **D ● ✦**	*Frequent orientation may help improve client's sense of orientation.*
• When speaking to the client, use his/her name. **D ● ✦**	*Use of the client's name during communication decreases potential for misunderstanding.*
• Place familiar objects and personal belongings of the client in his/her room. **D ●/✦**	*Having familiar objects in the client's room increases client's sense of security and comfort level in a strange environment.*

THERAPEUTIC INTERVENTIONS	RATIONALE
• When interacting with the client, maintain a calm demeanor, speak slowly, and maintain eye contact. **D** ● ✦	These actions improve potential for client understanding and demonstrates respect.
• Give client information and/or directions in a simple manner. Provide only one piece of information at a time.	Clients' ability to process information decreases as the disease progresses. They are unable to process more than one piece of information at a time.
• Refer to current events when interacting with the client. **D** ● ✦	Discussion of current events grounds client in the present and helps decrease disorientation, because client is not focusing on unreal events.
• Allow client time to formulate responses to questions and during interactions. Allow for periods of silence by the client. **D** ● ✦	Allowing time for client responses demonstrates respect; encourages a response; and helps improve communication. With progression of the disease, the client may have difficulty processing information and formulating an appropriate response.
• Use attentive listening when interacting with the client even when what is being said is confusing or gibberish. **D** ● ✦	
• Allow hoarding of objects as long as they will not be harmful to the client. **D** ● ✦	Allowing client to horde objects provides a sense of security.
• Allow client to interact with other patients, while monitoring client for inappropriate behavior.	Allows the nurse to observe client's social interaction
• Monitor for cyclic changes in cognition and behaviors (e.g., wandering, hoarding items, evening confusion, picking at clothing).	Cyclic changes in cognition indicate client may be experiencing "sundowner" syndrome.
• Maintain client on an appropriate schedule for sleep and rest. Turn off lights when client is in bed. Use a nightlight if needed. **D** ✦	Maintaining a schedule for the client decreases incidence of fatigue and promotes a sense of well-being.

Nursing Diagnosis IMPAIRED HOME MAINTENANCE NDx

Definition: Inability to maintain a safe and growth-promoting immediate environment

Related to:
• Degeneration in cognitive functioning
• Inability to make decisions

CLINICAL MANIFESTATIONS

Subjective	Objective
Expression of difficulty in maintaining household; family member request for assistance in caring for the client in their home	Household temperature too hot or too cold; inability to completely dress self or choose clothing to wear; lack of personal hygiene; offensive body odors; disorganized surroundings; becomes disoriented in familiar surroundings; tendency to wander; inability to provide appropriate meals for self

RISK FACTORS
• Inappropriate decision-making
• Deteriorating cognitive functioning
• Decreased fine and/or gross motor skills
• Memory deficits

DESIRED OUTCOMES

The client will not experience impaired home maintenance as evidenced by:
   a. Maintains a clean and safe home
   b. Dresses with appropriate clothing
   c. Maintains adequate nutritional status

NOC OUTCOMES

Family functioning; safety behavior; home physical environment; self-care: instrumental activities of daily living

NIC INTERVENTIONS

Family support; self-care assistance; home maintenance assistance

---

NDx = NANDA-I Diagnosis   **D** = Delegatable Action   ● = UAP   ✦ = LVN/LPN   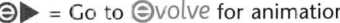 = Go to evolve for animation

Continued...

NURSING ASSESSMENT	RATIONALE
Assess client's sensory, motor, and cognitive functioning.	*Early recognition of signs and symptoms that client is not able to independently maintain his/her household without assistance allows for prompt intervention.*
Assess client's ability to maintain a safe household (e.g., ability to lock doors at night, smell smoke, recognize safety hazards).	
Assess frequency of client's wandering or becoming disoriented in home or familiar surroundings.	
Assess ability of family to support client in the home environment.	

THERAPEUTIC INTERVENTIONS	RATIONALE

Independent Actions

Develop a plan for home maintenance with family and client:

- Implement measures to maintain client safety in his/her home:
  - Encourage family to install smoke detectors, a security system, and easy-to-use door locks.
- Encourage client to wear a medic alert bracelet.
- Assist client and family to develop an exercise schedule.

- Assist client and family to develop a sleep/rest schedule.

- Encourage client and family members to identify safety concerns in the home (e.g., lots of throw rugs, poor lighting).
- Install child safety devices to prevent client from wandering into areas where injury might occur (e.g., decks, swimming pools, stairs).
- Assist family and client to develop a plan to obtain assistance in case the client becomes lost.
- Assist family in identifying community support services (e.g., Meals on Wheels, adult day care, support groups, respite services).

RATIONALE (right column):

This equipment provides security and may decrease wandering activities.

Helps client be quickly identified if client becomes lost

Exercise may decrease wandering activities and increase ability to sleep.

Schedules help decrease client's fatigue, which may increase client's coping abilities.

These actions help protect the client from injury.

Developing a plan form when a client becomes lost allows family to quickly obtain assistance in locating the client.

Community support assists caregivers in caring for the client and promotes client independence.

Nursing Diagnosis | RISK FOR CAREGIVER ROLE STRAIN NDx

Definition: Difficulty in performing family caregiver role

Related to:

- Duration of care
- Complexity of care
- Level of illness experienced by the client

CLINICAL MANIFESTATIONS

Subjective	Objective
Care giving: Verbalized apprehension about care of client if caregiver is unable to provide care; verbalized apprehension about the future regarding care receiver's health; verbalization about the future regarding caregiver's ability to provide care	**Caregiving:** Difficulty providing care; preoccupation with care routine
Emotional: Verbalization of feeling depressed; verbalization of feelings of anger	**Emotional:** Disturbed sleep; frustration; impatience; increased nervousness; increased emotional lability; lack of time to meet personal needs
	Socioeconomic: Changes in leisure activities; low work productivity; refuses career advancement; withdraws from social life
	Caregiver Health Status: Cardiovascular disease; diabetes; fatigue; gastrointestinal upset; headache; hypertension; rash; weight change

RISK FACTORS

- Financial status
- Support for the caregiver
- Caregiver's age
- Caregiver's health

DESIRED OUTCOMES

The caregiver will not experience role strain as evidenced by:

a. Feelings of being supported in the care of the client
b. Maintenance of his/her own physical and mental health
c. Accessing community resources and respite care
d. Expresses self-confidence in dealing with the complexity of client care

NOC OUTCOMES

Caregiver well-being; caregiver-patient relationship; caregiver role endurance

NIC INTERVENTIONS

Caregiver support

NURSING ASSESSMENT

Assess caregiver's relationship with the client.

Assess caregiver's understanding of required client care.

Assess caregiver's emotional and physical health and how the caregiver deals with stress.

Assess caregiver's support resources (e.g., respite care, community services, family support)

RATIONALE

Early recognition of signs and symptoms of caregiver role strain allows for prompt intervention.

THERAPEUTIC INTERVENTIONS

Independent Actions

Implement measures to support individual in the caregiver role:

- Collaboratively identify community resources to support caregiver (e.g., respite care, social services, community resources, support groups, adult day care, home health services).
- Assist caregiver in identifying ways to maintain his/her own mental and physical well-being.
- Educate caregiver on disease progression and management of care.
- Collaborate with caregiver to determine family members and friends who may support caregiver and/or assist with client care.
- Encourage caregiver to discuss issues and concerns in caring for client.

RATIONALE

Community resources provide continuum of care once discharged from the hospital. Respite care can give caregiver time away from client while knowing client is taken care of.

Self-care is important for caregiver to maintain ability to care for client.

Provides knowledge of the disease process and what is required to appropriately care for the client

These actions provide mental and physical support for the caregiver.

Provides caregiver an informed and safe resource in which to express feelings and receive information regarding client care.

ADDITIONAL NURSING DIAGNOSES

IMPAIRED SOCIAL INTERACTIONS NDx

Related to:

- Alterations in cognition
- Memory deficits
- Impaired judgment
- Inappropriate, hostile, and bizarre behaviors

DISTURBED SENSORY PERCEPTION NDx

Related to:

- Altered sensory integration
- Altered sensory reception
- Excessive environmental stimuli

GRIEVING NDx

Related to awareness of disease and disease progression

CEREBROVASCULAR ACCIDENT

A cerebrovascular accident (CVA, stroke, brain attack) is the result of an interruption in the blood flow in areas of the brain and is characterized by the sudden development of neurological deficits that last for at least 24 hours. These deficits range from mild symptoms such as tingling, weakness, and slight speech impairment to more severe symptoms such as hemi-

NDx = NANDA-I Diagnosis   **D** = Delegatable Action   ● = UAP   ✦ = LVN/LPN   ⊖▶ = Go to ⊖volve for animation

Continued...

plegia, aphasia, dysphagia, loss of portions of the visual field, spatial-perceptual changes, altered cognitive function, and loss of consciousness. Clinical manifestations depend on factors such as the area(s) of the brain affected, the adequacy of collateral cerebral circulation, and the extensiveness of subsequent cerebral edema.

CVAs are classified according to etiology. The major classifications are ischemic and hemorrhagic. Ischemic CVAs are most frequently the result of a thrombosis (which is usually associated with atherosclerosis) or an embolus. Conditions most often associated with a hemorrhagic CVA are extreme hypertension, cerebral aneurysm, or arteriovenous malformation. Treatment after a CVA is determined by the etiology and the neurological deficits that are present.

This care plan focuses on the adult client hospitalized with signs and symptoms of a CVA. Much of the information is also applicable to clients receiving follow-up care in an extended care or rehabilitation facility or home setting. This care plan focuses on the more common problems that occur as a result of a CVA. The reader should refer to neurological texts for additional information about specific speech, motor, and sensory deficits that can occur.

OUTCOME/DISCHARGE CRITERIA

The client will:

1. Have improved cerebral tissue perfusion
2. Have improved or stable neurological function
3. Experience optimal control of urinary elimination
4. Have no signs or symptoms of complications
5. Communicate an awareness of ways to decrease the risk of a recurrent CVA
6. Identify ways to manage sensory and speech impairments and disturbed thought processes
7. Identify ways to improve ability to swallow
8. Identify ways to manage urinary incontinence
9. Demonstrate measures to facilitate the performance of activities of daily living and increase physical mobility
10. Communicate an awareness of signs and symptoms to report to the health care provider and share thoughts and feelings about the effects of the CVA on lifestyle, roles, and self-concept
11. Communicate knowledge of community resources that can assist with home management and adjustment to changes resulting from the CVA
12. Communicate an understanding of and a plan for adhering to recommended follow-up care including future appointments with health care provider and therapists and medications prescribed.

Collaborative Diagnosis

DECREASED INTRACRANIAL ADAPTIVE CAPACITY RELATED TO TRAUMA/NEUROLOGICAL ILLNESS

Definition: Intracranial fluid dynamic mechanisms that normally compensate for increases in intracranial volumes are compromised, resulting in repeated disproportionate increases in intracranial pressure (ICP) in response to a variety of noxious and non-noxious stimuli

Related to: Changes in the CNS blood flow associated with thrombus, bleeding, decreased blood pressure, and hypoxia

CLINICAL MANIFESTATIONS

Subjective	Objective
Report of headache	Increases in ICP for greater than 5 minutes after stimuli; baseline ICP greater than 10 mm Hg; altered level of consciousness (early); changes in vital signs/cardiac rhythm (late), changes in papillary response, generalized weakness; Positive Babinski sign, seizures

RISK FACTORS

- Intracranial bleeding
- Cerebral ischemia or infarction
- Brain injury

DESIRED OUTCOMES

Stable ICP as evidenced by improved neurological status

NOC OUTCOMES

Neurological status

NIC INTERVENTIONS

ICP monitoring; neurological monitoring; cerebral edema management

NURSING ASSESSMENT	RATIONALE
Assess client for changes in intracranial pressure:	As ICP increases, neurological assessment will change.
• Reports of headache	Most sensitive indicator of increased ICP is level of consciousness.
• Increased ICP following stimuli	
• Cushing's triad	Changes in respiratory patterns, widening pulse pressure, and decreased heart rate are late signs of increased ICP.
• Changes in level of consciousness	
• Changes in pupillary response	Elevations of ICP can indicate deterioration in neurological status.
• Positive babinski	
• Generalized weakness	

THERAPEUTIC INTERVENTIONS	RATIONALE
Independent Actions	
Implement measures to maintain or decrease increased intra-cranial pressure.	Elevations in $Paco_2$ can lead to cerebral vasodilation, which further increases ICP.
• Maintain patent airway.	
• Maintain neutral neck position. Elevate head of bed 30 degrees. **D** ✦	Neutral head position and head elevation both facilitate venous drainage of head and aid in lowering ICP.
• Do not group caregiving activities such as bathing, suctioning, and dressing changes. **D** ● ✦	Spacing activities minimizes sustained elevations in ICP.
• Institute seizure precautions.	Seizures are possible with elevated ICP, and client safety must be considered.
Dependent/Collaborative Actions	
Administer medications such as osmotic diuretics, loop diuretics, and corticosteroids.	Medications act to reduce swelling of cerebral tissues or volume of cerebrospinal fluid (CSF), thereby decreasing ICP.
Drain CSF fluid via ventriculostomy as ordered.	Draining CSF fluid via ventriculostomy reduces the volume of CSF fluid in the head, lowering ICP.
Consult physician if signs and symptoms of increased intra-cranial pressure persist.	Notifying the physician allows for modification of the treatment plan

Nursing Diagnosis RISK FOR INEFFECTIVE AIRWAY CLEARANCE NDx

Definition: Inability to clear secretions from the respiratory tract to maintain patent airway

Related to:
• Stasis of secretions associated with decreased activity
• Poor cough effort due to fatigue, changes in neuromuscular functioning

CLINICAL MANIFESTATIONS

Subjective	Objective
Reports of shortness of breath (dyspnea)	Dyspnea; orthopnea; diminished breath sounds; adventitious breath sounds (crackles, rhonchi, wheezes); ineffective cough; difficulty vocalizing; restlessness; changes in respiratory rate, rhythm; late sign: cyanosis; decreasing pulse oximetry readings

RISK FACTORS

Excessive mucus production
Presence of artificial airway
Neuromuscular dysfunction
Infection
Smoking

DESIRED OUTCOMES

The client will maintain a clear, open airway as evidence by:
  a. Normal breath sounds
  b. Normal rate and depth of respirations
  c. Absence of dyspnea

NDx = NANDA-I Diagnosis   **D** = Delegatable Action   ● = UAP   ✦ = LVN/LPN   ⊖▶ = Go to ⊖volve for animation

Continued...

NOC OUTCOMES	NIC INTERVENTIONS
Respiratory status: airway patency	Monitor respirator function; artificial airway management; airway suctioning; chest physiotherapy; cough enhancement

NURSING ASSESSMENT	RATIONALE
Assess airway patency.	*Airway patency is priority especially with acute neurological dysfunction. Tongue obstruction may occur with altered levels of consciousness.*
Auscultate breath sounds: • Wheezes, crackles, rhonchi • Diminished breath sounds Assess respiratory rate, depth, and quality. Assess for cough effectiveness.	*Changes in the characteristics of breath sounds may be due to airway obstruction, mucous plugs, or retained secretions in larger airways.* *Altered neurological status may impact effective respiratory effort.* *Muscle fatigue/weakness may impair effective clearance of secretions.*
Assess for changes in vital signs and/or mental status.	*Increased work of breathing or hypoxia may cause tachycardia and/or hypertension along with restlessness, confusion, or irritability.*
Assess pulse oximetry and/or arterial blood gas values.	*Decreasing oxygen saturation, elevated partial pressure of carbon dioxide in arterial blood ($PaCO_2$), and/or decreased partial pressure of oxygen in arterial blood (PaO_2) indicate possible respiratory failure.*

THERAPEUTIC INTERVENTIONS	RATIONALE
Independent Actions Assist the patient to perform deep breathing, coughing, or "huffing" exercises and use of incentive spirometry. • Incentive spirometry **D** ● ✦	*Deep breathing helps clear the airways by loosening secretions and promoting more effective coughing. Coughing or "huffing" accelerates airflow through the airways, which helps mobilize and clear mucus and foreign matter from the respiratory tract. Use of incentive spirometry helps expand lung tissue and aids in the prevention of atelectasis.*
Instruct or assist client to change position frequently. **D** ● ✦	*Frequent position changes help in mobilization of secretions and promotes lung expansion.*
Implement measures to thin secretions: • Humidify inspired air. • Encourage adequate oral intake. **D** ✦	*Adequate hydration and humidification of inspired air help thin secretions, which facilitates mobilization and expectoration of secretions. These actions also help reduce dryness of the respiratory mucous membrane, which helps enhance mucociliary clearance.*
Dependent/Collaborative Actions Perform nasotracheal suctioning for ineffective cough. **D** ✦	*Suctioning removes secretions from airways while also promoting active cough effort.*
Administer medications (e.g., expectorants bronchodilators, expectorants). **D** ✦	*Bronchodilators increase the patency of the airways and enhance bronchial airflow.* *Expectorants reduce the viscosity of sputum, making it easier to remove it by coughing or suctioning.*
Consult respiratory therapy for chest physiotherapy and nebulizer treatments.	*Notification of the appropriate healthcare provider allows for modification of the treatment plan*

Nursing Diagnosis **RISK FOR ASPIRATION** NDx

Definition: At risk for entry of gastrointestinal secretions, oropharyngeal secretions, solids, or fluids into tracheobronchial passages

Related to: Changes in neuromuscular functioning

CLINICAL MANIFESTATIONS

Subjective	Objective
N/A	Cough; tachypnea; dyspnea; tachycardia; dull percussion noted over affected lung area; presence of food in aspirate

RISK FACTORS

- Reduced level of consciousness
- Depressed cough and gag reflexes
- Impaired swallowing in an acute neurological insult

DESIRED OUTCOMES

The client will not aspirate secretions or foods/fluids as evidenced by:
- a. Clear breath sounds
- b. Resonant percussion over lungs
- c. Absence of cough, tachypnea, and dyspnea

NOC OUTCOMES

Aspiration control; respiratory status: ventilation

NIC INTERVENTIONS

Aspiration precautions; respiratory monitoring; swallowing therapy; airway suctioning

NURSING ASSESSMENT

Assess level of consciousness.

Assess for the presence of a cough or gag reflex.
Assess for the presence of nausea or vomiting.

Assess respiratory system for signs and symptoms of aspiration of secretions or foods/fluids:
- Auscultate breath sounds for wheezes or crackles.
- Monitor chest radiograph results.

RATIONALE

Alterations in level of consciousness place a patient at risk for aspiration.
Lack of protective reflexes places patient at risk for aspiration.
Increases the risk of aspiration of gastric contents in the setting of an acute neurological even
Early recognition of objective assessment findings allows for prompt treatment and recognition.

Evidence of pulmonary infiltrates on chest radiograph results can indicate that aspiration has occurred.

THERAPEUTIC INTERVENTIONS

Independent Actions
Implement measures to reduce the risk for aspiration
- Keep suction equipment readily available at bedside.
- Place conscious, impaired patient in a side-lying position unless contraindicated. **D** ● ✦
- Position patient in high-Fowler's position before initiating feeding. Maintain patient in an upright position 30 to 45 minutes after eating. **D** ● ✦
- Supervise administration of oral intake. **D** ✦

- Offer foods with a thicker consistency, which facilitates swallowing. **D** ✦
- Place foods/medications on unaffected side of the mouth. **D** ● ✦
- Encourage eat slowly and to client to thoroughly chew food. **D** ✦
  - Provide oral care after feedings.
  - Inspect for "pocketing" of food. **D** ● ✦

Dependent/Collaborative Actions
Administer antiemetics as ordered. **D** ✦
Consult appropriate health care provider for swallowing difficulties.

RATIONALE

Necessary to maintain patency of airway
Oral secretions accumulate in the mouth, allowing for easier expectoration or removal by suctioning.
This position uses gravity to facilitate movement of food/fluids through the pharynx into the esophagus.

Supervision allows for observation of potential swallowing difficulty and implementation of actions to improve swallowing.
Semisolid foods are more readily swallowed. Thin fluids are difficult for patients with dysphagia to manage.
Chewing on the unaffected side of the mouth facilitates effective swallowing of food.
Taking adequate time to eat, thoroughly chewing food, makes food easier to swallow and decreases incidence of aspiration.
Good oral hygiene and inspection of the oral cavity after meals results in removal of any remaining food that could enter the pharynx and be aspirated into the lungs.

Antiemetics reduce the risk of nausea and vomiting.
Dysphagia assessment can establish techniques to prevent aspiration in patients with impaired swallowing.

INEFFECTIVE TISSUE PERFUSION: CEREBRAL NDx

Definition: Decrease in oxygen resulting in the failure to nourish cerebral tissues at the capillary level

Related to:
- Decreased cerebral blood flow associated with thrombus
- Embolus cerebral hemorrhage
- Hypotension and/or subsequent spasm
- Compression of cerebral vessels

CLINICAL MANIFESTATIONS

Subjective	**Objective**
May not be able to self-report symptoms; only presenting symptoms may be objective.	Altered mental status; changes in motor response; behavioral changes; changes in pupillary reactions; difficulty swallowing

RISK FACTORS
- Trauma
- Change in circulatory status

DESIRED OUTCOMES

The client will improve cerebral tissue perfusion as evidenced by:
  a. Absence of or reduction in dizziness, visual disturbances, and speech impairments
  b. Improved mental status
  c. Improved sensory and motor function

NOC OUTCOMES

Neurological status; tissue perfusion: cerebral.

NIC INTERVENTIONS

Cerebral edema management; cerebral perfusion pressure promotion; intracranial pressure monitoring

NURSING ASSESSMENT	**RATIONALE**
Assess neurological status hourly during acute phase (e.g., dizziness, visual disturbances, aphasia, irritability, restlessness, decreased level of consciousness, paresthesias, weakness, and paralysis).	*Provides baseline assessment data and determines signs of decreased tissue perfusions. Changes may be reflective of increased intracranial pressure.*
Assess vital signs hourly during the acute phase.	*Vitals signs must be maintained at a level that supports adequate oxygenation and perfusion of cerebral tissues.*

THERAPEUTIC INTERVENTIONS	**RATIONALE**

Independent Actions
Perform actions to prevent increased intracranial pressure (e.g., encourage client to not cough, elevate head of bed 30 degrees unless contraindicated to improve cerebral venous drainage).

Increased intracranial pressure reduces blood flow to the brain because of the closed nature of the skull. Coughing causes an increase in intracranial pressure, while elevation of the HOB improves venous drainage and reduces intracranial pressure.

Dependent/Collaborative Actions
Implement measures to improve cerebral tissue perfusion:
- Maintain blood pressure (B/P) within optimum range using antihypertensive, sympathomimetics, and/or fluid therapy.
- Administer calcium channel blockers.

- Administer thrombolytic therapy.

- Prepare client for emergency surgery.

B/P must be maintained within optimum range to keep cerebral perfusion pressure at a level that promotes oxygenation of cerebral tissues. Exact values may vary.
Calcium channel blockers reduce cerebral vasospasm, which improves perfusion to the cerebral tissues.
Thrombolytic therapy reduces or prevents clot formation, which restores blood flow to the brain.
Accumulation of blood or bleeding into the brain requires prompt surgical intervention.

Nursing Diagnosis DISTURBED SENSORY PERCEPTION NDx (AUDITORY, KINESTHETIC, VISUAL, TACTILE)

Definition: Change in the amount or patterning of incoming stimuli accompanied by a diminished, exaggerated, distorted, or impaired response to such stimuli

Related to: Ischemia within the sensory transmission pathways of the brain

CLINICAL MANIFESTATIONS

Subjective	Objective
Reported change in sensory acuity: photosensitive, hyperesthesia, altered sense of taste, inability to sense position of body parts (proprioception)	Measured change in sensory acuity (visual, auditory, tactile); mood swings; exaggerated emotional responses; disorientation to person, place, time; change in behavioral patterns; restlessness; irritability; hallucinations

RISK FACTORS

- Compression of the nerves
- Edema

DESIRED OUTCOMES

The client will experience a reduction in and/or demonstrate beginning adaptation to disturbed sensory perception as evidenced by:
  a. Communication of same
  b. Increased participation in activities

NOC OUTCOMES

Sensory function: proprioception; sensory function: vision

NIC INTERVENTIONS

Environmental/sensation management

NURSING ASSESSMENT	RATIONALE
Assess for visual impairments: • Homonymous hemianopsia • Diplopia Assess for kinesthetic impairments: • Ability to maintain balance • Ability to determine position of body parts Assess tactile sensation: • Ability to sense light touch • Ability to sense temperature Assess for auditory impairments: • Ability to hear	*Determines visual field deficits that can interfere with ability to perform activities of daily living and increases client's risk for injury.* *Spatial-perceptual deficits increase the patient's risk for injury.* *Tactile deficits increase the risk of injury in affected patients because they have a decreased ability to sense pain or temperature.*

THERAPEUTIC INTERVENTIONS	RATIONALE
Independent Actions Implement measures to assist client to adapt to changes in sensory functioning. Reorient client to person, place, and time as necessary. **D** ● ✦ • Speak clearly and distinctly • Face client when speaking Implement measures that address visual field deficits: • Provide eye patch for diplopia. • Approach client from unaffected side. • Verbally acknowledge client prior to touching him/her or if approaching on the affected side.	*Maximizes the current level of function* *Frequent orientation helps client's awareness of surroundings.* *Use of an eye patch aids client in adapting to visual field deficits, enhancing independence and safety.* *These actions decrease risk of startling client.*

Continued...

THERAPEUTIC INTERVENTIONS	RATIONALE
Implement measures to assist client to adapt to changes in kinesthetic functioning:	
• Perform regular skin inspections.	
• Reposition patient frequently, padding bony prominences. **D** ✦	*Inability to sense pressure increases the risk of skin breakdown. Changes in position and padding bony prominences help improve circulation to the skin.*
• Provide tactile stimulation to affected limbs.	*Tactile stimulation to affected limbs aids patient in recognizing different sensations.*
• Provide active/passive range of motion. **D** ● ✦	*Range-of-motion exercises aid in circulatory enhancement.*
• If client is experiencing kinesthetic impairments, place him/her in front of a full-length mirror during activities when possible after condition has stabilized.	*Viewing his/her reflection may help the client identify body position and vertical and horizontal planes.*
• Arrange client's environment to optimize functional abilities and prevent injury (physical obstacles, thermal injury prevention). **D** ● ✦	*Modification of the physical environment optimizes client safety.*
• After condition has stabilized, place items on affected side to promote environmental scanning. **D** ● ✦	*Encourages client to adapt to visual field deficits; helps compensate for visual field loss*
Dependent/Collaborative Actions	
Consult physical therapist/occupational therapist to facilitate adaptation to altered sensory perceptions.	*Aids client in learning adaptive skills and facilitates performance of self-care activities*

Nursing Diagnosis UNILATERAL NEGLECT NDx

Definition: Impairment in sensory and motor response, mental representation, and spatial attention of the body, and the corresponding environment characterized by inattention to one side and overattention to the opposite side; left side neglect is more severe and persistent than right side neglect

Related to: Ischemia primarily of the parietal lobe of the nondominant cerebral hemisphere

CLINICAL MANIFESTATIONS

Subjective	Objective
Reports feeling as though one part of the body does not belong to own self	Inattention to stimuli applied to affected side; lack of awareness of affected side/inattention to safety; failure to use the affected side after being reminded to do so; failure to notice people approaching from the neglected side; marked deviation of the eyes to the non-neglected side to stimuli and activities on that side

RISK FACTORS	DESIRED OUTCOMES
• Stroke	The client will experience a reduction in and/ or demonstrate beginning adaptation to unilateral neglect as evidenced by:
• Smoking	a. Awareness of stimuli on affected side
• Hypertension	b. Awareness of the affected side of the body

NOC OUTCOMES	NIC INTERVENTIONS
Self-care activities of daily living; self-initiated body positioning	Unilateral neglect management; sensory function: vision; vision compensation behavior

NURSING ASSESSMENT	RATIONALE
Assess for presence of unilateral neglect:	*Determines extent of impairment and how the patient acknowledges senses on the affected side*
• Client responses to sensory stimuli bilaterally (visual, tactile)	

NURSING ASSESSMENT	RATIONALE
• Distorted spatial-perceptual relationships • Denial of body parts Have patient point to body parts.	*Determines the lack of recognition of body parts or distorted awareness of body parts; important to identify to plan safe care of the patient*

THERAPEUTIC INTERVENTIONS	RATIONALE

Independent Actions

If unilateral neglect is present:

• Ensure affected extremities are positioned properly at all times. **D** ● ✦	*Protects extremities from development of contractures*
• Protect affected extremities from pressure/injury/burns. **D** ● ✦	*Lack of extremity recognition increases risk of injury.*
• Provide active/passive range of motion.	*Range-of-motion activities promote circulation in affected extremities.*
• Touch and move affected extremities. **D** ● ✦	*Provision of sensory stimulation can help client experience normal movement patterns.*
• Approach patient from unaffected side during acute phase. **D** ● ✦	*Diminishes fear and anxiety in a client with difficulty in interpreting the environment in its entirety*
• Place familiar items on affected side/affected extremities. **D** ● ✦	*Placing items on the affected side assists the client to recognize that the extremities are part of his/her body.*
• Provide mirror for client during self-care activities. **D** ◑ ✦	*Use of a mirror helps to improves recognition of affected side.*

Dependent/Collaborative Actions

Consult physical therapy/occupational therapy as appropriate.	*PT/OT can prescribe exercises that aid the client in client development of adaptive skills.*

Nursing Diagnosis IMPAIRED VERBAL COMMUNICATION NDx

Definition: Decreased, delayed, or absent ability to receive, process, transmit, and use a system of symbols

Related to: Damage to Broca's motor (expressive) or Wernicke's (receptive) speech centers in the brain

CLINICAL MANIFESTATIONS

Subjective	Objective
Reports difficulty expressing self	Unable to speak dominant language; speaks or verbalizes with difficulty; cannot speak; slurring/stuttering; difficulty forming words and sentences; difficulty in comprehending statements

RISK FACTOR	DESIRED OUTCOME
• Injury	The client will communicate needs and desires effectively.

NOC OUTCOMES	NIC INTERVENTIONS
Communication: receptive; communication: expressive	Communication enhancement: speech deficit; active listening

NURSING ASSESSMENT	RATIONALE
Assess for motor speech impairment or difficulty forming words (expressive).	*Provides a baseline assessment of client's impairment*
Assess for inability to understand words (receptive). Assess for total loss of ability to comprehend and speak (global aphasia).	*Type of impairment will depend on area of the brain involved.*

NDx = NANDA-I Diagnosis   **D** = Delegatable Action   ● = UAP   ✦ = LVN/LPN   ⊖▶ = Go to ⊖volve for animation

Continued...

THERAPEUTIC INTERVENTIONS	RATIONALE

Independent Actions
Implement measures to facilitate communication:

- Approach communication with client as an adult. **D ● ✦**

  Approaching the client in this manner prevents startling the client.

- Ask questions that require short answers and allow time for the patient to respond. **D ● ✦**

  The client will need more time to process information. Short, simple answers will reduce client's frustration, allowing for easier communication.

- Face client when speaking, using short statements, speaking slowly, and presenting one thought at a time. **D ● ✦**

  Facing the client when speaking enhances understanding and allows client to concentrate on one thing at a time.

- Create a calm, quiet environment. **D ＊ ●**

  In a quiet environment, the client can concentrate on communication efforts, does not have to speak loudly, and is able to hear others more clearly.

  Rest periods help conserve client's energy to maximize communication ability during therapy.

- Provide rest periods before speech therapy.
- Provide assistive communication aids such as pad/pencil, computer, word cards, or picture boards. **D ● ✦**

  Communication aids help facilitate communication.

- Encourage family to communicate with patient. **D ✦**

  Family involvement will reinforce consistency of communication measures.

Dependent/Collaborative Actions
Consult speech pathologist.

Multidisciplinary plan of care can be developed.

Nursing Diagnosis ### SELF-CARE DEFICIT NDx (BATHING, FEEDING, DRESSING, TOILETING)

Definition: Inability to perform or complete feeding, bathing/hygiene, dressing and grooming, or toileting activities for oneself

Related to:
- Impaired physical mobility
- Visual and spatial-perceptual impairments
- Apraxia
- Unilateral neglect
- Disturbed thought processes

CLINICAL MANIFESTATIONS

Subjective	Objective
N/A	Inability to prepare food, handle or use containers and/or utensils; inability to handle a glass or cup; inability to bathe or access the bathtub or shower; inability to dress self, use button closures; inability to get to the toilet or manipulate clothing; inability to provide appropriate personal hygiene

RISK FACTORS
- Weakness
- Loss of neuromuscular activity
- Bed rest

DESIRED OUTCOME
The client will perform self-care activities within cognitive and physical limitations.

NOC OUTCOMES
Self-care: activities of daily living

NIC INTERVENTIONS
Self-care assistance: activities of daily living; exercise therapy; muscle control

NURSING ASSESSMENT	RATIONALE
Assess the client's ability to perform activities of daily living: • Dressing • Toileting • Preparing food • Eating • Providing hair and/or nail care.	*Identification of client's self-care deficits will guide the nurse in the development of the plan of care.*

THERAPEUTIC INTERVENTIONS	RATIONALE

Independent Interventions

Implement additional measures to facilitate client's ability to perform self-care activities:

- If apraxia is present, explain and demonstrate use of items such as toothbrush, comb, and washcloth as often as necessary.

  Demonstrating the skill while explaining it will help the client in relearning skills for activities of daily living.

- Encourage client to wear eyepatch or opaque lens if diplopia is present.

  Without an eyepatch client will be unable to correctly focus on and/or have difficulty in using objects necessary for activities of daily living.

- Perform actions to enable client to feed self:
  - Place foods/fluids within client's visual field until client learns to effectively use scanning techniques. **D** ● ✦

    Food should be placed where client can easily see it.

  - Place only a few items on the tray at one time if spatial-perceptual deficits are present. **D** ● ✦

    When there are too many items on the tray, the client is unable to focus on a specific item.

  - Identify where items are placed on the plate and tray and open containers, cut meat, and butter bread as indicated. **D** ● ✦

    The client should know where each item is placed. Cutting food into small sizes helps prevent overfilling of the mouth, thus reducing the risk for choking.

- Perform actions to enable client to dress self:

    These actions help the client maintain a degree of independence.

  - Encourage use of assistive devices such as button hooks, long-handled shoehorns, and pull loops for pants.
  - Encourage client to select clothing that is easy to put on and remove (e.g., shirts with zippers or Velcro closures rather than buttons, loose-fitting clothing, pants with an elastic waistband or Velcro closures, shoes with Velcro fasteners or elastic laces).
  - If client has difficulty distinguishing right from left, mark outer aspect of shoes with tape.
- Perform actions to increase mobility (e.g., turn every 2 hours, perform active and passive range of motion, ambulate client as able). **D** ● ✦

  Increasing mobility and exercise further facilitates the client's ability to perform self-care activities.

- Reinforce exercises and activities recommended by the occupational therapist to improve fine motor skills.

Assist the client with activities he/she is unable to perform independently. **D** ● ✦

Inform significant others of client's abilities to perform own care. Explain importance of encouraging and allowing client to maintain an optimal level of independence.

Encouraging client's family to allow the client to care for his or her self, helps the client maintain some degree of independence.

Dependent/Collaborative Interventions

Implement additional measures to facilitate client's ability to perform self-care activities:

- Consult with occupational therapist about assistive devices available (e.g., broad-handled utensils, rocker knife, nonslip tray mat, plate guard); reinforce use of these devices.

  Provides multidisciplinary approach to care

NDx = NANDA-I Diagnosis   **D** = Delegatable Action   ● = UAP   ✦ = LVN/LPN   ⊖▶ = Go to ⊖volve for animation

ACUTE AND CHRONIC CONFUSION NDx

Definition

Acute: Abrupt onset of reversible disturbances of consciousness, attention, cognition, and perception

Chronic: Irreversible, long-standing, and/or progressive deterioration of intellect and personality characterized by decreased ability to interpret environmental stimuli and decreased capacity for intellectual thought processes; manifested by disturbances of memory, orientation, or behavior

Related to: Damage to cerebral tissue

CLINICAL MANIFESTATIONS

Subjective	Objective
N/A	Inaccurate interpretation of environment and time; memory loss; altered mood states (e.g., lability, hostility, irritability, inappropriate affect); inability to make decisions or problem solve; changes in attention span; disorientation; inappropriate social behavior

RISK FACTOR	DESIRED OUTCOMES
• Cerebral edema	The client will experience less confusion as evidence by: a. Improved attention span, memory, and problem-solving abilities b. Improved level of orientation c. Reduction in instances of inappropriate responses

NOC OUTCOMES	NIC INTERVENTIONS
Information processing; neurological status: consciousness; cognitive ability; disoriented thought self-control; memory; mood equilibrium	Reality orientation; cognitive stimulation; dementia management; presence; behavior management

NURSING ASSESSMENT	RATIONALE
Assess client for changes in level of confusion and orientation (e.g., shortened attention span, impaired memory, decreased ability to problem solve, confusion, inappropriate response, mood changes). Ascertain from significant others client's usual level of cognitive and emotional functioning.	*Early recognition of signs and symptoms of confusion allows for prompt intervention.*

THERAPEUTIC INTERVENTIONS	RATIONALE

Independent Actions
If client shows evidence of confusion and/or disorientation:

• Reorient to person, place, and time as necessary. **D ● ✦**	*These techniques help keep client oriented to environment, self, others, and current reality.*
• Address client by name. **D ● ✦**	*Helps client recognize self*
• Place familiar objects, clock, and calendar within client's view. **D ● ✦**	*Having familiar things surrounding the client increases his/her comfort level.*
• Face client when conversing with client. **D ● ✦**	*These techniques will help decrease client's frustration when communicating with others.*
• Approach client in a slow, calm manner; allow adequate time for communication. **D ● ✦**	
• Repeat instructions as necessary using clear, simple language and short sentences. **D ● ✦**	*Repetition of information helps client process information when thinking is impaired.*
• Keep environmental stimuli to a minimum but avoid sensory deprivation. **D ● ✦**	*Overstimulation may cause the client to become anxious or aggressive.*

THERAPEUTIC INTERVENTIONS	RATIONALE
• Maintain a consistent and fairly structured routine. **D** ● ✦	Maintenance of a structured routine helps the client maintain orientation and sense of reality.
• Provide written or taped information whenever possible for client to review as often as necessary.	Written or taped instructions provide a resource for the client concerning appropriate care.
• Have client perform only one activity at a time and allow adequate time for performance of activities. **D** ● ✦	Prevents client from being frustrated with many activities at one time
• Encourage client to make lists of planned activities, questions, and concerns.	Provides a mechanism for the client to organize thoughts
• Implement measures to stop emotional outbursts and inappropriate responses if they occur (e.g., provide distraction by clapping hands, handing client an object to look at or hold, or turning on the radio or television). **D** ● ✦	These techniques help the client refocus and decreases inappropriate responses.
• Maintain realistic expectations of client's ability to learn, comprehend, and remember information provided.	Don't ask clients to do things beyond their ability. Reinforce information as needed.
• Encourage significant others to be supportive of client; instruct them in methods of dealing with client's disturbed thought processes.	Significant others need to learn coping mechanisms and how to work with client.
• Discuss physiological basis for disturbed thought processes with client and significant others; inform them that cognitive and emotional functioning may improve gradually during the next 6 to 12 months.	Understanding what occurred helps the client and significant others work toward improving cognitive and emotional functioning.
Dependent/Collaborative Interventions	
Consult physician if disturbed thought processes worsen.	Notifying the physician allows for modification of the treatment plan.

DISCHARGE TEACHING/CONTINUED CARE

Nursing Diagnosis

DEFICIENT KNOWLEDGE NDx; INEFFECTIVE FAMILY THERAPEUTIC REGIMEN MANAGEMENT NDx; OR INEFFECTIVE HEALTH MAINTENANCE* NDx

Definition: Absence or deficiency of cognitive information related to specific topic (lack of specific information necessary for clients/significant others) to make informed choices regarding condition/treatment/lifestyle changes; pattern of regulating and integrating into family processes a program for treatment of illness and the sequelae of illness that is unsatisfactory for meeting specific health goals; inability to identify, manage, and/or seek out help to manage health

CLINICAL MANIFESTATION

Subjective	Objective
Requests information; client statements reflect misunderstanding	Inadequate follow through of instruction; inappropriate or exaggerated behaviors

RISK FACTOR

• Cognitive limitations or unfamiliarity of situation

---

*The nurse should select the diagnostic label that is most appropriate for the client's discharge teaching.

NDx = NANDA-I Diagnosis   **D** = Delegatable Action   ● = UAP   ✦ = LVN/LPN   ⊖▶ = Go to ⊖volve for animation

Continued...

NOC OUTCOMES	NIC INTERVENTIONS
Knowledge: disease process; knowledge: treatment regimen; knowledge: health resources	Teaching: individual; teaching: disease process; teaching: psychomotor skills; teaching: prescribed activity

NURSING ASSESSMENT	RATIONALE
Assess for stroke-related factors that may impede the learning process.	*Client may not be emotionally or physically able to learn.*
Assess client/family understanding of disease process.	*The nurse's understanding of the client's and significant other's knowledge based aids in formulating an educational plan.*

THERAPEUTIC INTERVENTIONS	RATIONALE

Desired Outcome: The client will communicate an awareness of ways to decrease the risk of a recurrent CVA.

Independent Actions	
Assist client in recognizing factors that contributed to the stroke (e.g., hypertension, elevated serum lipids, diabetes, atrial fibrillation, use of oral contraceptives).	*Knowledge of disease process and how to decrease the impact of risk factors helps the client and family understand what lifestyle changes decrease the incidence of a recurrent CVA.*
Identify appropriate actions that client can take to decrease risk of a recurrent CVA (e.g., take medications as prescribed, decrease stress, stop smoking, modify diet, adhere to medical treatment, plan to control hypertension and diabetes, use another form of birth control if taking oral contraceptives).	

THERAPEUTIC INTERVENTIONS	RATIONALE

Desired Outcome: The client will identify ways to manage sensory and speech impairments and disturbed thought processes.

Independent Actions

Instruct client regarding ways to adapt to visual impairments:
- Use scanning techniques if visual field cut is present.
- Arrange home setting so that when in favorite chair or bed, stimuli other than wall or furniture are within visual fields.
- Wear eye patch or opaque lens if double vision persists.

These interventions reduce the risk of injury from a visual deficit.

Reinforce use of established communication techniques and continuation with speech therapy if indicated.

Continued use of established communication techniques helps the client maintain current level of functioning.

If client is experiencing spatial perceptual deficits and/or unilateral neglect, stress need for assistance with usual daily activities and strict adherence to safety measures.

Decreases client frustration and risk for injury.

Reinforce methods of adapting to impaired memory and shortened attention span (e.g., make lists of planned activities, review taped or written instructions frequently).

This helps foster independence and decreases client's frustration with changes due to illness.

THERAPEUTIC INTERVENTIONS	RATIONALE

Desired Outcome: The client will identify ways to improve ability to swallow.

Independent Actions

Reinforce instructions regarding appropriate swallowing techniques:
- Sit upright for meals and snacks.
- Tilt head and neck forward slightly when eating.
- Place food on unaffected side of mouth.

These techniques promote effective swallowing and reduce the risk of aspiration.

THERAPEUTIC INTERVENTIONS	RATIONALE

- Do not put a lot of food in the mouth at one time.
- Thicken foods to promote ease of swallowing.

Reinforce food selection/preparation of foods and fluids (e.g., avoid sticky foods, use "Thick It," gelatin, or baby cereal to thicken liquids that are thin; moisten dry foods with gravy or sauces).

THERAPEUTIC INTERVENTIONS	RATIONALE

Desired Outcome: The client will identify ways to manage urinary incontinence.

Independent Actions

Reinforce instructions regarding client's bladder training program, stressing the importance of adhering to the program

Demonstrate procedures that are included in client's bladder training program (e.g., intermittent catheterization, application of an external catheter.

Continue implementation of the bladder training program reduces the risk of incontinence and allows client a sense of independence.

Improves self-care abilities of the patient

THERAPEUTIC INTERVENTIONS	RATIONALE

Desired Outcome: The client will demonstrate measures to facilitate the performance of activities of daily living and increase physical mobility.

Independent Actions

Instruct on measures to increase ability to perform activities of daily living:
- Use of assistive devices and mobility aids
- Continue concentration on body positioning, balance and movement
- Participation in an exercise program

Increases client muscle tone and ability to perform activities of daily living.

THERAPEUTIC INTERVENTIONS	RATIONALE

Desired Outcome: The client will communicate an awareness of signs and symptoms to report to the health care provider.

Independent Actions

- Instruct client to report the development of or increase in these signs and symptoms:
  - Weakness or loss of sensation in extremities
  - Visual disturbances such as tunnel vision, blurred vision, or transient blindness
  - Lethargy, irritability or confusion
  - Difficulty chewing or swallowing
  - Difficulty speaking or understanding verbal and nonverbal communication
  - Difficulty maintaining balance
  - Seizures

These clinical manifestations may indicate a subsequent stroke.

Seizures can begin to occur months after the CVA as scar tissue forms in the ischemic area.

THERAPEUTIC INTERVENTIONS	RATIONALE

Desired Outcome: The client will communicate knowledge of community resources that can assist with home management and adjustment to changes resulting from the CVA.

NDx = NANDA-I Diagnosis   **D** = Delegatable Action   ● = UAP   ✦ = LVN/LPN   ⊖▶ = Go to ⊖volve for animation

Continued...

THERAPEUTIC INTERVENTIONS	RATIONALE

Independent Actions

Provide information about community resources that can assist client and significant others with home management and adjustment to impairments in motor and sensory function and disturbed thought processes resulting from the CVA (e.g., home health agencies, stroke support groups, meals on wheels, social and financial services, local chapter of the American Heart Association, local service groups that can help obtain assistive devices, individual and family counselors).

Most stroke clients and significant others s have some degree of disability that requires additional support.

THERAPEUTIC INTERVENTIONS	RATIONALE

Desired Outcome: The client will communicate an understanding of and a plan for adhering to recommended follow-up care including future appointments with health care.

Independent action

Reinforce the importance of keeping follow-up appointments with health care provider and physical, occupational, and speech therapy.

Teach client the rationale for, side effects of, drug-to-drug interactions, food-drug interactions, and importance of taking prescribed medications (e.g., anticoagulants, platelet aggregation inhibitors, antihypertensives).

Recovery from a stroke requires long-term activities to restore and improve health status.

Client's and significant others' understanding of medication regimen helps improve regimen adherence and reduces the risk of a subsequent stroke.

ADDITIONAL NURSING DIAGNOSES

IMBALANCED NUTRITION: LESS THAN BODY REQUIREMENTS NDx

Related to decreased oral intake associated with difficulty chewing, swallowing, and feeding self

RISK FOR CONSTIPATION NDx
Related to:
* Decreased gastrointestinal motility associated with decreased activity
* Decreased intake of fluids and foods high in fiber associated with difficulty chewing, swallowing, and feeding self
* Failure to respond to the urge to defecate associated with decreased level of consciousness or inability to recognize sensation of rectal fullness

SEXUAL DYSFUNCTION NDx
Related to:
* Alteration in usual sexual activities associated with impaired motor function
* Decreased libido and/or impotence associated with impaired motor and sensory function, fear of urinary incontinence, depression, disturbed self-concept, and fear of rejection by partner

FEAR/ANXIETY NDx
Related to:
* Impaired verbal communication and/or motor and sensory function unfamiliar environment

* Lack of understanding of diagnosis, diagnostic tests, and treatments
* Uncertain prognosis
* Disturbed thought processes
* Financial concerns
* Anticipated effect of the CVA on future lifestyle and roles

POTENTIAL COMPLICATIONS OF CVA
Related to:
* Increased intracranial pressure (ICP)
  * Accumulation of blood in the cerebral tissue (can occur if CVA resulted from conditions such as ruptured cerebral aneurysm)
  * Cerebral edema associated with increased capillary permeability of cerebral vessels and disruption of the sodium pump within the cells (both occur as a result of cerebral hypoxia)
  * Increase in cerebral vascular volume associated with vasodilation of the cerebral vessels
* Corneal irritation and abrasion related to inability to close eye on affected side if facial nerve paresis or paralysis has occurred
* Subluxation of shoulder related to muscle weakness in affected upper arm and shoulder and gravity pull on affected arm

GRIEVING NDx
Related to changes in motor and sensory function and thought processes and the effect of these changes on future lifestyle and roles

IMPAIRED SWALLOWING NDx
Related to weakness or paralysis of the swallowing muscles on the affected side and diminished or absent swallowing reflex

IMPAIRED PHYSICAL MOBILITY NDx
Related to:
- Activity limitations associated with decreased motor function and spatial-perceptual impairments
- Loss of muscle tone during period of flaccidity of affected extremities (flaccid paralysis is usually present during the first few days after a CVA)
- Hypertonia of affected extremities (as muscle tone returns after period of flaccidity, it often progresses to spasticity within about 6-8 weeks)
- Reluctance to move associated with fear of injuring self (occurs mainly with ischemia of the dominant hemisphere)
- Loss of muscle mass, tone, and strength associated with prolonged disuse

IMPAIRED URINARY ELIMINATION: INCONTINENCE NDx
Related to:
- Increased reflex activity of the bladder and loss of voluntary control of urinary elimination associated with upper motor neuron involvement if it has occurred
- Decreased ability to control urination associated with decreased level of consciousness or inability to recognize sensation of bladder fullness
- Inability to get to bedside commode or bathroom in a timely manner associated with:
  - Delay in obtaining assistance resulting from inability to communicate the urge to urinate
  - Impaired physical mobility

DISTURBED SELF-CONCEPT NDx
Related to:
- Change in appearance (e.g., hemiplegia, facial droop, ptosis)
- Lifestyle and role changes associated with motor and spatial-perceptual impairments and disturbed thought processes
- Impaired verbal communication
- Loss of self-control (e.g., automatic speech, emotional lability, inappropriate behavior) or exaggerated emotional responses
- Urinary incontinence
- Dependence on others to meet basic needs

INEFFECTIVE COPING NDx
Related to:
- Fear
- Anxiety
- Depression
- Decreased ability to communicate verbally
- Changes in motor and sensory function, thought processes, and future lifestyle and roles
- Need for lengthy rehabilitation

INTERRUPTED FAMILY PROCESSES NDx
Related to:
- Change in family roles and structure associated with a family member's verbal, motor, and sensory impairments
- Disturbed thought processes
- Need for lengthy rehabilitation

CRANIOCEREBRAL TRAUMA/CRANIOTOMY

The leading causes of craniocerebral trauma (head injury, traumatic brain injury) are motor vehicle accidents, falls, sports/recreational injuries, and assaults. Examples of skull and brain injury that can occur include skull fracture; dural tear; cerebral contusion, concussion, and laceration; diffuse axonal injury (DAI); brainstem damage; and intracranial hemorrhage. Brain damage can occur during the initial injury and as a result of subsequent cerebral damage resulting from factors such as cerebral hematoma, infection, and edema; seizure activity; and/or obstruction of the flow of cerebrospinal fluid (CSF).

A craniotomy is a surgical opening into the skull to gain access to the brain. Reasons for the surgery include removing a tumor, abscess, hematoma, bone fragments, or foreign object (e.g., bullet); controlling cerebrovascular bleeding; repairing a vascular abnormality (e.g., aneurysm, arteriovenous malformation); and improving ventricular drainage. A craniectomy (excision of a portion of the skull) is the usual method of entering the brain. If this portion of the skull is replaced (using the preserved bone or a synthetic substance), it can be done on completion of the surgery or sometime in the future after there are no longer concerns about increased intracranial pressure (ICP) and/or cerebral infection.

After craniocerebral trauma, a person may have a disturbance in consciousness ranging from a brief loss of contact with the environment to persistent coma. As the level of consciousness improves, clients often experience headache, dizziness, and alterations in thought processes. These signs and symptoms tend to subside gradually but can persist for weeks to years. Additional signs and symptoms after craniocerebral trauma vary depending on the area of the brain that has been affected. For example, tissue damage in the frontal lobe could result in loss of voluntary motor control, personality changes, and/or expressive aphasia; damage to the occipital lobe could cause visual disturbances; and damage to the temporal lobe could result in receptive aphasia and/or hearing impairment. Many of the disturbances noted above may also occur after a craniotomy.

Craniocerebral trauma is classified according to location (e.g., skull, epidural area, brainstem), effect (e.g., concussion, DAI, depressed fracture of the skull, contusion, subdural hematoma), and/or severity. The severity of trauma ranges

---

NDx = NANDA-I Diagnosis   **D** = Delegatable Action   ● = UAP   ✦ = LVN/LPN   ⊖▶ = Go to ⊖volve for animation

Continued...

from minor (usually a concussion with no alteration in consciousness or a loss of consciousness lasting 5 minutes or less) to severe, in which extensive contusion and/or laceration of brain tissue and possible brainstem injury occurs. Severe craniocerebral trauma usually involves a period of prolonged unconsciousness and results in permanent neurological impairments that require extensive rehabilitation and long-term care.

A craniotomy is described in relation to the approach (i.e., supratentorial, infratentorial) and the location of the pathology (e.g., temporal, occipital, parietal). The neurological deficits that can occur after the surgical procedure depend primarily on the areas of the brain that are disrupted to gain access to the desired area (e.g., speech may be impaired after a temporal approach, ataxia is expected after a cerebellar approach) and the amount and location of the brain tissue that is excised or traumatized at the site of the pathology.

This care plan focuses on the adult client hospitalized after craniocerebral trauma and/or surgery. It deals mainly with nursing and collaborative diagnoses appropriate for a client who has regained consciousness after sustaining a moderate injury or undergoing an uncomplicated craniotomy. Much of the information is also applicable to clients receiving follow-up care in an extended care or rehabilitation facility or home setting. Nursing care and discharge teaching need to be individualized according to the areas of the brain affected and the extensiveness of the *tissue damage. If the client has sustained more severe craniocerebral trauma, refer also to the Care Plan on Cerebrovascular Accident.*

OUTCOME/DISCHARGE CRITERIA

The client will:

1. Have improved cerebral tissue perfusion
2. Have improved or stable neurological function
3. Have an adequate nutritional status
4. Have no signs or symptoms of complications
5. Identify ways to adapt to neurological deficits that may persist after craniocerebral trauma and/or surgery
6. Identify ways to reduce headache
7. State signs and symptoms to report to the health care provider
8. Share thoughts and feelings about residual neurological impairments
9. Identify community resources that can assist with home management and adjustment to changes resulting from craniocerebral trauma and/or craniotomy
10. Verbalize an understanding of and a plan for adhering to recommended follow-up care including future appointments with health care provider and therapists and medications prescribed
11. Use in conjunction with Preoperative and Postoperative Care Plan if the patient underwent surgery.

Nursing Diagnosis   **DECREASED INTRACRANIAL ADAPTIVE CAPACITY** NDx

Definition: Intracranial fluid dynamic mechanisms that normally compensate for increases in intracranial volume are compromised, resulting in repeated disproportionate increases in intracranial pressure (ICP) in response to a variety of noxious and nonnoxious stimuli

Related to:
- Cerebral hemorrhage resulting from laceration of blood vessels at the time of injury or loss of integrity of the ligated vessels
- Compression of cerebral vessels resulting in hematoma formation, cerebral edema, or accumulation of blood in cerebral hemispheres
- Spasm of the cerebral vessels resulting from trauma to and/or stretching of the vessels during surgery
- Hypotension resulting from hypovolemia and peripheral pooling of blood

CLINICAL MANIFESTATIONS

Subjective	Objective
Complaint of headache	Decreased level of consciousness; increased ICP greater than 10 mm Hg; changes in movement; vomiting; confusion; agitation; inappropriate affect; lethargy; speech impairment; pupil changes and asymmetry; cerebral perfusion pressure less than 70 mm Hg; PaO_2 less than 70 mmHg.

RISK FACTORS
- Mitral valve insufficiency
- Hypertension
- Smoking

DESIRED OUTCOME

The client will maintain adequate cerebral adaptation as evidenced by:
- a. Absence or reduction of neurological deficits
- b. Improved sensory and motor function
- c. Improved mental status

NOC OUTCOMES

Fluid balance; neurological status

NIC INTERVENTIONS

Cerebral edema management; neurological monitoring; ICP monitoring

NURSING ASSESSMENT	RATIONALE
Assess client for signs and symptoms of changes in cerebral perfusion:	*Early recognition of signs and symptoms of changes in cerebral perfusion allows for prompt intervention.*
• Level of consciousness	*Use a coma scale such as the Glasgow Coma Scale to assess eye opening, position and movement, pupil size and changes, and consciousness/mental status. Low scores in persons with severe head injury indicate impaired cerebral perfusion requiring prompt intervention.*
• Orientation to person, place, and time	
• Pupil size and reaction to light	
• Motor function	
• Paresthesias	*Abnormal movements, posturing, and abnormal flexion of extremities indicate diffuse cerebral damage.*
• Decreased motor movement	
• Altered reflexes	
• Posturing	
• Variability in B/P	*Changes in B/P impact cerebral perfusion pressure. Mean arterial pressure above 90 mm Hg is necessary to maintain adequate cerebral perfusion pressure.*
• ICP	*ICP greater than 15 mm Hg indicates compromise of cerebral perfusion.*
• Speech and thought processes	*Impaired thought process indicates damage to the cerebral cortex.*
• PaO$_2$ less than 70 mmHg	*Hypoxemia causes cerebrovascular dilation.*

THERAPEUTIC INTERVENTIONS	RATIONALE
Independent Actions	
Implement measures to improve cerebral tissue perfusion:	
• Elevate head of bed 30 degrees unless contraindicated.	*Elevating head of bed 30 degrees decreases ICP while maintaining adequate cerebral pressure.*
• If surgery was performed using the infratentorial approach, head of bed is usually kept flat postoperatively.	*Keeping the head of bed flat after surgery reduces the pressure on the brainstem.*
• Position client on side not operated on if bone flap and/or large mass was removed.	*This helps prevent an increase in ICP and venous congestion in the operative area.*
• Align head and neck in the midline position; avoid flexion, extension, and rotation of head and neck.	*Maintaining the head in midline position maximizes venous return.*
• Prevent hip flexion of 90 degrees or more.	*Hip flexion of 90 degrees or greater may maintain blood in the abdominal space, thus increasing abdominal and intrathoracic pressure, which reduces venous outflow from the head.*
Perform actions to prevent cerebral hypoxia and the subsequent vasodilation and cerebral edema:	
• Implement measures to maintain patent airway and suction if necessary.	*Decreases agitation, helping to stabilize ICP*
• Reorient to staff and environment. **D** ● ✦	*Relieves anxiety and helps maintain or lower ICP*
• Instruct client to avoid activities that result in isometric muscle contractions (e.g., pushing feet against footboard, tightly gripping side rails).	*Isometric exercises increase ICP.*

NDx = NANDA-I Diagnosis   **D** = Delegatable Action   ● = UAP   ✦ = LVN/LPN   ⊖▶ = Go to ⊖volve for animation

Continued...

THERAPEUTIC INTERVENTIONS	RATIONALE
Dependent/Collaborative Actions Implement measures to improve cerebral tissue perfusion: • Administer osmotic and/or loop diuretics.	*Osmotic diuretics lower ICP by creating an osmotic force in the cerebral vasculature that draws edematous fluid out of the brain. Loop diuretics decrease body fluid volume, which helps decrease cerebral edema. Corticosteroids decrease inflammation.*
• Administer a laxative, antitussive, and/or antiemetic if ordered.	*Prevents straining, coughing, or vomiting that can increase the intrathoracic pressure, which subsequently impedes venous return from the brain.*
• Administer central nervous system depressants judiciously; hold medication and consult physician if respiratory rate is less than 12 breaths/min.	*Hypoxemia increases cerebral vasodilation causing increased ICP.*
• Administer calcium channel blockers if ordered.	*Reduces cerebral vasospasm (the calcium that is released by the injured neural cells can cause vasospasm).*
• Administer oxygen as ordered and before and after tracheal suctioning.	*Administration of oxygen decreases cerebral hypoxia. It is not routine to hyperventilate the client before suctioning; however, hyperventilation that maintains $PaCO_2$ between 30 and 35 mm Hg may be used to prevent cerebral hypoxia.*
• If the client is hypotensive, administer sympathomimetic agents and maintain intravenous fluid therapy.	*Sympathomimetics and IV fluid therapy help maintain adequate blood pressure, which is required to maintain cerebral perfusion. Improves cerebral blood flow.*

If signs and symptoms of increased ICP are present:
 • Initiate seizure precautions.
 • Prepare client for:
   • Insertion of ICP monitoring device
   • Surgical intervention (i.e., ligation of bleeding vessels, repair of blocked shunt, removal of bone flap or hematoma)
	Protects client from injury
	
	 Provides direct measurement of ICP, which guides treatment plan
	 Decreases ICP and prevents further compromise of cerebral tissue

Nursing Diagnosis   ACUTE PAIN NDx (HEADACHE)

Definition: Unpleasant sensory and emotional experience arising from actual or potential tissue damage or described in terms of such damage (International Association for the Study of Pain); sudden or slow onset of head pain of any intensity from mild to severe with an anticipated or predictable end and a duration of less than 6 months

Related to:
• Trauma to the cerebral tissue associated with the surgical procedure
• Stretching or compression of cerebral vessels and tissue associated with increased ICP if it occurs
• Irritation of the meninges associated with bleeding from meningeal vessels into the cerebrospinal fluid (CSF) and/or inflammation of the meninges

CLINICAL MANIFESTATIONS

Subjective	**Objective**
Verbalization of a headache	Restlessness; irritability; grimacing; rubbing head; avoidance of bright lights and noises; reluctance to move

RISK FACTORS
• Edema
• Positioning
• Hypertension
• Trauma

DESIRED OUTCOMES

The client will obtain relief from headache as evidenced by:
   a. Verbalization of same
   b. Relaxed facial expression and body positioning

NOC OUTCOMES	NIC INTERVENTIONS
Comfort level; pain control	Pain management; analgesic administration

NURSING ASSESSMENT	**RATIONALE**
Assess for signs and symptoms of headache: • Statements of same • Restlessness • Irritability • Grimacing • Rubbing head • Avoidance of bright lights and noises • Reluctance to move	*Early recognition of signs and symptoms of a headache allows for prompt interventions.*
Assess client's perception of the severity of the headache using a pain intensity rating scale.	*An awareness of the severity of pain being experienced helps determine the most appropriate interventions for pain management. Use of a pain intensity rating scale gives the nurse a clearer understanding of the pain being experienced and promotes consistency when communicating with others about the client's pain experience.*
Assess the client's pain pattern (e.g., location, quality, onset, duration, precipitating factors, aggravating factors, alleviating factors).	*Knowledge of the client's pain pattern assists in the identification of effective pain management interventions.*

THERAPEUTIC INTERVENTIONS	**RATIONALE**

Independent Actions

Implement measures to relieve headache: • Perform actions to reduce fear and anxiety about the pain experience (e.g., assure client that the need for headache relief is understood, plan methods for relieving pain with client). • Assure client that staff members are nearby; respond to call signal as soon as possible.	*Fear and anxiety decrease a clients threshold for pain.*
• Perform actions to minimize environmental stimuli (e.g., provide a quiet environment, limit number of visitors and their length of stay, dim lights).	*Decreased environmental stimuli promotes relaxation and subsequently increases the client's threshold and tolerance for pain*
• Avoid jarring bed or startling client.	*Minimizes risk of sudden movements*
• Perform actions to prevent and treat increased ICP (e.g., elevate head of bed 30 degrees unless contraindicated; keep head and neck in neutral midline position).	*Prevents pain by preventing increased ICP via mechanisms that are nonsedating*
• Provide or assist with nonpharmacologic measures for headache relief (e.g., cool cloth to forehead, progressive relaxation exercise).	*Nonpharmacologic measures provide relief of pain without sedation.*

Dependent/Collaborative Actions

Implement measures to relieve headache: • Administer analgesics before activities and procedures that can cause headache and before headache becomes severe.	*Analgesics prevent pain from becoming too severe, which may prevent client from participating in activities and procedures.*
• Administer nonnarcotic analgesics or codeine if ordered.	*Opioid narcotics are usually contraindicated because they have a greater depressant effect on the central nervous system.*
• Administer osmotic diuretics, loop diuretics, and/or corticosteroids as ordered.	*Osmotic diuretics lower ICP by creating an osmotic force in the cerebral vasculature that draws edematous fluid out of the brain. Loop diuretics decrease body fluid volume, which helps decrease cerebral edema. Corticosteroids decrease inflammation.*
Consult appropriate health care provider (e.g., physician, pharmacist, pain management specialist) if above measures fail to provide adequate pain relief.	*Notifying the appropriate health care provider allows for modification of the treatment plan.*

NDx = NANDA-I Diagnosis   **D** = Delegatable Action   ● = UAP   ✦ = LVN/LPN   ⊝▶ = Go to ⊝volve for animation

Collaborative/Nursing Diagnosis | RISK FOR ACUTE CONFUSION NDx

Definition: Abrupt onset of reversible disturbances of consciousness, attention, cognition, and perception that develop over a short period of time

Related to: Damage to cerebral tissue associated with cerebral edema

CLINICAL MANIFESTATIONS

Subjective	Objective
N/A	Inaccurate interpretation of environment and time; memory loss; altered mood states (e.g., lability, hostility, irritability, inappropriate affect); inability to make decisions or problem solve; changes in attention span; disorientation; inappropriate social behavior

RISK FACTORS

- Trauma
- Smoking
- Hypertension

DESIRED OUTCOMES

The client will experience less confusion as evidence by:
a. Improved attention span, memory, and problem-solving abilities
b. Improved level of orientation
c. Reduction in instances of inappropriate responses

NOC OUTCOMES

Information processing; neurological status: consciousness; cognitive ability; disoriented thought self-control; memory; mood equilibrium

NIC INTERVENTIONS

Reality orientation; cognitive stimulation; dementia management; presence; behavior management

NURSING ASSESSMENT	RATIONALE
Assess client for changes in level of confusion and orientation (e.g., shortened attention span, impaired memory, decreased ability to problem solve, confusion, inappropriate response. mood changes). Ascertain from significant others client's usual level of cognitive and emotional functioning.	*Early recognition of signs and symptoms of pain allows for prompt intervention.*

THERAPEUTIC INTERVENTIONS	RATIONALE

Independent Actions

If client shows evidence of confusion and/or disorientation:

- Reorient to person, place, and time as necessary. **D** ● ✦
- Address client by name. **D** ● ✦
- Place familiar objects, clock, and calendar within client's view. **D** ● ✦
- Face client when conversing with client. **D** ● ✦
- Approach client in a slow, calm manner; allow adequate time for communication. **D** ● ✦
- Repeat instructions as necessary using clear, simple language and short sentences. **D** ● ✦
- Keep environmental stimuli to a minimum but avoid sensory deprivation. **D** ● ✦
- Maintain a consistent and fairly structured routine. **D** ● ✦
- Provide written or taped information whenever possible.

- Have client perform only one activity at a time and allow adequate time for performance of activities. **D** ● ✦

These techniques help keep client oriented to environment, self, others, and current reality

Facing the client when speaking helps improve communication with the client and decreases the client's stress concerning communication.

Repeating information helps client process information when thinking is impaired.

Overstimulation may cause the client to become anxious or aggressive and can block communication.

A structured routine helps client maintain orientation to place and time, and provides a sense of reality.

Written or taped instructions allow client to review information as often as necessary.

Prevents client from being frustrated with having to perform many activities at one time

THERAPEUTIC INTERVENTIONS	RATIONALE
• Encourage client to make lists of planned activities, questions, and concerns.	*Making lists provides a mechanism with which the client can organize thoughts.*
• Implement measures to stop emotional outbursts and inappropriate responses if they occur (e.g., provide distraction by clapping hands, handing client an object to look at or hold, or turning on the radio or television). **D ● ✦**	*Distraction helps client refocus and decreases inappropriate responses.*
• Maintain realistic expectations of client's ability to learn, comprehend, and remember information provided.	*Don't ask clients to do things beyond their ability.*
• Encourage significant others to be supportive of client; instruct them in methods of dealing with client's disturbed thought processes.	*Significant others need to learn coping mechanisms and how to deal with psychological change.*
• Discuss physiological basis for disturbed thought processes with client and significant others; inform them that cognitive and emotional functioning may improve gradually during the next 6 to 12 months.	*Understanding what occurred helps the client and significant others work toward improving cognitive and emotional functioning.*

Dependent/Collaborative Actions

Consult physician if symptoms worsen.	*Notifying the physician allows for modification of the treatment plan.*

Collaborative Diagnosis # RISK FOR MENINGITIS

Definition: Infection of the meninges

Related to:
• Irritation of the meninges associated with trauma to the meningeal vessels or presence of blood in the CSF
• Introduction of pathogens into the meninges or CSF associated with a tear in the dura (more likely to occur with a compound fracture of the skull, a linear fracture of the frontal or temporal bone, and/or penetration of the skull by an object such as a bullet) and presence of an intracranial monitoring devices and/or external ventricular drain

CLINICAL MANIFESTATIONS

Subjective	Objective
Report of persistent headache	Fever chills; nuchal rigidity; photophobia; positive Kernig's sign (inability to straighten knee when hip is flexed); positive Brudzinski's sign (flexion of hip and knee in response to forward flexion of the neck); cloudy CSF; elevated CSF pressure; CSF analysis showing increased white blood cell (WBC) count and protein levels

RISK FACTOR	DESIRED OUTCOMES
• Exposure to pathogens	The client will not develop meningitis as evidenced by: a. Absence of fever and chills b. Absence of nuchal rigidity and photophobia c. Negative Kernig's and Brudzinski's signs d. Normal CSF analysis

NURSING ASSESSMENT	RATIONALE
Assess for and report signs and symptoms of CSF leak:	*CSF leak indicates a tear in the dura and should be reported immediately.*
• Presence of glucose in clear drainage from nose, ear, or wound as shown by positive results on a glucose reagent strip	

Continued...

NURSING ASSESSMENT	RATIONALE

- Yellowish ring ("halo") around bloody serosanguineous drainage on dressing or pillowcase
- Constant swallowing

Assess for and report signs and symptoms of meningitis:

- Fever, chills
- Increasing or persistent headache
- Nuchal rigidity
- Photophobia
- Positive Kernig's sign (inability to straighten knee when hip is flexed)
- Positive Brudzinski's sign (flexion of hip and knee in response to forward flexion of the neck)
- Cloudy CSF
- Elevated CSF pressure
- CSF analysis showing increased WBC count and protein levels

Early recognition of signs and symptoms of meningitis allows for prompt intervention.

Pressure is often elevated with meningitis.
Indicates possible infection of the CSF

THERAPEUTIC INTERVENTIONS	RATIONALE

Independent Actions

Implement measures to prevent meningitis:

- Assist with thorough cleansing and debridement of head wound if indicated.
- Use sterile technique when changing dressings and working with ICP monitoring device and external ventricular drain.
- Instruct client to keep hands away from head wound, drainage tube(s), and dressing; apply wrist restraints or mittens if necessary.
- If a CSF leak is present:
  - Instruct client to avoid excessive movement and activity (bed rest is usually ordered).
  - Instruct client to avoid coughing, blowing nose, or straining to have a bowel movement).
  - If CSF is leaking from nose:
    (1) Position client with head of bed elevated at least 20 degrees unless contraindicated.
    (2) If client needs to sneeze, instruct to do so with mouth open.
    (3) Instruct client to avoid putting finger in nose.
    (4) Do not perform nasal suctioning or insert a nasogastric tube.
    (5) Do not attempt to clean nose unless ordered by physician.
  - If CSF is leaking from ear:
    (1) Position client on side of CSF leakage unless contraindicated.
    (2) Instruct client to avoid putting finger in ear.
    (3) Do not attempt to clean ear unless ordered by physician.
  - Do not pack dressing into area of CSF leakage (nose, ear, or wound).
  - Place a sterile pad over area of CSF leakage to absorb drainage and change pad as soon as it becomes damp.

These techniques and interventions prevent the introduction of bacteria into the brain tissue.

Prevention of excessive movement prevents further stress on the torn dura.
These activities raise ICP and can cause extension of the dural tear.

Elevating the head of the bed facilitates venous drainage.

Withholding a sneeze can force the bacteria backward through the torn dura and into the brain tissue.
These actions potentially introduce bacteria into the brain tissue.

This position allows the fluid to drain.

These actions potentially introduce bacteria into the brain tissue.

Packing the wound interferes with drainage of fluid.

This helps prevent bacteria from being introduced into the brain tissues.

THERAPEUTIC INTERVENTIONS	RATIONALE

If signs and symptoms of meningitis occur:
- Initiate seizure precautions.

- Provide a quiet environment with dim lighting.

Cerebral irritation can cause seizures. Seizure precautions help prevent client injury if a seizure does occur.
This reduces headaches and photophobia.

Dependent/Collaborative Actions
Implement measures to prevent meningitis:
- Assist with thorough cleansing and debridement of head wound if indicated.
- If a CSF leak is present:
  - Consult physician regarding an order for an antitussive, decongestant, and laxative if indicated.
  - Prepare client for surgical repair of the torn dura if the leak does not heal spontaneously.

If signs and symptoms of meningitis occur:
- Administer antimicrobials as ordered.

It is important to remove dead tissue so the wound does not become infected.

These medications decrease potential coughing, blowing the nose, and straining, which can increase ICP.
Prevents introduction of pathogens into the CNS

Treats and/or prevents infection

Collaborative Diagnosis RISK FOR INCREASED INTRACRANIAL PRESSURE (ICP)

Definition: Increase in cerebral pressure of 15 mm Hg or greater

Related to:
- Accumulation of blood in the cerebral tissue associated with trauma to the cerebral vessels
- Cerebral edema associated with:
  - Increased capillary permeability of cerebral vessels (occurs with cerebral hypoxia)
  - An increase in cellular volume resulting from disruption of the sodium pump within the cells (occurs as a result of cerebral hypoxia) and syndrome of inappropriate antidiuretic hormone (SIADH) if it occurs

CLINICAL MANIFESTATIONS

Subjective	Objective
Report of a sustained headache	Decreased level of consciousness; widening pulse pressure; neurogenic hyperventilation; bradycardia; small, sluggish pupils

RISK FACTORS
- Closed head injury
- Edema/trauma

DESIRED OUTCOMES
The client will not develop IICP as evidenced by:
a. Usual or improved level of consciousness
b. No reports of increased headache
c. Stable or improved motor and sensory function
d. Absence of vomiting, papilledema, and seizure activity
e. Usual pupillary size and reactivity
f. Stable vital signs

NURSING ASSESSMENT	RATIONALE

Assess for and report signs and symptoms of IICP:
- Increased restlessness, agitation, confusion, or lethargy
- Reports of increased headache
- Decreasing motor and sensory function
- Abnormal posturing (e.g., decerebrate, decorticate)
- Vomiting (usually without nausea)
- Papilledema
- Seizures
- Change in pupil size or reactivity

Early recognition of signs and symptoms of increased ICP leads to prompt intervention and prevention of deleterious consequences.

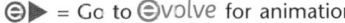

Continued...

NURSING ASSESSMENT	RATIONALE

- Altered respiratory pattern (e.g., shallow, slow respirations, periods of apnea, central neurogenic hyperventilation)
- Bounding, slow pulse
- Rise in systolic B/P with widening pulse pressure

THERAPEUTIC INTERVENTIONS	RATIONALE

Independent Actions
Implement measures to prevent increased ICP:
- Perform actions to promote adequate cerebral venous drainage:
  - Elevate head of bed 30 degrees unless contraindicated.
  - Keep head and neck in neutral, midline position; avoid flexion, extension, and rotation of the head and neck.
- Perform actions to maintain a patent airway (e.g., position client on side, suction if necessary).
- Perform actions to prevent excessive cerebral blood flow and/or dilation of cerebral vessels:
  - Observe for and control conditions that can cause or increase restlessness and agitation.
  - Instruct client to avoid activities that result in isometric muscle contractions (e.g., pushing feet against footboard, tightly gripping side rails).
- Perform actions to prevent and treat meningitis (e.g., use sterile technique when changing dressings and working with ICP device monitoring; have client avoid coughing, blowing nose, or straining to have a bowel movement; if CSF leak noted from nose, do not insert nasogastric or nasotracheal tubes; elevate head of bed at least 20 degrees).
- Schedule care so activities that could raise ICP (e.g., suctioning, bathing, repositioning) are not grouped together.

These actions help decrease incidence of cerebral hypoxia and subsequent vasodilation and cerebral edema.

These actions may increase ICP

Prevents obstruction of the flow of CSF and an increase in metabolic rate (infection causes an increase in metabolic rate and subsequent increase in cerebral blood flow, which results in cerebral vasodilation)

Provides rest between activities so the increased ICP does not significantly increase

Dependent/Collaborative Actions
Implement measures to prevent increased ICP:
- Administer laxative, antitussive, and antiemetic if ordered.

Laxatives prevent straining during bowel movements, antitussives prevent/decrease coughing, and antiemetics decrease vomiting, all of which can cause an increase in intrathoracic pressure and subsequently impede venous return from the brain.

- Administer central nervous system depressants judiciously; hold medication and consult physician if respiratory rate is less than 12 breaths/min.

Depression of the CNS can lead to hypoxia, which causes cerebrovascular vasodilation, which increases ICP.

- Administer oxygen as ordered and before and after tracheal suctioning.

Maintains tissue oxygenation

Collaborative Diagnosis **RISK FOR SEIZURES**

Definition: Transient, uncontrolled electrical activity in the brain that may be exhibited in physical and/or psychological signs and symptoms

Related to: Altered activity of the cerebral neurons associated with irritation of the brain tissue resulting from the injury, surgery, increased intracranial pressure (ICP), and/or meningitis

CLINICAL MANIFESTATIONS

Subjective	Objective
Report of feelings of general discomfort and feeling "out of sorts" (i.e., Malaise), headache, or sense of depression (prodromal)	Dependent upon the type of seizure: focal/motor; temporal lobe or psychomotor; grand mal Excessive muscle tone phase (tonic); alternating contraction/relaxation of muscles (clonic)

RISK FACTORS
- Edema
- Tissue irritation

DESIRED OUTCOME

The client will not experience seizure activity or injury if seizures occur.

NURSING ASSESSMENT

Assess for and report signs and symptoms of seizure activity (e.g., twitching [usually of face or hands], clonic-tonic movements).

RATIONALE

Cerebral irritation places the patient at risk for seizure activity. Risks for seizures are greater with head injuries.

THERAPEUTIC INTERVENTIONS

RATIONALE

Independent Actions
Implement measures to prevent seizures:
- Perform actions to prevent and treat increased ICP and meningitis (e.g., maintain fluid restrictions, elevated head of bed 30 degrees, keep head and neck in neutral position).

Increased ICP and meningitis are associated with seizures.

Initiate and maintain seizure precautions:
- Have oral airway and suction equipment readily available.
- Pad side rails with blankets or soft pads.
- Keep bed in low position with side rails up when client is in bed.

Placing the client on seizure precautions helps to prevent injury if and when seizures occur.

If seizures do occur:
- Implement measures to decrease risk of injury:
  - Ease client to the floor if client is sitting in chair or ambulating at onset of seizure.
  - Remain with but do not restrain client during seizure activity.
  - Do not force any object between clenched teeth or try to pry mouth open.
  - Clear area of objects that may cause injury.
  - Place towel under client's head if client is on floor.
  - As seizure activity subsides, perform actions to maintain a client's airway (e.g., turn client on side, insert an oral airway, suction as needed).
- Observe for and report characteristics of seizures (e.g., progression, time elapsed).

These measures help to protect the client from further injury.

Dependent/Collaborative Actions
Implement measures to prevent/treat seizures:
- If seizures are occurring, administer IV anticonvulsants (i.e., Benzodiazepines or diazepam).
- To prevent reoccurrence of seizures:
  - Administer antiepileptic medications (i.e., carbamazepine, phenytoin, valproic acid).

IV anticonvulsants decreases seizure activity.

Medication prescribed depends on the type of seizures experienced by the client.

Collaborative Diagnosis **RISK FOR CRANIAL NERVE DAMAGE**

Definition: Damage to one or all the cranial nerves

Related to: Trauma to the nerves during injury, before or after surgery and/or compression of the nerves associated with a cerebral hematoma or edema

CLINICAL MANIFESTATIONS

Subjective	Objective
Reports of sensory dysfunction of any of the sensory cranial nerves	Motor dysfunction of any of the 12 motor cranial nerves

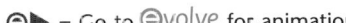

NDx = NANDA-I Diagnosis   **D** = Delegatable Action   ● = UAP   ✦ = LVN/LPN   ⊖▶ = Go to ⊖volve for animation

Continued...
RISK FACTORS

* Edema
* Nerve compression

DESIRED OUTCOME

> The client will not experience cranial nerve damage or will adapt to cranial nerve damage if it occurs.

NURSING ASSESSMENT	RATIONALE
Assess for and report signs and symptoms of damage to the following cranial nerves: • Olfactory (e.g., decreased or absent sense of smell) • Optic, oculomotor, trochlear, or abducens (e.g., diplopia, visual field cut, decreased visual acuity, abnormal extra-ocular movements) • Trigeminal (e.g., decreased or absent corneal reflex, difficulty chewing, pain when chewing) • Vagus or glossopharyngeal (e.g., loss of gag reflex, difficulty swallowing, hoarseness, inability to speak clearly) • Hypoglossal (e.g., difficulty chewing, swallowing, or speaking) • Facial (e.g., facial ptosis, impaired sense of taste)	*Early recognition of changes in functioning of cranial nerves allows for prompt intervention.*

THERAPEUTIC INTERVENTIONS	RATIONALE
Independent Actions Implement measures to help the client compensate for cranial nerve damage if it has occurred:	*Increased ICP increases compression of the cranial nerves. If the compression is not relieved, damage to the cranial nerves may occur.*
• If the olfactory nerve is affected, provide meals that are visually appealing.	*Damage to the olfactory nerve decreases the sense of smell. Increasing visual appeal of meals may improve the clients desire to eat.*
• If vision is impaired, provide an eye patch or opaque lens, instruct client in visual scanning techniques (if experiencing visual field cut), and assist client with self-care and ambulation if indicated.	*The eye patch helps reduce double vision.*

• If the corneal reflex is absent or the client is unable to close his/her eye, instruct the client to:
  • Avoid rubbing the eye
  • Reduce exposure to dust, powder, and smoke
  • Instill isotonic eye drops frequently
	These actions protect the client's cornea from dryness, irritation, and or trauma.

• If the trigeminal, hypoglossal, vagus, and/or glossopharyngeal nerves are affected: • Withhold oral foods/fluids until gag reflex returns and client is better able to chew and swallow.	*These actions decrease the risk of aspiration of food and fluids.*
• Provide parenteral nutrition or tube feedings if indicated.	
• Place client in high-Fowler's position during and for at least 30 minutes after meals and snacks.	
• Instruct client to avoid laughing and talking while eating and drinking.	
• Assist client with oral hygiene after eating.	*Ensures that food particles do not remain in the mouth.*
• Avoid serving sticky foods such as peanut butter and bananas.	*These foods decrease the client's ability to swallow.*
• Assist client to select foods that require little or no chewing and are easily swallowed.	
• Serve thick fluids or thicken thin fluids with substances such as "Thick-It" or gelatin.	
• Maintain quiet environment.	*These actions facilitate communication.*
• Provide pad and pencil, Magic Slate, computer, or word cards.	
• Listen carefully when client speaks.	

THERAPEUTIC INTERVENTIONS	RATIONALE
• If the sensory component of the facial nerve is affected, instruct client to add extra sweeteners or seasonings to food/fluids if desired.	*Sweeteners or seasoning improves taste of foods*

Dependent/Collaborative Actions
Implement measures to help the client compensate for cranial nerve damage if it has occurred:
• If the trigeminal, hypoglossal, vagus, and/or glossopharyngeal nerves are affected:
    • Consult speech pathologist about additional ways to facilitate swallowing and communication.

Provides for multidisciplinary treatment

Collaborative Diagnosis   # RISK FOR DIABETES INSIPIDUS

Definition: A condition in which kidneys are unable to conserve water from impaired release of antidiuretic hormone (ADH)

Related to: Decreased production and/or impaired release of ADH associated with trauma to the hypothalamus and/or the posterior lobe of the pituitary gland (can occur as a result of trauma or postoperative edema or hematoma in that area)

CLINICAL MANIFESTATIONS

Subjective	Objective
Report Continuous thirst and frequent urination	Polyuria; nocturia; polydipsia; low urine specific gravity; low urine osmolality; high serum plasma osmolality

RISK FACTORS

• Trauma
• Edema

DESIRED OUTCOMES

The client will not experience diabetes insipidus as evidenced by:
  a. Absence of polyuria
  b. Absence of intense thirst (polydipsia)

NURSING ASSESSMENT	RATIONALE
Assess for and report signs and symptoms of diabetes insipidus: • Polyuria (urine output can range from 4 to 10 L/day or more) • Reports of intense thirst (if oral fluids are allowed and tolerated, the client's intake is often an amount that corresponds to the high volume of urine output) • A decrease in urine specific gravity (often 1.005 or less)	*Signs and symptoms of hypovolemia and decreased urine specific gravity indicate diabetes insipidus and require prompt treatment to prevent further impact on other systems in the body.*
Assess for and report signs and symptoms of water deficit: • Decreased skin turgor • Dry mucous membranes • Weight loss of 2% or greater over a short period • Postural hypotension and/or low B/P • Weak, rapid pulse • Elevated serum sodium level and osmolality	*Early recognition of signs and symptoms of water deficit allows for prompt intervention.*

THERAPEUTIC INTERVENTIONS	RATIONALE
Dependent/Collaborative Actions If signs and symptoms of diabetes insipidus occur: • Maintain fluid intake equal to output.	*Decreases edema of the hypothalamus, pituitary gland, and surrounding tissue and subsequently reduces the risk of the development of diabetes insipidus*

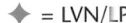

NDx = NANDA-I Diagnosis   **D** = Delegatable Action   ● = UAP   ✦ = LVN/LPN   ⊖▶ = Go to ⊖volve for animation

Continued...

THERAPEUTIC INTERVENTIONS	RATIONALE
• Administer an ADH replacement (e.g., vasopressin, desmopressin [DDAVP]) if ordered.	*Administration of vasopressin and desmopressin provide replacement for absent endogenous ADH.*

Collaborative Diagnosis | RISK FOR SYNDROME OF INAPPROPRIATE ANTIDIURETIC HORMONE (SIADH)

Definition: A condition in which ADH is not released appropriately

Related to:
• Increased production and/or release of ADH associated with altered function of the hypothalamus or the posterior lobe of the pituitary gland as a result of trauma and/or postoperative edema or hematoma in that area
• Stimulation of ADH output associated with pain, trauma, and/or stress

CLINICAL MANIFESTATIONS

Subjective	Objective
Report of loss of appetite, headaches, nausea	Hyponatremia; hypoosmolarity; concentrated urine; anorexia; dyspnea on exertion; fatigue, vomiting; diarrhea; cramping; hostility, confusion; lethargy; muscle twitching, change in level of consciousness and/or convulsions

RISK FACTORS	DESIRED OUTCOMES
• Pain • Trauma • Stress	The client will not develop SIADH as evidenced by: a. Stable weight b. Balanced intake and output c. Stable or improved mental status d. Stable or improved muscle strength e. Absence of cellular edema, abdominal cramping, nausea, vomiting, and seizure activity f. Urine and serum sodium and osmolality levels within normal limits

NURSING ASSESSMENT	RATIONALE
Assess for and report signs and symptoms of SIADH: • Weight gain of 2% or greater over a short period • Intake greater than output • Increased irritability or confusion • Increasing muscle weakness • Reports of persistent or increased headache • Fingerprint edema over sternum (reflects cellular edema) • Abdominal cramping, nausea, or vomiting • Seizures • Elevated urine sodium and osmolality levels • Low serum sodium and osmolality levels	*Early recognition of the signs and symptoms of SIADH allows for prompt intervention.*

THERAPEUTIC INTERVENTIONS	RATIONALE
Independent Actions Implement measures to reduce the risk for the development of SIADH: • Perform actions to reduce pain. • Perform actions to reduce fear and anxiety (e.g., assure client that staff members are nearby, respond to call signal as soon as possible).	*Pain, fear, and anxiety increase the production of ADH.*

THERAPEUTIC INTERVENTIONS	RATIONALE

Dependent/Collaborative Actions

Implement measures to reduce the risk for the development of SIADH:

* Administer osmotic diuretics (e.g., mannitol), loop diuretics (e.g., furosemide), and/or corticosteroids (e.g., dexamethasone) if ordered.

Osmotic diuretics decrease cerebral edema, which may decrease pressure on the pituitary and hypothalamus, thus decreasing SIADH; loop diuretics decrease circulating fluid volume; corticosteroids decrease swelling reducing pressure on the hypothalamus, pituitary gland, and surrounding tissue.

If signs and symptoms of SIADH occur:

* Maintain fluid restrictions if ordered (typically this is a restriction of free water).

Fluid restriction helps decrease vascular fluid volume.

* Encourage intake of foods/fluids high in sodium (e.g., tomato juice, cured meats, processed cheese, canned soups, catsup, canned vegetables, dill pickles, bouillon) if oral intake is allowed and tolerated.

A high sodium intake improves the sodium and vascular fluid (water) balance and increases fluid osmolality.

* Initiate seizure precautions.
* Administer the following if ordered:
* Diuretics (usually furosemide)

Loop diuretics promote water excretion and retention of sodium, thus improving the sodium/vascular fluid (water)balance.

* Intravenous infusion of a hypertonic saline solution
* Demeclocycline

Improves vascular fluid (water)/sodium balance
Demeclocycline increases urine output, thus decreasing free water and improving sodium/vascular fluid (water)balance.

Collaborative Diagnosis **RISK FOR GASTROINTESTINAL (GI) BLEEDING**

Definition: Bleeding in the esophagus, stomach, or duodenum

Related to:

* The development of an ulcer (often referred to as a stress-induced ulcer, stress-related mucosal damage, or Cushing's ulcer) associated with:
  * Gastric ischemia resulting from vasoconstriction (occurs with sympathetic nervous system stimulation that can result from cerebral injury)
  * Hypersecretion of hydrochloric acid resulting from parasympathetic nervous system stimulation that can occur with cerebral injury and stress

CLINICAL MANIFESTATIONS

Subjective	Objective
Report of abdominal pain and fullness	Bloody vomitus (bright red or coffee ground); black, tarry stools; frank bright red blood from the rectum; trace amounts of blood in gastric secretions

RISK FACTORS

* Trauma
* Stress

DESIRED OUTCOMES

The client will not experience GI bleeding as evidenced by:
  a. No reports of epigastric discomfort and fullness
  b. Absence of frank and occult blood in stool and gastric contents
  c. B/P and pulse within normal range for client
  d. Red blood cell (RBC) count, hematocrit (Hct), and hemoglobin (Hgb) levels within normal range

---

NDx = NANDA-I Diagnosis   **D** = Delegatable Action   ● = UAP   ✦ = LVN/LPN   ⊖▶ = Go to ⊖volve for animation

Continued...

NURSING ASSESSMENT	RATIONALE
Assess for and report signs and symptoms of GI bleeding (e.g., reports of epigastric discomfort or fullness; frank or occult blood in stool or gastric contents; decreased B/P; increased pulse; decreasing RBC count, Hct, and Hgb levels).	*Early recognition of signs and symptoms of GI bleeding allows for prompt intervention.*

THERAPEUTIC INTERVENTIONS	RATIONALE

Independent Actions
Implement measures to prevent ulceration of the gastric and duodenal mucosa:

- Perform actions to decrease fear and anxiety (e.g., assure client that staff members are nearby, respond to call signal as soon as possible).   *Fear and anxiety increase gastric acid production.*
- When oral intake is allowed:
- Instruct client to avoid coffee; caffeine-containing tea and colas; spices such as black pepper, chili powder, and nutmeg.   *These foods/fluids stimulate hydrochloric acid secretion or directly irritate the gastric mucosa.*

Dependent/Collaborative Actions
Implement measures to prevent ulceration of the gastric and duodenal mucosa:

- When oral intake is allowed:
  - Administer ulcerogenic medications (e.g., corticosteroids, phenytoin) with meals or snacks.   *Decreases gastric irritation, which can occur when taking certain medications on a empty stomach*
  - Administer histamine$_2$-receptor antagonists (e.g., ranitidine, famotidine), proton-pump inhibitors (e.g., omeprazole, rabeprazole), antacids, and/or cytoprotective agents (e.g., sucralfate)if ordered. **D** ✦   *Histamine receptor antagonists and proton-pump inhibitors suppress secretion of gastric acid. Antacids neutralize stomach acid and cytoprotective agents create a protective barrier against stomach acid and pepsin.*

If signs and symptoms of GI bleeding occur:

- Insert nasogastric tube and maintain suction as ordered. **D** ✦   *Insertion of an HG tube and suction removes gastric acid and pressure on the gastric lining.*
- Administer blood products and/or volume expanders if ordered.   *Hypotension may occur. Administration of blood and/or volume expanders may be needed to maintain adequate blood pressure and tissue perfusion.*
- Assist with measures to control bleeding (e.g., gastric lavage, endoscopic electrocoagulation) if planned.   *These interventions decrease or stop GI bleeding.*

Nursing Diagnosis **DEFICIENT KNOWLEDGE** NDx; **INEFFECTIVE HEALTH MAINTENANCE** NDx*; **OR INEFFECTIVE FAMILY THERAPEUTIC REGIMEN MANAGEMENT** NDx

Definition: Absence or deficiency of cognitive information related to specific topic (lack of specific information necessary for clients/significant others) to make informed choices regarding condition/treatment/lifestyle changes; inability to identify, manage, and/or seek out help to manage health; pattern of regulating and integrating into family processes a program for treatment of illness and the sequelae of illness that is unsatisfactory for meeting specific health goals

---

*The nurse should select the diagnostic label that is most appropriate for the client's discharge teaching.

CLINICAL MANIFESTATIONS

Subjective	Objective
Verbalizes inability to manage illness; verbalizes inability to follow prescribed regimen	Inaccurate follow through with instructions; inappropriate behaviors; experience of preventable complications of spinal cord injury

RISK FACTORS

- Cognitive deficit
- Financial concerns
- Failure to take action to reduce risk factors
- Inability to care for oneself
- Difficulty in modifying personal habits and integrating treatments into lifestyle

NOC OUTCOMES

Knowledge: treatment regimen; knowledge: health behavior; knowledge: health resources

NIC INTERVENTIONS

Health system guidance; teaching: individual; teaching: prescribed activity/exercise; teaching: prescribed medications

NURSING ASSESSMENT	RATIONALE
Assess client's willingness to learn and knowledge related to the disease process.	*The client's willingness to learn and knowledge base provides the basis for education.*
Assess for indications that the client may be unable to effectively manage the therapeutic regimen.	*Early recognition of inability to understand disease process or self-care allows for change in the teaching plan.*

THERAPEUTIC INTERVENTIONS	RATIONALE

Desired Outcome: The client will identify ways to adapt to neurological deficits that may persist after craniocerebral trauma and/or surgery

Independent Actions

Instruct client in ways to adapt to neurological deficits resulting from craniocerebral trauma:

These techniques provide a mechanism that helps the client adapt to neurological changes while maintaining as much independence as possible.

- Wear an eye patch or opaque lens if double vision is a problem.

Eye patch alleviates double vision

- Use scanning techniques if visual field cut is present.

Visual scanning techniques provide a more complete view of the environment for a client with a visual deficit.

- Use paper and pencil, Magic Slate, computer, pictures, and gestures to express self if verbal communication is impaired.

These techniques help improve communication.

- Make lists, write or record messages and reminders, and refer to written instructions repeatedly if experiencing difficulty concentrating or remembering.

Helps maintain activities of daily living when client experiences difficulty in concentrating and remembering

- Request assistance when problem solving and setting priorities, and seek validation of decisions if reasoning ability is impaired.

Client is able to validate decision making.

- Continue with techniques and exercises to improve swallowing if indicated.

Improves swallowing ability and decreases risk of aspiration.

- Prepare meals that are visually appealing to help stimulate appetite if senses of smell and/or taste are impaired.

This helps maintain adequate nutritional status when sense of smell and/or taste are impaired.

- Use assistive devices (e.g., broad-handled eating utensils, plate guard) and mobility aids (e.g., wheelchair, cane, walker) if motor function is impaired.

Use of assistive devices help client maintain as much independent functioning as possible.

- Plan daily activities to allow for adequate rest periods.

Planning daily activities reduces irritability that often occurs after craniocerebral trauma and/or surgery

Continued...

THERAPEUTIC INTERVENTIONS	RATIONALE

Desired Outcome: The client will identify ways to protect the surgical site from injury (if required).

Independent Actions

Instruct the client in ways to protect the surgical site from injury:

- Wear a scarf, turban, hat, or cap until hair has grown back.
- Do not shampoo hair until the incision has healed (usually 7-10 days after surgery).
- When shampooing hair, avoid vigorous scrubbing; pat surgical site dry rather than rubbing.
- Avoid use of hair dryer on hot setting, curling iron, and hot curlers at or near surgical site until hair has grown back.
- Avoid scratching the surgical site; if it itches as the incision heals and the hair grows back, apply light pressure to the surgical site or distract self with activities like taking a walk or watching television.
- If the bone flap was not replaced, avoid bumping or putting excessive pressure on the surgical site (if the skull depression is large, client may need to wear a protective helmet as level of activity increases).

These techniques aid in the promotion of healing and decrease the potential of infection.
Prevents sunburn and irritation to the scalp
Prevents fluid and soap from getting into the surgical area

Vigorous scrubbing may irritate and scratch scalp

Direct heat can burn the unprotected scalp.

Scratching the surgical site can increase risk of infection. Use of light surgical site pressure and distractions can help decrease urge to scratch the surgical site.

Prevents further client injury.

THERAPEUTIC INTERVENTIONS	RATIONALE

Desired Outcome: The client will identify ways to reduce headaches.

Independent Actions

Instruct client in ways to reduce headache, which may persist for months after injury/surgery:

- Dim environmental lighting if possible or wear sunglasses when light is bright.
- Reduce environmental noise whenever possible (e.g., lower volume on TV and radio).
- Avoid situations that increase stress.
- Advise client to take analgesics as prescribed.

These techniques decrease incidence of headaches and pain experienced.

THERAPEUTIC INTERVENTIONS	RATIONALE

Desired Outcome: The client will state signs and symptoms to report to the health care provider.

Independent Actions

Instruct client to report the following signs and symptoms:

- Increased drowsiness unrelated to a significant increase in activity or decrease in amount of sleep obtained
- Increased irritability or restlessness
- Changes in behavior, increased difficulty remembering or concentrating
- New or increased weakness of extremities
- Decreased sensation in extremities
- Severe headache
- Difficulty speaking or understanding what others are saying
- Difficulty chewing or swallowing

All of these signs may indicate increased ICP and should be reported to a health care provider immediately.

THERAPEUTIC INTERVENTIONS	RATIONALE

- Changes in vision (e.g., double vision, blurred vision, visual field cut)
- Increased dizziness, difficulty maintaining balance
- Seizures
- Bloody, yellowish, or clear drainage from nose or ear — *May indicate a leak of CSF*
- Stiff neck — *May indicate an irritation of the meninges*
- Sudden weight gain or loss, excessive thirst, and/or unusual increase or decrease in amount of urination — *Indicative of SIADH or diabetes insipidus.*
- Unexplained fever — *May indicate an infection*
- Exaggerated startle response; angry outbursts; diminished interest or participation in significant activities; feeling of detachment from others; and recurrent, intrusive, disturbing images and thoughts of the event that resulted in the craniocerebral trauma/surgery — *These are signs and symptoms of posttraumatic stress disorder (PTSD) that may occur for weeks to months after involvement in a traumatic event.*

THERAPEUTIC INTERVENTIONS	RATIONALE

Desired Outcome: The client will identify community resources that can assist with home management and adjustment to changes resulting from craniocerebral trauma or surgery.

Independent Actions

Inform client and significant others of community resources that can assist with home management and adjustment to changes resulting from craniocerebral trauma (e.g., home health agencies, Meals on Wheels, social and financial services, brain injury support groups, local service groups that can help obtain assistive devices, individual and family counseling services).
Initiate a referral if indicated.

Provides for continuum of care postdischarge from the acute care facility

THERAPEUTIC INTERVENTIONS	RATIONALE

Desired Outcome: The client will verbalize an understanding of and a plan for adhering to recommend follow-up care including future appointments with health care provider, therapists, and prescribed medication regimen.

Independent Actions

Reinforce the importance of keeping follow-up appointments with health care provider and physical, occupational, and speech therapists.

Keeping follow-up appointments helps the client have continued progress in improving health status.

Teach client the rationale for, side effects of, schedule for taking, and importance of taking medications prescribed (e.g., anticonvulsants, analgesics, antimicrobials). Inform client of pertinent food and drug interactions.

Knowledge of the medication regimen and the impact of these medications on the system, as well as how the medication regimen can be incorporated into the client's lifestyle, allows the client some mechanism of control of his/her disease and the ability to have an active part in treatment and care.

Implement measures to improve client compliance:
- Include significant others in teaching sessions if possible. — *Significant others may be able to assist client as needed.*
- Encourage questions and allow time for reinforcement and clarification of information provided. — *Helps significant others learn what ways they can assist the client*
- Provide written instructions on scheduled appointments with health care provider and occupational, physical, and speech therapists; medications prescribed; and signs and symptoms to report. — *An informed client and family are better able to adhere to a treatment regimen.*

Continued...

ADDITIONAL NURSING DIAGNOSES

RISK FOR IMBALANCED BODY TEMPERATURE NDx

Related to direct trauma to the hypothalamus and/or pressure on the hypothalamus associated with hematoma formation or edema of the surrounding tissue

IMPAIRED PHYSICAL MOBILITY NDx

Related to:

* Motor and spatial-perceptual impairments if present
* Activity restrictions imposed by the treatment plan
* Reluctance to move because of headache

SELF-CARE DEFICIT NDx

Related to:

* Impaired physical mobility
* Disturbed thought processes
* Visual impairments if present

FEAR/ANXIETY* NDx

Related to:

* Impaired motor and/or sensory function
* Disturbed thought processes
* Uncertainty as to permanence of neurological deficits
* Unfamiliar environment
* Lack of understanding of diagnostic tests, diagnosis, and treatments

RISK FOR POSTTRAUMA SYNDROME NDx

Related to having experienced a situation that resulted in physical injury and involved intense feelings of fear and helplessness

RISK FOR INJURY: FALLS, BURNS, AND LACERATIONS NDx

Related to:

* Dizziness
* Motor, visual, and/or spatial-perceptual impairments if present
* Quick, impulsive behavior (can occur with injury involving the nondominant cerebral hemisphere)
* Ataxia (can occur with cerebellar injury)

DISTURBED SELF-CONCEPT† NDx

Related to:

* Change in appearance (e.g., periocular edema and ecchymosis, loss of hair on head if an area was shaved for surgery or to repair lacerations)
* Changes in motor and sensory function
* Dependence on others to meet basic needs
* Anticipated changes in lifestyle and roles associated with sensory and motor impairments and disturbed thought processes

INEFFECTIVE COPING NDx

Related to:

* Persistent headache
* Changes in motor and sensory function and thought processes
* Possibility of lengthy rehabilitation and changes in future lifestyle and roles

INTERRUPTED FAMILY PROCESSES NDx

Related to change in family roles and structure associated with a family member's motor and sensory impairments, disturbed thought processes, and possible need for lengthy rehabilitation

⊖▶ SPINAL CORD INJURY

Spinal cord injury (spinal cord trauma) is most often the result of sudden, external trauma (e.g., motor vehicle accident, fall, sports or recreational injury, act of violence), although it can be caused by a tumor or conditions affecting the vertebrae (e.g., stenosis, pathologic fractures). Spinal cord injury is classified according to the cause of cord injury (e.g., contusion, compression, transection), direction of movement of the vertebrae or mechanism of injury (e.g., flexion, hyperextension, rotation), level of injury (e.g., cervical, sacral), stability of the vertebral column (i.e., stable, unstable), and/or degree of cord involvement (i.e., complete, incomplete).

Immediately after traumatic injury to the spinal cord, spinal shock (loss of motor, sensory, autonomic, and reflex activity below the level of the injury) occurs. Spinal shock usually lasts between 1 and 6 weeks but can persist for months. The neurological impairments that remain after the period of spinal shock depend upon the level of the cord injury (the

higher the level, the greater the loss of body function) and the degree of cord involvement (if complete, there is total loss of sensory function and voluntary motor function below the level of the injury; if incomplete, some of the motor and/or sensory fibers below the level of injury are able to function).

This care plan focuses on the adult client hospitalized with a complete injury of the spinal cord at the level of the fifth cervical vertebra (C5).

After the period of spinal shock, a client with a complete cord injury at the C5 level experiences loss of voluntary motor function below the clavicles; however, full neck, upper shoulder, and some bicep control and elbow flexion are retained. Sensory function is intact above the clavicles and in certain areas of the deltoids and forearms. With rehabilitation, the client may be able to do things such as operate an electric wheelchair and a manual wheelchair with hand rim projec-

---

*The nurse should select the diagnostic label that is most appropriate based on the client's clinical manifestations.
†This diagnostic label includes the nursing diagnoses of Disturbed body image, Low self-esteem, and Ineffective role performance. The nurse should select the diagnostic label that is most appropriate based on the client's clinical manifestations.

tions (quad pegs), feed self using assistive devices, use reflex activity to achieve an erection and stimulate bowel and bladder elimination, accomplish some change in body position, and operate some equipment (e.g., computer, telephone) using assistive devices.

Much of the information provided in this care plan is also applicable to spinal cord–injured clients in extended care, rehabilitation, and home settings.

Although the focus is on injury at the C5 level, the information can easily be individualized to plan nursing care for clients with injury to other segments of the spinal cord.

OUTCOME/DISCHARGE CRITERIA

The client will:
1. Have clear, audible breath sounds throughout lungs
2. Have no evidence of tissue irritation or breakdown
3. Have an adequate nutritional status
4. Experience optimal control of urinary and bowel elimination
5. Direct own care and perform or participate in self-care when possible
6. Have adequate tissue perfusion and thermoregulation
7. Have no signs and symptoms of complications resulting from the spinal cord injury and decreased mobility
8. Identify ways to prevent complications associated with spinal cord injury and decreased mobility
9. Demonstrate the ability to correctly use and maintain assistive devices
10. Identify ways to manage altered bowel and bladder function
11. State signs and symptoms to report to the health care provider
12. Identify resources that can assist with financial needs, home management, and adjustment to changes resulting from spinal cord injury
13. Share thoughts and feelings about the effects of spinal cord injury on self-concept, lifestyle, and roles
14. Verbalize an understanding of and a plan for adhering to recommended follow-up care including future appointments with health care provider and occupational and physical therapists and medications prescribed

---

Nursing Diagnosis **RISK FOR INEFFECTIVE CEREBRAL TISSUE PERFUSION** NDx

⊖▶ Definition: Risk for a decrease in cerebral tissue circulation

Related to:
- Decreased cardiac output associated with:
  - Bradycardia resulting from loss of sympathetic nervous system activity and subsequent unopposed action of the parasympathetic nervous system on the heart
  - Decreased venous return resulting from vasodilation below the level of the injury (the vasodilation occurs because of loss of sympathetic nervous system activity below the level of cord injury)
- Peripheral pooling of blood associated with vasodilation below the level of the injury and loss of muscle tone in extremities resulting from paralysis of extremities and decreased mobility

CLINICAL MANIFESTATIONS

Subjective	Objective
Reports of confusion	Decreased B/P; restlessness; cool extremities; pallor or cyanosis of extremities; diminished or absent peripheral pulses; slow capillary refill; edema; oliguria

RISK FACTOR
- Spinal trauma

DESIRED OUTCOMES

The client will maintain adequate tissue perfusion as evidenced by:
a. B/P within normal range for client
b. Usual mental status
c. Extremities warm with absence of pallor and cyanosis
d. Palpable peripheral pulses
e. Capillary refill time less than 2 to 3 seconds
f. Absence of edema
g. Urine output at least 30 mL/h

NDx = NANDA-I Diagnosis   **D** = Delegatable Action   ● = UAP   ✦ = LVN/LPN   ⊖▶ = Go to ⊖volve for animation

Continued...

NOC OUTCOMES	NIC INTERVENTIONS
Circulation status; vital signs status	Circulatory care: venous insufficiency; circulatory care: arterial insufficiency; vital signs monitoring

NURSING ASSESSMENT	RATIONALE
Assess for and report signs and symptoms of diminished tissue perfusion (e.g., decreased B/P, restlessness, confusion, cool extremities, pallor or cyanosis of extremities, diminished or absent peripheral pulses, slow capillary refill, edema, oliguria).	*Early recognition of signs and symptoms of decreased tissue perfusion allows for prompt intervention.*

THERAPEUTIC INTERVENTIONS	RATIONALE

Independent Actions

Implement measures to maintain adequate tissue perfusion:

- Avoid activities that cause vagal stimulation (e.g., suctioning) unless absolutely necessary. **D** ✦

  Decreased heart rate and B/P can occur with vagal stimulation, causing a greater decrease in tissue perfusion and potential injury.

- Perform actions to prevent peripheral pooling of blood and/or increase venous return:
  - Perform passive range-of-motion exercises at least three times a day. **D** ● ✦

    These interventions prevent blood from pooling in the lower extremities and contractures.

  - Avoid positions that compromise blood flow in the lower extremities (e.g., crossing legs, pillows under knees, sitting for long periods). **D** ● ✦
  - Apply thigh-high elastic stockings as ordered. **D** ● ✦
  - Apply/maintain a sequential compression device to lower extremities if ordered. **D** ● ✦
  - Apply an abdominal binder if ordered before placing client in a sitting or upright position. **D** ● ✦

    The binder reduces pooling of blood in the abdominal/pelvic vessels.

- Perform actions to allow time for remaining autoregulatory mechanisms to adjust to position changes:
  - Change client's position slowly. **D** ● ✦

    Changing positions slowly helps decrease the incidence of orthostatic hypotension.

  - Gradually progress client to a sitting or upright position using a recliner wheelchair or tilt table when allowed and tolerated.

    Increases the client's ability to remain upright and provides stretch of the muscles

Dependent/Collaborative Actions

Implement measures to maintain adequate tissue perfusion:

- Administer the following medications if ordered:
  - Anticholinergics (e.g., atropine)

    Anticholinergics are given to increase heart rate.

  - Sympathomimetics (e.g., dopamine)

    Sympathomimetics are given to increase cardiac output and maintain arterial pressure.

Nursing Diagnosis　# INEFFECTIVE THERMOREGULATION NDx

Definition: Temperature fluctuation between hypothermia and hyperthermia

Related to:

- Interruption in the feedback system between the area below the level of cord injury and the hypothalamus, and loss of vasomotor tone below the level of the injury (these conditions result in the loss of compensatory responses to temperature changes [i.e., vasodilation, sweating, vasoconstriction, shivering, and piloerection])
- Reduction in heat generation associated with limited body movement (especially during period of spinal shock)

CLINICAL MANIFESTATIONS

Subjective	Objective
Reports feeling too warm or too cold	Excessively warm or cool skin below the level of injury; temperature above or below normal range; tachycardia; hypotension/hypertension; shivering; skin cool to touch; pallor; slow capillary refill; cyanotic nail beds; piloerection; warm to touch; flushed skin; hypercapnia; seizures

RISK FACTORS

- Environmental temperature
- Edema
- Trauma

DESIRED OUTCOMES

The client will experience effective thermoregulation as evidenced by:
  a. Verbalization of comfortable body temperature
  b. Absence of excessively warm or cool skin below the level of the injury
  c. Temperature within normal range

NOC OUTCOMES

Thermoregulation

NIC INTERVENTIONS

Temperature regulation: environmental management

NURSING ASSESSMENT

Assess for signs and symptoms of ineffective thermoregulation (e.g., reports of feeling too warm or too cold, excessively warm or cool skin below the level of the injury, temperature above or below normal range).

RATIONALE

Early recognition of the signs and symptoms of inefficient thermoregulation allows for prompt intervention.

THERAPEUTIC INTERVENTIONS

RATIONALE

Independent Actions
Implement measures to maintain effective thermoregulation:
- Perform actions to prevent hypothermia:
  - Maintain room temperature at 70° F.
  - Provide extra clothing and bedding as necessary. **D** ● ✦
  - Protect client from drafts. **D** ● ✦
  - Provide warm liquids for client to drink. **D** ● ✦
  - Avoid taking client outdoors when it is very cold. **D** ● ✦
- Perform actions to prevent hyperthermia:
  - Maintain room temperature at 70°F . **D** ● ✦
  - Avoid use of excessive clothing and bedding. **D** ● ✦
  - Remove extra clothing during physical and occupational therapy sessions.
  - Avoid taking client outdoors when it is very hot (especially if the humidity is high). **D** ● ✦

The client is not able to regulate body temperature due to loss of sympathetic control. These interventions focus on keeping the client's temperature as close to normal as possible.

Dependent/Collaborative Actions
Implement measures to maintain effective thermoregulation:
- Apply warming and cooling blanket as ordered. **D** ● ✦
Consult physician if above measures fail to maintain effective thermoregulation.

Notifying the physician allows for modification of the treatment plan.

NDx = NANDA-I Diagnosis   **D** = Delegatable Action   ● = UAP   ✦ = LVN/LPN   ⊝▶ = Go to ⊝volve for animation

Nursing Diagnosis   RISK FOR IMPAIRED TISSUE INTEGRITY NDx

Definition: Damage to mucous membrane, corneal, integumentary of subcutaneous tissue

Related to:

• Accumulation of waste products and decreased oxygen and nutrient supply to the skin and subcutaneous tissue associated with reduced blood flow from prolonged pressure on the tissues as a result of decreased mobility and/or presence of an external device (e.g., halo vest, wrist splint) that is improperly applied or does not fit properly
• Damage to the skin or subcutaneous tissue associated with friction or shearing
• Increased fragility of the skin associated with dependent edema and decreased tissue perfusion
• Frequent contact with irritants if client is incontinent of urine

CLINICAL MANIFESTATIONS

Subjective	Objective
Not applicable	Pallor, redness, or breakdown of skin in edematous areas or bony prominences

RISK FACTORS

• Immobility
• Loss of body functions

DESIRED OUTCOMES

The client will maintain tissue integrity as evidenced by:
  a. Absence of redness and irritation
  b. No skin breakdown

NOC OUTCOMES

Tissue integrity: skin and mucous membranes

NIC INTERVENTIONS

Skin surveillance; pressure management; positioning: wheelchair; bed rest care; pressure ulcer prevention; skin care: topical treatments; traction/immobility care

NURSING ASSESSMENT	RATIONALE
Determine risk for skin breakdown using a risk assessment tool (e.g., Norton Scale, Braden Scale, Gosnell Scale).	*Identification of clients at risk for skin breakdown allows for implementation of nursing interventions to prevent breakdown from occurring. Use of a scale provides for more accurate assessment.*
Inspect the skin (especially bony prominences, dependent and/or edematous areas, perineum, area underneath halo vest, and areas of sensory loss) for pallor, redness, and breakdown.	*Early recognition of signs and symptoms of skin impairment allows for prompt intervention .*

THERAPEUTIC NURSING INTERVENTIONS	RATIONALE

Independent Actions
Implement additional measures to prevent tissue breakdown:

• Perform actions to maintain adequate tissue perfusion (e.g., turn client every 2 hours; position properly using pillows, foam, or specialized beds; massage reddened areas every 2 hours; keep bed linens dry and wrinkle free; protect skin from contact with urine and feces). **D** ● ✦

Turning client allows for appropriate circulation to tissues. Massage of reddened areas increases circulation. Use of assist devices and specialized beds reduces prolonged pressure on tissues, decreasing potential for tissue ischemia and pressure sores.

• If client is wearing a halo vest:
  • Ensure that vest lining and skin beneath it are kept clean and dry.
  • Make sure that clothing worn under the vest is clean, dry, wrinkle-free, and made of cotton (some physicians allow client to wear a T-shirt under the vest; others do not because they feel the shirt promotes slippage of the vest).

Skin will become macerated from accumulation of moisture on the vest lining.

  • Cover all rough vest edges with foam tape.

Rough edges on the vest can cause lacerations of the skin.

THERAPEUTIC NURSING INTERVENTIONS	**RATIONALE**

Perform actions to prevent urinary incontinence:

- Attempt to initiate voiding periodically by stimulating trigger zones of the reflex sacral arc (e.g., tap suprapubic area, stroke inner thigh, perform anal sphincter stretching, pull pubic hair); if voiding occurs, repeat stimulus as necessary to empty bladder. **D ✦**

  Preventing urinary incontinence will help keep the skin and perineal area clean and dry and will help prevent skin breakdown. These techniques will promote urination.

- If possible, place client on bedside commode or toilet when triggering voiding reflex or performing intermittent catheterization. **D ✦**

  Placing client on bedside commode allows gravity to help facilitate complete bladder emptying.

- Instruct client to space fluid intake evenly throughout the day rather than drinking a large quantity at one time.

  If the bladder fills rapidly and frequency of emptying is not increased, bladder distention occurs.

- Instruct client to limit intake of alcohol and beverages containing caffeine.

  Alcohol and caffeine have a mild diuretic effect and act as irritants to the bladder; increased urine production can result in bladder distention if the frequency of bladder emptying is not also increased, and the bladder irritation can trigger bladder spasms and subsequent incontinence.

- Limit oral fluid intake in the evening. **D ● ✦**

  Limiting evening oral intake is important so that the bladder does not become overdistended during the night. As rehabilitation progresses, most clients do not perform intermittent catheterization or attempt to trigger voiding during the night.

- Instruct client and others to avoid stimulating the voiding reflex trigger zones at times other than during bladder care.

  Stimulation of the voiding reflex trigger zones increases the risk of incontinence.

Perform actions to decrease spasticity:

- Instruct client in and assist with active and active-passive resistance exercises of neck, shoulders, and biceps if indicated.

  Spasms can cause movement and subsequent friction and make it difficult to keep client positioned properly.

- Ensure that wheelchair is not too small for client and that it is adequately cushioned. **D ● ✦**

  Pressure from the sides of the wheelchair can increase incidence of pressure ulcers.

- Be sure that client wears shoes or sturdy slippers when in wheelchair. **D ● ✦**

  Important to protect the feet from trauma

- If fade time (length of time it takes for reddened areas to fade after pressure is removed) is greater than 15 minutes, increase frequency of position changes and/or provide more effective methods of cushioning, padding, and positioning.

  Increased fade time indicates decreased circulation. If this occurs, implement interventions to relieve pressure on the skin and improve circulation.

Dependent/Collaborative Actions

Implement actions to prevent urinary incontinence:

- Perform intermittent catheterization.

  Intermittent emptying of the bladder decreases the incidence of incontinence.

Implement additional measures to prevent tissue breakdown:

- If client is wearing a halo vest:
  - Consult physician and orthotist about having the vest readjusted if it is placing excessive pressure on any skin area.

    Provides multidisciplinary approach to preventing tissue breakdown

If skin breakdown occurs:

- Notify appropriate health care provider (e.g., wound care specialist, physician).

  Wound care specialists can provide individualized treatment to improve healing of skin breakdown.

- Perform care of involved areas as ordered or per hospital standard.

  Hospital standard of care should be implemented to improve healing of skin breakdown.

NDx = NANDA-I Diagnosis   **D** = Delegatable Action   ● = UAP   ✦ = LVN/LPN   ⊖▶ = Go to ⊖volve for animation

Nursing Diagnosis **SELF-CARE DEFICIT** NDx **(BATHING, DRESSING, FEEDING, AND TOILETING)**

Definition: Impaired ability to perform or complete feeding, bathing, hygiene, dressing and grooming, or toileting activities for oneself

Related to: Impaired physical mobility associated with quadriplegia, spasticity, decreased motivation, pain, weakness, and activity restrictions imposed by treatment plan

CLINICAL MANIFESTATIONS

Subjective	Objective
Complaints of pain and/or weakness	Inability to move upper and/or lower extremities due to injury; muscle spasticity

DESIRED OUTCOME

The client will demonstrate increased participation in self-care activities within the limitations imposed by the treatment plan and effects of the spinal cord injury.

NOC OUTCOMES	NIC INTERVENTIONS
Self-care: activities of daily living	Self-care assistance

NURSING ASSESSMENT	RATIONALE
Assess readiness to engage in self-care activities. Determine level of motivation and family support.	*The level of client interest, motivation, and family support will determine when and how much self-care the client can assume.*

THERAPEUTIC INTERVENTIONS	RATIONALE

Independent Actions

With client, develop a realistic plan for meeting daily physical needs. Inform client that with rehabilitation and use of assistive devices, he/she may be able to accomplish activities such as:
- Feeding self once meal has been set up
- Washing face and chest
- Combing front and sides of hair, brushing teeth, and shaving with an electric razor
- Participating in dressing upper body **D ● ✦**

Engaging client in self-care activities will demonstrate to client that he or she will be able to care for self after discharge.

Schedule care at a time when client is most likely to be able to participate (e.g., when analgesics are at peak effect, after rest periods, not immediately after physical therapy sessions or meals).

Keep objects client can use independently within easy reach. **D ● ✦**

Allow adequate time for accomplishment of self-care activities. **D ● ✦**

Encourage client to perform as much of self-care as possible within physical limitations and activity restrictions imposed by the treatment plan. **D ● ✦**

Perform for client the self-care activities that he/she is unable to accomplish. **D ● ✦**

Inform significant others of client's abilities to participate in own care.

If the client is tired or experiencing pain, he/she will not be able to participate in activities of daily living, which may cause a decrease in morale if client has been previously successful in completing tasks.

Provides the client a way to be independent will improve morale and decrease recovery time.

Be sure not to rush the client. Learning new ways of caring for self may require additional time.

Allows client the ability to see that he/she can care for self, and promotes self-confidence

Explain the importance to significant others of encouraging and allowing client to achieve an optimal level of independence.

Dependent/Collaborative Actions

When condition stabilizes and physician allows, implement measures to facilitate client's ability to perform self-care activities:

THERAPEUTIC INTERVENTIONS	RATIONALE
• Perform actions to increase mobility (e.g., tilt table, active and passive range of motion [ROM]).	These actions increase client's ability to become more mobile and to perform self-care activities.
• Consult occupational therapist regarding assistive devices available; reinforce use of these devices, which may include:	Consulting an occupational therapist allows for interdisciplinary care and use of tools and techniques to improve and enhance self-care abilities.
• Rocker feeder, overhead sling, plate guard, sandwich holder, and broad-handled and/or swivel utensils for feeding self	
• Flexor-hinge splint or universal cuff to aid in brushing teeth, combing hair, and shaving with electric razor	
• Bath mitt for bathing face and chest	
• Velcro fasteners to facilitate dressing upper body	

Nursing Diagnosis   RISK FOR INJURY NDx

Definition: At risk for injury as a result of environmental conditions interacting with the individual's adaptive and defensive resources

Related to:

- **Falls** related to loss of motor function, use of kinetic bed, altered sitting balance if wearing a halo device (the structure and weight of the device alter the client's center of gravity), and unexpected body movements resulting from spasticity
- **Burns** related to loss of motor and sensory function and unexpected body movements resulting from spasticity

RISK FACTORS	DESIRED OUTCOME
• Changes in balance	The client will not experience falls or burns.
• Weakness	
• Loss of neuromuscular functioning	

NOC OUTCOMES	NIC INTERVENTIONS
Fall prevention behavior	Fall prevention; environmental management; surveillance: safety; peripheral sensation management

NURSING ASSESSMENT	RATIONALE
Assess for signs and symptoms that client is at risk for injury.	Early recognition of signs and symptoms that place the client at risk for injury allow for prompt intervention.

THERAPEUTIC INTERVENTIONS	RATIONALE

Independent Actions
Implement measures to reduce the risk for injury:
• Perform actions to prevent falls:
    • If client is in a standard hospital bed, keep bed in low position with side rails up. **D** ● ✦
    • If client is in a kinetic bed, use safety measures such as safety straps and padded side pieces. **D** ● ✦
    • Keep safety belts securely fastened when client is on a stretcher or in a wheelchair. **D** ● ✦
    • Obtain adequate assistance when moving client; follow instructions from physical therapist on correct transfer techniques. **D** ● ✦
    • Implement measures to increase client's stability when in a wheelchair (e.g., use wheelchair equipped with an antitipping device, fasten safety belt around upper body and chair to stabilize trunk, use H-straps to keep legs positioned properly).
	These actions will decrease the client's risk for falls and potential injury.

NDx = NANDA-I Diagnosis   **D** = Delegatable Action   ● = UAP   ✦ = LVN/LPN   ⊖▶ = Go to ⊖volve for animation

Continued...

THERAPEUTIC INTERVENTIONS	RATIONALE
• Do not rush client; allow adequate time for the accomplishment of transfers and position changes. **D** ● ✦	
• Perform actions to prevent burns:	
• Let hot foods and fluids cool slightly before serving. **D** ● ✦	*Client may accidentally spill liquids; without ability to feel hot or cold, client may inadvertently cause a burn.*
• Supervise client while smoking; do not place ashtray on client's lap.	*The cigarette could roll off the ashtray onto the client's clothing causing a fire and subsequent burns.*
• Assess temperature of bath water before and during use. **D** ● ✦	*The client has lost sense of feeling and may not be aware that water is too hot and can cause burning.*
• When client is in a wheelchair, instruct the client to avoid placing self next to sources of heat (e.g., heater, stove).	*This will cause the sides of the wheelchair to become hot and burn the client's skin..*
• Encourage client to request assistance whenever needed; have a specially adapted call signal available to client at all times.	*Stretching to reach a call light may cause the client to lose balance and fall out of bed.*
• Perform actions to decrease spasticity (e.g., avoid stimulating extremities or muscle groups; assist client to change position and perform ROM activities).	*It is important to reduce the risk of unexpected body movements to prevent injury.*
Include client and significance others in planning and implementing measures to prevent injury.	*Significant others should be informed on how to help prevent client injury.*
If injury does occur, initiate appropriate first aid and notify physician.	*Notification of the physician allows for modification of the treatment plan.*

Nursing Diagnosis | RISK FOR AUTONOMIC DYSREFLEXIA NDx

Definition: Life-threatening, uninhibited sympathetic response of the nervous system, post spinal shock, in an individual with spinal cord injury or lesion at T6 or above (has been demonstrated in clients with injuries at T7 and T9)

Related to:

Related to loss of autonomic nervous system control below the level of the cord injury (can occur once reflect activity returns after period of spinal shock):

- **Cardiopulmonary stimuli**—Deep vein thrombosis and pulmonary emboli
- **Gastrointestinal stimuli**—Bowel distention, constipation, digital stimulation, enemas, esophageal reflux, Fecal impaction, gall stones, gastric ulcers, Hemorrhoids, suppositories
- **Musculoskeletal-integumentary stimuli**—Cutaneous stimulation , pressure over bony prominences, pressure over genitalia, range-of-motion exercises, spasm, sunburns, wounds
- **Neurological stimuli**—irritating stimuli below of injury, painful stimuli below level of injury
- **Regulatory stimuli**—Extreme environmental temperatures, temperature fluctuations
- **Reproductive stimuli**—Ejaculation, labor and delivery, menstruation, pregnancy
- **Situational stimuli**—Constrictive clothing, drug reactions, narcotic/opiate withdrawal, positioning, surgical procedures
- **Urological stimuli**—Bladder distension and spasm, calculi, catheterization, cystitis, Epididymitis, surgery, urinary tract infection

CLINICAL MANIFESTATIONS

Subjective	Objective
Complaint of a sudden pounding headache; complaint of blurred vision; nausea; report of feelings of apprehension	Sudden onset of severe hypertension; bradycardia; flushing above the lesion; pale extremities below the level of the lesion; profuse diaphoresis above level of injury; piloerection

RISK FACTORS

- Trauma
- Any stimulus that irritates or increases pressure below the level of injury

DESIRED OUTCOMES

The client will not experience autonomic dysreflexia as evidenced by:
  a. Vital signs within normal range for client
  b. Skin dry and usual color above the level of the injury
  c. No reports of pounding headache, nasal congestion, and blurred vision

NOC OUTCOMES

Symptom severity

NIC INTERVENTIONS

Dysreflexia management

NURSING ASSESSMENT

Assess for signs and symptoms of autonomic dysreflexia:
- Sudden rise in B/P (systolic pressure may go as high as 300 mm Hg)
- Bradycardia
- Flushing and profuse diaphoresis above level of injury
- Pounding headache
- Nasal congestion
- Blurred vision

RATIONALE

Autonomic dysreflexia is considered a medical emergency that may occur after the resolution of spinal shock. Early recognition of the signs and symptoms of autonomic dysreflexia allows for prompt intervention.

THERAPEUTIC INTERVENTIONS

RATIONALE

Independent Actions

Implement measures to prevent stimulation of the sympathetic nervous system below the level of the cord injury to prevent autonomic dysreflexia.
- Perform actions to prevent distention of the bladder and bowel:

  Problems with the bladder and bowel are the two most frequent causes of autonomic dysreflexia.
  These interventions promote regular bladder and bowel emptying.

  - Attempt to initiate voiding periodically by stimulating the trigger zones of the reflex sacral arc (e.g., tap suprapubic area, stroke inner thigh, perform anal sphincter stretching, pull pubic hair); if voiding occurs, repeat stimulus as necessary to empty the bladder.
  - If possible, place client on bedside commode or toilet when triggering voiding reflex.

    Gravity promotes emptying of the bladder.

  - Instruct client to space fluid intake evenly throughout the day rather than drinking a large quantity at one time.

    If the bladder fills rapidly and frequency of emptying is not increased, bladder distention occurs.

  - Instruct client to limit intake of alcohol and beverages containing caffeine such as colas, coffee, and tea.

    Alcohol and caffeine have a mild diuretic effect and act as irritants to the bladder; the increased urine production can result in bladder distention if the frequency of bladder emptying is not also increased, and the bladder irritation can trigger bladder spasms and subsequent incontinence.

  - Limit oral fluid intake in the evening. **D** ● ✦

    Limiting oral intake in the evening prevents the bladder from becoming overdistended during the night. As rehabilitation progresses, most clients do not perform intermittent catheterization or attempt to trigger voiding during the night.

  - Instruct client and others to avoid stimulating the voiding reflex trigger zones at times other than during bladder care.

    This reduces the risk of incontinence.

- Implement measures to prevent constipation:
  - Encourage client to drink hot liquids before scheduled bowel evacuation.

    Drinking hot liquids prior to a bowel evacuation helps to stimulate peristalsis.

  - Assist client to eat at scheduled times and adhere to a routine time for defecation; follow client's preinjury pattern if possible. **D** ● ✦

    A scheduled eating and defecation routine helps maintain continence.

NDx = NANDA-I Diagnosis   **D** = Delegatable Action   ● = UAP   ✦ = LVN/_PN   ⊖▶ = Go to ⊖volve for animation

Continued...

THERAPEUTIC INTERVENTIONS	RATIONALE
• Perform actions to prevent pressure on any area of the client's body below the level of the cord injury.	*Pressure below the level of injury may stimulate autonomic dysreflexia.*
• Instruct and assist client to change positions frequently.	*These actions decrease pressure on the non-innervated areas of the body.*
• Ensure that overbed tray is not resting on chest. **D** ● ✦	
• Ensure that clothing is not constrictive and shorts are not too tight.	
• Perform good nail care.	*Long fingernails may stimulate the sympathetic nervous system.*

Dependent/Collaborative Actions

- Perform actions that prevent pressure on any area of the client's body below the level of cord injury.
- Perform intermittent catheterization or insert indwelling catheter as ordered.
- Maintain patency of indwelling catheters. **D** ✦
- Apply a topical anesthetic agent to any existing pressure ulcer.
- Apply a local anesthetic (e.g., Nupercainal ointment) if ordered before performing actions that can result in an exaggerated sympathetic response (e.g., urinary catheterization, removal of a fecal impaction, administration of an enema, care of any wound below the level of the injury).

If signs and symptoms of autonomic dysreflexia occur:

- Immediately implement measures to promote venous pooling and subsequent decrease in B/P (e.g., raise head of bed and lower client's legs unless contraindicated; remove abdominal binder, antiembolism stockings, and intermittent pneumatic compression device if present).
- Administer antihypertensives (e.g., diazoxide, hydralazine, nitroprusside) as ordered.
- Monitor B/P and pulse frequently (usually every 3 to 5 minutes until treatments and/or medication take effect).
- Notify physician immediately if signs and symptoms persist or if complications resulting from severe hypertension occur (e.g., seizures, intraocular hemorrhage, cerebrovascular accident, myocardial infarction).
- Notify all persons participating in client's care of the episode of autonomic dysreflexia because such episodes can reoccur.

These actions prevent the bladder from becoming distended and placing the client at increased risk for autonomic dysreflexia.

Use anesthetic ointment to decrease the risk of aggravating the autonomic dysreflexia.

Immediate treatment is important to prevent a hypertensive stroke. These actions decrease B/P.

Antihypertensive medications decrease blood pressure, which is important in stroke prevention.

These complications can have a very deleterious impact on the body and should be treated immediately to prevent further insult to the body.

The client's treatment plan may need to be altered to address other effects of autonomic dysreflexia.

Collaborative Diagnosis ▪ **RISK FOR ASCENDING SPINAL CORD INJURY**

Definition: Extension of damage from the original spinal cord injury that ascends up the spinal cord

Related to: Further damage to and/or ischemia of the cord above the C5 level associated with vasospasm of damaged vessels, progressive edema, bleeding, compression of cord by hematoma or bone fragments, and/or ineffective immobilization of an unstable cord injury

CLINICAL MANIFESTATIONS

Subjective	Objective
Report of shortness of breath	Increased dyspnea; shallow respirations; dusky or cyanotic skin color; drowsiness; confusion; decreased B/P and heart rate; progressive loss of sensory and motor function

RISK FACTORS

- Trauma
- Changes in hemodynamic status

DESIRED OUTCOMES

The client will not experience spinal cord injury above the level of C5 as evidenced by:
   a. Stable respiratory status
   b. Stable B/P and pulse
   c. No further loss of motor and sensory function

NURSING ASSESSMENT

Assess for and report signs and symptoms of ascending spinal cord injury:
- Respiratory failure (e.g., rapid, shallow respirations; dusky or cyanotic skin color; drowsiness; confusion)
- Significant decrease in B/P and pulse
- Further loss of motor and sensory function

RATIONALE

Early recognition of signs and symptoms of ascending spinal cord injury allows for prompt intervention.

THERAPEUTIC INTERVENTIONS

Implement measures to prevent spinal cord injury above the level of C5:
- Perform actions to maintain immobilization of the spine until stabilization has been accomplished:
   - Do not release or adjust skeletal traction or halo device unless ordered.

   - If skeletal traction is present, keep traction rope and weights hanging freely.
   - Always use turn sheet and adequate assistance when repositioning client.
   - Never use the rods of the halo device as handles. **D** ● ✦
   - Check pin sites of halo or traction device every shift; notify physician if pins are loose. **D** ✦
   - If immobilization device fails (e.g., pins fall out, traction weights drop, rods on halo device disconnect):
      (1) Stabilize client's head, neck, and shoulders with hands, sandbags, or cervical collar.
      (2) Notify physician immediately.

- Use the jaw thrust method rather than hyperextending client's neck if respiratory distress occurs.
- Perform actions to prevent ascending spinal cord ischemia:
   - Implement measures to maintain adequate tissue perfusion.
   - Prepare client for decompression of the spinal cord (e.g., removal of hematoma or bone fragments) if planned.
   - Prepare client for surgical stabilization (e.g., fusion) if planned.

   - Administer corticosteroids and calcium channel blockers if ordered.

If signs and symptoms of ascending spinal cord injury occur, be prepared to assist with intubation or tracheostomy and mechanical ventilation.

RATIONALE

Appropriate healing should occur before changes/adjustments in traction occur, because the changes may extend the area of spinal cord injury.
If weights are not hanging freely, the level of traction changes and may further the spinal cord injury.
Use of a turn sheet helps maintain the spine in proper alignment when repositioning the client.
Use of rods on the halo device to move a client places undue stress on the spinal cord and may further spinal cord injury.
Changes in the tightness of the halo pins or traction devices may extend the area of spinal cord injury.
Stabilize the client's head, neck and shoulders with any means possible to prevent further injury.

The physician must be notified to reestablish traction as soon as possible, thus preventing further injury.
Hyperextending the client's neck may extend the spinal cord injury.

Anything that alters spinal cord tissue perfusion may cause spinal cord ischemia.
Decreases pressure on the spinal cord and improves circulation.

Administration of high doses of methylprednisolone within the first 8 hours after spinal cord injury appears to be the most effective way of slowing the development of ischemia above the level of injury.
Calcium channel blockers decrease vasospasms.

Ascending spinal cord injuries may compromise the client's neurological stimulation to the lungs. Emergency care may be necessary to prevent death.

Collaborative Diagnosis **RISK FOR PARALYTIC ILEUS**

Definition: Paralysis of the intestines resulting in blockage of the intestines

Related to: Absence of neural stimulation of the intestine associated with absence of autonomic nervous system and reflex activity below the level of the spinal cord injury during period of spinal shock

CLINICAL MANIFESTATIONS

Subjective	Objective
Verbal reports of persistent abdominal pain and cramping	Firm, distended abdomen; absent bowel sounds; failure to pass flatus; abdominal x-ray showing distended bowel

RISK FACTORS
* Inability to follow treatment regimen
* Lack of fiber and food in diet

DESIRED OUTCOMES

The client will not develop a paralytic ileus as evidenced by:
  a. Absence or resolution of abdominal pain and cramping
  b. Soft, nondistended abdomen
  c. Gradual return of bowel sounds
  d. Passage of flatus

NURSING ASSESSMENT	RATIONALE
Assess for and report signs and symptoms of paralytic ileus: • Development of or persistent abdominal pain and cramping • Firm, distended abdomen • Absent bowel sounds • Failure to pass flatus	*Early recognition of signs and symptoms of a paralytic ileus allows prompt intervention.*
Monitor results of abdominal x-ray.	*An abdominal x-ray that demonstrates distended bowel and may be indicative of a paralytic ileus.*

THERAPEUTIC INTERVENTIONS	RATIONALE
Collaborative/Dependent Actions If signs and symptoms of paralytic ileus occur: • Withhold all oral intake. • Insert nasogastric tube and maintain suction as ordered. **D ✦**	*Paralytic ileus results in cessation of normal peristalsis. The client should have nothing by mouth (NPO) and have a nasogastric tube in place to facilitate gastric decompression until the ileus is resolved.*
Perform actions to maintain adequate tissue perfusion: • Administer gastrointestinal stimulants (e.g., metoclopramide) if ordered. **D ✦**	*Gastrointestinal stimulants help maintain adequate blood supply to the bowel.*

Collaborative Diagnosis **RISK FOR DEEP VEIN THROMBUS**

Definition: A clot that forms in a vessel wall in the extremities

Related to:
* Venous stasis associated with decreased mobility and decreased vasomotor tone below the level of the injury
* Hypercoagulability associated with increased blood viscosity (if fluid intake is inadequate) and increased levels of calcium in the blood from bone demineralization (can result from prolonged immobility)

CLINICAL MANIFESTATIONS

Subjective	Objective
Verbal reports of pain or tenderness in an extremity	Increase in circumference of extremity; distention of superficial vessels in extremity; unusual warmth of extremity; positive Homans' sign (not always a reliable indicator)

RISK FACTORS

- Changes in cardiovascular status
- Decreased activity

DESIRED OUTCOME

Client will not develop a deep vein thrombosis.

NURSING ASSESSMENT

Assess for and report signs and symptoms of a deep vein thrombus:
- Pain or tenderness in extremity
- Increase in circumference of extremity
- Distention of superficial vessels in extremity
- Unusual warmth of extremity
- Positive Homans' sign (not always a reliable indicator)

RATIONALE

Early recognition of signs and symptoms of deep vein thrombus allows for prompt intervention.

THERAPEUTIC INTERVENTIONS

Independent Actions

Implement measures to maintain adequate blood flow in legs to reduce the risk for thrombus formation and prevent a pulmonary embolism (e.g., maintain adequate fluid intake, use of thromboembolic disorder [TED] hose, position firm pillow between client's legs if spasms tend to cause legs to cross; instruct client to obtain assistance to reposition legs properly, if they do cross).

If signs and symptoms of a deep vein thrombus occur:
- Maintain client on strict bed rest in a semi- to high-Fowler's position.
- Do not exercise, check for Homans' sign in, or massage any extremity known to have a thrombus.

- Caution client to avoid activities that create a Valsalva response (e.g., holding breath while moving up in bed).
- Perform actions to prevent autonomic dysreflexia:
  - Perform measures to decrease incidence of a distended bladder and/or bowel.
  - Prevent pressure on any area of the client's body below the level of cord injury because this may lead to autonomic dysreflexia.

Collaborative/Dependent Actions

Implement measures to prevent deep vein thrombus formation:
- Apply mechanical devices designed to increase venous return in the immobile patient:
  - Sequential compression devices
  - Thromboembolic (TED) stockings **D** ✦
- Maintain a minimum fluid intake of 2500 mL/day (unless contraindicated). **D** ✦

If signs and symptoms of a deep vein thrombus occur:
- Administer anticoagulants:
  - Low- or adjusted-dose heparin
  - Fondaparinux

RATIONALE

Adequate blood flow in the legs reduces the risk for thrombus formation and prevents a thromboembolus from occurring.

Avoid putting pressure on the posterior knees because this action will compress the leg veins, increasing turbulent blood flow, and increasing the risk of thrombus formation. If a thrombus is suspected, elevate the affected extremity and do not massage the area because of the danger of dislodging the thrombus.

Valsalva response changes pressure in the chest cavity, which may dislodge a venous thrombus.

A full bladder or bowel is a major precipitator of autonomic dysreflexia.

Autonomic dysreflexia changes systemic B/P and may dislodge a clot from a vessel wall.

These sequential compression devices and TED stockings decrease venous stasis in the lower extremities and increase venous return through the deep leg veins, which are prone to the formation of a thrombus.

Adequate hydration helps reduces blood viscosity and decreases the incidence of deep vein thrombus.

Anticoagulants, if indicated, help suppress the formation of clots.

NDx = NANDA-I Diagnosis   **D** = Delegatable Action   ● = UAP   ✦ = LVN/LPN   ⊖▶ = Go to ⊖volve for animation

Continued...

THERAPEUTIC INTERVENTIONS	RATIONALE
• Warfarin • Low-molecular-weight heparin • Prepare client for diagnostic studies (e.g., venography, duplex ultrasound, impedance plethysmography). • Maintain oxygen therapy as ordered. **D** ✦	*Additional studies may be indicated to confirm the presence of a deep vein thrombus so the appropriate interventions can be implemented.* *Supplemental oxygen helps maintain adequate tissue oxygenation.*

Collaborative Diagnosis   # RISK FOR PULMONARY EMBOLISM

Definition: A clot that detaches from the vessel wall and circulates within the blood, becoming lodged in the pulmonary vasculature

Related to:

* Venous stasis associated with decreased activity, positioning during and after surgery, increased blood viscosity (can result from deficient fluid volume), and abdominal distention (the distended intestine may put pressure on the abdominal vessels)
* Hypercoagulability associated with increased release of tissue thromboplastin into the blood (occurs as a result of surgical trauma) and hemoconcentration and increased blood viscosity (can occur as a result of deficient fluid volume)
* Trauma to vein walls during surgery

CLINICAL MANIFESTATIONS

Subjective	Objective
Verbal reports of sudden chest or shoulder pain or shortness of breath	Dyspnea; tachypnea; tachycardia; apprehension; low partial pressure of oxygen in arterial blood (PaO_2)

RISK FACTORS
* Hypercoagulability
* Immobility

DESIRED OUTCOMES

The client will not experience a pulmonary embolism as evidenced by:
  a. Absence of sudden chest or shoulder pain
  b. Unlabored respirations at 12 to 20 breaths/min
  c. Pulse rate 60 to 100 beats/min
  d. Arterial blood gas values within normal range

NURSING ASSESSMENT	RATIONALE
Assess for and report signs and symptoms of a pulmonary embolism: • Sudden chest or shoulder pain • Dyspnea • Tachypnea • Tachycardia • Apprehension • Low PaO_2	*Early recognition of signs and symptoms of a pulmonary embolism allows for prompt intervention.*
Monitor continuous pulse oximetry.	*Pulse oximetry is an indirect measure of arterial oxygen saturation (SaO_2). Monitoring pulse oximetry (SaO_2) allows for early detection of hypoxia and implementation of the appropriate interventions.*
Monitor arterial blood gas values.	*Pulmonary embolism is suggested if arterial blood gas values indicate hypoxemia (PaO_2 <80 mm Hg) and hyperventilation (low partial pressure of carbon dioxide in arterial blood [$PaCO_2$]).*
Monitor D-dimer laboratory results for abnormalities.	*Elevated levels of D-dimer in the blood in combination with computed tomography (CT) pulmonary angiography results are indicative of pulmonary embolism.*
Monitor results of perfusion scan and/or CT pulmonary angiography.	

THERAPEUTIC INTERVENTIONS	RATIONALE

Independent Actions

Implement measures to prevent a pulmonary embolism:

- Perform actions to prevent and treat a deep vein thrombus.
  - Do not exercise, check for Homans' sign in, or massage any extremity known to have a thrombus.

  - Caution client to avoid activities that create a Valsalva response:
    (1) Straining to have bowel movement
    (2) Holding breath while moving up in bed

If signs and symptoms of a pulmonary embolism occur:

- Maintain client on strict bedrest in semi- to high Fowler's position.

The most common sources of pulmonary emboli are dislodged thrombi from the deep veins in the thighs.
If a venous thromboembolism is suspected, actions should be implemented to prevent dislodgment of an existing thrombi.
Pressure on the legs may dislodge a thrombus
Valsalva response changes pressure in the chest cavity, which may dislodge a venous thrombus.

Dependent/Collaborative Actions

If signs and symptoms of a pulmonary embolism occur:

- Maintain oxygen therapy as ordered. **D** ✦

Supplemental oxygen is indicated to correct the hypoxemia associated with a pulmonary embolism. The concentration of oxygen administered should be guided by pulse oximetry and/or arterial blood gas analysis.

- Prepare client for diagnostic tests:
  - Arterial blood gases
  - D-dimer level
  - Ventilation-perfusion lung scan
  - Pulmonary angiography
- Administer anticoagulants: **D** ✦
  - Heparin
  - Warfarin

- Prepare client for surgical intervention:
  - Vena caval interruption device (vena cava filter).
  - Embolectomy

Diagnosis of a pulmonary embolism is confirmed using a combination of tests.

Anticoagulants, if indicated, help suppress the formation of clots. The best action is to prevent the formation of thromboemboli in those at risk.
A vena caval interruption device helps prevent further pulmonary emboli. An embolectomy removes the clot from the body.

Collaborative Diagnosis   RISK FOR GASTROINTESTINAL BLEEDING

Definition: Bleeding that occurs in the gastrointestinal (GI) tract

Related to:
- Erosions of the gastric and duodenal mucosa (can develop as a result of the increased output of hydrochloric acid that occurs with stress)
- Irritation of the gastric mucosa associated with side effect of certain medications (e.g., corticosteroids)

CLINICAL MANIFESTATIONS

Subjective	Objective
Verbalization of shoulder pain, abdominal pain	Frank/occult blood in stool or gastric contents; decreased B/P, increased heart rate; decreasing red blood cell (RBC) count, hemoglobin (Hgb) and hematocrit (Hct) levels

Continued...

RISK FACTORS	DESIRED OUTCOMES
• Stress • Anxiety • Medication regimen	The client will not experience GI bleeding as evidenced by: a. No reports of shoulder pain b. Absence of frank and occult blood in stool and gastric contents c. B/P and pulse within normal range for client d. RBC count, Hct and Hgb levels within normal range

NURSING ASSESSMENT	RATIONALE
Assess for and report signs and symptoms of GI bleeding (e.g.. reports of shoulder pain [referred]; frank or occult blood in stool or gastric contents; decreased B/P; increased pulse rate; decreasing RBC count, Hct and Hgb levels).	*Early recognition of signs and symptoms of GI bleeding allows for prompt intervention.*

THERAPEUTIC INTERVENTIONS	RATIONALE

Independent Actions

Implement measures to prevent ulceration of the gastric and duodenal mucosa:

• Perform actions to decrease fear and anxiety (e.g., introduce client to staff, place call bell within client's hand, answer call promptly).	*These actions decrease fear, anxiety, and stress, thus decreasing the release of endogenous steroids.*
• Instruct client to avoid acidic foods/fluids that stimulate hydrochloric acid secretions or irritate the gastric mucosa (e.g., coffee, caffeine-containing tea and colas; spices such as black pepper, chili powder, and nutmeg).	*Acidic foods/fluids increases acidity in the GI tract and risk for GI bleeding.*

Dependent/Collaborative Actions

Implement measures to prevent ulceration of the gastric and duodenal mucosa:

• Administer histamine$_2$-receptor antagonists, proton-pump inhibitors, antacids, and/or cytoprotective agents, if ordered.	*Histamine receptor antagonists and proton-pump inhibitors suppress secretion of gastric acid. Antacids neutralize stomach acid and cytoprotective agents create a protective barrier against stomach acid and pepsin.*

If signs and symptoms of GI bleeding occur:

• Insert nasogastric tube and maintain suction as ordered.	*Insertion of an NG tube to facilitate suction removes gastric acid and pressure on the gastric lining.*
• Administer blood products and/or volume expanders if ordered.	*Hypotension may occur; administration of blood and/or volume expanders may be needed to maintain adequate blood pressure and tissue perfusion.*
• Assist with measures to control bleeding (e.g., gastric lavage, endoscopic electrocoagulation) if planned.	*These interventions decrease or stops GI bleeding.*

Collaborative Diagnosis ▪ **RISK FOR CONTRACTURES**

Definition: The permanent shortening of muscles or tendon

Related to:

• Muscle atrophy and lack of joint movement associated with prolonged immobility and quadriplegia
• Prolonged periods of hip flexion associated with use of wheelchair
• Difficulty putting joints through full range of motion associated with severe spasticity if it occurs and/or heterotopic ossification (excessive bone formation that can begin to develop around joints of paralyzed limbs as early as 1 month after the spinal cord injury)

CLINICAL MANIFESTATIONS

Subjective	Objective
Statements of shoulder pain or stiffness	Limited range of motion; stiffness; redness, unusual warmth, and swelling of joints in paralyzed limbs

RISK FACTOR

- Ineffective passive/active range of motion

DESIRED OUTCOME

The client will not develop contractures as evidenced by normal or expected range of motion.

NURSING ASSESSMENT	RATIONALE
Assess for and report the following: • Statements of shoulder joint stiffness • Limitations in range of motion • Redness, unusual warmth, and swelling of joints in paralyzed limbs (can be indicative of heterotopic ossification, which can cause restricted movement of the involved joint)	*Early recognition of signs and symptoms of developing contractures allows for prompt intervention.*

THERAPEUTIC INTERVENTIONS	RATIONALE
Independent Actions Implement measures to reduce the risk of contracture: • Perform actions to reduce spasticity (e.g., perform and assist the client with active and active-resistance exercises, instruct client and assist with use of mobility devices, implement exercise plan). **D** ✦	*Movement and exercise of limbs help reduce muscle spasticity and prevent contractures.*
• Position client in prone or supine position routinely unless contraindicated. **D** ✦	*Use of these positions counteract prolonged periods of hip flexion resulting from wheel chair use.*
Dependent/Collaborative Actions Implement measures to reduce the risk of contracture: • Administer etidronate if ordered. • Prepare client for surgical removal of abnormal bone formation around joints if planned.	*Etidronate is used to prevent or treat heterotopic ossification.* *Removal of abnormal bone formation around the joints helps maintain joint mobility.*

Nursing Diagnosis ## RISK FOR SEXUAL DYSFUNCTION NDx

Definition: The state in which an individual experiences a change in sexual function during the sexual response phases of desire, excitation, and/or orgasm that is viewed as unsatisfying, unrewarding, or inadequate

Related to:
- Decreased libido associated with:
  - Loss of sensory and voluntary motor function below the level of spinal cord injury
  - Presence of a urinary catheter and/or fear of urinary and bowel incontinence
  - Depression, disturbed self-concept
  - Fear of rejection by partner
  - Fear of autonomic dysreflexia (genital stimulation can cause dysreflexia)
- Decreased ability to control and maintain an erection associated with loss of ability to have a psychogenic erection (only reflexogenic erection is possible)
- Altered ejaculatory flow associated with impaired nerve function in the bladder neck (can result in retrograde ejaculation)

CLINICAL MANIFESTATIONS

Subjective	Objective
Verbalization of sexual dysfunction; stated inability to achieve sexual satisfaction or feelings of being sexually unattractive	Limitations imposed by quadriplegia specific to sexual dysfunction

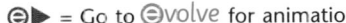

NDx = NANDA-I Diagnosis   **D** = Delegatable Action   ● = UAP   ✦ = LVN/LPN   ⊖▶ = Go to ⊖volve for animation

Continued...

RISK FACTORS

- Fear
- Trauma
- Loss of control of body

DESIRED OUTCOMES

The client will demonstrate beginning acceptance of changes in sexual functioning as evidenced by:
  a. Verbalization of a perception of self as sexually acceptable and adequate
  b. Statements reflecting beginning adjustment to the effects of the spinal cord injury on sexual functioning
  c. Maintenance of relationship with significant other

NOC OUTCOMES

Sexual identity; sexual functioning

NIC INTERVENTIONS

Sexual counseling

NURSING ASSESSMENT	RATIONALE
Assess for signs and symptoms of sexual dysfunction (e.g., verbalization of sexual concerns or inability to achieve sexual satisfaction, alteration in relationship with significant other, limitations imposed by quadriplegia).	*Recognition that the spinal cord injury patient will experience sexual dysfunction will alert the nurse to assess for both physical and mental alterations.*

THERAPEUTIC INTERVENTIONS	RATIONALE

Independent Actions
Implement measures to promote an optimal level of sexual functioning:

- Facilitate communication between client and partner; focus on the feelings the couple share and assist them to identify changes that affect their sexual relationship.

  Communication between partners about how the physical changes will affect their sexual relationship is important.

- Discuss ways to be creative in expressing sexuality (e.g., massage, fantasies, cuddling).

  Client will require education on ways that he or she can express sexuality.

- Suggest alternative methods of sexual gratification and use of assistive devices if appropriate; encourage partner to explore erogenous areas on the client's lips, neck, and ears.

  Learning different ways of maintaining a sexual relationship will take time.

- Arrange for uninterrupted privacy if desired by the couple.
  D ✦

  Arranging time for couples to explore their sexual relationship fosters closeness between partners.

- Inform male client and his partner of techniques for eliciting and maintaining reflexogenic erection (e.g., stimulate genitalia, stroke inner thigh, pull on pubic hairs, stimulate the rectum, manipulate the urinary catheter).

  Sexual activity in clients with spinal cord injury requires different approaches and the possible use of assistive devices.

- If client has difficulty maintaining an erection, encourage him to discuss various treatment options (e.g., vacuum erection aids, penile prosthesis) with physician if desired.

- If client experiences episodes of autonomic dysreflexia, instruct client to consult physician about ways to prevent it during sexual activity (e.g., have partner apply a local anesthetic to client's genitalia).

  To decrease the incidence of autonomic dysreflexia during sex, the client should be instructed to have the partner apply a local anesthetic to client's genitalia.

- Inform female client that vaginal lubrication can occur by local stimulation or can be enhanced by using a water-soluble lubricant.

  Female clients may need to use a water-soluble lubricant.

- If incontinence of urine is a concern, instruct client to:
  - Limit fluid intake 2 to 4 hours before sexual activity.
  - Have bladder emptied immediately before sexual activity.

  These actions limit urinary incontinence during sexual activity.

- Instruct client to perform bowel care several hours before sexual activity.

  This action reduces the risk of bowel incontinence if anal or rectal stimulation occurs during sexual activity.

THERAPEUTIC INTERVENTIONS	RATIONALE
• If appropriate, involve partner in care of client.	*Involvement of partner of client helps the partner adjust to the changes in the client's appearance and body functioning and subsequently decreases the possibility of partner's rejection of the client.*
• Encourage client to rest before sexual activity.	*The client needs to conserve energy before sexual activity to avoid fatigue.*
• Instruct client and partner to establish a relaxed, unhurried atmosphere for sexual activity.	*Providing an unhurried atmosphere for sexual activity allows the client and partner to explore what activities will provide sexual gratification including varying positions, use of explicit films and assist devices.*
• Discuss positions that may facilitate sexual activity (e.g., lying on side, client in supine position).	
• Provide explicit films and literature if desired by client and/or partner.	
• Include partner in above discussions and encourage continued support of the client.	*Changes in the client's functioning has a great impact on the partner, and to improve chances of a positive sexual relationship, the partner should be included in discussions on sexual activity.*

Dependent/Collaborative Actions

Consult appropriate health care provider (e.g., sex counselor, physician) when client is ready for sexual counseling and/or sexual counseling appears indicated.

The expertise of a sexual counselor will provide a multidisciplinary approach to a client's sexual activity.

Nursing Diagnosis INTERRUPTED FAMILY PROCESSES NDx

Definition: Change in family relationships and/or functioning

Related to:
• Change in family roles and structure associated with a family member's sudden, catastrophic injury, permanent disability, and need for extensive rehabilitation

CLINICAL MANIFESTATIONS

Subjective	Objective
Statements of being unable to accept client's quadriplegia or paraplegia	Disruptive family interactions; inability to use coping strategies; refusal to participate in client's care

RISK FACTOR
• Poor coping mechanisms

DESIRED OUTCOMES

The family members* will demonstrate beginning adjustment to changes in functioning of a family member and family roles and structure as evidenced by:
a. Meeting client's needs
b. Verbalization of ways to adapt to required role and lifestyle changes
c. Active participation in decision-making and client's rehabilitation
d. Positive interactions with one another

NOC OUTCOMES

Family coping; family functioning; family resiliency; family normalization

NIC INTERVENTIONS

Family involvement promotion; family integrity promotion; family process maintenance; family support; family mobilization; support system enhancement

*The term "family members" is being used here to include client's significant others.

NDx = NANDA-I Diagnosis   **D** = Delegatable Action   ● = UAP   ✦ = LVN/LPN   ⊖▶ = Go to ⊖volve for animation

Continued...

NURSING ASSESSMENT	RATIONALE
Assess for signs and symptoms of interrupted family processes (e.g., inability to meet client's needs, statements of not being able to accept client's quadriplegia or make necessary role and lifestyle changes, inability to make decisions, inability or refusal to participate in client's rehabilitation, negative family interactions).	*Early recognition of signs and symptoms of interrupted family processes allows for prompt intervention.*
Identify components of the family and the patterns of communication and role expectations.	

THERAPEUTIC INTERVENTIONS	RATIONALE

Independent Actions

Implement measures to facilitate family members' adjustment to client's diagnosis, changes in client's functioning within the family system, and altered family roles and structure:

- Encourage verbalization of feelings about the client's quadriplegia and its effect on family structure; actively listen to each family member and maintain a nonjudgmental attitude about feelings shared.

  Verbalization of feelings promotes communication and support for family members and may positively impact coping.

- Reinforce physician's explanations of the effects of the injury and planned treatment and rehabilitation.

  Information helps the client's family understand what is happening and keeps them informed of the management of care.

- Assist family members to gain a realistic perspective of client's situation, conveying as much hope as appropriate.

  Keep the family informed concerning what is occurring, answer questions as needed, assist in their understanding of a spinal cord injury while maintaining hope for the future.

- Provide privacy for the client and family and stress the importance of and facilitate the use of good communication techniques.

  It is important that the client and family share feelings as they deal with the client's body changes.

- Assist family members to progress through their own grieving process; explain that they may encounter times when they need to focus on meeting their own needs rather than the client's needs.

  The client's injury has a major impact on the life of the family, and family members will go through a grieving process. They need to be reassured as they work through the changes that have occurred in the family processes.

- Emphasize the need for family members to obtain adequate rest and nutrition and to identify and use stress management techniques.

  Family members need to take care of themselves so that they are better able to emotionally and physically deal with the changes and losses experienced.

- Encourage and assist family members to identify coping strategies for dealing with the client's body changes and the effects on the family.

  Reinforce family members' regular coping mechanisms and implement new techniques as needed.

- Assist family members to identify realistic goals and ways of reaching those goals.

  The setting of realistic goals will help the family feel that they have some control over the situation and their ability to care for the client once discharged.

- Include family members in decision-making about the client and care; convey appreciation for their input and continued support of client.

  Including the family in the care of the client and decision-making helps to improve family members' confidence in their ability to care for the client.

- Encourage and allow family members to participate in client's care and rehabilitation.

- Assist family members in identifying resources that can assist them in coping with their feelings and meeting their immediate and long-term needs (e.g., counseling and social services; caregiver assistance programs; pastoral care; service, church, and spinal cord injury groups); initiate a referral if indicated.

  Community resources can provide mental support, respite care, and information that can help the family reach rehabilitation goals.

Dependent/Collaborative Actions

Consult appropriate health care provider (e.g., psychiatric nurse clinician, physician) if family members continue to demonstrate difficulty adapting to changes in client's functioning and family structure.

Consultation with other health care providers may increase the family members' success in adapting to changes in the client's functioning and in the family structure.

DISCHARGE TEACHING/CONTINUED CARE

Nursing Diagnosis # DEFICIENT KNOWLEDGE NDx; INEFFECTIVE FAMILY THERAPEUTIC REGIMEN MANAGEMENT NDx; OR INEFFECTIVE HEALTH MAINTENANCE*† NDx

Definition: Absence or deficiency of cognitive information related to specific topic (lack of specific information necessary for clients/significant others) to make informed choices regarding condition/treatment/lifestyle changes; inability to identify, manage, and/or seek out help to manage health; pattern of regulating and integrating into family processes a program for treatment of illness and the sequelae of illness that is unsatisfactory for meeting specific health goals

CLINICAL MANIFESTATIONS

Subjective	Objective
Verbalizes inability to manage illness; verbalizes inability to follow prescribed regimen	Inaccurate follow through with instructions; inappropriate behaviors; experience of preventable complications of spinal cord injury

RISK FACTORS

- Cognitive deficit
- Financial concerns
- Failure to take action to reduce risk factors for complications of spinal cord injury
- Inability to care for oneself
- Difficulty in modifying personal habits and integrating treatments into lifestyle

NOC OUTCOMES

Knowledge: treatment regimen; knowledge: health behavior; knowledge: health resources; knowledge: treatment procedure(s)

NIC INTERVENTIONS

Teaching: individual; teaching: prescribed activity/exercise; teaching: psychomotor skills; health system guidance; financial resource assistance; support system enhancement

NURSING ASSESSMENT

Assess the client's ability to learn and readiness to learn. Assess the client's understanding of teaching.

RATIONALE

Learning is more effective when the client is motivated and understands the importance of what is to be learned. Readiness to learn changes based on situations, physical and emotional challenges.

THERAPEUTIC INTERVENTIONS

Desired Outcome: The client will identify ways to prevent complications associated with spinal cord injury and decreased mobility.

RATIONALE

*The nurse should select the diagnostic label that is most appropriate for the client's discharge teaching needs.
†Although the client will not be able to perform many of the following actions independently, he/she must be knowledgeable about them in order to provide proper instruction to significant others and attendant and maintain an active role in the rehabilitation process.

NDx = NANDA-I Diagnosis   **D** = Delegatable Action   ● = UAP   ✦ = LVN/LPN   ⊖▶ = Go to ⊖volve for animation

Continued...

THERAPEUTIC INTERVENTIONS	RATIONALE

Independent Actions

Instruct client in ways to prevent complications associated with spinal cord injury:

- Position firm pillow between legs if spasms tend to cause legs to cross.
- Wear an abdominal binder when changing from a reclining to a sitting position and take vasoconstrictor drugs if prescribed to prevent dizziness and fainting.
- Elevate legs periodically during the day.

- Implement measures to reduce severe spasticity (e.g., avoid fatigue and chills, change position at least every 2 hours, take muscle relaxants as prescribed).
- Use full-length and long-handled mirrors to examine all skin surfaces in the morning and the evening; increase pressure relief measures if any areas of redness or pallor develop.
- Obtain a kinetic bed for home use if possible.
- Wear shoes when in wheelchair.
- Avoid putting items such as coins, keys, and wallet in skirt or pant pockets.
- Avoid wearing tight-fitting belts, clothing, shoes, and jewelry; make sure that urine collection leg bag straps are not too tight.
- Replace wheelchair cushions when they become worn-out.
- Implement measures to prevent hyperthermia (e.g., avoid excessive clothing and bedding, limit length of time in direct sunlight in hot weather, wear a wide-brimmed hat when in direct sun, park your car or van in the shade in hot weather and open the doors to let the vehicle cool down before getting inside).
- Implement measures to prevent hypothermia (e.g., wear adequate amounts of clothing, wear a hat when in a cold environment, drink warm liquids).
- Implement measures to prevent falls (e.g., always use safety belt during transfers and when in chair, be certain to have adequate assistance for transfer activity).
- Implement measures to prevent burns:
  - Always check temperature of shower or bath water before use (can use bath water thermometer or have attendant check water temperature).
  - Never smoke when alone; do not place ashtray in lap.
  - Let hot foods/fluids cool slightly before attempting to feed self.
  - Never position self next to a stove, heater, or other major source of heat; be aware of where feet and legs are in relation to car heater when it is on.
  - Never use an electric heating pad or electric blanket.
- Implement measures to prevent autonomic dysreflexia:
  - Continue with effective bladder and bowel programs to prevent urinary retention and constipation/impaction.
  - Change position frequently.
  - Seek medical attention at first sign of infection, persistent pressure area, or ingrown toenail.

Use of firm pillows between legs helps prevent thrombus formation and adduction contractures

An abdominal binder supports the abdominal muscles and helps prevent injury.

Elevation of the legs prevents blood from pooling in the lower extremities and decreases the incidence of orthostatic hypotension.

These actions improve mobility and prevent contractures.

Daily skin assessment helps identify pressure areas to prevent skin breakdown

Use of a kinetic bed helps to prevent skin breakdown

Wearing shoes helps prevents injury to feet.

These items can cause pressure on underlying skin areas when placed in skirt or pants pockets.

These actions assure that there is no unnecessary pressure on the skin that may lead to skin breakdown.

The client is unable to maintain body temperature. These interventions help prevent hyperthermia injuries.

These actions help the client maintain appropriate body temperature.

These interventions help prevent client injuries.

These actions help prevent hyperthermia injuries.

Autonomic dysreflexia is a life-threatening emergency requiring immediate treatment. These actions help prevent autonomic dysreflexia. Bladder and bowel distention are the primary causes of dysreflexia and should be prevented.

THERAPEUTIC INTERVENTIONS	RATIONALE
• Apply a local anesthetic (e.g., Nupercainal ointment) to area being stimulated before procedures/activities that have previously resulted in episodes of autonomic dysreflexia (e.g., urinary catheterization, administration of an enema, sexual activity).	
Demonstrate the following procedures to client, significant others, and attendant: • Assisted coughing technique (quad-cough) • Heimlich maneuver • Skin care • Proper positioning and padding • Transfer techniques • Active and passive range-of-motion exercises • Application of elastic stockings, abdominal binder, and heel and elbow protectors • Emergency treatment of autonomic dysreflexia (e.g., elevate head of bed and lower client's legs, alleviate causative factor, administer an antihypertensive agent) Allow time for questions, clarification, and return demonstration.	*The client's family members should provide a return demonstration on client care and prevention of injuries so that they are able to perform these correctly and may help the client maintain functional status.*

THERAPEUTIC INTERVENTIONS	RATIONALE

Desired Outcome: The client will demonstrate the ability to correctly use and maintain assistive devices.

Independent Actions

Reinforce instructions from physical and occupational therapists regarding use of assistive devices. Allow time for questions, clarification, and return demonstration.	*Clarification of information and understanding of how to improve health status*
Instruct and demonstrate for client proper maintenance of assistive devices (e.g., replace parts that are worn-out or broken, clean wheel hubs and crossbars of wheelchairs per manufacturer's instructions, keep wheelchair tires properly inflated).	*Assist devices need to be kept in good working order to prevent client injury and help the client maintain independence and self-care.*

THERAPEUTIC INTERVENTIONS	RATIONALE

Desired Outcome: The client will identify ways to manage altered bowel and bladder function.

Independent Actions

Reinforce bladder and bowel training programs.	*Proper bladder and bowel elimination are important in preventing autonomic dysreflexia and other possible complications.*
Demonstrate bowel care (e.g., digital stimulation, insertion of suppositories, administration of enemas) and bladder care (e.g., stimulation techniques, intermittent catheterization, application of leg bag and bedside drainage bag, emptying of urinary collection bag). Allow time for questions, clarification, and return demonstration.	

THERAPEUTIC INTERVENTIONS	RATIONALE

Desired Outcome: The client will state signs and symptoms to report to the health care provider.

NDx = NANDA-I Diagnosis   **D** = Delegatable Action   ● = UAP   ✦ = LVN/LPN   ⊖▶ = Go to ⊖volve for animation

Continued...

THERAPEUTIC INTERVENTIONS	RATIONALE

Independent Actions

Instruct the client to report the following:

- Cloudy or foul-smelling urine
- Nausea and vomiting
- Cough productive of purulent, green, or rust-colored sputum
- Difficulty breathing or increased shortness of breath with activity
- Sudden or persistent shoulder pain (this can be a referred pain)
- Fever
- Chills or profuse sweating (can occur above the level of the injury)
- Increase in spasticity (could indicate an infection below the level of the injury)
- Unsuccessful bowel and/or bladder programs
- Redness in any extremity
- Swelling that appears suddenly, occurs only in one extremity, or does not subside overnight
- Increased restriction of any joint motion
- Persistent swelling over a joint
- Signs and symptoms of autonomic dysreflexia (e.g., pounding headache, sudden rise in B/P, blurred vision, slow pulse, flushing and sweating above level of injury, nasal congestion) that do not subside once the stimulus is removed
- Any area of persistent skin irritation or breakdown
- Indications of pregnancy (stress that appropriate prenatal care should be initiated as soon as possible)

Client and significant others should be instructed on the clinical manifestations of infections and other changes in health status and to inform their health care practitioner to prevent further injury or decline in health status.

THERAPEUTIC INTERVENTIONS	RATIONALE

Desired Outcome: The client will identify resources that can assist with financial needs, home management, and adjustment to changes resulting from spinal cord injury.

Independent Actions

Inform client and significant others about resources that can assist with financial needs, home management, and adjustment to changes resulting from spinal cord injury (e.g., spinal cord injury support and social groups; state and federally funded financial programs; home health agencies; community health agencies; local service groups; financial, individual, family, and vocational counselors).

Initiate a social service referral if indicated.

Community resources may provide the client and family with multiple levels of assistance (e.g., financial, social support, counseling).

A referral may be required for the client and family to access community resources.

THERAPEUTIC INTERVENTIONS	RATIONALE

Desired Outcome: The client will verbalize an understanding of plan for adhering to recommended follow-up care including future appointments with health care provider and occupational and physical therapists, and medications prescribed.

THERAPEUTIC INTERVENTIONS	RATIONALE

Independent Actions

Reinforce the importance of keeping scheduled follow-up visits with health care provider, occupational and physical therapists.

Explain the rationale for, side effects of, drug-to-drug and drug-to-food interactions, and importance of taking medications as prescribed.

Implement measures designed to improve client adherence:
- Include significant others and caregivers in teaching sessions.
- Encourage questions and allow time for reinforcement and clarification of information provided.
- Provide written instructions on scheduled appointments with health care provider and occupational and physical therapists, medications prescribed, and signs and symptoms to report.

The client requires life-long care and follow-up appointments help maintain health status.

Knowledge of the medication regimen and the impact of these medications on the system, as well as how the medication regimen can be incorporated into the client's lifestyle, allows the client some mechanism of control of his/her disease and the ability to have an active part in treatment and care.

An informed client and family are better able to adhere to a treatment regimen.

Understanding the impact of medications on the individual will allow the client to recognize changes and inform his/her health care practitioner as needed.

ADDITIONAL NURSING DIAGNOSES

FEAR AND ANXIETY NDx
Related to:
- Extensive loss of motor and sensory function
- Application of immobilization device to stabilize and align the cervical spine
- Lack of understanding of diagnostic tests, diagnosis, and treatment
- Unfamiliar environment
- Financial concerns
- Anticipated effects of the spinal cord injury on lifestyle and roles

INEFFECTIVE BREATHING PATTERN NDx
Related to:
- Decreased depth of respirations associated with:
  - The depressant effect of some medications (e.g., narcotic [opioid] analgesics, centrally acting muscle relaxants)
  - Weakness, fatigue, and decreased activity
  - Restricted chest expansion resulting from:
    (1) Loss of abdominal and intercostal muscle function (innervation of these muscles occurs at the thoracic level)
    (2) Impaired function of the diaphragm (the diaphragm is innervated by the phrenic nerve, which travels through segments 3 to 5 of the cervical spine)
    (3) Upward pressure on the diaphragm (can occur as a result of gastric distention if paralytic ileus develops during period of spinal shock)
    (4) Recumbent positioning (in this position, full expansion of the lungs is restricted by the bed surface and the abdominal contents pushing up against the diaphragm)
    (5) Improper fit or application of halo vest or abdominal binder

- Decreased rate of respirations associated with the depressant effect of some medications (e.g., narcotic [opioid] analgesics, centrally acting muscle relaxants)

INEFFECTIVE AIRWAY CLEARANCE NDx
Related to stasis of secretions associated with:
- Decreased mobility
- Decreased effectiveness of cough resulting from diminished lung/chest wall expansion, depressant effect of certain medications (e.g., narcotic [opioid] analgesics, centrally acting muscle relaxants), and possible tenacious secretions if fluid intake is inadequate

ACUTE/CHRONIC PAIN NDx
- Headache related to contractures of the neck muscles (can occur in response to stress and/or neck pain)
- Neck pain related to nerve root irritation at the site of spinal cord injury, muscle stiffness while immobilization device is in place, and muscle strain associated with increased use of neck muscles after removal of immobilization device
- Upper arm and shoulder pain related to muscle strain associated with increased use of biceps and shoulders as activity progresses

IMBALANCED NUTRITION: LESS THAN BODY REQUIREMENTS NDx
Related to:
- Decreased oral intake associated with:
  - Dietary restrictions during period of spinal shock if paralytic ileus develops
  - Anorexia resulting from fatigue, depression and social isolation, the effect of negative nitrogen balance, and early satiety that occurs with decreased gastrointestinal motility

Continued...

- Difficulty swallowing resulting from neck hyperextension and/or horizontal body position during the time that the cervical spine is immobilized
- Difficulty feeding self
- Increased nutritional needs associated with an imbalance in the rate of catabolism and anabolism (catabolic processes occur at a faster rate than anabolic processes in persons who have sustained a spinal cord injury and in those who are immobile)

DISTURBED SENSORY PERCEPTION NDx
- Visual related to decreased ability to move head associated with presence of immobilization device and recumbent position
- Tactile related to loss of integrity of ascending spinal pathways at the level of the cord injury

RISK FOR ASPIRATION NDx
Related to:
- Decreased ability to clear tracheobronchial passages associated with inability to cough forcefully resulting from weakness of the diaphragm and paralysis of the abdominal and intercostal muscles
- Difficulty swallowing associated with neck hyperextension and/or horizontal body positioning during the time that the cervical spine is immobilized.

RISK FOR POWERLESSNESS NDx
Related to:
- Quadriplegia
- Dependence on others
- Changes in roles, relationships, and future plans

GRIEVING NDx
Related to extensive loss of motor and sensory function and the effects of this loss on future lifestyle and roles

RISK FOR LONELINESS NDx
Related to inability to participate in usual activities, decreased contact with significant others and friends while in the hospital and extended care or rehabilitation facility, depression, and withdrawal from others

IMPAIRED PHYSICAL MOBILITY NDx
Related to:
- Activity limitations associated with quadriplegia and immobilization of the spine
- Spasticity after the period of spinal shock associated with stimulation of the reflex arcs below the level of the injury
- Decreased motivation associated with fatigue and the physiological response to the extensive motor and sensory losses that have occurred
- Pain
- Loss of muscle mass, tone, and strength in areas of existing motor function (biceps, upper shoulders, and neck) associated with prolonged disuse (more likely to occur when client is in skeletal traction and must remain in bed)
- Contractures (if they develop)

SELF-CARE DEFICIT NDx
Related to impaired physical mobility associated with quadriplegia, spasticity, decreased motivation, pain, weakness, and activity restrictions imposed by treatment plan

IMPAIRED UNRINARY ELIMINATION NDx
Retention related to:
- Atony of bladder wall during period of spinal shock
- Spasticity of the external urinary sphincter and/or loss of ability to coordinate bladder contraction and relaxation of the external urinary sphincter after period of spinal shock
- Incomplete bladder emptying associated with horizontal positioning (in this position, the gravity needed for complete bladder emptying is lost)
Incontinence related to :
- Spasticity of the bladder after period of spinal shock and loss of ability to contract the external urinary sphincter voluntarily (incontinence can occur if the bladder contracts strongly when the external urinary sphincter is relaxed)
- Inadvertent stimulation of the voiding reflex

RISK FOR CONSTIPATION NDx
Related to:
- Decreased gastrointestinal motility associated with:
  - Loss of autonomic nervous system function below the level of the injury during period of spinal shock
  - Decreased activity
- Lack of awareness of stool in rectum associated with sensory loss below the level of the injury
- Loss of central nervous system control over defecation reflex
- Decreased gravity filling of lower rectum associated with horizontal positioning
- Decreased intake of fluids and foods high in fiber

RISK FOR INFECTION NDx
- Pneumonia related to:
  - Stasis of secretions associated with decreased activity and decreased ability to clear tracheobronchial passages (client is unable to cough forcefully as a result of weakness of the diaphragm and paralysis of the abdominal and intercostal muscles)
  - Aspiration of foods/fluids (impaired swallowing can occur as a result of neck hyperextension and/or horizontal body positioning during the time that the cervical spine is immobilized)
- Urinary tract infection related to:
  - Growth and colonization of pathogens associated with urinary stasis
  - Introduction of pathogens associated with presence of an indwelling catheter and/or performance of intermittent catheterizations
- Skull pin site infection related to introduction of pathogens during or after insertion of skull pins

RISK FOR INJURY NDx
- Falls related to loss of motor function, use of kinetic bed, altered sitting balance if wearing a halo device (the struc-

ture and weight of the device alter the client's center of gravity)
- Burns related to loss of motor and sensory function and unexpected body movements resulting from spasticity

DISTURBED SELF-CONCEPT* NDx
Related to:
- Dependence on others to meet self-care needs
- Feelings of powerlessness
- Change in appearance associated with temporary presence of devices to immobilize the spine, necessity of wheelchair use, and spasticity after period of spinal shock
- Infertility (in males) associated with:
  - Possibility of retrograde ejaculation (can result from impaired nerve function in the bladder neck)

- Decreased sperm formation and viability resulting from testicular atrophy and impaired temperature regulation in the testes
- Changes in body functioning, lifestyle, and roles

INEFFECTIVE COPING NDx
Related to:
- Depression, fear, anxiety, feelings of powerlessness, and ongoing grieving associated with spinal cord injury and its effects on body functioning, lifestyle, and roles
- Dependence on others to meet basic needs
- Lack of personal resources to deal with spinal cord injury and its effects
- Need for extensive rehabilitation

PARKINSON'S DISEASE

Parkinson's disease (PD) is a degenerative disease of the central nervous system that leads to impairment of an individual's motor functioning. PD affects approximately 1 million individuals in the United States and about 4 million worldwide. It is slightly more prevalent in whites than other ethnic groups, with men affected slightly more than women. The diagnosis usually occurs after the age of 50 years; however, although rare, PD may affect individuals at a much younger age. Approximately 5% to 10% of individuals with PD are younger than 40. PD affects about 1 in 20 individuals older than 80 year of age. The cause of PD is unknown, but several risk factors are associated with its development. They include age, heredity, gender, exposure to toxins, and head trauma.

The symptoms of PD develop from an imbalance of acetylcholine and dopamine in the brain. Injury to the dopamine-producing neurons in the substantia nigra and the basal ganglia lead to loss of dopamine. In normal movement, there is a balance between dopamine, an inhibitory neurotransmitter, and acetylcholine, an excitatory neurotransmitter. When this balance is lost, the individual with PD experiences the classic clinical manifestations of tremors, rigidity, akinesia or bradykinesia, and postural changes. During the early stage of PD, these manifestations may develop alone or in combination; however, as the disease progresses, all of these manifestations are usually present. PD has an insidious onset that makes the diagnosis of the disease difficult until more pronounced symptoms appear. Other clinical manifestations seen as the disease progresses include shuffling gait; postural changes; loss of facial expressions; slurred speech; difficulty writing, eating, chewing, and swallowing; drooling; gastric retention; constipation; orthostatic hypotension; and urinary retention. Depression is often seen in individuals with PD.

There is no specific test to confirm the diagnosis of PD. The diagnosis is based on the client history and clinical mani-

festations. PD may be diagnosed when a client has at least two of the characteristic symptoms. The diagnosis of PD is confirmed when there is a positive response to medications.

There is no cure for PD. The standard treatment focuses on correcting the imbalance of neurotransmitters with medication. The medications approved for treatment of PD focus on improving the release of dopamine or blocking the effects of acetylcholine. The categories of medications used in PD are anticholinergics, dopamine precursors, dopamine agonists, monoamine oxidase B inhibitors, and catechol-O-methyltransferase inhibitors. Additional treatment may include exercise to maintain the client's health status as long as possible. Specific exercises may be prescribed to maintain muscle tone, decrease rigidity, and improve the ability to swallow and speak. Even with treatment, the disease is progressive, and ultimately clients will lose the ability to care for themselves.

This care plan focuses on the adult client hospitalized with signs and symptoms of PD. Much of the information is also applicable to clients receiving follow-up care in an extended care or rehabilitation facility or home setting.

OUTCOME/DISCHARGE CRITERIA

The client will:
1. Participate in activities of daily living
2. Engage in a regular exercise program to maintain strength
3. Maintain optimal nutritional status to meet caloric needs
4. Engage in appropriate social interaction with others.

---

*This diagnostic label includes the nursing diagnoses of Disturbed body image, Low self-esteem, and Ineffective role performance. The nurse should select the diagnostic label that is most appropriate based on the client's clinical manifestations.

NDx = NANDA-I Diagnosis   **D** = Delegatable Action   ● = UAP   ✦ = LVN/LPN   ⊖▶ = Go to ⊖volve for animation

Nursing Diagnosis IMPAIRED PHYSICAL MOBILITY NDx

Definition: Limitation in independent, purposeful physical movement of the body or of one or more extremities.

Related to: Physiological changes associated with Parkinson's disease

CLINICAL MANIFESTATIONS

Subjective	Objective
Reports of pain; discomfort; fatigue	Decreased reaction time; rigidity of muscles with movement; tremors of upper extremities; limited ability to perform gross and fine motor skills; limited range of motion; intentional movement–induced tremor; postural instability; uncoordinated movements

RISK FACTORS
- Lack of motivation
- Weakness
- Depression

DESIRED OUTCOMES

The client will improve mobility as evidenced by:
a. Increased physical activity
b. Movement of affected limb or limbs
c. Participation in activities of daily living
d. Demonstration of appropriate use of assistive devices to improve movement

NOC OUTCOMES

Activity tolerance; fall prevention behavior; endurance

NIC INTERVENTIONS

Ambulation; joint mobility; fall precautions; exercise therapy

NURSING ASSESSMENT	RATIONALE
Assess client's movement ability and activity tolerance. Use a tool such as the *"Assessment Tool for Safe Patient Handling and Movement* or the *Functional Independence Measures (FIM)*.	*Assessment of mobility is used to best determine how to facilitate movement. Assessment of activity tolerance provides a baseline for patient strength and endurance with movement.*
Assess for hallmark signs of PD:	
• Tremors	*Tremors are more prominent at rest or during emotional stress. Tremors are due to a central nervous system imbalance between acetylcholine and dopamine.*
• Changes in handwriting, "pill-rolling," shaking of the head	
• Rigidity	
• Jerky quality of movement with passive range of motion	*May be observed unilaterally or bilaterally*
• Bradykinesia	
• Decreased movement in blinking of eyelids, decreased movement of the arms while ambulating, difficulty with swallowing saliva, decreased facial expressions and movements of the hands, changes in posture	
Assess emotional response to immobility.	*Determine client's acceptance of limitations. This impacts implementation of therapeutic interventions.*
Assess need for assistive devices.	*Determine client's needs for assistive devices as well as proper use of wheelchairs, walkers, cane, etc., to reduce incidence of falls.*

THERAPEUTIC INTERVENTIONS	RATIONALE

Independent Actions
Encourage and implement strength-training activities:
- Active and/or passive range of motion
- Ambulation
- Activities of daily living **D** ● ✦

Inactivity contributes to muscle weakening. Regular exercise decreases muscle rigidity and contractures while maintaining joint mobility and physical strength.

THERAPEUTIC INTERVENTIONS	RATIONALE
Use assistive devices to help client with movement: • Crutches • Gait belt • Walker **D** ● ✦	*Assistive devices help caregivers decrease the potential for falls and/or injuries.*
Cluster treatments and care activities to allow for uninterrupted periods of rest. **D** ● ✦	*Adequate rest increases client's tolerance and strength for activities.*
Encourage patient with positive reinforcement during activities. **D** ● ✦	*A positive approach to activities supports the client's accomplishment and engagement in new activities, and improves self-esteem.*
Implement falls protocol. • Maintain the bed in low position and keep side rails up. **D** ● ✦	*These actions help prevent client falls.*
Use sequential compression devices or antiembolic stockings. **D** ● ✦	*These devices improve venous circulation and help prevent the development of thrombophlebitis in lower extremities.*
Implement measures to maintain healthy, intact skin (e.g., keep skin lubricated, clean, and dry; instruct or assist client to turn every 2 hours; keep bed linens dry and wrinkle-free). **D** ● ✦	*These actions help client maintain healthy, intact skin and reduce the risk of pressure sores and infection.*
Maintain an optimal nutritional status: • Increase protein intake.	*Adequate nutrition is needed to maintain adequate energy level.*
• Increase fluid intake to 2000 to 3000 mL/day unless contraindicated.	*Increased fluid intake maintains adequate hydration and helps prevent constipation and hardening of the stool.*
Encourage coughing and deep breathing exercises and use of incentive spirometry.	*Prevents buildup of secretions and promotes lung expansion.*

Dependent/Collaborative Actions

Consult appropriate health care provider: • Dietitian and physician and occupational therapists.	*These individuals provide specific activities and exercise programs to improve strength and mobility.*
• Administer pain medications before activities.	*Pain medications reduce muscle stiffness and tension, allowing the client to participate in activities.*

Nursing Diagnosis ## IMBALANCED NUTRITION: LESS THAN BODY REQUIREMENTS NDx

Definition: Inadequate intake or insufficient nutrition to meet the body's metabolic needs

Related to:
• Decreased oral intake associated with anorexia and nausea
• Loss of nutrients associated with vomiting if present
• Difficulty in swallowing

CLINICAL MANIFESTATIONS

Subjective	Objective
Report of lack of appetite; fatigue; difficulty swallowing	Choking episodes; vomiting of food or fluids through the nares; loss of weight with adequate food intake; body weight 20% or more under ideal weight; capillary fragility; pale conjunctiva and mucous membranes; constipation; poor muscle tone; increased blood urea nitrogen (BUN) and serum creatinine levels; decreased serum albumin and prealbumin levels; decreased Hct, Hgb levels, and white blood cell (WBC) count

RISK FACTORS
• Lack of appetite
• Fatigue
• Depression

Continued...

NOC OUTCOMES	NIC INTERVENTIONS
Appropriate appetite; positive body image; bowel elimination; compliance with prescribed diet; adequate hydration; weight maintenance behavior	Nutritional monitoring; nutritional counseling; nutritional management; aspiration precautions; weight management

NURSING ASSESSMENT	RATIONALE
Assess for and report signs and symptoms of malnutrition:	*Early recognition and reporting of signs and symptoms of malnutrition allow for prompt intervention.*
• Weight significantly below client's usual weight or below normal for client's age, height, and body frame	
• Decreased BUN and serum albumin, prealbumin, Hct, Hgb. and lymphocyte levels	
• Weakness and fatigue	
• Sore, inflamed oral mucous membrane	
• Pale conjunctiva	
Assess for physical difficulty with eating:	*Physical changes resulting from PD can lead to malnutrition.*
• Difficulty swallowing	
• Decreased gag reflex	
• Choking episodes	
• Vomiting from nares	
Monitor percentage of meals and snacks client consumes. Report a pattern of inadequate intake.	*An awareness of the amount of foods/fluids the client consumes alerts the nurse to deficits in nutritional intake. Reporting an inadequate intake allows for prompt intervention.*
Perform or assist with anthropometric measurements such as skinfold thickness, body circumferences (e.g., hip, waist, mid-upper arm), and bioelectrical impedance analysis if indicated. Report results that are lower than normal.	*Anthropometric measurements provide information about the amount of muscle mass, body fat, and protein reserves the client has. These assessments assist in evaluating the client's nutritional status.*

THERAPEUTIC INTERVENTIONS	RATIONALE
Independent Actions	
Implement measures to prevent choking and/or vomiting (e.g., eliminate noxious sites and odors). **D ● ✦**	*Choking and vomiting result in actual loss of nutrients.*
Implement measures to improve oral intake:	
• Perform actions to reduce nausea, pain, fear, and anxiety if present. **D ● ✦**	*Nausea, pain, fear, and anxiety all decrease client's appetite and oral intake.*
• Perform actions to relieve gastrointestinal distention if present (e.g., encourage and assist client with frequent ambulation unless contraindicated). **D ● ✦**	*Distention of the gastrointestinal tract (especially the stomach and duodenum) can result in stimulation of the satiety center and subsequent inhibition of the feeding center in the hypothalamus. This effect, along with the discomfort that occurs with distention, decreases appetite.*
• Increase activity as allowed and tolerated. **D ● ✦**	*Activity usually promotes a general feeling of well-being, which can result in improved appetite.*
• Maintain a clean environment and a relaxed, pleasant atmosphere. **D ● ✦**	*Noxious sites and odors can inhibit the feeding center in the hypothalamus. Maintaining a clean environment helps prevent this from occurring. In addition, maintaining a relaxed, pleasant atmosphere can help reduce the client's stress and promote a feeling of well-being, which tends to improve appetite and oral intake.*
• Encourage a rest period before meals if indicated. **D ● ✦ ✦**	*The physical activity of eating requires some expenditure of energy. Fatigue can reduce the client's desire and ability to eat.*
• Provide oral hygiene before meals. **D ●**	*Oral hygiene moistens the oral mucous membrane, which may make it easier to chew and swallow. It freshens the mouth and removes unpleasant tastes. This can improve the taste of foods/fluids, which helps stimulate appetite and increase oral intake.*

THERAPEUTIC INTERVENTIONS	RATIONALE
• Serve foods/fluids that are appealing to the client and adhere to personal and cultural (e.g., religious, ethnic) preferences whenever possible. **D** ● ✦	*Foods/fluids that appeal to the client's senses (especially sight and smell) and are in accordance with personal and cultural preferences are most likely to stimulate appetite and promote interest in eating.*
• Serve frequent, small meals rather than large ones if client is weak, fatigues easily, and/or has a poor appetite. **D** ● ✦	*Providing small rather than large meals can enable a client who is weak or fatigues easily to finish a meal. A client who has a poor appetite is often more willing to attempt to eat smaller meals because they seem less overwhelming than larger ones. If smaller meals are served, the number of meals per day should be increased to help ensure adequate nutrition.*
• Encourage significant others to bring in client's favorite foods unless contraindicated and eat with him/her if client desires.	*A client's favorite foods/fluids tend to stimulate his/her appetite more than institutional foods/fluids. The presence of significant others during meals helps create a familiar social environment that can stimulate appetite and improve oral intake. In addition, relieving dyspnea decreases the client's anxiety about and preoccupation with breathing efforts and increases the ability to focus on eating and drinking.*
• Place client in a high-Fowler's position for eating and drinking.	*Placing client in a high-Fowler's position to eat reduces the risk for aspiration.*
• Provide foods that can be easily chewed and provide thickened liquids.	*These actions improve the client's ability to swallow foods and decrease incidence of choking and potential for aspiration.*
• Allow adequate time for meals; reheat foods/fluids if necessary. **D** ● ✦	*A client who feels rushed during meals tends to become anxious, lose his/her appetite, stop eating, and possibly choke.*
• Limit fluid intake with meals unless the fluid has a high nutritional value. **D** ● ✦	*When the stomach becomes distended, its volume receptors stimulate the satiety center in the hypothalamus and the clients reduces his/her oral intake. Drinking liquids with meals distends the stomach and may cause satiety before an adequate amount of food is consumed.*
• Ensure that meals are well balanced and high in essential nutrients.	*The client must consume a diet that is well balanced and high in essential nutrients in order to meet his/her nutritional needs. Dietary supplements are often needed to help accomplish this.*
• Allow the client to assist in the selection of foods/fluids that meet nutritional needs.	*The client who is actively involved in menu planning is more likely to adhere to the diet plan. Involvement in meal selection increases the client's sense of control, which promotes a feeling of well-being and can lead to an increased oral intake.*

Dependent/Collaborative Actions

Implement measures to improve oral intake and nutritional status:

• Administer medications that may be ordered to improve client's nutritional status (e.g., antiemetics, antidiarrheals, gastrointestinal stimulants, and vitamins and minerals). **D** ✦	*Medications such as antiemetic, antidiarrheals, and gastrointestinal stimulants may relieve vomiting, diarrhea, and distention of the gastrointestinal tract, which decreases the discomfort that occurs with each of these signs and symptoms. Vitamins and minerals are needed to maintain metabolic functioning. If the client's dietary intake does not provide adequate amounts of them, oral and/or parenteral supplements may be necessary.*
• Obtain a dietary consult if necessary.	*A dietitian is best able to evaluate whether the foods/fluids selected will meet the client's nutritional needs.*
• Obtain a speech therapy consult.	*Speech therapists can work with the client to improve his/her ability to swallow.*
• Perform a calorie count if ordered. Report information to the dietitian and physician.	*A calorie count provides information about the caloric and nutritional value of the foods/fluids the client consumes. The information obtained helps the dietitian and physician determine whether an alternative method of nutritional support is needed.*
Consult the physician about an alternative method of providing nutrition (e.g., parenteral nutrition, tube feeding) if client does not consume enough food or fluids to meet nutritional needs.	*If the client's oral intake is inadequate, an alternative method of providing nutrients needs to be implemented.*

NDx = NANDA-I Diagnosis   **D** = Delegatable Action   ● = UAP   ✦ = LVN/LPN   ☺▶ = Go to ℰvolve for animation

Nursing Diagnosis | RISK FOR ASPIRATION NDx

◒▶ **Definition:** At risk for entry of gastrointestinal secretions, oropharyngeal secretions, solids, or fluids into tracheobronchial passages

Related to:
- Impaired swallowing
- Decreased gag reflex
- Decreased facial muscle tone

CLINICAL MANIFESTATIONS

Subjective	Objective
N/A	Cough; tachypnea; dyspnea; tachycardia; dull percussion noted over affected lung area; presence of foods in aspirate

RISK FACTORS
- Weakness
- Eating too fast

DESIRED OUTCOMES

The client will not aspirate secretions or foods/fluids as evidenced by:
  a. Clear breath sounds
  b. Resonant percussion note over lungs
  c. Absence of cough, tachypnea, and dyspnea

NOC OUTCOMES

Aspiration prevention; body positioning: self initiated; gastrointestinal function; nausea and vomiting control; respiratory status; swallowing status

NIC INTERVENTIONS

Aspiration precautions; respiratory monitoring; swallowing therapy; airway suctioning

NURSING ASSESSMENT	RATIONALE
Assess for and report signs and symptoms of aspiration of secretions or foods/fluids: • Rhonchi • Dull percussion note over affected lung area • Cough • Tachypnea • Dyspnea • Tachycardia • Presence of tube feeding in tracheal aspirate Assess for difficulty in swallowing and a decreased gag reflex.	*Early recognition of signs and symptoms of aspiration allows for prompt intervention.* *Allows for interventions to be implemented to decrease risk of aspiration*
Assist with diagnostic studies to determine whether aspiration is occurring during swallowing (e.g., videofluoroscopy).	*Aspiration of foods/fluids during swallowing process is evident on studies such as videofluoroscopy. Knowing when aspiration occurs during the swallowing process aids in the development of an individualized plan of care to prevent further aspiration.*
Monitor chest radiograph results. Report findings of pulmonary infiltrate.	*Evidence of pulmonary infiltrate on chest radiograph can indicate that aspiration has occurred.*

THERAPEUTIC INTERVENTIONS	RATIONALE

Independent Actions
Perform actions to decrease the risk of aspiration:
- Keep suction equipment readily available at bedside.
- Position patient in high-Fowler's position before initiating feeding.
- Maintain patient in an upright position 30 to 45 minutes after eating. **D ● ✦**

This equipment is necessary to maintain patency of airway.
This position uses gravity to facilitate movement of food/fluids through the pharynx into the esophagus.
Allows for observation of potential swallowing difficulty

THERAPEUTIC INTERVENTIONS	RATIONALE
• Supervise administration of oral intake. • Offer foods with a thicker consistency, which facilitates swallowing.	Semisolid foods are more readily swallowed. Watery fluids are difficult for patients with dysphagia to manage.
• Encourage client to chew each bite slowly and completely, and to eat slowly during meals. **D** ● ✦	Complete mastication of food products improves the client's ability to swallow food.
• Place foods/medications on unaffected side of the mouth. **D** ● ✦	This action facilitates effective swallowing of food.
• Provide oral care after feedings. **D** ● ✦	Good oral hygiene after meals results in removal of any remaining food that could enter the pharynx and be aspirated into the lungs.
• If client is receiving tube feedings, check tube placement before each feeding or on a routine basis if tube feeding is continuous.	Verification of feeding tube placement ensures that the tube feeding solution goes into the alimentary tract rather than the lungs.

Dependent/Collaborative Actions
Perform actions to decrease the risk of aspiration:

• Monitor chest radiograph results.	Evidence of pulmonary infiltrates on chest radiograph can indicate that aspiration has occurred.
• Administer antiemetics as ordered to prevent vomiting. **D** ✦	Antiemetics reduce the risk of vomiting.
• Consult appropriate speech therapist for swallowing difficulties.	Dysphagia assessment can establish techniques to prevent aspiration in patients with impaired swallowing.

Nursing Diagnosis ## CONSTIPATION NDx

Definition: Decrease in normal frequency of defecation accompanied by difficult or incomplete passage of stool and/or passage of excessively hard, dry stool

Related to: Physiological changes that alter normal bowel functioning

CLINICAL MANIFESTATIONS

Subjective	Objective
Reports of straining with defecation; feeling of rectal fullness or pressure; inability to pass stool; headache; indigestion	Infrequent bowel movements; dry, hard, formed stool; hyperactive/hypoactive bowel sounds; distended abdomen; percussed abdominal dullness; severe flatus; hypoactive or hyperactive bowel sounds; palpable abdominal mass; oozing liquid stool

RISK FACTORS

- Lack of fiber in diet
- Abdominal muscle weakness
- Physical inactivity
- Decreased fluid intake
- Side effects of medications

DESIRED OUTCOMES

The client will maintain usual bowel elimination pattern as evidenced by:
  a. Usual frequency of bowel movements
  b. Passage of soft, formed stool
  c. Absence of abdominal distention and pain, feeling of rectal fullness or pressure, and straining during defecation

NOC OUTCOMES

Bowel elimination; gastrointestinal function; hydration; symptom control

NIC NTERVENTIONS

Constipation/impaction management

NDx = NANDA-I Diagnosis   **D** = Delegatable Action   ● = UAP   ✦ = LVN/LPN   ⊖▶ = Go to ⊖volve for animation

Continued...

NURSING ASSESSMENT	RATIONALE
Ascertain client's usual bowel elimination habits.	*Knowledge of the client's usual bowel elimination habits is essential in determining whether constipation is present because the frequency of defecation varies among individuals.*
Assess for signs and symptoms of constipation: • Decrease in frequency of bowel movements • Passage of hard, formed stools • Anorexia • Abdominal distention and pain • Feeling of fullness or pressure in rectum • Straining during defecation	*Early recognition of signs and symptoms of constipation allows for prompt intervention.*
Assess bowel sounds. Report a pattern of decreasing bowel sounds.	*Bowel sounds are produced by peristaltic activity. A pattern of decreasing bowel sounds indicates a decrease in bowel motility, which can lead to and be present with constipation.*

THERAPEUTIC INTERVENTIONS	RATIONALE

Independent Actions

Implement measures to promote optimum bowel elimination:

• Encourage client to defecate whenever the urge is felt. **D** ● ✦	*Repeated inhibition of the defecation reflex results in progressive weakening of the reflex. In addition, when the defecation reflex is inhibited, feces remain in the colon longer and water continues to be absorbed from the feces, making the stool drier, harder, and subsequently more difficult to evacuate.*
• Assist client to toilet or bedside commode or place in high-Fowler's position on bedpan for bowel movements unless contraindicated. **D** ● ✦	*A sitting position aids in the expulsion of stool by taking advantage of gravity. This position also enhances the client's ability to perform the Valsalva maneuver, which increases intra-abdominal pressure and forces the fecal contents downward and into the rectum where the defecation reflex is then elicited.*
• Encourage client to relax, provide privacy, and have call signal within reach during attempts to defecate. **D** ● ✦	*If the client is able to relax during attempts to defecate, he/she will be able to relax the levator ani muscle and external anal sphincter, thus facilitating the passage of stool.*
• Encourage the client to establish a regular time for defecation, preferably within an hour after a meal. **D** ✦	*Attempting to have a bowel movement within an hour after a meal, particularly breakfast, takes advantage of mass peristalsis, which occurs only a few times a day and is strongest after meals. Mass peristalsis is stimulated by the gastrocolic reflex, which is initiated by the presence of foods/fluids in the stomach and duodenum.*
• Instruct client to increase intake of foods high in fiber (e.g., bran, whole grain breads and cereals, fresh fruits and vegetables) unless contraindicated.	*Foods high in fiber provide bulk to the fecal mass and keep the stool soft because of the ability of fiber to absorb water. The increased bulkiness (mass) of the stools stimulates peristalsis, which promotes more rapid movement of stool through the colon.* *The shorter the time that feces remains in the intestine, the less water is absorbed from it, which helps prevent the formation of hard, dry stools that are difficult to expel.*
• Encourage client to drink hot liquids (e.g., coffee, tea) upon arising in the morning. • Encourage client to maintain regular exercise. • Encourage client to perform isometric abdominal strengthening exercises unless contraindicated.	*These interventions can stimulate peristalsis.*

Dependent/Collaborative Actions

Implement measures to promote optimum bowel elimination:

• Instruct client to maintain a minimal fluid intake of 2500 mL/day unless contraindicated.	*Inadequate fluid intake reduces the water content of feces, which results in hard, dry stool that is difficult to evacuate.*

THERAPEUTIC INTERVENTIONS	RATIONALE
• Increase activity as allowed and tolerated. **D** ● ✦	*Ambulation stimulates peristalsis, which promotes the passage of stool through the intestines.*
• When appropriate, encourage the use of nonnarcotic rather than narcotic (opioid) analgesics for pain management.	*Narcotic analgesics slow peristalsis, which delays transit of intestinal contents. This delay also results in increased absorption of fluid from the fecal mass with the subsequent formation of hard, dry stool.*
• Administer laxatives as ordered. **D** ✦	*Laxatives/cathartics act in a variety of ways to soften the stool, increase stool bulk, stimulate bowel motility, and/or lubricate the fecal mass and thereby promote the evacuation of stool.*
• Administer cleansing and/or oil retention enemas if ordered. **D** ● ✦	*A cleansing enema stimulates peristalsis and evacuation of stool by distending the colon with a large volume of solution and/or by irritating the colonic mucosa. An oil retention enema facilitates the passage of stool by softening the fecal mass and lubricating the rectum and anal canal.*
• Consult physician about checking for an impaction and digitally removing stool if the client has not had a bowel movement in 3 days, if the client is passing liquid stool, or if other signs and symptoms of constipation are present.	*An impaction prohibits the normal passage of feces. Digital removal of an impacted fecal mass may be necessary before normal passage of stool can occur.*

Nursing Diagnosis IMPAIRED VERBAL COMMUNICATION NDx

Definition: Decreased, delayed, or absent ability to receive, process, transmit, and use a system of symbols

Related to:
- Decreased tone in facial muscles
- Slow and/or slurred speech
- Decreased facial expression
- Decreased mobility of the tongue
- Decreased tone of voice

CLINICAL MANIFESTATIONS

Subjective	Objective
Reports difficulty of expressing self	Unable to speak dominant language; speaks or verbalizes with difficulty; cannot speak; slurring/stuttering; difficulty forming words and sentences

RISK FACTORS	DESIRED OUTCOME
• Depression • Embarrassment • Change in muscle tone	The client will maintain positive interactions with others.

NOC OUTCOMES	NIC INTERVENTIONS
Communication: expressive	Communication enhancement: speech deficit; active listening

NURSING ASSESSMENT	RATIONALE
Assess for motor speech impairment or difficulty forming words.	*Provides a baseline assessment of client's status and allows for the implementation of appropriate interventions.*

THERAPEUTIC INTERVENTIONS	RATIONALE

Independent Actions
Implement measures to maintain positive communication:

• Approach communication with client as an adult. **D** ● ✦	*Inability to communicate can be frustrating. The client should be treated with dignity.*

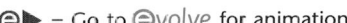

Continued...

THERAPEUTIC INTERVENTIONS	RATIONALE
• Ask questions that require short answers and allow time for the patient to respond. **D** ● ✦	*The client will need more time to express himself/herself. Short, simple answers will reduce client's frustration, allowing for easier communication.*
• Face client and maintain eye contact when client is speaking. **D** ● ✦	*In a calm, quiet environment the client can concentrate on communication efforts and can hear others more clearly.*
• Create a calm, quiet environment.	
• Provide rest periods before speech therapy. **D** ● ✦	
• Encourage client to routinely perform face and tongue exercises.	*These actions help the client maintain muscle tone, reduces rigidity and helps facilitate communication while decreasing frustration with the process.*
• Encourage client to sign or read out loud to self or family members.	
• Provide assistive communication aids such as pad/pencil, computer, word cards, or picture boards. **D** ● ✦	
• Encourage family to communicate with client. **D** ✦	*Family involvement will reinforce consistency of communication measures.*

Dependent/Collaborative Actions

Implement measures to maintain positive communication:	*Multidisciplinary plan of care can be developed.*
• Consult speech pathologist.	

Nursing Diagnosis # DISTURBED SELF-CONCEPT*

Definition

Disturbed body image NDx: Confusion in mental picture of one's physical self

Low self-esteem NDx: Development of a negative perception of self-worth in response to a current situation

Ineffective role performance NDx: Patterns of behavior and self-expression that do not match the environmental context, norms, and expectations

Related to:
• Loss of independent functioning
• Difficulty in communication

CLINICAL MANIFESTATIONS

Subjective	Objective
Verbalization of negative feelings about self	Lack of participation in activities of daily living; withdrawal from significant others; lack of planning to adapt to necessary changes in lifestyle

RISK FACTORS

• Changes in physical appearance
• Poor self-esteem

DESIRED OUTCOMES

The client will demonstrate beginning adaptation to changes in appearance, body functioning, and lifestyle as evidenced by:
  a. Verbalization of feelings of self-worth
  b. Maintenance of relationships with significant others -
  c. Active participation in activities of daily living
  d. Verbalization of a beginning plan for integrating changes in appearance and body functioning into lifestyle

NOC OUTCOMES

Body image; personal autonomy; self-esteem; psychosocial adjustment: life change

NIC INTERVENTIONS

Body image enhancement; self-esteem enhancement; emotional support; support system enhancement; role enhancement; counseling

---

*This diagnostic label includes the nursing diagnoses of Disturbed body image, Low self-esteem, and Ineffective role performance.

NURSING ASSESSMENT	RATIONALE
Assess for signs and symptoms of a disturbed self-concept (e.g., verbalization of negative feelings about self, withdrawal from significant others, lack of participation in activities of daily living, lack of plan for adapting to necessary changes in lifestyle).	*Early recognition of signs and symptoms of a disturbed self-concept allows for prompt treatment.*
Determine the meaning of changes in appearance, body functioning, and lifestyle to the client by encouraging verbalization of feelings and by noting nonverbal responses to the changes experienced.	*An understanding of what the change means to the client provides a basis for planning care.*

THERAPEUTIC INTERVENTIONS	RATIONALE
Independent Actions	
Be aware that client may grieve the loss of normal body functioning and change in appearance. Provide support during the grieving process.	*Allows client and significant others to grieve loss of normal body functioning; helps client work through changes that are occurring*
Discuss client's feelings about disease symptoms.	*Discussion of feelings about the disease process helps the client in dealing with his/her physiological changes.*
Instruct client in ways to maintain health status as long as possible:	
• Maintain regular exercise program.	*These actions help the client maintain health status, decrease muscle rigidity, and improve muscle strength.*
• Maintain optimal diet.	
• Maintain performance of activities of daily living.	
Encourage significant others to allow client to do what he/she is able.	*This improves client's confidence in ability to care for self and enhances client's feelings of self-worth and assists with the development of a positive self-concept.*
Assist client's and significant others' adjustment by listening, facilitating communication, and providing information.	*These actions facilitate client and family acceptance of changes and changes in lifestyle.*
Encourage visits and support from significant others.	
Encourage client to pursue usual roles and interests and to continue involvement in social activities as much as possible.	*Pursuit of usual roles and activities helps the client maintain independence and social interaction as long as possible.*
Refer client and family to support groups	*Support groups may help client and family work through changes related to the disease process.*
Refer client and family to community organizations.	*Allows for continuity of care and support once discharged from an acute care facility*

Nursing Diagnosis	**DEFICIENT KNOWLEDGE** NDx**; INEFFECTIVE FAMILY THERAPEUTIC REGIMEN MANAGEMENT** NDx**; OR INEFFECTIVE HEALTH MAINTENANCE** NDx*†

Definition: Absence or deficiency of cognitive information related to specific topic (lack of specific information necessary for clients/significant others) to make informed choices regarding condition/treatment/lifestyle changes; inability to identify, manage, and/or seek out help to manage health; pattern of regulating and integrating into family processes a program for treatment of illness and the sequelae of illness that is unsatisfactory for meeting specific health goals

*The nurse should select the diagnostic label that is most appropriate for the client's discharge teaching needs.
†Although the client will not be able to perform many of the following actions independently, he/she must be knowledgeable about them in order to provide proper instruction to significant others and attendant and maintain an active role in the rehabilitation process.

NDx = NANDA-I Diagnosis   **D** = Delegatable Action   ● = UAP   ✦ = LVN/LPN   ⊖▶ = Go to ⊖volve for animation

Continued...

CLINICAL MANIFESTATIONS

Subjective	Objective
Verbalizes inability to manage illness; verbalizes inability to follow prescribed regimen	Inaccurate follow through with instructions; inappropriate behaviors; experience of preventable complications of Parkinson's Disease

RISK FACTORS

- Cognitive deficit
- Financial concerns
- Failure to take action to reduce risk factors for complications of Parkinson's Disease
- Inability to care for oneself
- Difficulty in modifying personal habits and integrating treatments into lifestyle

NOC OUTCOMES	NIC INTERVENTIONS
Knowledge: treatment regimen; knowledge: health behavior; knowledge: health resources; knowledge: treatment procedure(s)	Teaching: individual; teaching: prescribed activity/exercise; teaching: psychomotor skills; health system guidance; financial resource assistance; support system enhancement

NURSING ASSESSMENT	RATIONALE
Assess the client's ability to learn and readiness to learn Assess the client's understanding of teaching	*Learning is more effective when the client is motivated and understands the importance of what is to be learned. Readiness to learn changes based on situations, physical and emotional challenges.*

THERAPEUTIC INTERVENTIONS	RATIONALE

Desired Outcome: The client will understand disease process and prognosis.

Independent Actions

Reinforce information concerning the disease and treatment modalities.	*Knowledge of disease process and treatment helps the client and family understand the changes that are occurring and the importance of treatment in maintaining health status as long as possible. This improves client's adherence to treatment regimen and allows client to maintain a level of independence for as long as possible.@@@Knowledge of the disease process may help with the client's ability to cope with physical changes.*

THERAPEUTIC INTERVENTIONS	RATIONALE

Desired Outcome: The client will verbalize an understanding of the rationale for and components of the recommended diet and the importance of maintaining optimal nutritional status.

Independent Actions

Provide instructions regarding ways to maintain an optimal nutritional status:

• Maintain an adequate diet with the appropriate mix of nutrients.	*Adequate nutritional status is required for the body to work efficiently and maintain optimal muscle strength and energy to perform activities of daily living as long as possible.*
• Reinforce instructions related to taking small bites and chewing food thoroughly.	*These actions improve the client's ability to swallow foods and decreases the risk of aspiration.*
• Inform client that eating small, frequent meals rather than three large meals may help achieve the recommended calorie intake.	
• Reinforce the benefits of eating when rested and in a relaxed atmosphere.	*Eating in a relaxed environment improves the clients ability to maintain nutritional status and decreases risk of aspiration. When a client is anxious or rushed, there is an increased risk for aspiration.*

THERAPEUTIC INTERVENTIONS	RATIONALE

Desired Outcome: The client will verbalize ways to maintain optimal muscle tone.

Independent Actions

Instruct client in ways that will maintain muscle strength for as long as possible:

- Maintain a regular exercise routine.
- Encourage client to maintain exercises that work the facial muscles (i.e., sing or read aloud, stick out tongue, move tongue from side to side).

Regular exercise including exercise of the facial muscles, improves balance, maintains muscle strength, and improves flexibility and mobility and the client's ability to verbally communicate.

THERAPEUTIC INTERVENTIONS	RATIONALE

Desired Outcome: The client will verbalize an understanding of medication regimen, including rationale, food and drug interactions, side effects, schedule for taking, and importance of taking as prescribed.

Independent Actions

Explain the rationale for, side effects of, food and drug interactions, and the importance of taking medications as prescribed. The client should understand which side effects require notification of the health care provider.

Reinforce importance of taking medications as prescribed.

Types of medications to treat PD include:

- Anticholinergics
- Dopamine agonists
- Monoamine oxidase B inhibitor
- Catechol-O-methyltransferase inhibitor

Instruct client to inform physician before taking other prescription and nonprescription medications.

Knowledge of medications and how they impact the system improves client adherence and helps enhance the client's understanding of the importance of adhering to the prescribed medication regimen. The client must be able to recognize alterations in functioning related to medication administration.
Missing doses of medications or not taking them as prescribed may adversely impact mobility.

Anticholinergics help control muscle activity.
Dopamine agonists, monoamine oxidase B inhibitors and catechol-O-methyl-transferase inhibitors increase the amount of CNS dopamine available for use, which decreases muscle rigidity and tremors.
Over-the-counter (OTC) medications may impact prescription medications and should not be taken without a health care provider's approval.

THERAPEUTIC INTERVENTIONS	RATIONALE

Desired Outcome: The client will identify resources that can assist in the adjustment to changes resulting from PD and its treatment.

Independent Actions

Provide information about resources that can assist the client and significant others in adjusting to PD and its effects (e.g., local support groups, Parkinson's disease foundations, counseling services).

Client may need assistance from community organizations for both emotional and financial support once discharged from the acute care facility.

THERAPEUTIC INTERVENTIONS	RATIONALE

Desired Outcome: The client will verbalize an understanding of and a plan for adhering to recommended follow-up care including future appointments with health care provider and activity level.

Independent Actions

Reinforce importance of keeping follow-up appointments with health care provider.

Implement measures to improve client's compliance:

- Include significant others in teaching sessions if possible.

PD is a chronic illness and requires appropriate follow-up with health care providers.

Support from client's significant others is important in maintaining adherence to the therapeutic regimen.

NDx = NANDA-I Diagnosis   **D** = Delegatable Action   ● = UAP   ✦ = LVN/LPN   ⊜▶ = Go to ⊜volve for animation

Continued...

THERAPEUTIC INTERVENTIONS	RATIONALE
• Encourage questions and allow time for reinforcement and clarification of information provided.	*Improves client's and family's understanding of disease process and what to do to remain healthy*
• Provide written instructions on future appointments with health care provider, medications prescribed, signs and symptoms to report, and future laboratory studies.	*Written instructions allow the client to refer to them after discharge as needed.*

ADDITIONAL NURSING DIAGNOSES

ACTIVITY INTOLERANCE NDx
Related to muscle weakness and fatigue

RISK FOR INJURY: FALLS NDx
Related to altered gait and muscle weakness

CAREGIVER ROLE STRAIN NDx
Related to:
• Level of illness experienced by the client
• Duration of care required
• Complexity of care
• Caregiver isolation

SELF-CARE DEFICIT NDx
Related to:
• Muscle weakness
• Tremors
• Rigidity of movements

ANTICIPATORY GRIEVING NDx
Related to awareness of disease and disease progression

See Bibliography at the back of the book.

The Client with Alterations in Hematologic and Immune Function

HUMAN IMMUNODEFICIENCY VIRUS (HIV) INFECTION AND ACQUIRED IMMUNE DEFICIENCY SYNDROME (AIDS)

Acquired immune deficiency syndrome (AIDS) is an infectious disease of the immune system and is considered to be the last phase of the clinical spectrum of infection by the human immunodeficiency virus (HIV). HIV is a retrovirus that affects the cells in the body that have a CD4 receptor on their surface. The types of cells that have the CD4 receptor and can be infected by the virus include lymphocytes, monocytes, macrophages, glial cells, bone marrow progenitors, and gut-associated lymphoid tissue. The CD4+ T lymphocytes (also called T4 or T-helper cells) have the greatest number of CD4 receptors and are consequently the major target of HIV. These lymphocytes are ultimately destroyed by HIV, which results in severely impaired cell-mediated immunity in the host. Humoral immune function is also impaired because the B lymphocytes are unable to respond appropriately to the presence of a new antigen without the help of normal CD4+ T lymphocytes. The effect of HIV on the monocyte and macrophage further depresses immune system function.

HIV has been isolated from all body fluids, but at this point, transmission has been associated only with blood, semen, amniotic fluid, vaginal secretions, and breast milk. The known routes of transmission are by intimate sexual contact, mucous membrane or percutaneous exposure to infected blood or blood products, and perinatal transmission from mother to child. The four high-risk groups for acquiring HIV infection are heterosexuals with multiple sexual partners, men who have sex with men, intravenous drug users, and recipients of blood/blood products. Treating HIV-infected women during pregnancy with an antiretroviral agent (e.g., zidovudine) has significantly reduced the transmission of HIV from mother to child.

Infection with HIV tends to follow a particular course, with the clinical expression being attributed to either the effects of the virus itself or the consequences of CD4+ T-lymphocyte depletion. The initial event in the course of the disease is acute retroviral infection, which occurs about 1 to 6 weeks after exposure to HIV. The person experiences symptoms such as fever, headache, myalgias, lymphadenopathy, rash, fatigue, and sore throat that may persist for a week or longer. Then, the HIV-infected person enters the chronic infection stage. In the early period of chronic infection, the person may be asymptomatic or continue to experience mild symptoms such as fatigue, headache, and lymphadenopathy. This early period often lasts as long as 10 to 12 years, depending on the rate of viral replication and the rapidity of CD4+ T-lymphocyte destruction. The symptomatic stage of HIV infection develops when the CD4+ T-lymphocyte count drops below 500 cells/mm^3 and the HIV viral load rises above 10,000 copies/mL. In the early symptomatic stage, the person has various nonspecific symptoms (e.g., unexplained fever and weight loss, fatigue, night sweats, peripheral neuropathy, persistent diarrhea) and persistent, localized viral or fungal infections. AIDS is the last stage of HIV infection. In addition to the symptoms experienced in the previous stage, AIDS is heralded by immune suppression (serologically defined as a CD4+ T-lymphocyte count <200 cells/mm^3) and the presence of a condition that meets the criteria for definition of an AIDS case as specified by the Centers for Disease Control and Prevention (CDC). These AIDS-indicator conditions include HIV-related encephalopathy, HIV wasting syndrome, opportunistic infections (e.g., *Pneumocystis jiroveci* pneumonia [formerly known as *pneumocystis carinii* PCP]; candidiasis of esophagus or bronchi, trachea, or lungs; *Mycobacterium tuberculosis*, *Mycobacterium avium* complex [MAC]; extrapulmonary cryptococcosis; cytomegalovirus infection; *Toxoplasma* encephalitis; coccidioidomycosis), and AIDS-related cancers (e.g., Kaposi's sarcoma, non-Hodgkin's lymphoma, invasive cervical cancer).

At this time, there is no cure for HIV infection. However, there have been significant advances in antiretroviral therapy and prevention of opportunistic infections that have increased the long-term survival of persons with HIV infection. Earlier treatment and the use of highly active antiretroviral therapy (HAART), which consists of a combination of at least three antiretroviral agents, have made significant differences in sustaining viral suppression, slowing disease progression, and reducing drug resistance. Because of the side effects of the antiretroviral agents and lack of adherence to the drug regimen, current federal guidelines suggest that treatment be offered early, but that it can be delayed until higher levels of immune suppression are observed.

The antiretroviral agents used to control viral replication of HIV include nucleoside reverse transcriptase inhibitors (e.g., zidovudine, lamivudine, zalcitabine, abacavir, didanosine, stavudine), protease inhibitors (e.g., saquinavir,

Continued...

ritonavir, indinavir, amprenavir, nelfinavir), nonnucleoside reverse transcriptase inhibitors (e.g., nevirapine, delavirdine, efavirenz), and fusion inhibitors (e.g., enfuvirtide). Chemoprophylactic therapy to prevent AIDS-defining opportunistic infections has also led to a significant decline in the incidence of certain diseases such as PCP, MAC, tuberculosis, and toxoplasmosis.

This care plan focuses on the adult client with HIV infection hospitalized for treatment of a probable opportunistic infection. Much of the information is applicable to clients receiving follow-up care in an extended care facility or home setting.

OUTCOME/DISCHARGE CRITERIA

The client will:
1. Have an adequate respiratory status
2. Have an adequate or improved nutritional status
3. Be able to perform activities of daily living without undue fatigue or dyspnea
4. Demonstrate evidence that opportunistic infection is resolving
5. Be effectively managing the signs and symptoms of neurological dysfunction
6. Have discomfort at a manageable level
7. Show evidence that skin and oral mucous membranes are intact or healing appropriately
8. Have fewer episodes of diarrhea
9. Identify ways to prevent the spread of HIV
10. Identify ways to decrease the risk for developing opportunistic infections
11. Verbalize ways to maintain an optimal nutritional status
12. State signs and symptoms to report to the health care provider
13. Share feelings about changes in mental and physical functioning and the social isolation and loneliness that may result from having AIDS
14. Identify resources that can assist with financial needs and adjustment to changes resulting from the diagnosis of AIDS
15. Verbalize an understanding of and a plan for adhering to recommended follow-up care including regular laboratory studies, future appointments with health care providers, and medications prescribed.

Nursing Diagnosis   IMPAIRED RESPIRATORY FUNCTION*

Definition: Inspiration and/or expiration that does not provide adequate ventilation; inability to clear secretions or obstructions from the respiratory tract to maintain a clear airway

Ineffective breathing pattern NDx related to:
- Decreased depth of respirations associated with fear, anxiety, weakness, fatigue, and chest pain if present
- Increased rate of respirations associated with fear, anxiety, and the increase in metabolic rate that occurs with infection

Ineffective airway clearance NDx related to:
- Increased production of secretions associated with some opportunistic infections of the lungs
- Stasis of secretions associated with decreased activity and poor cough effort resulting from fatigue and pain

Impaired gas exchange NDx related to a decrease in effective lung surface associated with:
- The presence of infiltrates and/or cavities in the lung tissue resulting from opportunistic infection of the lungs (e.g., PCP, pneumococcal pneumonia, tuberculosis, histoplasmosis)
- Compression and/or replacement of lung tissue if an AIDS-related cancer such as Kaposi's sarcoma or non-Hodgkin's lymphoma is present

CLINICAL MANIFESTATIONS

Subjective	Objective
Reports of difficulty vocalizing; verbal reports of restlessness	Dyspnea; orthopnea; diminished breath sounds; adventitious breath sounds; cough; change in respiratory rate and rhythm

RISK FACTORS
- Pulmonary infection
- Immunosuppression
- *Pneumocystis jiroveci* pneumonia
- Mycobacterium tuberculosis

DESIRED OUTCOMES

The client will experience adequate respiratory function as evidenced by:
  a. Normal rate and depth of respirations
  b. Decreased dyspnea
  c. Improved breath sounds
  d. Symmetrical chest excursion
  e. Usual mental status
  f. Oximetry results within normal range
  g. Arterial blood gas values within normal range

*This diagnostic label includes the following nursing diagnoses: ineffective breathing pattern, ineffective airway clearance, and impaired gas exchange.

NOC OUTCOMES

Respiratory status: airway patency; respiratory status: ventilation; respiratory status: gas exchange

NIC INTERVENTIONS

Respiratory monitoring; airway management; chest physiotherapy; cough enhancement; ventilation assistance; oxygen therapy; medication administration

---

NURSING ASSESSMENT

Assess for and report signs and symptoms of impaired respiratory function:
- Rapid, shallow respirations
- Dyspnea, orthopnea
- Use of accessory muscles when breathing
- Abnormal breath sounds (e.g., diminished, bronchial, crackles [rales], wheezes)
- Asymmetrical chest excursion
- Cough (can be productive or dry and nonproductive depending on the opportunistic disease present)

Monitor arterial blood gas values, chest x-ray results.

RATIONALE

Early recognition of signs and symptoms of impaired respiratory function allows for prompt intervention.

THERAPEUTIC INTERVENTIONS

RATIONALE

Independent Actions

Implement measures to improve respiratory status: **D** ✦
- Place client in a semi- to high-Fowler's position unless contraindicated; position with pillows to prevent slumping.
- Instruct client to breathe slowly if hyperventilating.
- If client must remain flat in bed, assist with position change at least every 2 hours.
- Instruct client to deep breathe or use incentive spirometer every 1 to 2 hours.
- Perform actions to promote removal of pulmonary secretions.
- Instruct and assist client to cough or "huff" every 1 to 2 hours.

- Discourage smoking.

High-Fowler's position allows for maximum diaphragmatic excursion and lung expansion. Prevention of slumping is essential because slumping causes abdominal contents to be pushed up.
Repositioning helps to mobilize secretions.
Deep breathing and use of an incentive spirometer promote maximal inhalation and lung expansion.

Coughing or "huffing" accelerates airflow through the airways, which helps mobilize and clear mucus and foreign matter from the respiratory tract.
The irritants in smoke increase mucus production, impair ciliary function, and can cause damage to the bronchial and alveolar walls; the carbon monoxide decreases oxygen availability.

Dependent/Collaborative Actions

Implement measures to improve respiratory status:
- Maintain activity restrictions as ordered to reduce oxygen needs.
- Assist with positive airway pressure techniques (e.g., continuous positive airway pressure [CPAP], bilevel positive airway pressure [BiPAP], flutter/positive expiratory pressure [PEP] device) if ordered
- Perform actions to promote removal of pulmonary secretions:
  - Implement measures to thin tenacious secretions and reduce dryness of the respiratory mucous membrane:
    - Maintain a fluid intake of at least 2500 mL/day unless contraindicated.
    - Humidify inspired air as ordered.
  - Assist with administration of mucolytics (e.g., acetylcysteine) and diluent or hydrating agents (e.g., water, saline) via nebulizer if ordered.
  - Assist with or perform postural drainage therapy (PDT) if ordered.
  - Perform suctioning if ordered.
  - Administer expectorants (e.g., guaifenesin) if ordered.

Positive pressure airway techniques increase intrapulmonary (alveolar) pressure, which helps reexpand alveoli and prevent further alveolar collapse.

Adequate hydration and humidified inspired air help thin secretions, which facilitates the mobilization and expectoration of secretions.

Mucolytics and diluent or hydrating agents are mucokinetic substances that reduce the viscosity of mucus, thus making it easier for the client to mobilize and clear secretions from the respiratory tract.

NDx = NANDA-I Diagnosis   **D** = Delegatable Action   ● = UAP   ✦ = LVN/LPN   ⊖▶ = Go to ⊖volve for animation

Continued...

THERAPEUTIC INTERVENTIONS	RATIONALE
• Perform actions to reduce pain and fatigue: • Administer analgesics before activities and procedures that can cause pain and before pain becomes severe.	*Reducing pain enables the client to breathe more deeply and participate in activities to improve respiratory status.*
• Maintain oxygen therapy as ordered. **D** ✦	
• Administer central nervous system depressants judiciously; hold medication and consult physician if respiratory rate is less than 12 breaths/min.	*Central nervous system depressants such as opioid narcotics cause depression of the respiratory center and cough reflex. This can result in stasis of secretions and hypoventilation with impaired gas exchange.*
• Administer the following medications if ordered: • Bronchodilators	*Bronchodilators dilate terminal airways, improving oxygen delivery and ventilation.*
• Antimicrobials	*Antimicrobials may be given to prevent pneumonia.*
• Corticosteroids	*Corticosteroids decrease pulmonary inflammation and are usually reserved for moderate to severe cases of PCP because of the risk for further immunosuppression.*
Consult appropriate health care provider (e.g., respiratory therapist, physician) if signs and symptoms of impaired respiratory function persist or worsen.	*Consulting the appropriate health care provider allows for modification of the treatment plan.*

Nursing Diagnosis   ACUTE/CHRONIC PAIN NDx

Definition: Pain is whatever the experiencing person says it is, existing whenever the person says it does. It is an unpleasant sensory and emotional experience arising from actual or potential tissue damage. Acute pain has a duration of less than 6 months, while chronic pain recurs at intervals for months or years

Oral, pharyngeal, and/or esophageal pain related to the presence of aphthous ulcers in the mouth and/or infections involving the oropharyngeal and esophageal mucosa (e.g., candidiasis, herpes simplex)

Abdominal pain related to nonspecific gastritis and opportunistic infection or neoplastic involvement of the intestine

Neuropathic pain related to the effect of HIV, some opportunistic infections, and some medications (e.g., didanosine, zalcitabine, isoniazid) on the peripheral nerves

Headache related to:
- Cranial inflammation/pressure associated with an opportunistic infection involving the sinuses or brain or the presence of a cerebral neoplasm
- Vasoactive cytokines that are present with HIV infection

Chest pain related to:
- Inflammation of the parietal pleura associated with an opportunistic infection of the lungs
- Muscle strain associated with excessive coughing if present

Skin and local tissue pain related to:
- Skin lesions associated with opportunistic infection and/or Kaposi's sarcoma
- Skin breakdown in perianal area associated with diarrhea

CLINICAL MANIFESTATIONS

Subjective	Objective
Verbal report of pain identifying the level of intensity using a pain rating scale; loss of appetite	Inability to breathe deeply, ambulate, sleep, or perform activities of daily living; crying; muscle rigidity; diaphoresis; blood pressure (B/P) or pulse changes; increase in the rate and depth of breathing

RISK FACTORS
- Chronic physical disability
- Chronic psychosocial disability
- Injury agents

DESIRED OUTCOMES

The client will experience diminished pain as evidenced by:
a. Verbalization of a decrease in or absence of pain
b. Relaxed facial expression and body positioning
c. Increased participation in activities
d. Stable vital signs

NOC OUTCOMES	NIC INTERVENTIONS
Comfort level; pain control; pain: disruptive effects	Pain management; environmental management: comfort; analgesic administration

NURSING ASSESSMENT

Assess for and report signs and symptoms of pain:
- Verbalization of pain
- Grimacing
- Reluctance to move or breathe deeply
- Rubbing head
- Reluctance to eat
- Restlessness
- Diaphoresis
- Increased B/P
- Tachycardia

Assess client's perception of the severity of pain using a pain intensity rating scale.

Assess the client's pain pattern:
- Location
- Quality
- Onset
- Duration
- Precipitating factors
- Aggravating factors
- Alleviating factors

Ask the client to describe previous pain experiences and methods used to manage pain effectively.

RATIONALE

Early recognition of signs and symptoms of acute or chronic pain allows for prompt intervention.

THERAPEUTIC INTERVENTIONS

Independent Actions

Implement measures to reduce pain: **D** ✦
- Perform actions to reduce fear and anxiety about the pain experience:
  - Assure client the need for pain relief is understood.
  - Plan methods for achieving pain control with client.
- Perform actions to reduce fear and anxiety:
  - Instruct client in relaxation techniques and encourage participation in diversional activities.
- Administer analgesics before activities and procedures that can cause pain and before pain becomes severe.
- Perform actions to reduce fatigue:
  - Organize nursing care to allow for uninterrupted periods of rest.
- Provide or assist with nonpharmacological methods for pain relief.
  - Position change
  - Progressive relaxation exercises
  - Guided imagery
  - Restful environment
  - Diversional activities such as watching television, reading, or conversing
- Plan methods for achieving pain control with client.
- Perform actions to prevent and treat oral mucous membrane and skin lesions:
  - Lubricate lips frequently
  - Have client rinse mouth frequently with salt and warm water.

RATIONALE

Actions help promote relaxation and subsequently increase the client's threshold and tolerance for pain.

Actions help to increase the client's threshold and tolerance for pain.

Collaborating with clients regarding pain control strategies can assist them in maintaining a sense of control over the pain experience.

NDx = NANDA-I Diagnosis   **D** = Delegatable Action   ● = UAP   ✦ = LVN/LPN   ⊖▶ = Go to ⊖volve for animation

Continued...

THERAPEUTIC INTERVENTIONS	RATIONALE

Dependent/Collaborative Actions

Implement measures to reduce pain:

- Administer the following if ordered:
  - Nonopioid (nonnarcotic) analgesics such as salicylates and other nonsteroidal anti-inflammatory agents
  - Opioid (narcotic) analgesics

  - Tricyclic antidepressants (e.g., amitriptyline) and/or anticonvulsants (e.g., carbamazepine, gabapentin)
  - Topical anesthetic/analgesic ointments (e.g., capsaicin)

  - Oral anesthetic and/or protective agents (e.g., sucralfate, viscous xylocaine mixed with diphenhydramine elixir and a magnesium or aluminum antacid)
  - Corticosteroids

  - Antimicrobials and/or antineoplastic agents

Consult appropriate health care provider if adequate pain relief cannot be achieved with the above measures.

Nonopioid analgesics are thought to interfere with the transmission of pain impulses by inhibiting prostaglandin synthesis

Opioid analgesics act by altering the clients perception of pain and emotional response to the pain experience

Tricyclic antidepressants are used to treat painful neuropathies.

Topical anesthetics help alleviate skin and superficial neuropathic pain.

Anesthetic agents help control pain by inhibiting the initiation and conduction of pain impulses along sensory pathways.

Corticosteroids may be utilized to relieve pain associated with some central nervous system lesions, sinusitis, and peripheral neuropathies.

These agents may be given to treat HIV infection and/or opportunistic disease(s) causing the pain.

Consulting the appropriate health care provider allows for modification of the treatment plan.

Nursing Diagnosis   IMBALANCED NUTRITION: LESS THAN BODY REQUIREMENTS NDx

Definition: Intake of nutrients insufficient to meet metabolic demands

Related to:

- **Decreased oral intake** associated with:
  - Anorexia resulting from malaise, fatigue, fear, anxiety, pain, depression, increased levels of certain cytokines that depress appetite (e.g., tumor necrosis factor [TNF]), and some antiretroviral agents
  - Nausea, dyspnea, and cognitive impairment if present
  - Oral pain and/or dysphagia resulting from opportunistic lesions in the mouth, pharynx, and esophagus
- **Impaired utilization of nutrients** associated with:
  - Accelerated and inefficient metabolism of nutrients resulting from an increased resting energy expenditure that occurs with infection and increased levels of certain cytokines (e.g., TNF, interleukin-1)
  - Decreased absorption of nutrients if HIV and/or opportunistic infection involve the intestine
- **Loss of nutrients associated with persistent diarrhea and vomiting** if present

CLINICAL MANIFESTATIONS

Subjective	Objective
Self report of inadequate food intake; reported lack of food; aversion to eating; lack of interest in food	Body weight 20% or more under ideal body weight; loss of weight with adequate food intake; weakness of muscles required for swallowing or chewing; sore, inflamed buccal cavity; hyperactive bowel sounds; diarrhea; excessive hair loss

RISK FACTORS

- Inability to digest food
- Inability to absorb nutrients
- Biological factors

DESIRED OUTCOMES

The client will maintain an adequate nutritional status as evidenced by:
   a. Weight within normal range for client
   b. Normal blood urea nitrogen (BUN) and serum albumin, prealbumin, hematocrit (Hct), and hemoglobin (Hgb) levels and lymphocyte count
   c. Usual strength and activity tolerance
   d. Healthy oral mucous membranes

NOC OUTCOMES	NIC INTERVENTIONS
Appetite; nutritional status	Nutritional monitoring; nutritional management; nutritional therapy; exercise promotion: strength training; nausea management

NURSING ASSESSMENT	RATIONALE

Assess for and report signs and symptoms of malnutrition:
• Weight significantly below client's usual weight or below normal for client's age, height, and body frame
• Weakness and fatigue
• Sore, inflamed oral mucous membrane
• Pale conjunctiva
• Lower-than-normal anthropometric measurements:
  • Skinfold thickness
  • Body circumferences (e.g., hip, waist, mid-upper arm)
  • Bioelectrical impedance analysis
Monitor percentage of meals and snacks client consumes. Report a pattern of inadequate intake.
	Early recognition of signs and symptoms of malnutrition allows for prompt intervention.

Monitor BUN, serum prealbumin, albumin, Hct, and Hgb levels	*Abnormal BUN, low serum prealbumin, albumin, Hct, and Hgb levels may indicate malnutrition. Because of the long (20 day) half-life of albumin, the value is a late indicator of malnutrition. Prealbumin has a half-life of 2 days and is a more timely, sensitive indicator of protein status.*

THERAPEUTIC INTERVENTIONS	RATIONALE

Independent Actions
Implement measures to maintain an adequate nutritional status:
• Perform actions to improve oral intake:
  • Implement measures to prevent breakdown of the oral mucous membrane and promote healing of existing lesions:
    • Lubricate lips frequently. **D** ✦
    • Rinse mouth frequently with salt and warm water; baking soda and warm water; or a solution of salt, baking soda, and warm water. **D** ✦
  • Implement measures to reduce nausea:
    • Encourage client to eat dry foods when nauseated.
    • Avoid serving foods with an overpowering aroma.
  • Implement measures to reduce pain.
  • Increase activity as tolerated.
  • If client is having difficulty swallowing, assist him/her to select foods that are easily chewed and swallowed (e.g., eggs, custard, macaroni and cheese, baby foods) and avoid serving foods that are sticky (e.g., peanut butter, soft bread).
  • Encourage a rest period before meals to minimize fatigue.
  • Maintain a clean environment and a relaxed, pleasant atmosphere. **D** ●
  • Provide oral hygiene before meals. **D** ●
  • Serve frequent, small meals rather than large ones if client is weak, fatigues easily, and/or has a poor appetite.
  • If client is dyspneic, place in a high-Fowler's position for meals and provide supplemental oxygen therapy during meals.
  • If client's sense of taste is altered, suggest adding extra sweeteners and flavorings/seasonings to foods.
	Actions help to reduce oral/pharyngeal pain and improve swallowing.
	
	Activity promotes a sense of well-being, which can improve appetite.
	
	Oral hygiene moistens the mouth, which may make it easier to chew and swallow; it also removes unpleasant tastes, which often improves the taste of foods/fluids.

NDx = NANDA-I Diagnosis   **D** = Delegatable Action   ● = UAP   ✦ = LVN/_PN   ⊖▶ = Go to ⊖volve for animation

Continued...

THERAPEUTIC INTERVENTIONS	RATIONALE
• Encourage significant others to bring in client's favorite foods and eat with him/her. • Assist client with meals if indicated. **D** ● • Allow adequate time for meals; reheat foods/fluids as necessary. • Perform actions to control diarrhea: • Instruct client to avoid foods/fluids that may stimulate or irritate the bowel or cause the stool to be more liquid.	*Action will assist client in selecting foods/fluids that meet nutritional needs, are appealing, and adhere to personal and cultural preferences.*

Dependent/Collaborative Actions

Implement measures to maintain an adequate nutritional status:
• Perform actions to improve oral intake:
  • Administer prescribed antiemetics.
  • Obtain a dietary consult if necessary.
• Ensure that meals are well balanced and high in essential nutrients; offer high-protein, high-calorie dietary supplements:
  • Elemental formulas
  • Nutrient-dense candy bars and soups if indicated
• Administer the following if ordered:
  • Vitamins and minerals
  • Appetite stimulants
  • Anabolic agents
  • Cytokine inhibitors (e.g., Thalidomide)
	Decreases nausea
	
	Cytokine inhibitors help to improve appetite and promote weight gain by suppressing TNF-α production (use of thalidomide is reserved for persons with severe HIV-related wasting).

Perform a calorie count if ordered. Report information to dietitian and physician. Consult physician or physical therapist about a progressive exercise program. Consult physician about an alternative method of providing nutrition if client does not consume enough food or fluids to meet nutritional needs: • Parenteral nutrition • Tube feedings	*Exercise is necessary to promote the maintenance/buildup of lean body mass and help prevent wasting.* *Consulting the appropriate health care provider allows for modification of the treatment plan.*

Nursing Diagnosis   ## RISK FOR IMBALANCED FLUID VOLUME NDx AND RISK FOR ELECTROLYTE IMBALANCE NDx

Definition: At risk for decrease, increase, or rapid shift from one to the other of intracellular, interstitial and/or extracellular fluid; at risk for imbalance of electrolytes

Related to:

- **Deficient fluid volume NDx** related to:
  - Excessive loss of fluid associated with diarrhea, diaphoresis, and vomiting if present
  - Decreased oral intake associated with anorexia, weakness, nausea, and oropharyngeal pain
- **Hypokalemia** related to:
  - Excessive loss of potassium associated with diarrhea and vomiting if present
  - Decreased oral intake
- **Hyponatremia** related to:
  - Excessive loss of sodium associated with diarrhea, profuse diaphoresis, and vomiting if present
  - Excessive loss of sodium associated with diarrhea, profuse diaphoresis, and vomiting if present
  - Water retention associated with increased antidiuretic hormone (ADH) output resulting from opportunistic disease involvement of the lungs or central nervous system

CLINICAL MANIFESTATIONS

Subjective	**Objective**
Verbal reports of weakness; confusion	Change in mental status; decreased skin turgor; postural hypotension; weak, rapid pulse; decreased urine output; cardiac dysrhythmias; nausea and vomiting; absent bowel sounds

RISK FACTORS

- Abdominal ascites
- Sepsis

DESIRED OUTCOMES

The client will maintain fluid and electrolyte balance as evidenced by:
  a. Normal skin turgor
  b. Moist mucous membranes
  c. Stable weight
  d. B/P and pulse within normal range for client and stable with position change
  e. Capillary refill time less than 2 to 3 seconds
  f. Usual mental status
  g. Balanced intake and output
  h. Usual muscle strength
  i. Soft, nondistended abdomen with normal bowel sounds
  j. Absence of nausea, vomiting, abdominal cramps, and seizure activity
  k. BUN, Hct, and serum potassium and sodium levels within normal range

NOC OUTCOMES

Fluid balance; hydration; electrolyte and acid-base balance

NIC NTERVENTIONS

Fluid management; electrolyte management: hypokalemia; electrolyte management: hyponatremia

NURSING ASSESSMENT

Assess for and report signs and symptoms of:
- Deficient fluid volume:
  - Decreased skin turgor, dry mucous membranes, thirst
  - Weight loss of 2% or greater over a short period
  - Postural hypotension and/or low B/P
  - Weak, rapid pulse
  - Capillary refill time greater than 2 to 3 seconds
  - Change in mental status
  - Decreased urine output (reflects an actual rather than potential fluid deficit)
- Hypokalemia
  - Cardiac dysrhythmias
  - Postural hypotension
  - Muscle weakness
  - Nausea and vomiting
  - Abdominal distention
  - Hypoactive or absent bowel sounds
- Hyponatremia
  - Nausea and vomiting
  - Abdominal cramps
  - Lethargy
  - Confusion
  - Weakness
  - Seizures
Monitor serum electrolyte, BUN, creatinine levels

RATIONALE

Early recognition of signs and symptoms of imbalanced fluid and electrolytes allow for prompt intervention.

NDx = NANDA-I Diagnosis   **D** = Delegatable Action   ● = UAP   ✦ = LVN/_PN   ⊖▶ = Go to ⊖volve for animation

Continued...

THERAPEUTIC INTERVENTIONS	RATIONALE

Independent Actions
Implement measures to prevent or treat imbalanced fluid and electrolytes:
• Perform actions to control diarrhea:
  • Instruct client to avoid foods/fluids that may stimulate or irritate the bowel or cause the stool to be more liquid.
• Perform actions to improve oral intake (e.g., prevent breakdown of oral mucous membrane).
• Perform actions to reduce fever (e.g., tepid sponge bath, cool cloths to groin and axillae).
• Encourage intake of foods/fluids high in potassium:
  • Bananas
  • Avocado
  • Potatoes
  • Raisins
  • Cantaloupe
• Encourage intake of foods/fluids high in sodium
  • Processed cheese
  • Canned soups
  • Canned vegetables
  • Bouillon
	Persistent or severe diarrhea results in excessive loss of gastrointestinal fluid.
	Foods or fluids that stimulate the bowel lead to increased intestinal motility and excessive mucous production that increases the liquidity of the intestinal contents.

Dependent/Collaborative Actions Implement measures to prevent or treat imbalanced fluid and electrolytes: • Administer antiemetics if ordered to control vomiting. • Maintain a fluid intake of at least 2500 mL/day unless contraindicated; if oral intake is inadequate or contraindicated, maintain intravenous and/or enteral therapy as ordered. • Administer electrolyte replacements if ordered.	*Nausea often causes the client to have decreased fluid intake. Preventing vomiting results in excessive loss of fluid.* *Adequate fluid intake needs to be provided to ensure adequate hydration.* *Serum electrolytes such as sodium and potassium, with narrow therapeutic ranges, must be kept within normal limits for normal body functions to occur.*
Consult physician if signs and symptoms of imbalanced fluid and electrolytes persist or worsen.	*Consulting the appropriate health care provider allows for modification of the treatment plan.*

Nursing Diagnosis HYPERTHERMIA NDx

Definition: Body temperature elevated above normal range

Related to: Stimulation of the thermoregulatory center in the hypothalamus by endogenous pyrogens that are released in an infectious process

CLINICAL MANIFESTATIONS

Subjective	Objective
Verbal reports of headache	Increase in body temperature above normal range; flushed skin; warm to touch; increased respiratory rate; tachycardia; seizures; convulsions

RISK FACTORS
• Increased metabolic rate
• Illness
• Medications
• Dehydration

DESIRED OUTCOMES

The client will experience resolution of hyperthermia as evidenced by:
  a. Skin usual temperature and color
  b. Pulse rate between 60 and 100 beats/min
  c. Respiratory rate 12 to 20 breaths/min
  d. Normal body temperature

NOC OUTCOMES	NIC INTERVENTIONS
Thermoregulation	Fever treatment

NURSING ASSESSMENT	**RATIONALE**
Assess for signs and symptoms of hyperthermia: • Warm, flushed skin • Tachycardia • Tachypnea • Elevated temperature	*Early recognition of signs and symptoms of hyperthermia allows for prompt intervention.*
Monitor and record all sources of fluid loss.	*Excessive fluid loss that may occur with hyperthermia can potentiate the loss of fluid and electrolytes.*
Monitor laboratory studies: • Arterial blood gas values • Serum electrolyte levels • Urinalysis • Chest x-ray results	*Hyperthermia may be a symptom of infection. Monitoring laboratory studies helps to identify possible contributing factors.*

THERAPEUTIC INTERVENTIONS	**RATIONALE**

Independent Actions

Implement measures to reduce fever:
- Perform actions to resolve the infectious process:
  - Implement measures to promote rest.
  - Implement measures to maintain an adequate nutritional status.
  - Implement measures to promote removal of pulmonary secretions if a respiratory infection is present.
- Administer tepid sponge bath and/or apply cool cloths to groin and axillae if indicated.
- Use a room fan to provide cool circulating air. **D** ●
- Apply cooling blanket if ordered. **D** ✦

While hyperthermia/fever is an important defense mechanism, the stress of fever is great. Fever increases demands on the cardiorespiratory system. A prolonged fever may weaken a client by exhausting energy stores. If the source of the fever is a potential respiratory infection, appropriate interventions that mobilize secretions must be implemented.

Dependent/Collaborative Actions

Implement measures to reduce fever:
- Perform actions to resolve the infectious process:
  - Maintain a fluid intake of at least 2500 mL/day unless contraindicated.
  - Administer antimicrobials as ordered.
- Administer antipyretics if ordered.

Fever may be accompanied by diaphoresis, which can result in excessive loss of fluid.

Consult physician if temperature remains higher than 38.5°C.

Consulting the appropriate health care provider allows for modification of the treatment plan.

Nursing Diagnosis   **FATIGUE** NDx

Definition: An overwhelming sustained sense of exhaustion and decreased capacity for physical and mental work at usual level

Related to:
- Difficulty resting and sleeping
- Increased energy utilization associated with the elevated metabolic rate that is present with infection
- Malnutrition
- Tissue hypoxia associated with:
  - Impaired alveolar gas exchange if respiratory infection is present
  - Anemia resulting from:
    - HIV or opportunistic disease involvement of erythroid precursors in the bone marrow
    - Treatment with medications that can cause bone marrow depression or red blood cell (RBC) hemolysis (e.g., zidovudine, antineoplastic agents, trimethoprim-sulfamethoxazole [TMP-SMX])
    - Vitamin B_{12} or folate deficiency (a result of malabsorption if intestinal involvement is present)
- Overwhelming emotional demands associated with the diagnosis of AIDS
- Side effects of some medications client may be receiving (e.g., narcotic [opioid] analgesics, antiemetics, antianxiety or antipsychotic agents)

NDx = NANDA-I Diagnosis   **D** = Delegatable Action   ● = UAP   ✦ = LVN/LPN   ⊖▶ = Go to ⊖volve for animation

Continued...

CLINICAL MANIFESTATIONS

Subjective	Objective
Verbalization of overwhelming lack of energy; tired; increase in physical complaints; compromised libido; inability to restore energy even after sleep	Lethargic or listless; drowsy; compromised concentration; disinterest in surroundings; decreased performance

RISK FACTORS

- Stress
- Depression
- Anemia
- Malnutrition

DESIRED OUTCOMES

The client will experience a reduction in fatigue as evidenced by:
  a. Verbalization of feelings of increased energy
  b. Ability to perform usual activities of daily living
  c. Increased interest in surroundings and ability to concentrate

NOC OUTCOMES

Endurance; energy conservation; rest; psychomotor energy

NIC INTERVENTIONS

Energy management; exercise promotion: strength training; nutrition management; sleep enhancement; mood management

NURSING ASSESSMENT

Assess for signs and symptoms of fatigue:
- Verbalization of lack of energy and inability to maintain usual routines
- Lack of interest in surroundings
- Decreased ability to concentrate
- Lethargy

Assist client to identify personal patterns of fatigue:
- Time of day
- After certain activities

RATIONALE

Early recognition and reporting of signs and symptoms of fatigue allow for prompt intervention.

THERAPEUTIC INTERVENTIONS

Independent Actions

Inform client that a feeling of persistent fatigue is not unusual and is a result of the disease itself as well as a side effect of certain medications the client may be taking.

Plan activities so that times of great fatigue are avoided.

Implement measures to increase strength and reduce fatigue:

D ✦ ●

- Perform actions to promote rest and/or conserve energy:
  - Maintain activity restrictions if ordered.
  - Minimize environmental activity and noise.
    - Organize nursing care to allow for periods of uninterrupted rest.
  - Assist client with self-care activities as needed.
  - Keep supplies and personal articles within easy reach.
  - Instruct client in energy-saving techniques:
    - Using shower chair when showering
    - Sitting to brush teeth or comb hair
  - Implement measures to reduce fear and anxiety and assist the client to adjust to and cope with the diagnosis of AIDS.
  - Implement measures to reduce pain.

RATIONALE

Any physical illness that causes pain or discomfort can result in fatigue. A client needs to be reassured that this is not unusual.

Do not plan activities for nursing convenience such as evening hours.

Schedule activities, treatments, or procedures for times when the client is awake in order to maximize the client's participation

THERAPEUTIC INTERVENTIONS	RATIONALE

- Implement measures to promote sleep:
  - Encourage relaxing diversional activities in the evening.
  - Allow client to continue usual sleep practices unless contraindicated.
  - Reduce environmental stimuli.
- Increase client's activity as allowed and tolerated.
- Perform actions to resolve the infectious process.
  - Encourage rest periods before meals to minimize fatigue.
- Perform actions to maintain adequate nutritional status.
- Perform actions to improve respiratory status:
  - Maintain activity restrictions as ordered to reduce oxygen needs.
  - Position the client for effective ventilation:
  - Sitting upright in bed propped with pillows
  - Discourage smoking and excessive intake of beverages high in caffeine such as coffee, tea, and colas.

Infection is a great source of stress and should be resolved to reduce the incidence of fatigue.
Adequate nutrition is needed to maintain optimal function of the immune system.

Clients with respiratory disorders should be positioned to promote effective breathing.
Nicotine and caffeine can increase cardiac workload and myocardial oxygen utilization, thereby decreasing oxygen availability.

Dependent/Collaborative Actions

Implement measures to increase strength and reduce fatigue:
- Perform actions to promote rest and/or conserve energy:
  - Administer prescribed sedative-hypnotics.

- Administer the following if ordered to treat anemia:
  - Packed red blood cells
  - Erythropoiesis-stimulating growth factor to stimulate RBC production (e.g., epoetin alfa)

- Administer stimulants if ordered (e.g., dextroamphetamine).

Consult appropriate health care provider (e.g., rehabilitation therapist, psychiatric nurse clinician, physician) if signs and symptoms of fatigue worsen.

Sedatives/hypnotics are central nervous system depressants that promote sleep.
Adequate sleep can reduce the incidence of fatigue.
Anemia is a reduction of the number of circulating erythrocytes or a decrease in the quality or quantity of hemoglobin. With anemia, oxygen-carrying capacity of the blood is reduced causing tissue hypoxia, resulting in symptoms of weakness and fatigue.
Stimulants act by stimulating the central nervous system. Stimulants may be used to prevent or reverse fatigue or sleep.
Consulting the appropriate health care provider allows for modification of the treatment plan.

Nursing Diagnosis **DISTURBED THOUGHT PROCESSES** NDx

Definition: Disruption in cognitive operations and activities

Related to: HIV encephalopathy associated with:
- AIDS dementia complex resulting from a direct effect of HIV on the central nervous system
- Opportunistic infections and/or neoplasms involving the central nervous system (e.g., toxoplasmic encephalitis, cryptococcal meningitis, progressive multifocal leukoencephalopathy, cytomegalovirus [CMV] encephalitis, primary central nervous system lymphoma)
- Imbalanced fluid and electrolytes and hypoxemia if present

CLINICAL MANIFESTATIONS

Subjective	Objective
Verbalization of hallucinations; delusions; memory deficit/problems	Inaccurate interpretation of the environment; distractibility; inappropriate social behavior; decreased ability to make decisions

Continued...

RISK FACTOR

- Cerebral abscess

DESIRED OUTCOMES

> The client will experience improvement in thought processes as evidenced by:
> a. Improved verbal response time
> b. Longer attention span

NOC OUTCOMES

Cognitive orientation; cognition; information processing

NIC INTERVENTIONS

Dementia management; behavior modification; medication administration

NURSING ASSESSMENT

Assess client for disturbed thought processes:
- Slowed verbal responses
- Decreased ability to concentrate
- Impaired memory
- Poor reasoning
- Apathy
- Agitation
- Hallucinations
- Confusion

Ascertain from significant others client's usual level of cognitive and emotional functioning.

RATIONALE

Early recognition and reporting of signs and symptoms of disturbed thought processes allow for prompt intervention.

THERAPEUTIC INTERVENTIONS

Independent Actions

If client shows evidence of altered thought processes:
- Reorient client to person, place, and time as necessary; avoid repeatedly asking questions about orientation that client cannot answer.
- Address client by name.
- Place familiar objects, clock, and calendar within client's view.
- Approach client in a slow, calm manner; allow adequate time for communication.
- Repeat instructions as necessary using clear, simple language and short sentences.
- Keep environmental stimuli to a minimum
- Avoid touch and proximity if this appears to increase anxiety.
- Maintain a consistent and fairly structured routine and write out schedule of activities for client to refer to if desired.
- Have client perform only one activity at a time and allow adequate time for performance of activities
- Encourage client to make lists of planned activities, questions, and concerns.
- Use distraction rather than confrontation to manage negative behavior.
- Set limits on negative behavior and avoid arguing about the established limits.
- If client is confused or experiencing hallucinations, allow significant others to remain with client in order to provide constant reassurance.
- Encourage significant others to be supportive of client; instruct them in methods of dealing with client's disturbed thought processes.

RATIONALE

Actions help to maintain a safe and therapeutic environment.

THERAPEUTIC INTERVENTIONS	RATIONALE

- Discuss physiological basis for disturbed thought processes with client and significant others; inform them that cognitive and emotional functioning may improve with drug therapy

Dependent/Collaborative Actions
- Implement measures to improve client's thought processes:
  - Perform actions to improve tissue oxygenation.

- Perform actions to prevent or treat imbalanced fluid and electrolytes.
- Administer the following medications if ordered:
  - Antimicrobials to treat HIV and opportunistic infections
  - Antineoplastic agents to treat neoplastic conditions affecting the central nervous system
  - Antipsychotic agents (e.g., haloperidol, perphenazine, risperidone, chlorpromazine) to reduce restlessness, agitation, or hallucinations
  - Antimania/mood-stabilizing agents (e.g., lithium; anticonvulsants such as carbamazepine, valproic acid, and gabapentin)
  - Central nervous system stimulants (e.g., dextroamphetamine sulfate, methylphenidate [Ritalin]) to reduce apathy and withdrawn behavior
- Toxoplasma and cryptococcal serology studies
- Cerebrospinal fluid analysis
- Brain biopsy
- Neuropsychological tests
Consult appropriate health care provider (e.g., psychiatric nurse clinician, physician) if disturbed thought processes persist or worsen.

Decreased tissue oxygenation to the cerebral tissues can lead to alterations in normal thought processes.
Electrolyte imbalances such as alterations in normal sodium levels can cause alterations in normal thought processes.

Diagnostic studies may be done to determine the cause of disturbed thought processes.

Consulting the appropriate health care provider allows for modification of the treatment plan.

Nursing Diagnosis ## RISK FOR INFECTION NDx (OPPORTUNISTIC INFECTION OR SEPSIS)

Definition: At increased risk for being invaded by pathogenic organisms

Related to:
- Decreased resistance to infection associated with:
  - Cellular and humoral immune deficiencies present in HIV infection
  - Inadequate nutritional status
  - Depletion of immune mechanisms resulting from presenting infection and treatment with antimicrobial agents
  - Myelosuppression resulting from certain medications (e.g., zidovudine, antineoplastic agents, trimethoprim-sulfamethoxazole, ganciclovir, pyrimethamine)
- Stasis of respiratory secretions and/or urinary stasis if mobility is decreased
- Break in integrity of skin associated with frequent venipunctures or placement of a central venous catheter
- Impaired integrity of skin or mucous membranes if present

CLINICAL MANIFESTATIONS*

Subjective	Objective
Verbal reports of pain at areas of impaired skin integrity	Fever, chills, tachycardia, warm discharge over areas of impaired skin integrity

*Specific objective and subjective symptoms will depend on site of infection and causative organism.

NDx = NANDA-I Diagnosis   **D** = Delegatable Action   ● = UAP   ✦ = LVN/LPN   ⊝▶ = Go to ⊝volve for animation

Continued...

DESIRED OUTCOMES

The client will remain free of additional opportunistic infection and sepsis as evidenced by:

1. Return of temperature toward client's normal range
2. Decrease in episodes of chills and diaphoresis
3. B/P within normal limits and pulse rate returning toward normal range
4. Normal or improved breath sounds
5. Absence or resolution of dyspnea
6. Stable or improved mental status
7. Voiding clear urine without reports of frequency, urgency, and burning
8. Absence or resolution of painful, pruritic skin lesions
9. Stable or gradual increase in body weight
10. No reports of increased weakness and fatigue
11. Absence of visual disturbances
12. Absence or resolution of heat, pain, redness, swelling, and unusual drainage in any area
13. Absence or resolution of oral mucous membrane irritation and ulceration
14. Ability to swallow without difficulty
15. White blood cell (WBC) and differential counts returning toward normal range
16. Negative results of cultured specimens

NOC OUTCOMES

Immune status; infection severity

NIC INTERVENTIONS

Infection control; infection protection

NURSING ASSESSMENT

Assess for and report signs and symptoms of additional opportunistic infection and sepsis (be alert to subtle changes in client since the signs of infection may be minimal as a result of immunosuppression; also be aware that some signs and symptoms vary depending on the site of infection, the causative organism, and the age of the client):

- Increase in temperature above client's usual level
- Increase in episodes of chills and diaphoresis
- Hypotension (a symptom of sepsis)
- Increased pulse rate
- Development or worsening of abnormal breath sounds
- Development or worsening of dyspnea
- Development or worsening of cough
- Decline in mental status
- Cloudy urine
- Reports of frequency, urgency, or burning when urinating
- Urinalysis showing a WBC count greater than 5, positive leukocyte esterase or nitrites, or presence of bacteria
- Vesicular lesions particularly on face, lips, and perianal area
- New or increased reports of pain in and/or itching of skin lesions and surrounding tissue
- Further increase in weight loss, fatigue, or weakness
- Visual disturbances
- New or increased heat, pain, redness, swelling, or unusual drainage in any area
- New or increased irritation or ulceration of oral mucous membrane
- Development of or increased dysphagia
- Significant change in WBC count and/or differential
- Positive results of cultured specimens (e.g., urine, vaginal drainage, stool, sputum, blood, drainage from lesions)

Assess results of complete blood cell count (CBC) with differential, and of all cultured specimens for positive results.

RATIONALE

Early recognition of signs and symptoms of infection allows for prompt intervention.

THERAPEUTIC INTERVENTIONS	RATIONALE

Independent Actions

Implement measures to prevent further infection:

- Use good hand hygiene and encourage client to do the same.
- Protect client from others with infection.
- Maintain sterile technique during all invasive procedures:
  - Urinary catheterization
  - Venous and arterial punctures
  - Injections

The use of sterile technique reduces the risk of introduction of pathogens into the body.

- Change peripheral intravenous line sites according to hospital policy.
- Anchor catheters/tubings:
  - Urinary
  - Intravenous

Securing catheters and tubings helps to reduce trauma to the tissues and the risk for introduction of pathogens associated with the in-and-out movement of the tubing.

- Change equipment, tubings, and solutions used for treatments such as intravenous infusions, respiratory care, irrigations, and enteral feedings according to hospital policy.
- Maintain a closed system for drains (e.g., urinary catheter) and intravenous infusions whenever possible.
- Provide a low-microbe diet (e.g., thoroughly cooked foods, fruits and vegetables that have been washed thoroughly).
- Perform actions to prevent stasis of respiratory secretions:
  - Assist client to turn, cough, and deep breathe.
  - Increase activity as allowed and tolerated.
- Instruct and assist client to perform good perineal care routinely and after each bowel movement.
- Perform actions identified in this care plan to reduce stressors, such as discomfort, dyspnea, and fear and anxiety.

Reducing stress helps to prevent an increase in secretion of cortisol (cortisol interferes with some immune responses).

- Perform actions to prevent breakdown of oral mucous membrane and promote healing of existing lesions:
  - Have client rinse mouth frequently with salt and warm water; baking soda and warm water; or a solution of salt, baking soda, and warm water.

Salt water/baking soda mouth rinses help to alkalinize the mouth, which reduces bacteria, as bacteria thrive in acidic environments.

- Perform actions to prevent or treat skin breakdown.

Healthy, intact skin reduces the risk of infection.

- Implement measures to relieve pruritus.
- If client has open lesions, perform actions to prevent wound infection:
  - Maintain sterile technique during wound care.
  - Instruct client to avoid touching wounds.
- Perform actions to prevent urinary retention:
  - Instruct client to urinate when the urge is first felt.
  - Promote relaxation during voiding attempts.

A client experiencing urinary retention is at increased risk for a urinary tract infection because the accumulated urine creates an environment conducive to the growth and colonization of organisms.

- If client has a central venous catheter, instruct and assist the client with proper care of the exit site.

Dependent/Collaborative Actions

Implement measures to prevent further infection:

- Administer the following if ordered:
  - Antiretroviral agents
  - Immunomodulating agents (e.g., interleukin-2, colony-stimulating factors such as filgrastim and sargramostim)

Agents to reduce the rate of replication of HIV
Agents to stimulate production/enhance activity of the WBCs

  - Antimicrobial agents (prophylaxis for *Pneumocystis carinii* pneumonia, *Mycobacterium tuberculosis*, toxoplasmosis, and *Mycobacterium avium* complex is recommended for all patients with a CD4+ cell count below a critical level)

Agents to treat current infection or prevent additional opportunistic infection

Continued...

THERAPEUTIC INTERVENTIONS	RATIONALE

- Vaccines (e.g., hepatitis A, hepatitis B, pneumococcal pneumonia, influenza)
- Maintain a fluid intake of at least 2500 mL/day unless contraindicated.
- Perform actions to maintain an adequate nutritional status:
  - Obtain a dietary consult if necessary to assist client in selecting foods/fluids that meet nutritional needs.

DISCHARGE TEACHING/CONTINUED CARE

Nursing Diagnosis | # DEFICIENT KNOWLEDGE NDx; INEFFECTIVE FAMILY THERAPEUTIC REGIMEN MANAGEMENT; OR INEFFECTIVE HEALTH MAINTENANCE* NDx

Definition: Absence or deficiency of cognitive information related to specific topic (lack of specific information necessary for clients/significant others to make informed choices regarding condition/treatment/lifestyle changes); pattern of regulating and integrating into family processes a program for treatment of illness and the sequelae of illness that is unsatisfactory for meeting specific health goals; inability to identify, manage, and/or seek out help to manage health

CLINICAL MANIFESTATIONS

Subjective	Objective
Verbalization of the desire to manage illness; verbalization of difficulty with prescribed regimen	Failure to include treatment in daily routines; failure to take action to reduce risk factors; makes choices in daily living ineffective for meeting health goals; inadequate follow through of instruction

RISK FACTORS

- Cognitive limitations
- Lack of recall
- Unfamiliarity with information, resources

NOC OUTCOMES	NIC INTERVENTIONS
Knowledge: disease process; knowledge: treatment regimen; knowledge: health behavior; knowledge: health resources; knowledge: infection control	Health system guidance; teaching: disease process; teaching: prescribed diet; teaching: prescribed medication; communicable disease management; financial resource assistance

*The nurse should select the diagnostic label that is most appropriate for the client's discharge teaching needs.

NURSING ASSESSMENT	RATIONALE
Assess the client's baseline understanding of: • Disease process • Therapeutic regimen • Health prevention measures	*Understanding the client's baseline knowledge allows for implementation of the appropriate interventions.*
Assess the client's access to resources to help with successful implementation of the treatment plan.	*Early identification of barriers to therapeutic regimen management allows for implementation of the appropriate interventions.*

THERAPEUTIC INTERVENTIONS	RATIONALE

Desired Outcome: The client will identify ways to prevent the spread of HIV.

Independent Actions

Instruct client in ways to prevent the spread of HIV to others:

HIV is a fragile virus that can be transmitted only under specified conditions in which a client comes in contact with infected body fluids including blood, vaginal secretions, and breast milk. HIV is transmitted through sexual intercourse with an infected partner, exposure to infected blood or blood products, and perinatal transmission during pregnancy, at the time of delivery, or through breast-feeding.

- If a spill of blood or other body fluids occurs, cleanse area with hot, soapy water or a household detergent and then disinfect with a solution of 1 part bleach to 10 parts water.

HIV is inactivated rapidly after being exposed to commonly used chemical germicides such as household bleach.

- Dispose of water used to clean up body fluid spills in the toilet.
- Do not share eating utensils, toothbrushes, razors, enema equipment, or sexual devices.
- Avoid getting pregnant, but if pregnancy occurs, consult health care provider about antiretroviral therapy (e.g., zidovudine) to reduce the risk of perinatal transmission of HIV to infant.
- Do not breast-feed infant.
- Do not donate blood, sperm, or body organs.
- If an intravenous drug user:
  - Get involved in a needle and syringe exchange program.
  - Do not share drug-injecting equipment (e.g., needles, syringes, cookers, cotton, rinse water).
  - Discard disposable needles and syringes after one use or clean them with household bleach and rinse thoroughly with water.

Drug use in and of itself does not cause HIV.
The major risk for HIV infection with drug use is the sharing of drug paraphernalia that may contain the blood of an infected individual.

- If sexually active with a partner:
  - Avoid multiple sexual partners and partners with risky sexual behaviors; be honest with desired partner about HIV infection.
  - Modify techniques so that both partners are protected from contact with body fluids.
  - Avoid unsafe sexual practices:
    - Sharing sex toys
    - Allowing ejaculate to come in contact with broken skin or mucous membranes
    - Intercourse without a condom
    - Any activity that could cause tears in lining of vagina, rectum, or penis
    - Mouth contact with penis, vagina, or anal area
  - Avoid vaginal intercourse during menstruation (the contact with blood increases the risk of HIV transmission).

Safe sexual activity eliminates the risk of exposure to HIV in semen and vaginal secretions. Abstinence is the most effective method.

Continued...

THERAPEUTIC INTERVENTIONS	RATIONALE
Instruct the client in effective use of condoms: • Always use a barrier (male and/or female condom) during anal, vaginal, and oral penetration (condom should be applied before time a body orifice is entered because HIV is found in preseminal fluid). • Use latex or polyurethane condoms (HIV can penetrate other types of materials). • Use condoms with a receptacle tip to reduce the risk of spillage of semen; if that type is unavailable, create a receptacle for ejaculate by pinching tip of condom as it is rolled on erect penis. • Lubricate outside of condom and area to be penetrated to minimize possibility of condom breakage. • Avoid lubricants made of mineral oil or petroleum distillates such as Vaseline or baby oil (these products weaken latex). • Hold condom at base of penis during withdrawal and use caution during removal of condom to prevent spillage of semen (penis should be withdrawn and condom removed before the penis has totally relaxed). • Dispose of condom immediately after use (a new one should be used for subsequent sexual activity). • Store condoms in a cool place to prevent them from drying out and breaking during use. • Do not use a condom if the expiration date on the package has passed, the package looks worn or punctured, or if the condom looks brittle or discolored or is sticky.	*Barriers should be used when engaging in insertive sexual activity. The effectiveness of male condoms is 80% to 90%.*

THERAPEUTIC INTERVENTIONS	RATIONALE
Desired Outcome: The client will identify ways to decrease the risk for developing opportunistic infections. **Independent Actions** Instruct client in ways to decrease risk for developing an opportunistic infection: • Cleanse kitchen and bathroom surfaces regularly with a disinfectant to prevent growth of pathogens. • If respiratory equipment (e.g., inhalers, humidifier) is used at home, cleanse it as instructed and change water in humidifier daily. • Wear gloves when gardening and when in contact with human or pet excreta (e.g., cleaning litter boxes, bird cages, and aquariums). • Avoid exposure to body fluids during sexual activity and use latex or polyurethane condoms during sexual intercourse. • Reduce the risk of food-borne illness. • Thoroughly wash hands and food preparation items and surfaces (e.g., knives, cutting board, countertop) before and after cooking, especially when working with raw meat, poultry, and fish.	*HIV disease progression may be delayed by promoting a healthy immune system.* *Actions that result in avoiding exposure to new infections are useful.*

THERAPEUTIC INTERVENTIONS	RATIONALE

- Avoid intake of foods/fluids with a high microorganism content (e.g., raw or undercooked poultry, seafood, meats, or eggs; unwashed fruits and vegetables; unpasteurized dairy products or fruit juices; raw seed sprouts; soft cheeses; anything that has passed its expiration date).
- Cook leftover foods or ready-to-eat foods (e.g., hot dogs) until steaming hot before eating.
- Avoid foods from delicatessen counters (e.g., prepared meats, salads, cheeses) and refrigerated pâtés and other meat spreads, or reheat these foods until steaming before eating.
- Do not drink water directly from lakes or rivers.
- Boil water for a full minute if a community "boil water" advisory is issued.

- Avoid activities such as cleaning, remodeling, or demolishing old buildings; exploring caves; disturbing soil beneath bird-roosting sites or cleaning chicken coops; being around disturbed native soil at building excavation sites or dust storms.

  Old buildings, damp areas may be source of molds or environmental contaminants. Other areas may be considered to be endemic areas for histoplasmosis and coccidioidomycosis.

- Wash hands after handling pets and avoid contact with reptiles (e.g., snakes, lizards, turtles), baby chickens, and ducklings.

  Action reduces the risk of exposure to environmental contaminants that may lead to viral or bacterial infection.

- Avoid swimming in lakes, rivers, and public pools.
- Keep living quarters well ventilated and change furnace filters regularly to reduce exposure to airborne disease.
- Avoid contact with persons who have an infection and those who have been recently vaccinated.

  Many vaccines are composed of live viruses and create a health risk for those with compromised immune systems.

- Maintain an adequate balance between activity and rest.
- Inform all health care providers of HIV infection so that drugs that further suppress the immune system (e.g., corticosteroids, immunosuppressants) will not be prescribed unnecessarily.
- Drink at least 10 glasses of liquid each day unless contraindicated.

THERAPEUTIC INTERVENTIONS	RATIONALE

Desired Outcome: The client will verbalize ways to maintain optimal nutritional status.

Independent Actions
Provide instructions regarding ways to maintain an optimal nutritional status:

Proper nutrition is essential to maintain body mass and ensure the necessary levels of vitamins and nutrients.

- Eat foods that are high in protein and calories.
- Try to eat a snack or a small meal, or drink a nutritional supplement every 2 to 3 hours.
- Take prescribed vitamins, appetite stimulants (e.g., megestrol acetate), and anabolic agents (e.g., oxandrolone).
- Participate in a progressive exercise program if possible.

THERAPEUTIC INTERVENTIONS	RATIONALE

Desired Outcome: The client will state signs and symptoms to report to the health care provider.

Continued...

THERAPEUTIC INTERVENTIONS	RATIONALE

Independent Actions

Stress importance of notifying the health care provider if the following signs and symptoms occur or if these existing signs and symptoms worsen:

- Persistent fever or chills
- Night sweats
- Persistent headache or different type of headache
- Swollen glands
- Skin lesions or significant rash
- Reddish purple patches or nodules on any body area
- Ulcerations or white patches in the mouth
- Difficulty swallowing
- Persistent diarrhea or vomiting
- Perianal or vulvovaginal itching and/or pain
- Frequency, urgency, or burning on urination
- Cloudy or foul-smelling urine
- Dry cough or a cough productive of purulent, green, or rust-colored sputum
- Progressive shortness of breath
- Increasing weakness, fatigue, or weight loss
- Change in vision, spots that appear to drift in front of eye (floaters)
- Decline in mental function or level of consciousness
- Loss of strength and coordination in extremities
- Inability to maintain an adequate fluid intake
- Yellow discoloration of skin
- Bleeding from rectum that is not related to hemorrhoids
- Severe depression or anxiousness or feeling of being a danger to self or others
- Seizures

Clients must notify the health care provider of signs and symptoms of disease progression or the development of opportunistic infections so the treatment plan can be modified.

THERAPEUTIC INTERVENTIONS	RATIONALE

Desired Outcome: The client will identify resources that can assist with financial needs and adjustment to changes resulting from the diagnosis of AIDS.

Independent Actions

Provide information to client and significant others about state and federally funded financial programs and resources that can assist in adjustment to the diagnosis of AIDS (e.g., American Foundation for AIDS Research, National Association of People with AIDS, hospice programs, community support groups, CDC National AIDS Hotline, Project Inform, counselors).

Initiate referral for state and federally funded financial programs if indicated.

Provides client and family with knowledge of resources to sustain therapeutic regimen during times of financial crisis.

THERAPEUTIC INTERVENTIONS	RATIONALE

Desired Outcome: The client will verbalize an understanding of and a plan for adhering to recommended follow-up care including regular laboratory studies, future appointments with health care providers, and prescribed medications.

THERAPEUTIC INTERVENTIONS	RATIONALE

Independent Actions

Stress the importance of adhering to the prescribed treatment regimen.

Reinforce the importance of keeping scheduled follow-up appointments for laboratory studies and with health care providers.

Explain the rationale for, side effects of, and importance of taking medications prescribed (e.g., antiretroviral agents, antimicrobial agents, hematopoietic agents, anabolic agents, appetite stimulants). Inform client of pertinent food and drug interactions.

Reinforce the importance of strictly adhering to the antiretroviral regimen prescribed (usually consists of a combination of at least three antiretroviral agents). Explain that not adhering to the prescribed regimen will limit the effectiveness of subsequent regimens.

Explain the importance of taking the full dose of any antimicrobial agents prescribed. Reinforce the possibility that lifelong treatment with antimicrobials (e.g., trimethoprim-sulfamethoxazole [TMP-SMX]) may be necessary to prevent some opportunistic infections if the CD4+ cell count is critically low.

Implement measures to improve client compliance:
- Include significant others in teaching sessions if possible.
- Encourage questions and allow time for reinforcement and clarification of information provided.
- Provide written instructions regarding scheduled appointments with health care providers and laboratory, medications prescribed, signs and symptoms to report, and ways to prevent infection.

Adherence to the prescribed regimen can reduce hospitalization, improve outcomes, and aid in maintaining optimal health status.

ADDITIONAL NURSING DIAGNOSES

DIARRHEA NDx
Related to:
- A direct effect of HIV on the intestine or opportunistic disease involvement of the intestine (e.g., Mycobacterium avium-intracellulare, Cryptosporidium, Salmonella, cytomegalovirus, Escherichia coli, Clostridium difficile, Entamoeba histolytica, Giardia, Kaposi's sarcoma)
- Side effect of some antiretroviral agents (e.g., protease inhibitors, didanosine)

ALTERED COMFORT: CHILLS AND EXCESSIVE DIAPHORESIS
Related to persistent or recurrent fever associated with HIV and opportunistic infections

ALTERED COMFORT: PRURITUS
Related to:
- Dry skin associated with deficient fluid volume (can occur as a result of decreased oral intake, excessive diaphoresis, and/or persistent diarrhea)
- Pruritic folliculitis (e.g., staphylococcal folliculitis, eosinophilic folliculitis)

- Dermatological disorders such as seborrheic dermatitis, photodermatitis, and psoriasis
- Side effect of some antimicrobials (e.g., TMP-SMX).
- Vulvovaginal candidiasis

IMPAIRED ORAL MUCOUS MEMBRANE NDx
Related to:
- Malnutrition and deficient fluid volume
- Infections such as candidiasis, herpes simplex, oral hairy leukoplakia, and bacterial gingivitis/periodontitis
- Kaposi's sarcoma or lymphoma in the oral cavity

ACTUAL/RISK FOR IMPAIRED SKIN INTEGRITY NDx
Related to:
- Presence of cutaneous infections such as folliculitis, herpes zoster or simplex, bullous impetigo, bacillary angiomatosis, molluscum contagiosum, and/or abscesses
- Presence of certain skin disorders (e.g., seborrheic dermatitis, photodermatitis, psoriasis)
- Skin lesions associated with Kaposi's sarcoma if present
- Excessive scratching associated with pruritus (can occur with certain skin disorders or as a side effect of some medications such as TMP-SMX)
- Increased skin fragility associated with malnutrition
- Persistent contact with irritants associated with diarrhea

Continued...
- Damage to the skin and/or subcutaneous tissue associated with prolonged pressure on tissues, friction, or shearing if mobility is decreased

RISK FOR INJURY NDx
Falls related to:
- Weakness and fatigue
- Decline in cognitive, behavioral, and/or motor function resulting from HIV-associated involvement of the brain and spinal cord (e.g., AIDS dementia complex, vacuolar myelopathy) and/or opportunistic infection or neoplastic involvement of the central nervous system (CNS)
- Visual impairment if present (can result from cytomegalovirus retinitis or from an infection and/or neoplasm involving the CNS)

Burns related to:
- Diminished sensation associated with peripheral neuropathy if present (can be a result of the effect of HIV and some opportunistic infections on the peripheral nerves and/or a side effect of some antiretroviral agents)

FEAR/ANXIETY NDx
Related to:
- Threat of permanent worsening of health status and possible disability and death
- Threat to self-concept associated with changes in physical and mental functioning (e.g., wasting syndrome, gait difficulty, poor coordination, dementia)
- Stigma associated with having AIDS
- Financial concerns
- Separation from support system
- Possibility of transmitting disease to others

INEFFECTIVE COPING NDx
Related to:
- Depression, fear, anxiety, and ongoing grieving associated with the diagnosis of AIDS and poor prognosis
- Need for permanent change in lifestyle associated with impaired immune system functioning and potential for disease transmission to others
- Uncertainty of disease course and feelings of powerlessness over course of disease
- Need for disclosure of diagnosis with possibility of subsequent rejection and/or distancing by others and loss of employment and health benefits
- Guilt associated with past behavior (if it was a factor in contracting HIV) and/or possibility of having transmitted HIV to others
- Lack of personal resources to deal with disability and premature death associated with youth (a significant number of clients are in their 20s or 30s and are not developmentally prepared to acknowledge and cope with disability and their own mortality)
- Multiple losses (e.g., death of close friends with AIDS; loss of normal body functioning, family support, financial security, and/or usual lifestyle and roles)
- Chronic symptoms (e.g., pain, diarrhea, fatigue) if present

RISK FOR LONELINESS NDx
Related to:
- Fear of associating with others because of possibility of contracting an infection
- Stigma and discrimination associated with the diagnosis of AIDS and others' fear of contracting HIV
- Decreased participation in usual activities because of weakness, pain, fatigue, and fear of falls
- Withdrawal from others associated with fear of embarrassment resulting from decline in physical and mental functioning

INTERRUPTED FAMILY PROCESSES NDx
Related to:
- Diagnosis of terminal, communicable disease in family member
- Fear of disclosure of diagnosis with subsequent rejection of family unit
- Change in family roles and structure associated with progressive disability and eventual death of family member
- Financial burden associated with extended illness and progressive disability of client
- Fear of contracting disease from client
- Decisions made by client and his/her partner about such issues as treatment plan, life support, and disposition of property that may be in conflict with the client's family of origin
- Anticipatory grief

SELF-CARE DEFICIT NDx
Related to:
- Cognitive and/or motor impairments if present (can result from HIV or opportunistic disease involvement of the CNS)
- Fatigue, weakness, and dyspnea
- Depression
- Visual impairment if present (can result from cytomegalovirus retinitis or from an infection and/or neoplasm involving the CNS)

DISTURBED SLEEP PATTERN NDx
Related to fear, anxiety, depression, frequent assessments and treatments, pain, diarrhea, pruritus, chills, night sweats, coughing and dyspnea (may occur if respiratory infection is present), unfamiliar environment, and the effect of some medications (e.g., zidovudine)

INEFFECTIVE SEXUALITY PATTERNS NDx
Related to:
- Rejection by desired partner associated with his/her fear of contracting AIDS
- Need to disclose to new partner(s) the diagnosis of AIDS
- Decreased sexual desire associated with fatigue, pain, weakness, anxiety, depression, and fear of transmitting or contracting disease

RISK FOR POWERLESSNESS NDx

Related to:

- The disabling and terminal nature of AIDS
- Increasing dependence on others to meet basic needs
- Changes in roles, relationships, and future plans

GRIEVING NDx

Related to:

- Having an incurable illness with an uncertain course and a high probability of premature death
- Changes in body functioning, appearance, lifestyle, and roles associated with the disease process

SEPSIS

Sepsis is a systemic response to infection. It is defined by the American College of Chest Physicians and Society of Critical Care Medicine as a documented infection with a finding of at least two of the four systemic inflammatory response criteria (i.e., temperature >38°C or below 36°C; heart rate >90 beats/min; respiratory rate >20 breaths/min or partial pressure of carbon dioxide in arterial blood [$PaCO_2$] <32 mm Hg; white blood cell [WBC] count >12,000/mm^3, <4000/mm^3, or >10% immature neutrophils).

Sepsis has become a leading cause of death in the United States. The increase in the number of cases of sepsis is attributed to a number of factors including the increased number of elderly persons and persons who are immunocompromised as a result of HIV infection, more aggressive treatment with chemotherapy and radiation for cancer, and treatment with corticosteroids and immunosuppressive agents. The increased use of invasive diagnostic and therapeutic procedures has also led to increased exposure to pathogens. In addition, the emergence of resistant organisms is making infections more difficult to treat.

Gram-positive bacteria (e.g., *Staphylococcus aureus, Staphylococcus epidermidis, enterococci, Streptococcus pneumoniae*) and gram-negative bacteria (e.g., *Escherichia coli, Haemophilus influenzae, Klebsiella pneumoniae, Pseudomonas aeruginosa, Serratia, Proteus, Enterobacter, Neisseria meningitides*) are the primary organisms that cause sepsis. The most common sites of infection that lead to sepsis are the lungs, blood, abdominal/pelvic cavity, and the urinary tract.

Once the causative organism enters the blood (referred to as septicemia or bacteremia), the toxins produced by the pathogens initiate a widespread inflammatory and immune response commonly referred to as the systemic inflammatory response syndrome (SIRS). This inflammatory response is designed to be a protective process but if uncontrolled, triggers the release of many inflammatory mediators that subsequently cause widespread vasodilation, injury to the endothelium, and increased capillary permeability. This chain of events can lead to maldistribution of circulating blood with hypotension, hypoperfusion, and organ dysfunction. Septic shock, disseminated intravascular coagulation (DIC), and multiple organ dysfunction syndrome (MODS) can develop if this chain of events is not reversed.

This care plan focuses on care of the adult client hospitalized for treatment of sepsis.

OUTCOME/DISCHARGE CRITERIA

The client will:

1. Demonstrate evidence that the infection is resolving
2. Have stable vital signs and evidence of adequate organ perfusion
3. Have no signs and symptoms of complications
4. Verbalize an understanding of ways to promote continued resolution of the existing infection
5. Identify ways to reduce the risk for recurrent infections
6. State signs and symptoms to report to the health care provider
7. Verbalize an understanding of and a plan for adhering to recommended follow-up care including future appointments with health care provider, medications prescribed, and activity limitations.

| Nursing Diagnosis | # IMPAIRED GAS EXCHANGE NDx |

Definition: Excess or deficit in oxygenation and/or carbon dioxide elimination at the alveolar capillary membrane

Related to: Decreased pulmonary blood flow associated with a reduction in systemic tissue perfusion resulting from inflammatory-mediated vasodilation, the fluid shift that occurs with increased capillary permeability, and selective vasoconstriction

- Loss of effective lung surface associated with:
  - Atelectasis resulting from hypoventilation and the decrease in surfactant production that occurs when blood flow to the lungs is diminished
  - Accumulation of secretions in the lungs resulting from decreased mobility, poor cough effort, and an increased production of secretions if a respiratory tract infection is present
  - Accumulation of fluid in the lungs resulting from the generalized endothelial damage and increase in capillary permeability that occur with a systemic inflammatory response to severe infection

---

NDx = NANDA-I Diagnosis   **D** = Delegatable Action   ● = UAP   ✦ = LVN/LPN   ⊖▶ = Go to ⊖volve for animation

Continued...

CLINICAL MANIFESTATIONS

Subjective	Objective
Verbal reports of shortness of breath; visual disturbances; headache upon awakening	Confusion; restlessness; dyspnea; irritability; somnolence; abnormal arterial blood gas values; abnormal skin color; abnormal rate and depth of breathing; tachycardia; diaphoresis; polycythemia

RISK FACTORS

- Alveolar capillary membrane changes
- Ventilation perfusion abnormalities

DESIRED OUTCOMES

The client will experience adequate oxygen/carbon dioxide exchange as evidenced by:
  a. Usual mental status
  b. Unlabored respirations at 12 to 20 breaths/min
  c. Oximetry results within normal range
  d. Arterial blood gas values within normal range

NOC OUTCOMES

Respiratory status: gas exchange

NIC INTERVENTIONS

Respiratory monitoring; cough enhancement; chest physiotherapy; oxygen therapy

NURSING ASSESSMENT	RATIONALE
Assess for and report signs and symptoms of impaired gas exchange: - Restlessness, irritability - Confusion, somnolence - Tachypnea, dyspnea - Significant decrease in oximetry results - Decreased partial pressure of arterial oxygen (PaO_2) and/or increased partial pressure of arterial carbon dioxide ($PaCO_2$) Monitor pulse oximetry results. Monitor arterial blood gas values.	*Early recognition of signs and symptoms of impaired gas exchange allows for prompt intervention.*

THERAPEUTIC INTERVENTIONS	RATIONALE

Independent Actions

Implement measures to improve gas exchange: **D** ✦

- Place client in a semi- to high-Fowler's position unless contraindicated.

  Improves lung expansion

- Instruct and assist client to change position, deep breathe, and cough at least every 2 hours.
- Discourage smoking.

  The irritants in smoke increase mucus production, impair ciliary function, and can damage the bronchial and alveolar walls; the carbon monoxide decreases oxygen availability.

Dependent/Collaborative Actions

Implement measures to improve gas exchange:

- Perform actions to maintain adequate tissue perfusion:

  Maintaining adequate tissue perfusion helps to ensure adequate pulmonary blood flow.

  - Administer intravenous fluids (colloids/crystalloids) as ordered.

    The massive vasodilation that occurs during sepsis results in a relative hypovolemia or distributive shock. Adequate volume replacement must occur first. If B/P remains low after volume has been replaced, vasopressors and/or inotropes may be added to support circulation. Adequate tissue perfusion promotes delivery of oxygen at the tissue level.

  - Administer vasopressors and positive inotropic agents if ordered to maintain adequate perfusion pressure and cardiac output.

- Assist with positive airway pressure techniques (e.g., continuous positive airway pressure [CPAP], bilevel positive airway pressure [BiPAP], flutter/positive expiratory pressure [PEP] device) if ordered.

  All actions help to open up terminal airways/alveoli, increasing the surface area available for gas exchange to occur, resulting in improved oxygenation.

THERAPEUTIC INTERVENTIONS	RATIONALE
• Maintain activity restrictions as ordered; increase activity gradually as allowed and tolerated.	*Restricting activity lowers the body's oxygen requirements.*
• Administer antimicrobial agents as ordered.	*Antimicrobial agents help to resolve the infectious process and control the systemic inflammatory response.*
Consult appropriate health care provider (respiratory therapist, physician) if signs and symptoms of impaired gas exchange persist or worsen.	*Allows for modification of the treatment plan*

Nursing Diagnosis INEFFECTIVE TISSUE PERFUSION NDx

Definition: Decrease in oxygen resulting in failure to nourish the tissues at the capillary level. NANDA International identifies five types of ineffective tissue perfusion: renal, gastrointestinal, peripheral, cerebral, and cardiopulmonary

Related to:
- Maldistribution of circulating blood associated with vasodilation, fluid shift that occurs with increased capillary permeability, and selective vasoconstriction that occur in response to inflammatory mediators (e.g., cytokines, complement, histamine, kinins) released in a serious infection
- Hypovolemia associated with deficient fluid volume resulting from decreased fluid intake, excessive loss of fluid (can occur with diaphoresis, hyperventilation, vomiting, and/or diarrhea if present), and the fluid shift that occurs with increased capillary permeability
- Decreased cardiac output (occurs late in severe sepsis and shock) associated with the depressant effect of acidosis, myocardial depressant factor, and some inflammatory mediators (e.g., cytokines) on myocardial contractility

CLINICAL MANIFESTATIONS

Subjective	Objective
Restlessness	Decreased B/P; confusion; cool extremities; pallor or cyanosis of extremities; diminished or absent peripheral pulses; slow capillary refill; edema; oliguria

RISK FACTORS
- Smoking
- Hyperlipidemic
- Sedentary lifestyle

DESIRED OUTCOMES

The client will maintain adequate tissue perfusion as evidenced by:
  a. B/P within normal range for client
  b. Usual mental status
  c. Extremities warm with absence of pallor and cyanosis
  d. Palpable peripheral pulses
  e. Capillary refill time less than 2 to 3 seconds
  f. Absence of edema
  g. Urine output at least 30 mL/h

NOC OUTCOMES

Circulation status; tissue perfusion: abdominal organs; tissue perfusion: cardiac; tissue perfusion: cerebral; tissue perfusion: peripheral; tissue perfusion: pulmonary

NIC INTERVENTIONS

Circulatory care: arterial insufficiency; circulatory care: venous insufficiency; cerebral perfusion promotion; hypovolemia management; cardiac care: acute

NURSING ASSESSMENT

Assess for and report signs and symptoms of diminished tissue perfusion:
- Decreased B/P
- Confusion
- Cool extremities
- Pallor or cyanosis of extremities

RATIONALE

Early recognition of signs and symptoms of ineffective tissue perfusion allows for prompt intervention.

Continued...

NURSING ASSESSMENT	RATIONALE

- Diminished or absent peripheral pulses
- Slow capillary refill
- Edema
- Oliguria

Monitor hemodynamic status:
- Vital signs
- Urine output
- Central venous pressure (if applicable)

THERAPEUTIC INTERVENTIONS	RATIONALE

Dependent/Collaborative Actions

- Perform actions to maintain adequate tissue perfusion:
  - Administer intravenous fluids (colloids/crystalloids) as ordered.
  - Administer vasopressors and positive inotropic agents if ordered to maintain adequate perfusion pressure and cardiac output.
- Perform actions to prevent or treat deficient fluid volume:
  - Control diarrhea if present.
  - Reduce nausea and vomiting if present.
- Administer antimicrobial agents as ordered.

Consult appropriate health care provider if signs and symptoms of diminished tissue perfusion persist or worsen.

Maintaining adequate tissue perfusion helps to ensure adequate pulmonary blood flow. The massive vasodilation that occurs during sepsis results in a relative hypovolemia or distributive shock. Adequate volume replacement must occur first. If B/P remains low after volume has been replaced, vasopressors and/or inotropes may be added to support circulation. Adequate tissue perfusion promotes delivery of oxygen at the tissue level.

Antimicrobial agents help to resolve the infectious process and control the systemic inflammatory response.
Allows for modification of the treatment plan

Nursing Diagnosis   RISK FOR DEFICIENT FLUID VOLUME NDx

Definition: At risk for experiencing vascular, cellular, or intracellular dehydration

Related to:
- Decreased oral intake associated with anorexia, fatigue, and nausea if present
- Increased insensible fluid loss associated with diaphoresis and hyperventilation if present
- Excessive loss of fluid associated with vomiting and/or diarrhea if present with initial infection or as a side effect of antimicrobial therapy
- Fluid shifting from the intravascular to extravascular space associated with the increased capillary permeability that occurs with a systemic inflammatory response

CLINICAL MANIFESTATIONS

Subjective	Objective
N/A	Decreased B/P; decreased pulse pressure; decreased skin turgor; dry mucous membranes; increased pulse rate; elevated Hct; increased body temperature; decreased urine output; increased urine concentration

DESIRED OUTCOMES

The client will not experience deficient fluid volume as evidenced by:
  a. Normal skin turgor
  b. Moist mucous membranes
  c. Stable weight
  d. B/P and pulse rate within normal range for client and stable with position change

  e. Usual mental status
  f. BUN and Hct values within normal range
  g. Balanced intake and output
  h. Urine specific gravity within normal range

NOC OUTCOMES	NIC INTERVENTIONS
Fluid balance; hydration	Fluid monitoring; fluid management; hypovolemia management; intravenous therapy; fever treatment; diarrhea management; nausea management

NURSING ASSESSMENT	RATIONALE
Assess for and report signs and symptoms of deficient fluid volume: • Decreased skin turgor • Dry mucous membranes, thirst • Weight loss of 2% or greater over a short period • Postural hypotension and/or low B/P • Weak, rapid pulse • Neck veins flat when client is supine • Change in mental status • Decrease in urine output with increased specific gravity Monitor BUN, Hct values.	*Early recognition of signs and symptoms of deficient fluid volume allows for prompt intervention.*

THERAPEUTIC INTERVENTIONS	RATIONALE

Dependent/Collaborative Actions
Implement measures to prevent or treat deficient fluid volume:
• Perform actions to reduce nausea and vomiting if present:
  • Administer antimicrobial agents with food unless contraindicated.
  • Administer prescribed antiemetics.
• Perform actions to control diarrhea if present:
  • Consult physician about another antimicrobial agent if onset of diarrhea seems related to initiation of antimicrobial therapy.
  • Administer prescribed antidiarrheal agents.
• Perform actions to reduce fever.
 	
• Administer antimicrobial agents as ordered to treat the infection and decrease the release of inflammatory mediators.
• Maintain a fluid intake of at least 2500 mL/day unless contraindicated; if oral intake is inadequate or contraindicated, maintain intravenous fluid therapy as ordered.
	
	Actions help to reduce insensible fluid loss associated with diaphoresis and hyperventilation.
	Decreasing the release of inflammatory mediators associated with infection decreases capillary permeability and the resultant fluid shift.

Nursing Diagnosis ## HYPERTHERMIA NDx

Definition: Body temperature elevated above normal range as a result of either fever or hyperthermia

Related to: Stimulation of the thermoregulatory center in the hypothalamus by endogenous pyrogens that are released in an infectious process

CLINICAL MANIFESTATIONS

Subjective	Objective
Report of chills	Flushed skin; increase in body temperature; tachycardia; tachypnea; warm to touch

---

Continued...

RISK FACTORS

- Illness
- Increased metabolic rate
- Dehydration

DESIRED OUTCOMES

The client will experience resolution of hyperthermia as evidenced by:
  a. Skin usual temperature and color
  b. Pulse rate between 60 and 100 beats/min
  c. Respiratory rate 12 to 20 breaths/min
  d. Normal body temperature

NOC OUTCOMES

Thermoregulation

NIC INTERVENTIONS

Fever treatment

NURSING ASSESSMENT	RATIONALE
Assess for signs and symptoms of hyperthermia: • Warm, flushed skin • Tachycardia • Tachypnea • Elevated temperature	*Early recognition and reporting of signs and symptoms of hyperthermia allow for prompt intervention.*

THERAPEUTIC INTERVENTIONS	RATIONALE

Independent Actions

Implement measures to reduce fever:
- Perform actions to resolve the infectious process: **D** ✦
  - Implement measures to promote rest (assist client with activities of daily living, provide uninterrupted rest periods, limit visitors).
  - Encourage client to eat a well-balanced diet high in essential nutrients. — *Helps to fight off infection*
- Administer tepid sponge bath and/or apply cool cloths to groin and axillae if indicated. — *Decreases hyperthermia*
- Use a room fan to provide cool, circulating air.

Dependent/Collaborative Actions

Implement measures to reduce fever:
- Perform actions to resolve the infectious process:
  - Maintain a fluid intake of at least 2500 mL/day unless contraindicated.
  - Administer antimicrobials as ordered. — *Treats/prevents infection*
- Apply cooling blanket if ordered — *Decreases fever*
- Administer antipyretics if ordered.
- Consult physician if temperature remains higher than 38.5°C. — *Allows for prompt alteration in interventions*

Nursing Diagnosis **RISK FOR INFECTION** NDx **(SUPERINFECTION)**

Definition: At risk for being invaded by pathogenic organisms

Related to:
- Decreased resistance to infection associated with depletion of immune mechanisms resulting from the current infection and treatment with antimicrobial agents
- Stasis of respiratory secretions and/or urinary stasis if mobility is decreased
- Break in skin integrity associated with frequent venipunctures or presence of invasive lines (e.g., intravenous catheter, hemodynamic monitoring devices)

CLINICAL MANIFESTATIONS

Subjective	Objective
Verbal reports of pain at areas of impaired skin integrity	Increased body temperature; redness, warmth discharge over areas of impaired skin integrity

DESIRED OUTCOMES

The client will have resolution of existing infection and remain free of superinfection as evidenced by:

a. Return of temperature toward normal range
b. Decrease in episodes of chills and diaphoresis
c. Pulse rate returning toward normal range
d. Normal or improved breath sounds
e. Absence or resolution of dyspnea and cough
f. Stable or improved mental status
g. Voiding clear urine without reports of frequency, urgency, and burning
h. No reports of increased weakness and fatigue
i. Absence or resolution of heat, pain, redness, swelling, and unusual drainage in any area
j. Absence of oral mucous membrane lesions and ulceration
k. Absence or resolution of diarrhea and abdominal pain and cramping
l. WBC and differential counts returning toward normal range
m. Negative results of cultured specimens

NOC OUTCOMES

Immune status; infection severity

NIC INTERVENTIONS

Infection control; infection protection

NURSING ASSESSMENT	RATIONALE
Assess for and report signs and symptoms of superinfection (be alert to subtle changes in client since the signs of infection may be minimal as a result of immunosuppression; also be aware that some signs and symptoms vary depending on the site of the infection, the causative organism, and the age of the client):	*Early recognition of signs and symptoms of an infection allows for prompt intervention.*

- Increase in temperature
- Increase in episodes of chills and diaphoresis
- Increased pulse rate
- Development or worsening of abnormal breath sounds
- Development or worsening of dyspnea and/or cough
- Decline in mental status
- Cloudy urine; reports of frequency, urgency, burning when urinating
- Further increase in fatigue or weakness
- New or increased heat, pain, redness, swelling, or unusual drainage in any area
- Development or worsening of lesions or ulceration of oral mucous membrane
- New or increased episodes of diarrhea and abdominal cramping or pain

Monitor CBC with differential; culture results; urinalysis; chest x-ray results.

THERAPEUTIC INTERVENTIONS	RATIONALE

Independent Actions
Implement measures to prevent superinfection:

- Use good hand hygiene and encourage client to do the same.

  Prevents spread of infection

- Protect client from others with infection.

  Decreases client's potential for infection

- Encourage client to eat a well-balanced diet high in essential nutrients; provide dietary supplements if indicated.

  Necessary to produce cells that fight infection

- Maintain sterile technique during all invasive procedures.

  Prevents entrance of pathogens into the body

- Change intravenous insertion sites according to hospital policy.

  Decreases potential for infection

- Anchor catheter/tubings securely.
- Change equipment, tubings, and solutions used for treatments such as intravenous infusions, respiratory care, irrigations, and enteral feedings according to hospital policy.

  Securely anchoring tubes/catheters reduces trauma to the tissues and the risk for introduction of pathogens associated with the in-and-out movement of the tubing.

NDx = NANDA-I Diagnosis   **D** = Delegatable Action   ● = UAP   ✦ = LVN/LPN   ⊖▶ = Go to ⊖volve for animation

Continued...

THERAPEUTIC INTERVENTIONS	RATIONALE
• Maintain a closed system for drains (e.g., urinary catheter) and intravenous infusions whenever possible.	*Prevents introduction of pathogens into the body*
• Perform actions to prevent stasis of respiratory secretions:	
• Assist client to turn, cough, and deep breathe.	*Improves lung expansion and motility of secretions*
• Increase activity as allowed and tolerated.	
• Perform actions to prevent urinary retention/stasis:	
• Urinate when urge is felt.	*Prevents stasis of urine, which increases the potential for infection*
• Promote relaxation when voiding.	*Prevents contamination from bacteria from the rectum*
• Instruct and assist client to perform good perineal care routinely and after each bowel movement.	
• If client has open lesions or wound drains, perform actions to prevent wound infection:	
• Maintain sterile technique during wound care.	
• Instruct client to avoid touching wounds.	

Dependent/Collaborative Actions
Implement measures to prevent superinfection:

• Maintain a fluid intake of 2500 mL/day unless contraindicated.	
• Consult physician about discontinuing urinary catheter if one is present.	
• Consult physician about:	
• Enteral feeding rather than total parenteral nutrition (TPN) if nutritional replacement is necessary	*Maintains nutritional status. TPN has a high glucose content, which provides a rich medium for bacterial growth.*
• Use of sucralfate rather than antacids and histamine$_2$-receptor antagonists	
• Administer antimicrobial agents as ordered.	*These agents increase the pH of the stomach contents, which promotes bacterial overgrowth; aspiration of gastric contents with a high bacteria content increases the risk for pneumonia.*

POTENTIAL COMPLICATIONS OF SEPSIS

COLLABORATIVE DIAGNOSIS

SEPTIC SHOCK

Definition: Sepsis-induced hypotension or the requirement for vasopressors or inotropes to maintain B/P despite adequate fluid volume resuscitation along with the presence of perfusion abnormalities that may include lactic acidosis, oliguria, or acute alteration in mental status

Related to: Systemic hypoperfusion associated with maldistribution of circulating blood, deficient fluid volume, and decreased myocardial contractility resulting from an uncontrolled systemic inflammatory response to severe infection

CLINICAL MANIFESTATIONS

Subjective	**Objective**
Reports of confusion	Low arterial pressure; low systemic vascular resistance; systemic edema; tachycardia; temperature instability

DESIRED OUTCOMES

The client will not develop septic shock as evidenced by:
a. Systolic B/P equal to or higher than 90 mm Hg
b. Usual mental status
c. Urine output at least 30 mL/h
d. Extremities warm and usual color
e. Capillary refill time less than 2 to 3 seconds
f. Palpable peripheral pulses

NURSING ASSESSMENT	RATIONALE

Assess for and report signs and symptoms of septic shock:
• Hyperdynamic or compensatory phase
  • Widened pulse pressure with the diastolic pressure dropping and little change in the systolic pressure
  • Restlessness
  • Tachycardia
  • Warm, flushed skin
• Hypodynamic or progressive phase
  • Systolic B/P less than 90 mm Hg or a reduction of greater than 40 mm Hg from baseline
  • Cool, clammy skin
  • Change in level of consciousness
  • Decreased urine output
  • Rapid, shallow breathing
  • Rapid, thready pulse
Monitor serum lactate levels.
	Early recognition of signs and symptoms of septic shock allows for prompt intervention.

THERAPEUTIC INTERVENTIONS	RATIONALE
Dependent/Collaborative Actions Implement measures to maintain adequate tissue perfusion: • Administer intravenous fluids (crystalloids/colloids) as ordered. If signs and symptoms of septic shock occur: • Maintain intravenous fluid therapy as ordered. • Maintain oxygen therapy as ordered. • Administer antimicrobials as ordered. • Administer vasopressors and positive inotropic agents as ordered to maintain adequate perfusion pressure and cardiac output. • Prepare client for transfer to critical care unit.	*Maintains intravascular volume* *Treatment for septic shock focuses on the expansion of circulating volume to improve tissue perfusion. Oxygenation and perfusion must be maintained to prevent extreme lactic acidosis. The patient often requires transfer to a critical care unit for invasive monitoring of hemodynamic status (Swan Ganz catheter; central venous pressure; arterial line.)*

COLLABORATIVE DIAGNOSIS

RISK FOR DISSEMINATED INTRAVASCULAR COAGULATION (DIC)

Definition: A systemic thrombohemorrhagic disorder seen in association with well-defined clinical situations and laboratory evidence

Related to: Widespread inflammation and the resulting endothelial damage associated with sepsis results in inappropriate triggering of the coagulation cascade due to the presence of tissue factor that is released by damaged or dead tissues

CLINICAL MANIFESTATIONS

Subjective	Objective
Reports of restlessness; agitation; confusion	Bleeding: rapid development of oozing from venipuncture sites, arterial lines, surgical wounds; ecchymotic lesions; bleeding in conjunctiva, nose, and gums
	Thrombosis: cyanosis of fingers/toes, nose, breast; symptoms of organ failure

DESIRED OUTCOMES

The client will not develop DIC as evidenced by:
a. Absence of petechiae, ecchymoses, and frank or occult bleeding
b. Usual color and temperature of extremities
c. Usual mental status
d. Fibrin degradation products (FDP) and D-dimer results within normal range
e. Fibrinogen level, platelet count, activated partial thromboplastin time (APTT), prothrombin time (PT), and thrombin time within normal range

Continued...

NURSING ASSESSMENT	RATIONALE
Assess for and report signs and symptoms of DIC: • Petechiae, ecchymoses • Frank or occult bleeding (e.g., oozing from venipuncture sites or surgical incisions, epistaxis, hematuria, gingival bleeding) • Cool, mottled extremities • Restlessness, agitation, confusion Monitor results of PT/PTT; FDP; fibrinogen level, D-dimer.	*Early recognition of signs and symptoms of DIC allows for prompt intervention.*

THERAPEUTIC INTERVENTIONS	RATIONALE

Independent Actions

If DIC occurs:
* Implement safety precautions to prevent further bleeding:
  * Avoid injections.
  * Avoid invasive procedures.
  * Discontinue any invasive lines with extreme caution.
  * Use electric rather than straight-edge razor for shaving.

The body has depleted its clotting factors; thus, after any invasive procedure, excessive bleeding may occur.

Dependent/Collaborative Actions

Implement measures to control infection and reduce the risk for an uncontrolled systemic inflammatory response in order to reduce the risk for DIC:
* Administer antimicrobial agents as ordered.
* Perform actions to reduce the risk for superinfection.

Treat/prevent infections

If DIC occurs:
* Administer fresh frozen plasma, platelets, and/or cryoprecipitate if ordered.
* Administer medications to interrupt clotting:
  * Heparin
  * Antithrombin III

Improves blood's clotting ability
Blood products identified help to enhance clotting and stop bleeding.

Heparin is contraindicated if platelet count is less than 50,000.

COLLABORATIVE DIAGNOSIS

RISK FOR ORGAN ISCHEMIA/DYSFUNCTION (MULTIPLE ORGAN DYSFUNCTION SYNDROME)
Definition: The progressive dysfunction of two or more organ systems resulting from an uncontrolled inflammatory response to severe illness or injury

Relation to:
* Hypoperfusion of major organs associated with shock
* Microvascular thrombosis associated with DIC

CLINICAL MANIFESTATIONS

Subjective	Objective
N/A	Low-grade fever; tachycardia; dyspnea; altered mental status; individual organ failure

RISK FACTORS

- Malnutrition
- Corticosteroids
- Bowel infarction
- Inadequate or delayed resuscitation
- Multiple blood transfusions
- Persistent infection
- Significant tissue injury
- Burns
- Trauma
- Acute pancreatitis
- Circulatory shock
- Adult respiratory distress syndrome
- Necrotic tissue

DESIRED OUTCOMES

The client will not develop organ ischemia/dysfunction as evidenced by:

a. Usual mental status
b. Urine output at least 30 mL/h
c. Unlabored respirations at 12 to 20 breaths/min
d. Audible breath sounds without an increase in adventitious sounds
e. Absence of new or increased abdominal pain, distention, nausea, vomiting, and diarrhea
f. BUN, creatinine, aspartate aminotransferase (AST), alanine aminotransferase (ALT), and lactate dehydrogenase (LDH) levels within normal range

NURSING ASSESSMENT

Assess for and report signs and symptoms of:

- Cerebral ischemia (e.g., change in mental status)
- Urine output less than 30 mL/h (elevated BUN and creatinine levels)
- Acute respiratory distress syndrome (e.g., dyspnea, increase in respiratory rate, low arterial oxygen saturation [SaO_2], crackles)
- Gastrointestinal ischemia (e.g., hypoactive or absent bowel sounds, abdominal pain and distention, nausea, vomiting, diarrhea, hematemesis, blood in stool)
- Liver dysfunction (e.g., increased AST, ALT, and LDH levels; jaundice)

Monitor results of chest x-ray and complete metabolic panel.

RATIONALE

Early recognition of signs and symptoms of multiple organ dysfunction syndrome (MODS) allows for prompt intervention.

THERAPEUTIC INTERVENTIONS

Dependent/Collaborative Actions

Implement measures to reduce the risk for organ ischemia/dysfunction:

- Perform actions to maintain adequate tissue perfusion.
- Perform actions to prevent and treat DIC.
- Administer recombinant activated protein C (drotrecogin alfa [Xigris]) if ordered.

If signs and symptoms of organ ischemia/MODS occur:

- Maintain oxygen therapy.
- Prepare client for transfer to critical care unit.

RATIONALE

This medication has been found to have antithrombotic, anti-inflammatory, and profibrinolytic activity and may reduce the risk of MODS; it is only used in persons with severe sepsis who are not having symptoms of DIC. Because of the risks associated with this drug and the patient's critical state, transfer to intensive care is indicated.

ADDITIONAL NURSING DIAGNOSES

FEAR/ANXIETY NDx

Related to:

- Unfamiliar environment
- Separation from significant others
- Severity of current condition
- Threat of death

DEFICIENT KNOWLEDGE NDx; INEFFECTIVE THERAPEUTIC REGIMEN MANAGEMENT NDx; OR INEFFECTIVE HEALTH MAINTENANCE* NDx

---

*The nurse should select the diagnostic label that is most appropriate for the client's discharge teaching needs.

NDx = NANDA-I Diagnosis   **D** = Delegatable Action   ● = UAP   ✦ = LVN/LPN   ⊖▶ = Go to ⊖volve for animation

⊖▶ SPLENECTOMY

Splenectomy is the surgical removal of the spleen. The most common indication for the surgery is rupture of the spleen. Causes of rupture include penetrating or blunt trauma to the spleen, operative trauma to the spleen during surgery on nearby organs, and damage to the spleen as a result of disease (e.g., mononucleosis, tuberculosis of the spleen). A splenectomy may also be indicated if the spleen is removing excessive quantities of platelets, erythrocytes, or leukocytes from the circulation (hypersplenism). Conditions associated with hypersplenism include leukemia, idiopathic thrombocytopenic purpura, Felty's syndrome, thalassemia major, lymphoma, and hereditary spherocytosis. Additionally, splenectomy may be performed to treat splenic cysts and neoplasm. When feasible, a partial splenectomy is performed so that some of the spleen's immunological function is maintained.

This care plan focuses on the adult client hospitalized for a splenectomy. The care plan will need to be individualized according to the client's underlying disease process or the extensiveness of abdominal trauma necessitating the surgery.

OUTCOME/DISCHARGE CRITERIA

The client will:
1. Have surgical pain controlled
2. Have evidence of normal healing of surgical wound
3. Have no signs and symptoms of infection
4. Have no signs and symptoms of postoperative complications
5. Identify appropriate safety measures to follow because of increased risk for infection
6. State signs and symptoms to report to the health care provider
7. Verbalize an understanding of and a plan for adhering to recommended follow-up care including future appointments with health care provider, medications prescribed, wound care, and activity level.

For a full, detailed care plan on this topic, go to http://evolve. elsevier.com/Haugen/careplanning/.

See Bibliography at the back of the book.

8

The Client with Alterations in Metabolic Function

DIABETES MELLITUS

Diabetes mellitus is a chronic multisystem disease characterized by alterations in carbohydrate, fat, and protein metabolism resulting from abnormal insulin production, impaired insulin utilization, or both. The hallmark of this metabolic disorder is hyperglycemia.

Diabetes* is often complicated by structural and functional abnormalities in the blood vessels and nerves. The atherosclerotic changes that frequently occur in the large vessels (macroangiopathy) affect the cardiac, cerebral, and peripheral circulation. Thickening of the basement membrane of the capillaries (microangiopathy) can also occur and is especially significant when it involves the vessels in the eyes and kidneys. The neurological involvement can be manifested in a wide variety of ways and is referred to as diabetic neuropathy. Several different mechanisms are thought to contribute to the development of diabetic neuropathy. These include reduced blood flow to the nerves as a result of angiopathies and a metabolic defect in the polyol pathway resulting in accumulation of sorbitol in the nerves, which subsequently alters nerve function. The most common neuropathy is peripheral sensorimotor polyneuropathy, which has a gradual onset of sensory manifestations such as numbness and tingling, burning or shooting pain sensations, and/or hyperesthesia. Neuropathy of the autonomic nervous system is also common.

Parasympathetic involvement often occurs earlier and is more profound than sympathetic nervous system involvement, and manifestations vary depending on the system involved.

The two major types of diabetes are type 1 and type 2. Individuals with type 1 diabetes have an absolute insulin deficiency and are dependent on insulin replacement. The insulin deficiency is usually due to an immune-mediated destruction of the pancreatic beta-cells in a person with a genetic predisposition and a triggering environmental insult (e.g., viral infection). Individuals with type 2 diabetes have a relative deficiency of insulin caused by decreased tissue responsiveness to insulin (insulin resistance), a defect in insulin secretion, and inappropriate hepatic glucose production. Heredity plays a role in development of type 2 diabetes. Additional risk factors for type 2 diabetes include a history of

gestational diabetes mellitus or impaired glucose tolerance, increasing age, obesity, and a sedentary lifestyle.

A sequence of pathophysiological events occurs in diabetes. When an insulin deficiency exists, glucose cannot be transported into the cells for energy metabolism. As a result, glucose accumulates in the blood and starts to spill into the urine once the level exceeds the renal threshold (>180 mg/dL). The high blood glucose acts as an osmotic diuretic, which leads to excessive diuresis and subsequent deficient fluid volume. Because the glucose cannot be used as an energy source by many cells, fat and protein are broken down to provide a source of energy for the starving cells. The free fatty acids that are mobilized from adipose tissue are converted by the liver to ketones to be used as an energy source. The ketones are strong acids and eventually deplete the body's buffer system and respiratory compensatory ability, leading to a state of metabolic acidosis. The simultaneous increase in glucagon and epinephrine release that occurs with an insulin deficiency exacerbates the hyperglycemia and ketogenesis. Continuation of these metabolic derangements leads to life-threatening imbalances.

This care plan focuses on the adult client who has had diabetes for many years and is being hospitalized because of difficulty stabilizing blood glucose levels. Many of the long-term vascular and neurological complications have been included in this care plan and should be individualized based on the client's current status. Much of the information in this care plan is applicable to clients receiving follow-up care in an extended care facility or home setting.

This care plan should be used in conjunction with the care plans on Heart Failure, Myocardial Infarction, Cerebrovascular Accident, Hypertension, and/or Chronic Renal Failure if the client is also being treated for one of these vascular complications of diabetes.

OUTCOME/DISCHARGE CRITERIA

The client will:
1. Have blood glucose stabilized within a desired range
2. Have signs and symptoms of vascular and neurological complications at a manageable level

---

*Diabetes mellitus will be referred to as *diabetes* throughout the care plan.

NDx = NANDA-I Diagnosis   **D** = Delegatable Action   ● = UAP   ✦ = LVN/LPN   ⊜▶ = Go to ⊜volve for animation   485

Continued...

3. Verbalize a basic understanding of diabetes mellitus
4. Verbalize an understanding of medications ordered and demonstrate the ability to correctly draw up and administer insulin if prescribed
5. Verbalize an understanding of the principles of dietary management and be able to calculate and plan meals within the prescribed caloric distribution
6. Demonstrate the ability to perform blood glucose and urine tests correctly and interpret results accurately
7. Verbalize an understanding of the role of exercise in the management of diabetes
8. Identify health care and hygiene practices that should be integrated into lifestyle
9. Identify appropriate safety measures to follow because of the diagnosis of diabetes
10. State signs and symptoms of hypoglycemia and ketoaci-

dosis and appropriate actions for prevention and treatment
11. State signs and symptoms to report to the health care provider
12. Share feelings and concerns about diabetes and its effect on lifestyle
13. Identify resources that can assist in the adjustment to and management of diabetes
14. Verbalize an understanding of and a plan for adhering to recommended follow-up care including future appointments with health care provider and for laboratory studies.

Collaborative Diagnosis ▪ **RISK FOR UNSTABLE BLOOD GLUCOSE LEVEL** NDx

Definition: Risk for variation of blood glucose/sugar levels from the normal range

Related to:

- Inadequate insulin production
- Insulin resistance that may lead to generalized vascular disease and neuropathy
- Inability of the client to adhere to the diabetic regimen
- Lack of knowledge of diabetes management
- Inappropriate dietary intake
- Inadequate medication management
- Inadequate physical exercise

CLINICAL MANIFESTATIONS

Subjective	Objective
Complaints of fatigue, weakness, and paresthesias	Fasting blood glucose level >126 mg/dL; oral glucose tolerance test (2-hour sample) blood glucose level ≥200 mg/dL; hemoglobin A_{1C}/glycosylated hemoglobin level >7%; polyuria; polydipsia; weight loss; metabolic acidosis; acetone breath; tachycardia

RISK FACTORS

- Stress
- Obesity
- Weight loss

DESIRED OUTCOMES

The client will experience normal or near-normal blood glucose levels as evidenced by:
  a. Blood glucose levels <180 mg/dL at all times
  b. Fasting blood glucose levels <110 mg/dL
  c. Hemoglobin A_{1C} <7%
  d. Capillary refill <3 seconds
  e. Pedal pulses >2+
  f. Client adherence to therapeutic regimen

NOC OUTCOMES

Tissue perfusion: cardiac; tissue perfusion: cerebral; tissue perfusion: abdominal organs; tissue perfusion: peripheral tissue integrity; skin and mucous membranes

NIC INTERVENTIONS

Circulator care: arterial insufficiency; circulatory care: venous insufficiency; vital signs monitoring; laboratory data interpretation; neurological monitoring; hypovolemia management; nausea management; foot care; pressure management; skin surveillance

NURSING ASSESSMENT	RATIONALE
Assess blood glucose levels before meals and at bedtime.	*Monitoring the client's blood glucose levels determines effectiveness of glucose control and allows for prompt treatment as needed.*
Assess for increased blood pressure (B/P).	*Hypertension is frequently associated with diabetes. Control of B/P is associated with decreased incidence of or limited development of heart disease, stroke, retinopathy, and nephropathy.*
Assess for capillary refill, temperature, peripheral pulses, and color.	*Monitors adequate peripheral vascular perfusion and aids in detection of peripheral vascular disease*
Assess for increased or decreased urine output and excessive complaints of thirst and hunger.	*Indicators that the individual may be experiencing increased blood glucose levels*

THERAPEUTIC INTERVENTIONS	RATIONALE

Independent Actions

Perform actions to maintain blood glucose at a near-normal level:

- Monitor blood glucose levels regularly. Report values <60 mg/dL, >180 mg/dL, or outside the parameters specified by physician. **D** ✦
- Monitor percentage of meals and snacks client consumes.
- Report a pattern of inadequate or excessive intake. **D** ✦
- Achieve ideal weight, and provide necessary nutrients.
- Encourage client to adhere to the diabetic diet as prescribed, and assist with appropriate selection of foods.
- Provide meals and snacks at evenly spaced intervals.
- Encourage the client to exercise on a regular basis.

Protect skin and extremities from injury. **D** ✦

Teach client to avoid crossing of knees, application of pressure at the back of the knees, and wearing of tight clothing, and to monitor skin integrity of the lower extremities.

Maintaining blood glucose at a near-normal level may prevent or delay development of some of the vascular complications from diabetes.

Pattern of inadequate or excessive intakes will indicate need for further dietary teaching.

These actions are important to maintain a balance between adequate nutrition and insulin and glucose levels.

Clients may experience decreased sensation in their extremities because of peripheral vascular disease.

These actions could cause venous stasis and a decrease in arterial perfusion. The client should monitor skin integrity as lower extremity sensation may be decreased.

Dependent/Collaborative Actions

Implement measures to maintain blood glucose at a near-normal level, achieve ideal weight, and provide necessary nutrients:

- Consult dietitian to develop a diet/meal plan and/or reinforce dietary education.
- Consult personal trainer to develop an individualized exercise routine for the client.
- ⊖▶ Administer insulin and hypoglycemic agents as ordered.

- Perform a calorie count if ordered.

Improves clients' ability to care for themselves and maintain appropriate blood glucose levels

Exercise improves the utilization of glucose. Clients are more likely to adhere to a plan that they like and feel they can do.

Hypoglycemia agents enhance cellular utilization of glucose and prevent abnormal metabolism of fats and proteins.

A calorie count helps to determine appropriate volume of calories needed to maintain adequate nutrition and blood glucose levels

---

Nursing Diagnosis # IMPAIRED COMFORT NDx (BURNING, ACHING, CRAMPING, HYPERESTHESIA, NUMBNESS, AND/OR TINGLING [PARTICULARLY IN LOWER EXTREMITIES])

Definition: Perceived lack of ease, relief, and transcendence in physical, psychospiritual, environmental, and social dimensions

Related to:
- Peripheral polyneuropathy and/or peripheral vascular insufficiency

Continued...

CLINICAL MANIFESTATIONS

Subjective	**Objective**
Complaints of burning, pain, numbness, tingling and/or increased sensitivity to sensory stimuli	Cool skin; decreased or absent lower extremity pulses; delayed capillary refill; restlessness; diaphoresis; hypertension; tachycardia

RISK FACTORS

- Consistently high blood glucose levels
- Wearing tight shoes or constrictive clothing

DESIRED OUTCOMES

The client will experience diminished discomfort in extremities as evidenced by:
  a. Verbalization of no discomfort
  b. Relaxed facial expression and body positioning
  c. Increased participation in activities
  d. Stable vital signs

NOC OUTCOMES

Comfort level; pain control

NIC INTERVENTIONS

Pain management; environmental management; analgesic administration; hyperglycemia management

NURSING ASSESSMENT	**RATIONALE**

Assess for:
- Signs and symptoms of peripheral neuropathy (e.g., reports of persistent burning; sharp, shooting pain; numbness; tingling; or increased sensitivity to sensory stimuli [hyperesthesia])
- Signs and symptoms of peripheral vascular insufficiency (e.g., reports of cramping in calves precipitated by ambulation [intermittent claudication], delayed capillary refill, cold feet, dependent rubor, diminished or absent pulses)
- Nonverbal signs of discomfort (e.g., grimacing, guarding of affected area, reluctance to move, restlessness, diaphoresis, increased B/P, tachycardia)

Assess client's perception of the severity of the discomfort using an intensity rating scale.

Assess the client's pattern of discomfort (e.g., location, quality, onset, duration, precipitating factors, aggravating factors, alleviating factors).

Ask the client to describe the methods used to manage the discomfort effectively.

Early recognition of signs and symptoms of peripheral neuropathy and vascular insufficiency allows for prompt intervention.

Provides a baseline to measure changes in discomfort pattern. May indicate worsening of neuropathies.

THERAPEUTIC INTERVENTIONS	**RATIONALE**

Independent Actions
Implement measures to reduce discomfort:
- Perform actions to reduce fear and anxiety about discomfort (e.g., assure client that the need for relief of discomfort is understood; plan methods for control of discomfort with client).
- Perform actions to reduce stress (e.g., explain procedures, maintain a calm environment).
- If client has hyperesthesia, provide a bed cradle. **D** ● ✦

- Assist client with ambulation if walking relieves discomfort. **D** ● ✦
- If client is experiencing intermittent claudication, encourage short, more frequent walks.

These actions promote relaxation and subsequently increases client's threshold and tolerance for discomfort.

Use of a bed cradle keeps bedding off affected extremities to decrease pressure on the skin.
Walking often relieves lower extremity discomfort associated with neuropathies.
Longer walks exacerbate pain associated with vascular insufficiency.

THERAPEUTIC INTERVENTIONS	RATIONALE
• Provide or assist with additional nonpharmacologic measures for relief of discomfort (e.g., position change, relaxation exercises, guided imagery, quiet conversation, restful environment).	*Use of nonpharmacologic measures provides relief of pain without sedation.*

Dependent/Collaborative Actions

Implement measures to reduce discomfort:

• Perform actions to maintain blood glucose at a near-normal level (e.g., appropriate diet, exercise, blood glucose monitoring).	*Maintaining optimal glycemic control can actually alleviate or reduce neuropathic discomfort and the progression of neuropathy.*
• Administer the following medications if ordered to control discomfort:	*Provides pain relief through a variety of mechanisms:*
• Analgesics	*Analgesics and tricyclic antidepressants work via the central*
• Tricyclic antidepressants	*nervous system (CNS).*
• Anticonvulsants (i.e., gabapentin or carbamazepine	*These anticonvulsants have been used to treat sharp or stabbing superficial burning pain.*
• Capsaicin cream	*Capsaicin cream is useful in treatment of superficial pain.*
• Hemorrheologic agents (e.g., pentoxifylline)	*Hemorrheologic agents can improve peripheral blood flow and reduce discomfort associated with intermittent claudication.*
• Skeletal muscle relaxants or quinine sulfate	*Quinine sulfate can be used to treat leg cramps.*
• Consult appropriate health care provider (e.g., pharmacist, pain management specialist, physician) if above measures fail to provide adequate relief of discomfort.	*If pain relief is inadequate, consultation with other member of the health care team provides a multidisciplinary approach to pain management.*

Nursing Diagnosis RISK FOR DYSFUNCTIONAL GASTROINTESTINAL MOTILITY NDx

Definition: Risk for increased, decreased, ineffective, or lack of peristaltic activity within the gastrointestinal system

Related to: Delayed emptying of the stomach associated with autonomic neuropathy involving the gastrointestinal tract

CLINICAL MANIFESTATIONS

Subjective	Objective
Complaints of abdominal gas, heart burn, fullness, bloating, and nausea	Palpable distended abdomen; decreased or absent bowel sounds

RISK FACTORS	DESIRED OUTCOMES

• Stress
• Consistently elevated blood glucose levels
• Lack of exercise
	The client will experience a reduction in gastric discomfort as evidenced by:
	  a. Verbalization of same
	  b. Relaxed facial expression and body positioning

NOC OUTCOMES	NIC INTERVENTIONS
Comfort level; symptom control	Environmental management: comfort; nausea management; hyperglycemia management

NURSING ASSESSMENT	RATIONALE
Assess client for: • Verbal reports of gastric discomfort (e.g., gastric fullness, postprandial bloating, nausea) • Nonverbal signs of discomfort (e.g., grimacing, rubbing upper abdomen, restlessness, reluctance to move)	*Early recognition of signs and symptoms of gastric discomfort allows for prompt intervention.*

Continued...

THERAPEUTIC INTERVENTIONS	RATIONALE
Independent Actions Implement measures to reduce gastric discomfort: • Perform actions to reduce the accumulation of gas and fluid in the stomach:	
• Encourage and assist client with frequent position changes and ambulation as tolerated.	*Activity stimulates gastrointestinal motility.*
• Have client sit up during meals and for 1 to 2 hours after meals. **D ● ✦**	*Gravity promotes passage of food and fluid through the gastrointestinal tract.*
• Provide small, frequent meals rather than three large ones; instruct client to ingest foods and fluids slowly.	*Small, frequent meals decrease abdominal fullness after meals.*
• Instruct client to avoid foods high in fat.	*Foods high in fat delay gastric emptying.*
• Instruct client to avoid activities such as chewing gum, drinking through a straw, and smoking.	*Avoiding these activities decreases air swallowing.*
• Instruct client to avoid intake of carbonated beverages and gas-producing foods (e.g., cabbage, onions, beans).	*Avoiding these foods/fluids reduces production of gas.*
• Encourage client to eructate whenever the urge is felt. **D ● ✦**	*Burping helps to remove gas from the stomach.*
• Perform actions to reduce nausea if present:	
• Encourage client to take deep, slow breaths when nauseated.	*Slow, deep breaths help to alleviate nausea.*
• Instruct client to avoid foods/fluids that irritate the gastric mucosa (e.g., spicy foods; caffeine-containing beverages such as coffee, tea, and colas).	*Foods that irritate the gastric mucosa increase the incidence of esophageal reflux and heartburn.*
• Eliminate noxious sights and odors from the environment. **D ● ✦**	*Noxious stimuli can cause stimulation of the vomiting center.*
• Instruct and assist client to change positions slowly. **D ● ✦**	*Rapid movement can result in stimulation of the chemoreceptor trigger zone and subsequent excitation of the vomiting center.*
• Avoid serving foods with an overpowering aroma; remove lids from hot foods before entering room. **D ● ✦**	*Powerful smells may stimulate the nausea center.*
• Instruct client to eat dry foods (e.g., toast, crackers) and avoid drinking liquids with meals when feeling nauseated.	*These actions help to settle the client's stomach when nauseated.*
• Perform actions to maintain blood glucose at a near-normal level. (e.g., establishing an exercise routine, adhering to a diabetic diet).	*Maintaining optimal glycemic control seems to improve gastric emptying.*
Dependent/Collaborative Actions Implement measures to reduce gastric discomfort: • Perform actions to reduce the accumulation of gas and fluid in the stomach:	
• Administer medications that enhance gastric motility (e.g., metoclopramide) if ordered. **D ✦**	*Metoclopramide stimulates gastric motility, which improves gastric emptying.*
• Perform actions to reduce nausea if present:	
• Administer antiemetics as ordered. **D ✦**	*Antiemetics decrease nausea and emesis.*
Consult physician if gastric discomfort persists or worsens.	*Notification of the physician allows for modification of the treatment plan.*

Nursing Diagnosis **DISTURBED SENSORY PERCEPTION NDx (VISUAL)**

Definition: Change in amount or patterning of incoming stimuli accompanied by a diminished, exaggerated, distorted, or impaired response to such stimuli

Related to:
• Osmotic swelling of the lens associated with hyperglycemia
• Changes in the retinal vessels (retinopathy)
• Presence of cataracts (there is an increased incidence of cataract formation in persons with diabetes)

CLINICAL MANIFESTATIONS

Subjective	Objective
Reports of blurred vision and/or partial or total loss of vision; complaints of floaters, spots, or flashing lights	N/A

RISK FACTOR

- Consistently elevated blood glucose levels

DESIRED OUTCOMES

The client will not experience further progression of visual disturbances and will demonstrate adaptation to existing ones.

NOC OUTCOMES

Vision compensation behavior; risk control: visual impairment

NIC INTERVENTIONS

Communication enhancement: visual deficit; environmental management

NURSING ASSESSMENT

Assess for visual disturbances (e.g., reports of blurred vision; partial or total loss of vision; the presence of "floaters," spots, or flashing lights).

RATIONALE

Diabetes is the number one cause of blindness in the United States. Early recognition and treatment may prevent or delay visual changes from occurring.

THERAPEUTIC INTERVENTIONS

RATIONALE

Independent Actions

Implement measures to maintain blood glucose at a near-normal level (e.g., diet, exercise, glucose monitoring) in order to reduce further progression of visual disturbances.

Studies show that the incidence and progression of changes in the eye can be reduced by optimal glycemic control.

If vision is impaired:

- Implement measures to reduce the risk for injury (e.g., orient client to surroundings and identify obstacles during ambulation, instruct client to ambulate in well-lit areas and use handrails if available).

These actions reduce anxiety, allowing the client to maintain appropriate autonomy while reducing risk for injury.

- Avoid startling client (e.g., speak client's name and identify yourself when entering room and before any physical contact, describe activities and reasons for various noises in the room). **D** ● ✦

These actions reduce the client's fear related to being in a new environment.

- Assist with personal hygiene that client is unable to perform independently. **D** ● ✦
- If client has glasses, make sure they are clean and within reach. **D** ● ✦

Having clean, accessible eyewear decreases the client's risk of falls.

- Identify where items are placed on plate and tray, cut food, open packages, and feed client if necessary. **D** ● ✦

These actions promote client independence and maintains nutritional status.

- Assist with activities such as filling out menus and reading mail and legal documents as needed.
- Instruct client in use of appropriate self-help devices (e.g., magnifier for insulin syringe, syringe with a plunger lock, insulin pen that delivers fixed amount of insulin, needle guide for insulin vial, glucometer that displays blood glucose values in bold numbers); monitor client's accuracy in testing blood glucose and administering insulin.

Appropriate self-help devices allow client to care for self and maintain a level of independence.

- Provide auditory rather than visual diversionary activities.

Promotes quality of life.

- Inform client of resources available if he/she desires additional information about visual aids (e.g., American Federation for the Blind).

Community resources provide for continuum of care.

- Encourage client to discuss options available for treatment of retinopathy (e.g., laser photocoagulation) and cataracts with physician.

Visual changes that occur with diabetes require ongoing health care.

Collaborative Diagnosis **RISK FOR DIABETIC KETOACIDOSIS (DKA)**

Definition: A life-threatening complication of diabetes in which there is inadequate insulin, resulting in increased blood glucose levels, acidosis, and ketone bodies

Related to: Hyperglycemia and accelerated ketogenesis associated with the combined effect of severe insulin deficiency and excess secretion of counterregulatory hormones such as glucagon and epinephrine

CLINICAL MANIFESTATIONS

Subjective	Objective
Complaints of weakness, nausea, or abdominal pain	Hypotension—fluid volume deficit; weakness; lethargy; vomiting; acetone odor on breath; Kussmaul respirations; blood glucose level >250 mg/dL; ketones in blood and urine; metabolic acidosis

RISK FACTORS

- Administration of inadequate amounts of insulin and/or the presence of stressors such as illness, trauma, or infection
- Inability to manage treatment regimen
- Non-adherence to dietary restrictions

DESIRED OUTCOMES

The client will not experience ketoacidosis as evidenced by:
  a. Stable vital signs
  b. Usual skin temperature and color
  c. Absence of unusual weakness, lethargy, nausea, vomiting, abdominal pain, and fruity odor on breath
  d. Unlabored respirations at 12 to 20 breaths/min
  e. Blood glucose level <250 mg/dL
  f. Absence of ketones in blood and urine
  g. Blood pH and bicarbonate level within normal range

NURSING ASSESSMENT	RATIONALE
Assess for and report signs and symptoms of ketoacidosis (clients at greatest risk have type 1 [insulin-dependent] diabetes): • Evidence of deficient fluid volume (e.g., hypotension; weak, rapid pulse; warm, flushed skin; thirst) • Weakness, lethargy • Nausea, vomiting, abdominal pain • Acetone (fruity) odor on breath • Kussmaul respirations • Blood glucose >250 mg/dL • Ketones in blood and urine • Low blood pH and bicarbonate level	*Early recognition of signs and symptoms of diabetic ketoacidosis allows for prompt treatment.*

THERAPEUTIC INTERVENTIONS	RATIONALE
Independent Actions Implement measures to prevent or treat hyperglycemia in order to prevent ketoacidosis: • Encourage client to adhere to the diabetic diet prescribed (e.g., consistent carbohydrate diet, exchange list, Food Guide Pyramid). • Minimize client's exposure to emotional and physiological stress. If signs and symptoms of ketoacidosis occur: • Maintain client on bed rest.	*An appropriate diet is helpful in preventing DKA.* *Stress causes an increased output of epinephrine, glucagon, and cortisol, all of which increase blood sugar.* *Bed rest reduces risk of injury as client may be weak, lethargic, and confused.*

THERAPEUTIC INTERVENTIONS	RATIONALE

Dependent/Collaborative Actions

Implement measures to prevent or treat hyperglycemia in order to prevent ketoacidosis:

- Administer insulin as ordered and in an area where maximum absorption will occur; if client has an insulin pump, maintain prescribed infusion rate and ensure that client receives preprandial boluses as ordered.

  The absorption of insulin can be erratic if it is administered in an area where tissue is hypertrophied.

- If client is hypotensive, consult health care provider about administering insulin intravenously rather than subcutaneously.

  Regular insulin is the only insulin that can be given intravenously. Subcutaneous insulin absorption will be delayed if client's B/P is low enough to cause inadequate tissue perfusion.

- If client is receiving continuous intravenous insulin, do not discontinue the infusion until subcutaneous insulin has been administered and had time to reach its onset of action.

  Discontinuing the intravenous insulin infusion before subcutaneous insulin has had time to reach its onset of action would increase the level of hyperglycemia, extending the time frame for resolution.

If signs and symptoms of ketoacidosis occur, administer the following if ordered:

- Insulin (regular insulin is administered intravenously in the initial phase of treatment)

  Regular insulin is the only insulin to be given intravenously.

- Intravenous fluid and electrolyte replacement based on lab value findings

  Intravenous fluids are rapidly infused until B/P is stabilized and urine output is adequate.

  - Infuse isotonic or half-strength normal saline
  - Provide supplemental potassium chloride or potassium phosphate

    Hypokalemia and hypophosphatemia result from osmotic diuresis and a shift of potassium and phosphorus into the cells during insulin therapy.

  - Combination saline and glucose solutions once blood glucose level falls to 250 to 300 mg/dL

    A saline and glucose solution prevents hypoglycemia that can result with a rapid drop in blood glucose.

  - Administer sodium bicarbonate if the serum pH drops to ≤7.0; if bicarbonate is administered, it should be discontinued when the pH reaches 7.1 to 7.2.

    Reversing acidosis too quickly has harmful physiological effects.

Collaborative Diagnosis

RISK FOR HYPERGLYCEMIC HYPEROSMOLAR NONKETOTIC COMA (SYNDROME)

Definition: A life-threatening complication of diabetes characterized by hyperglycemia, hyperosmolarity, and dehydration

Related to: Coma related to severe dehydration associated with sustained osmotic diuresis resulting from uncontrolled hyperglycemia

CLINICAL MANIFESTATIONS

Subjective	Objective
Complaints of hunger, thirst; blurred vision, fatigue, dry mouth, or itchy skin	Weight loss; dehydration; poor wound healing; dry skin; "fruity" smelling breath; impotence; Kussmaul respirations; stupor; coma

RISK FACTORS

- Inadequate insulin administration
- Antibiotic medications
- Inability to adhere to dietary regimen

DESIRED OUTCOMES:

The client will not experience hyperglycemic hyperosmolar nonketotic coma as evidenced by:
  a. Stable vital signs
  b. Usual skin temperature and color
  c. Absence of motor and sensory deficits and seizure activity
  d. Blood glucose level <600 mg/dL

NDx = NANDA-I Diagnosis   **D** = Delegatable Action   ● = UAP   ✦ = LVN/LPN   ⊝▶ = Go to ⊝volve for animation

Continued...

NURSING ASSESSMENT	RATIONALE

Assess for and report signs and symptoms of hyperglycemic hyperosmolar nonketotic coma (at greatest risk are clients >60 years; clients with type 2 [non–insulin-dependent] diabetes; clients with inadequate fluid intake or excessive fluid loss; those who are experiencing unusual emotional or physical stress [e.g., acute illness, infection, surgery]; and clients receiving corticosteroids, diuretics, hyperalimentation, or dialysis treatments):

Early recognition of the signs and symptoms of hyperglycemic hyperosmolar nonketotic coma allows for prompt intervention.

- Evidence of deficient fluid volume (e.g., hypotension; weak, rapid pulse; warm, flushed skin; decreased skin turgor; thirst)
- High serum osmolality (>320 mOsm/L)
- Neurological signs such as hemiparesis, aphasia, lethargy, disorientation, and seizures
- Blood glucose >600 mg/dL with absent or only slight elevation of ketones in urine and serum

Hyperglycemia promotes osmotic diuresis, which involves water movement from the intracellular to the extracellular compartment and excessive diuresis, both of which lead to serum hyponatremia.

THERAPEUTIC INTERVENTIONS	RATIONALE

Dependent/Collaborative Actions

Implement measures to prevent hyperglycemic hyperosmolar nonketotic coma:

- Perform actions to prevent or treat hyperglycemia (e.g., diet, exercise, self blood glucose control).
- Notify physician if client is unable to take in an adequate amount of oral fluids, develops signs and symptoms of infection, has persistent diarrhea or vomiting, or is experiencing unusual emotional stress.

Appropriate actions to maintain blood glucose control prevent hyperosmolarity and subsequent osmotic diuresis.
Notification of physician allows for alterations in the treatment plan.

If signs and symptoms of hyperglycemic hyperosmolar nonketotic coma occur, administer the following if ordered:

- Fluid replacement (isotonic or half-strength saline is infused rapidly until B/P is stabilized and urine output is adequate; once blood sugar falls to 250 to 300 mg/dL, 5% glucose is added)
- Insulin (regular insulin is administered intravenously in the initial phase of treatment)

- Intravenous potassium chloride or potassium phosphate

Fluid replacement helps to maintain blood pressure and urine output.

Administration of insulin promotes glucose entry into the cells and prevents hypoglycemia that can result from the rapid drop in blood glucose levels.
Hypokalemia and hypophosphatemia result from osmotic diuresis and a shift of potassium and phosphorus into the cells during insulin therapy.

Nursing Diagnosis INEFFECTIVE FAMILY THERAPEUTIC REGIMEN MANAGEMENT NDx

Definition: Pattern of regulating and integrating into family processes a program for treatment of illness and its sequelae that is unsatisfactory for meeting specific health goals

CLINICAL MANIFESTATIONS

Subjective	Objective
Statements about inability to manage care at home; statements reflecting a lack of understanding of factors that contribute to acute and chronic complications; statements about unwillingness or inability to modify personal habits and integrated treatments into lifestyle; statements reflecting a view that diabetes is curable or that the situation is hopeless and adherence will not improve health	Refusing medications; nonadherence to dietary restrictions

RISK FACTORS

- Lack of understanding of the implications of not following the prescribed treatment plan
- Feeling of lack of control over disease progression despite efforts to follow prescribed treatment plan
- Difficulty modifying personal habits and integrating necessary treatments and dietary regimen into lifestyle
- Insufficient financial resources

DESIRED OUTCOMES

The client will demonstrate the probability of effective therapeutic regimen management as evidenced by:
  a. Willingness to learn about and participate in treatments and care
  b. Statements reflecting ways to modify personal habits and integrate treatments into lifestyle
  c. Statements reflecting an understanding of the implications of not following the prescribed treatment plan

NOC OUTCOMES

Compliance behavior; diabetes self-management; treatment behavior: illness or injury; knowledge: treatment regimen; health beliefs: perceived resources; health beliefs: perceived ability to perform

NIC INTERVENTIONS

Self modification assistance; medication management; values clarification; teaching: disease process; teaching: prescribed diet; weight reduction assistance; financial resource assistance; support system enhancement

NURSING ASSESSMENT

Assess for indications that client may be unable to effectively manage the therapeutic regimen or may require further education:

- Statements reflecting inability to manage care at home
- Failure to adhere to treatment plan (e.g., refusing medications, not adhering to dietary restrictions)
- Statements reflecting a lack of understanding of factors that contribute to acute and chronic complications
- Statements reflecting an unwillingness or inability to modify personal habits and integrate necessary treatments into lifestyle
- Statements reflecting the view that diabetes is curable or that the situation is hopeless and that efforts to comply with treatments are useless

RATIONALE

Provides a baseline for client and family teaching and what specific concerns, lack of understanding, or level of acceptance is being experienced.

THERAPEUTIC INTERVENTIONS

Independent Actions

Implement measures to promote effective therapeutic management:

- Determine client's understanding of diabetes; clarify misconceptions and stress that diabetes is a chronic condition and adherence to the treatment plan may delay and/or prevent complications; caution the client that some complications may occur despite strict adherence to treatment plan.

- Encourage client to participate in assessment and treatments (e.g., blood glucose monitoring, selection of diet, insulin administration).

- Provide client with written instructions about future appointments with health care provider, diet, medications, exercise, signs and symptoms to report, and foot care.

- Discuss with client the difficulties of incorporating treatments into lifestyle; assist client in identifying ways to modify lifestyle rather than completely change it.

- Encourage client to discuss concerns about the cost of medications, food, and supplies; obtain a social service consult to assist with financial planning and obtain financial aid if indicated.

RATIONALE

Adherence to the treatment regimen will preserve the client's health for a longer period and may prevent some complications from occurring.

Through observation of the client's adherence to treatment regimen, the nurse can determine client's ability to care for self.

Written instructions provide the client an information resource once discharged.

Portrays a true picture of diabetes management and allows the client to determine what lifestyle modifications are feasible. This improves the client's ability to adhere to the treatment regimen.

Diabetes can have a significant financial impact on clients and their families and should be discussed openly to assist clients with treatment management.

Continued...

THERAPEUTIC INTERVENTIONS	RATIONALE
• Encourage client to attend follow-up diabetic education classes.	*Continued education improves client's understanding about diabetes and interventions to improve health.*
• Provide information about and encourage utilization of resources that can assist client to make necessary lifestyle changes (e.g., diabetes support groups, counseling services, American Diabetes Association, diabetic cookbooks, and publications).	*Provides for continuum of care once discharged from the acute care facility*
• Reinforce behaviors suggesting future compliance with the therapeutic regimen (e.g., participation in the treatment plan, statements reflecting plans for integrating treatments into lifestyle).	*Provides client feedback and can increase confidence in client's ability to care for self and adhere to treatment regimen*
• Include significant others in explanations and teaching sessions and encourage their support; reinforce the need for client to assume responsibility for managing as much of care as possible.	*Informed family members can support the client in lifestyle changes and treatment regimen management.*

Nursing Diagnosis DEFICIENT KNOWLEDGE NDx OR INEFFECTIVE SELF HEALTH MANAGEMENT* NDx

Definition: Absence or deficiency of cognitive information related to specific topic (lack of specific information necessary for clients/significant others) to make informed choices regarding condition/treatment/lifestyle changes; pattern of regulating and integrating into daily living a therapeutic regime for treatment of illness and its sequelae that is unsatisfactory for meeting specific health goals

CLINICAL MANIFESTATIONS

Subjective	Objective
Verbalization of inability to manage illness or inability to follow prescribed regimen	Inaccurate follow-through with instructions; inappropriate behaviors; experience of preventable complications of diabetes

RISK FACTORS
• Cognitive deficit
• Financial concerns
• Failure to take action to reduce risk factors for complications of Parkinson's disease
• Inability to care for oneself
• Difficulty in modifying personal habits and integrating treatments into lifestyle

NOC OUTCOMES	NIC INTERVENTIONS
Knowledge: treatment regimen; knowledge: health behavior; knowledge: health resources; knowledge: treatment procedure(s)	Teaching: individual; teaching: prescribed activity/exercise; teaching: psychomotor skills; health system guidance; financial resource assistance; support system enhancement

NURSING ASSESSMENT	RATIONALE
Assess client's ability to learn and readiness to learn. Assess client's understanding of teaching. Assess client's ability for self care.	Learning is more effective when client is motivated and understands the importance of what is to be learned. Readiness to learn changes based on situations and physical and emotional challenges.

*The nurse should select the diagnostic label that is most appropriate for the client's discharge teaching needs.

THERAPEUTIC INTERVENTIONS	RATIONALE

Desired Outcome: The client will verbalize a basic understanding of diabetes and of medications ordered and demonstrate the ability to correctly administer insulin if prescribed.

Independent Actions

Determine client's understanding of diabetes mellitus.

Clarify misconceptions and reinforce teaching as necessary. Use available teaching aids (e.g., pamphlets, videotapes).

Explain the rationale for, side effects of, storage and care of, method of administration of, and importance of taking medications prescribed.

Provide instructions if client is to self-administer insulin.

If client is discharged with an insulin pump device, provide instructions regarding its management (e.g., changing the insertion site, filling syringes, changing batteries in pump).

Allow time for practice and return demonstration.

Instruct client to consult pharmacist or health care provider before taking other prescription and nonprescription medications (e.g., over-the-counter cold preparations).

Instruct client to inform all health care providers of medications being taken.

Baseline understanding is important in developing client teaching plan.

A variety of teaching methods are more effective, as individuals have varying styles of learning.

Knowledge of medications and how they impact the system improves client adherence. Help enhance the client's understanding of the importance of adhering to the prescribed medication regimen. The client must be able to recognize alterations in functioning related to medication administration.

Client and family members should be taught how to correctly administer insulin.

Client should not leave health care institution without an understanding of how to appropriately use the insulin pump to prevent or decrease the number of hyperglycemic and hypoglycemic events.

Demonstration provides the nurse time to provide client feedback and improves client's confidence in ability to care for self.

Over-the-counter medications may affect the hypoglycemic agent taken by the client.

This action prevents drug interactions when health care provider is prescribing new medications.

THERAPEUTIC INTERVENTIONS	RATIONALE

Desired Outcome: The client will verbalize an understanding of the principles of dietary management and be able to calculate and plan meals within the prescribed caloric distribution.

Independent Actions

Reinforce dietary instructions regarding the prescribed diabetic diet and methods of calculating the foods/fluids allowed (e.g., exchange list, consistent carbohydrate diet, Food Guide Pyramid).

Have client plan sample menus before discharge to ensure that he/she is able to calculate the diet correctly.

Explain the purpose of weight reduction if client has been placed on a caloric restriction to reduce weight. Reinforce need to avoid fasting and fad diets.

Instruct client on appropriate dietary adjustments that should be made if meal schedule or activity level has been significantly altered.

Reinforce the following principles of good dietary management:

* Eat three meals each day about 4 to 5 hours apart and close to the same time each day; do not skip meals.
* Limit intake of concentrated sweets (e.g., sugar, candy, syrups, jams, jellies, cakes, pies, pastries, fruits packed in heavy syrup).

Knowledge of dietary instructions helps the client to determine appropriate foods to eat and to maintain proper blood glucose levels and nutritional status.

Planning sample menus provides client with an understanding of diet regulations and the ability to care for self.

Fasting or fad diets may impact client's ability to prevent hyperglycemic or hypoglycemic events.

Dietary adjustments help control blood glucose levels while maintaining adequate nutritional status.

Eating regularly timed meals helps to prevent large variations in blood glucose levels.

An intake of concentrated sweets may precipitate a hyperglycemic event.

Continued...

THERAPEUTIC INTERVENTIONS	RATIONALE
• Avoid foods high in saturated fat and cholesterol (e.g., butter, cheese, eggs, ice cream, red meat) and *trans* fats (e.g., stick margarine and shortening and foods such as commercial baked goods that are prepared with these products).	*Foods high in saturated fat increase the development of atherosclerosis, hypertension, and coronary artery disease.*
• Increase intake of foods high in soluble fiber (e.g., fruits, whole-grain cereals, green leafy vegetables).	*A high-fiber diet decreases blood glucose levels.*
• Read food/fluid labels and limit intake of those that contain significant amounts of sugar, honey, and nutritive sweeteners such as xylitol, sorbitol, and fructose (nutritive sweeteners are usually labeled as "sugar free" but are only "sucrose free," not carbohydrate free; however, they are not digested and absorbed as well as other carbohydrates and therefore contribute only 2 kcal/g as compared with 4 kcal/g of other carbohydrates).	*Client needs to understand what is in foods to prevent inadvertent increases in blood glucose levels.*
• Use artificial (nonnutritive or noncaloric) sweeteners such as saccharin (e.g., Sweet and Low), acesulfame (e.g., Sunette), and aspartame (e.g., Equal, NutraSweet) when possible.	*Client can use a sweetener without an increase in blood glucose levels.*
• Eat an afternoon carbohydrate snack (e.g., fresh fruit, ½ bagel, 1 cup skim milk) if taking an intermediate-acting insulin in the morning, and a snack at bedtime that includes protein and carbohydrate (e.g., milk and graham crackers, ½ meat sandwich, cheese and crackers) if taking an oral glucose-lowering agent or insulin in the evening.	*Appropriate snacks help to maintain adequate blood glucose levels.*
• If alcoholic beverages are consumed:	
• Drink alcohol with food.	*Alcohol can decrease blood glucose levels shortly after drinking and for 8 to 12 hours afterwards. Alcohol can also block effects of diabetic medications.*
• Avoid liqueurs, sweet wines, wine coolers, and sweet mixes that contain large amounts of carbohydrates.	*Wines with high levels of carbohydrates will increase blood sugar levels without any nutritional value.*
• Do not substitute alcohol for anything in prescribed diet.	*Alcohol is not an adequate exchanger for any food type in a prescribed diet.*
	Alcohol may interfere with the liver's ability to produce glucose. If on a weight-control diet, client should avoid alcohol because it adds calories without any nutritional value.
• Limit alcohol intake to two drinks per day for men and one drink per day for women (a "drink" is considered to be 1½ oz of liquor, 12 oz of beer, or 5 oz of wine).	*If a client chooses to drink, he/she should drink only the recommended amount for client's with diabetes.*

THERAPEUTIC INTERVENTIONS	RATIONALE
Desired Outcome: The client will demonstrate the ability to perform blood glucose and urine tests correctly and interpret results accurately.	
Independent Actions	
Review with client how and when to perform a blood glucose measurement and calibrate and maintain a glucose monitoring device.	*Reinforces what client knows and provides an opportunity to expand client's understanding.*
Have client demonstrate blood glucose measurement. Reinforce teaching as necessary.	*Client demonstration of blood glucose measurement provides clients with confidence that they can appropriately monitor blood glucose levels and allows the nurse time to reinforce teaching.*
Instruct client to keep a record of test results and take the record of results to appointments with the health care provider.	*Maintenance of a test results record can provide the health care provider with a long-term view of client's adherence to therapeutic regimen and control of blood glucose level.*

THERAPEUTIC INTERVENTIONS	RATIONALE
Provide instructions on actions client should take when test results are abnormal (some clients are instructed to adjust insulin dose and dietary intake; others are instructed to notify appropriate health care provider)	*Written instructions provide an ongoing resource for client to use in controlling blood glucose level.*

THERAPEUTIC INTERVENTIONS	RATIONALE

Desired Outcome: The client will verbalize an understanding of the role of exercise in the management of diabetes.

Independent Actions

Explain how exercise affects blood sugar levels.	*Exercise improves insulin's effectiveness, lowers hemoglobin A_{1c}, promotes weight loss, and decreases cardiovascular risk factors.*
Provide the following instructions about exercise and diabetes management:	
• Maintain a regular exercise program, making sure to start exercise slowly and build up gradually.	*A regular program gives client an indication of how exercise affects blood glucose levels before increasing exercise intensity and length of time.*
• Avoid exercising during insulin peak action time.	*This may precipitate a severe hypoglycemic episode.*
• Try to exercise about 1 hour after a meal and about the same time of the day.	*Promotes better processing of glucose through increased insulin sensitivity.*
• Avoid giving insulin in a site that will be heavily exercised.	*Increased circulation to the injection area will increase utilization of insulin, potentially causing a hypoglycemic event.*
• Adjust insulin dosage before exercise according to physician's instructions.	*Adjusting the dosage helps to decrease the potential for a hypoglycemic event during exercise.*
• Consume extra carbohydrates before vigorous exercise and supplement carbohydrate intake (15 to 30 g) at 30- to 60-minute intervals during vigorous prolonged exercise.	*Extra carbohydrate before vigorous exercise helps to prevent the potential for a hypoglycemic event.*
• Maintain adequate hydration during periods of intense exercise.	*Adequate hydration is needed to prevent dehydration.*
• Consume an extra bedtime snack on days that exercise has been prolonged or unusually vigorous.	*Doing so helps prevent hypoglycemic events.*
• Do not exercise in extreme heat or cold.	*Hot and cold weather affect how the body uses insulin.*
• Do not exercise at times when blood sugar is >250 mg/dL and ketones are present in urine or if blood sugar is >300 mg/dL.	*Strenuous exercise is perceived by the body as a stressor, leading to an increased output of counterregulatory hormones and a further increase in blood glucose.*
• Perform blood glucose tests more frequently during periods of significant variation in activity level.	*More frequent blood glucose testing during exercise helps to prevent large variations in blood glucose level.*
• Carry a rapid-acting carbohydrate source (e.g., hard candy, glucose tablets) during exercise (especially if using insulin and if exercise is expected to be prolonged or vigorous).	*Doing so helps to prevent hypoglycemic events.*
• Stop any activity that causes extreme weakness, trembling, incoordination, or nausea.	*Client should be aware of clinical manifestations of hypoglycemia and stop exercising.*

THERAPEUTIC INTERVENTIONS	RATIONALE

Desired Outcome: The client will identify health care and hygiene practices that should be integrated into lifestyle.

Independent Actions

Reinforce the importance of adhering to the following health care practices:	
• Perform oral hygiene including brushing and flossing at least twice a day.	*Individuals with diabetes are at higher risk for cavities, gum diseases, and oral infections. Good oral hygiene and regular dental appointments help to prevent these from occurring.*
• Have regular dental appointments at least every 6 months.	
• Have annual eye examinations (beginning 5 years after onset for type 1 and at onset for type 2 diabetes).	*Diabetes is the number one cause of blindness in the United States. Regular eye examinations allow for early recognition and treatment of changes and potentially decrease deleterious effects of diabetes.*
• Avoid smoking.	*Smoking increases the risk for cardiovascular disease.*

Continued...

THERAPEUTIC INTERVENTIONS	RATIONALE
• Have feet examined by health care provider annually.	*Early identification of peripheral vascular changes helps to prevent neuropathies, foot ulcers, and risk of infection.*

Provide instructions about foot care:
• Inspect feet daily for cuts, redness, cracks, blisters, corns, and calluses; use a mirror to check bottoms of feet if necessary.	*Daily foot inspection allows for early identification of alterations that increase the risk of infections that may lead to amputation.*
• Wash feet daily with a mild soap and warm water and dry gently but thoroughly.	*Doing so prevents breakdown of skin, particularly between toes.*
• Apply lanolin or other lubricating lotion to feet (except between toes) daily.	*Lubricants replace moisture lost from the skin. Lotion should have a low alcohol content to prevent skin dryness.*
• Keep feet dry by wearing cotton socks and avoiding shoes with rubber or plastic soles.	*Cotton socks absorb moisture from perspiration, decreasing risk of fungal infection. Shoes with rubber or plastic soles cause the feet to sweat.*
• Cut nails after a bath or shower; cut them straight across and smooth them with an emery board after cutting.	*The skin is softer after a shower, and proper cutting of nails helps to prevent injury to the feet, decreasing the risk for infection.*
• See a podiatrist rather than using home remedies to treat corns, calluses, and ingrown nails or if help is needed with routine nail care.	*Professional foot care helps to prevent injury and decrease the risk for infection.*
• Avoid wearing socks, stockings, or garters that are tight.	*These garments may further compromise peripheral blood flow.*
• Buy shoes that fit well and break them in gradually; it is best to buy shoes in the late afternoon when feet are at their largest.	*Peripheral neuropathy and loss of sensation increase the risk of foot injury from ill-fitting shoes.*
• Do not wear open-toed shoes, sandals, high heels, or thongs.	*These types of shoes increase the risk for trauma.*
• Do not walk barefoot; wear shoes or slippers when walking.	*Wearing shoes or slippers prevents foot injury.*
• Do not use a heating pad or hot water bottle on feet; test bath water with bath thermometer, wrist, or elbow before immersing feet (temperature should be 30°C to 32°C [84°F to 90°F]).	*Peripheral neuropathy and loss of pain and temperature sensation increase the risk for burns and other injuries.*
• Protect feet from extreme cold to prevent vasoconstriction and possible frostbite.	

THERAPEUTIC INTERVENTIONS	RATIONALE
Desired Outcome: The client will identify appropriate safety measures to follow because of the diagnosis of diabetes.	

Independent Actions
Teach client the following safety precautions:
• Always carry an identification card or wear a medical alert bracelet or tag identifying self as a diabetic patient; identification card should have the name of health care provider, the type and dose of insulin and/or oral agent(s), and measures to take if found behaving abnormally or unconscious.	*Carrying identification allows for prompt and appropriate treatment if client is alone and unable to speak.*
• Always carry a rapid-acting carbohydrate such as glucose tablets or instant glucose gel.	*A rapid-acting carbohydrate is necessary to reverse hypoglycemic events.*
• If insulin-dependent, always have insulin readily available (carry in purse or briefcase).	*Insulin is necessary to reverse hyperglycemic events.*
• If traveling by plane, bus, or train:	
• Carry a letter from health care provider indicating the necessity of having syringes, blood glucose monitoring equipment, and medication.	*A letter from a health professional prevents problems with security when traveling with syringes and other supplies.*
• Keep snack items, a quick-acting source of carbohydrate, a full day's supply of food, blood glucose monitoring equipment, and an extra supply of insulin, injection equipment, and oral agents in carry-on luggage.	*These supplies are necessary to maintain adequate nutrition and appropriate blood glucose levels.*

THERAPEUTIC INTERVENTIONS	RATIONALE
• Consult physician about plans for pregnancy and maintain close prenatal supervision.	*Pregnancy impacts the way a client controls diabetes, and this should be monitored by a health care practitioner.*
• Keep a glucagon kit readily available and know how and when to use it; make sure significant other is also trained in how to use it.	*A glucagon kit can be used for severe hypoglycemic events*
• If ill but able to tolerate some foods/fluids:	
• Take usual dose of insulin or oral glucose-lowering agent unless blood glucose is low.	
• Check blood glucose every 4 hours or a minimum of four times a day.	*Illness places an additional stress on blood glucose levels. To maintain adequate control, blood glucose levels need to be monitored more frequently.*
• If blood glucose is >240 mg/dL, test urine for ketones.	*Testing for ketones with a blood glucose >240 mg/dL provides early detection of diabetic ketoacidosis.*
• Drink 8 to 12 oz of caffeine- and alcohol-free fluid (e.g., broth, fruit juice, regular or diet soda, water, Gatorade) every hour.	*Caffeine and alcohol increase urine output and may increase risk for dehydration.*
• If not able to tolerate solid foods, substitute liquids and easily digested soft foods.	*Liquids and soft food can provide adequate nutrition.*
• Do not exercise.	*Exercise may cause hypoglycemia.*
• Notify physician if:	
• Unable to eat for >24 hours	*Not eating or vomiting may significantly decrease blood glucose levels and increases client's risk for injury*
• Vomiting or severe diarrhea persists for >4 hours	
• Blood glucose level is >300 mg/dL or ketones are present in urine	*Increased blood glucose levels with presence of ketones in the urine may indicate diabetic ketoacidosis.*
• Having difficulty breathing or a change in mental status occurs	*These signs and symptoms are indicative of diabetic ketoacidosis and should be treated immediately.*
• Symptoms of dehydration such as unusual thirst, dry mouth, or fever occur	
• Inform all health care providers of diabetic conditions.	*This helps the health care team provide the most appropriate care in a timely manner.*

THERAPEUTIC INTERVENTIONS	RATIONALE

Desired Outcome: The client will state signs and symptoms of hypoglycemia and ketoacidosis and appropriate actions for prevention and treatment.

Independent Actions

Reinforce the following information about hypoglycemia:

• Factors that precipitate hypoglycemia (e.g., too much insulin or oral hypoglycemic agent, insufficient oral intake, excessive exercise, excessive alcohol intake)	*The client should be able to identify clinical manifestations of hyperglycemic or hypoglycemic events and the treatment necessary to regain appropriate blood glucose levels.*
• Signs and symptoms of hypoglycemia (e.g., shakiness, nervousness, weakness, hunger, sweating, nightmares, early-morning headache, incoordination, blood glucose <70 mg/dL)	
• Actions to take if signs and symptoms of hypoglycemia occur:	
• Test blood glucose if possible and if <70 mg/dL (or if symptoms are present but glucose testing is not possible), take 15 g of rapid-acting carbohydrate (e.g., half a glass of regular [sugar-containing] soft drink, three glucose tablets, half a tube of instant glucose); if taking acarbose (Precose) or miglitol (Glyset), only the glucose tablets or instant glucose will correct hypoglycemia quickly.	*The client needs to base interventions on blood glucose levels.*

Continued...

THERAPEUTIC INTERVENTIONS	RATIONALE
• Retest glucose level in 15 minutes, and if still <70 mg/dL, take another 15 g of rapid-acting carbohydrate; if blood glucose level remains <70 mg/dL and/or symptoms persist for >30 minutes, consult health care provider.	*Retesting of glucose levels provides follow-up information so client may determine next actions based on blood glucose levels.*
• After the hypoglycemic episode, consume a snack (e.g., graham crackers and a glass of milk, half a sandwich and half a glass of milk) if it will be longer than 30 minutes until the next meal.	*Eating appropriate foods is important to maintain blood glucose level after the hypoglycemic event and prevent continued variations in blood glucose levels.*
Teach significant others how to treat hypoglycemia:	*Family members should know what to do in a hypoglycemic event if client is unable to care for self.*
• If client is awake but groggy, put corn syrup, honey, cake icing, or instant glucose in client's mouth between cheek and gum.	
• If client loses consciousness, administer glucagon injection.	
Reinforce the following information about ketoacidosis:	
• Factors that precipitate ketoacidosis (e.g., emotional stress, infection, failure to take insulin or oral glucose-lowering agent)	*Helps client avoid situations in which client is at increased risk for ketoacidosis.*
• Signs and symptoms of impending or actual ketoacidosis (e.g., unusual thirst; excessive urination; weakness; warm, flushed skin; blood glucose level >250 mg/dL; ketones in urine; abdominal pain; nausea and vomiting)	*If client and family are able to recognize signs and symptoms of ketoacidosis, they will be able to seek treatment early and prevent negative effects of ketoacidosis.*
• Immediate actions to take if signs and symptoms of ketoacidosis occur:	
• Drink a cup or more of broth or sugar-free liquid if able to tolerate it.	*Immediate actions decrease the level of blood glucose and improve recovery time frame from ketoacidosis.*
• Administer insulin (if previously instructed in insulin coverage based on blood glucose results).	
• Contact health care provider.	

THERAPEUTIC INTERVENTIONS	RATIONALE
Desired Outcome: The client will state signs and symptoms to report to the health care provider.	
Independent Actions	
Instruct client to report the following:	*These events should be reported to the client's health care practitioner to prevent further complications and for prompt implementation of therapeutic interventions.*
• Unexplained episodes of hypoglycemia and ketoacidosis	
• Unusual variations in blood glucose results	
• A cut, scratch, or burn that becomes red, swollen, or tender or does not start to heal within 24 hours	
• Nausea and vomiting or severe diarrhea that lasts >4 hours	
• Temperature elevation that lasts >2 days	
• Change in vision	
• Development or worsening of symptoms that are indicative of long-term complications (e.g., burning or aching pain in extremity, decreased sensation in extremity, persistent gastric discomfort, frequent urination of small amounts, impotence, gait disturbances, chest pain, extreme fatigue, persistent dizziness or lightheadedness)	

THERAPEUTIC INTERVENTIONS	RATIONALE
Desired Outcome: The client will identify resources that can assist in the adjustment to and management of diabetes.	

THERAPEUTIC INTERVENTIONS	RATIONALE

Independent Actions

Provide information about resources that can assist client and significant others in adjustment to and management of diabetes (e.g., American Diabetes Association, diabetic education classes, weight loss programs, diabetes support groups, counseling services, publications such as *Diabetes Forecast*, Internet sites [www.diabetes.org]). Initiate a referral if indicated.

Giving client resources provides for a continuum of care once client is discharged from the acute care facility.

THERAPEUTIC INTERVENTIONS	RATIONALE

Desired Outcome: The client will verbalize an understanding of and a plan for adhering to recommended follow-up care including future appointments with health care provider and for laboratory studies.

Independent Actions

Reinforce the importance of keeping follow-up appointments with health care provider and for laboratory studies.

Follow-up appointments allow for early recognition and treatment to help prevent or delay the macrovascular and microvascular complications of diabetes.

ADDITIONAL CARE PLANS

DIARRHEA NDx

Related to: Effects of autonomic neuropathy on intestinal motility

RISK FOR INJURY NDx

Falls related to:
- Gait abnormalities (may result from impaired proprioception and muscle weakness and loss of normal structure of the foot) and muscle weakness and diminished reflexes in one or more lower extremity associated with motor and sensory neuropathies that may be present
- Dizziness and syncope associated with postural hypotension that may be present as a result of autonomic neuropathy
- Diminished visual acuity

Burns related to:
- Decreased sensation in extremities (may be present as a result of peripheral polyneuropathy)

SEXUAL DYSFUNCTION NDx

Related to: Autonomic neuropathy and angiopathies that may occur (men may experience impotence and ejaculatory changes; women may experience changes in arousal pattern, vaginal lubrication, and orgasm)

INEFFECTIVE COPING NDx

Related to:
- Fear of complications and inability to manage them
- Discomfort
- Need to alter lifestyle
- Feeling of powerlessness
- Knowledge that condition is chronic and will require life-long medical supervision, dietary regulation, and medication therapy

RISK FOR DEFICIENT FLUID VOLUME NDx

Related to: Excessive loss of fluid associated with the osmotic diuresis that can result from hyperglycemia

IMBALANCED NUTRITION: LESS THAN BODY REQUIREMENTS NDx

Related to:
- Decreased cellular uptake and utilization of glucose and a compensatory increase in metabolism of fat and protein stores associated with insulin deficiency
- Decreased oral intake associated with nausea and feeling of fullness resulting from delayed gastric emptying if diabetic gastroparesis is present

URINARY RETENTION NDx

Related to: Loss of bladder sensation and diminished contractility of the detrusor muscle associated with autonomic neuropathy involving the genitourinary system

CONSTIPATION NDx

Related to: Colonic atony or dilatation associated with autonomic neuropathy involving the large bowel

RISK FOR INFECTION NDx

Related to:
- Decreased efficiency of leukocyte function in a hyperglycemic environment
- Delayed healing of any break in skin integrity associated with decreased tissue perfusion and altered nutritional status (there is diminished protein synthesis and tissue repair when insulin is deficient)

NDx = NANDA-I Diagnosis   **D** = Delegatable Action   ● = UAP   ✦ = LVN/_PN   ⊖▶ = Go to ⊖volve for animation

HYPERTHYROIDISM/THYROIDECTOMY

Hyperthyroidism is a condition in which the thyroid gland has a sustained increase in synthesis and release of thyroid hormones. The increased levels of thyroid hormone—triiodothyronine (T_3), thyroxine (T_4), or both—exaggerate normal body functions, causing a hypermetabolic state and increased activity of the sympathetic nervous system. Graves' disease accounts for approximately 75% of the cases of hyperthyroidism. It is an autoimmune disease in which antibodies are made and attach to the thyroid-stimulating hormone (TSH) receptors, causing increased hormone production. The most common clinical manifestations of hyperthyroidism/Graves' disease include hyperactivity, trouble sleeping, fatigue, frequent bowel movements, irritability, heat sensitivity, weight loss without dieting, increased sweating, muscular weakness, blurred or double vision, palpitations and/or tachycardia, hand tremors, diffuse goiter, and exophthalmos. Exophthalmos is seen when the tissues of the ocular orbit swell and push the eye forward.

Thyrotoxicosis (also called thyrotoxic crisis or thyroid storm) is an acute exacerbation of increased thyroid hormone levels. This is a life-threatening situation and is almost always fatal unless treatment is rapid and aggressive. Clinical manifestations include fever, tachycardia, hypertension, and neurological and gastrointestinal abnormalities. If left untreated, hypertension leads to heart failure, hypotension, and shock. Precipitating factors include emotional stress, infection, abrupt withdrawal of antithyroid medications, thyroid surgery (occurs afterward), and trauma.

Diagnostic studies to determine alterations in the levels of thyroid hormones include measurement of TSH and free triiodothyronine (FT_3) and free thyroxine (FT_4) levels. Decreased TSH and elevated FT_3 or FT_4 levels are indicative of hyperthyroidism. Hyperthyroidism may be treated medically or surgically. Medical treatment involves the use of antithyroid medications that block thyroid hormone production. Iodine preparations, which decrease blood flow through the thyroid, are also used to reduce the synthesis and release of thyroid hormones. The effects of medical treatment are not seen for several weeks after initiation because medications do not impact the large amounts of stored thyroid hormones that continue to be released. During medical treatment, the client should be closely monitored because antithyroid medications may cause hypothyroidism.

Thyroidectomy is the surgical removal of the thyroid gland. It may be performed to treat a benign or malignant tumor, an unusually large goiter, or hyperthyroidism that has been refractory to medical treatment. A subtotal thyroidectomy (i.e., removal of up to 90% of the thyroid gland) is the preferred procedure unless the surgery is being done to treat a malignancy, in which case a total thyroidectomy will usually be performed. After a subtotal thyroidectomy, the remaining gland tissue usually hypertrophies enough to eventually supply adequate amounts of thyroid hormone.

The client is often given antithyroid agents for 6 to 8 weeks before hospitalization for a thyroidectomy in order to achieve a euthyroid state and minimize the risk of thyroid crisis. Iodine preparations may also be administered for 7 to 10 days before surgery to reduce the vascularity of the thyroid gland and the risk for hemorrhage in the intraoperative and postoperative period. During this presurgical period, it is also important that an optimal nutritional state and cardiovascular status be attained.

This care plan focuses on the adult client with hyperthyroidism whose condition is being stabilized before surgery and who will subsequently be hospitalized for a thyroidectomy.

OUTCOME/DISCHARGE CRITERIA

PREOPERATIVE
The client will:
1. Maintain adequate cardiovascular status
2. Maintain appropriate weight for height
3. Maintain appropriate activity level and sleep patterns

POSTOPERATIVE
The client will:
1. Have surgical pain controlled
2. Have evidence of normal healing of the surgical wound
3. Have no signs and symptoms of complications
4. Verbalize an understanding of range-of-motion exercises for the neck
5. State signs and symptoms to report to the health care provider
6. Verbalize an understanding of and a plan for adhering to recommended follow-up care including future appointments with health care provider, medications prescribed, dietary recommendations, activity level, and wound care.

Nursing Diagnosis   **RISK FOR DECREASED CARDIAC OUTPUT** NDx

Definition: Inadequate amount of blood pumped by the heart to meet metabolic demands of the body

Related to:
- Increased cardiac workload
- Changes in heart rate, rhythm, and conduction
- Fear, anxiety, and restlessness

CLINICAL MANIFESTATIONS

Subjective	Objective
Complaints of fear and anxiety; complaints of fatigue	Hypertension; tachycardia; dysrhythmias; restlessness; dyspnea; increased appetite

RISK FACTOR

- Hypermetabolic state

DESIRED OUTCOMES

The client will maintain adequate cardiac output as evidenced by:
  a. B/P within normal limits
  b. Apical pulse with regular rate and rhythm and 60 to 100 beats/min
  c. Normal heart sounds
  d. Absence of gallop rhythms
  e. Absence of fatigue and weakness
  f. Client's normal respiratory rate and rhythm, and clear breath sounds

NOC OUTCOMES

Tissue perfusion: cardiac; tissue perfusion: cellular; energy conservation; vital signs; respiratory status: gas exchange

NIC INTERVENTIONS

Cardiac care: acute; cardiac precautions; dysrhythmia management; hypovolemia management

NURSING ASSESSMENT	RATIONALE
Assess for and report signs and symptoms of decreased cardiac output: • Variations in B/P (may be increased because of compensatory vasoconstriction; may be decreased when compensatory mechanisms and pump fail) • Tachycardia • Presence of gallop rhythm • Fatigue and weakness • Restlessness, change in mental status	*Early recognition of signs and symptoms of decreased cardiac output allows for prompt intervention.*

THERAPEUTIC INTERVENTIONS	RATIONALE
Independent Actions Monitor electrocardiogram (ECG) readings and report significant abnormalities.	*ECG readings provide data regarding functioning of the heart's electrical conduction system. Tachycardia in a hypermetabolic state may reflect cardiac stimulation by thyroid hormones. Dysrhythmias may occur.*
Monitor heart sounds and changes, noting changes including gallops, extra heart sounds, and murmurs.	*Murmurs have been associated with changes in cardiac function associated with a hypermetabolic state.*
Monitor respiratory rate, rhythm, and breath sounds.	*Changes in rate and rhythm and increased adventitious sounds may be signs of pulmonary congestion related to heart failure.*
Monitor B/P while sitting, standing, and in supine position.	*Orthostatic hypotension may indicate vascular dilation.*
Weigh daily. **D** ✦ ●	*A hypermetabolic state may lead to excessive weight loss, even with an increased caloric intake.*
Encourage client to rest and limit unnecessary activities.	*Rest and limiting activities conserve client energy, potentially reducing fatigue.*
Dependent/Collaborative Actions Administer the following medications if ordered: **D** ✦ • Antithyroid medications to decrease levels of thyroid hormones; examples include the following: • Thyroid hormone antagonists	
	Thyroid hormone antagonists work through different mechanisms to prevent synthesis and/or block conversion of T_4 to T_3.
• Iodine solution	*Iodine inhibits synthesis of T_3 and T_4 and blocks their release into the circulatory system.*

NDx = NANDA-I Diagnosis   **D** = Delegatable Action   ● = UAP   ✦ = LVN/LPN   ⊖▶ = Go to ⊖volve for animation

Continued...

THERAPEUTIC INTERVENTIONS	RATIONALE
• Radioactive iodine	*Radioactive iodine damages or destroys thyroid gland tissue, thus limiting production and hormone secretion.*
• Beta-blockers	*Beta-blockers control tachycardia and decrease heart rate and cardiac workload.*
• Diuretics	*Diuretics decrease fluid volume overload and are used if client experiences heart failure.*
• Corticosteroids	*Corticosteroids reduce peripheral conversion of T_4 to T_3 and decrease hyperthermia.*

Nursing Diagnosis   RISK FOR IMBALANCED NUTRITION: LESS THAN BODY REQUIREMENTS NDx

Definition: Intake of nutrients insufficient to meet metabolic needs

Related to:
• Nausea, vomiting, diarrhea
• Increased volume of activity

CLINICAL MANIFESTATIONS

Subjective	Objective
Verbalization of increase appetite and thirst	Excessive weight loss; increased peristalsis, diarrhea, increased bowel sounds, hair loss

RISK FACTORS
• Inadequate intake
• Hypermetabolic state

DESIRED OUTCOMES

The client will maintain adequate nutritional status as evidenced by:
  a. Weight within normal range for client
  b. Normal blood urea nitrogen (BUN) and serum albumin levels
  c. Usual strength
  d. Healthy oral mucous membrane

NOC OUTCOMES

Appropriate appetite; positive body image; bowel elimination; compliance with prescribed diet; adequate hydration; weight maintenance behavior

NIC INTERVENTIONS

Nutritional monitoring; nutritional counseling; nutrition management; nutrition therapy; weight management

NURSING ASSESSMENT	RATIONALE
Assess for and report signs and symptoms of malnutrition: • Weight significantly below client's usual weight or below normal for client's age, height, and body frame • Abnormal BUN and low serum albumin levels • Weakness and fatigue • Sore, inflamed oral mucous membrane • Pale conjunctiva	*Early recognition of signs and symptoms of malnutrition allows for prompt intervention.*
Monitor percentage of meals and snacks client consumes. Report a pattern or inadequate intake.	*An awareness of the amount of foods/fluids the client consumes alerts the nurse to deficits in nutritional intake. Reporting an inadequate intake allows for prompt intervention.*
Perform or assist with anthropometric measurements such as skinfold thickness, body circumferences (e.g., hip, waist, mid-upper arm), and bioelectrical impedance analysis if indicated. Report results that are lower than normal.	*Anthropometric measurements provide information about the amount of muscle mass, body fat, and protein reserves the client has. These assessments assist in evaluating the client's nutritional status.*

THERAPEUTIC INTERVENTIONS	RATIONALE

Independent Actions

Provide client with high-caloric, high-protein diet including finger foods and high nutrient and caloric drinks. **D** ✦ ●

Hyperthyroidism causes a hypermetabolic state in which the client will need to consume a high-caloric diet.

Weigh daily **D** ✦ ●

Client should be weighed daily at the same time with the same amount of clothing to determine whether diet is effective in maintaining client's normal weight.

Implement measures to prevent vomiting if indicated (e.g., eliminate noxious sights and odors). **D** ✦ ●

Vomiting results in actual loss of nutrients.

Implement measures to control diarrhea if present (e.g., discourage intake of spicy foods and foods high in fiber or lactose).

Increased intestinal motility causes diarrhea, which results in a decreased absorption of nutrients in the bowel. Spicy foods and foods high in fiber increase gastric irritation and motility.

Implement measures to improve oral intake:

* Perform actions to reduce nausea, pain, fear, and anxiety if present.

Fear, anxiety, nausea, and pain will decrease client's appetite and caloric intake.

* Maintain a clean environment and a relaxed, pleasant atmosphere. **D** ✦ ●

Noxious sights and odors can inhibit the feeding center in the hypothalamus. Maintaining a clean environment helps prevent this from occurring. Maintaining a relaxed, pleasant atmosphere can help reduce the client's stress and promote a feeling of well-being, which tends to improve appetite and oral intake.

* Provide oral hygiene before meals. **D** ✦ ●

Oral hygiene moistens the oral mucous membrane, which may make it easier to chew and swallow. It also freshens the mouth and removes unpleasant tastes.

* Serve foods/fluids that are appealing to the client and adhere to personal and cultural (e.g., religious, ethnic) preferences whenever possible.

Foods/fluids that appeal to the client's senses (especially sight and smell) and are in accordance with personal and cultural preferences.

* Serve frequent, small meals rather than large ones if client is weak, fatigues easily, and/or has a poor appetite. **D** ✦ ●

Providing small rather than large meals can enable a client who is weak or fatigues easily to finish a meal. If smaller meals are served, the number of meals per day should be increased to help ensure adequate nutrition.

* Limit fluid intake with meals unless the fluid has a high nutritional value.

When the stomach becomes distended, its volume receptors stimulate the satiety center in the hypothalamus and the client reduces his/her oral intake. Drinking liquids with meals distends the stomach and may cause satiety before an adequate amount of food is consumed.

* Ensure that meals are well balanced and high in essential nutrients. Offer dietary supplements if indicated.

The client must consume a diet that is well balanced and high in essential nutrients in order for nutritional needs to be met. Dietary supplements are often needed to help accomplish this.

* Allow the client to assist in the selection of foods/fluids that meet nutritional needs.

The client who is actively involved in menu planning is more likely to adhere to the diet plan. In addition, the involvement increases the client's sense of control, which promotes a feeling of well-being and can lead to an increased oral intake.

Dependent/Collaborative Actions

Administer medications that may be ordered to improve client's nutritional status (e.g., antiemetics, antidiarrheals, gastrointestinal stimulants, and vitamins and minerals). **D** ✦

Medications may relieve vomiting, diarrhea, and distention of the gastrointestinal tract, which decreases the discomfort that occurs with each of these signs and symptoms. Vitamins and minerals are needed to maintain metabolic functioning. If the client's dietary intake does not provide adequate amounts of vitamins and minerals, oral and/or parenteral supplements may be necessary.

Obtain a dietary consult if necessary.

A dietitian is best able to evaluate whether the foods/fluids selected will meet the client's nutritional needs.

Perform a calorie count if ordered. Report information to the dietitian and physician.

A calorie count provides information about the caloric and nutritional value of the foods/fluids the client consumes. The information obtained helps the dietitian and physician determine whether an alternative method of nutritional support is needed.

Continued...

THERAPEUTIC INTERVENTIONS	RATIONALE
Consult the physician about an alternative method of providing nutrition (e.g., parenteral nutrition, tube feeding) if the client does not consume enough food or fluids to meet nutritional needs.	*If the client's oral intake is inadequate, an alternative method of providing nutrients needs to be implemented.*

Nursing Diagnosis   **ACTIVITY INTOLERANCE** NDx

Definition: Insufficient physiological or psychological energy to endure or complete required daily activities

Related to:
* Heat intolerance
* Inadequate caloric intake

CLINICAL MANIFESTATIONS

Subjective	Objective
Verbal report of fatigue or weakness	Abnormal heart rate or B/P response to activity; exertional discomfort or dyspnea; ECG changes reflecting dysrhythmias or ischemia

RISK FACTOR
* Hypermetabolic state and increased energy requirements

DESIRED OUTCOMES

The client will demonstrate an increased tolerance for activity as evidenced by:
  a. Verbalization of feeling less fatigued and weak
  b. Ability to perform activities of daily living without exertional dyspnea, chest pain, diaphoresis, dizziness, and significant changes in vital signs

NOC OUTCOMES

Activity tolerance; discomfort; endurance; fatigue level; nutritional energy status

NIC INTERVENTIONS

Activity therapy; energy management; nutrition management; sleep enhancement; cardiac care

NURSING ASSESSMENT	RATIONALE
Assess for signs and symptoms of activity intolerance: • Statements of fatigue or weakness • Exertional dyspnea, chest pain, diaphoresis, or dizziness • Abnormal heart rate response to activity (e.g., increase in rate of 20 beats/min above resting rate, rate not returning to preactivity level within 3 minutes after stopping activity, change from regular to irregular rate) • A significant change (15 to 20 mm Hg) in B/P with activity	*Early recognition of signs and symptoms of activity intolerance allows for prompt intervention.*

THERAPEUTIC INTERVENTIONS	RATIONALE
Independent Actions Implement measures to improve activity tolerance: **D** ✦ ● • Conserve energy. • Maintain prescribed activity restrictions. • Minimize environmental activity and noise. • Provide uninterrupted rest periods. • Instruct client in energy-saving techniques (e.g., using a shower chair when showering, sitting to brush teeth or comb hair).	*Cells use oxygen and fat, protein, and carbohydrate to produce the energy needed for all body activities. Rest and activities that conserve energy result in a lower metabolic rate, which preserves nutrients and oxygen for necessary activities.*

THERAPEUTIC INTERVENTIONS	RATIONALE
• Discourage smoking and intake of beverages high in caffeine such as coffee, tea, and colas.	*Both nicotine and excessive caffeine intake can increase cardiac workload and myocardial oxygen utilization, thereby decreasing the amount of oxygen necessary for energy production.*
Instruct client to report a decreased tolerance for activity and to stop any activity that causes chest pain, shortness of breath, dizziness, or extreme fatigue or weakness.	*These symptoms indicate that insufficient oxygen is reaching the tissues and that activity has been increased beyond a therapeutic level.*

Dependent/Collaborative Actions

Implement measures to improve activity tolerance:

• Implement measures to increase cardiac output (e.g., administer positive inotropic agents, vasodilators, or antiarrhythmics as ordered; elevate the head of the bed) if decreased cardiac output is contributing to the client's activity intolerance.	*Positive inotropic agents, vasodilators, or anti-dysrhythmic agents improve cardiac output.* *Sufficient cardiac output is necessary to maintain an adequate blood flow and oxygen supply to the tissues. Adequate tissue oxygenation promotes more efficient energy production, which subsequently improves client's activity tolerance.*
• Implement measures to reduce fever if present (e.g., administer tepid sponge bath, administer antipyretics as ordered). **D** ✦ ●	*An elevated temperature increases the metabolic rate, with subsequent depletion of available energy and a decrease in the ability to tolerate activity.*
• Implement measures to maintain an adequate nutritional status (e.g., provide a diet high in essential nutrients, provide dietary supplements as indicated, administer vitamins and minerals as ordered). **D** ✦	*Metabolism is the process by which nutrients are transformed into energy. If nutrition is inadequate, energy production is decreased, which subsequently reduces one's ability to tolerate activity.*
Implement measures to treat anemia if present (e.g., administer prescribed iron, folic acid, and/or vitamin B$_{12}$; administer packed red blood cells [RBCs] as ordered). **D** ✦	*Iron, folic acid, and vitamin B$_{12}$ are all necessary for RBC production. Packed RBCs provide immediate improvement in tissue oxygenation.*
Administer supplemental oxygen **D** ✦	*An oxygen deficiency results in anaerobic metabolism, which is less efficient than the aerobic mechanism of energy supply.* *Supplemental oxygen helps to alleviate hypoxia and restore the more efficient aerobic metabolism, thereby improving energy levels and activity tolerance.*

Nursing Diagnosis   ## DISTURBED SLEEP PATTERN NDx

Definition: Time-limited disruption of sleep (natural, periodic suspension of consciousness) amount and quality

Related to:
• Anxiety
• Excessive sympathetic nervous system stimulation

CLINICAL MANIFESTATIONS

Subjective	Objective
Verbal reports of difficulty falling asleep and staying asleep; awakening earlier than desired; not feeling well rested; anxiety; and agitation	Hyperactivity, restlessness, irritability

RISK FACTOR
• Hypermetabolic state

DESIRED OUTCOMES

The client will attain optimal amounts of sleep as evidenced by:
a. Statements of feeling well rested
b. Ability to perform normal daily activities

NOC OUTCOMES

Rest; sleep; personal well-being

NIC INTERVENTIONS

Sleep enhancement; energy management

NDx = NANDA-I Diagnosis   **D** = Delegatable Action   ● = UAP   ✦ = LVN/LPN   ⊖▶ = Go to ⊖volve for animation

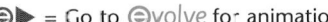

Continued...

NURSING ASSESSMENT	RATIONALE
Assess for signs and symptoms of a disturbed sleep pattern (e.g., statements of difficulty falling asleep, sleep interruptions, or not feeling well rested).	Early recognition of signs and symptoms of a disturbed sleep pattern allows for prompt intervention.
Determine client's usual sleep habits.	Knowledge of the client's usual sleep-wake cycle and routines that help induce and maintain sleep helps the nurse plan interventions aimed at preventing a sleep pattern disturbance.

THERAPEUTIC INTERVENTIONS	RATIONALE

Independent Actions

Discourage long periods of sleep during the day unless signs and symptoms of sleep deprivation exist or daytime sleep is usual for client. **D** ✦ ●	Long periods of sleep during the day are often a change in client's usual sleep-wake cycle and cause desynchronization of client's circadian rhythm. This can result in a poorer quality of sleep.
Implement measures to reduce fear and anxiety (e.g., maintain a calm, confident manner when working with client; assist client to identify specific stressors and ways to cope with them). **D** ✦	Fear and anxiety stimulate the sympathetic nervous system, which increases alertness and makes it difficult for the client to fall asleep. Sympathetic nervous system stimulation is also believed to shorten the duration of nonrapid eye movement (NREM) and REM sleep, which results in a poorer quality of sleep.
Encourage participation in relaxing diversional activities during the evening.	Involvement in relaxing activities in the evening helps the client fall asleep more easily.
Discourage intake of foods/fluids high in caffeine (e.g., chocolate, coffee, tea, colas) in the evening.	Caffeine acts as a central nervous system stimulant and can interfere with relaxation and subsequent sleep induction. Caffeine also acts as a diuretic, which can cause an interruption in sleep if the client awakens in response to the urge to urinate.
Offer client an evening snack that includes milk unless contraindicated. **D** ✦ ●	Milk contains the amino acid L-tryptophan, which is believed to help induce and maintain sleep.
Allow client to continue usual sleep practices (e.g., position; time; presleep routines such as reading, watching television, listening to music, and meditating) whenever possible.	Adherence to usual sleep practices promotes mental and physical relaxation that assists the client to maintain his/her usual sleep-wake cycle.
Reduce environmental distractions (e.g., close door to client's room; use night light rather than overhead light whenever possible; lower volume of paging system; keep staff conversations at a low level and away from client's room; close curtains between clients in a semiprivate room or ward; keep beepers and alarms on low volume; provide client with "white noise" such as a fan, soft music, or tape-recorded sounds of the ocean or rain; have sleep mask and earplugs available for client if needed).	Environmental activity, noise, and light can interfere with the client's ability to fall asleep and stay asleep. Reducing stimuli helps prevent a sleep pattern disturbance.
Encourage client to avoid drinking alcohol in the evening.	Although alcohol can induce drowsiness, which promotes sleep induction, it is known to interfere with REM sleep. Alcohol also inhibits the release of antidiuretic hormone (ADH), which can cause an interruption in sleep if the client awakens in response to the urge to urinate.
Encourage client to avoid smoking before bedtime.	Nicotine is a stimulant that can interfere with sleep by making it difficult for the client to relax and fall asleep and to stay asleep.
Implement measures to reduce interruptions during sleep (e.g., restrict visitors, group care whenever possible) so that client is able to sleep undisturbed for 70- to 100-minute intervals. **D** ✦	One sleep cycle takes about 70 to 100 minutes to complete. Each time the cycle is interrupted, it begins again with NREM stage 1 sleep so the client loses portions of NREM and/or REM sleep. When the client is deprived of NREM sleep, lethargy and depression occur. Loss of REM sleep results in irritability and anxiety. Reducing the frequency of sleep interruptions helps ensure that the client progresses through all of the sleep stages and does not experience a sleep pattern disturbance.

THERAPEUTIC INTERVENTIONS	RATIONALE

Dependent/Collaborative Actions

If possible, administer medications that can interfere with sleep (e.g., steroids, diuretics) early in the day rather than late afternoon or evening. **D** ✦

Administer prescribed sedative-hypnotics if indicated. **D** ✦

Consult appropriate health care provider if signs and symptoms of sleep deprivation (e.g., irritability, lethargy, agitation, inability to concentrate) occur and persist or worsen.

Administering these medications as early as possible during the day helps prevent nighttime insomnia and/or frequent awakenings.

Sedative-hypnotics are central nervous system depressants that promote sleep by reducing anxiety, shortening sleep induction, and/or reducing arousal level (wakefulness). These medications should be used for only a short time because they interfere with the length of REM sleep and can actually create a disturbance in client's sleep-wake cycle.

Notifying the appropriate health care provider allows for modification of treatment plan.

PREOPERATIVE—USE IN CONJUNCTION WITH PREOPERATIVE CARE PLAN

Nursing Diagnosis **DEFICIENT KNOWLEDGE** NDx

Definition: Absence or deficiency of cognitive information related to specific topic (lack of specific information necessary for clients/significant others) to make informed choices regarding condition/treatment/lifestyle changes

CLINICAL MANIFESTATIONS

Subjective	Objective
Expressions of anxiety/fear about potential surgery	Multiple questions related to proposed procedure

NOC OUTCOMES	NIC INTERVENTIONS
Knowledge: treatment regimen; knowledge: prescribed activity	Teaching individual; teaching: preoperative; teaching: prescribed activity/exercise

NURSING ASSESSMENT	RATIONALE
• Assess client's ability and readiness to learn • Assess client's fear and anxiety level	*Learning is most effective when client is calm and able to comprehend what is being taught.*

THERAPEUTIC INTERVENTIONS	RATIONALE

Desired Outcomes: The client will:

a. Verbalize an understanding of the surgical procedure, preoperative care, and postoperative sensations and care

b. Demonstrate the ability to perform activities designed to prevent postoperative complications

Independent Actions

Inform client that assessments for voice changes will be done routinely after surgery. Explain that hoarseness is expected for a few days and unnecessary talking should be avoided during that time.

Client will be hoarse after surgery because of irritation to the throat and vocal cords from intubation as well as edema from the surgical site.

Continued...

THERAPEUTIC INTERVENTIONS	RATIONALE
Provide instructions on ways to prevent complications after a thyroidectomy:	
• Instruct client on ways to minimize stress on the suture line:	
• Support head and neck with hands when turning head and coughing for first few days after surgery.	*Head and neck need to be supported to prevent opening of the suture line.*
• Avoid turning head abruptly and hyperextending the neck.	*Hyperextension of the next stretches the suture line increasing the risk of opening the suture line.*
Inform client of the need to do neck range-of-motion exercises beginning 2 to 4 days after surgery; demonstrate flexion, extension, rotation, and lateral movement of head and neck.	*These activities decrease neck stiffness and pain after surgery.*

POSTOPERATIVE—USE IN CONJUNCTION WITH THE STANDARDIZED POSTOPERATIVE CARE PLAN

Nursing Diagnosis RISK FOR INEFFECTIVE AIRWAY CLEARANCE NDx

Definition: Inability to clear secretions or obstructions from the respiratory tract to maintain a clear airway

Related to:
• Occlusion of the pharynx in the immediate postoperative period associated with relaxation of the tongue resulting from the effect of anesthesia and some medications (e.g., narcotic [opioid] analgesics)
• Stasis of secretions associated with:
  • Decreased activity
  • Poor cough effort resulting from the depressant effect of anesthesia and some medications (e.g., narcotic [opioid] analgesics), pain, weakness, and fear of disrupting incision
• Increased secretions associated with irritation of the respiratory tract (can result from inhalation anesthetics and endotracheal intubation)
• Tracheal compression associated with swelling and/or bleeding in the surgical area

CLINICAL MANIFESTATIONS

Subjective	Objective
Verbal report of dyspnea and difficulty coughing	Dyspnea, orthopnea; diminished breath sounds; adventitious breath sounds (crackles, rhonchi, wheezes); cough, ineffective or absent sputum production; difficulty vocalizing; wide-eyed; restlessness; changes in respiratory rate and rhythm; cyanosis

RISK FACTORS
• Surgical procedure
• Anesthetic agents

DESIRED OUTCOMES

The client will maintain clear, open airways as evidenced by:
  a. Normal breath sounds
  b. Normal rate and depth of respirations
  c. Absence of dyspnea

NOC OUTCOMES

Aspiration prevention; mechanical ventilation response: adult artificial airway; respiratory status: airway patency; respiratory status: ventilation

NIC INTERVENTIONS

Respiratory monitoring; airway management; airway suctioning; chest physiotherapy; cough enhancement

NURSING ASSESSMENT	RATIONALE
Assess for signs and symptoms of ineffective airway clearance: • Abnormal breath sounds • Rapid, shallow respirations • Dyspnea • Cough	*Early recognition of signs and symptoms of ineffective airway clearance allows for prompt intervention.*

THERAPEUTIC INTERVENTIONS	RATIONALE

Independent Actions

Implement measures to decrease pain if present:
- Splint chest or abdominal incisions with pillow when coughing and deep breathing. **D** ✦

Pain often interferes with client's willingness to move, cough, and deep breathe. Pain reduction enables client to increase activity and cough and deep breathe more effectively, all of which promote effective airway clearance.

Instruct and assist client to change position, deep breathe, and cough or "huff" every 1 to 2 hours.

Repositioning helps mobilize secretions.

Deep breathing helps clear the airways by loosening secretions and promoting a more effective cough. Coughing or "huffing" (a forced expiration technique) accelerates airflow through the airways, which helps mobilize and clear mucus and foreign matter from the respiratory tract.

Perform suctioning if needed. **D** ✦

Suctioning removes secretions from the large airways. It also stimulates coughing, which helps clear airways of mucus and foreign matter.

Implement additional measures to promote effective airway clearance:
- Keep head of bed elevated at least 30 degrees.
- Apply cooling pad or ice packs to neck if ordered.

These actions minimize swelling in surgical area and subsequently reduces pressure on the trachea

Dependent/Collaborative Actions

Implement measures to decrease pain:
- Administer prescribed analgesics before planned activity. **D** ✦

Pain often interferes with a client's willingness to move, cough, and deep breathe. Pain reduction enables the client to increase activity and cough and deep breathe more effectively, all of which promote effective airway clearance.

Increase activity as allowed and tolerated. **D** ✦ ●

Activity helps to mobilize secretions and promote deeper breathing. Deep breathing can help loosen secretions and enhance the effectiveness of coughing.

Implement measures to thin secretions and maintain adequate moisture of the respiratory mucous membranes:
- Maintain a fluid intake of 2500 mL/day.
- Humidify inspired air.

Adequate hydration and humidified inspired air help thin secretions, which facilitates the mobilization and expectoration of secretions.

- Assist with the administration of mucolytics (e.g., acetylcysteine) and diluting or hydrating agents (e.g., water, saline) via nebulizer as ordered.

Mucolytics, diluents, and/or hydrating agents are mucokinetic substances that reduce the viscosity of mucus, thus making it easier for the client to mobilize and clear secretions from the respiratory tract.

- Administer expectorants if ordered (e.g., guaifenesin, dornase alfa).

Expectorants reduce the viscosity of sputum, making it easier to be removed by coughing or suctioning.

Administer the following medications if ordered: **D** ✦
- Bronchodilators
  - Methylxanthines (e.g., theophylline, aminophylline, oxtriphylline)
  - Sympathomimetic (adrenergic) agents (e.g., albuterol, terbutaline, metaproterenol, salmeterol)
  - Anticholinergic agents (e.g., ipratropium)

These medications increase the patency of the airways and enhance bronchial airflow.

Methylxanthines and sympathomimetics produce bronchodilation by relaxing the bronchial smooth muscle.

Anticholinergic agents block cholinergic reflex constriction of the bronchioles and decrease mucus production.

- Corticosteroids
  - Prednisone
  - Methylprednisolone
  - Beclomethasone

Corticosteroids and leukotriene modifiers reduce inflammation in the airways, which results in decreased bronchial hyperactivity and constriction and mucus production.

NDx = NANDA-I Diagnosis   **D** = Delegatable Action   ● = UAP   ✦ = LVN/_PN   ⊜▶ = Go to ⊜volve for animation

Continued...

THERAPEUTIC INTERVENTIONS	RATIONALE

• Flunisolide
• Triamcinolone
• Budesonide
• Leukotriene modifiers
  • Montelukast
  • Zafirlukast	

Administer central nervous system depressants judiciously.	*Central nervous system depressants suppress the cough reflex, which can result in stasis of secretions.*
Assist with or perform postural drainage therapy if ordered.	*Postural drainage therapy techniques (e.g., vibration, percussion, postural drainage) use the forces of motion and gravity to mobilize secretions from the periphery of the lungs to the larger central airways, where they can be removed by coughing or suctioning.*
Consult the appropriate health care provider (e.g., physician, respiratory therapist) if signs and symptoms of ineffective airway clearance persist.	*Notifying the appropriate health care provider allows for modification of the treatment plan.*

Collaborative Diagnosis   RISK FOR HEMORRHAGE

Definition: Excessive bleeding

Related to: Surgery in a highly vascular area

CLINICAL MANIFESTATIONS

Subjective	Objective
Verbalization of fullness or pressure in the neck; difficulty swallowing or feeling of choking	Increasing tightness of neck dressing; excessive blood on the dressing or pillow; dyspnea; decreased B/P

RISK FACTORS
- Stress on suture lines
- Rupture of suture lines

DESIRED OUTCOMES

> The client will not have excessive bleeding in the surgical area as evidenced by:
> a. Absence of feeling of tightness of neck dressing and sensation of pressure of fullness in incision site
> b. Expected amount of drainage on dressing
> c. Increasing ease of swallowing
> d. Absence of choking sensation and respiratory distress
> e. Stable vital signs

NURSING ASSESSMENT	RATIONALE
Assess for and report signs and symptoms of hemorrhage (e.g., increased tightness of neck dressing; complaints of fullness or pressure in neck; excessive bloody drainage on dressing, pillow, or back of neck; statements of persistent or increased difficulty swallowing or a choking sensation; difficulty breathing; tachycardia; decrease in B/P).	*Early recognition of signs and symptoms of hemorrhage leads to prompt interventions.*

THERAPEUTIC INTERVENTIONS	RATIONALE
Independent Actions Implement measures to reduce the risk of hemorrhage: • Maintain pressure dressing over incision site as ordered.	*Pressure dressing supports the suture line and decreases edema in the surgical area, venous pressure, and swelling of the suture line.*

THERAPEUTIC INTERVENTIONS	RATIONALE
• Maintain head and neck in proper alignment using pillows or sandbags if necessary.	*These actions prevent excessive pulling on the suture line, which may lead to increased bleeding at the surgical site.*
• Support client's head and neck during position change until client is able to do so independently.	
• Reinforce preoperative instructions about supporting head and neck and remind client to avoid turning head abruptly and hyperextending the neck.	*Movements of the head and neck with vomiting may lead to suture line rupture and increased bleeding.*
• Perform actions to prevent nausea and vomiting (e.g., apply cool cloth to head, place basin under neck, change positions slowly).	*These actions decrease pressure in the surgical area.*
• Keep head of bed elevated at least 30 degrees.	
• Discourage vigorous coughing.	

Dependent/Collaborative Actions
If signs and symptoms of bleeding occur:
- Loosen dressing.
- Assist with suture/staple removal and drainage of hematoma if indicated.
- Assist with emergency tracheostomy if respiratory distress develops.
- Prepare client for surgical intervention (e.g., ligation of bleeding vessels) if planned.

These actions promote drainage of blood and reduce risk of respiratory distress.

A tracheostomy provides maintenance of a patent airway

Collaborative Diagnosis   # RISK FOR RESPIRATORY DISTRESS

Definition: Inability of the client to maintain a patent airway

Related to:
- Airway obstruction associated with:
- Tracheal compression resulting from swelling and/or bleeding in the surgical area
- Closure of the glottis resulting from paralysis of the vocal cords (can occur with injury to the bilateral recurrent laryngeal nerves) or laryngeal spasm that can occur with calcium deficiency

CLINICAL MANIFESTATIONS

Subjective	Objective
Verbalization of being unable to breathe and feelings of suffocation	Increased swelling of the neck; rapid and/or labored respirations; stridor; use of accessory muscles; significant decrease in oximetry results; abnormal arterial blood gas values

RISK FACTORS
- Surgical procedure
- Anesthetic agents

DESIRED OUTCOMES

The client will not experience respiratory distress as evidenced by:
  a. Unlabored respirations at 12 to 20 breaths/min
  b. Absence of stridor and sternocleidomastoid muscle retraction
  c. Usual mental status
  d. Usual skin color
  e. Oximetry results within normal range
  f. Arterial blood gas values within normal range

Continued...

NURSING ASSESSMENT	RATIONALE
Assess for and immediately report: • Increased swelling of the neck or bulging of the wound • Persistent or increased difficulty swallowing or choking sensation • Signs and symptoms of respiratory distress (e.g., rapid and/or labored respirations, stridor, sternocleidomastoid muscle retraction, restlessness, agitation, cyanosis) • Significant decrease in oximetry results • Abnormal arterial blood gas values	*Early recognition of signs and symptoms of respiratory distress allows for prompt intervention.*

THERAPEUTIC INTERVENTIONS	RATIONALE
Independent Actions Have oxygen and staple or suture removal, tracheostomy, and suction equipment readily available if the client experiences respiratory distress.	*Swelling of the surgical area may cause occlusion of the trachea.*
Perform actions to minimize swelling in the surgical area: • Keep head of bed elevated 30 degrees. • Apply cooling pad or ice packs to neck if ordered.	*These actions decrease swelling at the surgical site.*
Dependent/Collaborative Actions If signs and symptoms of respiratory distress occur: • Place client in high-Fowler's position unless hypotension is present. • Loosen dressing on the neck. • Maintain oxygen therapy as ordered. • Suction client if indicated. • Assist with emergency tracheostomy if performed.	*These actions improve the client's ability to maintain a patent airway and decrease symptoms of respiratory distress*

Collaborative Diagnosis RISK FOR HYPOCALCEMIA

Definition: Decreased serum calcium levels

Related to:
• Disruption of blood supply to parathyroid gland(s)
• Damage to or inadvertent removal of the parathyroid gland(s) during surgery

CLINICAL MANIFESTATIONS

Subjective	Objective
Verbalization of numbness or tingling of fingers, toes, or circumoral area	Positive Chvostek's and Trousseau's sign; muscle twitching; seizures

RISK FACTOR
• Surgical procedure

DESIRED OUTCOMES

The client will experience resolution of hypocalcemia if it occurs, as evidenced by:
  a. Absence of numbness and tingling in fingers, toes, and circumoral area
  b. Negative Chvostek's and Trousseau's signs
  c. Absence of muscle twitching and spasms and seizure activity
  d. Serum calcium level within normal range

NURSING ASSESSMENT	RATIONALE
Assess for signs and symptoms of hypocalcemia: • Numbness or tingling of fingers, toes, or circumoral area • Positive Chvostek's and Trousseau's signs • Muscle twitching or spasms • Seizures • Low calcium level	*Early recognition of signs and symptoms of hypocalcemia allows for prompt intervention.*

THERAPEUTIC INTERVENTIONS	RATIONALE
Dependent/Collaborative Actions If signs and symptoms of hypocalcemia occur: • Institute seizure precautions. • Administer calcium preparations (e.g., intravenous calcium gluconate, calcium carbonate) as ordered.	*These actions allow for prompt treatment and decrease the risk of laryngeal spasms and client injury.*

Collaborative Diagnosis RISK FOR THYROID STORM (THYROTOXIC CRISIS)

Definition: A life-threatening condition in which an excessive amount of thyroid hormone in the circulation causes an exacerbated physiological response

Related to: Excessive amounts of thyroid hormone in the blood associated with surgical manipulation of a hyperactive thyroid gland

CLINICAL MANIFESTATIONS

Subjective	Objective
Verbalization of fatigue, weakness, anxiety, heat intolerance	Hyperactivity; tachycardia; dysrhythmias; hypertension; warm, moist skin; agitation; change in level of consciousness; shaking; sweating, fever

RISK FACTOR
• Inadequate management of care preoperatively

DESIRED OUTCOMES
The client will not develop thyroid storm as evidenced by:
    a. Stable vital signs
    b. Usual mental status
    c. Absence of tremors, nausea, and vomiting

NURSING ASSESSMENT	RATIONALE
Assess for and report signs and symptoms of thyroid storm: • Temperature >38° C (100.4° F) • Marked increase in client's usual pulse rate • Increasing restlessness, agitation, irritability, tremors • Nausea, vomiting • Delirium, coma	*Early recognition of the signs and symptoms of thyroid storm allows for prompt intervention.*

THERAPEUTIC INTERVENTIONS	RATIONALE
Dependent/Collaborative Actions If signs and symptoms of thyroid storm occur: • Use hypothermia techniques (e.g., cooling blanket, tepid sponge bath). • Maintain intravenous fluid and electrolyte therapy as ordered. • Maintain oxygen therapy as ordered.	*Reduction of fever decrease hypermetabolic state.* *These actions help maintain vascular volume.* *Oxygen therapy improves oxygenation of tissues and decreases respiratory distress if present.*

Continued...

THERAPEUTIC INTERVENTIONS	RATIONALE
• Institute appropriate safety measures if client is irrational, delirious, or comatose.	*Implementation of safety measures decreases potential for client injury.*
• Administer the following medications if ordered:	
• Antipyretics (avoid aspirin)	*Antipyretics reduce fever. Avoid aspirin because it increases free thyroid hormone levels.*
• Antithyroid agents (e.g., propylthiouracil, methimazole) and iodine preparations (e.g., sodium iodide)	*These agents suppress production and release of thyroid hormone from the remaining thyroid tissue; propylthiouracil also blocks the peripheral conversion of T4 to T3.*
• Glucocorticoids (e.g., dexamethasone)	*Steroids aid the body in handling stress, replenish endogenous glucocorticoids that have probably been depleted by the increased metabolism, and block the peripheral conversion of T_4 to T_3.*
• Adrenergic inhibiting agents (e.g., propranolol)	*These agents reduce severity of many of the cardiac manifestations.*
• Anti–atrial fibrillation agents	*Atrial fibrillation may occur in thyroid storm as a result of excessive stimulation of the heart.*

Collaborative Diagnosis RISK FOR LARYNGEAL NERVE DAMAGE

Definition: Damage to the nerves of the larynx

Related to: Trauma to the nerve(s) during surgery and/or pressure on the nerve(s) associated with swelling and/or bleeding in the surgical area

CLINICAL MANIFESTATIONS

Subjective	Objective
Verbalization of difficulty or choking with swallowing, and difficulty with speaking	Hoarseness; weak, whispery voice; inability to speak; dyspnea

RISK FACTOR
• Surgical procedure

DESIRED OUTCOMES

The client will experience resolution of laryngeal nerve damage if it occurs as evidenced by:
  a. Improved tone and quality of voice
  b. Gradual resolution of hoarseness
  c. Absence of dysphagia
  d. Absence of respiratory distress

NURSING ASSESSMENT	RATIONALE
Assess for indications of laryngeal nerve damage: • Voice changes (e.g., hoarseness; weak, whispery voice; inability to speak) • Statements of difficulty swallowing and/or coughing or choking when eating • Respiratory distress	*Early recognition of signs and symptoms of laryngeal nerve damage allows for prompt intervention.*

THERAPEUTIC INTERVENTIONS	RATIONALE
Independent Actions If signs and symptoms of laryngeal nerve damage occur: • Implement swallowing precautions (e.g., place client in a high Fowler's position when drinking and eating, introduce fluids and foods cautiously, instruct client to avoid putting too much fluid/food in mouth at one time, provide thick rather than thin fluids).	*These actions decrease stress and pressure on the throat and the laryngeal nerve.*

THERAPEUTIC INTERVENTIONS	RATIONALE
• Encourage client to avoid unnecessary talking.	*These actions provide rest of the vocal cords.*
• Implement measures to facilitate communication (e.g., ask questions that require a short answer or nod of head, provide materials such as Magic Slate or pad and pencil, answer call signal in person rather than using intercommunication system).	
• Notify physician immediately if signs and symptoms of respiratory distress occur; client is unable to speak; or hoarseness, voice changes, or swallowing difficulties worsen.	*Notification of the physician allows for modification of the treatment plan.*

DISCHARGE TEACHING/CONTINUED CARE

Nursing Diagnosis ## DEFICIENT KNOWLEDGE NDx; INEFFECTIVE SELF-HEALTH MANAGEMENT NDx; OR INEFFECTIVE HEALTH MAINTENANCE* NDx

Definition: Absence or deficiency of cognitive information related to specific topic (lack of specific information necessary for clients/significant others) to make informed choices regarding condition/treatment/lifestyle changes; inability to identify, manage, and/or seek out help to maintain health; pattern of regulating and integrating into daily living a therapeutic regimen for treatment of illness and the sequelae of illness that is unsatisfactory for meeting specific health goals

CLINICAL MANIFESTATION

Subjective	Objective
Requests for information; client statements reflect misunderstanding	Inadequate follow-through of instruction; inappropriate or exaggerated behaviors

RISK FACTORS
• Cognitive limitations or unfamiliarity of situation

NOC OUTCOMES	NIC INTERVENTIONS
Knowledge: treatment regimen; knowledge: health behavior; knowledge: health resources	Health system guidance; teaching: individual; teaching: prescribed activity/exercise; teaching: prescribed medications

NURSING ASSESSMENT	RATIONALE
Assess client's willingness to learn and knowledge related to the disease process.	*Client's willingness to learn and knowledge base provides the basis for education.*
Assess for indications that client may be unable to effectively manage the therapeutic regimen.	*Early recognition of inability to understand disease process or self-care allows for change in the teaching plan.*

THERAPEUTIC INTERVENTIONS	RATIONALE
Desired Outcome: The client will verbalize understanding of range-of-motion exercises of the neck.	
Independent Actions	
Reinforce preoperative teaching about range-of-motion exercises of the neck. Instruct client to do exercises as prescribed by physician (exercises are usually begun 2 to 4 days after surgery and are done three to four times per day for a few weeks).	*Range-of-motion exercises will strengthen the neck, improve circulation to the area, and improve healing.*

*The nurse should select the diagnostic label that is most appropriate for the client's discharge teaching.

NDx = NANDA-I Diagnosis   **D** = Delegatable Action   ● = UAP   ✦ = LVN/LPN   ⊖▶ = Go to ⊖volve for animation

Continued...

THERAPEUTIC INTERVENTIONS	RATIONALE
Allow time for client demonstration and for questions and clarification of information provided.	*Client should provide a return demonstration of the range-of-motion activities so nurse knows client is able to perform them correctly.*

THERAPEUTIC INTERVENTIONS	RATIONALE

Desired Outcome: The client will state signs and symptoms to report to the health care provider

Independent Actions:

Instruct client to report the following signs and symptoms:

• Persistent low-grade fever (temperature >100° F); feeling unusually anxious or agitated; warm, flushed skin; or nausea and vomiting	*These may indicate thyroid crisis and should be treated immediately.*
• Difficulty breathing	*Difficulty breathing and chest pain should be reported immediately because they require prompt treatment.*
• Chest pain	
• Cough productive of purulent, green, or rust-colored sputum	*A productive cough of abnormally colored sputum indicates a respiratory infection.*
• Increasing weakness or inability to tolerate prescribed activity level	*Weakness and difficulty with activities may indicate decreased calcium levels.*
• Increasing discomfort or discomfort not controlled by prescribed medications and treatments	*Increasing discomfort may indicate that pain is not being adequately treated.*
• Increasing abdominal distention and/or discomfort	*Abdominal distention or pain may indicate paralytic ileus.*
• Increased feeling of fullness or tightness in neck or separation of wound edges	*May indicate edema, infection, or excessive exercise and should be treated immediately to decrease potential respiratory problems and wound scarring.*
• Unexplained weight gain, persistent fatigue, drowsiness, constipation, cold intolerance	*These indicate inadequate thyroid hormone replacement or progressive thyroid failure in clients who had a partial thyroidectomy.*
• Numbness or tingling of toes or fingers or around mouth, muscle twitching, or spasms	*These symptoms are indicative of hypocalcemia.*
• Increasing redness, warmth, pain, or swelling around wound	
• Unusual or excessive drainage from the surgical wound	*These clinical manifestations may indicate an infection of the surgical area.*
• Pain or swelling in calf of one or both legs	*Pain or swelling in the calf indicates a possible deep vein thrombosis and requires prompt treatment.*
• Urine retention; frequency, urgency, or burning on urination; cloudy or foul-smelling urine	*These symptoms are indications of possible urinary tract infection.*

THERAPEUTIC INTERVENTIONS	RATIONALE

Desired Outcome: The client will verbalize an understanding of and a plan for adhering to recommended follow-up care including future appointments with health care provider, medications prescribed, dietary recommendations, activity level, and wound care

Independent Actions:

• Teach client the rationale for, side effects of, schedule for taking, and importance of taking medications prescribed (e.g., thyroid hormone, calcium supplements, vitamin D). Inform client of pertinent food and drug interactions.	*Knowledge of the medication regimen and the impact of these medications on the system, as well as how the medication regimen can be incorporated into the client's lifestyle, allows the client some mechanism of control of his/her disease and the ability to have an active part in treatment and care.*

If client had a subtotal thyroidectomy:

• Explain that thyroid hormone replacement will probably not be given unless symptoms of hypothyroidism develop.	*In a patient who has had a subtotal thyroidectomy, the gland will continue to produce thyroid hormones. If synthetic hormones are given, it may delay the regeneration of the remaining thyroid gland.*
• Instruct client to maintain an adequate iodine intake (e.g., use iodized salt, eat seafood one to two times a week).	*Adequate iodine intake promotes thyroid hormone production by the remaining thyroid tissue.*
• Instruct client to avoid excessive intake of foods that contain thyroid-inhibiting substances (goitrogens) such as turnips, rutabagas, peanuts, and soybeans.	*This will delay the regeneration of the remaining thyroid tissues.*

THERAPEUTIC INTERVENTIONS	RATIONALE
• Encourage client to maintain a low-calorie diet.	*A low-calorie diet helps to prevent weight gain while the remaining thyroid tissue is regenerating.*
• Encourage client to participate in a regular exercise program.	*Exercise helps to maintain an optimal weight and stimulate regeneration of remaining thyroid tissue.*
• Allow time for questions and clarification of information provided.	*These actions help to improve understanding of required care and client adherence to therapeutic regimen.*
• Demonstrate wound care to client and allow for client demonstration of care.	*Client should provide a return demonstration of wound care so the nurse knows that they are able to perform this correctly.*

HYPOTHYROIDISM/MYXEDEMA

Hypothyroidism is a condition in which the thyroid gland has sustained underproduction and/or undersecretion of thyroid hormones. The decreased levels of thyroid hormones, thyroxine (T_4) and triiodothyronine (T_3), slow down all body functions causing a hypometabolic state. This decrease in metabolism affects most tissues and organs. In the individual, cellular energy is decreased and metabolites build up in the system. The edema found in individuals with hypothyroidism is due to the metabolic compounds that build up in the cell. These compounds cause systemic nonpitting edema, which is noted particularly around the eyes and in the hands and feet. Other areas that may be impacted are the tongue and larynx, which leads to voice changes. Overall physiological functioning is decreased, and this may be demonstrated by increased hours of sleep, fatigue, lethargy, cold intolerance, anorexia, irregular or heavy menses, constipation, depression, impaired memory, slowed speech, and paresthesias.

Myxedema coma is a rare but serious complication of hypothyroidism. It usually occurs because of untreated or poorly treated hypothyroidism but may also occur with infections, trauma, and surgery. Myxedema coma should be treated as a medical emergency in which the individual may experience increased mental sluggishness, drowsiness, and lethargy possibly leading to loss of consciousness and coma. Hypotension, hypovolemia, and subnormal temperature are indicators that the individual is experiencing myxedema coma. Treatment of this condition requires support of the individual's vital signs and thyroid hormone replacement.

Diagnosis of hypothyroidism includes a combination of laboratory findings and a review of clinical manifestations. Serum thyroid-stimulating hormone and free T_4 levels are correlated with the signs and symptoms found in a health history and the findings on physical examination.

This care plan focuses on the adult client with hypothyroidism whose condition is being stabilized. Much of the information in this care plan is applicable to clients receiving long-term therapy in an extended care facility or home setting.

OUTCOME/DISCHARGE CRITERIA

The client will:
1. Maintain a euthyroid state
2. Maintain a positive self-image
3. Maintain normal client weight
4. Verbalize an understanding of the disease process
5. State signs and symptoms to report to the health care provider
6. Verbalize an understanding of and a plan for adhering to recommended follow-up care including future appointments with health care provider and medication regimen.

Nursing Diagnosis	**IMBALANCED NUTRITION: MORE THAN BODY REQUIREMENTS** NDx

Definition: Intake of nutrients that exceeds metabolic needs

Related to: Decreased metabolism rate, lethargy, and activity intolerance

CLINICAL MANIFESTATIONS

Subjective	Objective
Complaint of fatigue	Weight gain; decreased activity level

Continued...

RISK FACTORS

* Lack of exercise
* Lack of thyroid hormone production
* Inadequate treatment regimen

DESIRED OUTCOMES

> The client will maintain adequate nutritional status as evidenced by:
> a. Weight within normal range for client
> b. Usual activity tolerance

NOC OUTCOMES

Nutritional status: food and fluid intake; nutritional status: nutrient intake; weight control

NIC INTERVENTIONS

Nutrition management; teaching: prescribed diet; weight management

NURSING ASSESSMENT

Assess for and report signs and symptoms of weight gain:
* Weight significantly above client's usual weight or above normal for client's age, height, and body frame

Measure body mass index (BMI).

Perform or assist with anthropometric measurements such as skinfold thickness, body circumferences (e.g., hip, waist, mid-upper arm), and bioelectrical impedance analysis if indicated. Report results that are lower than normal.

RATIONALE

Early recognition of signs and symptoms of weight gain allows for prompt intervention.

BMI >25 is associated with increased morbidity and mortality.

Anthropometric measurements provide information about the amount of muscle mass, body fat, and protein reserves the client has. These assessments assist in evaluating the client's nutritional status.

THERAPEUTIC INTERVENTIONS

Independent Actions

Monitor dietary intake noting what type and volume, and caloric content of food eaten. **D ● ✦**

Provide client with a diet high in protein and low in calories.

Limit client's intake of empty calories found in nondiet sodas, candy, etc.

Limit client's intake of sodium either through fluids or foods.

Encourage client to eat foods high in fiber.

Encourage client to increase activities and regular exercise.

Include family and significant others in education about dietary requirements.

Dependent/Collaborative Actions

Administer vitamin supplements as ordered. **D ✦**

RATIONALE

A client in a hypometabolic state should monitor intake to prevent excessive weight gain.

A high-protein diet helps client to maintain current weight while maintaining nutritional status.

In a hypometabolic state, empty calories may cause significant weight gain.

Sodium causes edema through fluid retention.

Fiber promotes gastric motility, which aids in elimination, which may be decreased due to the client's hypometabolic state.

Exercise helps client to maintain appropriate weight during the hypometabolic state.

Client's ability to eat an appropriate diet during the metabolic state increases with assistance from family/significant others.

Supplements ensure that client maintains appropriate intake of vitamins.

Nursing Diagnosis   **ACTIVITY INTOLERANCE** NDx

Definition: Insufficient physiological or psychological energy to endure or complete required or desired daily activities

Related to:
* Weakness and fatigue related to hypometabolic state
* Depression or lack of motivation
* Shortness of breath on exertion related to hypermetabolic state

CLINICAL MANIFESTATIONS

Subjective	Objective
Verbal report of fatigue or weakness; depression	Abnormal heart rate or B/P in response to activity; exertional discomfort or dyspnea; electrocardiographic (ECG) changes reflecting dysrhythmias or ischemia; unable to speak with physical activity

RISK FACTORS

- Decreased production of thyroid hormone
- Inadequate hormone replacement

DESIRED OUTCOMES

The client will demonstrate an increased tolerance for activity as evidenced by:
- a. Verbalization of feeling less fatigued and weak
- b. Ability to perform activities of daily living without exertional dyspnea, chest pain, diaphoresis, dizziness, and significant changes in vital signs

NOC OUTCOMES

Endurance: activity tolerance; fatigue level; self-care status; energy conservation; vital signs

NIC INTERVENTIONS

Activity therapy; energy management; oxygen therapy; nutrition management; sleep enhancement; cardiac care; cardiac rehabilitation; teaching regarding prescribed activity

NURSING ASSESSMENT	RATIONALE

Assess for signs and symptoms of activity intolerance:
- Statements of fatigue or weakness
- Exertional dyspnea, chest pain, diaphoresis, or dizziness
- Abnormal heart rate response to activity (e.g., increase in rate of 20 beats/min above resting rate, rate not returning to preactivity level within 3 minutes after stopping activity, change from regular to irregular rate)
- A significant change (15-20 mm Hg) in B/P with activity

Early recognition of signs and symptoms of activity intolerance allow for prompt intervention.

THERAPEUTIC INTERVENTIONS	RATIONALE

Independent Actions
Implement measures to improve activity tolerance:
- Conserve energy.
- Maintain prescribed activity restrictions.
- Minimize environmental activity and noise. **D** ✦ ●
- Provide uninterrupted rest periods. **D** ✦ ●
- Assist with care. **D** ✦ ●
- Keep supplies and personal articles within easy reach. **D** ✦ ●
- Limit the number of visitors.
- Instruct client in energy-saving techniques (e.g., using a shower chair when showering, sitting to brush teeth or comb hair).
- Implement measures to promote sleep (e.g., quiet, dark environment; discourage napping). **D** ● ✦
- Discourage smoking and excessive intake of beverages high in caffeine such as coffee, tea, and colas.

- Implement measures to improve respiratory status (e.g., encourage use of incentive spirometer; elevate head of bed; assist with turning, coughing, and deep breathing) if ineffective breathing pattern, ineffective airway clearance, or impaired gas exchange is contributing to client's activity intolerance.

Cells use oxygen and fat, protein, and carbohydrate to produce the energy needed for all body activities. Rest and activities that conserve energy result in a lower metabolic rate, which preserves nutrients and oxygen for necessary activities.

Both nicotine and excessive caffeine intake can increase cardiac workload and myocardial oxygen utilization, thereby decreasing the amount of oxygen necessary for energy production.
Altered respiratory function can lead to inadequate tissue oxygenation, which results in less efficient energy production and a reduced ability to tolerate activity. Improving respiratory status increases the amount of oxygen available for energy production. It also eases the work of breathing, which reduces energy expenditure.

Continued...

THERAPEUTIC INTERVENTIONS	RATIONALE
Instruct client to report a decreased tolerance for activity and to stop any activity that causes chest pain, shortness of breath, dizziness, or extreme fatigue or weakness.	*These symptoms indicate that insufficient oxygen is reaching the tissues and that activity has been increased beyond a therapeutic level.*
Dependent/Collaborative Actions Implement measures to improve activity tolerance:	
• Implement measures to increase cardiac output (e.g., administer positive inotropic agents, vasodilators, or antiarrhythmics as ordered; elevate the head of the bed) if decreased cardiac output is contributing to the client's activity intolerance.	*Sufficient cardiac output is necessary to maintain an adequate blood flow and oxygen supply to the tissues. Adequate tissue oxygenation promotes more efficient energy production, which subsequently improves client's activity tolerance.*

Nursing Diagnosis   **CONSTIPATION** NDx

Definition: A decrease in normal frequency of defecation accompanied by difficult or incomplete passage of stool and/or passage of excessively hard, dry stool

Related to:
• Decreased activity level
• Decreased fiber/fluid intake

CLINICAL MANIFESTATIONS

Subjective	**Objective**
Complaints of abdominal discomfort; complaints of straining with defecation; anorexia	Infrequent defecation; dry, hard formed stools; hypoactive bowel sounds; nausea and/or vomiting

RISK FACTORS
• Decreased hormone production
• Inadequate hormone replacement
• Hypometabolic state, which decreases gastrointestinal activity

DESIRED OUTCOMES

The client will maintain usual elimination pattern as evidenced by:
  a. Usual frequency of bowel movement
  b. Passage of soft, formed stool

NOC OUTCOMES

Bowel elimination; hydration

NIC INTERVENTIONS

Constipation/impaction management; bowel management; fluid management; nutrition management; medication administration

NURSING ASSESSMENT	RATIONALE
Assess client's usual bowel elimination habits.	*Knowledge of the client's usual bowel elimination habits is essential in determining whether constipation is present because frequency of defecation varies among individuals.*
Assess for signs and symptoms of constipation: • Decrease in frequency of bowel movements • Passage of hard formed stool • Feeling of fullness or pressure in rectum • Straining during defecation	*Early recognition of signs and symptoms of constipation allows for prompt intervention.*
Assess bowel sounds. Report a pattern of decreasing bowel sounds.	*Decreased bowel sounds indicate a decrease in peristalsis/motility, which can lead to and be present with constipation.*

THERAPEUTIC INTERVENTIONS	RATIONALE
Independent Actions Instruct client to increase intake of foods high in fiber (e.g., bran, whole-grain breads and cereals, fresh fruits and vegetables) unless contraindicated.	*Foods high in fiber provide bulk to the fecal mass and increases its ability to absorb water. Increased bulkiness of the stool stimulates peristalsis, which promotes more rapid movement of the stool through the colon.*

THERAPEUTIC INTERVENTIONS	RATIONALE
Instruct the client to maintain a minimal fluid intake of 2500 mL/day unless contraindicated.	*Inadequate fluid intake reduces the water content of feces, which results in a hard, dry stool that is difficult to evacuate.*
Encourage client to drink hot liquids (e.g., coffee or tea) upon arising in the morning. **D** ● ✦	*Ingestion of hot fluids can stimulate peristalsis.*
Increase activity as tolerated. **D** ● ✦	*Ambulation stimulates peristalsis, which promotes the passage of stool through the intestines.*

Dependent/Collaborative Actions

Administer laxatives or cathartics (e.g., stool softeners, bulk-forming agents, irritants/stimulants, lubricant agents) as ordered.	*Laxatives/cathartics act in a variety of ways to soften the stool, increase stool bulk, stimulate bowel motility, and/or lubricate the rectum and anal canal.*
Administer cleansing and/or oil retention enemas if ordered.	*A cleansing enema stimulates peristalsis and evacuation of the stool. An oil retention enema facilitates stool passage by softening the fecal mass and lubricating the rectum and anal canal.*

Collaborative Diagnosis | RISK FOR MYXEDEMA COMA

Definition: A life-threatening condition in which the body's thyroid hormone level becomes excessively low and the symptoms of hypothyroidism are exacerbated

Related to:
- Inadequate response to treatment
- Infection
- Discontinuing medication regimen

CLINICAL MANIFESTATIONS

Subjective	Objective
Complaints of feeling cold	Hypotension; bradycardia; decreased cardiac output; hypoventilation; hypoxia; hypothermia; hypoglycemia; altered mental status; decreasing level of consciousness; coma

RISK FACTORS

- Response to prolonged radiation therapy for hyperthyroidism
- Surgery
- Lack of pituitary release of thyroid stimulating hormone (TSH)
- Medications (e.g., opioids, tranquilizers, barbiturates)
- Exposure to cold
- Trauma

DESIRED OUTCOMES

The client will not experience myxedema coma as evidenced by:
a. Usual mental status
b. Usual vital signs
c. Usual temperature

NOC OUTCOMES

Safety status: physical injury

NIC INTERVENTIONS

Risk identification: emergency care

NURSING ASSESSMENT	RATIONALE
Assess for signs and symptoms of myxedema coma: - Hypotension - Bradycardia - Decreased cardiac output - Hypoventilation - Hypoxia	*Early recognition of signs and symptoms of myxedema coma allows for prompt interventions.*

NDx = NANDA-I Diagnosis   **D** = Delegatable Action   ● = UAP   ✦ = LVN/LPN   ⊖▶ = Go to ⊖volve for animation

Continued...

NURSING ASSESSMENT	RATIONALE

- Hypothermia
- Hypoglycemia
- Deterioration in mental status
- Decreasing level of consciousness
- Coma

THERAPEUTIC INTERVENTIONS	RATIONALE

Independent Actions

Monitor for changes in vital signs and mental status in clients who have hypothyroidism and are undergoing surgery or experiencing an infection.	*These events may precipitate myxedema coma in individuals with hypothyroidism.*
Monitor client for deterioration in mental status.	*Deterioration of mental status is a cardinal sign of myxedema coma.*
Monitor blood glucose and serum sodium levels.	*During myxedema coma, sodium may decrease to <137 mEq/L, and glucose may decrease to <80 mg/dL.*

Dependent/Collaborative Actions

Monitor levels of thyroid hormones during treatment and hospitalization.	*Monitoring ensures maintenance of adequate thyroid hormone levels.*
If myxedema coma occurs:	
• Administer intravenous (IV) thyroid hormone replacement.	*IV administration of thyroid hormones rapidly increases level of circulating thyroid hormone*
• Administer IV fluids, possibly hypertonic saline as ordered.	*IV administration of hypertonic saline corrects hypovolemia and hyponatremic state.*
• Administer IV glucose and hydrocortisone.	*Administration of glucose corrects glucose level. Hydrocortisone decreases incidence of hyperadrenalism, which can occur with IV administration of thyroid hormones.*
• Administer cardiac medications as ordered.	*Cardiac medications are given to maintain adequate B/P and heart rate.*
• Apply a warming blanket if required.	*A warming blanket increases body core temperature.*
• Provide mechanical ventilation if indicated.	*Mechanical ventilation provides for adequate respiratory status when the client has lost the ventilatory drive.*

DISCHARGE TEACHING/CONTINUED CARE

Nursing Diagnosis ## DEFICIENT KNOWLEDGE NDx; INEFFECTIVE HEALTH MAINTENANCE NDx; OR INEFFECTIVE SELF-HEALTH MANAGEMENT* NDx

Definition: Absence or deficiency of cognitive information related to specific topic (lack of specific information necessary for clients/significant others) to make informed choices regarding condition/treatment/lifestyle changes; inability to identify, manage, and/or seek out help to maintain health; pattern of regulating and integrating into daily living a therapeutic regimen for treatment of illness and the sequelae of illness that is unsatisfactory for meeting specific health goals

CLINICAL MANIFESTATIONS

Subjective	Objective
Verbalizes inability to manage illness; verbalizes inability to follow prescribed regimen	Inaccurate follow-through with instructions; inappropriate behaviors; experience of preventable complications of spinal cord injury

*The nurse should select the diagnostic label that is most appropriate for the client's discharge teaching needs.

RISK FACTORS

- Cognitive deficit
- Financial concerns
- Inability to care for oneself or maintain medication regimen

NOC OUTCOMES	NIC INTERVENTIONS
Knowledge: treatment regimen	Health system guidance: teaching individual

NURSING ASSESSMENT	RATIONALE
Assess client's ability to learn and readiness to learn Assess client's understanding of teaching	*Learning is more effective when the client is motivated and understands the importance of what is to be learned. Readiness to learn changes based on situations, physical and emotional challenges.*

THERAPEUTIC INTERVENTIONS	RATIONALE

Desired Outcome: The client will verbalize an understanding of medication regimen including rationale, food and drug interactions, side effects, schedule for taking, and importance of taking as prescribed

Independent Actions

Teach client rationale for, side effects of, schedule for, and importance of taking medications as prescribed. Inform client of pertinent food and drug interactions.	*Knowledge of medication(s) and how they impact the system improves client adherence. Help enhance client's understanding of the importance of adhering to the prescribed medication regimen. Client must be able to recognize alterations in functioning related to medication administration.*
Instruct client on importance of not discontinuing the medication without permission of a health care provider.	*Client must understand the importance of continued medication administration to prevent incidence of myxedema coma.*
Instruct client at the beginning of treatment to expect frequent blood draws while medication levels are being titrated to provide adequate blood levels of thyroid hormones.	*Treatment is individualized and is based on client's serum thyroid hormone levels and clinical manifestations.*

THERAPEUTIC INTERVENTIONS	RATIONALE

Desired Outcome: The client will state signs and symptoms to report to the health care provider

Independent Actions

Instruct client to report the following signs and symptoms to the health care provider:

- Depression - Difficulty breathing	*Depression and difficulty breathing may indicate myxedema coma and should be treated immediately.*
- Cough productive of purulent, green, or rust-colored sputum	*This symptom indicates an infection, which may precipitate myxedema coma.*
- Increasing weakness or inability to tolerate prescribed activity level - Continued weight gain - Increasing abdominal distention and/or discomfort - Unexplained weight gain, persistent fatigue, drowsiness, constipation, cold intolerance	*These clinical manifestations may indicate appropriate thyroid hormone levels have not been reached by medication regimen.*
- Nervousness, restlessness, significant weight loss, tachycardia, diarrhea, anxiety, or insomnia	*These signs and symptoms may indicate hyperthyroidism and overmedication with thyroid hormones*

THERAPEUTIC INTERVENTIONS	RATIONALE

Desired Outcome: The client will verbalize an understanding of and a plan for adhering to recommended follow-up care including future appointments with health care provider and treatment regimen

Continued...

THERAPEUTIC INTERVENTIONS	RATIONALE

Independent Actions

Encourage client to maintain a low-calorie, high-protein, high-fiber diet until thyroid hormone levels have stabilized.

Treatment is individualized and may take some time to regulate adequate levels of thyroid hormones in the system. This type of diet helps to prevent excessive weight gain.

Encourage client to participate in a regular exercise program to maintain an optimal weight.

An exercise plan helps client lose any weight gained before hormone replacement.

Stress the importance of follow-up visits with a health care provider.

Hypothyroidism is a chronic illness and requires mentoring by a health care provider for the client to maintain optimum wellness.

See Bibliography at the back of the book.

The Client with Alterations in the Gastrointestinal Tract

ABDOMINAL TRAUMA

Abdominal trauma involves injury to the body structures located between the diaphragm and the pelvis. Injury to abdominal contents occurs from a direct impact or movement of organs within the body as a result of rapid deceleration, causing rupture, lacerations, and/or tears in organs or blood vessels. Organs injured with abdominal trauma include the spleen, liver, stomach, large and small intestines, pancreas, kidneys, and urinary bladder. The large vessels in the abdomen, the aorta and vena cava, may also be injured.

Abdominal trauma occurs as the result of blunt or penetrating trauma. Blunt trauma is the result of motor vehicle accidents, assaults, sports injuries, or falls. In blunt trauma injury, the liver and spleen are the most commonly affected organs. Liver and splenic injuries can lead to profuse bleeding because these organs are highly vascular. The client with injuries to these organs may have upper right quadrant pain, abdominal rigidity and guarding with rebound tenderness, loss of bowel sounds, signs of hemorrhagic shock, and Kehr's sign, which is seen with splenic rupture. Injury to the intestines leads to leakage of intestinal contents, leading to abdominal distention, pain, peritonitis, and sepsis, and may lead to multiple organ dysfunction syndrome. Other injuries that may be seen in individuals with abdominal trauma include pancreatic trauma, diaphragmatic rupture, urinary bladder rupture, tears in the great vessels, renal injury, and stomach and intestinal rupture.

Penetrating abdominal trauma can be caused by stabbing, gunshot, or impalement. In an individual with a penetrating injury it is important to determine the entry and exit point or the trajectory of a stab wound. The external injury may mask extensive internal injury.

A person admitted to the emergency department with an abdominal trauma is assessed using the "ABCDE" method: airway, breathing, circulation, and exposure disability. Life-threatening injuries are identified and treated. Emergency care focuses on establishing or maintaining a patent airway, establishing or maintaining an effective breathing pattern, pain relief, fluid replacement, and prevention of shock and other potential complications. The initial resuscitation phase focuses on maintaining hemodynamic stability. An exploratory laparotomy with repairs of injuries is required in hemodynamically unstable clients who have a penetrating abdominal injury. Diagnosis of the specific organ or vessel injured may include liver function tests, ultrasound of the abdomen, and computed tomography scan, which can reveal organ-specific damage. After stabilization of the client, care focuses on structural healing and prevention of complications.

This care plan focuses on the adult client hospitalized for treatment of abdominal trauma. Some of the information is applicable to clients receiving follow-up care at home.

OUTCOME/DISCHARGE CRITERIA

The client will:
1. Have evidence of normal healing of trauma and/or surgical wound
2. Have clear, audible breath sounds
3. Tolerate prescribed diet
4. Have surgical pain controlled
5. Have no signs and symptoms of complications
6. State signs and symptoms to report to the health care provider
7. Verbalize an understanding of and a plan for adhering to recommended follow-up care including future appointments with health care provider, medications prescribed, activity level, and wound care.

Nursing Diagnosis   **INEFFECTIVE BREATHING PATTERN** NDx

Definition: Inspiration and/or expiration that does not provide adequate ventilation

Related to:
- Increased rate of respirations associated with:
  - Fear and anxiety
  - Pressure on the diaphragm from abdominal distention
- Decreased rate of respirations associated with injury and/or the depressant effect of anesthesia and some medications (e.g., narcotic [opioid] analgesics, some antiemetics)
- Decreased depth of respirations associated with:
  - Reluctance to breathe deeply because of pain
  - Fear, anxiety, weakness, and fatigue
  - Restricted chest expansion resulting from positioning and elevation of the diaphragm if abdominal distention is present

CLINICAL MANIFESTATIONS

Subjective	Objective
Complaints of shortness of breath	Dyspnea; orthopnea; increased respiratory rate; decreased depth of breathing; decreased minute ventilation; decreased vital capacity; nasal flaring; use of accessory muscles to breathe; altered chest excursion; pursed-lip breathing; decreased oxygen saturation; arterial blood gas (ABG) values: respiratory acidosis

RISK FACTOR	DESIRED OUTCOMES
• Abdominal injury	The client will maintain an effective breathing pattern as evidenced by: a. Normal rate and depth of respirations b. Absence of dyspnea

NOC OUTCOMES	NIC INTERVENTIONS
Respiratory status: ventilation	Ventilation assistance; respiratory monitoring

NURSING ASSESSMENT	RATIONALE
Assess for signs and symptoms of an ineffective breathing pattern: • Shallow or slow respirations • Limited chest excursion • Tachypnea or dyspnea • Use of accessory muscles when breathing	*Early recognition of signs and symptoms of an ineffective breathing pattern allows for prompt intervention.*
Assess/monitor pulse oximetry (arterial oxygen saturation [SaO_2]), ABG values as indicated.	*Monitoring continuous SaO_2 readings allows for the early detection of hypoxia.* *Assessment of ABG values allows for a more direct measurement of both the partial pressure of oxygen in arterial blood (PaO_2) and the partial pressure of carbon dioxide in arterial blood ($PaCO_2$), both of which reflect the adequacy of ventilation.*

THERAPEUTIC INTERVENTIONS	RATIONALE

Independent Actions
Implement measures to improve breathing pattern:
- Perform actions to reduce fear and anxiety:
  - Promote a calm environment.
- Perform actions to reduce pain:
  - Reposition client for comfort.
  - Instruct client to support incision with hands or a pillow when moving or coughing.
  - Instruct client to bend knees while coughing and deep breathing.

Reducing fear and anxiety helps to prevent shallow and/or rapid breathing.

Reducing pain helps to increase the client's willingness to move and breathe more deeply.

Relieves tension on abdominal muscles and incision

THERAPEUTIC INTERVENTIONS	RATIONALE
• Perform actions to reduce the accumulation of gas and fluid in the gastrointestinal tract: • Maintain patency of nasogastric, gastric, or intestinal tubes if present.	*Reducing the accumulation of gas in the gastrointestinal tract decreases pressure on the diaphragm, facilitating more effective ventilation.*
• Have client deep breathe or use incentive spirometer every 1 to 2 hours.	*Deep breathing and use of an incentive spirometer promotes maximal inhalation and lung expansion.*
• Instruct client to breathe slowly if hyperventilating.	*Hyperventilation is an ineffective breathing pattern that can lead to respiratory alkalosis.* *Clients can often slow breathing rate if they concentrate on doing so.*
• Place client in a semi- to high-Fowler's position unless contraindicated.	*A semi- to high-Fowler's position allows for maximal diaphragmatic excursion and lung expansion.*
If client develops signs and symptoms of respiratory distress and impaired gas exchange (e.g., restlessness, confusion, significant decrease in oximetry results, decreased PaO_2 and increased $PaCO_2$ levels):	*Improves tissue oxygenation.*
• Prepare client for intubation and mechanical ventilation.	

Dependent/Collaborative Actions

Implement measures to improve breathing pattern:

• Maintain oxygen as ordered.	*Improves oxygen saturation if the client is unable to maintain normal oxygen saturation.*

• Assist with positive airway pressure techniques if ordered:
   • Continuous positive airway pressure (CPAP)
   • Bilevel positive airway pressure (BiPAP)
   • Flutter/positive expiratory pressure (PEP) device
	Positive airway pressure techniques increase intrapulmonary (alveolar) pressure, which helps reexpand collapsed alveoli and prevent further alveoli collapse.

• Administer central nervous system depressants judiciously: • Hold medication and consult physician if respiratory rate is less than 12 breaths/min.	*Central nervous system depressants cause depression of the respiratory center in the brainstem, which can result in a decreased rate and depth of respiration.*
• Perform actions to reduce pain: • Administer analgesics before activities and procedures that can cause pain and before pain becomes severe.	*Reducing pain helps to increase the client's willingness to move and breathe more deeply.*

Nursing Diagnosis   **RISK FOR IMBALANCED FLUID VOLUME** NDx**; RISK FOR ELECTROLYTE IMBALANCE*** NDx

Definition: Risk for developing an imbalance of electrolytes and fluids in the intracellular and extracellular compartments of the body.

Related to:

- **Deficient fluid volume** NDx related to excessive blood loss, loss of fluid associated with vomiting and nasogastric tube drainage (if present)
- **Hypokalemia and metabolic alkalosis** related to loss of electrolytes and hydrochloric acid associated with blood loss, vomiting, and nasogastric tube drainage

CLINICAL MANIFESTATIONS

Subjective	Objective
Reports of nausea; headache	Hypotension; tachycardia; prolonged capillary refill >2 to 3 seconds; decreased urine output; vomiting; abnormal serum electrolyte levels; flat neck veins when client is flat; increased urine specific gravity; increased blood urea nitrogen (BUN) and hematocrit (Hct) values

---

*The nurse should select the diagnostic label that is most appropriate based on the assessment of the client.

Continued...

RISK FACTORS

- Injury
- Possible surgical procedure
- Ineffective fluid level and electrolyte replacement therapy

DESIRED OUTCOMES

The client will maintain fluid and electrolyte balance as evidenced by:

   a. Blood pressure (B/P) and pulse within normal range for client and stable with position change

   b. Capillary refill time less than 2 to 3 seconds

   c. Usual mental status

   d. Balanced intake and output

   e. Urine specific gravity within normal range

   f. Soft, nondistended abdomen with active bowel sounds

   g. Absence of cardiac dysrhythmias, muscle weakness, paresthesias, twitching, spasms, and dizziness

   h. BUN, Hct, serum electrolyte, and ABG values within normal range

NOC OUTCOMES

Fluid balance; electrolyte and acid-base balance

NIC INTERVENTIONS

Fluid management; electrolyte management: hypokalemia; electrolyte management: hypocalcemia; acid-base management: metabolic acidosis

NURSING ASSESSMENT

Assess for and report signs and symptoms of deficient fluid volume:

- Postural hypotension and/or low B/P
- Weak, rapid pulse
- Capillary refill time longer than 2 to 3 seconds
- Neck veins flat when client is supine
- Change in mental status
- Decreased urine output with increased specific gravity (reflects an actual rather than potential fluid deficit)
- Significant increase in BUN and Hct above previous levels
- Hypokalemia (e.g., cardiac dysrhythmias, postural hypotension, muscle weakness, nausea and vomiting, abdominal distention, hypoactive or absent bowel sounds
- Metabolic acidosis (e.g., drowsiness; disorientation; stupor; rapid, deep respirations; headache; nausea and vomiting; cardiac dysrhythmias; low pH and carbon dioxide [CO_2] content)

RATIONALE

Early recognition of signs and symptoms of fluid and electrolyte imbalance allows for prompt treatment.

THERAPEUTIC INTERVENTIONS

Dependent/Collaborative Actions

Implement measures to treat fluid volume deficit:

- Perform actions to improve hypovolemia associated with recent abdominal injury:
  - Rapidly infuse warmed fluids.
  - Administer blood and blood products as ordered.

- Perform actions to prevent nausea and vomiting (e.g., medicate as needed for pain relief)
- If a nasogastric tube is present and needs to be irrigated frequently and/or with large volumes of solution, irrigate it with normal saline rather than water.
- When oral intake is allowed and tolerated, assist client to choose foods/fluids high in potassium (e.g., bananas, orange juice, potatoes, raisins, cantaloupe, tomato juice).

RATIONALE

Clients who experience abdominal injuries often experience excessive bleeding. Replacement fluids are necessary to maintain vascular volume.

Replaces lost blood volume and improves oxygenation to the tissues.

Decreases loss of electrolytes.

Irrigation of an NG Tube with normal saline decreases the loss of electrolytes.

Maintains fluid volume and increases potassium intake.

THERAPEUTIC INTERVENTIONS	RATIONALE
• After initial fluid volume resuscitation, maintain a fluid intake of at least 2500 mL/day unless contraindicated.	*Maintains vascular fluid volume status.*
• Monitor intake and output (I&O) and administer replacements as ordered.	*Maintains vascular fluid volume.*
• Administer electrolyte replacements (e.g., magnesium sulfate, sodium bicarbonate, potassium) if ordered.	*Helps prevent fluid volume deficit and maintains electrolyte levels.*
If signs and symptoms of hypovolemic shock occur:	
• Place the client flat in bed with legs elevated unless contraindicated.	*Placing client flat on the bed and elevating the legs increases fluid return to the heart to maintain cardiac output.*
• Monitor vital signs frequently.	*Changes in vital signs indicate improvement or worsening of hypovolemic shock.*
• Administer oxygen as ordered.	*Improves tissue oxygenation.*
• Administer blood products and/or volume expanders as ordered.	*Replaces fluid and/or blood cells, which improves cardiac output and tissue oxygenation.*
• Prepare client for insertion of hemodynamic monitoring devices (e.g., central venous catheter, intra-arterial catheter) if planned.	*Improves ability to monitor hemodynamic changes.*
• Administer vasopressor medications as ordered.	*Improves B/P and reduces heart rate.*

Nursing Diagnosis INEFFECTIVE PERIPHERAL TISSUE PERFUSION NDx

Definition: Decrease in blood circulation to the periphery that may compromise health

Related to:
• Hypovolemia secondary to blood loss due to injury and/or subsequent surgical procedure

CLINICAL MANIFESTATIONS

Subjective	**Objective**
Complaint of nausea, abdominal pain, or tenderness; complaint of dizziness and lightheadedness	Hypoactive or absent bowel sounds; nausea; abdominal distention; abdominal pain or tenderness; tachycardia; hypotension; cyanotic, pale skin; oliguria; capillary refill time greater than 2 to 3 seconds; elevated BUN and serum creatinine level; decreasing oxygen saturation

RISK FACTORS
• Decreased cardiac output
• Trauma
• Inadequate therapeutic regimen

DESIRED OUTCOMES

The client will maintain adequate tissue perfusion as evidenced by:
 a. B/P within normal range and stable with position change
 b. Usual mental status
 c. Extremities warm with absence of pallor and cyanosis
 d. Palpable peripheral pulses
 e. Capillary refill time less than 2 to 3 seconds
 f. BUN and serum creatinine levels within normal limits
 g. Urine output at least 30 mL/h

NOC OUTCOMES

Circulation status; tissue perfusion: abdominal organs; tissue perfusion: cardiac; tissue perfusion: cerebral; tissue perfusion: peripheral; tissue perfusion: pulmonary

NIC NTERVENTIONS

Circulatory care: arterial insufficiency; circulatory care: venous insufficiency; cerebral perfusion promotion; hypovolemia

 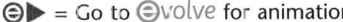

Continued...

NURSING ASSESSMENT	RATIONALE
Assess for and report signs and symptoms of diminished tissue perfusion: • Significant decreased B/P • Restlessness, confusion, or other change in mental status • Reports of dizziness or lightheadedness or occurrence of syncopal episodes • Cool, pale, or cyanotic skin • Diminished or absent peripheral pulses • Increasing abdominal girth • Capillary refill time greater than 2 to 3 seconds • Elevated BUN and serum creatinine levels • Oliguria	*Early recognition of signs and symptoms of diminished gastrointestinal tissue perfusion allows for prompt intervention.*

THERAPEUTIC INTERVENTIONS	RATIONALE
Dependent/Collaborative Actions Implement measures to maintain adequate tissue perfusion: • Administer intravenous fluids and blood as ordered.	*IV fluids and blood help to maintain adequate circulatory status and tissue perfusion.*
• Apply thromboembolism deterrent (TED) hose or a sequential compression device.	*Prevents pooling of blood in the extremities.*
• If the client is hypothermic, apply warming blankets to increase temperature.	*Hypothermia inhibits platelet function and decreases coagulation.*
• Administer coagulation factors as ordered.	*Coagulation factors improves body's ability to clot blood and decrease bleeding.*
• Administer supplemental oxygen.	*Helps to improve tissue oxygenation.*
• Prepare client for surgery to further control the bleeding.	

Nursing Diagnosis ACUTE PAIN NDx

Definition: Unpleasant sensory and emotional experience arising from actual or potential tissue damage or described in terms of such damage (International Association for the Study of Pain); sudden or slow onset of any intensity from mild to severe with an anticipated or predictable end and a duration of less than 6 months

Related to:
• Injury
• Surgery

CLINICAL MANIFESTATIONS

Subjective	Objective
Verbal report of pain	Grimacing; diaphoresis; changes in B/P; tachypnea; tachycardia; restlessness; grading behaviors

RISK FACTORS	DESIRED OUTCOMES
• Abdominal trauma, bleeding into the abdomen, and surgical intervention	The client will experience diminished pain as evidenced by: a. Verbalization of decrease in or absence of pain b. Relaxed facial expression and body positioning c. Increased participation in activities d. Stable vital signs.

NOC OUTCOMES	NIC INTERVENTIONS
Pain control: comfort level	Analgesic administration; pain management; patient-controlled analgesia (PCA) assistance

NURSING ASSESSMENT	RATIONALE
Assess for signs and symptoms of pain (e.g., verbalization of pain, grimacing, reluctance to move, restlessness, diaphoresis, increased B/P, tachycardia).	*Early recognition of signs and symptoms of pain allows for prompt intervention and improved pain control.*
Assess client's perception of the severity of pain using a pain intensity rating scale.	
Assess specific area of pain (e.g., location and quality); note that a finding of pain radiating to the left shoulder may indicate splenic bleeding (Kehr's sign).	

THERAPEUTIC INTERVENTIONS	RATIONALE
Independent Actions	
Implement measures to reduce fear and anxiety (e.g., assure client that the need for pain relief is understood; plan methods for achieving pain control with client; provide a calm environment).	*Fear and anxiety are experienced after a traumatic event. Reassurance that the client's issues are understood will help to control pain.*
Dependent/Collaborative Actions	
Administer analgesics as ordered.	*Pharmacological therapy is an effective method of reducing or relieving pain. Use opioids with care because they decrease gastric motility.*
Postoperative pain: consult physician about an order for PCA if indicated.	*The use of PCA allows the client to self-administer analgesics within parameters established by the physician. This method facilitates pain management by ensuring prompt administration of the drug when needed, providing more continuous pain relief and increasing the client's control over the pain.*
Consult appropriate health care provider (e.g., physician, pharmacist, pain management specialist) if above measures fail to provide adequate pain relief.	*Allows for alterations in treatment plan.*

Collaborative Diagnosis | RISK FOR PERITONITIS

Definition: Inflammation of the peritoneum

Related to:
- Release of intestinal contents into the peritoneal cavity resulting from abdominal trauma
- Exposure of abdominal contents to pathogens associated with a penetrating abdominal wound

CLINICAL MANIFESTATIONS

Subjective	Objective
Verbalization of increasing abdominal pain, rebound tenderness, and nausea	Temperature above 38°C; rigid abdomen; diminished or absent bowel sounds; tachycardia; hypotension; tachypnea; elevated white blood cell (WBC) count

RISK FACTOR
- Exposure to pathogens

DESIRED OUTCOMES

The client will not develop peritonitis as evidenced by:
- a. Temperature stable and less than 38°C
- b. Soft, nondistended abdomen
- c. No increase in abdominal pain and tenderness, nausea, and vomiting
- d. Normal bowel sounds
- e. Stable vital signs

 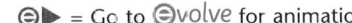

Continued...

NURSING ASSESSMENT	RATIONALE
Assess for and report signs and symptoms of peritonitis (e.g., further increase in temperature or temperature above 38°C; distended, rigid abdomen; increase in severity of abdominal pain; rebound tenderness; increased nausea and vomiting; diminished or absent bowel sounds; tachycardia; tachypnea; hypotension; a WBC count greater than 15,000/mm³).	*Early recognition of signs and symptoms of peritonitis allows for prompt intervention.*

THERAPEUTIC INTERVENTIONS	RATIONALE

Dependent/Collaborative Actions

Implement measures to prevent peritonitis:

- Administer antimicrobials as ordered.

  Prevents and/or treats infections.

- Perform actions to prevent inadvertent removal of wound drain if present:
  - Use caution when changing dressings surrounding drain. **D** ✦

    Prevents accidental dislodgment of a drain if present.

  - Provide extension tubing if necessary. **D** ✦

    Use of extension tubing enables client to move without placing tension on the drain.

  - Instruct client not to pull on drain and drainage tubing. **D** ✦

    Prevents accidental dislodgment of the drain.

- Maintain sterile technique during dressing changes and wound care. **D** ✦

  Prevents introduction of bacteria into the wound.

- Keep abdominal dressing clean and dry. **D** ✦

  Prevents stasis of drainage and decreases potential for infection.

If signs and symptoms of peritonitis occur:

- Withhold oral intake as ordered. **D** ✦

  Withholding oral intake decreases further increase in abdominal contents.

- Place client on bedrest in a semi-Fowler's position. **D** ✦

  Putting the client in a semi-Fowler's position assists in pooling or localizing gastrointestinal contents and urine in the pelvis rather than under the diaphragm.

- Prepare client for diagnostic tests (e.g., abdominal radiograph, peritoneal aspiration, computed tomography, ultrasonography) if planned.
- Insert a nasogastric tube and maintain suction as ordered. **D** ✦

  Decreases potential for gastrointestinal distention.

- Administer antimicrobials as ordered.

  Treats infection.

- Administer intravenous fluids and/or blood volume expanders if ordered to prevent or treat shock.

  Maintains circulatory volume and prevents the increased capillary permeability that occurs with inflammation and the subsequent escape of protein, fluid, and electrolytes from the vascular space into the peritoneal cavity.

- Prepare client for surgical intervention (e.g., drainage and irrigation of peritoneum) if indicated.

  Decreases client's fear and anxiety and promotes understanding of what is to happen.

Collaborative Diagnosis   RISK FOR SEPTIC SHOCK

Definition: A life-threatening medical condition that involves decreased tissue perfusion resulting from a systemic infection

Related to:

- Systemic hypoperfusion associated with maldistribution of circulating blood, deficient fluid volume, and decreased myocardial contractility resulting from uncontrolled systemic inflammatory response to severe infection

CLINICAL MANIFESTATIONS

Subjective	Objective
N/A	Hypotension; tachycardia; widening pulse pressure; restlessness; warm, flushed skin; change in level of consciousness; capillary refill greater than 2 to 3 seconds; significant decrease in pulse oximetry values; changes in arterial blood gas values

RISK FACTORS

- Trauma
- Infection
- Decreased cardiac output
- Failure of regulatory mechanisms

DESIRED OUTCOMES

The client will not develop septic shock as evidenced by:
a. Systolic B/P equal to or higher than 90 mm Hg
b. Usual mental status
c. Urine output at least 30 mL/h
d. Extremities warm and usual color
e. Capillary refill time less than 2 to 3 seconds
f. Palpable peripheral pulses

NURSING ASSESSMENT

Assess for and report signs and symptoms of septic shock:
- Hyperdynamic or compensatory phase (e.g., widened pulse pressure with the diastolic pressure dropping and little change in the systolic pressure; restlessness; tachycardia; warm, flushed skin)
- Hypodynamic or progressive phase (e.g., systolic B/P less than 90 mm Hg or a reduction of greater than 40 mm Hg from baseline; cool, clammy skin; change in level of consciousness; decreased urine output; rapid, shallow breathing; rapid, thready pulse)

RATIONALE

Early recognition of signs and symptoms of septic shock allows for prompt intervention.

THERAPEUTIC INTERVENTIONS

Dependent/Collaborative Actions

Implement measures to maintain adequate tissue perfusion in order to reduce the risk for septic shock:
- Administer intravenous fluids and blood as ordered.

- Apply TED hose or a sequential compression device.
- If the client is hypothermic, apply warming blankets to increase temperature.
- Administer coagulation factors as ordered.

- Administer supplemental oxygen.

If signs and symptoms of septic shock occur:
- Maintain intravenous fluid therapy as ordered.
- Maintain oxygen therapy as ordered.
- Administer antimicrobials as ordered.

- Administer vasopressors and positive inotropic agents (dopamine, dobutamine, norepinephrine) as ordered.

RATIONALE

IV fluids and administration of blood help maintain adequate circulatory status and tissue perfusion.
Prevents pooling of blood in the extremities.
Hypothermia inhibits platelet function and decreases coagulation.

Coagulation factors improve the body's ability to clot blood and decrease bleeding.
Helps to improve tissue oxygenation.

Helps maintain adequate perfusion, pressure and cardiac output.
Provides supplemental oxygen.
Treats infection, which helps decrease vasodilation caused by the systemic infection.
Vasopressors increase blood pressure and positive inotropic agents increase heart rate to maintain circulatory status.

Collaborative Diagnosis | # RISK FOR ORGAN ISCHEMIA/DYSFUNCTION (MULTIPLE ORGAN DYSFUNCTION SYNDROME [MODS])

Definition: A life-threatening syndrome in which the body is unable to maintain homeostasis without intervention

Related to:
- Hypoperfusion of major organs associated with septic shock
- Microvascular thrombosis associated with disseminated intravascular coagulation (DIC) if it occurs

CLINICAL MANIFESTATIONS

Subjective	Objective
N/A	Severe hypotension; tachycardia; urine output less than 30 mL/h; dyspnea, tachypnea; altered arterial blood gas values with low PaO_2; elevated BUN and serum creatinine levels; crackles throughout lungs; changes in mental status

---

NDx = NANDA-I Diagnosis   **D** = Delegatable Action   ● = UAP   ✦ = LVN/LPN   ⊝▶ = Go to ⊝volve for animation

Continued...

RISK FACTORS

- Decreased cardiac output
- Infection
- Decreased vascular fluid volume
- Failure of regulatory mechanisms

DESIRED OUTCOMES

> The client will not develop organ ischemia or dysfunction as evidenced by:
> a. Usual mental status
> b. Urine output at least 30 mL/h
> c. Unlabored respirations at 12 to 20 breaths/min
> d. Audible breath sounds without an increase in adventitious sounds
> e. Absence of new or increased abdominal pain, distention, and diarrhea
> f. BUN, creatinine, aspartate aminotransferase (AST), alanine aminotransferase (ALT), and lactate dehydrogenase (LDH) levels within normal range

NURSING ASSESSMENT

Assess for and report signs and symptoms of:
- Cerebral ischemia (e.g., change in mental status)
- Renal insufficiency (e.g., urine output <30 mL/h, elevated serum BUN and creatinine levels)
- Acute respiratory distress syndrome (e.g., dyspnea, increase in respiratory rate, low SaO_2, crackles)
- Gastrointestinal ischemia (e.g., hypoactive or absent bowel sounds, abdominal pain and distention, nausea, vomiting, diarrhea, hematemesis, blood in stool)
- Liver dysfunction (e.g., increased serum AST, ALT, and LDH levels; jaundice)

RATIONALE

Early recognition of signs and symptoms of MODS allows for prompt intervention.

THERAPEUTIC INTERVENTIONS

RATIONALE

Dependent/Collaborative Actions

Implement measures to reduce the risk for organ ischemia/ dysfunction:
- Administer antimicrobial agents as ordered.
- Maintain fluid intake of 2500 mL/day unless contraindicated.
- Use good hand hygiene.
- Maintain adequate nutritional status.
- Maintain sterile technique during all invasive procedures (e.g., urinary catheterization, venous and arterial punctures, injections).
- Consult physician about discontinuing urinary catheter if one is present.
- Anchor catheter/tubings securely.
- Change equipment, tubings, and solutions according to hospital policy.
- Maintain a closed system for drains (e.g., urinary catheter) and intravenous infusions whenever possible.
- Administer recombinant activated protein C (drotrecogin alfa) if ordered.

Prevents/treats infections.
Maintains adequate vascular fluid volume.

Decreases transmission of infectious agents.
Required for healing and to fight off infections.
Decreases transmission of infectious agents.

A urinary catheter is another avenue by which the body's defenses can be breached and increases the risk for infection.
Prevents accidental removal.
Decreases potential for infection.

Prevents introduction of infectious agents.

Drotrecogin alfa has antithrombotic, anti-inflammatory, and profibrinolytic activity and may reduce the risk of MODS.

DISCHARGE TEACHING/CONTINUED CARE

Nursing Diagnosis   # DEFICIENT KNOWLEDGE NDx; INEFFECTIVE FAMILY THERAPEUTIC REGIMEN MANAGEMENT NDx; OR INEFFECTIVE HEALTH MANAGEMENT* NDx

Definition: Absence or deficiency of cognitive information related to specific topic (lack of specific information necessary for clients/significant others) to make informed choices regarding condition/treatment/lifestyle changes; pattern of regulating and integrating into family processes a program for treatment of illness and the sequelae of illness that is unsatisfactory for meeting specific health goals; inability to identify, manage, and/or seek out help to maintain health

CLINICAL MANIFESTATION

Subjective	Objective
Requests information; client statements reflect misunderstanding	Inadequate follow through of instruction; inappropriate or exaggerated behaviors

RISK FACTORS
- Cognitive limitations or unfamiliarity of situation

NOC OUTCOMES	NIC INTERVENTIONS
Knowledge: treatment regimen; knowledge: health behavior; knowledge: health resources	Health system guidance; teaching: individual; teaching: prescribed activity/exercise; teaching: prescribed medications

NURSING ASSESSMENT	RATIONALE
Assess client's willingness to learn and knowledge related to the disease process.	*The client's willingness to learn and knowledge base provides the basis for education.*
Assess for indications that the client may be unable to effectively manage the therapeutic regimen.	*Early recognition of inability to understand disease process or self-care allows for change in the teaching plan.*

THERAPEUTIC INTERVENTIONS	RATIONALE

Desired Outcome: The client will identify ways to prevent post-operative infection.

Independent Actions
Instruct client in ways to prevent postoperative infection/injury:

- Continue with coughing and deep breathing every 2 hours while awake.	*These activities improve lung expansion.*
- Continue to use incentive spirometer if activity is limited.	
- Increase activity as ordered.	
- Avoid contact with persons who have infections.	*Decreases potential for infection.*
- Avoid crowds during flu and cold seasons.	
- Decrease or stop smoking.	*Nicotine intake can increase cardiac workload and myocardial oxygen use, thereby decreasing the amount of oxygen necessary to fight infection.*
- Drink at least 10 glasses of liquid per day unless contraindicated.	*Adequate hydration is necessary to maintain fluid balance.*
- Maintain a balanced nutritional intake.	*Balanced nutritional intake is required for healing.*
- Maintain proper balance of rest and activity.	*Promotes healing.*
- Maintain good personal hygiene (especially oral care, hand washing, and perineal care).	*These activities decrease the potential for an infection.*

*The nurse should select the diagnostic label that is most appropriate for the client's discharge teaching needs.

Continued...

THERAPEUTIC INTERVENTIONS	RATIONALE
• Avoid touching any wound unless it is completely healed. • Maintain sterile or clean technique as ordered during wound care.	*Prevents introduction of pathogens and decreases potential for infection.*

THERAPEUTIC INTERVENTIONS	RATIONALE

Desired Outcome: The client will state signs and symptoms to report to the health care provider.

Independent Actions

Instruct client to report the following signs and symptoms:
- Persistent low-grade fever or significantly elevated (≥38.3°C [101°F]) temperature
- Difficulty breathing
- Chest pain
- Productive cough of purulent, green, or rust-colored sputum
- Increasing weakness or inability to tolerate prescribed activity level
- Increasing discomfort or discomfort not controlled by prescribed medications and treatments
- Continued nausea or vomiting
- Increasing abdominal distention and/or discomfort
- Separation of wound edges
- Increasing redness, warmth, pain, or swelling around wound
- Unusual or excessive drainage from any wound site
- Pain or swelling in calf of one or both legs
- Urine retention
- Frequency, urgency, or burning on urination
- Cloudy or foul-smelling urine

Signs and symptoms indicate the client may be experiencing complications from the abdominal injury and/or surgery. Signs and symptoms indicate possible infection of the surgical area or other body systems and possible thromboembolism.

THERAPEUTIC INTERVENTIONS	RATIONALE

Desired Outcome: The client will verbalize an understanding of and a plan for adhering to recommended follow-up care including future appointments with health care provider, medications prescribed, activity level, and wound care.

Independent Actions

Reinforce importance of keeping scheduled follow-up appointments with the health care provider.

Reinforcing information improves understanding and adherence to treatment regimen and for follow-up care.

Reinforce physician's instructions on suggested activity level and treatment plan.

Maintenance of treatment plant is important for continued healing and maintenance of health.

Explain the rationale for, side effects of, and importance of taking medications as prescribed. Inform client of pertinent food and drug interactions.

Knowledge of medications and how they impact the system improves client adherence and helps enhance the client's understanding of the importance of adhering to the prescribed medication regimen. The client must be able to recognize alterations in functioning related to medication administration.

Include significant others in teaching sessions if possible.

Involvement of the client's significant others improves the client's potential for success in maintaining the treatment regimen.

Encourage questions and allow time for reinforcement and clarification of information provided.

Helps improves client's understanding of discharge information

Provide written instructions on scheduled appointments with health care provider, dietary modification, activity level, treatment plan, medications prescribed, and signs and symptoms to report.

Written instructions provide ongoing access to information once client is discharged from the acute care facility.

APPENDICITIS/APPENDECTOMY

Acute appendicitis is one of the most common indications for emergency abdominal surgery. The appendix is a small finger-like pouch that extends from the inferior part of the cecum and is usually located in the right iliac region. The most common cause of appendicitis is obstruction of the lumen by a fecalith, a foreign body, an appendiceal calculus, a tumor, or intramural thickening caused by lymphoid hyperplasia. Obstruction of the appendix leads to increased luminal pressure, vascular congestion, bacterial invasion, and ultimately, necrosis and perforation of the appendix.

An appendectomy is the surgical removal of the appendix. It can be done via a laparotomy or laparoscopy. A laparoscopic appendectomy offers the advantage of shorter hospitalization and decreased morbidity and mortality but is contraindicated in persons with extensive intraperitoneal adhesions or other intestinal problems that would impede mobilization and dissection of the appendix.

This care plan focuses on the adult client with suspected appendicitis who is hospitalized for a possible appendectomy.

OUTCOME/DISCHARGE CRITERIA

The client will:
1. Have evidence of normal healing of surgical wound
2. Have clear, audible breath sounds
3. Tolerate prescribed diet
4. Have surgical pain controlled
5. Have no signs and symptoms of postoperative complications
6. State signs and symptoms to report to the health care provider
7. Verbalize an understanding of and a plan for adhering to recommended follow-up care including future appointments with health care provider, medications prescribed, activity level, and wound care.

For a full, detailed care plan on this topic, go to http://evolve.elsevier.com/Haugen/careplanning/.

BOWEL DIVERSION: ILEOSTOMY

An ileostomy is the diversion of the ileum from the abdominal cavity through an opening created in the abdominal wall. It may be performed after abdominal trauma or to treat conditions such as familial polyposis, intestinal cancer, and most commonly, inflammatory bowel disease that is refractory to conservative management. An ileostomy can be temporary or permanent.

A temporary ileostomy is usually created to allow the bowel to heal after traumatic abdominal injury or to permit healing of a newly constructed ileoanal reservoir (pouch). The ileoanal reservoir is a treatment option for some persons with inflammatory bowel disease or familial polyposis. In the initial surgery, the diseased portion of the intestine is removed, a temporary ileostomy is performed, and a reservoir is created in the rectal area using a portion of the ileum. After 2 to 4 months, the ileostomy is closed and intestinal continuity is established between the remaining intestine and the ileoanal reservoir.

There are two types of permanent ileostomies. The conventional (Brooke) ileostomy is the most common one. It is created by bringing a portion of the terminal ileum through the abdominal wall, usually in the right lower quadrant. The ileostomy drains intermittently but, because it cannot be regulated, a collection device needs to be worn over the stoma at all times. Another type of permanent ileostomy is the continent ileostomy. In this procedure, the terminal ileum is used to construct an intra-abdominal reservoir (Kock pouch). Initially, the reservoir drains via a catheter that is placed through the stoma and a surgically constructed one-way valve. After the surgical area heals, the catheter is removed and the reservoir only needs to be drained periodically. If the system functions properly, the client does not need to wear a collection device over the stoma. The type of permanent ileostomy constructed depends on the client's age, underlying disease process, and preference and expertise of the surgeon. A proctocolectomy (removal of the colon, rectum, and anus) is often done at the same time as a permanent ileostomy to treat the disease process or to prevent future bowel changes that could occur. If a proctocolectomy is not performed, the rectal stump is sutured across the top; the rectum stays intact and secretes mucus that is expelled via the anus.

This care plan focuses on the adult client with inflammatory bowel disease hospitalized for bowel diversion with creation of a permanent ileostomy. Much of the postoperative information is applicable to clients receiving follow-up care in an extended care facility or home setting.

OUTCOME/DISCHARGE CRITERIA

The client will:
1. Have surgical pain controlled
2. Have evidence of normal healing of the surgical wound
3. Have a medium pink to red, moist stoma and intact peristomal and perianal skin
4. Have no evidence of fluid and electrolyte imbalances

5. Maintain an adequate nutritional status
6. Have no signs and symptoms of postoperative complications
7. Verbalize a basic understanding of the anatomical changes that have occurred as a result of the bowel diversion
8. Identify ways to maintain fluid and electrolyte balance
9. Verbalize ways to maintain an optimal nutritional status
10. Identify methods of controlling odor and sound associated with ileostomy drainage and gas
11. Demonstrate the ability to change the pouch system, maintain integrity of the peristomal and perianal skin, and maintain adequate stomal integrity
12. Demonstrate the ability to properly use, clean, and store ostomy products
13. Demonstrate the ability to drain and irrigate a continent ileostomy if present
14. Identify ways to prevent and treat blockage of the stoma
15. State signs and symptoms to report to the health care provider
16. Share thoughts and feelings about the effect of altered bowel function on self-concept and lifestyle
17. Identify appropriate community resources that can assist with home management and adjustment to changes resulting from the bowel diversion
18. Verbalize an understanding of and a plan for adhering to recommended follow-up care including future appointments with health care provider, wound care, activity level, and medications prescribed.

USE IN CONJUNCTION WITH STANDARDIZED PREOPERATIVE CARE PLAN

Nursing Diagnosis ## DEFICIENT KNOWLEDGE NDx

Definition: Absence or deficiency of cognitive information related to a specific topic

RISK FACTORS
- Lack of knowledge regarding the surgical procedure, physical preparation for the bowel diversion, sensations that normally occur after surgery and anesthesia, expected appearance and function of the ileostomy, and postoperative care and management of the ileostomy

NOC OUTCOMES	NIC INTERVENTIONS
Knowledge: treatment regimen; knowledge: treatment procedure(s)	Health system guidance; teaching: individual; teaching: procedure/treatment

NURSING ASSESSMENT	RATIONALE
Assess client's understanding of surgical procedure and outcome.	*Client's understanding of what may occur will decrease anxiety.*

THERAPEUTIC INTERVENTIONS	RATIONALE

Desired Outcome: The client will verbalize an understanding of the surgical procedure, preoperative care, and postoperative sensations and care of the ileostomy; verbalize an understanding of the appearance, function, and management of the ileostomy

Independent Actions
Provide information regarding specific preoperative care and postoperative sensations and care for clients having a bowel diversion with ileostomy:
- Explain the preoperative bowel preparation (e.g., low-residue or clear liquid diet, cleansing enemas, laxatives, antimicrobial therapy).

Improves client's understanding of what will occur during the operative procedure and what to expect during recovery. Information helps to decrease fear and anxiety and improve postoperative adherence to treatment regimen.

THERAPEUTIC INTERVENTIONS	RATIONALE

- If proctocolectomy is planned, inform client that:
- A perineal wound drain will be present after surgery.
  - Occasional feelings of pressure in the perineal area are expected after surgery and that these will subside as edema decreases.
- If a continent ileostomy is planned, inform client that:
  - A catheter will be inserted into the reservoir during surgery and will extend from the stoma and drain into an external collection device; stress that this is a temporary measure (usually for 2-4 weeks).

    This keeps the reservoir from becoming distended while the suture lines are healing.
  - The reservoir will need to be irrigated periodically (especially in the early postoperative period) to remove mucus that accumulates in the reservoir.

    The bowel used to construct the reservoir initially secretes quite a bit of mucus.
  - After removal of the stomal catheter, a catheter will be inserted into the stoma at regularly scheduled intervals.

    This is to drain the reservoir so that an external collection device will not be needed.

Allow time for questions and clarification of information provided.

Arrange for a visit with an enterostomal therapy (ET) nurse if available.

The client should be well informed about what will occur before the procedure and what to expect in the post operative period and subsequent changes that may occur following discharge.

Reinforce information provided by physician and/or ET nurse about the appearance and function of the ileostomy:
- The stoma will be medium pink to red and will be moist.
- The stoma will shrink in size as edema resolves during the first 6 weeks after surgery (final stoma height is usually 1.5-2.5 cm [about ½-1 inch] from the skin surface).
- Slight bleeding of the stoma is expected when it is wiped with tissue.
- For the first day or two after surgery, the stoma will drain a small amount of clear to white, blood-tinged fluid containing some mucus; after a few days, the color of the drainage will change to green and then light to medium brown as the diet progresses.
- When the ileostomy begins to function (usually 2-3 days after surgery), the drainage will be watery and high-volume (up to 1-2 L/day), but within a couple of weeks the amount will begin to decrease (expected amount of output after 2-3 months is 500-800 mL/day) and develop a thicker, pastelike consistency.

Provide basic information about peristomal skin care, ways to control intestinal gas and odor of the effluent, products the client will be using after surgery, and irrigation and drainage of the reservoir (if a continent ileostomy is planned).

Allows client more time to process information when given before surgery.

Provide visual aids and allow client to handle ileostomy appliances that will be used in the immediate postoperative period. Provide a pouch clamp so that client can practice putting it on and taking it off of an empty pouch.

The client should become familiar with how to use the appliances to decrease stress postoperatively when using the appliances.

Encourage client to try wearing a pouch system partially filled with water in order to experience how it feels and to determine whether the planned stoma site will be adequate for successful adhesion of the pouch.

Allows the client to know what the pouch will feel like when working with a full pouch.

Allow time for questions and clarification of information provided.

Nursing Diagnosis | **RISK FOR IMBALANCED FLUID VOLUME** NDx; **RISK FOR ELECTROLYTE IMBALANCE*** NDx

Definition: Risk for developing an imbalance of electrolytes and fluids in the intracellular and extracellular compartments of the body

Related to:

Deficient fluid volume NDx related to:
- Restricted oral fluid intake before, during, and after surgery
- Blood loss
- Loss of fluid associated with vomiting, nasogastric tube drainage, and/or high-volume ileostomy output

Hypokalemia, hypomagnesemia, and hypochloremia related to loss of electrolytes associated with vomiting, nasogastric tube drainage, decreased oral intake, and/or high-volume ileostomy output

Metabolic alkalosis related to:
- Loss of hydrochloric acid associated with vomiting and nasogastric tube drainage
- Loss of bicarbonate ions associated with high-volume ileostomy output (effluent contains bicarbonate ions that would normally be absorbed throughout the large intestine)

CLINICAL MANIFESTATIONS

Subjective	Objective
Verbal reports of weakness; confusion, nausea	Change in mental status; decreased skin turgor; postural hypotension; weak, rapid pulse; decreased urine output; cardiac dysrhythmias; nausea and vomiting; absent bowel sounds; decreased urine output; capillary refill ≤ 2-3 seconds; decreased electrolyte levels, decreased pH and CO_2 levels; positive Chvostek's and Trousseau's sign

RISK FACTORS
- Inadequate fluid replacement
- Surgery

DESIRED OUTCOMES

The client will not experience deficient fluid volume, hypokalemia, hypochloremia, hypomagnesemia, and acid-base imbalance as evidenced by:
   a. Normal skin turgor
   b. Moist mucous membranes
   c. Stable weight
   d. B/P and pulse rate within normal range for client and stable with position change
   e. Capillary refill time less than 2 to 3 seconds
   f. Usual mental status
   g. Balanced intake and output within 48 hours after surgery
   h. Urine specific gravity within normal range
   i. Return of peristalsis within expected time
   j. Usual mental status
   k. Absence of cardiac dysrhythmias, twitching, muscle weakness, paresthesias, dizziness, headache, nausea, and vomiting
   l. Negative Chvostek's and Trousseau's sign
   m. BUN, serum electrolyte, and arterial blood gas values within normal range

---

*The nurse should determine the most appropriate nursing diagnoses based on client assessment.

NOC OUTCOMES

Fluid balance; electrolyte and acid-base balance

NIC INTERVENTIONS

Fluid monitoring; electrolyte management: hypokalemia; electrolyte management: hypomagnesemia; fluid/electrolyte management; acid-base monitoring; acid-base management: metabolic alkalosis; acid-base management: metabolic acidosis

NURSING ASSESSMENT

Assess for and report signs and symptoms of deficient fluid volume, hypokalemia, hypochloremia, hypomagnesemia, and metabolic alkalosis:
- Decreased skin turgor, dry mucous membranes, thirst
- Weight loss of 2% or greater over a short period
- Postural hypotension and/or low B/P
- Capillary refill time greater than 2 to 3 seconds
- Neck veins flat when client is supine
- Change in mental status
- Continued low urine output 48 hours after surgery with a change in specific gravity

- Excessive ileostomy output (after bowel activity returns)
- Elevated BUN
- Changes in serum electrolyte levels
- Drowsiness
- Disorientation
- Stupor
- Rapid, deep respirations
- Headache
- Nausea and vomiting
- Low pH and CO_2

RATIONALE

Early recognition of signs and symptoms of fluid volume deficit and electrolyte imbalance allow for prompt intervention.

Specific gravity will usually increase with an actual fluid volume deficit but may be decreased depending on the cause of the deficit.

After bowel activity returns, expected output may be as high as 2000 mL/day, and then in 10 to 14 days it should begin to gradually decrease to 500 to 800 mL/day within 2 to 3 months.

THERAPEUTIC INTERVENTIONS

Independent Actions
Implement measures to prevent or treat fluid volume deficit:
- Perform actions to prevent nausea and vomiting (e.g., assist client to ingest food/fluid slowly, eliminate noxious sights and odors, medicate as needed for pain relief). **D** ✦
- If a nasogastric tube is present and needs to be irrigated frequently and/or with large volumes of solution, irrigate it with normal saline rather than water. **D** ✦
- When oral intake is allowed and tolerated, assist client to choose foods/fluids high in potassium (e.g., bananas, orange juice, potatoes, raisins, cantaloupe, tomato juice).
- Encourage intake of foods that may thicken effluent (e.g., applesauce, bananas, boiled rice, tapioca, pretzels, creamy peanut butter, pasta).
- Maintain a fluid intake of at least 2500 mL/day unless contraindicated. **D** ✦
- Monitor I&O and administer fluid replacements as ordered.
- Perform actions to reduce fever if present (e.g., sponge client with tepid water, remove excessive clothing or bedcovers). **D** ● ✦
- Instruct client to avoid excessive intake of foods/fluids that may cause diarrhea (e.g., raw fruits and vegetables; prune juice; fatty, spicy, or extremely hot or cold items; coffee).

RATIONALE

Nausea often causes the client to have decreased fluid volume intake. Persistent vomiting results in excessive loss of fluid.

Irrigation of the NG tube helps prevent fluid volume deficit and maintains electrolyte levels.

Helps to maintain electrolyte levels.

Foods that thicken fluid in the bowel help slow its progress through the bowel and allow for increased absorption of fluid and electrolytes.
Maintains fluid volume.

Monitoring I&O provides baseline for fluid volume replacement.
Reduction of a fever prevents diaphoresis and subsequent loss of fluid.

Foods high in fiber, those that are spicy, very hot or cold, or with caffeine may induce diarrhea.

NDx = NANDA-I Diagnosis   **D** = Delegatable Action   ● = UAP   ✦ = LVN/LPN   ⊖▶ = Go to ⊖volve for animation

Continued...

THERAPEUTIC INTERVENTIONS	RATIONALE
Dependent/Collaborative Actions Implement measures to prevent or treat fluid volume deficit: • Administer antipyretics. • Administer electrolyte replacements (e.g., magnesium sulfate, sodium bicarbonate, potassium) if ordered. • Administer antidiarrheal agents (e.g., loperamide, diphenoxylate hydrochloride) if ordered. **D** ✦ Consult physician if signs and symptoms of deficient fluid volume and electrolyte imbalances persist or worsen.	*Antipyretics are given to reduce fever.* *Electrolyte replacements help to normalize fluid and electrolyte levels.* *Antidiarrheal medications prevent/treat diarrhea.* *Notification of the physician allows for prompt alterations in the treatment plan.*

Nursing Diagnosis ACTUAL/RISK FOR IMPAIRED TISSUE INTEGRITY NDx

Definition: Damage to mucous membrane, corneal, integumentary, or subcutaneous tissues

Related to:
• Disruption of tissue associated with the surgical procedure
• Delayed wound healing associated with factors such as decreased nutritional status and inadequate blood supply to wound area
• Irritation of skin associated with:
  • Contact with wound drainage, ileostomy output (effluent is rich in proteolytic enzymes), soap residue and perspiration under the pouch, and/or mucus drainage from the anus (occurs if rectum was left intact)
  • Frequent or improper removal of tape, adhesives, or other substances used to secure pouch to the skin
  • Aggressive cleansing of peristomal area
  • Sensitivity to tape, pouch material, ostomy paste, and/or substances used to secure pouch to the skin (e.g., adhesive disk, skin barrier, adhesive spray)
  • Pressure from tubes, appliance belt, and/or pouch drainage valve or clamp

CLINICAL MANIFESTATIONS

Subjective	Objective
N/A	Redness of skin around suture line and stoma; redness of skin where tape or skin barrier had been removed; swelling of ileostomy stoma; drainage from wound

RISK FACTORS
• Surgical procedure
• Preoperative nutritional deficit
• Delayed nutritional therapy post-operatively

DESIRED OUTCOMES

The client will experience normal healing of surgical wounds as evidenced by:
  a. Gradual reduction in periwound swelling and redness
  b. Presence of granulation tissue if healing by secondary or tertiary intervention
  c. Intact, approximated wound edges if healing is by primary intention
The client will maintain integrity of peristomal and perianal skin and skin in contact with wound drainage, tape, and tubings as evidenced by:
  a. Absence of redness and irritation
  b. No skin breakdown

NOC OUTCOMES

Wound healing: primary intention; ostomy self-care; tissue integrity: skin and mucous membranes

NIC INTERVENTIONS

Skin surveillance; pressure management; skin care: topical treatments; incision site care; ostomy care

NURSING ASSESSMENT

RATIONALE

Assess for and report signs and symptoms of impaired wound healing (e.g., increasing periwound swelling and redness, pale or necrotic tissue in wounds healing by secondary or tertiary intention, separation of wound edges in wounds healing by primary intention).

Assess for signs and symptoms of:

- Peristomal irritation or breakdown (e.g., redness, inflammation, and/or excoriation of peristomal skin; reports of itching or burning under the pouch seal; inability to keep pouch on).
- Perianal irritation or breakdown (e.g., redness, inflammation, and/or excoriation of perianal skin; reports of itching or burning in perianal area).

Early recognition of signs and symptoms of impaired wound healing allows for prompt treatment.

THERAPEUTIC INTERVENTIONS

RATIONALE

Independent Actions

Implement measures to promote wound healing:

- Ensure that dressings are secure enough to keep them from rubbing and irritating wound.
- Carefully remove tape and dressings when performing wound care.
- Remind client to keep hands away from the wound.
- Instruct and assist client to support the surgical area when moving.
- Instruct and assist client to splint wound when coughing.
- Apply abdominal binder during periods of activity if ordered.
- Encourage the client to eat a diet with adequate amounts of protein. **D** ✦

Implement measures to prevent tissue irritation and breakdown in areas in contact with wound drainage, tape, and tubings:

- Inspect dressings, wounds, and areas around drains; cleanse wound and change dressings when appropriate.
- Maintain patency of drainage tubes.
- Apply a collection device over drains that are draining copiously.
- Apply a protective barrier product to skin that is likely to be in frequent contact with drainage.
- When positioning client, ensure that he/she is not laying on tubings. **D** ✦

- Anchor all tubing securely. **D** ✦

- Apply a water-soluble lubricant to external nares every 2 to 4 hours. **D** ✦
- Use Montgomery straps or tubular netting. **D** ✦

- When removing tape, pull it in the direction of hair growth; use adhesive solvents if necessary. **D** ✦

Implement measures to prevent peristomal irritation and breakdown:

- Shave or clip hair from peristomal skin if necessary. **D** ✦

- Patch test all products that will come in contact with the skin (e.g., sealant, ostomy paste, barrier, adhesive, and solvent) before initial use; do not use products that cause redness, rash, itching, or burning.

Secure dressings help protect the wound from mechanical injury.

These actions decrease stress on the surgical area and support wound healing.

These actions prevent wound drainage from contacting or remaining on the skin.

Pressure on the skin can compromise circulation to that area; if drainage tubing is occluded, there is an increased risk for leakage of drainage around the tubing.

Anchoring tubing prevents excessive movement of tubes against tissues.

Decreases irritation from nasogastric tube and nasal airway or cannula.

Using Montgomery straps or netting helps avoid repeated application and removal of tape if frequent dressing changes are anticipated.

Prevents irritation to skin when removing tape.

Helps achieve an adequate pouch seal and reduce irritation when the pouch system is removed.

The client may be allergic to products used against the skin. Patch testing them will prevent allergic reaction at the suture line or stoma site.

NDx = NANDA-I Diagnosis   **D** = Delegatable Action   ● = UAP   ✦ = LVN/LPN   ⊖▶ = Go to ⊖volve for animation

Continued...

THERAPEUTIC INTERVENTIONS	RATIONALE
• Change entire pouch system only when necessary (e.g., if pouch seal is leaking, if client reports burning or itching of the peristomal skin, when the stoma size changes); pouch system is usually changed every 3 days in early postoperative period and then should be able to remain in place for 5 to 7 days.	*Too frequent changes of the pouch system cause unnecessary irritation to the peristomal site.*
• Use a 2-piece pouch system (e.g., faceplate and pouch, wafer with flange and pouch) during the initial postoperative period.	*This type of system allows the pouch to be removed to assess the stoma without having to remove the adhesive from the skin.*
• Perform actions to reduce peristomal irritation during removal of the pouch:	
• Place drops of warm water or solvent where the pouch system adheres to the skin; allow time for adhesive to loosen before removing pouch.	*These actions facilitate the removal of the pouch and decrease potential for drainage to come in contact with the skin.*
• Remove pouch system gently and in direction of hair growth; hold skin adjacent to the skin barrier taut and push down slightly on skin.	
• Perform actions to prevent effluent from coming in contact with the skin when changing the pouch system or pouch or when the pouch system is on:	
• Change the pouch or pouch system when the ileostomy is least active (e.g., upon awakening in the morning, before meals, 2-4 hours after eating, before retiring at night).	
• Place a wick (rolled gauze pad or tampon) on the stoma opening when the pouch system or pouch is off.	
• Cleanse peristomal skin thoroughly with mild soap and water, rinse completely, and pat dry; use tepid rather than hot water.	*Prevents burning the skin.*
• Apply skin sealant to the clean, dry peristomal skin before applying the skin barrier.	*Protects skin from the irritating effects of the adhesive.*
• Always use a skin barrier (e.g., Reliaseal, Stomahesive). **D ✦**	*Protects skin from the proteolytic enzymes that are in the effluent.*
• Measure the diameter of the stoma; cut skin barrier the same size as stoma and select a pouch with an opening that is not more that 0.3 cm (⅛ inch) larger than the stoma (it may be necessary to create a pattern to use for cutting barrier and pouch openings if stoma has an irregular shape and cannot be measured using appliance manufacturer's standard measuring guide).	*Creates a barrier that is close to the size of the stoma, decreasing potential for contact between skin and proteolytic enzymes.*
• Implement measures to achieve an adequate pouch seal:	
(1) Avoid use of ointments or lotions on peristomal skin.	*Ointments and lotions can interfere with adequate adhesive bonding.*
(2) Follow manufacturer's instructions when applying skin products and pouch system.	*Prevents potential injury to skin and poor adhesive bonding.*
(3) Use products such as ostomy paste to skin in irregularities around stoma site before applying pouch system.	*Allows for an adequate seal in areas where there are body folds or scars.*
(4) Apply firm pressure and remove air pockets when applying pouch system; place client in a supine position.	*Increases tautness of skin surface during application and increases adequate pouch seal.*
• Empty pouch when it is one third full of effluent or inflated with gas. **D ✦**	*A heavy or inflated pouch can cause the pouch system to separate from the skin.*
• Position pouch so gravity flow facilitates drainage away from stoma and peristomal skin.	*Prevents effluent stasis or backflow, which increases the chance of irritation to the skin.*
• Rinse out bottom of drainable pouch after emptying it and then close pouch clamp securely.	*Prevents leakage of effluent*
• Use a drainable pouch, 2-piece pouch system, and/or pouch with a release valve if gas is a problem; never puncture or cut the pouch to release gas.	*These actions prevent effluent from seeping out of the pouch and can seep, causing skin irritation.*

THERAPEUTIC INTERVENTIONS	RATIONALE
• If a belted pouch system is used, fasten the belt so that two fingers can slip easily between belt and skin.	*Use of a belted pouch system prevents excessive pressure on the skin and potential skin irritation.*
• Instruct and assist client to check pouch periodically to ensure that pouch clamp is not placing pressure on the skin. **D** ✦	
Implement measures to prevent perianal irritation and breakdown:	
• Keep perianal area dry and clean.	*Prevents irritation and potential breakdown*
• Instruct client to regularly perform perineal exercises (e.g., relaxing and tightening perineal and gluteal muscles).	*Increases anal sphincter tone and reduces the risk of mucous leakage.*
• Place absorbent pads in client underwear if needed and change pads when they become damp.	*Prevents irritation of anal area and potential skin breakdown.*
• Apply moisture-barrier ointment to perianal area as ordered. **D** ● ✦	
If signs and symptoms of peristomal or perianal skin irritation or breakdown occur:	
• Cleanse areas gently with warm water.	*Decreases further skin irritation.*
• Avoid use of any product that may have caused the irritation or breakdown.	*Prevents adverse skin reactions.*
• Perform skin care as ordered or according to hospital procedure.	*Usual care may include exposing affected area to air for 20 to 30 minutes, applying an antifungal agent or corticosteroid preparation to affected skin, and/or covering all irritated skin with a solid skin barrier. This promotes skin healing.*
Consult appropriate health care provider (e.g., wound care specialist, ET nurse, physician) if area of irritation or breakdown does not improve within 48 hours.	*Allows for prompt alteration in treatment plan.*

 Collaborative Diagnosis # RISK FOR PERITONITIS

Definition: Inflammation of the peritoneum

Related to:
• Wound infection (a client with inflammatory bowel disease often has a decreased resistance to infection as a result of long-term preoperative corticosteroid use and decreased nutritional status)
• Leakage of intestinal contents into the peritoneum during surgery and/or postoperatively associated with loss of integrity of the sutures at sites of anastomoses or separation of the peristomal skin from the stoma (retraction of the stoma can occur as a result of slippage of sutures, impaired healing of surgical site, or shrinkage of the supporting tissues)
• Accumulation of wound drainage in the peritoneum

CLINICAL MANIFESTATIONS

Subjective	Objective
Reports of increasing abdominal pain; rebound tenderness	Hyperthermia, rigid abdomen, vomiting, tachycardia, tachypnea, hypotension, decreased or absent bowel sounds, increased WBC count or failure to decrease to normal levels

RISK FACTORS
• Surgery
• Exposure to pathogens
• Exposure to abdomen, to intestinal fluids and content

DESIRED OUTCOMES
The client will not develop peritonitis as evidenced by:
 a. Gradual resolution of abdominal pain
 b. Soft, nondistended abdomen
 c. Temperature declining toward normal
 d. Stable vital signs
 e. Absence of nausea and vomiting
 f. Gradual return of normal bowel sounds
 g. WBC count declining toward normal

Continued...

NURSING ASSESSMENT	RATIONALE
Assess for and report signs and symptoms of peritonitis (e.g., increase in severity of abdominal pain; rebound tenderness; distended, rigid abdomen; increase in temperature; tachycardia; tachypnea; hypotension; nausea; vomiting; continued or diminished or absent bowel sounds; WBC counts that increase or fail to decline toward normal).	*Early recognition of signs and symptoms of peritonitis allows for prompt intervention.*

THERAPEUTIC INTERVENTIONS	RATIONALE

Independent Actions

Implement measures to prevent peritonitis:
- Implement measures to prevent wound infection:
  - Maintain an optimal nutritional status.

    Adequate nutrition is needed to maintain normal function of the immune system.
  - Do not apply dressing too tight.

    Dressings that are too tight decrease circulation to the surgical area and decreasing healing.
  - Ensure dressings are secure enough to keep them from rubbing the wound.

    Prevents irritation to the wound.
  - Carefully remove tape from the wound.

    Decreases potential for injury to the stoma.
- Perform measures to maintain patency of wound drain if present:
  - Keep tubing free of kinks. **D** ✦

    Allows drainage to flow away from the wound and prevents distention of the conduit.
  - Empty collection device as often as necessary. **D** ✦

    Prevents stress on the wound and stasis of drainage and prevents distention of the conduit.
  - Maintain suction as ordered.

    Prevents stasis of secretions and prevents distention of conduit.
- Perform measures to prevent inadvertent removal of the tube:

    These actions prevent accidental dislodgement of a drain if present and enables the client to move without placing unnecessary tension on the drain.
  - Use caution when changing dressings surrounding drain. **D** ✦
  - Provide extension tubing if necessary. **D** ✦
  - Instruct client not to pull on drain and drainage tubing. **D** ✦

Dependent/Collaborative Actions

Implement measures to prevent peritonitis:
- Perform actions to prevent distention of the internal reservoir (if client has a continent ileostomy) or remaining segment of the ileum:

    Distention can cause strain on the suture lines and subsequent leakage of effluent into the peritoneal cavity.
  - Implement measures to prevent stomal obstruction:
    (1) Irrigate stoma if ordered.

    Removes excessive mucus that could block stoma.
    (2) Maintain a fluid intake of 2500 mL/day.

    Keeps effluent from becoming too thick and maintains fluid volume.
    (3) Administer oral medications crushed and mixed in water or in liquid or chewable form.

    Undigested pills can block stoma.
  - Instruct client to avoid activates such as drinking carbonated beverages, chewing gum, smoking, and eating gas-producing foods (e.g., cabbage, onions, broccoli, beans, cucumbers),

    Prevents accumulation of air and gas in the remaining intestine or internal reservoir.
  - Use only the prescribed amount of irrigating solution (e.g., 20-30 mL) when irrigating the stoma or internal reservoir.

    Prevents accumulation of fluid in the remaining intestine or internal reservoir

THERAPEUTIC INTERVENTIONS	RATIONALE
• Maintain patency of stomal catheter (e.g., keep stomal catheter and drainage bag below level of reservoir, keep catheter free of kinks, irrigate catheter as ordered).	*Promotes gravity drainage and prevents stasis or backflow of drainage.*
• Change pouch system carefully. **D** ✦	*Helps prevent unintentional dislodgment of the stomal catheter.*
• If client has a continent ileostomy and the stomal catheter is removed before discharge, assist client with drainage of the internal reservoir at scheduled intervals and when client feels increased abdominal pressure.	*Prevents accumulation of drainage in the internal reservoir.*
• Do not reposition the stomal catheter.	*Repositioning could disrupt the suture line.*
• If the peristomal skin separates from the stoma:	*Appropriate wound care facilitates the formation of granulation tissue in the affected area.*
• Perform wound care as ordered.	
• Prepare client for surgical reconstruction of the stoma if planned.	
• Administer antimicrobials if ordered.	*Antimicrobials prevents and treats infections.*
If signs and symptoms of peritonitis occur:	
• Withhold oral intake as ordered. **D** ✦	*Prevents increased pressure in the abdomen.*
• Place client on bedrest in a semi-Fowler's position. **D** ✦	*Positioning in a semi-Fowler's position assists in pooling or localizing gastrointestinal contents in the pelvis rather than under the diaphragm.*
• Prepare client for diagnostic tests (e.g., abdominal radiograph, peritoneal aspiration, computed tomography, ultrasonography) if planned.	*Decreases client's fear and anxiety.*
• Insert a nasogastric tube and maintain suction as ordered. **D** ✦	*Insertion of an NG tube to suction decreases potential for gastrointestinal distention.*
• Administer intravenous fluids and/or blood volume expanders if ordered to prevent or treat shock.	*Administration of IV fluids maintains circulatory volume and prevents the increased capillary permeability that occurs with inflammation and the subsequent escape of protein, fluid, and electrolytes from the vascular space into the peritoneal cavity.*
• Prepare client for surgical intervention (e.g., drainage and irrigation of peritoneum, repair of sites of anastomoses) if indicated.	*Decreases client's fear and anxiety.*

Collaborative Diagnosis   RISK FOR STOMAL CHANGES

Definition: Changes in the structure of the stoma

Related to:
Necrosis related to intraoperative and/or postoperative interruption of blood supply to the stoma
Excessive bleeding related to irritation associated with aggressive cleansing of stoma and/or improper fit or application of pouch system
Prolapse related to loss of integrity of the sutures or pressure around the stoma

CLINICAL MANIFESTATIONS

Subjective	Objective
N/A	Changes in color of stoma to pale or dark blue, black or purple; increased stoma height; increased stoma bleeding and/or edema

RISK FACTORS

- Surgery
- Preoperative poor skin integrity
- Inadequate or inappropriate stomal/skin therapy

DESIRED OUTCOMES

The client will maintain stomal integrity as evidenced by:
a Medium pink to red stomal coloring
b Expected stomal height
c Absence of excessive bleeding and increasing edema of the stoma

Continued...

NURSING ASSESSMENT	RATIONALE
Assess for and report signs and symptoms of impaired stomal integrity: • Pale, dark red, dusky blue, blue-black, or purple color of stoma • Increased height of stoma • Increased stomal edema or bleeding	*Early recognition of signs and symptoms of impaired stomal integrity allows for prompt treatment.*

THERAPEUTIC INTERVENTIONS	RATIONALE

Independent Actions
Use clear pouches during immediate postoperative period.
Implement measures to maintain integrity of stoma:
• Perform actions to maintain adequate stomal circulation:
  • Ensure that the openings of the skin barrier, faceplate, and pouch are not too small and that the stoma is centered in the openings.
  • Instruct client to avoid wearing clothing that puts pressure on the stoma.
• Apply pouch system securely. **D** ✦
• Cleanse stoma gently using a soft cloth, gauze, or tissue. **D** ✦
If signs and symptoms of impaired stomal integrity occur:
• Perform stomal care as ordered.
• Prepare client for surgical revision of stoma if indicated.
	Clear pouches allow for easy visibility and assessment of the stoma.
	Prevents pressure on and around the stoma.
	
	Prevents it from slipping and irritating or shearing stoma.
	These actions prevent skin irritation.

Collaborative Diagnosis   RISK FOR STOMAL OBSTRUCTION

Definition: Inability of fecal material to pass through the stoma

Related to:
• Stomal edema and/or blockage of stoma

Subjective	Objective
Report of abdominal cramping; nausea or increased feeling of fullness	Less than expected output; thin, watery effluent consistency

RISK FACTORS	DESIRED OUTCOMES
• Surgery • Inadequate flushing • Lack of peristalsis • Immobility	The client will not develop stomal obstruction as evidenced by: a. Expected amount and consistency of ileostomy output b. No reports of abdominal cramping, nausea, or increased feeling of fullness c. Absence of vomiting

NURSING ASSESSMENT	RATIONALE
Assess for and report signs and symptoms of stomal obstruction: • Less than expected amount of ileostomy output • Change in effluent consistency from a thicker consistency to a thin, watery liquid • Reports of abdominal cramping, nausea, or increased feeling of fullness • Vomiting	*Early recognition of signs and symptoms of stomal obstruction allows for prompt intervention.* *After return of peristalsis, output may be as high as 2000 mL/day and will gradually decrease to about 500 to 800 mL/day.* *Postoperatively, effluent gradually becomes thicker; a return to thin, watery consistency may indicate blockage of stoma.*

THERAPEUTIC INTERVENTIONS	RATIONALE

Independent Actions

Implement measure to prevent stomal obstruction:

- Irrigate stoma if ordered. **D** ✦

  Stomal irrigation removes excessive mucus that could block stoma.
  Undigested pills can block stoma.

- Administer oral medications crushed and mixed in water or in liquid or chewable form. **D** ✦
- When oral intake is allowed, perform actions to prevent blockage of stoma by food:
  - Encourage client to eat small, frequent meals rather than three large ones.

    Small meals help keep effluent from becoming too thick and allow body time to more fully digest smaller amounts of food.

  - Instruct client to chew food thoroughly.

    Chewing thoroughly will increase absorption of food.

  - Instruct client to avoid or eat only small amounts of foods that are high in fiber.

    Fibrous foods absorb water in the intestinal tract.

  - Instruct client to avoid or eat only small amounts of foods that are hard to digest (e.g., popcorn, coconut, raw vegetables, fruits with seeds, celery, bean sprouts, bamboo shoots, whole kernel corn, potato skins, bran, nuts, fruit skins).

    Hard-to-digest foods increase abdominal distention.

If food particles or mucus seem to be obstructing the stoma, implement measures to promote flow of effluent through the stoma:

- Perform action to relax the abdominal muscle that surrounds the stoma (e.g., apply warm compresses to the abdomen unless contraindicated, encourage participation in relaxing activities such as reading and listening to music).

  These actions decrease the stricture around the stoma from a contracted abdominal muscle.

- Perform actions to break up or shift foods or mucus:
  - Encourage fluid intake unless contraindicated.

    Adequate fluid intake liquefies secretions, improving effluent flow out of the stoma.

  - Instruct and assist client to assume a knee-chest position.

    Positioning in the knee-chest position may break up or shift stomal blockage.

  - Gently massage peristomal area unless contraindicated.

    Gentle massage may stimulate peristalsis to move fecal material through the colon.

  - Assist with or gently perform digital dilation of stoma if ordered.

    Provides manual removal of blockage.

  - Irrigate ileostomy if ordered.

    Irrigation of the ileostomy may flush out blockage.

Dependent/Collaborative Actions

- Maintain fluid intake of 2500 mL/day unless contraindicated.

  Keeps effluent from becoming too thick.

If stomal edema seems to be obstructing the stoma, consult physician about gently inserting a catheter through the stoma into the ileal segment.

If signs and symptoms of stomal obstruction persist:

- Withhold oral intake as ordered.

  Prevents food from further obstructing stoma.

- Maintain intravenous fluid therapy.

  Prevents fluid volume deficit and increased viscosity of effluent.

- Insert a nasogastric tube and maintain suction as ordered.

  An NG tube to suction removes contents from stomach.

- Prepare client for surgical intervention to remove obstruction if indicated.

  Decreases fear and anxiety.

Nursing Diagnosis ## RISK FOR INEFFECTIVE SEXUALITY PATTERNS NDx

Definition: Expression of concern regarding own sexuality

Related to:
- Decreased libido associated with feelings of loss of femininity/masculinity and sexual attractiveness
- Fear of offensive odor or leakage of effluent and gas
- Fear of rejection by partner
- Discomfort resulting from surgical incision
- Depression

NDx = NANDA-I Diagnosis   **D** = Delegatable Action   ● = UAP   ✦ = LVN/LPN   ⊕▶ = Go to ⊕volve for animation

Continued...

CLINICAL MANIFESTATIONS

Subjective	Objective
Verbalization of sexual concerns; expression of fear of rejection by partner	N/A

RISK FACTORS

- Changes in body
- Embarrassed by physical appearance

DESIRED OUTCOMES

The client will demonstrate beginning acceptance of changes in sexual functioning as evidenced by:
  a. Verbalization of a perception of self as sexually acceptable and adequate
  b. Statements reflecting beginning adjustment to the effects of the ileostomy on sexual functioning

NOC OUTCOMES

Body image; personal well-being; sexual functioning

NIC INTERVENTIONS

Body image enhancement; sexual counseling

NURSING ASSESSMENT	RATIONALE
Assess for signs and symptoms of sexual dysfunction (e.g., verbalization of sexual concerns, alteration in relationship with significant other, reports of anticipated changes in sexual activities or behaviors).	*Early recognition of signs and symptoms of changes in sexual functioning allows for prompt intervention.*

THERAPEUTIC INTERVENTIONS	RATIONALE

Independent Actions
Implement measures to promote optimal sexual functioning:

- Facilitate communication between client and partner; focus on the feelings the couple share and assist them to identify changes that may affect their sexual relationship.

  Allows client and partner to explore concerns and work through issues related to changes that affect their sexual relationship.

- Perform actions to promote a positive self-concept (e.g., use odor-proof pouches, change appliance regularly).

  Improves self-concept and self-esteem.

- Instruct client in ways to reduce risk of leakage of effluent during sexual activity:
  - Empty the pouch or drain internal reservoir (if present) before sexual activity.

    These actions prevent leakage.

  - Secure appliance seal with tape for added security.

    Prevents inadvertent dislodgment of the appliance and subsequent leakage.

- If client is concerned about odor, instruct client to:
  - Shower or bathe before sexual activity.
  - Use an odor-proof pouch or pouch deodorant.
  - Use cologne or perfume if desired.
  - Keep room well ventilated.

    These actions prevent odor from effluent from being noticed during sexual activity making the client less self-conscious.

- If client is concerned about the presence of the stoma and pouch system, discuss the possibility of:
  - Using opaque or patterned pouches or decorative pouch covers

    Makes client less self-conscious about wearing the appliance.

  - Wearing underwear with the crotch removed (for females), boxer shorts (for males), or a cummerbund or stretch tube top around abdomen during sexual activity

    Wearing crotchless underwear provides support for and covers the appliance during sexual activity.

THERAPEUTIC INTERVENTIONS	RATIONALE
• If client is concerned that operative site discomfort will interfere with usual sexual activity:	
• Assure client that discomfort is temporary and will diminish as the incision heals.	
• Encourage alternatives to intercourse or use of positions that decrease pressure on surgical site (e.g., side-lying).	*Decreases pressure on the surgical site or pressure from a partner on top of the client during sexual activity.*
• If appropriate, involve partner in ileostomy care.	*Facilitates partner's adjustment to the changes in client's appearance and body functioning and subsequently decreases the possibility of a partner's rejection of client.*
• Encourage client to obtain written information regarding sexual activity from the United Ostomy Association and from manufacturers of ostomy products.	*Provides for continuum of care and resources for the client once discharged from the acute care environment.*
• Include partner in above discussion and encourage continued support of the client.	*Allows client and partner to work through physical changes and emotional concerns together.*

Dependent/Collaborative Actions

Consult appropriate health care provider (e.g., ET nurse, psychiatric nurse clinician, sex therapist, physician) if counseling is indicated.	*Provides for a multidisciplinary approach to client care.*

Nursing Diagnosis   # DISTURBED SELF-CONCEPT*

Definition:

Disturbed body image: NDx Confusion in mental picture of one's physical self

Situational low self-esteem: NDx Development of a negative perception of self-worth in response to a current situation (specify)

Ineffective role performance: NDx Patterns of behavior and self-expression that do not match the environmental, context, norms, and expectations

Related to:

- Change in appearance associated with presence of stoma and pouch system
- Embarrassment associated with sounds and odor resulting from gas and effluent
- Dependence (usually temporary) on others for assistance with ileostomy management
- Loss of control over bowel elimination if client has conventional ileostomy
- Loss of ability to urinate normally
- Dependence (usually temporary) on others for assistance with ileostomy management
- Change in appearance associated with the presence of a stoma and appliance
- Changes in usual sexual functioning
- Possibility of impotence if nerve damage occurred during a proctocolectomy (use of nerve-sparing surgical techniques has greatly reduced the occurrence of nerve damage and subsequent impotence)

CLINICAL MANIFESTATIONS

Subjective	**Objective**
Verbalization of negative feelings about self	Lack of participation in activities of daily living; withdrawal from significant others; refusal to look at or touch stoma; lack of planning to adapt to necessary changes in lifestyle

---

*This diagnostic label includes the nursing diagnoses of Disturbed body image, Situational low self-esteem, and Ineffective role performance.

Continued...

RISK FACTORS

- Physical changes
- Depression
- Surgery
- Inability to perform perceived family role

DESIRED OUTCOMES

> The client will demonstrate beginning adaptation to changes in appearance, body functioning, and lifestyle as evidenced by:
> a. Verbalization of feelings of self-worth
> b. Maintenance of relationships with significant others
> c. Active participation in activities of daily living
> d. Verbalization of a beginning plan for integrating changes in appearance and body functioning into lifestyle

NOC OUTCOMES

Body image; personal autonomy; self-esteem; psychosocial adjustment: life change

NIC INTERVENTIONS

Body image enhancement; self-esteem enhancement; emotional support; support system enhancement; role enhancement; counseling

NURSING ASSESSMENT	**RATIONALE**
Assess for signs and symptoms of a disturbed self-concept (e.g., verbalization of negative feelings about self, withdrawal from significant others, lack of participation in activities of daily living, refusal to look at or touch stoma, lack of plan for adapting to necessary changes in lifestyle).	*Early recognition of signs and symptoms of a disturbed self-concept allows for prompt treatment.*
Determine the meaning of changes in appearance, body functioning, and lifestyle to the client by encouraging verbalization of feelings and by noting nonverbal responses to the changes experienced.	*An understanding of what the change means to the client provides a basis for planning care.*

THERAPEUTIC INTERVENTIONS	**RATIONALE**
Independent Actions	
Be aware that client may grieve the loss of usual bowel function and change in appearance. Provide support during the grieving process.	*Allow client and significant others to grieve loss of normal body functioning; helps to work through changes that are occurring.*
Emphasize the positive effects of the surgery on future lifestyle (e.g., the discomfort and frequent diarrhea associated with inflammatory bowel disease and the side effects of medications such as corticosteroids usually have had a disruptive effect on many aspects of the client's life).	*Unrealistic expectations may lead to difficulty in dealing with the physical changes that have occurred.*
Implement measures to promote optimal sexual functioning (e.g., ways to support stoma during sexual activity; proper positioning during sexual activity; ways to decrease odor from the stoma during sexual activity).	*Sexual activity may have a positive effect on self-esteem.*
Instruct and assist client in ways to reduce gas formation:	
• Avoid activities that can cause air swallowing (e.g., chewing gum, smoking).	*Prevents abdominal distention related to gas from air swallowing.*
• Limit intake of carbonated beverages and gas-producing foods (e.g., cabbage, onions, beans, radishes, broccoli, cucumbers).	*These foods cause gas production and abdominal distention.*
Instruct client in and assist with measures to reduce the odor of ileostomy drainage and/or gas:	*These interventions are effective in reducing noticeable pouch system odor.*
• Use odor-proof pouches and change appliance regularly.	
• Empty pouch regularly, rinse inside of pouch, and clean off any effluent before closing pouch.	
• Drain the reservoir of continent ileostomy at scheduled intervals and when it feels full to reduce possibility of leakage from stoma.	
• Use a disposable pouch and change it regularly, or clean reusable pouch thoroughly.	

THERAPEUTIC INTERVENTIONS	RATIONALE
• Perform actions to achieve an adequate pouch seal (e.g., patch test all products that come into contact with the skin, change/empty pouch when necessary, place a drop of warm water on the skin to increase adherence of the appliance, measure diameter of the stoma and cut skin barrier to prevent exposure to the effluent).	
• Limit intake of foods that cause effluent to have a strong odor (e.g., onions, fish, eggs, strong cheeses, asparagus).	
• Increase intake of foods/fluids that control odor (e.g., spinach, parsley, yogurt, buttermilk).	
• Change bed linens and clothing promptly if they become soiled.	
Inform client that pouch and clothing muffle sounds of bowel activity.	*Assures client that bowel sounds may not be noticed by others.*
Assure client that once stomal edema and discomfort associated with the surgery have resolved, the client will be able to dress as before with minor, if any, modifications.	*Realistic expectations about appearance and/or body functioning facilitate goal setting and are essential for positive adaptation to the changes experienced and integration of these changes into self-concept.*
Show client and significant others some of the attractive ileostomy products that are available (e.g., opaque or patterned pouches, pouch covers).	*Helps reduce client self-consciousness.*
Encourage participation in activities that can assist client to integrate physical changes that have occurred (e.g., ileostomy care, bathing).	*Supporting behaviors indicative of positive adaptation to changes encourages the client to repeat these behaviors. Repetition of positive adaptive behaviors facilitates the development of a positive self-concept.*
Demonstrate acceptance of client using techniques such as touch and frequent visits.	*Frequent visits and the use of touch convey a feeling of acceptance to the client. This enhances feelings of self-worth and assists with the development of a positive self-concept.*
Support behaviors suggesting positive adaptation to changes that have occurred (e.g., willingness to care for ileostomy, compliance with the treatment plan, verbalization of feelings of self-worth, maintenance of relationships with significant others).	*Improves client's confidence in ability to care for self. This enhances client's feelings of self-worth and assists with the development of a positive self-concept.*
Encourage significant others to allow client to do what he/she is able.	*Demonstrates to the client that independence can be reestablished and/or self-esteem redeveloped.*
Assist client's and significant others' adjustment by listening, facilitating communication, and providing information.	*Demonstrates acceptance of physical changes by significant others and enhances self-worth.*
Encourage visits and support from significant others.	
If acceptable to client, arrange for a visit with an ostomate of similar age and same sex who has successfully adjusted to an ileostomy.	*Demonstrates that client is not alone in the changes experienced and ability to have a positive future.*
Encourage client to pursue usual roles and interests and to continue involvement in social activities.	*The ability to pursue usual roles and activities has a positive effect on the client's self-esteem.*
Provide information about and encourage utilization of community agencies and support groups (e.g., ostomy groups; sexual, family, individual, and/or financial counseling).	*Provides for continuum of care once the client has been discharged from the acute care setting.*
If nerve damage that could result in impotence is believed to have occurred during a proctocolectomy, encourage client to discuss it and various treatment options (e.g., vacuum erection aids, penile prosthesis) with physician.	*Helps client realize there are options if nerve damage has occurred.*

Dependent/Collaborative Actions

Consult appropriate health care provider (e.g., psychologist, psychiatric nurse clinician, ET nurse, physician) if client seems unwilling or unable to adapt to changes resulting from the bowel diversion.	*Allows for multidisciplinary interventions.*

NDx = NANDA-I Diagnosis   **D** = Delegatable Action   ● = UAP   ✦ = LVN/_PN   ◉▶ = Go to ⊖volve for animation

DISCHARGE TEACHING/CONTINUED CARE

Nursing Diagnosis # DEFICIENT KNOWLEDGE NDx; INEFFECTIVE FAMILY THERAPEUTIC REGIMEN MANAGEMENT NDx; OR INEFFECTIVE SELF HEALTH MANAGEMENT* NDx

Definition: Absence or deficiency of cognitive information related to specific topic (lack of specific information necessary for clients/significant others) to make informed choices regarding condition/treatment/lifestyle changes; pattern of regulating and integrating into daily living and family processes a therapeutic regimen for treatment of illness and the sequelae of illness that is unsatisfactory for meeting specific health goals.

CLINICAL MANIFESTATIONS

Subjective	Objective
Verbalization of the problem	Inaccurate follow through of instructions; inappropriate behaviors

RISK FACTORS

- Denial of disease process and physical changes
- Cognitive deficiency
- Failure to participate in self-care while hospitalized

NOC OUTCOMES	NIC INTERVENTIONS
Knowledge: ostomy care; knowledge: treatment regimen; knowledge: diet	Health systems guidance; teaching: individual; teaching: disease process; teaching: prescribed diet; teaching: prescribed medication

NURSING ASSESSMENT	RATIONALE
Assess client's knowledge base related to the disease process. Assess for indications that the client may be unable to effectively manage the therapeutic regimen: • Statements reflecting inability to manage care at home • Failure to adhere to treatment plan	*The client's knowledge base provides the basis for education.* *Early recognition of inability to understand disease process or self-care allows for change in teaching modality.*

THERAPEUTIC INTERVENTIONS	RATIONALE
Desired Outcome: The client will verbalize a basic understanding of anatomical changes that have occurred as a result of the bowel diversion. **Independent Actions** Reinforce teaching regarding the anatomical changes that have occurred as a result of the bowel diversion. Use appropriate teaching aids (e.g., pictures, videotapes, anatomical models).	*Improves client's understanding of surgery and subsequent physical and lifestyle changes as a result of surgery.*

THERAPEUTIC INTERVENTIONS	RATIONALE
Desired Outcome: The client will identify ways to maintain fluid and electrolyte balance.	

---

*The nurse should select the diagnostic label that is most appropriate for the client's discharge teaching needs.

THERAPEUTIC INTERVENTIONS	RATIONALE
Instruct client to drink at least 10 glasses of liquid per day unless contraindicated and to increase fluid intake during hot weather, during and after intense physical activity, when perspiring profusely, if urine is dark yellow, and during episodes of diarrhea; inform client that pale yellow urine is a good indicator of adequate fluid intake.	*These actions provide client with methods to maintain adequate fluid volume during weather and physical changes.*
Instruct client to perform the following actions to prevent excessive ileostomy output:	*Excessive ileostomy output may cause changes in fluid and electrolyte balance. These actions help prevent increased and excessive ileostomy output.*
• Avoid excessive intake of foods/liquids that may cause diarrhea (e.g., raw fruits and vegetables, prune juice, fatty foods, spicy foods, coffee).	
• Do not take laxatives or excessive amounts of magnesium-containing antacids (e.g., Milk of Magnesia, Mylanta, Maalox).	
• Take antidiarrheal agents (e.g., loperamide, diphenoxylate hydrochloride) as prescribed.	
If ileostomy output increases or becomes more watery, instruct client to:	
• Increase intake of foods that may thicken effluent (e.g., applesauce, bananas, boiled rice, tapioca, pretzels, creamy peanut butter, pasta).	*Foods that thicken fluid in the bowel help to slow its progress and allow for more fluid and electrolytes to be absorbed.*
• Increase intake of foods/liquids such as fruit juices, Gatorade, potatoes (without skins), bananas, and bouillon.	*These actions help maintain electrolyte balance.*
• Drink a mixture of baking soda and water (usually ¼ to ½ teaspoon baking soda in 1 cup of water) if prescribed by physician.	

THERAPEUTIC INTERVENTIONS	RATIONALE
Desired Outcome: The client will verbalize ways to maintain an optimal nutritional status.	
Independent Actions Provide instructions regarding ways to maintain an optimal nutritional status:	
• Stress the importance of eating a well-balanced diet.	*Eating a well-balanced diet is necessary for postoperative healing and normal body functions.*
• Stress the need to chew food thoroughly.	*Thoroughly chewing foods enhances digestion and subsequent absorption of nutrients.*
• Stress the importance of taking vitamins and minerals as prescribed.	*Vitamin and mineral supplements enhance nutritional status.*

THERAPEUTIC INTERVENTIONS	RATIONALE
Desired Outcome: The client will identify methods of controlling odor and sound associated with ileostomy drainage and gas.	
Independent Actions Reinforce instructions regarding ways to reduce gas formation and odor associated with ileostomy drainage and gas (e.g., avoid activities that can cause air swallowing, limit intake of carbonated beverages, use odor-proof pouches, change pouch regularly).	*These actions prevent abdominal distention related to gas from air swallowing or intake of gas-producing foods. Reduction of odor and excessive bowel sounds helps improve client's self-esteem.*
Inform client that the ostomy pouch and clothing will muffle the sounds from the ileostomy.	

Continued...

THERAPEUTIC INTERVENTIONS	RATIONALE

Desired Outcome: The client will demonstrate the ability to change the pouch system, maintain integrity of the peristomal and perianal skin, and maintain adequate stomal integrity.

Independent Actions

Reinforce teaching regarding application of the pouch system, prevention of peristomal and perianal skin irritation and breakdown, and maintenance of adequate stomal integrity:

- Shave or clip hair from peristomal skin as necessary.

  Helps achieve an adequate pouch seal and reduces irritation when the pouch system is removed.

- Patch test all products to prevent irritation or allergic reaction when used.

  Helps prevent skin irritation surrounding the stoma.

- Change entire pouch system only when necessary.
- Place drops of warm water or solvent where the pouch system adheres to the skin.

  Facilitates removal of pouch system.

- Remove pouch system gently and in direction of hair growth; hold skin adjacent to the skin barrier taut and push down on skin slightly.

  Facilitates separation of pouch system and client's skin.

Support client's efforts to decrease odor of effluent and gas but discourage excessive changing and emptying of pouch or pouch system

Excessive pouch system changing and emptying causes skin and stoma irritation.

Instruct and assist client to establish a routine for emptying and changing pouch or emptying ileostomy.

A routine for emptying and changing the pouch system reduces the risk of leakage of effluent and skin irritation.

Instruct client to follow special precautions for products used (e.g., skin sealants should be used only on healthy peristomal skin).

Skin sealants used on reddened and excoriated skin can cause further irritation.

Allow time for questions, clarification, practice, and return demonstration of emptying the pouch, changing the pouch system, and performing appropriate stoma and skin care.

Improves client's self-confidence in ability to care for self.

THERAPEUTIC INTERVENTIONS	RATIONALE

Desired Outcome: The client will demonstrate the ability to properly use, clean, and store ostomy products.

Independent Actions

Instruct client regarding proper use of ostomy products that will be used after discharge.

Improves client's self-confidence in ability to care for self.

Demonstrate appropriate pouch system cleansing. Emphasize importance of:

These actions in caring for the pouch system help decease odors and prevent leakage of effluent onto the skin.

- Rinsing inside of pouch each time it is emptied
- Soaking reusable pouch according to manufacturer's instruction and allowing it to dry thoroughly before reusing

Instruct client to avoid reusing disposable products and to discard a reusable pouch if it retains an odor after thorough cleansing or it becomes brittle.

Discuss recommended methods of sorting ostomy products based on manufacturer's recommendations.

THERAPEUTIC INTERVENTIONS	RATIONALE

Desired Outcome: The client will demonstrate the ability to drain and irrigate a continent ileostomy if present.

Independent Actions

Explain the gradual and progressive clamping routine if catheter will still be in the stoma of a continent ileostomy at time of discharge.

Initially the reservoir will need to be drained for 5 to 15 minutes every 3 to 4 hours, but after about 6 months, it may need emptying only 2 to 3 times a day.

If the stomal catheter has been removed, demonstrate the correct method of and explain the schedule for stomal catheter insertion.

Demonstrate the correct technique for irrigating a continent ileostomy. Caution client to use only the prescribed amount of irrigant (usually 20-30 mL).

Avoids overdistending and damaging the internal reservoir.

THERAPEUTIC INTERVENTIONS	RATIONALE

Desired Outcome: The client will identify ways to prevent and treat blockage of the stoma.

Independent Actions

Instruct client in ways to prevent blockage of the stoma:
- Drink at least 10 glasses of liquid per day unless contraindicated.

Adequate hydration helps liquefy stool.

- Chew food thoroughly.

Thoroughly chewing food prevents food particles from blocking stoma.

- Avoid or eat only small amounts of foods that are high in fiber or hard to digest (e.g., popcorn, coconut, raw vegetables, bean sprouts, bamboo shoots, celery, caraway seeds, whole kernel corn, potato skins, fruit with seeds, nuts, fruit skins).

These foods can block the stoma.

- Ensure that skin barrier and pouch openings are large enough to prevent mechanical constriction of the stoma.

Appropriate sizing and placement of pouch system prevents the stoma from becoming blocked due to lack of appropriate drainage of effluent.

Instruct client in ways to unblock the stoma:
- Apply a warm compress to abdomen.
- Participate in relaxing activities (e.g., warm bath, reading).
- Assume a knee-chest position.
- Gently message the peristomal area.
- Irrigate the stoma or gently perform digital dilation of the stoma if prescribed.

These actions help relax abdominal muscles around the stoma and enhance removal of what is blocking the stoma.

Demonstrate techniques and have client provide a return demonstration of massage of the abdomen, irrigation of stoma, and digital dilation of stoma if appropriate.

Enhances client's self-esteem and confidence in ability to care for self.

THERAPEUTIC INTERVENTIONS	RATIONALE

Desired Outcome: The client will state signs and symptoms to report to the health care provider.

Independent Actions

Educate the client on signs and symptoms to report to the health care provider:
- Difficulty breathing
- Productive cough of discolored sputum
- Unusual or excessive drainage from the wound site
- Pain or swelling in the calf of one or both legs
- Unusual and continuous abdominal or pelvic pain

May indicate a thromboembolism.
May indicate an infection.

May indicate a deep vein thrombus.
May indicate that pain has not been well controlled or possible injury to the client.

Continued...

THERAPEUTIC INTERVENTIONS	RATIONALE
• Temperature above 38°C (100.4°F)	*May indicate an infection or dehydration.*
• Absence of or reduction in urinary output despite an adequate fluid intake	*May indicate a urinary tract infection.*
• Dark red, dusky blue, blue-black, purple, or pale stoma	*May indicate strangulation of the stoma.*
• Change in color, consistency, or odor of effluent that is not readily identified as a response to food or fluid intake	*May indicate a blockage in the bowel.*
• Unexplained change in shape, size, or height of stoma (use diagrams and descriptive terms so client does not confuse decreasing stoma size due to resolving edema with actual stomal retraction)	*May indicate injury, infection, or improper healing.*
• Excessive bleeding of stoma or bloody drainage from stoma	*May indicate injury.*
• Difficulty accomplishing ileostomy care	*May indicate lack of acceptance of physical changes or understanding of self-care.*
• Persistent skin irritation and breakdown	*May lead to an infection.*
• Bright red, bumpy, itchy rash or white-coated area on skin around stoma	*May indicate an allergic reaction or yeast infection.*
• Persistent thirst, dry mucus membranes, dizziness, or decreased urine output	*May indicate dehydration/inadequate fluid volume.*
• Irregular pulse, muscle weakness and cramping, nausea, and vomiting	*May indicate decreased serum potassium levels.*
• Headache, abdominal cramping, fatigue, and irritability	*May indicate decreased serum sodium levels.*
• Thin, watery ileostomy output; absence of ileostomy output; unusual foul odor of gas; abdominal distention and/or nausea and vomiting that does not resolve within 2 hours of implementing measures to relieve stomal blockage	*These indicate a possible blockage of bowel above the stoma.*
• Persistent leakage of pouch systems	*May indicate lack of understanding of self-care.*
• Persistent leakage of effluent from stoma if client has a continent ileostomy	
• Fever; pain or cramping in reservoir area; pain when draining the reservoir; and/or persistent watery, high-volume ileostomy output	*May indicate inflammation of the internal reservoir (pouchitis), which is a long-term complication that can develop in the client with a continent ileostomy.*
• Difficulty adjusting to changes in appearance and body functioning	*May indicate depression and place the client at risk for poor self-care.*

THERAPEUTIC INTERVENTIONS	RATIONALE
Desired Outcome: The client will identify appropriate community resources that can assist with home management and adjustment to changes resulting from the bowel diversion.	
Independent Actions	
Provide information about community resources that can assist the client and significant others with home management and adjustment to changes resulting from the bowel diversion (e.g., local ostomy support groups; community health agencies; ET nurse; home health agencies; financial, individual, and family counseling services).	*Provides for continuum of care once client is discharged from the acute care facility*

THERAPEUTIC INTERVENTIONS	RATIONALE

Desired Outcome: The client will verbalize an understanding of and a plan for adhering to recommended follow-up care including future appointments with health care provider, wound care, activity level, and medications prescribed.

Independent Actions

Reinforce physician's instructions regarding activity limitations:

- Avoid strenuous exercise and lifting objects more than 10 lb for at least 6 weeks.

Prevents potential injury to suture line and to stoma.

- Avoid participating in contact sports.

Provide client with a list of ostomy products he/she is using (including product name, size, and number) and where these supplies can be obtained.

Provides for continuum of care once client is discharged from acute care facility.

Explain the rationale for, side effects of, food and drug interactions, and the importance of taking medications as prescribed (e.g., electrolyte supplements, vitamins, antimicrobials).

Knowledge of medications and how they impact the system improves client adherence to treatment regimen and understanding of the importance of adhering to the prescribed medication regimen. The client must be able to recognize alterations in functioning related to medication administration and what clinical manifestations that should be reported to the health care provider.

Stress that oral medications should be crushed or in liquid, chewable, uncoated, or sugar-coated form rather than enteric-coated tablets or timed-release capsules.

Medications should be in liquid, chewable, crushed, uncoated, or sugar-coated so absorption can take place before the medication is excreted. Unabsorbed medications may cause stomal blockage.

ADDITIONAL NURSING DIAGNOSES

- Increased nutritional needs associated with the increased metabolic rate that occurs during wound healing

IMBALANCED NUTRITION: LESS THAN BODY REQUIREMENTS NDx

Related to:

- Decreased oral intake associated with prescribed dietary modifications; pain; weakness; fatigue; nausea; and fear of excessive ileostomy output, gas, and/or odor
- Inadequate nutrition replacement therapy
- Loss of nutrients associated with vomiting and excessive ileostomy output
- Decreased absorption of nutrients associated with loss of absorptive surface of the bowel resulting from surgical removal of a large portion of the intestine

INEFFECTIVE COPING NDx

Related to:

- Fear, anxiety, and depression associated with loss of control over bowel elimination (especially with a conventional ileostomy) and possibility of rejection by others
- Difficulty performing ileostomy care and incorporating the care into lifestyle
- Need for lifelong medical supervision

GRIEVING NDx

- Related to loss of usual manner of bowel elimination and change in appearance associated with the ileostomy

ENTERAL NUTRITION

Malnutrition, defined as an imbalance in the essential components of a healthy diet, is common in clients with acute and chronic illnesses cared for in both long-term and acute care settings. Left untreated, malnutrition can lead to compromise of the immune system, decreased respiratory ability, and muscle and adipose tissue wasting. Enteral nutrition, also known as tube feeding, is one method of providing nutritional support for malnourished clients who have a functioning gastrointestinal tract but are unable to take any or enough oral nourishment.

Categories of malnutrition include protein-calorie malnutrition (PCM), marasmus, and kwashiorkor. PCM can result from either primary or secondary factors. Primary PCM results from poor eating habits, whereas secondary PCM results from alterations in normal ingestion, digestion, absorption, or metabolism. Marasmus, which results from caloric and protein deficiencies, can lead to the loss of both muscle and body fat. Kwashiorkor results from a protein deficiency that occurs within the setting of a catabolic stress event such as surgery, burns, or infectious diseases.

Several diagnostic studies can assist in assessment of a client's nutritional state. Serum albumin, the most frequently assessed value, with a half-life of 20 to 22 days, is not the best indicator of a client's current state of malnutrition because the value lags behind a client's current protein deficiency by as much as 14 days. Serum prealbumin, with a half-life of approximately 2 days, is a much better indicator of a client's current nutritional state. Serum transferrin, blood

Continued...

urea nitrogen (BUN), hematocrit (Hct), and hemoglobin (Hgb) levels and the lymphocyte count provide additional values that assist in understanding a client's current nutritional state. Anthropometric measurements such as skinfold thickness, body circumferences, and bioelectrical impedance analysis can provide information about the amount of muscle mass, body fat, and protein reserves the client has.

Enteral nutrition is delivered via a nasogastric tube (short-term), or a tube placed in the duodenum or jejunum (long-term). Enteral nutrition can be delivered continuously or cyclically by pump, or intermittently by gravity or syringe bolus. The type of formula used for enteral nutrition varies depending upon the clinical diagnosis of the client.

This care plan focuses on the adult client undergoing enteral nutritional therapy in an acute care, extended care, or long-term care environment.

OUTCOME/DISCHARGE CRITERIA

The client will:
1. Progressively gain weight toward desired goal
2. Weigh within normal weight for height and age
3. Consume adequate nutrition to meet metabolic needs
4. Be free of signs of malnutrition
5. Maintain adequate fluid volume status
6. Recognize factors contributing to malnutrition/underweight
7. Be free of complications related to enteral feeding.

Nursing Diagnosis   RISK FOR ASPIRATION NDx

Definition: At risk for entry of gastrointestinal secretions, oropharynx secretions, solids, or fluids into the tracheobronchial passages

Related to:
- Decreased gastric motility
- Delayed gastric emptying
- Presence of a gastrointestinal tube
- Residual gastric volumes
- Impaired swallowing
- Decreased level of consciousness

CLINICAL MANIFESTATIONS

Subjective	Objective
N/A	Rhonchi; cough; dyspnea; tachycardia; presence of tube feeding in aspirate; dull percussion note over affected lung area

RISK FACTORS
- Presence of endotracheal tube
- Depressed cough and gag reflex
- Tracheostomy

DESIRED OUTCOMES

The client will
- Swallow and digest oral, nasogastric, or gastric feeding without aspiration
- Maintain patent airway and lung sounds

NOC OUTCOMES

Aspiration prevention

NIC INTERVENTIONS

Aspiration precautions; respiratory monitoring; swallowing therapy; airway suctioning

NURSING ASSESSMENT	RATIONALE
Assess client's level of consciousness, cough reflex, gag reflex, and swallowing ability. Assess for and report signs and symptoms of aspiration: • Crackles • Cough • Tachycardia • Presence of tube feeding aspirate • Dyspnea • Dull percussion note over affected area	*Reduced level of consciousness, depressed gag or cough reflexes, and alterations in normal swallowing increase the risk for aspiration.* *Early recognition of signs and symptoms of aspiration allows for prompt intervention.*

NURSING ASSESSMENT	RATIONALE
Assess client for signs of gastric retention: • Feelings of fullness • Nausea/vomiting • Abdominal distention	*Gastric retention can increase the risk for aspiration.*
Monitor chest radiograph results. Report findings of pulmonary infiltrate.	*Evidence of pulmonary infiltrate on chest radiograph can indicate that aspiration has occurred.*

THERAPEUTIC INTERVENTIONS	RATIONALE

Independent Actions

Confirm tube placement before each feeding or on a routine basis if tube feeding is continuous: • Aspirate stomach contents to verify tube placement.	*The greatest risks associated with enteral nutrition are malposition of feeding tubes and aspiration. Secondary marking of the tube after initial radiographic confirmation of proper placement allows for additional visual confirmation of tube placement before administering medications or feeding.*
• Check pH of gastric contents. • After radiographic confirmation of placement, mark the feeding tube with indelible ink at the exit site from the lip or naris.	*Measuring the pH of feeding tube aspirate is of limited benefit with continuous tube feedings because the feedings buffer gastric secretions.*
Implement measures during feeding to prevent aspiration: **D** ✦ • Elevate the head of the bead 30 degrees to 45 degrees at all times during feeding. • Keep head of the bed elevated for 30 to 60 minutes after intermittent feeding. • Discontinue feeding 30 to 60 minutes before placing the client in a supine position.	*Head-of-bed elevation helps to prevent the regurgitation of gastric contents.*
Check residual gastric volumes every 4 to 6 hours: **D** ✦ • Hold tube feeding if residual volume is greater than 200 mL or more than 110% to 120% of the hourly rate.	*Checking residual volumes helps to assess gastric emptying. Residual volumes increase with delayed gastric emptying. High gastric residual volumes increase the risk for aspiration of tube feeding formula.*

Dependent/Collaborative Actions

Obtain a chest radiograph to confirm placement of a nasogastric or orogastric feeding tube after insertion.	*Radiography is the "gold standard" for ruling out respiratory placement of blindly inserted enteral feeding tubes.*
If client has an artificial airway (e.g., tracheostomy or endotracheal tube), maintain proper cuff inflation.	*Maintaining adequate cuff pressure helps to secure the airway and prevent aspiration.*
Notify the appropriate health care provider if signs and symptoms of aspiration develop.	*Notifying the appropriate health care provider allows for modification of the treatment plan.*

Nursing Diagnosis

IMBALANCED NUTRITION: LESS THAN BODY REQUIREMENTS NDx

Definition: Intake of nutrients insufficient to meet metabolic needs

Related to: The presence of biological, economical, or psychological factors that prevent the ingestion, digestion, or absorption of nutrients sufficient to meet metabolic needs

CLINICAL MANIFESTATIONS

Subjective	Objective
Reports of abdominal cramping; abdominal pain; aversion to eating; lack of interest in food; perceived inability to eat food; altered taste sensation	Body weight 20% or more under ideal; diarrhea; hyperactive bowel sounds; weight loss with adequate food intake; poor muscle tone; pale mucous membranes; sore buccal cavity; capillary fragility; excessive hair loss

Continued...

RISK FACTOR	DESIRED OUTCOMES

• Stress of illness	The client will:
	  a. Progressively gain weight towards ideal body weight
	  b. Consume adequate nourishment
	  c. Be free of signs of malnutrition

NOC OUTCOMES	NIC INTERVENTIONS
Nutritional status: biochemical measures; nutritional status: energy	Nutritional therapy; nutritional monitoring; nutritional management

NURSING ASSESSMENT	**RATIONALE**
Assess for and report signs and symptoms of intolerance of enteral feeding: • Vomiting • Diarrhea • Abdominal pain/distention • Constipation • Absence of bowel sounds	*Early recognition of signs and symptoms of problems with enteral feeding allows for prompt intervention.*
Perform or assist with anthropometric measurements such as skinfold thickness if indicated. Report lower than normal values.	*Anthropometric measurements provide information about a client's muscle mass, body fat, and protein reserves.*
Monitor albumin, prealbumin, transferrin, BUN, Hct, and Hgb levels and lymphocyte counts, reporting abnormal values.	*Laboratory values assist in determining the nutritional status of the client.*
Monitor bedside glucose values.	*After initiation of tube feeding, a client is at risk for hyperglycemia. Bedside glucose checks should be assessed. Elderly clients often have difficulty handling high glucose loads and should be monitored closely.*
Assess daily weights.	*Daily weight values will determine whether adjustments to caloric intake are necessary.*

THERAPEUTIC INTERVENTIONS	**RATIONALE**
Independent Actions Ensure patency of enteral tube:	*Feeding tube occlusions are often caused by coagulation of protein-based formulas.*
• Irrigate with water before and after intermittent feedings. **D** ✦	*Routine water flushes with water are necessary to maintain tube patency.*
• Routinely flush tubes every 4 hours with 20 to 100 mL sterile water.	
Monitor client tolerance of tube feeding: • If gastric residual volume greater than 200 to 250 mL, hold tube feeding for 1 hour and recheck residual. **D** ✦	*Tube feedings should not be automatically discontinued because of a single elevated residual volume. The feeding should be held for 1 hour and the client assessed for symptoms of gastric distress. Gastric residual volumes less than 200 mL can be replaced. Any amount greater than 200 mL should be discarded and documented as output. Refer to institutional policy as to current practice regarding residual volumes, as protocols may vary.*
Dependent/Collaborative Actions Consult dietician to determine the number of calories and type of nutrients needed.	*Enteral formulas may vary based on client diagnose.*
Administer enteral feedings as ordered. Continuous feedings should be administered via a pump. **D** ✦	*Tube feedings are initiated slowly, increasing gradually during the first 24 to 48 hours to minimize side effects (e.g., nausea/diarrhea).*
Administer prokinetic agents. **D** ✦	*In the presence of high gastric volumes, prokinetic agents can be administered to promote gastric motility and prevent unnecessary cessation of tube feeding.*

THERAPEUTIC INTERVENTIONS	RATIONALE
Administer pancreatic enzyme solution if tube becomes clogged.	*Pancreatic enzyme solution with sodium bicarbonate has been successful in unblocking feeding tubes and in prolonging the time to occlusion. Other methods such as soft drinks and cranberry juice have not been consistently effective.*
Minimized interruptions to continuous tube feedings: • Maintain enteral feedings until the start of medical or diagnostic procedures. • Restart tube feeding within 1 hour unless contraindicated.	*Nutritional goals for enteral nutrition are often not met because of frequent interruption of feeding. Refer to institutional policy.*
If signs and symptoms of intolerance to tube feeding develop, consult appropriate health care provider.	*Notifying the appropriate health care provider allows for modification of the treatment plan.*

Nursing Diagnosis RISK FOR DEFICIENT FLUID VOLUME NDx

Definition: Decreased intravascular, interstitial, and/or intracellular fluid; this refers to dehydration: water loss alone without change in sodium

Related to: diarrhea, vomiting, or inadequate fluid intake

CLINICAL MANIFESTATIONS

Subjective	Objective
Verbalization of weakness	Change in mental status; decreased urine output; increased urine concentration; decreased capillary refill; increased body temperature; elevated Hct; decreased skin turgor; dry skin/mucous membranes; increased pulse rate; decreased B/P

RISK FACTORS
• Active fluid volume loss
• Failure of regulatory mechanisms

DESIRED OUTCOMES
The client will not experience a deficient fluid volume as evidenced by:
  a. Normal skin turgor
  b. Moist mucous membranes
  c. Stable weight
  d. B/P and pulse rate within normal range for client
  e. Capillary refill time less than 2 to 3 seconds
  f. Usual mental status
  g. BUN and Hct within normal limits
  h. Balanced intake and output

NOC OUTCOMES
Fluid balance

NIC NTERVENTIONS
Fluid monitoring; fluid management; hypovolemia management; intravenous therapy

NURSING ASSESSMENT	RATIONALE
Assess for and report signs and symptoms of deficient fluid volume: • Change in mental status • Decreased urine output • Increased urine concentration • Hyperthermia • Elevated Hct • Decreased skin turgor • Dry mucous membranes • Increased pulse rate • Decreased blood pressure	*Early recognition of signs and symptoms of deficient fluid volume allows for prompt intervention.*

Continued...

THERAPEUTIC INTERVENTIONS	RATIONALE

Independent Actions

Implement measures to decrease diarrhea:
- Check for medications that may contribute to diarrhea.
- Administer tube feeding at room temperature. ● ✦

- Decrease the risk of contamination of tube feeding formula:
  - Wash hands with an antimicrobial soap or alcohol-based hand rub for 10 seconds before preparing, handling, and assembling any portion of the tube feeding system.
  - Discard feedings that have been infusing more than 8 to 12 hours or follow manufacturer's guidelines. **D** ✦
  - Disinfect tube feeding container with 70% isopropyl alcohol, disinfecting the opening of the can and the rim before opening.
  - Refrigerate unused formula and record the date of opening.
  - Use closed systems when possible.
  - Change tubing every 24 hours.

Diarrhea is a common problem associated with enteral feeding. Feeding too fast, medications such as antibiotics, contamination of feeding formula, and type of formula can be contributing factors.

Contamination of tube feeding could introduce microbes, which could lead to development of diarrhea.

Dependent/Collaborative Actions

Implement measures to decrease diarrhea:
- Slow tube feeding rate or decrease the strength of the formula.

Implement measures to prevent dehydration:
- Increase supplemental fluids (water) via feeding tube or mouth as ordered.
- Monitor bedside glucose level upon initiation of feeding.

Consult the appropriate health care personnel (e.g., physician, dietician) if diarrhea persists, for a change in formula:
- Formula with more fiber content

Consult physician if signs and symptoms of deficient fluid volume persist or worsen.

The more calorically dense the formula, the greater the need for supplemental fluids.
Protein content greater than 16% can lead to dehydration.

Notifying the appropriate health care provider allows for modification of the treatment plan.

DISCHARGE TEACHING/CONTINUED CARE

Nursing Diagnosis **DEFICIENT KNOWLEDGE** NDx**; INEFFECTIVE FAMILY THERAPEUTIC REGIMEN MANAGEMENT** NDx**; OR INEFFECTIVE SELF HEALTH MANAGEMENT*** NDx

Definition: Absence or deficiency of cognitive information related to specific topic (lack of specific information necessary for clients/significant others) to make informed choices regarding condition/treatment/lifestyle changes; pattern of regulating and integrating into daily living and family processes a therapeutic regimen for treatment of illness and the sequelae that is unsatisfactory for meeting specific health goals

CLINICAL MANIFESTATIONS

Subjective	Objective
Verbalization of inability to follow prescribed regimen	Inaccurate follow through of instructions; inappropriate behaviors

*The nurse should select the nursing diagnostic label that is most appropriate for the client's discharge teaching needs

RISK FACTORS

- Denial of disease process
- Cognitive deficiency
- Failure to take action to reduce risk factors
- Lack of recall
- Information misinterpretation
- Unfamiliarity with information resources

NOC OUTCOMES	NIC INTERVENTIONS
Knowledge: treatment regimen; knowledge: infection control	Teaching: individual; teaching: psychomotor skill

NURSING ASSESSMENT	RATIONALE
Assess client's readiness and ability to learn. Assess meaning of nutritional therapy to client.	*Early recognition of readiness to learn and meaning of nutritional therapy to client allows for implementation of the appropriate teaching interventions.*

THERAPEUTIC INTERVENTIONS	RATIONALE

Desired Outcome: The client will be able to demonstrate proper technique in mixing and handling of solutions and administration sets.

Independent Actions

Instruct client and family on the proper way to mix, handle, and store enteral feedings. • Allow time for return demonstration.	*Enteral feeding should be refrigerated to prevent bacterial growth.*
Instruct client and family on proper care of enteral feeding administration sets: • Discard enteral feeding sets every 24 hours. • Allow time for return demonstration.	*Changing administration sets every 24 hours helps to prevent bacterial growth.*

THERAPEUTIC INTERVENTIONS	RATIONALE

Desired Outcome: The client will be able to demonstrate proper care of gastrostomy or jejunostomy tube.

Independent Actions

Instruct the client and family to inspect the skin surrounding the feeding tube site on a daily basis.	*The skin surrounding the feeding tube site may become irritated by gastric juices. The client should be instructed to report any redness or maceration.*
Instruct client and family on protective skin care measures around the feeding tube site: • Initially rinse with sterile water and dry. • After healed, the client may wash with mild soap and water. • A protective ointment may be used around the insertion site (zinc oxide, Karaya paste) until site is healed. • Site should be kept clean and dry.	*Actions help to protect the skin surrounding the feeding tube, preventing breakdown and infection.*
Instruct client to report the following signs and symptoms to health care provider: • Diarrhea • Vomiting • Constipation • Redness or purulent drainage around gastrostomy or jejunostomy site • Dislodgment of the tube	*These signs and symptoms may be a result of infection, contaminated formula, inappropriate formula, or signs of an infection at the feeding tube insertion site. The appropriate health care provider must be notified to determine whether a change in formula is necessary or whether an infection has developed.*

RISK FOR CONSTIPATION NDx

Related to:

- Poor fluid intake
- Formula components

RISK FOR INFECTION NDx

Related to:

- Bacterial contamination of tube feeding formula during preparation or administration
- Bacterial contamination of tube feeding delivery system
- Skin breakdown around jejunostomy or gastrostomy feeding tube site

⊖▸ GASTRECTOMY

Gastrectomy is the surgical removal of all or part of the stomach. A total gastrectomy involves removal of the entire stomach and anastomosis of the esophagus to the jejunum (esophagojejunostomy). It may be considered as treatment for advanced stomach cancer or Zollinger-Ellison syndrome that is not controlled by more conservative measures. However, a total gastrectomy is performed infrequently because it is so difficult to maintain an adequate nutritional status postoperatively. The more common type of gastrectomy performed is a partial gastrectomy. This less extensive surgery is most often done to treat peptic ulcer disease that continues to be symptomatic despite conservative management or to treat complications that develop as a result of the disease (e.g., perforation, gastric outlet obstruction, hemorrhage). A partial gastrectomy may also be performed to resect lesions that are believed to be precancerous.

A partial gastrectomy usually involves excision of 40% to 75% of the distal stomach including the antrum (which contains the gastrin-secreting cells) and a portion of the body of the stomach that contains much of the parietal cell mass. Gastrointestinal continuity is reestablished by anastomosis of the remaining stomach to the duodenum (gastroduodenostomy or Billroth I) or jejunum (gastrojejunostomy or Billroth II). In the latter procedure, the duodenal stump is left intact so that bile and pancreatic secretions can enter the jejunum. The decreased output of gastric secretions that results from a partial gastrectomy can be enhanced by a vagotomy (truncal, selective, or highly selective), which is often performed concurrently to further reduce stimulation of gastric secretions. A truncal vagotomy (resection of the vagal nerve trunks at the level of the esophageal hiatus) is the most effective in reducing gastric secretions; however, the extensive denervation also greatly suppresses gastric motility and impairs normal functioning of the pancreas, gallbladder, and small intestine.

Because of this, a selective vagotomy (which preserves the hepatic and celiac branches of the vagus nerve) or highly selective vagotomy (which only affects the parietal cell mass) is performed more frequently.

This care plan focuses on the adult client who is hospitalized for a partial gastrectomy. Much of the postoperative information is applicable to clients receiving follow-up care in an extended care facility or home setting.

OUTCOME/DISCHARGE CRITERIA

The client will:

1. Have surgical pain controlled
2. Have evidence of normal healing of the surgical wound
3. Have clear, audible breath sounds throughout lungs
4. Have no signs and symptoms of postoperative complications
5. Tolerate prescribed diet
6. Verbalize an understanding of ways to maintain an adequate nutritional status
7. Identify ways to control postvagotomy diarrhea if it occurs
8. Identify ways to manage dumping syndrome if it occurs
9. State signs and symptoms to report to the health care provider
10. Verbalize an understanding of and a plan for adhering to recommended follow-up care including future appointments with health care provider, medications prescribed, activity level, and wound care.

For a full, detailed care plan on this topic, go to http://evolve.elsevier.com/Haugen/careplanning/.

GASTRIC REDUCTION/BARIATRIC SURGERY

Gastric reduction or bariatric surgery is a procedure performed to control obesity. The methods most frequently used to accomplish gastric reduction are vertical banded gastroplasty and gastric bypass. Both involve reducing the capacity of the stomach to 30 to 50 mL by partitioning off a small portion of the stomach distal to the gastroesophageal junction to form a gastric pouch. A narrow outlet is then created for the gastric pouch so that it does not empty quickly. As a result of the decreased gastric capacity and delayed pouch emptying, it is expected that the client will experience early satiety and subsequently decrease his/her oral intake and lose weight.

Gastroplasty and gastric bypass differ with regard to the path the ingested food/fluid takes after it enters the gastric pouch. With a vertical banded gastroplasty, the gastric pouch is formed on the lesser curvature side of the stomach by the placement of two adjacent rows of vertical staple lines. The narrow channel created between the pouch and remaining stomach is reinforced with a ring of mesh or plastic to reduce the risk of channel widening. Food/fluid then passes from the pouch, through the channel, into the remaining stomach, and through the intestinal tract. Gastric bypass also incorporates gastric partitioning, but in this method of gastric reduction, the gastric pouch is created by the placement of horizontal rows of staples or by actual surgical transection of the stomach. A gastrojejunostomy (Roux-en-Y) is then performed so that foods/fluids pass from the pouch directly into the jejunum.

Clients are carefully screened physically and psychologically and must meet certain criteria before undergoing gastric reduction surgery. The criteria usually include massive obesity for at least 5 years, inability to reduce weight using other forms of treatment, weight that is at least 100 lb or 100% or more over ideal body weight, and obesity that results from a caloric intake greater than the body's needs rather than an underlying metabolic disorder. The client must also be emotionally stable, have no uncontrolled or severe major illness, verbalize a willingness to adhere to lifelong dietary modifications, and have access to adequate follow-up medical care.

This care plan focuses on the adult client hospitalized for gastric reduction surgery. Much of the information is relevant to the client receiving continued care in the home setting.

OUTCOME/DISCHARGE CRITERIA

The client will:
1. Have evidence of normal healing of surgical wounds
2. Have clear, audible breath sounds throughout lungs
3. Tolerate prescribed diet
4. Have no signs and symptoms of postoperative complications
5. Identify ways to prevent excessive stretching of the gastric pouch
6. Verbalize an understanding of ways to maintain an adequate nutritional status
7. Identify ways to reduce the risk of consuming excessive amounts of food, fluid, and calories
8. Demonstrate the ability to accurately calculate and measure the allotted amounts of food and fluid
9. State signs and symptoms to report to the health care provider
10. Identify community resources that can assist in the adjustment to prescribed dietary modifications and future changes in body image
11. Verbalize an understanding of and a plan for adhering to recommended follow-up care including future appointments with health care provider, activity level, medications prescribed, and wound care.

PREOPERATIVE USE IN CONJUNCTION WITH PREOPERATIVE AND POSTOPERATIVE CARE PLANS FOR ADDITIONAL DIAGNOSES

Nursing Diagnosis　DISTURBED SELF-CONCEPT*

Definition:
Disturbed body image NDx: Confusion in mental picture of one's physical self
Situational low self-esteem NDx: Development of a negative perception of self-worth in response to a current situation (specify)

Related to: Obesity and inability to lose weight by more conventional methods

CLINICAL MANIFESTATIONS

Subjective	Objective
Report of feelings or perceptions that reflect an altered view of one's body in appearance, structure, or function; verbally reports current challenge to self-worth; self-negating verbalizations; indecisive, nonassertive behavior	Lack of involvement in preoperative care or self-care

---

*This diagnostic label includes the nursing diagnoses of Disturbed body image and Chronic low self-esteem.

Continued...

RISK FACTORS

- Obesity
- Poor self-esteem
- Ineffective dieting

DESIRED OUTCOMES

The client will demonstrate a positive self-concept as evidenced by:
  a. Verbalization of feelings of self-worth
  b. Positive statements regarding anticipated effects of surgical procedure
  c. Maintenance of relationships with significant others
  d. Active participation in preoperative care and self-care

NOC OUTCOMES

Body image; self-esteem

NIC INTERVENTIONS

Body image enhancement; self-esteem enhancement; emotional support; support system enhancement

NURSING ASSESSMENT	**RATIONALE**
Assess for signs and symptoms of a disturbed self-concept: • Verbalization of negative feeling about self • Withdrawal from significant others • Lack of participation in preoperative care or self-care	*Early recognition of signs and symptoms of a disturbed self-concept allows for prompt intervention.*

THERAPEUTIC INTERVENTIONS	**RATIONALE**

Independent Actions

Implement measures to assist client to increase self-esteem (e.g., limit negative self-assessment, encourage positive comments about self, assist to identify strengths, give positive feedback about accomplishments, provide positive feedback about decision to have the surgery and lose weight).

Self-esteem is a major component of one's view of self. An increase in self-esteem has a positive effect on the client's self-concept.

Implement measures to reduce client's embarrassment about obesity:

- Obtain information from physician regarding client's height and weight so that oversized equipment and supplies (e.g., bed, chair, commode, B/P cuff, gowns, bathrobe) can be obtained before client is admitted.

If the equipment is obtained ahead of time, it helps the client feel more comfortable in the health care environment.

- Remove unnecessary furniture and equipment from room so client can move around easily. **D ● ✦**

Improves client's mobility.

- Provide privacy when weighing client. **D ● ✦**

Privacy while weighing the client decreases client embarrassment.

- Transfer client to and from operating room in own hospital bed rather than attempting to use a regular-sized stretcher.

Prevents embarrassment when trying to transfer client to a regular-sized stretcher.

Allow client to wear own clothes rather than hospital gown before and after surgery if desired.

Provides client some control over the situation

Assure client that he/she will be assisted with usual grooming and makeup habits after surgery if necessary.

Decreases anxiety concerning postoperative care.

Arrange for a visit from an individual who has achieved weight loss after gastric reduction surgery if client desires.

Provides client with an experiential perspective on postoperative care and lifestyle changes.

If client is expressing concerns about the amount of excess skin that will be present after the majority of weight loss occurs (usually after 1-1½ years), provide information about various clothing styles that may be most flattering (e.g., long-sleeved shirts or blouses) and reconstructive surgery that is available to remove excess skin from abdomen, breasts, upper arms, and thighs.

Decreases fear and anxiety concerning postoperative and lifestyle changes.

Dependent/Collaborative Interventions

Consult physician if client has unrealistic expectations of postoperative weight loss and dietary management.

Provides additional time for the physician to address client's concerns related to surgery and subsequent lifestyle changes,

POSTOPERATIVE: USE IN CONJUNCTION WITH THE STANDARDIZED POSTOPERATIVE CARE PLAN

Nursing Diagnosis # INEFFECTIVE BREATHING PATTERN NDx

Definition: Inspiration and/or expiration that does not provide adequate ventilation

Related to:

- Increased rate of respirations associated with fear and anxiety
- Decreased rate of respirations associated with the depressant effect of anesthesia (effect lasts longer in the obese client because adipose tissue more readily absorbs and stores anesthetic agents) and some medications (e.g., narcotic [opioid] analgesics, some antiemetics)
- Decreased depth of respirations associated with:
  - Depressant effects of anesthesia and some medications (e.g., narcotic [opioid] analgesics, some antiemetics)
  - Reluctance to breathe deeply because of pain and fear of dislodging tubes
  - Fear, anxiety, weakness, and fatigue
  - Restricted chest expansion resulting from:
    (1) Limited diaphragmatic excursion (occurs because of the large amount of abdominal adipose tissue and postoperative abdominal distention)
    (2) Decreased activity (chest expansion is restricted by the bed surface when client is lying in bed)
    (3) Increased weight of the chest wall of an obese client (especially in women with large, pendulous breasts)

CLINICAL MANIFESTATIONS

Subjective	Objective
Verbalization of shortness of breath	Limited chest excursion; tachypnea; dyspnea; use of accessory muscles when breathing; decreased pulse oximetry less than 85%

RISK FACTORS

- Surgical procedure
- Obesity
- Immobility

DESIRED OUTCOMES

The client will maintain an effective breathing pattern as evidenced by:
  a. Normal rate and depth of respirations
  b. Absence of dyspnea

NOC OUTCOMES

Respiratory status: ventilation

NIC INTERVENTIONS

Respiratory monitoring; ventilation assistance

NURSING ASSESSMENT	RATIONALE
Assess for and report signs and symptoms of an ineffective breathing pattern: • Complaints of feeling short of breath • Shallow or slow respirations • Limited chest excursion • Tachypnea • Dyspnea • Use of accessory muscles when breathing	*Early recognition of signs and symptoms of an ineffective breathing pattern allows for prompt intervention.*
Monitor for and report a significant decrease in oximetry results.	*Oximetry is a noninvasive method of measuring arterial oxygen saturation. The results assist in evaluating respiratory status.*

Continued...

THERAPEUTIC INTERVENTIONS	RATIONALE

Independent Actions

Implement measures to reduce chest or abdominal pain if present (e.g., splint incision with pillow during coughing and deep breathing). **D ● ✦**

Implement measures to decrease fear and anxiety (e.g., assure client that breathing deeply will not dislodge tubes or cause incision to break open, interact with client in a confident manner). **D ● ✦**

Implement measures to increase strength and activity tolerance if client is weak and fatigued (e.g., provide uninterrupted rest periods, maintain optimal nutrition). **D ● ✦**

Assist client to deep breathe or use incentive spirometer every 1 to 2 hours. **D ● ✦**

Instruct client to breathe slowly if hyperventilating.

Position client with head of bed elevated at least 30 degrees at all times. **D ● ✦**

Instruct and assist client to use overhead trapeze and turn at least every 2 hours.

Add extensions to tubings if necessary.

Instruct client to bend knees while coughing and deep breathing.

Instruct and assist client to splint incision with hands or pillow when coughing and deep breathing.

A client with upper abdominal pain often guards respiratory efforts and breathes shallowly in an attempt to prevent additional discomfort.

Fear and anxiety may cause a client to breathe shallowly or to hyperventilate.

Decreasing fear and anxiety allows the client to focus on breathing more slowly and taking deeper breaths.

An increase in strength and activity tolerance enables the client to breathe more deeply and participate in activities to improve breathing pattern.

Deep breathing and use of an incentive spirometer promote maximal inhalation and lung expansion.

Hyperventilation is an ineffective breathing pattern that can eventually lead to respiratory alkalosis. The client can often slow breathing rate by concentrating on doing so.

This position allows for maximal diaphragmatic excursion and lung expansion.

Repositioning promotes maximal chest wall and lung expansion.

Enables client to turn and move without fear of dislodging tubes.

Relieves tension on abdominal muscles and incision.

Provides support to the abdomen and helps to decrease discomfort when coughing and deep breathing.

Collaborative Diagnosis   # RISK FOR OVERDISTENTION OF THE GASTRIC POUCH

Related to:

- Accumulation of gas and fluid in the pouch associated with:
  - Decreased peristalsis and/or impaired functioning of nasogastric or gastrostomy tube
  - Obstruction of the pouch outlet (the channel between the pouch and distal stomach if gastroplasty performed or the opening between the pouch and jejunal loop if gastric bypass performed) resulting from edema and/or ingestion of medications or fluids that are too thick to pass through pouch outlet
- Excessive oral intake

CLINICAL MANIFESTATIONS

Subjective	Objective
Verbalization of frequent epigastric fullness and nausea	Vomiting

RISK FACTORS

- Physiological changes
- Inappropriate diet and intake

DESIRED OUTCOMES

The client will not experience overdistention of the gastric pouch as evidenced by:
  a. Decreased reports of epigastric fullness
  b. Absence of nausea and vomiting

NURSING ASSESSMENT	RATIONALE
Assess for and report signs and symptoms of overdistention of the gastric pouch (e.g., increasing reports of epigastric fullness, nausea, vomiting).	*Early recognition of signs and symptoms of overdistention of the gastric pouch allows for prompt intervention.*

THERAPEUTIC INTERVENTIONS	RATIONALE

Dependent/Collaborative Actions

Implement measures to prevent overdistention of the gastric pouch:

- Maintain patency of nasogastric or gastric tube; irrigate the tube only if ordered and with no more than prescribed amount of solution. **D** ✦

- Encourage and assist client with frequent position changes and ambulation as soon as allowed and tolerated. **D** ● ✦

- Instruct the client to avoid activities such as chewing gum and smoking.

- Do not change position of nasogastric or gastric tube unless ordered.

- When oral intake is allowed:
  - Adhere strictly to prescribed oral intake schedule (clients usually begin with hourly liquid feedings of 30 mL and, over at least 6 weeks, progress to 5 or 6 small [1-2 oz] liquid meals per day with 1-2 oz of water allowed periodically between meals).
  - Provide client with allotted amounts of fluids at the proper times; discard skipped "meals." **D** ● ✦
  - Instruct client to adhere to the liquid or blenderized diet as ordered.
  - Administer oral medication in liquid or chewable form or crushed thoroughly. **D** ● ✦

- Encourage client to eructate whenever the urge is felt.

- Encourage use of nonnarcotic analgesics once severe pain has subsided.

If signs and symptoms of overdistention occur:

Withhold all oral intake as ordered. **D** ● ✦

- Prepare client for upper abdominal radiographs to check placement of nasogastric or gastric tube if present.

- Assist physician with adjustment or reinsertion of the nasogastric or gastric tube if indicated.

Reduces gas and fluid accumulation during period of decreased peristalsis.

Activity stimulates peristalsis, which promotes passage of food through the gastrointestinal tract and decreases distention of the gastric pouch.
Reduces air swallowing.

The NG tube is usually positioned at the pouch outlet to help prevent obstruction of the opening into the distal stomach (if gastroplasty performed) or jejunal loop (if gastric bypass is performed).

The stomach size is reduced and the client will have to eat smaller meals to prevent overdistention of the stomach.

This is done so the client does not ingest feedings too close together, as this will cause overdistention of the stomach.
Oral intake that is too thick can block the pouch outlet, which may be narrower in the early postoperative period because of edema.
Prevents blockage of the pouch outlet.

Releases gas from the stomach
Narcotic (opioid) analgesics depress gastrointestinal motility.

Helps to reduce stomach distention
Determines appropriate placement of tubes and whether manipulation of them is required.

Collaborative Diagnosis RISK FOR PERITONITIS

Definition: Inflammation of the peritoneum.

Related to:

- Leakage of gastric contents into the peritoneum associated with disruption of the staple line (if gastroplasty performed) or proximal anastomosis (if gastric bypass performed)

CLINICAL MANIFESTATIONS

Subjective	Objective
Verbalization of abdominal pain	Nausea and vomiting; distended and rigid abdomen; diminished or absent bowel sounds; fever; tachypnea; increased WBC count

Continued...

RISK FACTORS

- Surgery
- Exposure to pathogens
- Exposure of abdominal contents to irritating fluids

DESIRED OUTCOMES

The client will not develop peritonitis as evidenced by:
  a. Gradual resolution of abdominal pain
  b. Soft, nondistended abdomen
  c. Temperature declining toward normal
  d. Stable vital signs
  e. Absence of nausea and vomiting
  f. Gradual return of normal bowel sounds
  g. WBC count declining toward normal

NURSING ASSESSMENT

Assess for and report signs and symptoms of peritonitis (e.g., increase in severity of abdominal pain; generalized abdominal pain; rebound tenderness; distended, rigid abdomen; increase in temperature; tachycardia; tachypnea; hypotension; nausea; vomiting; continued diminished or absent bowel sounds; WBC count that increases or fails to decline toward normal).

RATIONALE

Early recognition of signs and symptoms of peritonitis allows for prompt intervention.

THERAPEUTIC INTERVENTIONS

RATIONALE

Dependent/Collaborative Actions
Implement measures to prevent peritonitis:
- Implement measures to prevent wound infection:
  - Maintain an optimal nutritional status.
  - Administer vitamins and minerals as ordered. **D** ✦

  - Do not apply dressing too tight. **D** ✦
- Ensure dressings are secure enough to keep them from rubbing the wound.
  - Carefully remove tape from the wound. **D** ✦
  - Maintain adequate fluid volume of 2500 mL/day unless contraindicated. **D** ✦
- Perform measures to maintain patency of wound drain if present.
  - Keep tubing free of kinks. **D** ✦

  - Empty collection device as often as necessary. **D** ✦

  - Maintain suction as ordered. **D** ✦
- Perform measures to prevent inadvertent removal of the tube:
  - Use caution when changing dressings surrounding drain. **D** ✦
  - Provide extension tubing if necessary. **D** ✦
Instruct client not to pull on drain and drainage tubing. **D** ✦
- Perform actions to prevent stress on and subsequent leakage of gastric contents from the staple line or site of proximal anastomosis.
  - Implement measures to prevent overdistention of gastric pouch.
  - Implement measures to prevent nausea and vomiting (e.g., maintain patency of nasogastric or gastric tube, eliminate noxious sights and odors from the environment, instruct client to change positions slowly, administer antiemetics and/or gastrointestinal stimulants as ordered).
  - Do not adjust position of nasogastric or gastric tube unless ordered.

Adequate nutrition is needed to maintain normal function of the immune system. Vitamin and mineral supplements may be required to maintain nutritional status.
Tight dressings decrease circulation to the surgical site.
Applying secure dressings prevents wound irritation.
Prevents irritation of surgical site and damage to surrounding skin.

Maintains adequate circulatory volume.

Allows drainage to flow away from the wound and prevents distention of the conduit.
Prevents stress on the wound and stasis of drainage and prevents distention of the conduit.
Prevents stasis of secretions and prevents distention of conduit.

Prevents accidental dislodgment of a drain if present.

Enables client to move without placing tension on the drain
Prevents accidental dislodgment of the drain.

Distention can cause strain on the suture lines and subsequent leakage of gastric contents into the peritoneal cavity.
Prevents pressure and strain on the abdominal wound and the proximal anastomosis.

Adjustment of the nasogastric tube or gastric tube may cause disruption of staples or perforation at the site of proximal anastomosis.

THERAPEUTIC INTERVENTIONS	RATIONALE
If signs and symptoms of peritonitis occur:	
• Withhold oral intake and jejunostomy tube feedings as ordered.	*Prevents further leakage of food content into the abdominal cavity.*
• Place client on bedrest in a semi-Fowler's position.	*Assists in pooling or localizing gastric contents in the pelvis rather than under the diaphragm.*
• Prepare client for diagnostic test (e.g., abdominal radiograph, computed tomography, ultrasound).	*Decreases fear and anxiety.*
• Assist physician with insertion of nasogastric tube or gastric tube and maintain to suction as ordered.	*Removes secretions from the stomach*
• Administer antimicrobials as ordered.	*Treats infection.*
• Administer intravenous fluids and/or blood volume expanders if ordered.	*IV fluids/blood volume expanders prevents or treats shock, which can result from the increased capillary permeability that occurs with inflammation and the subsequent escape of protein, fluid, and electrolytes from the vascular space into the peritoneal cavity.*
• Prepare client for surgical intervention (e.g., repair of perforation) if planned.	*Decreases fear and anxiety.*

Collaborative Diagnosis

RISK FOR DEEP VEIN THROMBOSIS AND THROMBOEMBOLISM

Definition: A clot that detaches from the vessel wall and circulates within the blood, becoming lodged in a blood vessel

Related to:
• Venous stasis associated with decreased activity, increased blood viscosity (can result from deficient fluid volume), and pressure on abdominal vessels from excessive adipose tissue and abdominal distention
• Hypercoagulability associated with increased release of thromboplastin into the blood (occurs as a result of surgical trauma) and hemoconcentration and increased blood viscosity (can occur as a result of deficient fluid volume)
• Trauma to vein walls during surgery

CLINICAL MANIFESTATIONS

Subjective	Objective
Verbal reports of pain or tenderness in an extremity	Increase in circumference of extremity; distention of superficial vessels in extremity; unusual warmth of extremity; positive Homans' sign (not always a reliable indicator)

RISK FACTORS	DESIRED OUTCOMES
• Immobility	The client will not develop a deep vein thrombus as evidenced by:
• Inadequate fluid intake	a. Absence of pain, tenderness, swelling, and distended superficial vessels in extremities
• Ineffective treatment regimen	b. Usual temperature of extremities
	c. Negative Homans' sign

NURSING ASSESSMENT	RATIONALE
Assess for and report signs and symptoms of a deep vein thrombus:	*Early recognition of signs and symptoms of a deep vein thrombus allows for implementation of the appropriate interventions.*
• Pain or tenderness in extremity	
• Increase in circumference of extremity	
• Distention of superficial vessels in extremity	
• Unusual warmth of extremity	
• Positive Homans' sign (not always a reliable indicator)	
• Pain in area where thromboembolus lodged	

Continued...

THERAPEUTIC INTERVENTIONS	RATIONALE
Independent Actions	
Implement measures to prevent thrombus formation: **D** ✦	
• Perform actions to prevent peripheral pooling of blood such as leg exercises:	*Leg and ankle exercises help promote venous return and reduce the risk of venous thromboembolism.*
• Ankle rotation	*These actions facilitate venous return to the heart.*
• Alternate dorsiflexion and plantar extension of both feet	
If signs and symptoms of a deep vein thrombus occur: **D** ✦	
• Maintain client on bedrest until activity orders received.	*Avoid putting pressure on the posterior knees because this action will compress leg veins, increasing turbulent blood flow, and increase the risk of thromboembolism formation. If a thrombus is suspected, avoid activity, elevate the affected extremity, and do not massage the area because of the danger of dislodging the thrombus.*
• Elevate foot of bed 15 to 20 degrees above heart level if ordered.	
• Discourage positions that compromise blood flow (e.g., pillows under knees, crossing legs, sitting for long periods).	
Dependent/Collaborative Actions	
Implement measures to prevent thrombus formation:	
• Apply mechanical devices designed to increase venous return in the immobile patient: **D** ✦	*These devices decrease venous stasis in the lower extremities and increase venous return through the deep leg veins, which are prone to the formation of a thromboembolism. These devices should remain in place until the patient is ambulatory.*
• Sequential compression devices	
• Thromboembolic (elastic) stockings	
• Maintain a minimum fluid intake of 2500 mL/day (unless contraindicated).	*Adequate hydration helps to reduce blood viscosity, which may contribute to the formation of a thrombus.*
If signs and symptoms of a deep vein thrombus occur:	
• Administer anticoagulants:	*Anticoagulants, if indicated, help to suppress the formation of clots.*
• Low- or adjusted-dose heparin	
• Fondaparinux	
• Warfarin	
• Low-molecular-weight heparin	
Prepare client for diagnostic studies (e.g., venography, duplex ultrasound, impedance plethysmography).	*Additional studies may be indicated to confirm the presence of a thromboembolism so the appropriate interventions can be implemented.*

THERAPEUTIC INTERVENTIONS	RATIONALE
If signs and symptoms of embolism occur:	
• Maintain client on strict bedrest in a semi- to high-Fowlers position	*Improves lung expansion and provides supplemental oxygen.*
• Maintain oxygen therapy as ordered	
• Prepay client for diagnostic tests (e.g. blood gases, D-dimer level, ventilation-perfusion lung scan; pulmonary angiography)	
• Prepare client for the following if planned:	
• Venal caval interruption	*Decreases client fear/anxiety to prevent further pulmonary emboli*
• Embolectomy	*Removal of emboli*

DISCHARGE TEACHING/CONTINUED CARE

Nursing Diagnosis | # DEFICIENT KNOWLEDGE NDx; INEFFECTIVE FAMILY THERAPEUTIC REGIMEN MANAGEMENT NDx; OR INEFFECTIVE SELF-HEALTH MAINTENANCE= NDx

Definition: Absence or deficiency of cognitive information related to specific topic (lack of specific information necessary for clients/significant others) to make informed choices regarding condition/treatment/lifestyle changes; pattern of regulating and integrating into daily living and family processes a therapeutic regimen for treatment of illness and the sequelae of illness that is unsatisfactory for meeting specific health goals.

RISK FACTORS
- Financial concerns related to lifestyle change
- Cognitive difficult
- Inability to integrate exercise and diet into lifestyle

CLINICAL MANIFESTATIONS

Subjective
Verbalization of difficulty in implementing lifestyle changes; expressed financial concerns; refusal to participate in self-care

NOC OUTCOMES

Participation: health care decisions; compliance behavior; adherence behavior; health beliefs: perceived ability to perform; health beliefs: perceived control; knowledge: diet; knowledge: treatment regimen

NIC INTERVENTIONS

Self-modification assistance; weight reduction assistance; teaching: prescribed diet; behavior modification; support system enhancement; health system guidance; teaching: individual; teaching: prescribed diet; self-modification assistance; support system enhancement

NURSING ASSESSMENT

Assess for indications that the client may be unable to effectively manage the therapeutic regimen:
  Failure to adhere to treatment plan while in the hospital (e.g., not adhering to dietary modifications and fluid restrictions, refusing to increase activity)
  Statements reflecting a lack of understanding of dietary modifications and factors that will cause stretching of the gastric pouch
  Verbalization of an inability to integrate necessary dietary modifications and exercise program into lifestyle
  Statements reflecting the belief that the surgical procedure will result in continued weight loss even without adherence to the prescribed dietary modifications

RATIONALE

Early recognition of signs and symptoms of inability to effective manage the therapeutic regimen allows for prompt intervention.

THERAPEUTIC INTERVENTIONS

Desired Outcome: The client will verbalize an understanding of the lifestyle changes that need to be maintained as a result of gastric reduction surgery.
Explain the surgical procedure and importance of dietary modifications and a balanced exercise program in terms the client can understand; emphasize that adherence to the treatment program is necessary if an optimal weight is to be attained.

RATIONALE

Understanding of surgical procedure will help client maintain diet and exercise program, as these will help client meet weight reduction goals.

---

*The nurse should select the diagnostic label that is most appropriate for the client's discharge teaching needs.

NDx = NANDA-I Diagnosis **D** = Delegatable Action ● = UAP ✦ = LVN/LPN ⏵▶ = Go to ⏵volve for animation

Continued...

THERAPEUTIC INTERVENTIONS	RATIONALE
Inform the client that prescribed food and fluid modifications are not as strict after the surgical area has healed (usually 6-8 weeks).	*After 6 to 8 weeks, the client has more dietary choices than those available in the early postoperative period.*
Stress the positive effects of compliance with dietary modifications and exercise program (e.g., weight loss resulting in change in appearance; decreased risk of development or worsening of conditions such as diabetes mellitus, cardiovascular disease, respiratory problems, and arthritis).	*Compliance with dietary modification and exercise program is important to continued weight reduction and subsequent maintenance.*
Encourage activities other than eating to cope with stress (e.g., exercise).	*Stress eating will interfere with dietary regimen.*
Provide written instructions about future appointments with health care provider, dietary modifications, and signs and symptoms to report.	*Provides an information resource for the client once discharged from the acute care facility.*

THERAPEUTIC INTERVENTIONS	RATIONALE

Desired Outcome: The client will identify ways to prevent excessive stretching of the gastric pouch.

Independent Actions

Instruct client in ways to prevent excessive stretching of the gastric pouch:

- Decrease risk of blockage of the pouch outlet by:
  - Limiting oral intake to liquids and blenderized foods for about 6 to 8 weeks after surgery
  - Taking all prescription and nonprescription medications in liquid or chewable form or crushing them thoroughly
  - Chewing food thoroughly

- Do not exceed prescribed volume of food/fluid intake.

- Do not make up for skipped meals while on an hourly drinking/eating schedule.
- Eat and drink slowly.

- Avoid intake of carbonated beverages for 6 to 8 weeks after surgery and limit intake of these beverages after that time.
- When solid foods are allowed, consume fluids between rather than with meals.

Liquids and blenderized foods will move out of the stomach quicker than solid food.
Unabsorbed pills may block output from the pouch.

Thoroughly chewing food breaks it down into small particles, which improves digestion and helps the bolus move more quickly out of the stomach.
Limiting the volume of intake prevents over distention of the stomach.
Provides potential for overeating and stretching of the gastric pouch.
Eating and drinking slowly, increases satiety, as this occurs approximately 20 minutes after beginning a meal.
Carbonated beverages increase gas in the stomach and the potential for over distention.
Fluids will fill the stomach quickly and when combined with a meal can cause overdistention of the stomach.

THERAPEUTIC INTERVENTIONS	RATIONALE

Desired Outcome: The client will verbalize an understanding of ways to maintain an adequate nutritional status.

Independent Actions

Instruct client regarding ways to maintain an adequate nutritional state:

- Do not skip meals.

- Consume foods/fluids from each food group daily as diet advances.
- Consume adequate amounts of protein (e.g., blenderized drinks containing peanut butter, pureed meats and fish, cottage cheese) as diet advances.
- Take vitamin and mineral supplements as prescribed.

- Obtain dietary consult if indicated to assist client in planning meals.

Skipping meals will decrease caloric intake and can negatively affect nutritional status.
Daily consumption from all the food groups provides for nutritional balance in the diet.
Prevents over distention of the stomach while maintaining nutritional status.

Dietary supplements may be required to maintain nutritional status.
Meal planning should include foods the client likes while providing the appropriate nutrition.

THERAPEUTIC INTERVENTIONS	RATIONALE

Desired Outcome: The client will identify ways to reduce the risk of consuming excessive amounts of food, fluid, and calories through accurately calculating and measuring the allotted amounts of foods and fluid.

Independent Actions
Instruct client in ways to reduce the risk of consuming excessive amounts of food, fluid, and calories:

- Limit food/fluid intake to prescribed volume.

- Prepare food ahead of time, freeze in 1-oz portions using plastic ice cube trays or plastic bags, and then reheat only allowed amounts at mealtime.
- Have jars of prepared strained baby food products rather than high-calorie puddings and snacks on hand.
- Have only low-calorie drinks available (other than the required high-protein supplements).
- Decrease the risk of hunger by adhering to a schedule of 5 or 6 meals per day as diet advances (each meal will usually consist of 2-4 tablespoons of food).

- Serve food on a small plate.

- Eat and drink very slowly (use techniques such as putting fork down between bites of food and putting glass down between sips of fluid).
- If going out to dinner, order an appetizer and have it served with everyone else's entrée.
- Avoid excessive intake of high-calorie foods/fluids

- Demonstrate ways to measure foods/fluids accurately using measuring spoons and a cup with 1-oz markings.
- Allow time for questions, clarification, and return demonstration.

Consumption of excessive food/fluid and calories can lead to overdistention of the stomach and weight gain.
Helps with meal planning and for eating the appropriate amount of food.

These preparations are easily digested and won't overdistend the stomach.
Prevents increased caloric intake.

Adhering to a schedule for meals provides for adequate nutrition without client becoming hungry between meals.

Eating off of a small plate provides an illusion that meals are larger than they really are.
Allows satiety center of the brain to register fullness before overeating.

Allows the client to eat with party without feeling deprived.

It is possible to maintain or gain weight if only high-calorie substances are consumed.
These help the client understand the size of servings using common kitchen items.
Having a client do a return demonstration improves client's self-esteem and ability to be successful in lifestyle changes.

THERAPEUTIC INTERVENTIONS	RATIONALE

Desired Outcome: The client will state signs and symptoms to report to the health care provider.

Independent Actions
Educate the client on signs and symptoms to report to the health care provider:

- Difficulty breathing
- Productive cough of discolored sputum
- Unusual or excessive drainage from the wound site
- Pain or swelling in the calf of one or both legs
- Unusual and continuous abdominal or pelvic pain
- Temperature above 38°C (100.4°F)
- Absence of or reduction in urinary output despite an adequate fluid intake
- Nausea and vomiting after consuming prescribed amount of foods/fluids
- Inability to adhere to dietary modifications
- Weight gain
- Inability to lose weight or excessive weight loss (expected weight loss is usually about 10 lb per month for the first year or 30% of preoperative body weight by the end of the first year)

These clinical manifestations indicate a variety of complications from the surgery including: deep vein thrombosis, thromboembolism, infection, and dehydration.

Client may be experiencing dumping syndrome.

Increases potential weight gain.
Indicates problems maintaining lifestyle changes.

Continued...

THERAPEUTIC INTERVENTIONS	RATIONALE
• Abdominal cramping, flushing, palpitations, weakness, and/or dizziness within 30 minutes after eating	*May indicate dumping syndrome, which sometimes occurs after bypass when the client begins to eat solid food; if dumping syndrome does occur, symptoms are usually mild and self-limiting or easily controlled with minor dietary modifications.*
Reinforce the physician's instructions regarding need to adhere to a schedule of moderate exercise (clients are usually instructed to begin a walking program and should be walking 1-2 miles/day by the fourth week after discharge).	*Regular moderate exercise improves activity tolerance and weight loss.*

THERAPEUTIC INTERVENTIONS	RATIONALE

Desired Outcome: The client will identify community resources that can assist in the adjustment to prescribed dietary modifications and future changes to body image.

Independent Actions

Provide information about community resources that can assist the client with adjustment to prescribed dietary modifications and future changes in body image (e.g., weight reduction groups, counseling services, support groups of persons who have had the same or similar surgery).	*Provides for continuum of care once client is discharged from the acute care facility.*
Initiate a referral if needed.	

THERAPEUTIC INTERVENTIONS	RATIONALE

Desired Outcome: The client will verbalize an understanding of and a plan for adhering to recommended follow-up care including future appointments with health care provider, activity level, medications prescribed, and wound care.

Independent Actions

Reinforce the importance of follow-up appointments with the health care provider.	*Follow-up visits to the health care provider improve the potential for a client's adherence to treatment regimen and lifestyle changes.*
Include significant others in teaching sessions if possible.	*Knowledge of the required lifestyle changes improves the significant other's ability to support client's adherence to the treatment regimen.*
Encourage questions and allow for reinforcement and clarification of information provided about treatment regimen.	
Provide written instructions on scheduled appointments with health care provider, dietary modifications, activity level, treatment plan, medications, and signs and symptoms to report.	*Provides an information resource for the client after discharge from the acute care facility.*

ADDITIONAL NURSING DIAGNOSES:

IMBALANCED NUTRITION: LESS THAN BODY REQUIREMENTS NDx

Related to:
• Decreased oral intake associated with nausea, pain, weakness, fatigue, prescribed dietary modifications, and early satiety resulting from small gastric pouch and delayed pouch emptying
• Inadequate nutritional replacement therapy
• Increased nutritional needs associated with the increased metabolic rate that occurs during wound healing

ACTUAL/RISK FOR IMPAIRED TISSUE INTEGRITY NDx

Related to:
• Disruption of tissue associated with the surgical procedure
• Delayed wound healing associated with factors such as decreased nutritional status and inadequate blood supply to wound area
• Irritation of skin associated with contact with wound drainage, pressure from tubes, and use of tape

- Difficulty keeping deep skinfold areas dry
- Damage to the skin and/or subcutaneous tissue associated with:

- Friction or shearing when moving in bed
- Pressure on tissue as a result of excessive body weight and decreased activity

GASTROINTESTINAL BLEED, ACUTE

Upper gastrointestinal (GI) bleeding accounts for a significant number of hospital admissions each year. Ulcers in the stomach or duodenum are the major cause of GI bleeding. Other causes include esophageal varices, erosive esophagitis or gastritis, gastric cancer, Mallory-Weiss tears, regular use of ulcerogenic medications such as corticosteroids and nonsteroidal anti-inflammatory drugs (NSAIDs), vascular anomalies (e.g., angiodysplasia), and certain blood dyscrasias (e.g., leukemia, aplastic anemia).

The severity of the bleed ranges from slight oozing to frank, profuse hemorrhage and depends on whether the source is arterial, venous, or capillary. Significant bleeding is almost always arterial in nature. A massive GI bleed is generally considered to be a loss of more than 1500 mL of blood. Hematemesis of bright red or "coffee ground" vomitus is often the initial symptom of an upper GI bleed. Melena (dark, tarry stools) can also indicate upper GI bleeding that is occurring at a slower rate.

Most people who experience a GI bleed spontaneously stop bleeding. However, treatment is initiated immediately in cases of massive bleeding and consists of endoscopic hemostasis of the bleeding vessel. Vasoactive medications such as epinephrine, octreotide, or vasopressin may also be administered to help stop the bleeding. Gastric lavage may be done before endoscopy to remove blood from the stomach and improve endoscopic visualization. If bleeding continues, surgery may be necessary. Subsequent treatment to prevent rebleeding depends on the cause of the bleeding.

This care plan focuses on the adult client hospitalized with a massive upper GI bleed. It should be used in conjunction with the care plans on Peptic Ulcer and Cirrhosis if it is determined that the client's bleed is associated with either of these conditions.

OUTCOME/DISCHARGE CRITERIA

The client will:
1. Have adequate tissue perfusion
2. Tolerate prescribed activity without a significant change in vital signs, chest pain, dizziness, or extreme fatigue or weakness
3. Have no signs and symptoms of complications
4. Identify ways to reduce the risk for rebleeding
5. State signs and symptoms to report to the health care provider
6. Verbalize an understanding of and a plan for adhering to recommended follow-up care including future appointments with health care provider, medications prescribed, and dietary restrictions.

Nursing Diagnosis ## INEFFECTIVE PERIPHERAL TISSUE PERFUSION NDx

Definition: Decrease in blood circulation to the periphery that may compromise health

Related to:
Hypovolemia associated with GI bleeding

CLINICAL MANIFESTATIONS

Subjective	Objective
Complaint of nausea, abdominal pain or tenderness; complaint of dizziness and lightheadedness	Hypoactive or absent bowel sounds; nausea; abdominal distention; abdominal pain or tenderness; tachycardia; hypotension; cyanotic, pale skin; oliguria; capillary refill time greater than 2 to 3 seconds; elevated BUN and serum creatinine levels

NDx = NANDA-I Diagnosis **D** = Delegatable Action ● = UAP ✦ = LVN/LPN ⊖▶ = Go to ⊖volve for animation

Continued...

RISK FACTOR

* Inadequate fluid volume replacement

DESIRED OUTCOMES

The client will maintain adequate tissue perfusion as evidenced by:
a. B/P within normal range and stable with position change
b. Usual mental status
c. Extremities warm with absence of pallor and cyanosis
d. Palpable peripheral pulses
e. Capillary refill time less than 2 to 3 seconds
f. BUN and serum creatinine levels within normal limits
g. Urine output at least 30 mL/h

NOC OUTCOMES

Circulation status; tissue perfusion: abdominal organs; tissue perfusion: cardiac; tissue perfusion: cerebral; tissue perfusion: peripheral; tissue perfusion: pulmonary

NIC INTERVENTIONS

Circulatory care: arterial insufficiency; circulatory care: venous insufficiency; cerebral perfusion promotion; hypovolemia

NURSING ASSESSMENT

Assess for and report signs and symptoms of diminished tissue perfusion:
* Decreased B/P
* Decline in systolic B/P of more than 15 mm Hg when client changes from a lying to a sitting or standing position
* Restlessness, confusion, or other change in mental status
* Reports of dizziness or lightheadedness or occurrence of syncopal episodes
* Cool, pale, or cyanotic skin
* Diminished or absent peripheral pulses
* Capillary refill time greater than 2 to 3 seconds
* Elevated BUN and serum creatinine levels
* Oliguria

RATIONALE

Early recognition of signs and symptoms of diminished GI tissue perfusion allows for prompt intervention.

THERAPEUTIC INTERVENTIONS

Independent Actions
Implement measures to maintain adequate tissue perfusion:
* Maintain a minimum fluid intake of 2500 mL/day if able.
* Instruct client to change from a supine to an upright position slowly.
* Maintain a comfortable room temperature and provide client with adequate clothing and blankets. **D** ● ✦

Dependent/Collaborative Actions
Implement measures to maintain adequate tissue perfusion:
* Prepare client for measures that may be performed to control bleeding:
  * Endoscopic thermocoagulation, sclerotherapy, or banding of bleeding varices
  * Intra-arterial or intravenous administration of vasoactive medications (e.g., epinephrine, octreotide, vasopressin)
  * Surgery
* Administer intravenous fluids and blood as ordered.

RATIONALE

Maintains adequate circulatory volume and tissue perfusion.
Allows time for autoregulatory mechanisms to adjust to the change in distribution of blood associated with an upright position
Exposure to cold causes generalized vasoconstriction.

Processes that will obliterate bleeding varices.

Maintains adequate circulatory status and tissue perfusion.

THERAPEUTIC INTERVENTIONS	RATIONALE
• Administer the following medications if ordered to reduce the risk of rebleeding:	*These medications decrease acid production and irritation of the stomach lining.*
• Proton pump inhibitors (e.g., omeprazole, lansoprazole, pantoprazole, esomeprazole)	
• Histamine₂-receptor antagonists (e.g., famotidine, ranitidine, nizatidine) **D** ✦	*Histamine receptor antagonists and proton-pump inhibitors suppress secretion of gastric acid.*
Consult appropriate health care provider if signs and symptoms of diminished tissue perfusion persist or worsen.	*Allows for prompt alterations in interventions.*

Nursing Diagnosis RISK FOR IMBALANCED FLUID VOLUME NDx; RISK FOR ELECTROLYTE IMBALANCE* NDx

Definition: Risk for developing an imbalance of electrolytes and fluids in the intracellular and extracellular compartments of the body

Related to:
- **Deficient fluid volume NDx** related to blood loss, decreased oral intake, and loss of fluid associated with vomiting and nasogastric tube drainage
- **Hypokalemia, hypochloremia, and metabolic alkalosis** related to loss of electrolytes and hydrochloric acid associated with vomiting and nasogastric tube drainage

CLINICAL MANIFESTATIONS

Subjective	Objective
Complaint of nausea; headache	Poor skin turgor; dry, cracked mucous membranes; hypotension; weight loss; prolonged capillary refill greater than 2 to 3 seconds; decreased urine output; increased urine specific gravity; vomiting; positive Chvostek's and Trousseau's sign; abnormal serum electrolyte levels; metabolic acidosis

RISK FACTORS
- Chronic illness
- Stress
- Infection
- Inadequate therapeutic regimen

DESIRED OUTCOMES

The client will maintain fluid and electrolyte balance as evidenced by:
a. Normal skin turgor
b. Moist mucous membranes
c. Stable weight
d. B/P and pulse rate within normal range for client and stable with position change
e. Capillary refill time less than 2 to 3 seconds
f. Usual mental status
g. Balanced intake and output
h. Urine specific gravity within normal range
i. Soft, nondistended abdomen with normal bowel sounds
j. Absence of cardiac dysrhythmias, muscle weakness, paresthesias, twitching, spasms, and dizziness
k. BUN, Hct, serum electrolyte, and arterial blood gas values within normal range

NOC OUTCOMES

Fluid balance; electrolyte and acid-base balance

NIC INTERVENTIONS

Fluid management; electrolyte management: hypokalemia; electrolyte management: hypocalcemia; electrolyte management: hypomagnesemia; acid-base management: metabolic acidosis; diarrhea management

*The nurse should select the diagnostic label that is most appropriate for the client's discharge teaching needs.

 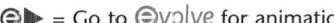

Continued...

NURSING ASSESSMENT	RATIONALE
Assess for and report signs and symptoms of deficient fluid volume: • Decreased skin turgor, dry mucous membranes, thirst • Weight loss of 2% or greater over a short period • Postural hypotension and/or low B/P • Weak, rapid pulse • Capillary refill time longer than 2 to 3 seconds • Neck veins flat when client is supine • Change in mental status • Decreased urine output with increased specific gravity (reflects an actual rather than potential fluid deficit) • Significant increase in BUN and Hct above previous levels • Hypokalemia (e.g., cardiac dysrhythmias, postural hypotension, muscle weakness, nausea and vomiting, abdominal distention, hypoactive or absent bowel sounds) • Hypomagnesemia and/or hypocalcemia (e.g., anxiousness; irritability; cardiac dysrhythmias; positive Chvostek's and Trousseau's signs; numbness or tingling of fingers, toes, or circumoral area; hyperactive reflexes; tetany; seizures) • Metabolic acidosis (e.g., drowsiness; disorientation; stupor; rapid, deep respirations; headache; nausea and vomiting; cardiac dysrhythmias; low pH and CO_2 content)	*Early recognition of signs and symptoms of electrolyte imbalance allows for prompt intervention.*

THERAPEUTIC INTERVENTIONS	RATIONALE

Dependent/Collaborative Actions
Implement measures to prevent or treat imbalanced fluid and electrolytes:
• Perform actions to prevent nausea and vomiting:
  • Insert nasogastric tube and maintain suction and/or perform gastric lavage if ordered.
  • Administer antiemetics if ordered. **D** ✦
	
	Maintaining an NG tube to suction removes blood from the stomach reducing the stimulus to vomit.
	Antiemetics decrease nausea and vomiting, which decreases fluid and electrolyte loss.

• If gastric lavage is being done or nasogastric tube is being irrigated frequently with large volumes of solution, consult physician about using saline rather than water. • Administer intravenous fluid and electrolytes as ordered. Once oral intake is allowed, maintain a fluid intake of at least 2500 mL/day unless contraindicated. **D** ✦ Consult physician if signs and symptoms of imbalanced fluid and electrolytes persist or worsen.	*Water is sometimes preferred because it breaks up clots better than saline, but irrigation with large volumes of water may create electrolyte imbalance.* *IV fluids maintain adequate circulatory balance.* *Maintains circulatory fluid volume status.* *Notification of the physician allows for prompt alteration in interventions.*

Nursing Diagnosis **RISK FOR ASPIRATION** NDx

Definition: At risk for entry of gastrointestinal secretions, oropharyngeal secretions, solids, or fluids into the tracheobronchial passages.

Related to: hematemesis and possible decreased level of consciousness

CLINICAL MANIFESTATIONS

Subjective	Objective
N/A	Rhonchi; dull percussion note over affected lung area; cough; tachypnea; dyspnea; tachycardia; chest radiograph results showing pulmonary infiltrate

RISK FACTORS

- Depressed gag reflex
- Increased gastric residual volume
- Increased intragastric pressure
- Impaired swallowing

DESIRED OUTCOMES

The client will not aspirate as evidenced by:
a. Clear breath sounds
b. Resonant percussion note over lungs
c. Absence of cough, tachypnea, and dyspnea

NOC OUTCOMES

Respiratory status: airway patency; respiratory status: gas exchange

NIC INTERVENTIONS

Respiratory monitoring; aspiration precautions; airway suctioning

NURSING ASSESSMENT

Assess for and report signs and symptoms of aspiration (e.g., rhonchi, dull percussion note over affected lung area, cough, tachypnea, dyspnea, tachycardia, chest radiograph results showing pulmonary infiltrate).

RATIONALE

Early recognition of signs and symptoms of aspiration allows for prompt intervention.

THERAPEUTIC INTERVENTIONS

RATIONALE

Independent Actions

Implement measures to reduce the risk for aspiration:

- Keep head of bed elevated at least 45 degrees if vital signs are stable, or position client on side (if client is hypotensive, elevating the head of bed is contraindicated).

This position uses gravity to facilitate movement of foods/fluids through the pharynx into the esophagus where the risk of aspiration is greatly reduced.

Dependent/Collaborative Actions

Implement measures to reduce the risk for aspiration:

- Perform actions to prevent nausea and vomiting (e.g., insert nasogastric tube, provide oral hygiene, eliminate noxious odors, administer antiemetics as needed). **D** ✦

Withhold oral foods/fluids as ordered. **D** ● ✦

- Perform oropharyngeal suctioning and provide oral hygiene as often as needed. **D** ● ✦

If signs and symptoms of aspiration occur:

- Perform tracheal suctioning.
- Withhold oral intake.
- Prepare client for chest radiograph.

These actions decrease incidence of nausea and vomiting thus decreasing the risk of aspiration.

Keeps the stomach empty, decreasing the chance of aspiration
Suctioning and frequent oral hygiene removes any blood and vomitus and keeps oral pharynx clean.

Removes aspirate
Keeps the stomach empty
Shows where the aspirate has lodged and potential damage to the lungs.

Nursing Diagnosis **RISK FOR ACTIVITY INTOLERANCE** NDx

Definition: Insufficient physiological or psychological energy to endure or complete required or desired daily activities

Related to:

- Hypoxia associated with anemia resulting from blood loss
- Difficulty resting and sleeping associated with assessment and treatments, fear, and anxiety

CLINICAL MANIFESTATIONS

Subjective	Objective
Verbalization of feeling tired; chest pain	Dyspnea on exertion; tachycardia with exertion; B/P increase with exertion

---

Continued...

RISK FACTORS

* Fatigue
* Shortness of breath
* Pain

DESIRED OUTCOMES

> The client will not experience activity intolerance as evidenced by:
> a. No reports of fatigue or weakness
> b. Ability to perform activities of daily living without exertional dyspnea, chest pain, diaphoresis, dizziness, and a significant change in vital signs

NOC OUTCOMES

Activity tolerance; energy conservation; self-care activities of daily living

NIC INTERVENTIONS

Energy management; oxygen therapy; sleep enhancement

NURSING ASSESSMENT	RATIONALE

Assess for signs and symptoms of activity intolerance:

* Statements of fatigue or weakness
* Exertional dyspnea, chest pain, diaphoresis, or dizziness
* Abnormal heart rate response to activity (e.g., increase in rate of 20 beats/min above resting rate, rate not returning to preactivity level within 3 minutes after stopping activity, change from regular to irregular rate)
* Significant change (15-20 mm Hg) in B/P with activity

Early recognition of signs and symptoms of activity intolerance allows for prompt intervention.

THERAPEUTIC INTERVENTIONS	RATIONALE

Independent Actions

Implement measures to prevent activity intolerance:

* Perform actions to promote rest and/or conserve energy:
  * Maintain prescribed activity restrictions.
  * Minimize environmental activity and noise. **D** ● ✦
  * Organize care to provide uninterrupted rest periods. **D** ● ✦
  * Assist with self-care activities. **D** ● ✦
  * Keep supplies and personal articles within easy reach. **D** ● ✦
  * Limit the number of visitors.
  * Instruct client in energy-saving techniques (e.g., using a shower chair when showering, sitting to brush teeth or comb hair).
  * Implement measures to promote sleep (e.g., allow client to continue usual sleep practices unless contraindicated, administer sedative-hypnotic as ordered).
* Discourage smoking and excessive intake of beverages high in caffeine such as coffee, tea, and colas.

Instruct client to report a decreased tolerance for activity and to stop any activity that causes chest pain, shortness of breath, dizziness, or extreme fatigue or weakness.

Cells use oxygen and fat, protein, and carbohydrate to produce the energy needed for all body activities. Rest and activities that conserve energy result in a lower metabolic rate, which preserves nutrients and oxygen for necessary activities.

Both nicotine and excessive caffeine intake can increase cardiac workload and myocardial oxygen utilization, thereby decreasing the amount of oxygen necessary for energy production.

These symptoms indicate that insufficient oxygen is reaching the tissues and that activity has been increased beyond a therapeutic level.

Dependent/Collaborative Actions

Implement measures to prevent activity intolerance:

* Administer the following if ordered to treat anemia if present:
  * Iron supplements
  * Packed red blood cells
* Maintain oxygen therapy as ordered. **D** ✦
* Implement measures to maintain an adequate nutritional status (e.g., provide a diet high in essential nutrients, provide dietary supplements as indicated, administer vitamins and minerals as ordered).

Anemia reduces the oxygen-carrying capacity of the blood. Resolution of anemia increases oxygen availability to the cells, which increases the efficiency of energy production and subsequently improves activity tolerance.

Provides supplemental oxygen.

Metabolism is the process by which nutrients are transformed into energy. If nutrition is inadequate, energy production is decreased, which subsequently reduces one's ability to tolerate activity.

Vitamins and minerals may be required to support nutritional status.

THERAPEUTIC INTERVENTIONS	RATIONALE
• Increase client's activity gradually as allowed and tolerated. **D ● ✦**	*A gradual increase in activity helps prevent a sudden increase in cardiac workload and myocardial oxygen consumption and the subsequent imbalance between oxygen supply and demand.*
Consult physician if signs and symptoms of activity intolerance persist.	*Notifying the physician allows for modification of the treatment plan.*

Collaborative Diagnosis **RISK FOR HYPOVOLEMIC SHOCK**

Definition: A form of shock in which the blood volume is so significantly decreased that the heart is unable to supply blood to the body

Related to:
• Excessive bleeding
• Lack of adequate fluid volume replacement

CLINICAL MANIFESTATIONS

Subjective	Objective
N/A	Changes in mental status; agitation; confusion; hypotension; tachycardia; cool skin; rapid respirations; pallor and cyanosis; oliguria; restlessness

RISK FACTORS
• Stress
• Rupture of varices

DESIRED OUTCOMES

The client will not develop hypovolemic shock as evidenced by:
  a. Usual mental status
  b. Stable vital signs
  c. Skin warm and usual color
  d. Palpable peripheral pulses
  e. Urine output at least 30 mL/h

NURSING ASSESSMENT	RATIONALE
Assess for and report signs and symptoms of hypovolemic shock: • Restlessness, agitation, confusion, or other change in mental status • Significant decrease in B/P • Postural hypotension • Rapid, weak pulse • Rapid respirations • Cool skin • Pallor, cyanosis • Diminished or absent peripheral pulses • Urine output less than 30 mL/h	*Early recognition of signs and symptoms of gastrointestinal bleeding allows for prompt intervention.*

THERAPEUTIC INTERVENTIONS	RATIONALE
Dependent/Collaborative Actions Implement measures to control bleeding (insert nasogastric tube and irrigate with saline; prepare client for endoscopic thermocoagulation, sclerotherapy, or banding of bleeding varices).	*These actions decrease blood loss and reduces the risk of hypovolemic shock.*
If signs and symptoms of hypovolemic shock occur: • Place the client flat in bed with legs elevated unless contraindicated.	*Increases vascular return to the heart to maintain cardiac output.*
• Monitor vital signs frequently.	*Changes in vital signs indicate improvement or worsening hypovolemic shock.*

NDx = NANDA-I Diagnosis   **D** = Delegatable Action   ● = UAP   ✦ = LVN/LPN   ⊖▶ = Go to ⊖volve for animation

Continued...

THERAPEUTIC INTERVENTIONS	RATIONALE
• Administer oxygen as ordered.	*Improves tissue oxygenation.*
• Administer blood products and/or volume expanders as ordered.	*Replaces fluid and/or blood cells, which improves cardiac output and tissue oxygenation.*
• Prepare client for insertion of hemodynamic monitoring devices (e.g., central venous catheter, intra-arterial catheter) if planned.	*Improves ability to monitor hemodynamic changes.*

DISCHARGE TEACHING/CONTINUED CARE

Nursing Diagnosis | # DEFICIENT KNOWLEDGE NDx; INEFFECTIVE FAMILY THERAPEUTIC REGIMEN MANAGEMENT NDx; or INEFFECTIVE SELF HEALTH MANAGEMENT* NDx

Definition: Absence or deficiency of cognitive information related to specific topic (lack of specific information necessary for clients/significant others) to make informed choices regarding condition/treatment/lifestyle changes; pattern of regulating and integrating into daily living and family processes a therapeutic regimen for treatment of illness and the sequelae that is unsatisfactory for meeting specific health goals

Subjective	Objective
Verbalizes inability to manage illness; verbalizes inability to follow prescribed regimen	Inaccurate follow through with instructions; inappropriate behaviors; unwillingness to participate in self care

RISK FACTORS
• Cognitive deficit
• Financial concerns
• Inability to care for oneself
• Difficulty in modifying personal habits and integrating treatments into lifestyle

NOC OUTCOMES	NIC INTERVENTIONS
Knowledge: disease process; knowledge: treatment regimen	Health system guidance; teaching: individual; teaching: disease process; teaching: prescribed diet; teaching: prescribed medication

NURSING ASSESSMENT	RATIONALE
Assess the client's ability to learn and readiness to learn. Assess the client's understanding of teaching.	*Learning is more effective when the client is motivated and understands the importance of what is to be learned. Readiness to learn changes based on situations, physical and emotional challenges.*

THERAPEUTIC INTERVENTIONS	RATIONALE

Desired Outcome: The client will identify ways to reduce the risk of bleeding.

Independent Interventions
Instruct client on how to reduce the risk for rebleeding:

• Drink decaffeinated or caffeine-free tea and colas rather than those containing caffeine	*These drinks/foods irritates GI lining, slow down healing and/or may cause re-ulceration.*

*The nurse should select the diagnostic label that is most appropriate for the client's discharge teaching.

THERAPEUTIC INTERVENTIONS	RATIONALE
• Avoid drinking coffee and alcohol or drink these beverages only in small amounts during or immediately following a meal	
• Avoid ingestion of foods that are known to irritate gastric mucosa directly or increase gastric acid production (e.g., whole grains, chocolate, rich pastries, spicy foods, meat extracts, extremely hot foods)	
• Avoid intake of any foods and fluids that cause gastric distress	*Neutralizes gastric acid.*
• Eat three regularly scheduled meals (moderate-sized, rather than large) and snacks each day; do not skip meals	*A large bolus of food causes an increased output of hydrochloric acid and pepsin.*
• Eat slowly and chew food thoroughly	*Decreases stress and production of gastric acid.*
• Maintain a calm, pleasant atmosphere at mealtime and whenever possible	
• Stop smoking	*Smoking may cause ulcers, lowers healing, and contributes to recccurrence.*
• Maintain a balance of physical activity and rest	*Reduces stress and promotes healing.*
• Avoid stressful situations whenever possible	*Stress increases gastric acid production.*
• Avoid ingestion of over-the-counter medications such as aspirin and ibuprofen; if it is necessary to take these or other ulcerogenic medications (e.g., corticosteroids), take them with antacids or food unless contraindicated and/or take enteric-coated or buffered preparations of the drugs if available	*Many medications cause gastric irritation and should be avoided or taken with antacids or food.*
• If it is necessary to take an NSAID, consult health care provider about taking it with a medication that helps protect the gastric mucosa (e.g., misoprostol, sucralfate) and/or switching to an NSAID that is known to be less irritating to the mucosa (e.g., a COX-2 inhibitor selective agent such as celecoxib, valdecoxib, and rofecoxib)	
• Take medications for ulcer treatment as prescribed	*Enhances ulcer healing and reduces recurrence.*

THERAPEUTIC INTERVENTIONS	RATIONALE

Desired Outcome: The client will state signs and symptoms to report to the health care provider.

Independent Actions
Instruct client to report:
• Blood or "coffee-ground" vomitus
• Black or tarry stools
• Persistent epigastric fullness or bloating, nausea and/or vomiting
• Abdominal distention
• Persistent or increased epigastric or abdominal pain
• Persistent weakness and fatigue

Indication of bleeding and should be reported immediately to allow for prompt intervention.

THERAPEUTIC INTERVENTIONS	RATIONALE

Desired Outcome: The client will verbalize an understanding of and a plan for adhering to recommended follow-up care including future appointments with health care provider, medications prescribed, and dietary restriction.

Independent Actions
Reinforce the importance of keeping follow-up appointments with health care provider.

The client should be monitored for a period of time to ensure adequate healing.

Continued...

THERAPEUTIC INTERVENTIONS	RATIONALE
Explain the rationale for, side effects of, and importance of taking prescriptions as prescribed. Inform client of pertinent food and drug interactions.	*Knowledge of the medication regimen and the impact of these medications on the system, as well as how the medication regimen can be incorporated into the client's lifestyle, allows the client some mechanism of control of his/her disease and the ability to have an active part in treatment and care.*
Reinforce physician's instruction regarding dietary restrictions such as caffeinated beverages, alcohol, and spicy foods.	*Irritants to the gastrointestinal tract may increase potential for rebleeding.*
Provide written instructions about future appointments with health care provider, prescribed medications, dietary restrictions, and signs and symptoms to report.	*Provides a resource for information once the client has been discharged from the acute care facility.*

ADDITIONAL NURSING DIAGNOSIS

FEAR/ANXIETY NDx
Related to:
- Presence of large amount of blood in vomitus and nasogastric tube drainage
- Concern that bleeding may not be controlled

- Lack of understanding of the cause of the bleeding, diagnostic tests, treatment plan, and prognosis
- Possible need to change lifestyle in order to prevent rebleeding

INFLAMMATORY BOWEL DISEASE: ULCERATIVE COLITIS AND CROHN'S DISEASE

Crohn's disease and ulcerative colitis are idiopathic chronic inflammatory bowel diseases, which are often jointly referred to as inflammatory bowel disease. These disorders have similarities but can usually be differentiated by clinical, radiological, and pathological findings.

The classic clinical manifestations of inflammatory bowel disease include diarrhea, abdominal pain and cramping, and fever. The severity and pattern of signs and symptoms depend on the portion(s) of the bowel affected and depth of bowel wall involvement. Ulcerative colitis primarily involves the mucosa of the bowel wall, extending to the submucosa only in severe cases. It typically starts in the rectum and sigmoid colon and progresses in a continuous pattern through the colon. It rarely involves the small intestine. Crohn's disease can occur anywhere in the gastrointestinal tract. The most frequent sites of involvement are the terminal ileum and right colon. The entire thickness of the bowel wall is involved, and it has a segmental, discontinuous pattern of progression.

Clients with either condition may experience a number of the same complications; however, those with ulcerative colitis have a higher incidence of toxic megacolon and bowel perforation, whereas clients with Crohn's disease have a higher incidence of perianal involvement and fistula formation. Some clients also experience extraintestinal manifestations such as liver and biliary involvement; kidney stones; arthritis; and skin, eye, and oral lesions. Clients with inflammatory bowel disease may require hospitalization during periods of exacerbation or if complications are suspected.

Cornerstones of medical treatment have traditionally included corticosteroids, sulfasalazine, nonsulfa-aminosalicy-

lates, and immunomodulator agents such as azathioprine and mercaptopurine. Research indicates that there may be a defect in immunoregulation of inflammation in Crohn's disease. This has led to the use of monoclonal antibodies that neutralize a cytokine (specifically tumor necrosis factor-alpha) to treat persons with Crohn's disease who have not been responsive to conventional therapy or who have draining enterocutaneous fistulas.

This care plan focuses on the adult client with severe abdominal pain and diarrhea who is hospitalized for medical management of inflammatory bowel disease. Much of the information is applicable to clients receiving follow-up care in an extended care facility or home setting.

OUTCOME/DISCHARGE CRITERIA

The client will:
1. Have decreased abdominal pain
2. Have fewer episodes of diarrhea
3. Tolerate prescribed diet and have an improved nutritional status
4. Be free of signs and symptoms of complications
5. Identify ways to reduce the incidence of disease exacerbation
6. Verbalize ways to maintain an optimal nutritional status
7. State ways to prevent perianal skin breakdown
8. Verbalize an understanding of medications ordered including rationale, food and drug interactions, side

effects, schedule for taking, and importance of taking as prescribed

9. State signs and symptoms to report to the health care provider

10. Identify resources that can assist in the adjustment to changes resulting from inflammatory bowel disease and its treatment

11. Share feelings and thoughts about the effects of inflammatory bowel disease on lifestyle and self-concept

12. Verbalize an understanding of and a plan for adhering to recommended follow-up care including future appointments with health care provider and activity level.

Nursing/Collaborative Diagnosis | ## RISK FOR IMBALANCED FLUID AND ELECTROLYTES*

Definition: Risk for developing an imbalance of electrolytes and fluids in the intracellular and extracellular compartments of the body

Related to:
- **Deficient fluid volume NDx, hypokalemia, hypomagnesemia,** and **hypocalcemia** related to:
  - Prolonged inadequate oral intake associated with pain, fatigue, prescribed dietary restrictions, and fear of precipitating an attack of abdominal cramping and diarrhea.
  - Impaired absorption of fluid and electrolytes associated with inflammation and scarring of the intestine
  - Excessive loss of fluid and electrolytes associated with persistent diarrhea (loss of potassium can occur as a result of treatment with corticosteroids)
- **Metabolic acidosis** related to excessive loss of bicarbonate associated with persistent diarrhea

CLINICAL MANIFESTATIONS

Subjective	Objective
Report of nausea; headache	Poor skin turgor; dry, cracked mucous membranes; hypotension; weight loss; prolonged capillary refill greater than 2 to 3 seconds; decreased urine output; increased urine specific gravity; vomiting; positive Chvostek's and Trousseau's sign; abnormal electrolytes; metabolic acidosis

RISK FACTORS

- Chronic illness
- Failure of regulatory mechanisms
- Inadequate diet and fluid intake

DESIRED OUTCOMES

The client will maintain fluid and electrolyte balance as evidenced by:
  a. Normal skin turgor
  b. Moist mucous membranes
  c. Stable weight
  d. B/P and pulse rate within normal range for client and stable with position change
  e. Capillary refill time less than 2 to 3 seconds
  f. Usual mental status
  g. Balanced intake and output
  h. Urine specific gravity within normal range
  i. Soft, nondistended abdomen with active bowel sounds
  j. Absence of cardiac dysrhythmias, muscle weakness, and seizure activity
  k. Absence of headache, nausea, and vomiting
  l. Negative Chvostek's and Trousseau's signs
  m. Decreased serum electrolytes and arterial blood gasses within normal range

NOC OUTCOMES

Fluid balance; electrolyte and acid-base balance

NIC INTERVENTIONS

Fluid management; electrolyte management: hypokalemia; electrolyte management: hypocalcemia; electrolyte management: hypomagnesemia; acid-base management: metabolic acidosis; diarrhea management

---

*The nurse should select the diagnostic label that is most appropriate for the client's discharge teaching needs.

NDx = NANDA-I Diagnosis   **D** = Delegatable Action   ● = UAP   ✦ = LVN/LPN   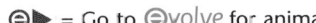 = Go to ⊖volve for animation

Continued...

NURSING ASSESSMENT	RATIONALE
Assess for and report signs and symptoms of deficient fluid volume: • Decreased skin turgor, dry mucous membranes, thirst • Weight loss of 2% or greater over a short period • Postural hypotension and/or low B/P • Weak, rapid pulse • Capillary refill time longer than 2 to 3 seconds • Neck veins flat when client is supine • Change in mental status • Decreased urine output with increased specific gravity (reflects an actual rather than potential fluid deficit) • Significant increase in BUN and Hct above previous levels • Hypokalemia (e.g., cardiac dysrhythmias, postural hypotension, muscle weakness, nausea and vomiting, abdominal distention, hypoactive or absent bowel sounds) • Hypomagnesemia and/or hypocalcemia (e.g., anxiousness; irritability; cardiac dysrhythmias; positive Chvostek's and Trousseau's signs; numbness or tingling of fingers, toes, or circumoral area; hyperactive reflexes; tetany; seizures) • Metabolic acidosis (e.g., drowsiness; disorientation; stupor; rapid, deep respirations; headache; nausea and vomiting; cardiac dysrhythmias; low pH and CO_2 content)	*Early recognition of signs and symptoms of electrolyte imbalance allows for prompt treatment.*

THERAPEUTIC INTERVENTIONS	RATIONALE

Independent Actions
Implement measures to prevent or treat imbalanced fluid and electrolytes:
• Perform actions to control diarrhea (e.g., restrict intake as needed, reduce stress, avoid milk and milk products, foods high in fat, those high in fiber or residue, high in caffeine, spicy foods, extremely hot or cold fluids). **D** ● ✦
• When oral intake is allowed:
  • Assist client to select foods/fluids within the prescribed dietary regimen that would replenish electrolytes (be aware that many foods/fluids high in potassium and magnesium are contraindicated on a low-residue diet) **D** ● ✦
  (1) Foods high in potassium (e.g., bananas, avocado, raisins, potatoes, cantaloupe)
  (2) Foods high in magnesium (e.g., seafood)
	Clients with Crohn's disease may have an intolerance to lactose-rich foods because of a deficiency of lactase.
	The foods listed stimulate the bowel and increase the incidence of diarrhea.
	Oral intake of foods high in potassium are necessary to maintain adequate electrolyte balance.

Dependent/Collaborative Actions
Implement measures to prevent or treat imbalanced fluid and electrolytes:
• Administer the following if ordered:
  • Maintain a fluid intake of at least 2500 mL/day unless contraindicated.
  • If oral intake is inadequate or contraindicated, maintain intravenous and/or enteral fluid therapy as ordered.
  • Electrolyte replacements (e.g., potassium chloride, magnesium sulfate, calcium gluconate, calcium carbonate)
  • Vitamin D preparations **D** ✦
If signs and symptoms of hypomagnesemia or hypocalcemia occur, institute seizure precautions. **D** ● ✦
Consult physician if signs and symptoms of imbalanced fluid and electrolytes persist or worsen.
	Required to prevent the client from becoming dehydrated.
	
	Replenishes electrolytes.
	
	Increases intestinal absorption of calcium.
	Low levels of magnesium and calcium have been associated with increased seizure activity.
	Notification of the physician allows for alterations in treatment plan.

Nursing Diagnosis   IMBALANCED NUTRITION: LESS THAN BODY REQUIREMENTS NDx

Definition: Inadequate intake or insufficient nutrition to meet the body's metabolic needs

Related to:
- Decreased oral intake associated with pain, fatigue, prescribed dietary restrictions, and the knowledge that eating often precipitates abdominal cramping and diarrhea
- Decreased absorption of nutrients associated with inflammation and scarring of the bowel
- Loss of nutrients associated with diarrhea and protein exudation from the inflamed bowel
- Impaired folate absorption associated with treatment with sulfasalazine
- Increased metabolism of nutrients associated with the increased metabolic rate that may be present during periods of exacerbation

CLINICAL MANIFESTATIONS

Subjective	Objective
Complaints of weakness and fatigue; lack of appetite; irritability; poor self-esteem	Weight significantly below client's usual weight or below normal for client's age, height, and body frame; abnormal BUN and low serum prealbumin, albumin, Hct, Hgb, and folate levels and low lymphocyte count; pale conjunctiva

RISK FACTORS
- Treatment regimen
- Inadequate/inappropriate diet

DESIRED OUTCOMES
The client will have an improved nutritional status as evidenced by:
- a. Weight approaching a normal range for client
- b. Improved BUN and serum prealbumin, albumin, Hct, Hgb, and folate levels and lymphocyte count
- c. Increased strength and activity tolerance
- d. Healthy oral mucous membranes

NOC OUTCOMES
Nutritional status

NIC INTERVENTIONS
Nutritional monitoring; nutrition management; nutrition therapy; total parenteral nutrition (TPN) administration; enteral tube feeding

NURSING ASSESSMENT	RATIONALE
Assess for signs and symptoms of malnutrition: • Weight significantly below client's normal or below normal for client's age, height, and body frame • Abnormal BUN and low serum prealbumin, albumin, Hct, Hgb, and folate levels and low lymphocyte count • Weakness and fatigue • Sore, inflamed oral mucous membrane • Pale conjunctiva	*Early recognition of signs and symptoms of imbalanced nutrition allows for prompt intervention.*

THERAPEUTIC INTERVENTIONS	RATIONALE
Independent Actions When oral intake is allowed, monitor the percentage of meals and snacks client consumes. **D** ● ✦ Report a pattern of inadequate intake. **D** ● ✦	*The client's intake should be monitored to ensure adequate amount of calories and nutrients.*
Dependent/Collaborative Actions Implement measures to improve nutritional status: • Administer TPN or enteral tube feeding if ordered.	*Provides adequate nutrition until oral intake may be resumed.*

NDx = NANDA-I Diagnosis   **D** = Delegatable Action   ● = UAP   ✦ = LVN/LPN   ⊖▶ = Go to ⊖volve for animation

Continued...

THERAPEUTIC INTERVENTIONS	RATIONALE
• Perform actions to reduce inflammation and hypermotility of the bowel (restrict intake; limit activity to bedrest as needed; limit milk and milk products, those high in fats, fiber, caffeine, spicy foods, extremely hot or cold foods/fluids).	*These actions reduce episodes of diarrhea and increase absorption of nutrients.*
• Maintain activity restrictions as ordered (usually bedrest with bedside commode or bathroom privileges)	*Reduces caloric requirements.*
• When food or fluid is allowed:	
• Provide elemental formulas (e.g., Vivonex, Criticare HN) if ordered.	*Helps rest the bowel; these formulas are high in calories and nutrients, free of lactose and fiber, and absorbed in the proximal small bowel.*
• Progress diet as tolerated (usual progression is from elemental formulas to a low-residue, high-calorie, high-protein diet). **D ● ✦**	
• Implement measures to reduce pain (e.g., encourage a rest period before meals). **D ● ✦**	*Minimizes fatigue.*
• Maintain a clean environment and a relaxed, pleasant atmosphere. **D ● ✦**	*Eliminates noxious odors, which may decrease appetite.*
• Provide oral hygiene before meals. **D ● ✦**	*Oral hygiene removes unpleasant tastes, which often improves the taste of foods/fluids.*
• Implement measures to improve the palatability of elemental formulas (e.g., offer a variety of flavors, serve chilled).	*A variety of measures help them to become more palatable.*
• Obtain a dietary consult if necessary to assist client in selecting foods/fluids that are appealing and adhere to personal and cultural preferences as well as the prescribed dietary modifications.	*Improves nutritional status while allowing individuals to eat foods that they like.*
• Serve frequent, small meals rather than large ones if client is weak, fatigues easily, or has a poor appetite. **D ● ✦**	*Small, frequent meals promote better nutritional status for the client who tires easily.*
• Allow adequate time for meals; reheat foods/fluids if necessary. **D ● ✦**	*Clients who feel rushed during meals tend to become anxious, lose their appetite, and stop eating. Appetite is also suppressed if foods/fluids normally served hot or warm become cold and then do not appeal to the client.*
• Administer the following if ordered:	
• Iron	*Oral iron preparations may not be effective during an acute attack because they may be poorly absorbed from the inflamed bowel.*
• Vitamin preparations (e.g., fat-soluble vitamins, vitamin B$_{12}$, folic acid)	*Supplements of these vitamins may be required because they may not be adequately absorbed from the inflamed bowel.*
Perform a calorie count if ordered. Report information to dietitian and physician. **D ✦**	*Monitors client's nutritional status.*
Consult physician and/or dietitian if nutritional status continues to decline.	*Notification of the physician allows for alterations in treatment plan.*

Nursing Diagnosis ACUTE/CHRONIC PAIN NDx

Definition: Unpleasant sensory and emotional experience arising from actual or potential tissue damage or described in terms of such damage (International Association for the Study of Pain); sudden or slow onset of any intensity from mild to severe, constant or recurring, without an anticipated or predictable end and a duration of greater than 6 months

Related to:
• **Abdominal pain and cramping** related to:
  • Inflammation and ulceration of the bowel
  • Interference with the flow of intestinal contents associated with narrowing of the intestinal lumen as a result of inflammation and hypertrophy and fibrosis of the bowel wall if present
• **Joint pain** related to extraintestinal involvement of the joints (peripheral arthritis, ankylosing spondylitis, and sacroiliitis are the most common joint disorders that occur)
• **Perianal pain** related to irritation and breakdown of the skin in the perianal area associated with persistent diarrhea and/or the presence of an anorectal abscess or fistula

CLINICAL MANIFESTATIONS

Subjective	Objective
Verbalization of reluctance to move; pain	Grimacing; rubbing abdomen, back, or joints; diaphoresis; increased B/P; tachycardia; restlessness

RISK FACTOR

- Chronic illness

DESIRED OUTCOMES

The client will experience diminished pain as evidenced by:
  a. Verbalization of same
  b. Relaxed facial expression and body positioning
  c. Increased participation in activities
  d. Stable vital signs

NOC OUTCOMES

Comfort level: pain control

NIC INTERVENTIONS

Environmental management: comfort; analgesic administration

NURSING ASSESSMENT	RATIONALE
Assess for signs and symptoms of pain (e.g., verbalization of pain, grimacing, reluctance to move, restlessness, diaphoresis, increased B/P, tachycardia).	*Early recognition of signs and symptoms of pain allows for prompt intervention and improved pain control.*
Assess client's perception of the severity of pain using a pain intensity rating scale.	*An awareness of the severity of pain being experienced helps determine the most appropriate interventions for pain management. Use of a pain intensity rating scale gives the nurse a clearer understanding of the pain being experienced and promotes consistency when communicating with others about the client's pain experience.*
Assess the client's pain pattern (e.g., location, quality, onset, duration, precipitating factors, aggravating factors, alleviating factors).	*Knowledge of the client's pain pattern assists in the identification of effective pain management interventions.*
Ask the client to describe previous pain experiences and methods used to manage pain effectively.	*Many variables affect a client's response to pain (e.g., age, sex, coping style, previous experience with pain, culture, cause of pain). Knowledge of the client's usual response to pain and methods previously used to manage pain effectively enables the nurse to evaluate the client's pain more accurately and facilitates the identification of effective strategies for pain management.*

THERAPEUTIC INTERVENTIONS	RATIONALE
Independent Actions	
Implement measures to reduce fear and anxiety (e.g., assure client that the need for pain relief is understood, plan methods for achieving pain control with client, provide a calm environment). **D** ● ✦	*Fear and anxiety can decrease the client's threshold and tolerance for pain and thereby heighten the perception of pain. In addition, pain management methods are not as effective if the client is tense and unable to relax.*
Implement measures to promote rest (e.g., minimize environmental activity and noise). **D** ● ✦	*Fatigue can decrease the client's threshold and tolerance for pain and thereby heighten the perception of pain. A well-rested client often experiences decreased pain and increased effectiveness of pain management measures.*
Perform actions to reduce inflammation and hypermotility of the bowel:	
• Perform actions to rest the bowel:	
• Restrict oral intake; maintain NPO during acute stage.	*Restricting intake and placing the client on NPO rests the bowel and conserves the individual's energy.*
• Maintain activity restrictions (initially may be limited to bedrest with bedside commode or bathroom privileges).	*Enhances healing of the bowel.*

NDx = NANDA-I Diagnosis   **D** = Delegatable Action   ● = UAP   ✦ = LVN/LPN   ⊖▶ = Go to ⊖volve for animation

Continued...

THERAPEUTIC INTERVENTIONS	RATIONALE
When oral intake is allowed, diet usually progresses from elemental formulas to a low-residue diet. **D** ● ✦	*Elemental formulas are absorbed in the proximal small bowel and thereby minimize stimulation of the bowel.*
• Instruct the client to avoid the following foods/fluids that may be poorly digested or can act as irritants to the inflamed bowel:	*Clients with Crohn's disease may have an intolerance to lactose-rich foods because of a deficiency of lactase.*
(1) Milk and milk products	*These foods cause an increase in the potential for diarrhea and irritation of the colon.*
(2) Foods high in fat (e.g., fried foods, gravies)	
(3) Foods high in fiber (e.g., whole-grain cereals, nuts, raw fruits and vegetables)	
(4) Foods high in caffeine (e.g., coffee, tea, colas)	
(5) Spicy foods	
(6) Extremely hot or cold foods/fluids	
Perform actions to relieve perianal pain if present:	*These actions help to decrease pain and irritation.*
• Clean perianal area with medication wipes such as "Tucks" after each bowel movement.	
• Apply protective ointment or cream to perianal area after each bowel movement. **D** ● ✦	
Instruct client to add new foods one at a time.	*Adding one food at a time allows client to determine which foods cause more discomfort*
Provide small, frequent meals rather than three large ones.	*Small, frequent meals are tolerated better than three large meals.*

Dependent/Collaborative Actions

Perform actions to relieve perianal pain if present:	
• Consult physician about order for sitz baths.	*These actions decrease pain experienced in the perianal area.*
• Apply anesthetic preparation (e.g., Nupercainal, Tronolane) to perianal area or into rectum as ordered.	
Consult physician regarding measures to help relieve joint pain if present (e.g., application of brace/splint to affected joint, application of heat to affected joints).	*Braces and splints support the joints and help to reduce pain.*
Perform actions to reduce inflammation and hypermotility of the bowel:	
• Administer anti-inflammatory medications:	
• Corticosteroids	*Corticosteroids and sulfasalazine or non–sulfa-aminosalicylates reduce bowel inflammation.*
• Sulfasalazine or non–sulfa-aminosalicylates	
• Antidiarrheal agents **D** ✦	*Antidiarrheal agents slow intestinal motility; however, these medications should be used with caution because of the risk of megacolon.*
Administer analgesics before activities and procedures that can cause pain and before pain becomes severe. **D** ✦	*The administration of analgesics before a pain-producing event helps minimize the pain that will be experienced. Analgesics are also more effective if given before pain becomes severe because mild to moderate pain is controlled more quickly and effectively than severe pain.*
Provide or assist with nonpharmacological methods for pain relief. Examples include:	*Nonpharmacological pain management includes a variety of interventions. It is believed that most of these are effective because they stimulate closure of the gating mechanism in the spinal cord and subsequently block the transmission of pain*
• Cutaneous stimulation measures (e.g., pressure, massage, heat and cold applications, transcutaneous electrical nerve stimulation [TENS], acupuncture)	*impulses. In addition, some interventions are thought to stimulate the release of endogenous analgesics (e.g., endorphins)*
• Relaxation techniques (e.g., progressive relaxation exercises, meditation, guided imagery)	*that inhibit the transmission of pain impulses and/or alter the client's perception of pain. Many of the nonpharmacological interventions also help decrease pain by promoting relaxation.*
• Distraction measures (e.g., listening to music, conversing, watching television, playing cards, reading)	*Pharmacological therapy is an effective method of reducing or relieving pain.*
• Position change	

THERAPEUTIC INTERVENTIONS	RATIONALE
Administer the following medications as ordered:	
• Opioid (narcotic) analgesics	Opioid analgesics act mainly by altering the client's perception of pain and emotional response to the pain experience.
• Nonopioid (nonnarcotic) analgesics such as acetaminophen and salicylates and other nonsteroidal anti-inflammatory agents (e.g., ketorolac, ibuprofen, naproxen)	Nonopioid analgesics are thought to interfere with the transmission of pain impulses by inhibiting prostaglandin synthesis.
• Anesthetic agents (e.g., bupivacaine, lidocaine)	Anesthetics help control pain by inhibiting the initiation and conduction of pain impulses along the sensory pathways at and near the infusion site.
Consult physician about an order for patient-controlled analgesia (PCA) if indicated.	The use of PCA allows the client to self-administer analgesics within parameters established by the physician. This method facilitates pain management by ensuring prompt administration of the drug when needed, providing more continuous pain relief and increasing the client's control over the pain.
Consult appropriate health care provider (e.g., physician, pharmacist, pain management specialist) if above measures fail to provide adequate pain relief.	Notifying the appropriate health care provider allows for modification of the treatment plan.

Nursing Diagnosis ## RISK FOR INFECTION NDx

Definition: At increased risk for being invaded by pathogenic organisms

Related to:
• Ulcerations in the bowel wall
• Lowered resistance to infection associated with malnutrition and treatment with corticosteroids and/or immunosuppressive agents
• Stasis of respiratory secretions and urine associated with decreased mobility if activity restrictions are prescribed

CLINICAL MANIFESTATIONS

Subjective	Objective
Chills; malaise; lethargy; confusion; complaints of frequency, urgency, or burning with urination	Fever; tachycardia; loss of appetite; abnormal breath sounds; productive cough of purulent, green, or rust-colored sputum; cloudy urine; urinalysis showing a WBC count greater than 5 per high-power field, positive leukocyte esterase or nitrites, or presence of bacteria; elevated WBC count and/or significant change in differential

RISK FACTORS

• Exposure to pathogens
• Treatment regimen
• Lack of exercise
• Inadequate fluid intake

DESIRED OUTCOMES

The client will remain free of infection as evidenced by:
a. Temperature declining toward normal
b. Absence of chills
c. Pulse rate within normal limits
d. Normal breath sounds
e. Usual mental status
f. Cough productive of clear mucus only
g. Voiding clear urine without reports of frequency, urgency, and burning
h. No increase in episodes of diarrhea and abdominal cramping and pain
i. Absence of heat, pain, redness, swelling, and usual drainage in any area
j. No reports of increased weakness and fatigue
k. WBC and differential counts returning toward normal
l. Negative results of cultured specimens

NDx = NANDA-I Diagnosis   **D** = Delegatable Action   ● = UAP   ✦ = LVN/LPN   ⊖▶ = Go to ⊖volve for animation
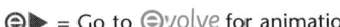

Continued...

NOC OUTCOMES	NIC INTERVENTIONS
Immune status; infection severity	Infection control; infection protection

NURSING ASSESSMENT	RATIONALE

Assess for and report signs and symptoms of infection (be aware that some signs and symptoms vary depending on the site of infection, the causative agent, and the age and immune status of the client):

- Elevated temperature
- Chills
- Increased pulse rate
- Malaise, lethargy, acute confusion
- Loss of appetite
- Abnormal breath sounds
- Productive cough of purulent, green, or rust-colored sputum
- Cloudy urine
- Reports of frequency, urgency, or burning when urinating
- Urinalysis showing a WBC count greater than 5 per high-power field, positive leukocyte esterase or nitrites, or presence of bacteria
- Heat, pain, redness, swelling, or unusual drainage in any area
- Elevated WBC count and/or significant change in differential

Early recognition of signs and symptoms of infection allows for prompt intervention.

Obtain specimens (e.g., urine, wound drainage, vaginal drainage, sputum, blood) for culture as ordered. Report positive results.

Cultures are done to identify the specific organism(s) causing the infection. Culture results provide information that helps determine the most effective treatment.

THERAPEUTIC INTERVENTIONS	RATIONALE

Independent Actions

Maintain a fluid intake of at least 2500 mL/day unless contraindicated. **D** ● ✦

Adequate hydration helps prevent infection by:
- *Helping maintain adequate blood flow and nutrient supply to the tissues*
- *Promoting urine formation and subsequent voiding, which flushes pathogens from the bladder and urethra*
- *Thinning respiratory secretions so that they can more easily be removed by coughing or suctioning (respiratory secretions provide a good medium for growth and colonization of microorganisms)*

Use good hand hygiene and encourage client to do the same. **D** ● ✦

Good hand hygiene removes transient flora, which reduces the risk of transmission of pathogens. Use of products such as an antibacterial soap, a chlorhexidine solution, or an alcohol-based handrub agent can actually inhibit the growth of or kill microorganisms, which further reduces infection risk.

Adhere to the appropriate precautions established to prevent transmission of infection to the client (standard precautions, transmission-based precautions on other clients, neutropenic precautions). **D** ● ✦

Adhering to the appropriate precautions that have been established to help prevent the transmission of microorganisms reduces the client's risk of infection.

Use sterile technique during invasive procedures (e.g., urinary catheterizations, venous and arterial punctures, injections, tracheal suctioning, wound care) and dressing changes.

Use of sterile technique reduces the possibility of introducing pathogens into the body.

Anchor catheters/tubings (e.g., urinary, intravenous, wound drainage) securely. **D** ● ✦

Catheters/tubings that are not securely anchored have some degree of in-and-out movement. This movement increases the risk of infection because it allows for the introduction of pathogens into the body. It can also cause tissue trauma, which can result in colonization of microorganisms.

THERAPEUTIC INTERVENTIONS	RATIONALE
Change equipment, tubings, and solutions used for treatments such as intravenous infusions, respiratory care, irrigations, and enteral feedings according to hospital policy. **D** ✦	*The longer that equipment, tubings, and solutions are in use, the greater the chance of colonization of microorganisms, which can then be introduced into the body.*
Maintain a closed system for drains (e.g., wounds, chest tubes, urinary catheters) and intravenous infusions whenever possible.	*Each time a drainage or infusion system is opened, pathogens from the environment have an opportunity to enter the body. Maintaining a closed system decreases this risk, which reduces the possibility of infection.*
Change peripheral intravenous line sites according to hospital policy.	*Peripheral intravenous line sites are changed routinely to reduce persistent irritation of one area of a vein wall and the resultant colonization of microorganisms at that site.*
Provide appropriate wound care (e.g., use dressing materials that maintain a moist wound surface, assist with debridement of necrotic tissue, use dressing materials that absorb excess exudate, protect granulating tissue from trauma and contamination, maintain patency of wound drains). **D** ✦	*Proper wound care facilitates wound healing and reduces the number of pathogens that enter or are present in the wound, which reduce the risk of the wound becoming infected.*
Protect client from others with infections. **D** ● ✦	*Protecting the client from others with infections reduces the client's risk of exposure to pathogens.*
Implement measures to maintain healthy, intact skin (e.g., keep skin lubricated, clean, and dry; instruct or assist client to turn every 2 hours; keep bed linens dry and wrinkle-free). **D** ● ✦	*Healthy, intact skin reduces the risk for infection by:* • *Providing a physical barrier against the introduction of pathogens into the body* • *Removing many of the microorganisms on the surface of the skin by means of the constant shedding of the epidermis* • *Inhibiting the growth of some bacteria on the surface of the skin (sebum contains fatty acids, which create a slightly acidic environment that inhibits the growth of some bacteria)*
Implement measures to reduce stress (e.g., reduce fear, anxiety, and pain; help client identify and use effective coping mechanisms). **D** ● ✦	*Stress causes an increased secretion of cortisol. Cortisol interferes with some immune responses, which subsequently increases the client's susceptibility to infection.*
Instruct and assist client to perform good perineal care routinely and after each bowel movement. **D** ● ✦	*The perineal area contains a large number of organisms. Routine cleansing of the area reduces the risk of colonization of organisms and subsequent perineal, urinary tract, and/or vaginal infection.*
Instruct and assist client to perform good oral hygiene as often as needed. **D** ● ✦	*Frequent oral hygiene helps prevent infection by removing most of the food, debris, and many of the microorganisms that are present in the mouth. It also helps maintain the integrity of the oral mucosa, which provides a physical and chemical barrier to pathogens.*
Implement measures to prevent urinary retention (e.g., instruct client to urinate when the urge is felt, promote relaxation during voiding attempts). **D** ✦	*A client experiencing urinary retention is at increased risk for urinary tract infection because:* • *The urine that accumulates in the bladder creates an environment conducive to the growth and colonization of microorganisms.* • *Voiding does not occur so microorganisms are not flushed from the mucous lining of the urethra; these microorganisms can colonize and ascend into the bladder.*
Implement measures to prevent stasis of respiratory secretions (e.g., assist client to turn, cough, and deep breathe; increase activity as allowed and tolerated; perform tracheal suctioning if indicated). **D** ✦	*Respiratory secretions provide a good medium for growth of microorganisms. By preventing stasis, there is less chance of colonization of microorganisms and a decreased risk for development of respiratory tract infection.*
Instruct client to receive immunizations (e.g., influenza vaccine, pneumococcal vaccine) if appropriate.	*Immunizations are often recommended to reduce the possibility of some infections in high-risk clients (e.g., those clients who are immunosuppressed, elderly, or have a chronic disease).*

Dependent/Collaborative Actions

Maintain an optimal nutritional status. Administer vitamins and minerals as ordered. **D** ✦	*Adequate nutrition is needed to maintain normal function of the immune system.*

Continued...

THERAPEUTIC INTERVENTIONS	RATIONALE
Perform actions to reduce inflammation of the bowel: • Administer corticosteroids, aminosalicylates, and/or immunomodulating agents as ordered.	*These medications are given to prevent further ulceration of the bowel and subsequently reduce the risk of intestinal infection*
Consult appropriate health care provider regarding initiation of antimicrobial therapy if indicated. Administer antimicrobials if ordered (antimicrobials are generally given only if surgery is planned or if the client has severe colitis and is at high risk for infection; however, metronidazole or ciprofloxacin may be prescribed by some practitioners for the relief of symptoms).	*Most antimicrobials disrupt cell wall synthesis, which halts the growth of or kills microorganisms. This can effectively reduce the client's risk for infection.*

Collaborative Diagnosis | RISK FOR RENAL CALCULI

Definition: Crystallized stones in the urinary tract.

Related to:
• Crystalline deposits in the urine associated with:
  • Increased serum oxalate levels (dietary oxalate normally binds with calcium in the intestine and is excreted in the stool; in clients with inflammatory bowel disease, calcium is bound with the poorly absorbed fat and oxalate becomes available for absorption)
  • Decreased flushing of solutes from the urinary tract if urine formation is reduced as a result of deficient fluid volume
  • Treatment with sulfasalazine

CLINICAL MANIFESTATIONS

Subjective	Objective
Verbalization of flank pain; verbalization of nausea	Hematuria; vomiting

RISK FACTORS
• Chronic disease
• Treatment regimen

DESIRED OUTCOMES

The client will not develop renal calculi as evidenced by:
  a. Absence of flank pain, hematuria, nausea, and vomiting
  b. Clear urine without calculi

NURSING ASSESSMENT	RATIONALE
Assess for and report signs and symptoms of renal calculi (e.g., dull, aching or severe, colicky flank pain; hematuria; nausea; vomiting).	*Early recognition of signs and symptoms of renal calculi allows for prompt intervention.*

THERAPEUTIC INTERVENTIONS	RATIONALE
Independent Actions Implement measures to prevent renal calculi: • Maintain a minimum fluid intake of 2500 mL/day unless contraindicated. **D ● ✦**	*Providing adequate hydration helps maintain adequate blood flow to the kidneys to maintain glomerular filtration rate.*
• Encourage client to decrease intake of foods/fluids high in oxalate (e.g., tea, instant coffee, peanuts, chocolate, spinach).	*Decreases absorption of oxalate from the intestine.*
• Encourage client to adhere to a low-fat diet.	*A low fat diet reduces the amount of fat available to bind calcium, thereby freeing calcium to bind with oxalate.*
Dependent/Collaborative Actions If signs and symptoms of renal calculi occur: • Strain all urine and save any calculi for analysis; report finding to physician.	*Straining the urine helps to determine whether the client has passed a renal calculi.*

THERAPEUTIC INTERVENTIONS	RATIONALE
• Maintain a minimum fluid intake of 2500 mL/day unless contraindicated.	*Helps to flush out the urinary tract and helps to pass a renal calculi.*
• Administer analgesics and antispasmodic agents (e.g., oxybutynin) as ordered.	*Analgesics and antispasmodic agents decrease/eliminate pain experienced with renal calculi.*
• Prepare client for removal of calculi (e.g., extracorporeal shock wave lithotripsy, percutaneous nephrolithotomy, ureteroscopy with lithotripsy and stone extraction) if planned.	*Explain procedures to client and provide required preprocedure or preoperative interventions.*
Implement measures to reduce inflammation of the bowel (e.g., administer corticosteroids, aminosalicylates, and/or immunomodulating agents as ordered).	*These agents decrease inflammation and are used to put the disease in remission.*

Collaborative Diagnosis   # RISK FOR PERIRECTAL, RECTOVAGINAL, ENTEROVESICAL, AND ENTEROENTERIC ABSCESSES AND FISTULAS

Definition: Fistula—ulceration or tear in the intestinal wall; abscess—an accumulation of puss in tissues or a body cavity

Related to: Extension of a mucosal fissure or ulcer through the intestinal wall

CLINICAL MANIFESTATIONS

Subjective	Objective
Verbalization of increased or constant abdominal pain; verbalization of rectal pain	Fever; perianal redness, swelling, and bleeding; foul-smelling vaginal discharge; increased WBC count

RISK FACTOR

• Chronic illness

DESIRED OUTCOMES

The client will have resolution of any abscesses and fistulas that develop as evidenced by:
  a. Temperature declining toward normal
  b. Resolution of abdominal pain
  c. Absence of perianal redness, swelling, and pain
  d. No unusual vaginal drainage
  e. Clear, yellow urine
  f. WBC count declining toward normal

NURSING ASSESSMENT	RATIONALE
Assess for and report signs and symptoms of abscess and/or fistula formation (e.g., further increase in temperature; increased or more constant abdominal pain; perianal redness, swelling, and pain; foul-smelling vaginal discharge or passage of stool from vagina; dysuria; fecaluria; further increase in WBC count).	*Early recognition of signs and symptoms of abscess and/or fistula formation allows for prompt intervention.* *Corticosteroids, aminosalicylates and/or immunomodulating agents reduce bowel inflammation.*

THERAPEUTIC INTERVENTIONS	RATIONALE
Dependent/Collaborative Actions Implement measures to reduce inflammation of the bowel (e.g., administer corticosteroids, aminosalicylates and/or immunomodulating agents as ordered).	*Promotes healing of the intestinal mucosa and subsequently decreases the risk for the development of abscesses and fistulas.*
If signs and symptoms of abscesses or fistulas occur: • Prepare client for diagnostic studies (e.g., computed tomography, ultrasonography, barium enema).	*Decreases client anxiety.*
• Administer the following medications if ordered:	
• Antimicrobial agents (e.g., metronidazole, ciprofloxacin)	*Antimicrobials treat/prevent infection.*
• Immunomodulator agents such as azathioprine, mercaptopurine, or a monoclonal antibody (e.g., infliximab)	*Decreases inflammation and promotes healing.*

NDx = NANDA-I Diagnosis   **D** = Delegatable Action   ● = UAP   ✦ = LVN/LPN   ⊖▶ = Go to ⊖volve for animation

Continued...

THERAPEUTIC INTERVENTIONS	RATIONALE
• If a cutaneous fistula is present, perform wound care as ordered.	
• Prepare client for surgical intervention (e.g., incision and drainage of abscess, resection of involved area) if planned.	*Explain procedures to client and provide required preoperative interventions.*

Collaborative Diagnosis   RISK FOR TOXIC MEGACOLON

Definition: A life-threatening complication of inflammatory bowel diseases in which there is segmental or total dilation of the colon as a result of inflammation or infection

Related to:
• Loss of colonic muscle tone associated with the effects of widespread inflammation in the bowel, use of some medications (e.g., opiates, anticholinergics), and hypokalemia

CLINICAL MANIFESTATIONS

Subjective	Objective
Verbalization of increasing abdominal pain and tenderness	Hypoactive or absent bowel sounds; abdominal percussion reveals tympany; sudden episodes of diarrhea; tachycardia; fever; increased WBC count

RISK FACTORS
• Chronic illness
• Treatment regimen

DESIRED OUTCOMES

The client will not develop toxic megacolon as evidenced by:
a. Absence of abdominal distention
b. Gradual resolution of abdominal pain
c. Active bowel sounds
d. Gradual resolution of diarrhea
e. Temperature and WBC count declining toward normal

NURSING ASSESSMENT	RATIONALE
Assess for and report signs and symptoms of toxic megacolon: • Abdominal distention and increased abdominal pain and tenderness • Hypoactive or absent bowel sounds with tympanic percussion note over abdomen • Sudden decrease in episodes of diarrhea • Fever (usually >38.6°C) and tachycardia • Increase in WBC count • Abdominal radiograph showing colonic dilation	*Early recognition of signs and symptoms of toxic megacolon allows for prompt intervention.*

THERAPEUTIC INTERVENTIONS	RATIONALE
Dependent/Collaborative Actions Implement measures to prevent development of toxic megacolon:	
• Perform actions to reduce inflammation of the bowel (e.g., administer corticosteroids, aminosalicylates, and/or immunomodulating agents as ordered).	*These medications reduce inflammation, which will help prevent toxic megacolon.*
• Administer medications that slow gastrointestinal motility (e.g., narcotic analgesics, antidiarrheal agents, anticholinergics) judiciously.	*Narcotics may cause constipation, thereby contributing to toxic megacolon.*
• Perform actions to prevent or treat hypokalemia (e.g., eat foods high in potassium, take potassium supplements).	*Helps prevent megacolon.*

THERAPEUTIC INTERVENTIONS	RATIONALE

If signs and symptoms of toxic megacolon occur:
- Withhold oral intake as ordered.
- Consult physician about discontinuing any medications that slow gastrointestinal motility (e.g., narcotic analgesics, antidiarrheal agents, anticholinergics).
- Insert nasogastric tube and maintain suction as ordered.
- Administer the following if ordered:
  - Intravenous fluids

  - Corticosteroids
  - Antimicrobials (e.g., metronidazole)

- Prepare client for surgical intervention (e.g., colectomy) if planned.
- Implement measures to reduce inflammation of the bowel (e.g., administer corticosteroids, aminosalicylates, and/or immunomodulating agents as ordered).

Withholding oral intake helps decompress the colon.
Increasing motility helps to decompress the colon.

Insertion of an NG tube provides decompression of the gastrointestinal tract.
IV fluids are given to maintain adequate vascular volume (third-space fluid shifting occurs as a result of increased capillary permeability associated with the inflammation and increased intraluminal pressure that are present with toxic megacolon).
Steroids reduce intestinal inflammation.
Antimicrobials help prevent infection, which is important because the risk of perforation is increased when toxic megacolon develops.
If above treatment is not effective in decompressing the colon, surgery is indicated.
These actions reduce intestinal narrowing and scar tissue formation.

Collaborative Diagnosis RISK FOR BOWEL OBSTRUCTION

Definition: Blockage within the colon that prevents materials from passing though and exiting the bowel

Related to: Narrowing of the intestinal lumen associated with inflammation and scar tissue formation in the bowel

CLINICAL MANIFESTATIONS

Subjective	Objective
Verbalization of increased abdominal pain and cramping; verbalization of nausea	Vomiting; change in bowel sounds to high-pitched and hyperactive or absent; abdominal radiograph showing partial or complete obstruction

RISK FACTORS
- Chronic illness
- Inadequate fluid intake

DESIRED OUTCOMES

The client will not develop a bowel obstruction as evidenced by:
a. Gradual resolution of abdominal pain
b. Absence of vomiting and abdominal distention
c. Gradual return of normal bowel sounds

NURSING ASSESSMENT	RATIONALE

Assess for and report signs and symptoms of a bowel obstruction:
- Increased abdominal cramping and pain
- Vomiting
- Abdominal distention
- Change in bowel sounds (bowel sounds can be high-pitched and more hyperactive if the bowel is partially obstructed, or they can be absent once there is complete obstruction)
- Abdominal radiograph showing partial or complete bowel obstruction

Early recognition of signs and symptoms of a bowel obstruction allows for prompt intervention.

Continued...

THERAPEUTIC INTERVENTIONS	RATIONALE

Dependent/Collaborative Actions

If signs and symptoms of a bowel obstruction occur:

- Withhold oral intake as ordered.
- Insert nasogastric tube and maintain suction as ordered.
- Administer intravenous fluids if ordered.

- Prepare client for endoscopic balloon dilatation of strictures or surgical intervention (e.g., stricturoplasty, bowel resection) if planned.

These actions provide decompression of the gastrointestinal tract.

Administration of IV fluids are required to maintain adequate vascular volume. Dehydration occurs with prolonged vomiting, and third-spacing occurs because of the increased capillary permeability that results from increased intraluminal pressure in a bowel obstruction.

Provide preprocedure or preoperative information as required by the client.

Collaborative Diagnosis   **RISK FOR PERITONITIS**

Definition: Inflammation of the peritoneum

Related to: Perforation of the bowel or leakage from an abscess or fistula

CLINICAL MANIFESTATIONS

Subjective	Objective
Verbalization of abdominal pain	Nausea and vomiting; distended and rigid abdomen; diminished or absent bowel sounds; fever; tachypnea; increased WBC count

RISK FACTORS	DESIRED OUTCOMES

• Exposure to pathogens
• Treatment regimen
	The client will not develop peritonitis as evidenced by:
	  a. Temperature declining toward normal
	  b. Soft, nondistended abdomen
	  c. Gradual resolution of abdominal pain
	  d. Gradual return of normal bowel sounds
	  e. Absence of nausea and vomiting
	  f. Stable vital signs
	  g. WBC count declining toward normal

NURSING ASSESSMENT	RATIONALE

Assess for and report signs and symptoms of peritonitis (e.g., increase in severity of abdominal pain; generalized abdominal pain; rebound tenderness; distended, rigid abdomen; increase in temperature; tachycardia; tachypnea; hypotension; nausea; vomiting; continued diminished or absent bowel sounds; WBC count that increases or fails to decline toward normal).

Early recognition of signs and symptoms of peritonitis allows for prompt intervention.

THERAPEUTIC INTERVENTIONS	RATIONALE

Dependent/Collaborative Actions

If signs and symptoms of peritonitis occur:

- Withhold oral intake as ordered.

- Place client on bedrest in a semi-Fowler's position.

- Prepare client for diagnostic tests (e.g., abdominal radiograph, computed tomography, ultrasonography) if planned.

Oral intake irritates the colon and increases pain associated with peritonitis.

These positions assist in pooling or localizing intestinal contents in the pelvis rather than under the diaphragm

Provide preprocedure information as required by the client.

THERAPEUTIC INTERVENTIONS	RATIONALE
• Insert nasogastric tube and maintain suction as ordered.	*Decompresses the gastrointestinal tract.*
• Administer antimicrobials (e.g., metronidazole) as ordered.	*Helps decrease infection in the gastrointestinal tract.*
• Administer intravenous fluids and/or blood volume expanders if ordered.	*IV fluids and/or blood volume expanders prevents or treats shock that can result from the increased capillary permeability that occurs with inflammation and the subsequent escape of protein, fluid, and electrolytes from the vascular space into the peritoneal cavity.*
• Prepare client for surgical intervention (e.g., repair of perforation, bowel resection) if planned.	

Nursing Diagnosis | # DEFICIENT KNOWLEDGE NDx; INEFFECTIVE FAMILY THERAPEUTIC REGIMEN MANAGEMENT NDx; OR INEFFECTIVE SELF HEALTH MANAGEMENT* NDx

Definition: Absence or deficiency of cognitive information related to specific topic (lack of specific information necessary for clients/significant others) to make informed choices regarding condition/treatment/lifestyle changes; Pattern of regulating and integrating into daily living and family processes a therapeutic regimen for treatment of illness and the sequelae of illness that is unsatisfactory for meeting specific health goals.

CLINICAL MANIFESTATIONS

Subjective	Objective
Verbalization of the problem	Inaccurate follow through of instructions; inappropriate behaviors

RISK FACTORS
• Denial of disease process
• Cognitive deficiency
• Failure to take action to reduce risk factors

NOC OUTCOMES	NIC INTERVENTIONS
Knowledge: diet; knowledge: medication; knowledge: treatment regimen	Health system guidance; teaching: individual; teaching: disease process; teaching: prescribed diet; teaching: prescribed medication

NURSING ASSESSMENT	RATIONALE
Assess client's ability and readiness to learn. Assess the client's understanding of teaching.	*Learning is more effective when the client is motivated and understands the importance of what is to be learned. Readiness to learn changes based on situations, physical and emotional challenges.*

THERAPEUTIC INTERVENTIONS	RATIONALE

Desired Outcome: The client will identify ways to reduce the incidence of disease exacerbation.

Independent Actions
Reinforce the importance of adhering to the prescribed treatment regimen.

---

*The nurse should select the diagnostic label that is most appropriate for the individual client's teaching needs.

Continued...

THERAPEUTIC INTERVENTIONS	RATIONALE
Instruct the client regarding ways to reduce bowel irritation: • Reduce intake of or avoid foods/fluids likely to be poorly digested or that may irritate the bowel (e.g., raw fruits and vegetables, whole-grain cereals, gravy, fried foods, spicy foods, milk and milk products, caffeine-containing beverages, extremely hot drinks, iced drinks, alcohol). • Avoid use of laxatives.	*Irritation of the bowel may cause nausea and vomiting as well as an exacerbation of the disease.*
Explain that stress can precipitate periods of exacerbation. Provide information about stress management classes and counseling services that may assist client to manage stress.	*Encourage client to find ways of reducing stress in his/her life as this will decrease exacerbations of the disease.*

THERAPEUTIC INTERVENTIONS	RATIONALE

Desired Outcome: The client will verbalize ways to maintain an optimal nutritional status.

Independent Actions

Provide instructions regarding ways to maintain an optimal nutritional status: • Reinforce instructions regarding prescribed diet (a low-residue, high-calorie, high-protein diet is often recommended). • Inform client that eating small, frequent meals rather than three large meals may help achieve the recommended high-calorie intake. • Reinforce the benefits of eating when rested and in a relaxed atmosphere. • Stress the importance of taking vitamins and minerals as prescribed..	*Maintenance of nutritional status and the appropriate diet is important in decreasing exacerbations of the disease and maintaining nutritional status.*

THERAPEUTIC INTERVENTIONS	RATIONALE

Desired Outcome: The client will state ways to prevent perianal skin breakdown.

Independent Actions

Provide the following instructions about ways to prevent perianal skin breakdown: • Use soft toilet tissue for wiping after each bowel movement. • Cleanse perianal area with a mild soap and warm water after each bowel movement; dry thoroughly. • Apply a protective ointment or cream to perianal area after skin has been cleansed.	*Each of these interventions prevents skin breakdown, which subsequently decreases the risk of infection and pain.*

THERAPEUTIC INTERVENTIONS	RATIONALE

Desired Outcome: The client will verbalize an understanding of medications ordered including rationale, food, and drug interactions, side effects, schedule for taking, and importance of taking as prescribed.

Independent Actions

Explain rationale for, side effects of, and importance of taking medications prescribed. Inform client of pertinent food and drug interactions. Examples: • Sulfasalazine • Corticosteroid	*Knowledge of the medication regimen and the impact of these medications on the system, as well as how the medication regimen can be incorporated into the client's lifestyle, allows the client some mechanism of control of his/her disease and the ability to have an active part in treatment and care.*

THERAPEUTIC INTERVENTIONS	RATIONALE
Instruct client to inform physician before taking other prescription and nonprescription medications.	*Over-the-counter medications may impact prescription medications and should not be taken without a health care provider's approval.*

THERAPEUTIC INTERVENTIONS	RATIONALE

Desired Outcome: The client will state signs and symptoms to report to the health care provider.

Independent Actions

Instruct client to report the following signs and symptoms:

- Recurrent episodes of diarrhea and abdominal pain and cramping
- Increasing abdominal distention
- Persistent vomiting
- Unusual rectal or vaginal drainage
- Burning on urination or brownish, foul-smelling urine
- Pain, swelling, or open sores in perianal area
- Continued weight loss
- Constipation
- Yellowing of skin, flank pain, change in vision, eye pain, or joint pain or swelling (can indicate extraintestinal involvement)

The client and significant others should be aware of what symptoms are associated with exacerbations of the disease or infection and to report these to the health care provider.

THERAPEUTIC INTERVENTIONS	RATIONALE

Desired Outcome: The client will identify resources that can assist in the adjustment to changes resulting from inflammatory bowel disease and its treatment.

Independent Actions

Provide information about resources that can assist the client and significant others in adjusting to inflammatory bowel disease and its effects (e.g., local support groups, Crohn's and Colitis Foundation of America, counseling services, stress management classes).

Client may require assistance from community organizations for both emotional and financial support once discharged from the acute care facility.

Reinforce importance of keeping follow-up appointments with health care provider.

Inflammatory bowel disease is a chronic illness and requires appropriate follow-up with health care providers.

THERAPEUTIC INTERVENTIONS	RATIONALE

Desired Outcome: The client will verbalize an understanding of and a plan for adhering to recommended follow-up care including future appointments with health care provider and activity level.

Independent Actions

Reinforce importance of frequent rest periods throughout the day.

Allows body to heal.

Implement measures to improve client compliance:

- Include significant others in teaching sessions if possible

Support from client's significant others is important in maintaining compliance to the therapeutic regimen.

- Encourage questions and allow time for reinforcement and clarification of information provided.

Improves client's and family's understanding of disease process and what to do to remain healthy.

- Provide written instructions on future appointments with health care provider, medications prescribed, signs and symptoms to report, and future laboratory studies.

Written instructions allow the client to refer to them after discharge as needed.

ADDITIONAL NURSING DIAGNOSIS

DISTURBED SLEEP PATTERN NDx
Related to frequent need to defecate, pain, fear, and anxiety

FEAR NDx

ANXIETY NDx
Related to:
- Symptoms being experienced (e.g., abdominal pain, persistent diarrhea, fever)
- Lack of understanding of diagnosis, diagnostic tests, and treatment
- Concern about need for surgery if disease condition cannot be medically controlled
- Anticipated changes in future lifestyle because of inability to control symptoms
- Concern about expense of hospitalization and treatment for a chronic disease

DISTURBED SELF-CONCEPT
Related to:
- Dependence on others to meet self-care needs
- Embarrassment associated with diarrhea
- Changes in sexual functioning associated with pain, fatigue, and weakness
- Changes in lifestyle associated with pain and chronic diarrhea

RISK FOR IMPAIRED TISSUE INTEGRITY NDx
Related to:
- Damage to the skin and/or subcutaneous tissue associated with prolonged pressure on the tissues, friction, and shearing that can occur when mobility decreased
- Frequent contact with irritants associated with persistent diarrhea
- Increased fragility of skin associated with malnutrition
- Hyperthermia related to stimulation of the thermoregulatory center in the hypothalamus by endogenous pyrogens that are released in an inflammatory process

ACTIVITY INTOLERANCE NDx
Related to:
- Inadequate nutritional status
- Difficulty resting and sleeping associated with pain, frequent need to defecate, fear, and anxiety
- Tissue hypoxia associated with anemia resulting from:
  - Blood loss from the ulcerated bowel
  - Decreased oral intake and impaired absorption of iron, vitamin B_{12}, and folate
- Increased energy expenditure associated with the increased metabolic rate that may be present during period of exacerbation

INTESTINAL OBSTRUCTION AND BOWEL RESECTION

Intestinal (bowel) obstruction is a condition in which the intestinal contents fail to move through the bowel. The obstruction can be partial or complete and can develop slowly or rapidly. It can occur as a result of any factor that narrows the lumen of the intestine or interferes with peristalsis. Narrowing of the lumen results in a mechanical obstruction and can be caused by factors such as adhesions, tumors, inflammatory bowel disease, hernias, fecal impaction, intussusception, a volvulus, and strictures. In a nonmechanical obstruction, the bowel lumen remains open but the intestinal contents are not propelled forward. Factors that can cause this paralytic (adynamic) ileus include abdominal surgery, effects of anesthesia and some medications (e.g., narcotic [opioid] analgesics, some antiemetics, anticholinergics, antidiarrheals), electrolyte imbalances such as hypokalemia, decreased blood flow to the intestine (can occur with conditions such as hypovolemia or blockage of mesenteric vessels as a result of an embolus, thrombus, or arteriosclerosis), spinal cord injury, and peritonitis.

Signs and symptoms of intestinal obstruction vary depending on the location, cause, and degree of the obstruction. Common clinical manifestations include abdominal pain and distention, nausea, and vomiting. Hyperactive, high-pitched bowel sounds are present early in the development of a mechanical obstruction. Bowel sounds are absent or hypoactive in nonmechanical obstruction and as mechanical obstruction worsens.

Treatment of intestinal obstruction is directed toward relieving symptoms, managing fluid and electrolyte imbalances, preventing complications, and determining and treating the cause of the obstruction. Most cases of nonmechanical obstruction do not necessitate surgery. Some mechanical obstructions can be treated nonsurgically (e.g., enemas and laxatives to remove fecal impaction, dilatation of obstructed portion of bowel via endoscopy, radiation or chemotherapy to reduce tumor size, gentle instillation of barium to resolve an intussusception or reverse a sigmoid volvulus). Surgical intervention (intestinal resection with reanastomosis or creation of an ileostomy or colostomy) is indicated when it is necessary to remove an obstruction that persists despite conservative management or to remove a segment of bowel that is strangulated or necrotic.

This care plan focuses on the adult client hospitalized with an intestinal obstruction and addresses what postoperative care is required if a bowel resection is required. Some of the information is applicable to clients receiving follow-up care in an extended care facility or home setting.

OUTCOME/DISCHARGE CRITERIA

The client who does not have surgery will:
1. Have absence of or minimal abdominal pain
2. Have gradual return of normal bowel function
3. Tolerate prescribed diet
4. Have no signs and symptoms of complications
5. Verbalize an understanding of ways to reduce the risk for recurrent intestinal obstruction
6. State signs and symptoms to report to the health care provider
7. Verbalize an understanding of and a plan for adhering to recommended diet, prescribed medications, ways to prevent recurrent intestinal obstruction, and future appointments with health care provider.

POSTOPERATIVE

The client will:
1. Have absence of or minimal abdominal postoperative pain
2. Have gradual return of normal bowel function
3. Tolerate prescribed diet
4. Have no signs and symptoms of postoperative complications
5. Have clear, audible breath sounds throughout lungs
6. Have evidence of normal healing of surgical wound(s)
7. Verbalize an understanding of ways to reduce the risk for recurrent intestinal obstruction
8. State signs and symptoms to report to the health care provider
9. Verbalize an understanding of and a plan for adhering to recommended diet, prescribed medications, ways to prevent recurrent intestinal obstruction, and future appointments with health care provider.

Nursing/Collaborative Diagnosis   **IMBALANCED FLUID AND ELECTROLYTES***

Definition: Risk for developing an imbalance of electrolytes and fluids in the intracellular and extracellular compartments of the body

Related to:
- **Deficient fluid volume NDx, hypokalemia, hypochloremia,** and **metabolic alkalosis** related to:
  - Decreased absorption of intestinal fluid into the vascular space associated with inflammation and distention of the bowel (the sequestering of fluid in the intestine is a major factor with obstructions of the small intestine and proximal portion of the large intestine)
  - Restricted oral intake
  - Excessive loss of fluid and electrolytes associated with vomiting and nasogastric tube drainage
- **Third-spacing** related to the increased capillary permeability that results from increased intraluminal pressure in the distended bowel

CLINICAL MANIFESTATIONS

Subjective	Objective
Complaint of nausea, headache, and abdominal pain	Poor skin turgor; dry, cracked mucous membranes; hypotension; weight loss; prolonged capillary refill greater than 2 to 3 seconds; decreased urine output; increased urine specific gravity; abdominal distention; vomiting; positive Chvostek's and Trousseau's signs; abnormal serum electrolyte levels; cardiac dysrhythmias, muscle weakness, paresthesias, twitching, spasms, and dizziness; increased BUN and Hct

---

*The nurse must determine the appropriate nursing diagnosis based on assessment of the client.

NDx = NANDA-I Diagnosis   **D** = Delegatable Action   ● = UAP   ✦ = LVN/LPN   ⊖▶ = Go to ⊖volve for animation

Continued...

RISK FACTORS

- Failure of regulatory mechanisms
- Inadequate fluid/food intake
- Immobility

DESIRED OUTCOMES

The client will maintain fluid and electrolyte balance as evidenced by:
  a. Normal skin turgor
  b. Moist mucous membranes
  c. Stable weight
  d. B/P and pulse rate within normal range for client and stable with position change
  e. Capillary refill time less than 2 to 3 seconds
  f. Usual mental status
  g. Balanced intake and output
  h. Urine specific gravity within normal range
  i. Abdomen less distended and bowel sounds returning toward normal
  j. Absence of cardiac dysrhythmias, muscle weakness, paresthesias, twitching, spasms, and dizziness
  k. BUN, Hct, serum electrolyte, and arterial blood gas values within normal range

NOC OUTCOMES

Fluid balance; electrolyte and acid-base balance

NIC INTERVENTIONS

Fluid management; electrolyte management: hypokalemia; electrolyte management: hypocalcemia; electrolyte management: hypomagnesemia; acid-base management: metabolic acidosis; diarrhea management

NURSING ASSESSMENT

Assess for and report signs and symptoms of deficient fluid volume:
- Decreased skin turgor, dry mucous membranes, thirst
- Weight loss of 2% or greater over a short period
- Postural hypotension and/or low B/P
- Weak, rapid pulse
- Capillary refill time longer than 2 to 3 seconds
- Neck veins flat when client is supine
- Change in mental status
- Decreased urine output with increased specific gravity (reflects an actual rather than potential fluid deficit)
- Significant increase in BUN and Hct above previous levels
- Hypokalemia (e.g., cardiac dysrhythmias, postural hypotension, muscle weakness, nausea and vomiting, abdominal distention, hypoactive or absent bowel sounds,
- Hypomagnesemia and/or hypocalcemia (e.g., anxiousness; irritability; cardiac dysrhythmias; positive Chvostek's and Trousseau's signs; numbness or tingling of fingers, toes, or circumoral area; hyperactive reflexes; tetany; seizures)
- Metabolic acidosis (e.g., drowsiness; disorientation; stupor; rapid, deep respirations; headache; nausea and vomiting; cardiac dysrhythmias; low pH and CO_2 content)
- Third-spacing
- Ascites
- Evidence of vascular depletion (e.g., postural hypotension, weak, rapid pulse; decreased urine output)

RATIONALE

Early recognition of signs and symptoms of electrolyte imbalance allows for prompt treatment.

THERAPEUTIC INTERVENTIONS

Independent Actions
Implement measures to prevent or treat imbalanced fluid and electrolytes:

RATIONALE

THERAPEUTIC INTERVENTIONS	RATIONALE
• Perform actions to reduce nausea and vomiting (e.g., eliminate noxious stimuli, have patient change positions slowly, provide oral hygiene after each meal). **D** ● ✦	*These interventions decrease nausea and vomiting, helping to maintain positive fluid and electrolyte imbalance.*
If a nasogastric tube is present and needs to be irrigated frequently and/or with large volumes of solution, irrigate it with normal saline rather than water. **D** ✦	*Provides decompression of the stomach, and irrigation with normal saline causes less irritation of the gastric mucosa.*
Dependent/Collaborative Actions Implement measures to prevent or treat imbalanced fluid and electrolytes:	
• Maintain intravenous fluid therapy as ordered.	*Prevents dehydration.*
• Administer electrolyte replacement as ordered.	*Helps to maintain appropriate electrolyte balance.*
• Administer albumin infusions if ordered.	*Increases colloid osmotic pressure and promotes mobilization of third-space fluid back into the vascular space.*
• When oral intake is allowed, assist client to select foods/fluids within the prescribed dietary regimen that would replenish electrolytes. **D** ✦	*Oral intake of foods high in potassium is necessary to maintain adequate electrolyte balance.*
Consult physician if signs and symptoms of imbalanced fluid and electrolytes persist or worsen.	*Notification of the physician allows for prompt alteration in the treatment plan.*

Nursing Diagnosis ACUTE PAIN NDx (ABDOMINAL)

Definition: Unpleasant sensory and emotional experience arising from actual or potential tissue damage or described in terms of such damage (International Association for the Study of Pain); sudden or slow onset of any intensity from mild to severe with an anticipated or predictable end and a duration of less than 6 months

Related to:
• Distention of the intestinal lumen associated with the accumulation of gas and fluid
• Inflammation of the intestine (can occur as a result of the underlying cause of the obstruction [e.g., inflammatory bowel disease])

CLINICAL MANIFESTATIONS

Subjective	**Objective**
Verbal or coded report of pain	Autonomic responses (e.g., diaphoresis; changes in B/P, respiration, pulse rate; pupillary dilatation); expressive behavior (e.g., restlessness, moaning, crying, vigilance, irritability, sighing); changes in appetite and eating; protective gestures; guarding behavior; facial mask; sleep disturbance (eyes lack luster, fixed or scattered movement, beaten look, grimace); self-focus; narrowed focus (altered time perception, impaired thought processes, reduced interaction with people and environment); distraction behavior (e.g., pacing, seeking out other people and/or activities, repetitive activities)

RISK FACTOR
• Chronic illness

DESIRED OUTCOMES

The client will experience diminished pain as evidenced by:
  a. Verbalization of same
  b. Relaxed facial expression
  c. Increased participation in activities
  d. Stable vital signs

NDx = NANDA-I Diagnosis **D** = Delegatable Action ● = UAP ✦ = LVN/LPN ⊝▶ = Go to ⊝volve for animation

Continued...

NOC OUTCOMES	NIC INTERVENTIONS
Pain control; minimizing pain's disruptive effects	Pain management; environmental management: comfort; analgesic administration

NURSING ASSESSMENT	RATIONALE
Assess for signs and symptoms of pain (e.g., verbalization of pain, grimacing, reluctance to move, restlessness, diaphoresis, increased B/P, tachycardia).	*Early recognition of signs and symptoms of pain allows for prompt intervention and improved pain control.*
Assess client's perception of the severity of pain using a pain intensity rating scale.	*An awareness of the severity of pain being experienced helps determine the most appropriate interventions for pain management. Use of a pain intensity rating scale gives the nurse a clearer understanding of the pain being experienced and promotes consistency when communicating with others about the client's pain experience.*
Assess the client's pain pattern (e.g., location, quality, onset, duration, precipitating factors, aggravating factors, alleviating factors).	*Knowledge of the client's pain pattern assists in the identification of effective pain management interventions.*
Ask the client to describe previous pain experiences and methods used to manage pain effectively.	*Many variables affect a client's response to pain (e.g., age, sex, coping style, previous experience with pain, culture, cause of pain). Knowledge of the client's usual response to pain and methods previously used to manage pain effectively enables the nurse to evaluate the client's pain more accurately and facilitates the identification of effective strategies for pain management.*

THERAPEUTIC INTERVENTIONS	RATIONALE

Independent Actions

Implement measures to reduce fear and anxiety (e.g., assure client that the need for pain relief is understood, plan methods for achieving pain control with client, provide a calm environment).	*Fear and anxiety can decrease the client's threshold and tolerance for pain and thereby heighten the perception of pain. In addition, pain management methods are not as effective if the client is tense and unable to relax.*
Perform actions to decrease the accumulation of intestinal gas and fluid (e.g., using a straw, chewing gum, sucking on ice or hard candy, and smoking). **D** ● ✦	*These actions reduce air swallowing and subsequent gas production.*
Implement measures to promote rest (e.g., minimize environmental activity and noise, provide care to allow for periods of interrupted rest). **D** ● ✦	*Fatigue can decrease the client's threshold and tolerance for pain and thereby heighten the perception of pain. A well-rested client often experiences decreased pain and increased effectiveness of pain management measures.*
When oral intake is allowed, advance diet slowly and instruct client to avoid intake of carbonated beverages and gas-producing foods (e.g., cabbage, onions, beans).	*Reduces gas in the gastrointestinal tract.*

Dependent/Collaborative Actions

Insert nasogastric tube and maintain suction as ordered.	*Provides decompression and prevents gas accumulation in the stomach*
Administer gastrointestinal stimulants (e.g., metoclopramide) if ordered. **D** ✦	*Promotes intestinal motility (may be ordered if obstruction is not complete or is the result of a paralytic ileus)*
Administer analgesics as ordered (the use of narcotic [opioid] analgesics is often avoided until the cause of the obstruction is determined). **D** ✦	*The administration of analgesics before a pain-producing event helps minimize the pain that will be experienced. Analgesics are also more effective if given before pain becomes severe because mild to moderate pain is controlled more quickly and effectively than severe pain.*

THERAPEUTIC INTERVENTIONS	RATIONALE
Provide or assist with nonpharmacological methods for pain relief. Examples include: • Cutaneous stimulation measures (e.g., pressure, massage, heat and cold applications, transcutaneous electrical nerve stimulation [TENS], acupuncture) • Relaxation techniques (e.g., progressive relaxation exercises, meditation, guided imagery) • Distraction measures (e.g., listening to music, conversing, watching television, playing cards, reading) • Position change Consult appropriate health care provider (e.g., physician, pharmacist, pain management specialist) if above measures fail to provide adequate pain relief.	*Nonpharmacological pain management includes a variety of interventions. It is believed that most of these are effective because they stimulate closure of the gating mechanism in the spinal cord and subsequently block the transmission of pain impulses. In addition, some interventions are thought to stimulate the release of endogenous analgesics (e.g., endorphins) that inhibit the transmission of pain impulses and/or alter the client's perception of pain. Many of the nonpharmacological interventions also help decrease pain by promoting relaxation.* *Notifying the appropriate health care provider allows for modification of the treatment plan.*

Nursing Diagnosis **NAUSEA** NDx

Definition: An unpleasant, wavelike sensation in the back of the throat, epigastrium, or throughout the abdomen that may or may not lead to vomiting

Related to:
• Stimulation of the vomiting center associated with:
  • Stimulation of the visceral afferent pathways resulting from inflammation and distention of the intestine
  • Stimulation of the cerebral cortex resulting from pain and stress

CLINICAL MANIFESTATIONS

Subjective	Objective
Complaints of nausea	N/A

RISK FACTORS
• Chronic illness
• Gastric irritation

DESIRED OUTCOMES

The client will experience relief of nausea and vomiting as evidenced by:
  a. Verbalization of relief of nausea
  b. Absence of vomiting

NOC OUTCOMES

Nausea and vomiting severity

NIC INTERVENTIONS

Nausea management; vomiting management; environmental management: comfort

NURSING ASSESSMENT	RATIONALE
Assess for nausea and vomiting. Determine: • Duration • Frequency • Severity	*Identification of the signs and symptoms of nausea and vomiting allows for prompt intervention.*

THERAPEUTIC INTERVENTIONS	RATIONALE
Independent Actions Implement measures to reduce nausea and vomiting: • Maintain food and oral fluid restrictions as ordered.	*Food/fluid restrictions and insertion of an NG tube decreases pressure within the abdomen.*

Continued...

THERAPEUTIC INTERVENTIONS	RATIONALE

Dependent/Collaborative Actions

- Insert nasogastric tube and maintain suction as ordered.
- Eliminate noxious sights and odors from the environment.
- Instruct client to change positions slowly. **D** ● ✦

Provide oral hygiene after each emesis. **D** ● ✦

Reduce pain via medications, positioning, or distractions. **D** ✦

- Perform actions to reduce fear and anxiety (e.g., assure client that staff are nearby; provide a calm, restful environment; explain all tests and procedures).

Encourage client to take deep, slow breaths when nauseated. **D** ● ✦

Noxious stimuli can cause stimulation of the vomiting center.
Rapid movements can result in chemoreceptor trigger zone stimulation and subsequent excitation of the vomiting center.
Oral hygiene removes the taste of emesis from the mouth and helps to decrease subsequent nausea.
Pain may stimulate chemoreceptor trigger zone and produce nausea.

Fear and anxiety may produce nausea.

Taking slow, deep breaths helps to relax the client and reduce stress.

Dependent/Collaborative Actions

Implement measures to reduce nausea and vomiting:
Administer antiemetics as ordered. **D** ✦

- When oral intake is allowed, advance diet slowly. Initially encourage bland floods such as jello, rice, broth, toast, and dry crackers.

Consult a physician or a pharmacist if nausea continues.

Antiemetics raise the threshold of the chemoreceptor trigger zone, thus decreasing nausea.
Oral intake helps maintain nutritional status and should be advanced slowly to decrease the incidence of nausea.

Allows for continued intervention to decrease/eliminate nausea.

Collaborative/Nursing Diagnosis   # RISK FOR PERITONITIS

 Definition: Inflammation of the peritoneum.

Related to: Release of intestinal contents into the peritoneal cavity associated with perforation of the bowel if it occurs

CLINICAL MANIFESTATIONS

Subjective	Objective
Verbalization of abdominal pain	Nausea and vomiting; distended and rigid abdomen; diminished or absent bowel sounds; fever; tachypnea; increased WBC count

RISK FACTORS

- Exposure to pathogens
- Chronic illness

DESIRED OUTCOMES

The client will not develop peritonitis as evidenced by:
   a. Temperature stable and less than 36°C
   b. Abdomen less distended and firm
   c. No increase in abdominal pain and tenderness, nausea, and vomiting
   d. Gradual return of normal bowel sounds
   e. Stable vital signs
   f. No increase in WBC count

NURSING ASSESSMENT	RATIONALE

Assess for and report signs and symptoms of peritonitis (e.g., further increase in temperature or temperature >38°C, abdomen more distended and firm, increase in severity of abdominal pain, rebound tenderness, increased nausea and vomiting, tachycardia, hypotension, increase in WBC count)

Early recognition of signs and symptoms of peritonitis allows for prompt intervention.

THERAPEUTIC INTERVENTIONS	RATIONALE

Dependent/Collaborative Actions

Implement measures to prevent peritonitis:
- Perform actions to reduce the risk for perforation of the bowel:
  - Implement measures to decrease the accumulation of intestinal gas and fluid (e.g., insert a nasogastric tube and attach to suction, avoid carbonated beverages, avoid gas-producing foods).
  - Continue with actions to treat the underlying cause of the obstruction (e.g., anti-inflammatory agents to treat inflammatory bowel disease, chemotherapeutic agents to reduce tumor size).
- Administer antimicrobials if ordered.

These actions maintain decompression of the gut.

Antimicrobials reduce/prevent infection.

If signs and symptoms of peritonitis occur:
- Withhold oral food and fluids as ordered.
- Place client on bedrest in semi-Fowler's position.

Decrease pressure within the abdomen.
Assists in pooling or localizing gastrointestinal contents in the pelvis rather than the diaphragm.

- Prepare client for diagnostic tests (e.g., abdominal radiograph, computed tomography) if planned.
- Administer antimicrobials as ordered.
- Administer fluids and/or blood volume expanders if ordered.

Decreases client's fear and anxiety

Antimicrobials reduce infection.
Fluid volume and/or blood expanders prevent or treat shock that can result from the increased capillary permeability that occurs with inflammation and the subsequent escape of protein, fluid, and electrolytes from the vascular space into the peritoneal cavity.

- Prepare client for surgery (e.g., drainage and irrigation of the peritoneum, bowel resection) if planned.

If infection is not controlled, a bowel resection may be required.

Collaborative Diagnosis | # RISK FOR INTESTINAL NECROSIS

Definition: Death of intestinal tissue

Related to:
- Obstruction of blood flow in the affected area associated with:
  - Inflammation and distention of the bowel lumen
  - Hypovolemia
  - Mesenteric vessel thrombosis or embolus (can be a cause of nonmechanical obstruction)
  - Strangulation of a portion of the intestine (especially if obstruction is a result of a hernia, strictures, adhesions, or a volvulus)

CLINICAL MANIFESTATIONS

Subjective	Objective
Verbalization of severe abdominal pain	Bloody diarrhea; increased WBC count

RISK FACTORS
- Exposure to pathogens
- Chronic illness
- Lack of exercise

DESIRED OUTCOMES
The client will not experience intestinal necrosis as evidenced by:
  a. Decreased abdominal pain
  b. Absence of bloody diarrhea
  c. No increase in WBC count

NDx = NANDA-I Diagnosis **D** = Delegatable Action ● = UAP ✦ = LVN/LPN ⊖▶ = Go to ⊖volve for animation

Continued...

NURSING ASSESSMENT	RATIONALE
Assess for and report signs and symptoms of intestinal necrosis (e.g., severe, continuous abdominal pain; bloody diarrhea; WBC count that increases or fails to decline toward normal).	*Early recognition of signs and symptoms of complications of intestinal obstruction allows for prompt intervention.*

THERAPEUTIC INTERVENTIONS	RATIONALE

Dependent/Collaborative Interventions

Implement measures to improve blood flow to the intestine in order to prevent intestinal necrosis:	
• Perform actions to prevent and treat deficient fluid volume (e.g., provide antiemetics for nausea and vomiting, insert nasogastric tube as needed, maintain intravenous fluids as ordered, administer electrolytes as needed).	*Maintenance of fluid volume is necessary to maintain adequate circulation to the gut.*
• Perform actions to reduce the accumulation of intestinal gas and fluid (e.g., instruct client not to chew gum, suck on ice or hard candy; insert nasogastric tube as needed; avoid carbonated beverages).	*Decreases intestinal gas and fluid, which may decrease intestinal blood flow.*
• Prepare client for treatment of the underlying cause of vascular obstruction (e.g., mesenteric thrombectomy or embolectomy; surgery to repair hernia, release adhesions, or correct volvulus) if planned.	*If obstruction is not resolved, surgery may be necessary. The type of surgical intervention depends upon the underlying cause of the obstruction.*
If signs and symptoms of intestinal necrosis occur:	
• Administer antimicrobials if ordered.	*Prevention of infection.*
• Prepare client for surgical resection of the affected bowel.	*Usually performed if the client has extensive tissue necrosis or gangrenous patches have developed.*

DISCHARGE INFORMATION IF CLIENT DOES NOT REQUIRE SURGERY

Nursing Diagnosis

DEFICIENT KNOWLEDGE NDx; INEFFECTIVE FAMILY THERAPEUTIC REGIMEN MANAGEMENT NDx; OR INEFFECTIVE SELF HEALTH MANAGEMENT* NDx

Definition: Absence or deficiency of cognitive information related to specific topic (lack of specific information necessary for clients/significant others) to make informed choices regarding condition/treatment/lifestyle changes; Pattern of regulating and integrating into daily living and family processes a therapeutic regimen for treatment of illness and the sequelae of illness that is unsatisfactory for meeting specific health goals.

CLINICAL MANIFESTATIONS

Subjective	Objective
Verbalizes inability to manage illness; verbalizes inability to follow prescribed regimen	Inaccurate follow through with instructions; inappropriate behaviors; experience of preventable complications of spinal cord injury

RISK FACTORS
• Cognitive deficit
• Financial concerns
• Failure to take action to reduce risk factors for complications of Parkinson's Disease
• Inability to care for oneself
• Difficulty in modifying personal habits and integrating treatments into lifestyle

*The nurse must determine the appropriate diagnosis based on client assessment.

NOC OUTCOMES	NIC INTERVENTIONS
Knowledge: disease process; knowledge: treatment regimen	Health system guidance; teaching: individual; teaching: disease process; teaching: prescribed diet; teaching: prescribed medication

NURSING ASSESSMENT	RATIONALE
Assess the client's ability to learn and readiness to learn Assess the client's understanding of teaching	*Learning is more effective when the client is motivated and understands the importance of what is to be learned. Readiness to learn changes based on situations, physical and emotional challenges.*

THERAPEUTIC INTERVENTIONS	RATIONALE

Desired Outcome: The client will state signs and symptoms to report to health care providers.

Independent Actions

Instruct client to report the following signs and symptoms: • Recurrent episodes of abdominal pain • Increasing abdominal distention • Nausea or vomiting • Constipation • Elevated temperature	*Client awareness of what changes require health care intervention will improve timeliness of treatment for complications.*

THERAPEUTIC INTERVENTIONS	RATIONALE

Desired Outcome: The client will verbalize an understanding of ways to minimize the risk of recurrence of intestinal obstruction.

Independent Actions

Reinforce physician's instructions regarding ways to prevent the risk for recurrent intestinal obstruction. For example: • Follow-up radiation and/or chemotherapy if obstruction was caused by a tumor • Dietary and medication management if obstruction was caused by inflammatory bowel disease • Bowel care regimen if obstruction was caused by a fecal impaction.	*Reinforcement of information provided by the physician allows for clients to ask questions and improve their understanding of the causes of recurrence of bowel obstruction, and the dietary interventions to help prevent further complications.*

THERAPEUTIC INTERVENTIONS	RATIONALE

Desired Outcome: The client will verbalize an understanding of and a plan for adhering to recommended follow-up care including recommended diet, prescribed medications, ways to prevent recurrent intestinal obstruction, and future appointments with health care provider.

Independent Actions

Reinforce the importance of keeping follow-up appointments with health care provider.	*Allows for health care provider to monitor progress and alter interventions as needed.*
Reinforce physician's instructions regarding dietary restrictions and advancement of diet.	*Important to maintain nutritional status and to promote healing.*
Reinforce physician's instructions regarding prescribed medications.	*Adherence to the regimen is increased with education about prescribed medications.*
Include significant others in teaching sessions if possible.	*Significant others may provide support to clients as they implement treatment regimen.*

Continued...

THERAPEUTIC INTERVENTIONS	RATIONALE
Encourage questions and allow time for reinforcement and clarification of information provided.	*Allows client to internalize information and clarify any areas of confusion.*
Provide written instructions on future appointments with health care provider, dietary restrictions, medications prescribed, and signs and symptoms to report.	*Allows quick reference once the client has been discharged.*

POSTOPERATIVE INTERVENTIONS

Nursing Diagnosis   INEFFECTIVE BREATHING PATTERN NDx

Definition: Inspiration and/or expiration that does not provide adequate ventilation

Related to:
- Reluctance to breathe deeply due to pain, weakness, and a large abdominal incision
- Decreased rate and depth of respirations associated with the depressant effect of anesthesia

CLINICAL MANIFESTATIONS

Subjective	Objective
Verbal report of difficulty breathing	Alterations in depth of breathing; altered chest excursion; bradypnea; decreased minute ventilation; use of accessory muscles to breathe; dyspnea

RISK FACTOR	DESIRED OUTCOMES

• Surgical procedure	The client will maintain an effective breathing pattern as evidenced by:
	  a. Normal rate and depth of respirations
	  b. Absence of dyspnea

NOC OUTCOMES	NIC INTERVENTIONS
Respiratory status: ventilation	Ventilation assistance; respiratory monitoring

NURSING ASSESSMENT	RATIONALE
Assess for signs and symptoms of an ineffective breathing pattern: • Shallow or slow respirations • Limited chest excursion • Tachypnea or dyspnea • Use of accessory muscles when breathing	*Early recognition of signs and symptoms of an ineffective breathing pattern allows for prompt intervention.*
Assess/monitor pulse oximetry (arterial oxygen saturation [SaO_2]) and arterial blood gas (ABG) values as indicated.	*Monitoring continuous SaO_2 readings allows for the early detection of hypoxia.* *Assessment of ABG values allows for a more direct measurement of both the partial pressure of oxygen in arterial blood (PaO_2) and the partial pressure of carbon dioxide in arterial blood ($PaCO_2$), both of which reflect the adequacy of ventilation.*

THERAPEUTIC INTERVENTIONS	RATIONALE
Independent Actions Implement measures to improve breathing pattern: • Perform actions to reduce fear and anxiety: • Promote a calm, restful environment.	*Reducing the client's fear and anxiety helps to prevent shallow and/ or rapid breathing.*

THERAPEUTIC INTERVENTIONS	RATIONALE

• Perform actions to reduce pain:
  • Reposition client for comfort.
  • Instruct client to support incision when moving or coughing.
	Reducing pain helps to increase the client's willingness to move and breathe more deeply.

• Perform actions to reduce the accumulation of gas and fluid in the gastrointestinal tract: • Maintain patency of nasogastric, gastric, or intestinal tubes if present.	*Reducing the accumulation of gas in the gastrointestinal tract decreases pressure on the diaphragm, facilitating more effective ventilation.*
• Perform actions to increase strength and improve activity tolerance (e.g., increase activity as tolerated; provide for periods of rest; maintain adequate nutrition): • Implement measures to conserve energy.	*Increasing activity tolerance enables the client to breathe more deeply and participate in activities to improve breathing pattern.*
• Have client deep breathe or use incentive spirometer every 1 to 2 hours. **D** ✦	*Deep breathing and use of an incentive spirometer promotes maximal inhalation and lung expansion.*
• Instruct client to breathe slowly if hyperventilating.	*Hyperventilation is an ineffective breathing pattern that can lead to respiratory alkalosis.* *A client can often slow breathing rate by concentrating on doing so.*
• Place client in a semi- to high-Fowler's position unless contraindicated.	*A semi- to high-Fowler's position allows for maximal diaphragmatic excursion and lung expansion.*

Dependent/Collaborative Actions

Implement measures to improve breathing pattern:

• Increase activity as allowed and tolerated.	*During activity, especially ambulation, the client usually takes deeper breaths, thus increasing lung expansion.*

• Assist with positive airway pressure techniques if ordered:
  • Continuous positive airway pressure (CPAP)
  • Bilevel positive airway pressure (BiPAP)
  • Flutter/positive expiratory pressure (PEP) device
	Positive airway pressure techniques increase intrapulmonary (alveolar) pressure, which helps reexpand collapsed alveoli and prevent further alveoli collapse.

• Administer central nervous system depressants judiciously. • Hold medication and consult physician if respiratory rate is less than 12 breaths/min.	*Central nervous system depressants cause depression of the respiratory center in the brainstem, which can result in a decreased rate and depth of respiration.*
• Perform actions to reduce pain: • Administer analgesics before activities and procedures that can cause pain and before pain becomes severe. **D** ✦	*Reducing pain helps to increase the client's willingness to move and breathe more deeply.*

Consult appropriate health care provider if:

• Ineffective breathing pattern continues. • Client develops signs and symptoms of impaired gas exchange such as restlessness, irritability, confusion, significant decrease in oximetry results, decreased PaO_2 and increased $PaCO_2$ levels.	*Notifying the appropriate health care provider allows for modification of treatment plan.*

Nursing Diagnosis ## INEFFECTIVE AIRWAY CLEARANCE NDx

Definition: Inability to clear secretions or obstructions from the respiratory tract to maintain a clear airway

Related to:
• Stasis of secretions associated with:
  • Decreased activity
  • Depressed ciliary function due to anesthesia
  • Inability to produce an effective cough effort due to abdominal incision and depressant effect of anesthesia and pain medications

---

Continued...

CLINICAL MANIFESTATIONS

Subjective	**Objective**
Verbal report of difficulty breathing	Dyspnea, orthopnea; diminished breath sounds; adventitious breath sounds (crackles, rhonchi, wheezes); cough, ineffective or absent sputum production; difficulty vocalizing; wide-eyed; restlessness; changes in respiratory rate and rhythm; cyanosis

RISK FACTORS

- Surgical procedure
- Positioning inactivity

DESIRED OUTCOMES

The client will maintain clear, open airways as evidenced by:
  a. Normal breath sounds
  b. Normal rate and depth of respirations
  c. Absence of dyspnea

NOC OUTCOMES

Respiratory status: ventilation; respiratory status: airway patency

NIC INTERVENTIONS

Respiratory monitoring; airway management; cough enhancement

NURSING ASSESSMENT	**RATIONALE**
Assess for signs and symptoms of ineffective airway clearance: • Abnormal breath sounds • Rapid, shallow respirations • Dyspnea • Cough	*Early recognition of signs and symptoms of ineffective airway clearance allows for prompt intervention.*
Assess/monitor pulse oximetry (SaO₂) and ABG values as indicated.	*Monitoring continuous SaO_2 readings allows for the early detection of hypoxia.* *Assessment of ABG values allows for a more direct measurement of both PaO_2 and $PaCO_2$, both of which reflect the adequacy of ventilation.*

THERAPEUTIC INTERVENTIONS	**RATIONALE**

Independent Actions

Implement measures to promote effective airway clearance: • Position client on side and/or insert an artificial airway if necessary.	*An artificial airway helps prevent obstruction of airway by the tongue.*

• Perform actions to reduce pain:
  • Reposition client for comfort. **D** ● ✦
  • Instruct client to support incision when moving or coughing.
	Reducing pain helps to increase the client's willingness to move and breathe more deeply.

Instruct and assist client to change position at least every 2 hours while in bed. **D** ● ✦	*Repositioning helps mobilize secretions.*
• Perform actions to promote the removal of secretions: • Assist client to deep breathe and cough every 1 to 2 hours.	*Deep breathing and coughing can help loosen secretions and enhance the effectiveness of coughing.*
• Support abdominal incision when coughing. **D** ✦	*Provides incisional support while coughing.*
• Discourage smoking.	*Irritants in smoke increase mucus production, impair ciliary function, and can cause inflammation and damage to the bronchial walls.*
• Perform suctioning if needed.	*Suctioning removes secretions from the large airways. It also stimulates coughing, which helps clear airways of mucus and foreign matter.*

THERAPEUTIC INTERVENTIONS	RATIONALE

Dependent/Collaborative Actions

Implement measures to promote effective airway clearance:

- Implement measures to thin tenacious secretions and reduce drying of the respiratory mucous membrane:
  - Maintain a fluid intake of at least 2500 mL/day unless contraindicated.
  - Humidify inspired air as ordered. **D** ✦
  - Assist with administration of mucolytics and diluent or hydrating agents via nebulizer if ordered:
    (1) Acetylcysteine
    (2) Water, saline
- Increase activity as allowed and tolerated. **D** ● ✦
- Administer central nervous system depressants judiciously.

Consult appropriate health care provider such as a physician or respiratory therapist if:

- Signs and symptoms of ineffective airway clearance persist
- Signs and symptoms of impaired gas exchange are present:
  - Restlessness
  - Irritability
  - Confusion
  - Significant decrease in oximetry results
  - Decreased PaO_2 and increased $PaCO_2$

Adequate hydration and humidified inspired air help thin secretions, which facilitates the mobilization and expectoration of secretions.

These actions also reduce dryness of the respiratory mucous membrane, which helps enhance mucociliary clearance.

Mucolytics and diluents or hydrating agents are mucokinetic substances that reduce the viscosity of mucus, thus making it easier for the client to mobilize and clear secretions from the respiratory tract.

Activity helps to mobilize secretions and promotes deeper breathing.

Central nervous system depressants depress the cough reflex, which can result in stasis of secretions.

Notifying the appropriate health care provider allows for modification of the treatment plan.

Nursing Diagnosis

IMBALANCED NUTRITION: LESS THAN BODY REQUIREMENTS NDx

Definition: Intake of nutrients insufficient to meet metabolic needs

Related to:

- Inability to ingest food due to lack of bowel sounds
- Decreased oral intake associated with pain, weakness, fatigue, and nausea
- Increased nutritional needs associated with increased metabolic rate that occurs during wound healing

CLINICAL MANIFESTATIONS

Subjective	Objective
Verbal reports of abdominal cramping or pain; aversion toward eating; lack of interest in food; altered taste sensation	Inadequate food intake; inability to ingest food; diarrhea; hypoactive or absent bowel sounds; weakness of muscles of mastication

RISK FACTORS

- Poor preoperative nutritional status
- Delayed postop nutritional therapy

DESIRED OUTCOMES

The client will maintain an adequate nutritional status as evidenced by:
  a. Weight within normal range for client
  b. Normal BUN and serum albumin, Hct, and Hgb levels and lymphocyte count
  c. Usual strength and activity tolerance
  d. Healthy oral mucous membrane

NOC OUTCOMES

Nutritional status

NIC INTERVENTIONS

Nutritional monitoring; nutrition management; nutrition therapy; diet staging

---

Continued...

NURSING ASSESSMENT	RATIONALE
Assess for and report signs and symptoms of malnutrition: • Weight significantly below client's usual weight or below normal for client's age, height, and body frame • Weakness and fatigue • Sore, inflamed oral mucous membrane • Pale conjunctiva	*Early recognition of signs and symptoms of malnutrition allows for prompt intervention.*
Assess for return of bowel function every 2 to 4 hours.	*Once the client begins to expel flatus, the physician should be notified so oral intake can be resumed as soon as possible.*
Monitor serum albumin, prealbumin, total protein, ferritin, transferrin, Hgb, Hct, and electrolyte levels as indicated.	*Serum albumin levels less than 3.5 g/100 mL are considered a risk for poor nutritional status. Early recognition of abnormal lab values reflective of the client's overall nutritional state allows for prompt intervention.*
When oral intake is allowed, monitor percentage of meals and snacks client consumes. Report pattern of inadequate intake.	*An awareness of the amount of foods/fluids a client consumes alerts the nurse to deficits in nutritional intake. Reporting inadequate intake allows for prompt intervention.*

THERAPEUTIC INTERVENTIONS	RATIONALE

Independent Actions

When food or oral fluids are allowed, implement measures to maintain an adequate nutritional status:
• Implement measures to prevent nausea and vomiting: **D ● ✦**
  • Eliminate noxious sights and odors from the environment.
  • Encourage the client to take deep, slow breaths when nauseated.
  • Instruct client to change positions slowly.
  • Apply a cold washcloth to the client's forehead.
	The presence of nausea can decrease the appetite. Preventing nausea and vomiting can improve the client's appetite. These actions reduce nausea.

• Implement measures to reduce pain: • Instruct client to support incision with movement. **D ✦**	*The presence of pain decreases the appetite.*

Implement measures to reduce the accumulation of gas and fluid in the gastrointestinal tract and prevent constipation. **D ✦**
  • Encourage frequent position changes.
  • Encourage ambulation.
	The subsequent feeling of fullness that accompanies gas accumulation leads to an early feeling of satiety. These actions stimulate peristalsis and move gas and fluid through the bowel.

• Encourage a rest period before meals.	*To conserve energy for consuming meals, rest periods before eating should be encouraged.*
• Provide nursing assistance during meals. **D ●**	
• Maintain a clean environment and a relaxed, pleasant atmosphere. **D ●**	*A pleasant environment helps to promote adequate intake.*
• Provide oral hygiene before meals. **D ●**	*Good oral hygiene enhances appetite. A moist oral mucosa makes chewing and swallowing easier. Oral hygiene can also remove unpleasant tastes, improving the taste of foods/fluids.*
Serve frequent, small meals rather than large ones if client is weak, fatigues easily, and/or has a poor appetite. **D ✦**	*Small, frequent meals are better tolerated in clients with a poor appetite.*
• Encourage significant others to bring in client's favorite foods unless contraindicated. **D ✦**	*Allowing a client to eat foods they prefer enhances intake and nutritional status.*
• Allow adequate time for meals; reheat foods/fluids if necessary. **D ●**	*Research has demonstrated that it takes 35 minutes to feed the client who is willing to eat.*
• Limit fluid intake with meals (unless the fluid has high nutritional value). **D ✦**	*A high fluid intake with meals promotes a feeling of fullness and early satiety that may decrease actual food intake.*

Dependent/Collaborative Actions

When food or oral fluids are allowed, implement measures to maintain an adequate nutritional status:
• Implement measures to prevent nausea and vomiting:
  • Administer antiemetics as ordered. **D ✦**
  • Implement measures to reduce pain:
	The presence of nausea can decrease the appetite. Preventing nausea and vomiting can improve the client's appetite.

THERAPEUTIC INTERVENTIONS	RATIONALE
Administer pain medications as ordered. **D** ✦	*The presence of pain decreases the appetite.*
• Increase activity as tolerated and allowed. **D** ●	*Activity promotes gastric emptying, which reduces the feeling of gastric fullness; it also usually promotes a sense of well-being, which can improve appetite.*
• Obtain a dietary consult if necessary to assist client in selecting foods/fluids that meet nutritional needs, are appealing, and adhere to personal and cultural preferences as well as the prescribed dietary modifications.	*A dietician or nutritional support team can help clients individualize their diet within prescribed dietary restrictions. Providing food in line with client's preferences can enhance adherence to prescribed diet.*
• Ensure that meals are well balanced and high in essential nutrients; offer dietary supplements if indicated.	*Dietary supplements have shown a positive relationship with weight gain, reduced mortality, and reduced length of hospitalization.*
• Administer vitamins and minerals if ordered. **D** ✦	*Vitamins and minerals are essential to many metabolic processes in the body.*
• Perform a calorie count if ordered. Report information to dietitian and physician. **D** ✦	*Information gathered from an accurate calorie count is used to determine the adequacy of a client's daily diet or the need for nutritional support.*
Consult physician about an alternative method of providing nutrition if client does not consume enough food or fluids to meet nutritional needs: • Enteral tube feedings • Parenteral nutrition	*Notifying the physician allows for modification of the treatment plan.*

POTENTIAL COMPLICATIONS AFTER SURGERY

Collaborative Diagnosis | # RISK FOR ATELECTASIS

Definition: Collapse of lung tissue caused by hypoventilated alveoli

Related to:
• Shallow respirations
• Stasis of secretions in the alveoli and bronchioles

CLINICAL MANIFESTATIONS

Subjective	Objective
Verbal reports of difficulty breathing	Diminished or absent breath sounds; dull percussion over affected area; increased respiratory rate; dyspnea; tachycardia; elevated temperature

RISK FACTORS
• Immobility
• Surgery
• Lack of adequate cough effort

DESIRED OUTCOMES
The client will not develop atelectasis as evidenced by:
a. Clear, audible breath sounds
b. Resonant percussion note over lungs
c. Unlabored respirations at 12 to 20 breaths/min
d. Pulse rate within normal range for client
e. Afebrile status

NURSING ASSESSMENT	RATIONALE
Assess for and report signs and symptoms of atelectasis: • Diminished or absent breath sounds • Dull percussion note over affected area • Increased respiratory rate • Dyspnea • Tachycardia • Elevated temperature	*Early recognition of signs and symptoms of atelectasis allows for implementation of the appropriate interventions.*

Continued...

NURSING ASSESSMENT	RATIONALE
Monitor pulse oximetry as indicated.	*Pulse oximetry is an indirect measure of arterial oxygen saturation (SaO₂. Monitoring pulse oximetry (SaO₂) allows for early detection of hypoxia and implementation of the appropriate interventions.*
Monitor chest radiograph results.	*Chest radiograph provides confirmation of atelectasis.*

THERAPEUTIC INTERVENTIONS	RATIONALE

Independent Actions

Implement measures to prevent atelectasis: **D** ✦	
• Perform actions to improve breathing pattern:	*Lack of movement places a client at risk for atelectasis. Changing positions frequently, coughing, and deep breathing help to expand the lungs, enhancing alveolar expansion.*
• Encourage client to deep breathe.	
• Incentive spirometry	
• Perform actions to promote effective airway clearance:	
• Turn, cough, and deep breath.	
If signs and symptoms of atelectasis occur:	
• Increase frequency of position change, coughing or "huffing," deep breathing, and use of incentive spirometer.	
Consult physician if signs and symptoms of atelectasis persist or worsen.	*Notifying the appropriate health care provider will allow for modification of the treatment plan.*

Collaborative Diagnosis   # RISK FOR THROMBOEMBOLISM

Definition: A clot that detaches from the vessel wall and circulates within the blood, becoming lodged in a blood vessel

Related to:
• Venous stasis associated with decreased activity
• Positioning during and after surgery
• Abdominal distention that may put pressure on the abdominal vessels
• Increased blood viscosity from deficient fluid volume

CLINICAL MANIFESTATIONS

Subjective	Objective
Verbal reports of pain or tenderness in an extremity	Increase in circumference of extremity; distention of superficial vessels in extremity; unusual warmth of extremity; positive Homans' sign (not always a reliable indicator)

RISK FACTORS	DESIRED OUTCOMES

• Immobility
• Inadequate fluid replacement
	The client will not develop a deep vein thrombus as evidenced by:
	  a. Absence of pain, tenderness, swelling, and distended superficial vessels in extremities
	  b. Usual temperature of extremities
	  c. Negative Homans' sign
	  d. Pain in area where thromboembolus lodged

NURSING ASSESSMENT	RATIONALE
Assess for and report signs and symptoms of a deep vein thrombus: • Pain or tenderness in extremity • Increase in circumference of extremity • Distention of superficial vessels in extremity • Unusual warmth of extremity • Positive Homans' sign (not always a reliable indicator)	*Early recognition of signs and symptoms of atelectasis allows for implementation of the appropriate interventions.*

THERAPEUTIC INTERVENTIONS	RATIONALE

Independent Actions

Implement measures to prevent thrombus formation: **D** ✦
- Use of sequential compression device during and after surgery until ambulatory
- Perform actions to prevent peripheral pooling of blood such as leg exercises:
  - Ankle rotation
  - Alternate dorsiflexion and plantar flexion of both feet

Sequential compression devices and leg and ankle exercises promote venous return and reduce the risk of venous thromboembolism.

If signs and symptoms of a deep vein thrombus occur: **D** ✦
- Maintain client on bedrest until activity orders received.
- Elevate foot of bed 15 degrees to 20 degrees above heart level if ordered.
- Discourage positions that compromise blood flow (e.g., pillows under knees, crossing legs, sitting for long periods).

Avoid putting pressure on the posterior knees as this action will compress leg veins, increasing turbulent blood flow, and increase the risk of thromboembolism formation. If a thrombus is suspected, elevate the affected extremity and do not massage the area because of the danger of dislodging the thrombus.

Dependent/Collaborative Actions

Implement measures to prevent thrombus formation:
- Apply mechanical devices designed to increase venous return in the immobile patient: **D** ✦
  - Sequential compression devices
  - Thromboembolic (elastic) stockings
- Maintain a minimum fluid intake of 2500 mL/day (unless contraindicated).

These devices decrease venous stasis in the lower extremities and increase venous return through the deep leg veins, which are prone to the formation of a thromboembolism. These devices should remain in place until the patient is ambulatory.
Adequate hydration helps to reduce blood viscosity, and decrease the incidence of a thromboembolism.

If signs and symptoms of a deep vein thrombus occur:
- Administer anticoagulants:
  - Low- or adjusted-dose heparin
  - Fondaparinux
  - Warfarin
  - Low-molecular-weight heparin

Anticoagulants, if indicated, help to suppress the formation of clots.

- Prepare client for diagnostic studies (e.g., venography, duplex ultrasound, impedance plethysmography).

Additional studies may be indicated to confirm the presence of a thromboembolism so the appropriate interventions can be implemented.

THERAPEUTIC INTERVENTIONS	RATIONALE

If signs and symptoms of embolism occur
- Maintain on strict bedrest in a semi- or high-Fowler's position

Improves lung expansion

- Maintain oxygen therapy as ordered

Provides supplemental oxygenation

- Prepare client for diagnostic tests (e.g., blood gases, D-dimer level, ventilation, perfusion lung scan; pulmonary angiography)
- Prepare client for the following, if planned
  - Venal caval interruption
  - Embolectomy

Decreases client fear/anxiety
Prevents further emboli
Removal of emboli

Collaborative Diagnosis # RISK FOR PARALYTIC ILEUS

Definition: Paralysis of the intestines resulting in blockage of the intestines

Related to:
- Manipulation of intestines during abdominal surgery
- Depressant effect of anesthesia and some medications on bowel motility

Continued...

CLINICAL MANIFESTATIONS

Subjective	Objective
Verbal reports of persistent abdominal pain and cramping	Firm, distended abdomen; absent bowel sounds; failure to pass flatus; abdominal radiograph showing distended bowel

RISK FACTORS

- Inadequate exercise
- Surgery

DESIRED OUTCOMES

The client will not develop a paralytic ileus as evidenced by:

  a. Absence or resolution of abdominal pain and cramping
  b. Soft, nondistended abdomen
  c. Gradual return of bowel sounds
  d. Passage of flatus

NURSING ASSESSMENT	RATIONALE
Assess for and report signs and symptoms of paralytic ileus: • Development of or persistent abdominal pain and cramping • Firm, distended abdomen • Absent bowel sounds • Failure to pass flatus Monitor results of abdominal radiograph.	*Early recognition of signs and symptoms of a paralytic ileus allows for prompt intervention.* *An abdominal radiograph that demonstrates distended bowel may be indicative of a paralytic ileus.*

THERAPEUTIC INTERVENTIONS	RATIONALE
Independent Actions Implement measures to prevent paralytic ileus: • Increase activity as soon as allowed and tolerated. • Perform actions to prevent hypokalemia.	*Early ambulation in a postoperative client promotes the return of peristalsis.* *Hypokalemia promotes atony of the intestinal wall, which results in a decrease in peristalsis.*
Dependent/Collaborative Actions If signs and symptoms of paralytic ileus occur: • Withhold all oral intake. • Insert nasogastric tube and maintain suction as ordered.	*Paralytic ileus results in cessation of normal peristalsis. The client should have nothing by mouth (NPO) and have a nasogastric tube in place to facilitate gastric decompression until the ileus is resolved.*
If signs and symptoms of paralytic ileus occurs: • Administer gastrointestinal stimulants (e.g., metoclopramide) if ordered.	*Gastrointestinal stimulants help to maintain adequate blood supply to the bowel.*

Collaborative Diagnosis # RISK FOR DEHISCENCE

Definition: Pulling apart of a surgical wound at the suture line

Related to:

- Inadequate wound closure
- Stress on incision line associated with persistent coughing
- Poor wound healing associated with decreased tissue perfusion of wound area and inadequate nutritional status

CLINICAL MANIFESTATIONS

Subjective	Objective
Verbal reports of something "popping" or "giving way" at the incision site	Separation of edges of the wound

RISK FACTORS
- Poor preoperative nutritional status
- Surgery
- Delayed post-operative nutritional therapy

DESIRED OUTCOME

The client will not experience dehiscence as evidenced by intact, approximated wound edges.

NURSING ASSESSMENT	RATIONALE
Assess for and report evidence of wound dehiscence: • Separation of edges of the wound Assess for and immediately report signs and symptoms of evisceration: • Sudden profuse drainage of serosanguineous fluid from wound • Protrusion of intestinal contents	*Early recognition of evidence of wound dehiscence allows for implementation of the appropriate interventions.* *Total separation of wound layers sometimes results in evisceration. This is an emergency situation that requires surgical intervention.*

THERAPEUTIC INTERVENTIONS	RATIONALE

Independent Actions
Implement measures to promote wound healing:
• Implement measures to reduce stress on the wound:
   • Limit movement of affected area.
   • If client has a chest or abdominal incision, instruct client to avoid coughing.
   • If client has an abdominal incision, place on bedrest in a semi-Fowler's position with knees slightly flexed.
	Proper wound healing decreases the risk of dehiscence.
	Decreasing stress on the incision reduces the risk of wound dehiscence.

Dependent/Collaborative Actions If dehiscence occurs: • Cover wound with a sterile, nonadherent dressing. • Apply skin closures (e.g., butterfly tape, Steri-Strips) to the incision line if appropriate. • Assist with resuturing the wound if indicated.	*A wound that has dehisced requires a sterile, nonadherent dressing. The choice of a dry dressing or wet dressing will depend upon the presence of evisceration.*

DISCHARGE TEACHING

Nursing Diagnosis **DEFICIENT KNOWLEDGE** NDx; **INEFFECTIVE FAMILY THERAPEUTIC REGIMEN MANAGEMENT** NDx; **OR INEFFECTIVE SELF HEALTH MANAGEMENT*** NDx

Definition: Absence or deficiency of cognitive information related to specific topic (lack of specific information necessary for clients/significant others) to make informed choices regarding condition/treatment/lifestyle changes; pattern of regulating and integrating into daily living and family processes a therapeutic regimen for treatment of illness and the sequelae of illness that is unsatisfactory for meeting specific health goals.

CLINICAL MANIFESTATIONS

Subjective	Objective
Verbalizes inability to manage illness; verbalizes inability to follow prescribed regimen	Inaccurate follow through with instructions; inappropriate behaviors; experience of preventable complications of spinal cord injury

*The nurse should select the diagnostic label that is most appropriate for the client's discharge teaching needs.

NDx = NANDA-I Diagnosis   **D** = Delegatable Action   ● = UAP   ✦ = LVN/LPN   ⊖▶ = Go to ⊖volve for animation

Continued...

RISK FACTORS

* Cognitive deficit
* Financial concerns
* Inability to care for oneself
* Difficulty in modifying personal habits and integrating treatments into lifestyle

NOC OUTCOMES	NIC INTERVENTIONS
Knowledge: treatment regimen	Teaching: individual; teaching: prescribed activity/exercise; teaching: prescribed medication; health system guidance

NURSING ASSESSMENT	RATIONALE
Assess the client's ability to learn and readiness to learn. Assess the client's understanding of teaching.	*Learning is more effective when the client is motivated and understands the importance of what is to be learned. Readiness to learn changes based on situations, physical and emotional challenges.*

THERAPEUTIC INTERVENTIONS	RATIONALE

Desired Outcome: The client will identify ways to prevent postoperative infection.

Independent Actions

Instruct client in ways to prevent postoperative infection:

* Continue with coughing (unless contraindicated) and deep breathing every 2 hours while awake.
* Continue to use incentive spirometer if activity is limited.
* Increase activity as ordered.
* Avoid contact with persons who have infections.
* Avoid crowds during flu and cold seasons.
* Decrease or stop smoking.

* Drink at least 10 glasses of liquid per day unless contraindicated.
* Maintain a balanced nutritional intake.
* Maintain proper balance of rest and activity.
* Maintain good personal hygiene (especially oral care, hand washing, and perineal care).
* Avoid touching any wound unless it is completely healed.
* Maintain sterile or clean technique as ordered during wound care.

These actions work to expand the lungs, mobilize secretions, and provide adequate oxygenation for healing.

Decreases client's exposure to infectious agents.

The irritants in smoke increase mucus production, impair ciliary function, and can cause inflammation and damage to the bronchial and alveolar walls; the carbon monoxide decreases oxygen availability.

Maintains adequate fluid for circulation.

Protein is required for appropriate wound healing.
Supports wound healing and recovery from surgery.
Prevents cross contamination, contamination of the surgical wound and potential for infection.

THERAPEUTIC INTERVENTIONS	RATIONALE

Desired Outcome: The client will demonstrate the ability to perform wound care.

Independent Actions

Discuss the rationale for, frequency of, and equipment necessary for the prescribed wound care.

Provide client with the necessary supplies (e.g., dressings, irrigating solution, tape) for wound care and with names and addresses of places where additional supplies can be obtained.

Demonstrate wound care and proper cleansing of any reusable equipment. Allow time for questions, clarification, and return demonstration.

Client adherence is improved if client understands what to do and how to use equipment as needed.

Improves adherence wound care.

Improves client's confidence in ability to care for self.

THERAPEUTIC INTERVENTIONS	RATIONALE

Desired Outcome: The client will state signs and symptoms to report to the health care provider.

Independent Actions

Instruct the client to report the following signs and symptoms:

- Persistent low-grade fever or significantly elevated (≥38.3° C [101° F]) temperature
- Difficulty breathing
- Chest pain
- Cough productive of purulent, green, or rust-colored sputum
- Increasing weakness or inability to tolerate prescribed activity level
- Increasing discomfort or discomfort not controlled by prescribed medications and treatments
- Continued nausea or vomiting
- Increasing abdominal distention and/or discomfort
- Separation of wound edges
- Increasing redness, warmth, pain, or swelling around wound
- Unusual or excessive drainage from any wound site
- Pain or swelling in calf of one or both legs
- Urine retention
- Frequency, urgency, or burning on urination
- Cloudy or foul-smelling urine

These clinical manifestations indicate complications that include infection, thromboembolism, and poor nutritional status.

May indicate increasing problems or tolerance to medication.

May indicate a recurrence of the bowel obstruction.

May indicate dehydration or urinary tract infection.

THERAPEUTIC INTERVENTIONS	RATIONALE

Desired Outcome: The client will verbalize an understanding of and a plan for adhering to recommended follow-up care including future appointments with health care provider, dietary modifications, activity level, treatments, and medications prescribed.

Independent Actions

Reinforce importance of keeping scheduled follow-up appointments with the health care provider.

Reinforce physician's instructions about dietary modifications. Obtain a dietary consult for client if needed.

Reinforce physician's instructions on suggested activity level and treatment plan.

Explain the rationale for, side effects of, and importance of taking medications prescribed.

Inform client of pertinent food and drug interactions.

Improves adherence to treatment regimen and for follow-up care.

Important for continued healing and maintenance of health.

Improves adherence if client understands what to do for self-care.

Knowledge of medications and how they impact the system improves client adherence to treatment regimen and understanding of the importance of adhering to the prescribed medication regimen. The client must be able to recognize alterations in functioning related to medication administration and what clinical manifestations that should be reported to the health care provider.

Implement measures to improve client compliance:

- Include significant others in teaching sessions if possible.

- Encourage questions and allow time for reinforcement and clarification of information provided.
- Provide written instructions on scheduled appointments with health care provider, dietary modifications, activity level, treatment plan, medications prescribed, and signs and symptoms to report.

Improves the ability of significant others to support client adherence to the treatment regimen.

Improves client understanding of discharge information.

Provides an information resource for the client after discharge from the acute care facility.

NDx = NANDA-I Diagnosis   **D** = Delegatable Action   ● = UAP   ✦ = LVN/LPN   ⊝▶ = Go to ⊝volve for animation

ADDITIONAL NURSING DIAGNOSES

IMPAIRED ORAL MUCOUS MEMBRANE NDx
Related to:
- Deficient fluid volume associated with restricted oral intake and fluid loss resulting from vomiting and nasogastric tube drainage
- Decreased salivation associated with deficient fluid volume, restricted oral intake, and the effect of some medications (e.g., narcotic [opioid] analgesics, some antiemetics)
- Mouth breathing when nasogastric tube is in place

RISK FOR CONSTIPATION NDx
Related to decreased gastrointestinal motility associated with manipulation of bowel during abdominal surgery, depressant effect of anesthesia and narcotic (opioid) analgesics, and decreased activity

DISTURBED SLEEP PATTERN NDx
Related to fear, anxiety, discomfort, inability to assume usual sleeping position, and frequent assessments and treatments

RISK FOR INFECTION NDx
Pneumonia related to stasis of pulmonary secretions and aspiration (if it occurs)
Wound infection related to:
- Contamination associated with introduction of pathogens during or after surgery
- Decreased resistance to infection associated with factors such as diminished tissue perfusion of wound area and inadequate nutritional status
Urinary tract infection related to:
- Increased growth and colonization of microorganisms associated with urinary stasis
- Introduction of pathogens associated with an indwelling catheter if present

RISK FOR FALLS NDx
Related to:
- Weakness and fatigue
- Dizziness or syncope associate with postural hypotension resulting from peripheral pooling of blood and blood loss during surgery
- Central nervous system depressant effect of some medications (narcotic [opioid] analgesics, some antiemetics)
- Presence of tubing or equipment

RISK FOR ASPIRATION NDx
Related to:
- Decreased level of consciousness and absent or diminished gag reflex associated with depressant effect of anesthesia and narcotic (opioid) analgesics
- Supine positioning
- Increased risk for gastroesophageal reflux associated with increased gastric pressure resulting from decreased gastrointestinal motility

FEAR/ANXIETY NDx
Related to:
- Unfamiliar environment
- Pain
- Lack of understanding of surgical procedure performed, diagnosis, and postoperative treatment plan
- Possible change to body image and roles
- Financial concerns

PARENTERAL NUTRITION

Early nutritional therapy, implemented within 48 hours of either hospital admission or surgery, is supported by various consensus statements and professional guidelines as critical to reducing patient morbidity and mortality. Early enteral nutrition, advocated for the preservation of the mucosal barrier of the gut, is associated with both lower hospital costs and shorter hospital lengths of stay. However, certain clinical conditions may interfere with the client's ability to ingest, digest, or absorb nutrients, resulting in the need for parenteral nutrition.

Parenteral nutrition is defined as the delivery of nutrients by a route other than the gastrointestinal system (e.g., bloodstream). The primary goal of parenteral nutrition is to provide the nutrients necessary to meet the metabolic needs of the client and allow for growth of new tissue. Clinical conditions that necessitate the use of parenteral nutrition include chronic, severe diarrhea and/or vomiting, complicated surgery or trauma, gastrointestinal obstruction, gastrointestinal tract anomalies, severe anorexia, severe malabsorption, and short bowel syndrome.

Parenteral nutrition is composed of both a base solution of dextrose and protein in the form of amino acids and pre-scribed levels of electrolytes, vitamins, and trace elements. The caloric intake requirement of clients in need of parenteral nutrition therapy far exceeds the 1200 to 1500 cal/day necessary to maintain normal physiological function. Carbohydrates in the form of dextrose and fat emulsions supply the calories that compose parenteral nutrition. While exact parenteral nutrition formulations are based upon individual client nutritional requirements, disease states, metabolic conditions, and medication use, there are accepted standard ranges of parenteral nutrition elements based on age and normal physiological requirements.

To minimize complications associated with nonfeeding, total caloric recommendations include 20 to 30 kcal/kg/day, daily protein of 1.5 to 2 g/kg/day, and fluid requirements of 30 to 40 mL/kg/day in clients who are stressed. Standard distribution of nonprotein calories includes 70% to 85% from carbohydrates and 15% to 30% supplied by fats. Fat content of parenteral solutions is not to exceed Food and Drug Administration recommendations of 2.5 g/kg/day. Fats are administered slowly over 12 to 24 hours using concentrations of 10%, 20%, or 30% fat emulsion solutions. Standard electrolyte requirements include 10 to 15 mEq calcium, 8 to

20 mEq magnesium, 20 to 40 mmol phosphorous, 1 to 2 mEq/kg sodium, 1 to 2 mEq/kg potassium, and chloride as needed to maintain acid-base balance.

A common metabolic complication associated with the administration of parenteral nutrition is hyperglycemia. Both hyperglycemia and insulin resistance can occur in clients receiving parenteral nutrition. Parenteral nutrition solutions have high glucose concentrations that range between 20% and 50%. As a result, clients receiving parenteral nutrition should have blood glucose levels checked every 4 to 6 hours, maintaining target blood glucose levels between 100 and 150 mg/dL or as indicated by institutional protocol. To avoid hypoglycemic episodes, parenteral infusions should not be abruptly discontinued for any reason.

Parenteral nutrition, prepared using strict aseptic techniques by a pharmacist, can be administered through a peripherally inserted catheter or centrally inserted device. Central administration is indicated for long-term support, or when the client has high protein and caloric requirements necessitating the administration of hypertonic solutions (>20% glucose concentration) that are caustic to peripheral veins. Parenteral nutrition administered through peripheral veins can be safely accomplished with minimal vein irritation using solutions with less than 20% glucose concentration.

Safe, effective preparation, administration, and storage of parenteral solutions requires a multidisciplinary health care team. Prescribing, preparing, and administering parenteral therapy require the expertise of physicians, pharmacists, dieticians, and nurses. **This care plan focuses on the adult client undergoing parenteral nutritional therapy in an acute care, extended care, or long-term care environment.**

OUTCOME/DISCHARGE CRITERIA

The client will:
1. Progressively gain weight toward desired goal
2. Weigh within normal weight for height and age
3. Consume adequate nutrition to meet metabolic needs
4. Be free of signs of malnutrition
5. Maintain adequate fluid volume status
6. Recognize factors contributing to malnutrition/underweight
7. Be free of complications related to parenteral feeding.

Nursing Diagnosis ## RISK FOR UNSTABLE BLOOD GLUCOSE LEVEL NDx

Definition: Risk for variation of blood glucose levels from normal range

Related to:
- Insulin resistance associated with the stress of illness and/or diabetes
- Administration of hypertonic parenteral solutions
- Interruption in administration of parenteral nutritional therapy
- Inadequate blood glucose monitoring

CLINICAL MANIFESTATIONS

Subjective	Objective
Verbal reports of hyperglycemia: thirst; dizziness; blurred vision; nausea	Hyperglycemia: polyuria; elevated serum glucose level; vomiting; dehydration
Verbal reports of hypoglycemia: hunger	Hypoglycemia: sweating; weakness; tremors

RISK FACTORS
- Physical health status
- Weight loss

DESIRED OUTCOME

The client will maintain blood glucose level between 90 and 130 mg/dL or close to 110 mg/dL in the critically ill client.

NOC OUTCOMES

Stable blood glucose levels; electrolyte and acid-base balance

NIC INTERVENTIONS

Hyperglycemia management; hypoglycemia management

NURSING ASSESSMENT

Assess client for signs and symptoms of hyper/hypoglycemia:
- Hyperglycemia: thirst, dizziness, blurred vision, polyuria, increased serum glucose level, nausea/vomiting, dehydration
- Hypoglycemia: hunger, weakness, sweating, tremors

RATIONALE

Early recognition of signs and symptoms of hyper/hypoglycemia allows for prompt intervention.

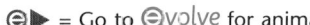

NDx = NANDA-I Diagnosis **D** = Delegatable Action ● = UAP ✦ = LVN/LPN ⊖▶ = Go to ⊖volve for animation

Continued...

NURSING ASSESSMENT	RATIONALE
Assess serum blood glucose every 4 to 6 hours during administration of parenteral nutrition.	*Because of the high dextrose concentration of most parenteral nutritional solutions, and possible insulin resistance in diabetic clients, blood glucose monitoring is warranted during therapy. Hypoglycemia may occur with abrupt cessation of parenteral nutrition because of the steady production of insulin by the pancreas in response to the high glucose concentration of parenteral solutions.*
	Assessment determines the patient's tolerance of the infusion.
Assess serum electrolyte levels for imbalances and report any deviations from normal.	*The exact amount of electrolytes needed in a parenteral solution will vary by client condition. Blood testing of serum electrolyte levels should occur several times a week to ensure electrolyte values remain therapeutic.*
	Refeeding syndrome, characterized by electrolyte imbalances and fluid retention, can be associated with long-standing malnutrition.

THERAPEUTIC INTERVENTIONS	RATIONALE

Independent Actions

Implement interventions to reduce the risk of hypoglycemia:

The pancreas becomes accustomed to producing insulin at a level necessary to keep blood glucose levels within a normal range.

Any abrupt cessation of an infusion of total parenteral nutrition places the client at risk for hypoglycemia.

- Administer infusion using an infusion pump.
- Ensure patency of infusion site (e.g., peripheral or central catheter).
- Monitor bedside serum glucose levels every 4 to 6 hours.
- Wean clients from parenteral nutrition therapy slowly.

Administration of parenteral nutrition using an infusion pump allows for appropriate hourly rate regulation and detection of interruption of infusion when/if infusion site becomes occluded or obstructed.

Implement measures to reduce the risk of hyperglycemia:
- Begin infusion slowly as prescribed.
- Monitor serum blood glucose levels frequently to assess tolerance to therapy.

Administration of parenteral nutritional therapy occurs gradually allowing the pancreas to adapt insulin production to the increased serum glucose levels.

Dependent/Collaborative Actions

Infuse a 10% or 20% dextrose solution (based on the amount in the parenteral solution) if the formula bag is empty before the next solution is available.

Administration of dextrose-containing solutions helps to prevent hypoglycemia in a client whose system has adjusted to the high levels of glucose in parenteral solutions.

Administer insulin as prescribed.

Supplemental insulin in accordance with a sliding scale may be necessary, as an increase in serum blood glucose level is expected after initiation of parenteral nutritional therapy.

Implement hypoglycemic protocol for blood glucose level less than 70 mg/dL:
- For the conscious patient, ingestion of 15 to 20 g of simple carbohydrate (e.g., 4-6 oz fruit juice)
- In acute care settings, or with patients who are unconscious, administer 20 to 50 mL of 50% dextrose intravenous (IV) push.
- Recheck blood glucose level 15 minutes after intervention and repeat treatment if client's blood glucose level remains less than 70 mg/dL.

The brain requires a constant supply of glucose to properly function. Untreated hypoglycemia can lead to loss of consciousness, seizures, coma, and/or death.

Notify the appropriate health care provider if signs and symptoms of hyperglycemia or hypoglycemia, or other electrolyte imbalances develop:
- Physician provider
- Dietician/nutritional consultant

Notifying the appropriate health care provider allows for modification of the treatment plan.

Nursing Diagnosis | **RISK FOR INFECTION** NDx

Definition: At risk for being invaded by pathogenic organisms

Related to:
- Administration of fluids that support bacterial growth
- Placement of central venous catheter (invasive procedure)
- Malnutrition
- Decreased defense mechanisms

CLINICAL MANIFESTATIONS

Subjective	Objective
Verbal reports of nausea; malaise; chills	Erythema, tenderness, and exudate at venous access site; increased temperature; increased white blood cell (WBC) count, abnormal differential count; positive blood and/or wound cultures

RISK FACTORS
- Chronic illness
- Inadequate immune response
- Exposure to pathogens

DESIRED OUTCOMES

The client will:
a. Remain free from symptoms of infection
b. Maintain WBC and differential count within normal range
c. Demonstrate appropriate care of infection-prone site
d. State signs and symptoms of infection of which to be aware

NOC OUTCOMES

Infection severity

NIC INTERVENTIONS

Infection control; infection protection

NURSING ASSESSMENT	**RATIONALE**
Assess client's venous access site for signs and symptoms of infection: - Nausea - Malaise - Erythema - Tenderness and exudate at venous access site - Chills - Fever - Increased WBC's - Abnormal differential count - Positive blood/wound cultures Monitor complete blood count, blood and wound culture results for abnormalities.	*Early recognition of signs and symptoms of infection allows for prompt intervention.*

THERAPEUTIC INTERVENTIONS	**RATIONALE**

Independent Actions
Wash hands before and after each patient encounter.
Maintain aseptic technique when administering solution:
- Administer parenteral solutions not containing fat emulsion through a 0.22-micron Millipore filter.
- Administer parenteral solutions containing fat emulsions through a 1.2-micron filter.
- Change filters and tubing as appropriate, marking the date and time of initiation of use:
  - Change every 24 hours if lipid emulsions are used.
  - Change every 72 hours if amino acids and dextrose is used.
	Parenteral nutritional therapy, because of the high glucose concentrations, provides an excellent environment for microbial growth.
	The use of in-line filters helps reduce or eliminate the infusion of particulates, microprecipitates, microorganisms, pyrogens, and air.

Continued...

THERAPEUTIC INTERVENTIONS	RATIONALE
Visually inspect solution before administration for any visual indication of precipitates, color changes (turbidity), or leaks.	*If any abnormalities are suspected, the solution should be returned to the pharmacy promptly for replacement.*
Change peripheral and central line IV sites and dressings in accordance with institutional policy/Centers for Disease Control and Prevention (CDC) guidelines for infection prevention.	*Catheter-related infection and septicemia can occur in patients receiving parenteral nutrition through both central and peripheral access devices.*
Complete all parenteral solution infusions at the ordered rate within 24 hours of initiation.	*At room temperature, parenteral solutions and fat emulsions provide a medium for bacterial growth.*

Dependent/Collaborative Actions

Obtain blood cultures as indicated.	
Obtain culture of venous access device catheter tip if discontinued.	
Notify physician provider if signs and symptoms of systemic or site infection develop.	*Notifying the appropriate health care provider allows for modification of the treatment plan.*

DISCHARGE TEACHING/CONTINUED CARE

Nursing Diagnosis   **DEFICIENT KNOWLEDGE** NDx; **INEFFECTIVE FAMILY THERAPEUTIC REGIMEN MANAGEMENT** NDx; **OR INEFFECTIVE SELF HEALTH MANAGEMENT*** NDx

Definition: Absence or deficiency of cognitive information related to specific topic (lack of specific information necessary for clients/significant others) to make informed choices regarding condition/treatment/lifestyle changes; pattern of regulating and integrating into daily living and family processes a therapeutic regimen for treatment of illness and the sequelae of illness that is unsatisfactory for meeting specific health goals.

CLINICAL MANIFESTATIONS

Subjective	Objective
Verbalizes inability to manage illness; verbalizes inability to follow prescribed regimen	Inaccurate follow through with instructions; inappropriate behaviors

RISK FACTORS
- Cognitive deficit
- Financial concerns
- Inability to care for oneself

NIC OUTCOMES	NOC INTERVENTIONS
Knowledge: treatment regimen; knowledge: infection management	Teaching: individual; teaching: psychomotor skill

NURSING ASSESSMENT	RATIONALE
Assess client's readiness and ability to learn. Assess meaning of nutritional therapy to client.	*Early recognition of readiness to learn and meaning of nutritional therapy to client allows for implementation of the appropriate teaching interventions.*

---

*The nurse should select the nursing diagnostic label that is most appropriate for the client's discharge teaching needs.

THERAPEUTIC INTERVENTIONS	RATIONALE

Desired Outcome: The client will demonstrate the proper technique when changing infusion tubing and parenteral solution bags.

Independent Actions

Instruct client and family on the proper way to mix, handle, and store parenteral feedings.
* Allow time for return demonstration.

Instruct client and family on proper care of parenteral solution administration sets:
* Administer solution using appropriate filter.
* Discard administration sets every 72 hours for solutions with amino acids/dextrose.
* Discard administration sets every 72 hours for solutions containing lipid emulsions.

Instruct client and family on the proper handling and storage of solutions:
* Solutions must be infused within 24 hours.
* Mixed solutions must be refrigerated until ½ hour before use.

Proper care of parenteral feedings is necessary to prevent contamination.

Given the high glucose concentration found in parenteral solutions, proper filtration and line maintenance is necessary to prevent bloodstream infections.

Parenteral nutritional therapy, because of the high glucose concentrations, provides an excellent environment for microbial growth.

The use of in-line filters helps reduce or eliminate the infusion of particulates, microprecipitates, microorganisms, pyrogens, and air At room temperature, parenteral solutions and fat emulsions provide a medium for bacterial growth.

THERAPEUTIC INTERVENTIONS	RATIONALE

Desired Outcome: The client will demonstrate proper care of venous access device.

Independent Actions

Instruct client and family on the proper method of changing central line or venous access dressings.

Allow time for return demonstration.

Sterile dressing care of long-term venous access devices is necessary to prevent the development of catheter line sepsis.

THERAPEUTIC INTERVENTIONS	RATIONALE

Desired Outcome: The client will verbalize signs and symptoms of infection to report to health care provider.

Independent Actions

Instruct client and family to report any signs and symptoms of systemic or localized (catheter site) infection to the health care provider immediately.

Notifying the appropriate health care provider allows for modification of the treatment plan.

RELATED CARE PLAN

INFECTION NDx

Related to:
* Bacterial contamination of parenteral solution during preparation or administration
* Catheter/venous access site infection

⊖▶ PEPTIC ULCER

A peptic ulcer is a break in the continuity of the gastrointestinal mucosa that is exposed to acidic digestive secretions. The areas most often involved are the stomach and duodenum. Erosion of these areas can result from direct damage to the mucosa or from an increase in mucosal permeability, which allows gastric acids to diffuse through the mucosal barrier into the underlying tissue. The two most common causes of peptic ulcers are infection with *Helicobacter pylori (H. pylori)* and use of aspirin or other nonsteroidal anti-inflammatory agents (NSAIDs). Other factors believed to have a role in ulcer development, exacerbation, and/or recurrence include ingestion of alcohol, coffee, certain foods and spices, and caffeine; medications such as corticosteroids and some chemotherapeutic agents; smoking; stress; hypovolemia (can result in ischemia of the gastrointestinal mucosa and subsequent alteration in mucosal permeability); certain disease conditions (e.g., Zollinger-Ellison syndrome, chronic obstructive pulmonary disease, pancreatitis, chronic renal failure); and genetic predisposition.

Peptic ulcers are usually classified by location (e.g., gastric, duodenal) and by the extensiveness of erosion (e.g., acute [superficial erosion with minimal inflammation], chronic [erosion of mucosa and submucosa with scar tissue formation]). Causative factors and the relationship between eating and occurrence of pain vary depending on the location and extensiveness of the ulcer. The characteristic symptom of a peptic ulcer is chronic, intermittent epigastric pain that is described as burning, aching, gnawing, or cramping.

Medical treatment of a peptic ulcer focuses on eradicating *H. pylori* infection if present, decreasing the degree of gastric acidity, and promoting mucosal integrity and regeneration. Surgical intervention (e.g., vagotomy, pyloroplasty, partial gastrectomy) may be indicated if symptoms cannot be medically controlled; if ulcers recur frequently; or if complications such as hemorrhage, perforation, or obstruction occur in the ulcerated area(s).

This care plan focuses on the adult client hospitalized for evaluation and medical treatment of a peptic ulcer that has become increasingly symptomatic. Much of the information presented here is applicable to clients receiving care in an extended care facility or home setting.

OUTCOME/DISCHARGE CRITERIA

The client will:
1. Have pain controlled
2. Have no signs and symptoms of complications
3. Verbalize a basic understanding of peptic ulcer disease and the importance of adhering to the prescribed treatment plan
4. Identify ways to promote healing of the existing ulcer and prevent recurrence of peptic ulcer
5. Verbalize an understanding of medications ordered including rationale, food and drug interactions, side effects, schedule for taking, and importance of taking as prescribed
6. State signs and symptoms to report to the health care provider
7. Verbalize an understanding of and a plan for adhering to recommended follow-up care including future appointments with health care provider

For a full, detailed care plan on this topic, go to http://evolve.elsevier.com/Haugen/careplanning/.

10 Nursing Care of the Client with Disturbances of the Liver, Biliary Tract, and Pancreas

CHOLECYSTECTOMY

A cholecystectomy is the surgical removal of the gallbladder. It is commonly performed to treat symptomatic cholecystitis or cholelithiasis, or both. A cholecystectomy can be done via laparoscopy or through a right subcostal incision (open cholecystectomy). A laparoscopic cholecystectomy is usually the procedure of choice because of the short hospitalization (<2 days), reduced pain, and a more rapid return to usual activities. An open cholecystectomy is warranted when the client is in the last trimester of pregnancy or has a gangrenous or perforated gallbladder, a suspected gallbladder malignancy, severe inflammation that obscures the structures of the hepatobiliary triangle, or large stones in the biliary ducts. An open cholecystectomy may also be performed when problems are encountered during a laparoscopic cholecystectomy. If stones are present in the common bile duct, they can often be extracted endoscopically, but a choledocholithotomy may be necessary if the stones are large. After a choledocholithotomy, a T tube is placed in the common bile duct to maintain adequate flow or drainage of bile until ductal edema subsides.

This care plan focuses on the adult client hospitalized for an open cholecystectomy with common bile duct exploration.

OUTCOME/DISCHARGE CRITERIA

The client will:
1. Have pain controlled
2. Tolerate prescribed diet
3. Have evidence of normal healing of surgical wound(s) and normal skin integrity around T-tube site
4. Have clear, audible breath sounds throughout lungs
5. Have no signs and symptoms of postoperative complications
6. Demonstrate the ability to appropriately care for T tube and surrounding skin if T tube is present
7. Verbalize an understanding of the rationale for and components of a low- to moderate-fat diet if prescribed
8. State signs and symptoms to report to the health care provider
9. Verbalize an understanding of and a plan for adhering to recommended follow-up care including future appointments with health care provider, wound care, medications prescribed, and activity level.

See Care Plan on Cholelithiasis/Cholecystitis and the Standardized Preoperative and Postoperative Care Plans for additional diagnoses.

Nursing Diagnosis | ## INEFFECTIVE BREATHING PATTERN NDx

Definition: Inspiration and/or expiration that does not provide adequate ventilation

Related to:
- Increased rate of respirations associated with fear and anxiety
- Decreased rate of respirations associated with the depressant effect of anesthesia and some medications (e.g., narcotic [opioid] analgesics, some antiemetics)
- Decreased depth of respirations associated with:
  - Depressant effect of anesthesia and some medications (e.g., narcotic [opioid] analgesics, some antiemetics)
  - Reluctance to breathe deeply because of pain
  - Fear, anxiety, weakness, and fatigue
  - Restricted chest expansion resulting from positioning and elevation of the diaphragm if abdominal distention is present

---

CLINICAL MANIFESTATIONS

Subjective	Objective
Complaints of shortness of breath	Dyspnea; orthopnea; increased respiratory rate; decreased depth of breathing; decreased inspiratory/expiratory pressure; decreased minute ventilation; decreased vital capacity; nasal flaring; use of accessory muscles to breathe; assumption of three-point position; altered chest excursion; pursed-lip breathing; prolonged expiration phases

RISK FACTORS

- Surgery
- Immobility

DESIRED OUTCOMES

The client will maintain an effective breathing pattern as evidenced by:
  a. Normal rate and depth of respirations
  b. Absence of dyspnea

NOC OUTCOMES

Respiratory status: ventilation

NIC INTERVENTIONS

Ventilation assistance; respiratory monitoring

NURSING ASSESSMENT	RATIONALE
Assess for signs and symptoms of an ineffective breathing pattern: • Shallow or slow respirations • Limited chest excursion • Tachypnea or dyspnea • Use of accessory muscles when breathing	*Early recognition of signs and symptoms of an ineffective breathing pattern allows for prompt intervention.*
Assess/monitor pulse oximetry (arterial oxygen saturation [SaO_2]), arterial blood gas (ABG) values as indicated.	*Monitoring continuous SaO_2 readings allows for the early detection of hypoxia.* *Assessment of ABG values allows for a more direct measurement of both the partial pressure of oxygen in arterial blood (PaO_2) and the partial pressure of carbon dioxide in arterial blood ($PaCO_2$), both of which reflect the adequacy of ventilation.*

THERAPEUTIC INTERVENTIONS	RATIONALE
Independent Actions Implement measures to improve breathing pattern: • Perform actions to reduce fear and anxiety: • Promote a calm, restful environment. **D ● ✦**	*Reducing fear and anxiety helps to prevent shallow and/or rapid breathing.*

• Perform actions to reduce pain:
  • Reposition client for comfort.
  • Instruct client to support incision with hands or a pillow when moving or coughing. **D ● ✦**
	Reducing pain helps to increase the client's willingness to move and breathe more deeply.

• Assist client to bend knees while coughing and deep breathing. **D ● ✦**	*Relieves tension on abdominal muscles and incision allowing for better chest expansion.*
• Perform actions to reduce the accumulation of gas and fluid in the gastrointestinal tract: • Maintain patency of nasogastric, gastric, or intestinal tubes if present. **D ✦**	*Reducing the accumulation of gas in the gastrointestinal tract decreases pressure on the diaphragm facilitating more effective ventilation.*
• Perform actions to increase strength and improve activity tolerance: • Implement measures to conserve energy. **D ● ✦**	*Increasing activity tolerance enables the client to breathe more deeply and participate in activities to improve breathing pattern.*
• Have client deep breathe or use incentive spirometer every 1 to 2 hours. **D ✦**	*Deep breathing and use of an incentive spirometer promotes maximal inhalation and lung expansion.*

THERAPEUTIC INTERVENTIONS	RATIONALE
• Instruct client to breathe slowly if hyperventilating. **D** ✦	*Hyperventilation is an ineffective breathing pattern that can lead to respiratory alkalosis.* *A client can often slow breathing rate by concentrating on doing so.*
• Place client in a semi- to high-Fowler's position unless contraindicated.	*A semi- to high-Fowler's position allows for maximal diaphragmatic excursion and lung expansion.*
• If client must remain flat in bed, assist with position change at least every 2 hours. **D** ●	*Compression of the thorax and subsequent limited chest wall expansion occur when the client lies in one position. Frequent repositioning promotes maximal chest wall and lung expansion.*

Dependent/Collaborative Actions

Implement measures to improve breathing pattern:

• Increase activity as allowed and tolerated.	*During activity, especially ambulation, the client usually takes deeper breaths, thus increasing lung expansion.*

• Assist with positive airway pressure techniques if ordered:
  • Continuous positive airway pressure (CPAP)
  • Bilevel positive airway pressure (BiPAP)
  • Flutter/positive expiratory pressure (PEP) device
	Positive airway pressure techniques increase intrapulmonary (alveolar) pressure, which helps reexpand collapsed alveoli and prevent further alveoli collapse.

• Administer central nervous system depressants judiciously: • Hold medication and consult physician if respiratory rate is less than 12 breaths/min.	*Central nervous system depressants cause depression of the respiratory center in the brainstem, which can result in a decreased rate and depth of respiration.*
• Perform actions to reduce pain: • Administer analgesics before activities and procedures than can cause pain and before pain becomes severe. **D** ✦	*Reducing pain helps to increase the client's willingness to move and breathe more deeply.*

Consult appropriate health care provider if:

• Ineffective breathing pattern continues. • Client develops signs and symptoms of impaired gas exchange such as restlessness, irritability, confusion, significant decrease in oximetry results, decreased PaO$_2$ and increased PaCO$_2$ levels.	*Notifying the appropriate health care provider allows for modification of treatment plan.*

Collaborative Diagnosis — # RISK FOR ABSCESS FORMATION

Definition: An accumulation of pus in any area of the body

Related to:
• Accumulation of drainage in the surgical area and subsequent invasion of the area by microorganisms and neutrophils

CLINICAL MANIFESTATIONS

Subjective	Objective
Verbalization of pain in the surgical area	Redness, swelling, and/or warmth in the surgical area; fever, tachycardia; increased white blood cell (WBC) count

RISK FACTORS

• Surgery
• Exposure to pathogens

DESIRED OUTCOMES

The client will not develop an abscess as evidenced by:
  a. Gradual resolution of abdominal pain
  b. Temperature declining toward normal
  c. WBC count declining toward normal

NURSING ASSESSMENT	RATIONALE
Assess for and report signs and symptoms of an abscess (e.g., increased or more constant abdominal pain, increase in temperature and pulse rate, further increase in WBC count).	*Early recognition of signs and symptoms of an abscess allows for prompt intervention.*

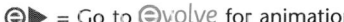

NDx = NANDA-I Diagnosis   **D** = Delegatable Action   ● = UAP   ✦ = LVN/LPN   ⊖▶ = Go to ⊖volve for animation

Continued...

THERAPEUTIC INTERVENTIONS	RATIONALE

Independent Actions

Implement measures to prevent accumulation of drainage in the surgical area:

- Perform actions to maintain patency of wound drain and/or T tube if present:
  - Implement measures to prevent stasis and reflux of drainage: **D** ✦
    - (1) Keep drainage tubing free of dependent loops and kinks (prevent kinking by placing a gauze roll under the drain tube and anchoring it to the skin or dressing with tape).
    - (2) Keep collection device(s) below drain insertion site(s) unless ordered otherwise (physician may order T tube collection device to be positioned just slightly below, level with, or above drain insertion site).
    - (3) Empty collection device(s) as often as necessary and at least every shift. **D** ● ✦

Implement measures to prevent inadvertent removal of wound drain and/or T tube:

- Instruct client not to pull on drain(s) and drainage tubing.
- Use caution when changing dressings surrounding drain(s).
- Attach collection device(s) securely to abdominal dressing.
- Maintain client in a semi- to high-Fowler's position as much as possible when in bed. **D** ✦

Promotes drainage of fluids from the wound, preventing stasis of fluids and reducing the risk for abscess formation.

Maintains appropriate drainage and prevents it from leaking into the abdomen.

Reduces loss of bile.

Prevents stasis of fluids.

These actions prevent the T tube from becoming dislodged, which can introduce bacteria into the body.

Improves lung expansion and promotes drainage of respiratory secretions.

Dependent/Collaborative Actions

If signs and symptoms of an abscess occur:

- Prepare client for diagnostic tests (e.g., ultrasonography, computed tomography).
- Administer antimicrobials if ordered.
- Prepare client for surgical intervention (e.g., incision and drainage of abscess) if planned.

Alleviates fear and anxiety.

Alleviate infections.
Alleviates fear and anxiety.

⊖▸ Collaborative Diagnosis **RISK FOR PERITONITIS**

Definition: Inflammation of the peritoneum

Related to: Escape of bile into the peritoneal cavity associated with surgical trauma to the gallbladder and biliary duct

CLINICAL MANIFESTATIONS

Subjective	Objective
Verbalization of abdominal pain	Nausea and vomiting; distended and rigid abdomen; diminished or absent bowel sounds fever; tachypnea; increased WBC count

RISK FACTORS

- Surgery
- Exposure to pathogens

DESIRED OUTCOMES

The client will not develop peritonitis as evidenced by:
  a. Gradual resolution of abdominal pain
  b. Soft, nondistended abdomen
  c. Temperature declining toward normal
  d. Stable vital signs
  e. Absence of nausea and vomiting
  f. Gradual return of normal bowel sounds
  g. WBC count declining toward normal

NURSING ASSESSMENT	RATIONALE
Assess for and report signs and symptoms of peritonitis (e.g., increase in severity of abdominal pain; generalized abdominal pain; rebound tenderness; distended, rigid abdomen; increase in temperature; tachycardia; tachypnea; hypotension; nausea; vomiting; continued diminished or absent bowel sounds; WBC count that increases or fails to decline toward normal).	*Early recognition of the signs and symptoms of peritonitis allows for prompt intervention.*

THERAPEUTIC INTERVENTIONS	RATIONALE

Dependent/Collaborative Actions

Implement measures to prevent peritonitis:

- Perform actions to maintain patency and prevent inadvertent removal of wound drain and/or T tube if present (keep tubes from kinking, keep device below the level of drainage). — *These actions reduce the risk for wound drainage and bile accumulating and leaking into the peritoneum.*
- Administer antimicrobials if ordered. — *Treats/prevents infection.*

If peritonitis occurs:

- Withhold oral intake as ordered.
- Place client on bed rest in a semi-Fowler's position. — *Positioning the client in a semi-Fowler's position assists in pooling or localizing gastrointestinal contents in the pelvis rather than under the diaphragm.*
- Prepare client for diagnostic tests (e.g., abdominal radiograph, computed tomography, ultrasonography). — *Alleviates fear and anxiety.*
- Insert a nasogastric tube and maintain suction as ordered. — *Insertion of NG tube and connecting it to section decompresses the stomach.*
- Administer antimicrobials as ordered. — *Antimicrobials treat and reduce the risk for infection.*
- Administer intravenous fluids and/or blood volume expanders if ordered to prevent or treat shock. — *Administration of IV fluids and volume expanders prevent and/or treat shock that can result from the increased capillary permeability that occurs with inflammation and the subsequent escape of protein, fluid, and electrolytes from the vascular space into the peritoneal cavity.*
- Prepare client for surgical intervention (e.g., drainage and irrigation of peritoneum, repair of leakage site) if planned. — *Alleviates fear and anxiety.*

Collaborative Diagnosis ### RISK FOR CONTINUED OBSTRUCTION OF BILE FLOW

Definition: Blockage of bile flow

Related to: Residual stones in the biliary duct system or persistent inflammation and/or strictures of the common bile duct associated with surgical trauma

CLINICAL MANIFESTATIONS

Subjective	Objective
Verbalization of continued abdominal pain and nausea	Increased drainage from T tube; yellow-tinged skin; clay colored stools; dark amber urine

RISK FACTOR

- Surgery

DESIRED OUTCOMES

The client will have resolution of bile flow obstruction within 7 to 10 days after surgery as evidenced by:
a. Decline in output of bile in T tube to less than 400 mL/day
b. Absence of pain, nausea, and feeling of fullness when T tube is clamped
c. Absence of jaundice, clay-colored stools, and dark amber urine

---

NDx = NANDA-I Diagnosis   **D** = Delegatable Action   ● = UAP   ✦ = LVN/LPN   ⊖▶ = Go to ⊖volve for animation

Continued...

NURSING ASSESSMENT	RATIONALE
Assess for and report signs and symptoms of continued bile flow obstruction (e.g., T tube draining more than 1000 mL in 24 hours; a marked increase in T-tube drainage after it has started to decline; persistent pain, nausea, or feeling of fullness when T tube is clamped; jaundice; clay-colored stools; dark amber urine).	*Early recognition of the signs and symptoms of bile flow obstruction allows for prompt intervention.*

THERAPEUTIC INTERVENTIONS	RATIONALE
Independent Actions Implement measures to maintain patency of T tube (e.g., keep free of kinks, keep device below the drainage level).	*These actions promote the drainage of bile.*
Dependent/Collaborative Actions If signs and symptoms of bile flow obstruction occur: • Leave T tube unclamped. • Prepare client for diagnostic tests (e.g., ultrasound, cholangiogram) if planned. • Prepare client for removal of residual stones (e.g., extraction via T tube, endoscopic sphincterotomy with basket removal of stones) or treatment of bile duct stricture (e.g., endoscopic or percutaneous balloon dilatation with or without stent placement, surgical resection of stricture site) if planned.	*This promotes drainage of bile.* *Alleviates fear and anxiety.*

DISCHARGE TEACHING/CONTINUED CARE

Nursing Diagnosis | # DEFICIENT KNOWLEDGE NDx; INEFFECTIVE FAMILY THERAPEUTIC REGIMEN MANAGEMENT NDx; OR INEFFECTIVE SELF-HEALTH MANAGEMENT* NDx

Definition: Absence or deficiency of cognitive information

Related to absence or deficiency of cognitive information related to specific topic (lack of specific information necessary for clients/significant others) to make informed choices regarding condition/treatment/lifestyle changes; pattern of regulating and integrating into daily living and family processes a therapeutic regimen for the treatment of illness and the sequelae that are unsatisfactory for meeting specific health goals

CLINICAL MANIFESTATIONS

Subjective	Objective
Verbalizes inability to manage illness; verbalizes inability to follow prescribed regimen	Inaccurate follow through with instructions; inappropriate behaviors; experience of preventable complications of surgery

---

*The nurse should select the diagnostic label that is most appropriate for the client's discharge teaching needs.

RISK FACTORS
- Cognitive deficit
- Financial concerns
- Failure to take action to reduce risk factors for complications of surgery (if performed)
- Inability to care for oneself
- Difficulty in modifying personal habits and integrating treatments into lifestyle

NOC OUTCOMES	NIC INTERVENTIONS
Knowledge: treatment regimen; knowledge: diet	Health system guidance; teaching: prescribed diet; teaching: procedure/treatment; teaching: prescribed medication

NURSING ASSESSMENT	RATIONALE
Assess the client's ability to learn and readiness to learn. Assess the client's understanding of teaching.	*Learning is more effective when the client is motivated and understands the importance of what is to be learned. Readiness to learn changes based on situations, physical and emotional challenges.*

THERAPEUTIC INTERVENTIONS / RATIONALE

Desired Outcome: The client will demonstrate the ability to appropriately care for T tube and surrounding skin if T tube is present.

Independent Actions

If the client is to be discharged with a T tube in place, instruct regarding care of the T tube and surrounding skin:

- Cleanse the skin around the T-tube insertion site daily and cover the site with a dry sterile dressing; apply zinc oxide cream to skin around insertion site if skin is irritated.
- Keep the T-tube drainage collection device in the position prescribed (usually slightly below the insertion site).
- Keep the tubing pinned to the dressing and avoid any kinks or tension on the tubing.
- Empty the drainage collection device at least twice daily or more often if needed; keep a record of the amount of drainage.
- When emptying the drainage collection device, check to see that the tube has not become dislodged (this can be easily monitored if the tube is marked at the skin line before discharge).
- Clamp T tube only as instructed.

Allow time for questions, clarification, and return demonstration of care of T tube and surrounding skin.

These actions help maintain drainage patency, promote drainage, and prevent infection.

Monitors output, noting changes in volume.

This can indicate a problem with drainage and/or tube placement/ blockage.

Clamping the T tube helps prevent bile leakage.
Improves client's confidence in ability to care for self.

Desired Outcome: The client will verbalize an understanding of the rationale for and components of a low- to moderate-fat diet if prescribed

Independent Actions

Explain the rationale for avoiding excessive fat intake for the first 4 to 6 weeks after surgery (many physicians instruct client to just avoid foods that cause epigastric discomfort).

Instruct client to increase fat intake gradually and introduce foods/fluids high in fat (e.g., butter, cream, whole milk, ice cream, fried foods, gravies, nuts) one at a time.

Fats cause gastric upset and gastric discomfort.

Gradual increase in fat intake allows the body to become used to absorbing fats, without severe epigastric discomfort.

Continued...

THERAPEUTIC INTERVENTIONS	RATIONALE

Desired Outcome: The client will state signs and symptoms to report to the health care provider.

Independent Actions

Instruct the client to report the following signs and symptoms to health care provider:

- Persistent low-grade fever or significantly elevated temperature (≥38.8° C [101° F])
- Difficulty breathing
- Chest pain
- Cough productive of purulent, green, or rust-colored sputum
- Increased weakness or inability to tolerate prescribed activity level
- Increasing discomfort or discomfort not controlled by prescribed medications and treatments

These clinical manifestations indicate that the client may be experiencing complications from surgery if performed. They indicate possible infection of the surgical area or other body systems and possible thromboembolism.

- Nausea and vomiting
- Decreased urine output
- Frequency, urgency, or burning on urination
- Cloudy or foul-smelling urine
- Urine retention

May indicate increased consumption of fatty foods.
Indicates a possible urinary tract infection

- Clay-colored stools or dark amber urine
- Development of increased itchiness or yellowing of skin
- When the T-tube drainage subsides or after the T tube has been removed, purulent drainage from the T tube or green-brown drainage around T tube or from wound site

These changes indicate bile leaking into the abdomen.

- A significant increase in or more than 500 mL/day of drainage from T tube

This change may indicate increased bile production or infection.

- A sudden marked decrease in T-tube drainage or increase in length of the T tube (may indicate that the T tube has become dislodged)

These changes may indicate T tube has become dislodged or is blocked.

- Abdominal distention or rigidity
- Persistent heartburn, feeling of bloating, or nausea
- Loose stools that continue for longer than 2 to 3 months

May indicate consumption of too many fatty foods.

Instruct client in ways to prevent postoperative infection:

- Continue with coughing unless contraindicated and deep breathing every 2 hours while awake.
- Continue to use incentive spirometer if activity is limited.

Coughing and deep breathing exercises help improve oxygenation to the tissues, expand the lungs, and prevent stasis of secretions.

- Increase activity as ordered.

These actions prevent thromboembolism and improves ability to resume normal activities.

- Avoid contact with persons who have infections.
- Avoid crowds during flu and cold seasons.

Prevents exposure of client to others who are ill and decreases the risk for an infection.

- Drink at least 10 glasses of liquid per day unless contraindicated.

Maintains adequate hydration and vascular fluid volume.

- Maintain a balanced nutritional intake.

An appropriate diet with adequate protein improves the body's ability to heal.

- Maintain proper balance of bedrest and activity.
- Maintain good personal hygiene (e.g., oral care, hand washing, and perineal care).
- Maintain sterile or clean technique as ordered during wound care.

These actions help prevent infection.

- Provide client with supplies necessary for wound care.

Improves client's adherence to treatment regimen and decreases potential for infection.

Instruct client to avoid heavy lifting for 4 to 6 weeks.

The client should not do any heavy lifting until approved by the health care provider. Lifting may cause a rupture of suture line.

THERAPEUTIC INTERVENTIONS	RATIONALE

Desired Outcome: The client will verbalize an understanding of and a plan for adhering to recommended follow-up care including future appointments with health care provider, wound care, medications prescribed, and activity level

Independent Actions

Explain the rationale for, side effects of, schedule for taking, and importance of taking medications prescribed. Inform client of pertinent food and drug interactions.

Knowledge of disease process and treatment helps the client and family understand the changes that are occurring and the importance of treatment in maintaining health status. This improves client's adherence to treatment regimen and allows client to maintain a level of independence for as long as possible. Appropriate positioning postoperatively helps relieve pain.

If the client has had a laparoscopic cholecystectomy, mild shoulder pain may persist for a week after surgery until the carbon dioxide used during surgery is completely absorbed. Tell client that lying on his/her left side with the right knee flexed may help relieve this pain.

CHOLELITHIASIS/CHOLECYSTITIS

Cholelithiasis refers to the presence of gallstones in the gallbladder. Factors that contribute to gallstone formation are abnormal bile composition; biliary stasis or slow emptying of the gallbladder resulting from factors such as fasting, pregnancy, prolonged parenteral nutrition, or an obstructive lesion in the biliary system; and inflammation of the gallbladder. Cholesterol stones are the most prevalent type of gallstone. They are most often associated with a high-cholesterol diet or cholesterol-lowering drugs and form when bile becomes supersaturated with cholesterol, which then precipitates and starts to form stones. Other components of bile that precipitate into stones are bile salts, bilirubin, calcium, and protein. Stones either remain in the gallbladder or migrate into the duct system where they may cause partial or complete obstruction. The severity of the client's symptoms depends on the degree of bile flow obstruction.

Cholecystitis is inflammation of the gallbladder wall. Most cases of cholecystitis result from bile stasis, which is most commonly due to obstruction of the cystic duct by a gallstone. The bile trapped in the gallbladder acts as a chemical irritant causing inflammation and edema of the gallbladder wall. Cholecystitis in the absence of stones (acalculous cholecystitis) is thought to result from a buildup of mucus or sludge in the gallbladder associated with biliary stasis. This stasis can result from factors such as prolonged fasting or total parenteral nutrition, ischemia of the gallbladder associated with vasculitis, or bacterial invasion of the gallbladder via the blood or lymph system. After the period of acute inflammation, scarring often develops, resulting in loss of normal gallbladder function.

In most cases, the treatment of choice for symptomatic cholelithiasis and cholecystitis is cholecystectomy and cho-

ledocholithotomy if stones have migrated into the biliary duct system. A percutaneous cholecystostomy may be done to relieve symptoms if the client has severe symptoms and is a poor surgical risk. Nonsurgical treatment of gallstones includes endoscopic sphincterotomy with basket removal of stones, dissolution of stones using oral bile acids, percutaneous or endoscopic instillation of a dissolution agent into the gallbladder, and extracorporeal shockwave lithotripsy. These nonoperative modalities are only performed on a small percentage of patients (e.g., high-risk surgical candidates, persons who refuse surgery) because of the high incidence of recurrence of gallstones with nonsurgical treatments and the increasing popularity of laparoscopic surgery.

This care plan focuses on the adult client hospitalized with probable cholelithiasis and/or cholecystitis.

OUTCOME/DISCHARGE CRITERIA

The client will:
1. Have relief of severe pain
2. Tolerate prescribed diet
3. Have no signs and symptoms of complications
4. Verbalize an understanding of ways to reduce the risk for recurrent gallbladder attacks
5. State signs and symptoms to report to the health care provider
6. Verbalize an understanding of and a plan for adhering to recommended follow-up care including future appointments with health care provider and medications prescribed.

For a full, detailed care plan on this topic, go to http://evolve.elsevier.com/Haugen/careplanning/.

CIRRHOSIS

Cirrhosis is a chronic disease of the liver that occurs as a result of extensive destruction of the parenchymal cells in the liver. These cells are eventually replaced by fibrous scar tissue with subsequent change in the structure and functioning of the liver. The structural changes impair portal blood flow, which results in venous congestion in other organs and systems such as the spleen and gastrointestinal tract.

There are numerous causes of cirrhosis. More than half of the cases of cirrhosis are associated with alcohol and chronic viral hepatitis. Other causes of cirrhosis include exposure to toxic chemicals or drugs, hereditary metabolic disorders (e.g., alpha$_1$-antitrypsin deficiency, Wilson's disease, hemochromatosis), heart failure, and conditions that cause persistent bile flow obstruction (e.g., primary biliary cirrhosis, primary sclerosing cholangitis). In approximately 15% to 20% of cases, no cause is identified.

All types of cirrhosis have similar signs and symptoms, which are manifestations of impaired liver function and the venous congestion that occurs with portal hypertension. Alcohol-related cirrhosis may have additional manifestations such as cerebral degeneration and demyelinating neuropathies that are thought to be a direct result of the toxic effects of alcohol or certain associated vitamin deficiencies. Treatment of cirrhosis is supportive and directed at slowing the progression of liver failure and reducing the incidence and/or severity of complications. The primary goals of treatment are to eliminate or manage the factors/conditions that contributed to the development of cirrhosis, provide a diet that is high in nutrients and will reduce the risk for further liver damage, and encourage rest to reduce the metabolic demands on the liver. A liver transplant may be indicated to treat end-stage liver disease.

This care plan focuses on the adult client with alcoholic (Laennec's) cirrhosis hospitalized for management of increasing ascites and peripheral edema. Much of the information is applicable to clients receiving follow-up care in an extended care facility or home setting.

OUTCOME/DISCHARGE CRITERIA

The client will:
1. Have an adequate nutritional intake
2. Perform activities of daily living without extreme fatigue or dyspnea
3. Have a reduction in or resolution of ascites and edema
4. Have no evidence of life-threatening complications
5. Identify ways to prevent further liver damage
6. Verbalize an understanding of the rationale for and components of the recommended diet
7. Identify ways to reduce stress on or trauma to the esophageal blood vessels
8. Identify ways to prevent bleeding
9. Identify ways to reduce the risk of infection
10. Identify ways to relieve pruritus
11. State signs and symptoms to report to the health care provider
12. Identify community resources that can assist with home management and adjustment to lifestyle changes necessary for effective management of cirrhosis
13. Share concerns and feelings about the diagnosis of cirrhosis; prognosis; and effects of the disease process and its treatment on self-concept, lifestyle, and roles
14. Verbalize an understanding of and a plan for adhering to recommended follow-up care including future appointments with health care provider, medications prescribed, and activity level.

Nursing Diagnosis   INEFFECTIVE BREATHING PATTERN NDx

Definition: Inspiration and/or expiration that does not provide adequate ventilation

Related to:
- Increased rate of respirations associated with fear and anxiety
- Decreased depth of respirations associated with:
  - Weakness and fatigue
  - Decreased lung compliance (distensibility) resulting from pleural effusion (hepatic hydrothorax) that occurs because of excess fluid volume and passage of ascitic fluid into the pleural space through a probable pressure-related defect in the diaphragm
  - Restricted chest expansion resulting from positioning and pressure on the diaphragm as a result of ascites

CLINICAL MANIFESTATIONS

Subjective	Objective
Complaints of shortness of breath	Dyspnea; orthopnea; increased respiratory rate; decreased depth of breathing; decreased inspiratory/expiratory pressure; decreased minute ventilation; decreased vital capacity; nasal flaring; use of accessory muscles to breathe; assumption of three-point position; altered chest excursion; pursed-lip breathing; prolonged expiration phases; increased anterior-posterior diameter

RISK FACTORS
- Chronic illness
- Failure of body's regulatory mechanisms

DESIRED OUTCOMES

The client will have an improved breathing pattern as evidenced by:
  a. Normal rate and depth of respirations
  b. Decreased dyspnea
  c. Symmetrical chest excursion

NOC OUTCOMES

Respiratory status: ventilation

NIC INTERVENTIONS

Ventilation assistance; respiratory monitoring

NURSING ASSESSMENT	RATIONALE
Assess for signs and symptoms of an ineffective breathing pattern: • Shallow or slow respirations • Limited chest excursion • Tachypnea or dyspnea • Use of accessory muscles when breathing	*Early recognition of signs and symptoms of an ineffective breathing pattern allows for prompt intervention.*
Assess/monitor pulse oximetry (arterial oxygen saturation [SaO_2]), arterial blood gas (ABG) values as indicated.	*Monitoring continuous SaO_2 readings allows for the early detection of hypoxia.* *Assessment of ABG values allows for a more direct measurement of both the partial pressure of oxygen in arterial blood (PaO_2) and the partial pressure of carbon dioxide in arterial blood ($PaCO_2$), both of which reflect the adequacy of ventilation.*

THERAPEUTIC INTERVENTIONS	RATIONALE

Independent Actions

Implement measures to improve breathing pattern:
- Perform actions to increase strength and activity tolerance (e.g., maintain activity restrictions, maintain a calm environment, organize nursing care to provide for periods of rest, limit number of visitors and their length of stay). **D ● ✦**

  These actions increase a client's willingness and ability to move, deep breathe, and use incentive spirometer.

- Perform actions to restore fluid balance:
  - Restrict sodium intake as ordered.
  - Maintain fluid restriction.

  Reduces fluid accumulation in the peritoneal cavity and pleural space.

- Encourage client to periodically rest in a recumbent position.

  Lying down reduces peripheral pooling of blood, which increases effective circulating volume and renal blood flow and subsequently promotes diuresis.

- Place client in a semi-Fowler's position (a high-Fowler's position is uncomfortable if ascites is severe). **D ● ✦**

  Places less compression on the diaphragm.

- Instruct client to deep breathe or use incentive spirometer every 1 to 2 hours.

  Deep breathing and use of an incentive spirometer promote maximal inhalation and lung expansion.

- Instruct client to avoid intake of gas-forming foods (e.g., beans, cauliflower, cabbage, onions), carbonated beverages, and large meals.

  Avoidance of gas forming foods prevents gastric distention and additional pressure on the diaphragm.

Dependent/Collaborative Actions

Implement measures to improve breathing pattern:
- Assist with positive airway pressure techniques (e.g., continuous positive airway pressure [CPAP], bilevel positive airway pressure [BiPAP], flutter/positive expiratory pressure [PEP] device) if ordered.

  Positive airway pressure techniques increase intrapulmonary (alveolar) pressure, which helps reexpand collapsed alveoli and prevent further alveoli collapse.

- Administer central nervous system depressants judiciously; hold medication and consult physician if respiratory rate is less than 12 breaths/min.

  Reducing pain helps to increase the client's willingness to move and breathe more deeply.

- Assist with thoracentesis and/or paracentesis if performed.

  To remove pleural and/or peritoneal fluid in order to allow increased chest and lung expansion.

NDx = NANDA-I Diagnosis   **D** = Delegatable Action   ● = UAP   ✦ = LVN/LPN   ⊖▶ = Go to ⊖volve for animation

Continued...

THERAPEUTIC INTERVENTIONS	RATIONALE
Consult appropriate health care provider (e.g., respiratory therapist, physician) if: • Ineffective breathing pattern continues. • Signs and symptoms of impaired gas exchange (e.g., restlessness, irritability, confusion, significant decrease in oximetry results, decreased PaO_2 and increased $PaCO_2$ levels) are present.	*Notifying the appropriate health care provider allows for prompt modification of treatment plan.*

Nursing/Collaborative Diagnosis   RISK FOR EXCESS FLUID VOLUME NDx AND THIRD-SPACING

Definition: Risk for developing an imbalance of electrolytes and fluids in the intracellular and extracellular compartments of the body

Related to:
• Sodium and water retention associated with an increased serum aldosterone level resulting from:
  • Inability of the liver to metabolize aldosterone
  • Activation of the renin-angiotensin-aldosterone mechanism as a result of decreased renal blood flow (occurs because of a decrease in intravascular volume that results from vasodilation and from third-spacing and sequestration of fluid in the splanchnic system)
• Low plasma colloid osmotic pressure associated with hypoalbuminemia (a result of decreased hepatic synthesis of albumin and prolonged inadequate nutrition)
  Increased pressure in the portal system and hepatic lymph system associated with blood flow backup resulting from structural changes in the liver

CLINICAL MANIFESTATIONS

Subjective	Objective
Shortness of breath	Jugular venous distention; decreased hemoglobin (Hgb) and hematocrit (Hct); weight gain over short period; dyspnea; intake exceeds output; pleural effusion; orthopnea; S_3 heart sound; pulmonary congestion; change in respiratory pattern; change in mental status; B/P changes; pulmonary artery pressure changes; oliguria; specific gravity changes; azotemia; altered serum electrolyte levels; restlessness; anxiety; abnormal breath sounds (crackles); edema, may progress to anasarca; increased central venous pressure; positive hepatojugular reflex

RISK FACTORS
• Hyperaldosteronism
• Poor nutritional status
• Portal hypertension

DESIRED OUTCOMES

The client will experience resolution of fluid and electrolyte imbalance fluid as evidenced by:
  a. Decline in weight toward client's normal weight
  b. B/P and pulse rate within normal range for client and stable with position change
  c. Absence or resolution of S_3 heart sound
  d. Balanced intake and output
  e. Usual mental status
  f. Serum sodium level returning toward normal range
  g. Decreased dyspnea, peripheral edema, and neck vein distention
  h. Improved breath sounds
  i. Resolution of ascites

NOC OUTCOMES	NIC INTERVENTIONS
Fluid balance; fluid overload severity; electrolyte and acid-base balance	Fluid monitoring; fluid/electrolyte management; electrolyte management: hyponatremia; electrolyte management: hypokalemia; hypervolemia management

NURSING ASSESSMENT	RATIONALE
Assess for and report:	
• Signs and symptoms of excess fluid volume:	*Early recognition of signs and symptoms of fluid and electrolyte imbalance allows for prompt treatment.*
• Weight gain of 2% or greater in a short period	
• Elevated B/P	*B/P may not be elevated if fluid has shifted out of the vascular space.*
• Development or worsening of S_3 heart sound	*Indicates vascular fluid overload.*
• Intake greater than output	*Causes retention of fluids.*
• Change in mental status	*May also reflect impending hepatic encephalopathy.*
• Low serum sodium level	*May also result from diuretic therapy and a low-sodium diet.*
• Dyspnea, orthopnea, crackles (rales), diminished or absent breath sounds	*Increased pulmonary congestion*
• Peripheral edema	
• Distended neck veins	
• Signs and symptoms of third-spacing:	*Early recognition of signs and symptoms of third-spacing allows for prompt treatment.*
• Ascites	
• Dyspnea and diminished or absent breath sounds	
• Evidence of vascular depletion (e.g., postural hypotension; weak, rapid pulse; decreased urine output)	
• Chest radiograph results showing pulmonary vascular congestion, pleural effusion, or pulmonary edema	
• Low serum albumin levels	*Results in fluid shifting out of the vascular space because albumin normally maintains plasma colloid osmotic pressure.*

THERAPEUTIC INTERVENTIONS	RATIONALE
Dependent/Collaborative Actions	
Implement measures to restore fluid balance:	
• Perform actions to reduce excess fluid volume:	
• Restrict sodium intake as ordered.	*Decreases fluid retention.*
• Maintain fluid restrictions if ordered.	
• Encourage client to rest periodically in a recumbent position. **D** ● ✦	*Lying down reduces peripheral pooling of blood, which increases effective circulating volume and renal blood flow and subsequently promotes diuresis.*
• Administer diuretics if ordered (e.g., potassium-sparing diuretics such as spironolactone and amiloride are often used initially). **D** ✦	*Diuretics reduce fluid volume by increasing urinary output.*
• Perform actions to promote mobilization of fluid back into the vascular space and to prevent further third-spacing:	*Improves renal blood flow, which increases water excretion and reduces activation of the renin-angiotensin-aldosterone mechanism.*
• Administer albumin infusions if ordered.	*Albumin infusions increase vascular colloid osmotic pressure and pulls fluid back into the vascular system.*
Consult physician if signs and symptoms of imbalanced fluid persist or worsen.	*Notifying the appropriate health care provider allows for prompt modification of treatment plan.*

Nursing/Collaborative Diagnosis **RISK FOR HYPOKALEMIA**

Definition: Below normal range for serum potassium levels

Related to: Excessive potassium loss associated with an increased aldosterone level (aldosterone causes potassium excretion) and diuretic therapy

---

NDx = NANDA-I Diagnosis   **D** = Delegatable Action   ● = UAP   ✦ = LVN/_PN   ⊜▶ = Go to ⊜volve for animation

Continued...

CLINICAL MANIFESTATIONS

Subjective	Objective
Verbalization of nausea and muscle weakness	Cardiac dysrhythmias; electrocardiogram (ECG) reading showing ST-segment depression, T-wave inversion or flattening, and presence of U waves; postural hypotension; vomiting; abdominal distention; hypoactive or absent bowel sounds; low serum potassium level

RISK FACTORS

- Chronic illness
- Failure of regulatory mechanisms
- Medication regimen

DESIRED OUTCOMES

The client will maintain a safe serum potassium level as evidenced by:
  a. Regular pulse at 60 to 100 beats/min
  b. B/P within normal range for client and stable with position change
  c. Usual muscle tone and strength
  d. Absence of nausea and vomiting
  e. Soft, nondistended abdomen with normal bowel sounds
  f. Normal ECG reading
  g. Serum potassium level within normal range

NURSING ASSESSMENT	RATIONALE
Assess for and report signs and symptoms of: • Hypokalemia (e.g., cardiac dysrhythmias; postural hypotension; muscle weakness; nausea and vomiting; abdominal distention; hypoactive or absent bowel sounds; ECG reading showing ST segment depression, T wave inversion or flattening, and presence of U waves	*Early recognition of signs and symptoms of hypokalemia allows for prompt intervention.*

THERAPEUTIC INTERVENTIONS	RATIONALE
Dependent/Collaborative Actions Implement measures to prevent or treat hypokalemia: • Administer intravenous and oral potassium replacements as ordered.	*Replacements for potassium; it is important to monitor serum potassium levels and urine output closely when giving supplemental potassium; consult physician if potassium level increases above normal and/or urine output is less than 30 mL/h.*
• If client is taking a potassium-depleting diuretic or if signs and symptoms of hypokalemia are present, encourage intake of foods/fluids high in potassium (e.g., bananas, potatoes, raisins, cantaloupe).	
• Administer antidysrhythmic agents if ECG changes are noted.	*Decreases incidence of dysrhythmias.*
Consult physician if signs and symptoms of hypokalemia persist or worsen.	*Notification of the physician allows for prompt modification of treatment regimen.*

Collaborative Diagnosis ## RISK FOR HYPONATREMIA

Definition: Below normal range for serum sodium levels

Related to: Hemodilution associated with excess fluid volume, sodium loss associated with diuretic therapy, and dietary sodium restriction

CLINICAL MANIFESTATIONS

Subjective	Objective
Verbalization of nausea and abdominal cramps; feelings of lethargy and weakness	Vomiting; confusion; seizures; decreased serum sodium level

RISK FACTORS

- Chronic illness
- Failure of regulatory mechanisms
- Medication regimen

DESIRED OUTCOMES

The client will maintain a safe serum sodium level as evidenced by:

    a. Absence of nausea, vomiting, and abdominal cramps

    b. Usual mental status

    c. Usual muscle strength

    d. Absence of seizure activity

    e. Serum sodium level within normal range

NURSING ASSESSMENT	RATIONALE
Assess for and report signs and symptoms of hyponatremia (e.g., nausea, vomiting, abdominal cramps, lethargy, confusion, weakness, seizures).	*Early recognition of signs and symptoms of hyponatremia allows for prompt treatment.*

THERAPEUTIC INTERVENTIONS	RATIONALE
Dependent/Collaborative Actions Implement measures to treat hyponatremia:	
- Maintain fluid restrictions if ordered.	*Decreases fluid volume, which decreases dilutional hyponatremia*
- Administer hypertonic saline solutions if ordered.	*Hypertonic solutions are not commonly given until hyponatremia is severe because of the risk of hypernatremia and intravascular volume overload; furosemide may be given concurrently to promote water excretion and reduce the risk for intravascular volume overload.*
Consult physician if signs and symptoms of hyponatremia persist or worsen.	*Notifying the physician allows for prompt modification of treatment plan.*

Nursing Diagnosis | IMBALANCED NUTRITION: LESS THAN BODY REQUIREMENTS NDx

Definition: Inadequate intake or insufficient nutrition to meet the body's metabolic needs

Related to:

- Decreased oral intake associated with dyspepsia, fatigue, dyspnea, dislike of the prescribed diet, and feeling of fullness from ascites
- Reduced metabolism and storage of nutrients by the liver associated with a reduction of functional liver tissue
- Malabsorption of fats and fat-soluble vitamins associated with impaired bile production and flow.

CLINICAL MANIFESTATIONS

Subjective	Objective
Verbalization of lack of appetite; fatigue; sore buccal membrane irritability; poor self-esteem	Loss of weight with adequate food intake; body weight 20% or more under ideal weight; inflamed buccal cavity; capillary fragility; pale conjunctiva and mucous membranes; poor muscle tone; excessive hair loss; amenorrhea

RISK FACTORS

- Chronic illness
- Anorexia
- Poor nutritional status
- Poor dietary habits

DESIRED OUTCOMES

The client will maintain an adequate nutritional status as evidenced by:

    a. Dry weight approaching normal for the client (dry weight achieved after fluid volume excess has been resolved)

    b. Normal BUN and serum albumin, prealbumin, Hct, and Hgb levels, and normal lymphocyte count

    c. Improved strength and activity tolerance

    d. Healthy oral mucous membrane

Continued...

NOC OUTCOMES	NIC INTERVENTIONS
Nutritional status	Nutritional monitoring; nutritional counseling; nutritional management; nutritional therapy

NURSING ASSESSMENT	RATIONALE
Assess for and report signs and symptoms of malnutrition: • Weight significantly below client's usual weight or below normal for client's age, height, and body frame • Decreased serum prealbumin, albumin, Hct, and Hgb levels and decreased lymphocyte count • Weakness and fatigue • Sore, inflamed oral mucous membrane • Pale conjunctiva	*Early recognition and reporting of signs and symptoms of malnutrition allows for prompt intervention.*
Monitor percentage of meals and snacks client consumes. Report a pattern of inadequate intake.	*An awareness of the amount of food/fluid the client consumes alerts the nurse to deficits in nutritional intake. Reporting an inadequate intake allows for prompt intervention.*

THERAPEUTIC INTERVENTIONS	RATIONALE

Independent Actions

Implement measures to improve nutritional status:

• Implement measures to reduce dyspepsia (e.g., keep head of bed elevated for 2 to 3 hours after eating; provide small, frequent meals; encourage client to ingest foods slowly; avoid carbonated beverages; do not use a straw). **D ● ✦**	*Elevation of the head of the bed after eating decreases pressure on abdomen, which may improve appetite. Small frequent meals. and non use of carbonated beverages or a straw decrease pressure in the abdomen.*
Encourages a rest period before meals. **D ● ✦**	*Minimizes fatigue.*
• Maintain a clean environment and a relaxed, pleasant atmosphere. **D ● ✦**	*Maintaining a clean environment and a relaxed, pleasant atmosphere can help reduce the client's stress and promote a feeling of well-being, which tends to improve appetite and oral intake.*
• Serve frequent, small meals rather than large ones if client is weak, fatigues easily, and/or has a poor appetite. **D ● ✦**	*Providing small rather than large meals can enable a client who is weak or fatigues easily to finish a meal. Also, a client who has a poor appetite is often more willing to attempt to eat smaller meals because they seem less overwhelming than larger ones. If smaller meals are served, the number of meals per day should be increased to help ensure adequate nutrition.*
• Elevate the head of bed as tolerated for meals. **D ● ✦**	*Helps reduce dyspnea and feeling of fullness (a high-Fowler's position may be too uncomfortable if ascites is severe).*
• Allow adequate time for meals; reheat foods/fluids if necessary. **D ● ✦**	*Appetite is also suppressed if foods/fluids normally served hot or warm become cold and do not appeal to the client.*
• Limit fluid intake with meals unless the fluid has a high nutritional value. **D ✦**	*Drinking liquids with meals distends the stomach and may cause satiety before an adequate amount of food is consumed.*
• Increase activity as allowed and tolerated. **D ● ✦**	*Activity usually promotes a sense of well-being, which can improve appetite.*
• Assist and instruct client to adhere to the following dietary recommendations: • Avoid skipping meals.	*Skipping meals reduces caloric intake.*
• Consume a diet high in calories (2000-3000 calories/day) and carbohydrates.	
• Limit protein intake with hepatic encephalopathy.	*Changes in the client's metabolism due to liver failure can cause hepatic encephalopathy, as ammonia is not metabolized and passes through the liver unchanged and can become a cerebral toxin.*
• Consume meals that are well balanced and high in essential nutrients.	*The client must consume a diet that is well balanced and high in essential nutrients in order to meet nutritional needs.*

THERAPEUTIC INTERVENTIONS	RATIONALE

Dependent/Collaborative Actions

Implement measures to improve nutritional status:

- Implement measures to restore fluid volume (e.g., restrict sodium intake; maintain fluid restrictions as ordered; administer diuretics as ordered).

Reduces fluid in the peritoneal cavity and subsequently reduces the feeling of fullness

- Administer vitamins and minerals (e.g., fat-soluble vitamins, thiamine, folic acid, iron) if ordered.

Vitamins and minerals are needed to maintain metabolic functioning. If the client's dietary intake does not provide adequate amounts of them, oral and/or parenteral supplements may be necessary.

- Instruct client to use herbs, spices, and salt substitutes (if approved by a physician).

Use of spices makes low-sodium diet more palatable.

- Obtain a dietary consult if necessary.

A dietitian is best able to evaluate whether the foods/fluids selected will meet the client's nutritional needs.

- Perform a calorie count if ordered. Report information to the dietitian and physician.

A calorie count provides information about the caloric and nutritional value of the foods/fluids the client consumes. The information obtained helps the dietitian and physician determine whether an alternative method of nutritional support is needed.

- Consult physician about an alternative method of providing nutrition (e.g., parenteral nutrition, tube feeding) if client does not consume enough food or fluids to meet nutritional needs.

If the client's oral intake is inadequate, an alternative method of providing nutrients needs to be implemented.

Nursing Diagnosis **IMPAIRED COMFORT** NDx **(PRURITUS)**

Definition: Perceived lack of ease, relief, and transcendence in physical, psychospiritual, environmental, and social dimensions

Related to: Stimulation of itch receptors in the skin by bile acid metabolites that accumulate in the blood as a result of bile flow obstruction

CLINICAL MANIFESTATIONS

Subjective	Objective
Complaint of skin itching	Persistent scratching or rubbing of skin

RISK FACTOR

- Chronic illness

DESIRED OUTCOMES

The client will experience relief of pruritus as evidenced by:
   a. Verbalization of same
   b. No scratching or rubbing of skin

NOC OUTCOMES

Comfort level; symptom control

NIC INTERVENTIONS

Pruritus management

NURSING ASSESSMENT	RATIONALE

Assess for the following:
- Reports of itchiness
- Persistent scratching or rubbing of skin

Early recognition of signs and symptoms of pruritus allows for prompt intervention.

NDx = NANDA-I Diagnosis   **D** = Delegatable Action   ● = UAP   ✦ = LVN/LPN   ⊖▶ = Go to ⊖volve for animation

Continued...

THERAPEUTIC INTERVENTIONS	RATIONALE

Independent Actions

Instruct client in and/or implement measures to relieve pruritus:

- Apply cool, moist compresses to pruritic areas. **D** ● ✦

  Cold/cool compresses provide a counter sensation that decreases the urge to rub or scratch the area.

- Apply emollient creams or ointments frequently. **D** ● ✦

  Creams and ointments prevent dryness.

- Add emollients, cornstarch, or baking soda to bath water. **D** ● ✦

  Adding these products to bath water decreases skin dryness and provides a protective barrier.

- Use tepid water and mild soaps for bathing. **D** ● ✦

  Use of tepid water and mild soaps decreases skin dryness.

- Pat skin dry after bathing, making sure to dry thoroughly. **D** ● ✦

  Rubbing of the skin with a towel after a bath can stimulate itching.

- Maintain a cool environment. **D** ● ✦

  A cool environment provides a counter sensation that decreases urge to rub or scratch.

- Encourage participation in diversional activity.
- Use relaxation techniques.

  Distracts client from focusing on the itch.

- Use cutaneous stimulation techniques (e.g., massage, pressure, vibration, stroking with soft brush) at sites of itching or acupressure points.

  Cutaneous stimulation blocks the neurotransmission of the itch sensation.

- Encourage client to wear loose cotton garments and avoid clothes or blankets made from wool.

  Wearing loose clothing and non-wool blankets decrease skin irritation.

Dependent/Collaborative Actions

Instruct client in and/or implement measures *to relieve pruritus:*

- Administer the following medications if ordered:
  - Antihistamines (e.g., diphenhydramine, hydroxyzine [Atarax])

    Antihistamines blocks histamine, which stimulates itchy sensations.

  - Bile acid–sequestering agents (e.g., cholestyramine).

    Bile acid sequestering agents bind with the bile acids in the intestines, prevents absorption and enhances elimination, thereby decreasing itch sensations.

Consult appropriate health care provider (e.g., clinical nurse specialist, physician) if above measures fail to alleviate pruritus or if the skin becomes excoriated.

Notification of the appropriate health care provider allows for prompt modification in treatment plan.

Nursing Diagnosis **IMPAIRED COMFORT** NDx **(DYSPEPSIA)**

Definition: Perceived lack of ease, relief, and transcendence in physical, psychospiritual, environmental, and social dimensions

Related to:

- Impaired fat digestion associated with bile flow obstruction
- Reflux of gastric contents associated with increased intra-abdominal pressure resulting from ascites
- Impaired gastrointestinal functioning associated with venous congestion in the gastrointestinal tract (portal hypertensive gastropathy)
- Esophagitis/gastritis associated with the irritant effect of chronic alcohol ingestion on the esophageal and gastric mucosa

CLINICAL MANIFESTATIONS

Subjective	Objective
Complaints of stomach discomfort; heartburn; nausea; or feeling of fullness or bloating	Frequent eructation

RISK FACTORS

- Impaired digestive processes
- Alcohol ingestion
- Portal hypertension

DESIRED OUTCOME

The client will verbalize relief of dyspepsia.

NOC OUTCOMES

Comfort level

NIC INTERVENTIONS

Flatulence reduction; nausea management

NURSING ASSESSMENT	**RATIONALE**
Assess client for signs and symptoms of dyspepsia (e.g., reports of epigastric discomfort, heartburn, nausea, or feeling of fullness or bloating; frequent eructation).	*Early recognition of signs and symptoms of dyspepsia allows for prompt intervention.*
Assess which foods/fluids contribute to dyspepsia (client usually reports an intolerance of fatty foods).	*Helps client determine which foods to avoid.*

THERAPEUTIC INTERVENTIONS	**RATIONALE**

Independent Actions

Implement measures to reduce gastroesophageal reflux:

• Keep head of bed elevated for 2 to 3 hours after meals. **D** ● ✦	*Elevation of the head of the bed uses gravity to decease reflux.*
• Provide small, frequent meals rather than large ones. **D** ● ✦	*Small, frequent meals reduce pressure in and distention of the stomach, thereby decreasing reflux.*
• Instruct client to ingest foods and fluids slowly. **D** ● ✦	*Eating slowly prevents rapid filling of the stomach and decreases incidence of reflux.*
• Encourage client not to smoke.	*Smoking stimulates the production of bile.*
• Encourage client to avoid the following foods/fluids:	
• Those high in fat (e.g., fried foods, gravies, butter, cream, ice cream)	*These foods produce excessive gas in the gastrointestinal tract; stimulates the production of bile.*
• Carbonated beverages	
• Gas-producing foods (e.g., beans, onions, cabbage)	*Causes gastric distention.*
• Those that may cause gastric irritation (e.g., spicy foods; caffeine-containing beverages such as coffee, tea, and colas; alcohol)	*Causes gastric irritation.*

Dependent/Collaborative Actions

Perform actions to restore fluid balance (e.g., restrict sodium intake; maintain fluid restrictions as ordered; administer diuretics as ordered).	*Restoration of fluid balance promotes the resolution of ascites and subsequently reduces abdominal pressure and the associated gastroesophageal reflux and feeling of fullness and bloating.*
Administer the following medications if ordered:	
• Antacids, histamine₂-receptor antagonists (e.g., famotidine, nizatidine, ranitidine), or proton pump inhibitors (e.g., omeprazole, lansoprazole, pantoprazole, esomeprazole)	*Antacids neutralize stomach acids. Histamine receptor antagonists and proton-pump inhibitors suppress secretion of gastric acid.*
• Cytoprotective agents (e.g., sucralfate, misoprostol)	*Cytoprotective agents create a protective barrier against stomach acid and pepsin.*
• Antiflatulents (e.g., simethicone)	*Antiflatulents relieves gas and decreases abdominal pressure.*
• Antiemetics (phenothiazines should be used cautiously)	*Antiemetics decrease incidence of nausea and/or vomiting.*
Consult clinical nurse specialist or physician if above measures fail to control dyspepsia.	*Notification of the physician allows for prompt alterations in the treatment plan.*

Nursing Diagnosis	**ACTIVITY INTOLERANCE** NDx

Definition: Insufficient physiological or psychological energy to endure or complete required or desired daily activities

Related to:

- Tissue hypoxia associated with anemia resulting from:
  - Decreased production of red blood cells (RBCs) resulting from a decreased intake and absorption of vitamins and minerals and an inability of the liver to store vitamins and minerals
  - Excessive RBC destruction resulting from hypersplenism (if venous congestion has resulted in splenomegaly, the spleen will destroy RBCs faster than usual)
  - Blood loss if bleeding has occurred
- Loss of muscle mass, tone, and strength associated with malnutrition and disuse if mobility has been limited for an extended period
- Decrease in available energy associated with inability of the liver to metabolize glucose, fats, and proteins properly
- Difficulty resting and sleeping associated with dyspnea, discomfort, frequent assessments and treatments, fear, anxiety, and unfamiliar environment

---

NDx = NANDA-I Diagnosis   **D** = Delegatable Action   ● = UAP   ✦ = LVN/LPN   ⊖▶ = Go to ⊖volve for animation

Continued...

CLINICAL MANIFESTATIONS

Subjective	Objective
Verbal report of fatigue or weakness	Abnormal heart rate or B/P response to activity; exertional discomfort or dyspnea; ECG changes reflecting dysrhythmias or ischemia; unable to speak during physical activity

RISK FACTORS

- Chronic illness
- Poor nutritional status
- Immobility
- Impaired digestive processes

DESIRED OUTCOMES

The client will demonstrate an increased tolerance for activity as evidenced by:
   a. Verbalization of feeling less fatigued and weak
   b. Ability to perform activities of daily living without exertional dyspnea, chest pain, diaphoresis, dizziness, and significant changes in vital signs

NOC OUTCOMES

Rest; energy conservation; activity tolerance

NIC INTERVENTIONS

Energy management; oxygen therapy; nutrition management; sleep enhancement

NURSING ASSESSMENT	RATIONALE
Assess for signs and symptoms of activity intolerance: • Statements of fatigue or weakness • Exertional dyspnea, chest pain • Diaphoresis, or dizziness • Abnormal heart rate response to activity (e.g., increase in rate of 20 beats/min above resting rate, rate not returning to preactivity level within 3 minutes after stopping activity, change from regular to irregular rate) • Significant change (15-20 mm Hg) in B/P with activity	*Early recognition of signs and symptoms of activity intolerance allows for prompt intervention.*

THERAPEUTIC INTERVENTIONS	RATIONALE

Independent Actions

Implement measures to improve activity tolerance:

- Perform actions to promote rest and/or conserve energy
  - Maintain prescribed activity restrictions.
  - Minimize environmental activity and noise. **D** ● ✦
  - Provide uninterrupted rest periods. **D** ● ✦
  - Assist with care. **D** ● ✦
  - Keep supplies and personal articles within easy reach. **D** ● ✦
  - Limit the number of visitors.
  - Instruct client in energy-saving techniques (e.g., using a shower chair when showering, sitting to brush teeth or comb hair).
- Implement measures to reduce fear and anxiety (e.g., assure client that staff are nearby, explain all tests and procedures, encourage verbalization of fear and anxiety).
- Implement measures to promote sleep (e.g., elevate head of bed and support arms on pillows to facilitate breathing; discourage intake of fluids high in caffeine, especially in the evening; encourage relaxing diversional activities in the evening).
- Implement measures to reduce discomfort (e.g., proper positioning). **D** ✦

Cells use oxygen and fat, protein, and carbohydrate to produce the energy needed for all body activities. Rest and activities that conserve energy result in a lower metabolic rate, which preserves nutrients and oxygen for necessary activities. These actions promote energy conservation and rest.

Fear and anxiety interfere with a client's ability to rest.

Increased hours of sleep improves the client's ability to increase level of activity.

Decreasing discomfort improves the client's ability to perform activities as needed.

THERAPEUTIC INTERVENTIONS	RATIONALE
• Discourage smoking and excessive intake of beverages high in caffeine such as coffee, tea, and colas.	*Both nicotine and excessive caffeine intake can increase cardiac workload and myocardial oxygen utilization, thereby decreasing the amount of oxygen necessary for energy production.*
• Implement measures to improve respiratory status (e.g., encourage use of incentive spirometer; elevate head of bed; assist with turning, coughing, and deep breathing) if ineffective breathing pattern, ineffective airway clearance, or impaired gas exchange is contributing to client's activity intolerance.	*Altered respiratory function can lead to inadequate tissue oxygenation, which results in less efficient energy production and a reduced ability to tolerate activity. Improving respiratory status increases the amount of oxygen available for energy production. It also eases the work of breathing, which reduces energy expenditure.*

Dependent/Collaborative Actions

Implement measures to improve activity tolerance:

• Implement measures to maintain an adequate nutritional status (e.g., provide a diet high in essential nutrients, provide dietary supplements as indicated, administer vitamins and minerals as ordered).	*Metabolism is the process by which nutrients are transformed into energy. If nutrition is inadequate, energy production is decreased, which subsequently reduces one's ability to tolerate activity.*
• Implement measures to treat anemia if present (e.g., administer prescribed iron, folic acid, and/or vitamin B$_{12}$; administer packed RBCs as ordered).	*Anemia reduces the oxygen-carrying capacity of the blood. Resolution of anemia increases oxygen availability to the cells, which increases the efficiency of energy production and subsequently improves activity tolerance.*
• Implement measures to promote sleep (e.g., maintain oxygen therapy during sleep, administer sleep aids and analgesics).	*Improves tissue oxygenation.* *Improves client's ability to rest/sleep.*
• Increase client's activity gradually as allowed and tolerated.	*Progressive activity helps strengthen the myocardium, which enhances cardiac output and improves activity tolerance.*
Instruct client to report a decreased tolerance for activity and to stop any activity that causes chest pain, a marked increase in shortness of breath, dizziness, or extreme fatigue or weakness.	
Consult physician if signs and symptoms of activity intolerance persist or worsen.	*Notification of the physician allows for prompt modification of the treatment plan.*

Collaborative/Nursing Diagnosis **ACUTE AND CHRONIC CONFUSION** NDx

Definition:

Acute: Abrupt onset of reversible disturbances of consciousness, attention, cognition, and perception

Chronic: Irreversible, long-standing, and/or progressive deterioration of intellect and personality characterized by decreased ability to interpret environmental stimuli; decreased capacity for intellectual thought processes; and manifested by disturbances of memory, orientation, or behavior

Related to:

Disturbances in central nervous system functioning associated with accumulation of toxic substances (e.g., ammonia) in the brain, toxic effects of long-term alcohol use, deficiencies of certain vitamins (e.g., thiamine), and hypoxia if anemia is moderate to severe.

CLINICAL MANIFESTATIONS

Subjective	Objective
N/A	Inaccurate interpretation of environment and time; memory loss; altered mood states (e.g., liability, hostility, irritability, inappropriate affect); inability to make decisions or problem solve; changes in attention span; disorientation; inappropriate social behavior

Continued...

RISK FACTORS
- Alcohol use
- Inability of body to remove toxins
- Poor nutritional status

DESIRED OUTCOMES

The client will demonstrate decreased confusion as evidenced by:
   a. Improved ability to grasp ideas
   b. Improved memory
   c. Longer attention span
   d. Absence or resolution of inappropriate behavior
   e. Oriented to person, place, and time

NOC OUTCOMES

Cognitive orientation; distorted thought process; neurological status; agitation; sleep level; safety behavior; information processing

NIC INTERVENTIONS

Environmental management; behavioral management

NURSING ASSESSMENT	**RATIONALE**
Assess for episodes of disorientation to person, place, and time; episodes of inappropriate behavior; impaired decision-making ability; impaired attention span	*Early recognition of signs and symptoms of confusion allows for prompt intervention.*

THERAPEUTIC INTERVENTIONS	**RATIONALE**

Dependent/Collaborative Actions
Implement measures to maintain optimal thought processes:

- Perform actions to improve nutritional status (e.g., provide a diet high in essential nutrients, provide dietary supplements as indicated, administer vitamins and minerals as ordered). **D** ✦

   Provides vitamins and minerals that are essential for normal neurological functioning and treatment of anemia

- Perform actions to prevent or manage hepatic coma (e.g., prevent constipation, decrease potential for gastrointestinal hemorrhage, maintain fluid and electrolytes).

   These actions eliminate or control levels of ammonia and other nitrogenous substances.

- Administer central nervous system depressants such as opioids (narcotics), sedative-hypnotics, and antianxiety agents with extreme caution; question any order for a normal adult dose of these medications. **D** ✦

   Liver damage associated with cirrhosis reduces normal drug metabolism and may lead to increased serum blood levels/ toxicity of these medications.

- Administer thiamine if ordered. **D** ✦

   Thiamine is essential for appropriate neurological functioning and binds with iron which helps to decrease the iron load on the liver.

- Maintain oxygen therapy as ordered.

   Helps maintain appropriate tissue oxygenation.

If client shows evidence of confusion or disorientation:
- Address client by name. **D ● ✦**

   The client may respond to name even when unable to recognize others.

- Reorient client to person, place, and time as necessary **D ● ✦**

   Frequent re-orientation may provide the client with a sense of security.

- Place familiar objects, clock, and calendar within client's view. **D ● ✦**

   Placing familiar objects helps to orient client and provides a sense of security.

- Approach client in a slow, calm manner; allow adequate time for communication. **D ● ✦**

   These actions help the client remain calm and increases appropriate communication.

- Repeat instructions as necessary using clear, simple language and short sentences.

   Repetition of information increases potential for client understanding.

- Maintain a consistent and fairly structured routine and write out a schedule of activities for client to refer to if desired.

   Structure provides a sense of security and ability to cope with cognitive changes.

- Have client perform only one activity at a time and allow adequate time for performance of activities. **D ● ✦**

   Decreases client's risk of becoming confused and subsequently frustrated in performing multiple activities.

- Encourage client to make lists of planned activities, questions, and concerns.

   Structure provides the client with a sense of security.

- Assist client to problem solve if necessary.

   Provides client some control over the situation.

- Maintain realistic expectations of client's ability to learn, comprehend, and remember information provided; provide client with a written copy of instructions.

   Decreases frustration of client, significant others, and nurses.

THERAPEUTIC INTERVENTIONS	RATIONALE
• Encourage significant others to be supportive of client. Instruct them in methods of dealing with client's confusion. • Inform client and significant others that cognitive and emotional functioning is likely to improve with treatment. Consult physician if disturbed thought processes worsen.	*Decreases frustration and agitation. Allows client's significant others to be involved in care and improves their understanding of the situation,* *Provides hope to client and significant others for the client's future cognitive abilities.* *Notification of the physician allows for prompt modification of the treatment plan.*

Nursing Diagnosis RISK FOR BLEEDING NDx

Definition: At risk for a decrease in blood volume that may compromise health

Related to:
• Decreased production of clotting factors associated with impaired liver function and decreased available vitamin K (can occur from malnutrition, antimicrobials that suppress activity of intestinal flora, and impaired absorption of vitamin K as a result of bile flow obstruction)
• Thrombocytopenia associated with hypersplenism (if venous congestion has resulted in splenomegaly, the spleen will destroy platelets faster than usual)

CLINICAL MANIFESTATIONS

Subjective	Objective
Verbalization of unusual joint pain	Petechiae, purpura, and ecchymoses; gingival bleeding; prolonged bleeding from puncture sites; epistaxis, hemoptysis; further increase in abdominal girth; frank or occult blood in the stool, urine, or vomitus; menorrhagia; restlessness, confusion; hypotension and tachycardia; decrease in Hct and Hgb levels

RISK FACTORS
• Poor nutritional status
• Lack of clotting factors
• Early destruction of blood cells

DESIRED OUTCOMES

The client will not experience unusual bleeding as evidenced by:
  a. Skin and mucous membranes free of petechiae, purpura, ecchymoses, and active bleeding
  b. Absence of unusual joint pain
  c. No further increase in abdominal girth
  d. Absence of frank and occult blood in stool, urine, and vomitus
  e. Usual menstrual flow
  f. Vital signs within normal range for client
  g. Stable or improved Hct and Hgb levels

NURSING ASSESSMENT	RATIONALE
Assess client for and report signs and symptoms of unusual bleeding: • Petechiae, purpura, ecchymoses • Gingival bleeding • Prolonged bleeding from puncture sites • Epistaxis, hemoptysis • Unusual joint pain • Further increase in abdominal girth • Frank or occult blood in the stool, urine, or vomitus • Menorrhagia • Restlessness, confusion • Decreasing B/P and increased pulse rate • Decrease in Hct and Hgb levels Monitor platelet count and coagulation test results (e.g., prothrombin time or international normalized ratio [INR], activated partial thromboplastin time, bleeding time). Report abnormal values.	*Early recognition of signs and symptoms of bleeding allows for prompt intervention.*

NDx = NANDA-I Diagnosis **D** = Delegatable Action ● = UAP ✦ = LVN/LPN ⊜▶ = Go to ⊜volve for animation

Continued...

THERAPEUTIC INTERVENTIONS	RATIONALE

Dependent/Collaborative Actions

Implement measures to reduce bleeding:

- Perform actions to reduce risk of bleeding from esophageal varices (e.g., reduce excess fluid volume; avoid straining to have a bowel movement, coughing, sneezing, lifting heavy objects; avoid spicy foods or ones that may cause trauma to the esophagus).

These actions reduce pressure or irritation on esophageal vessels.

- Avoid giving injections whenever possible; consult physician about prescribing an alternative route for medications ordered to be given intramuscularly or subcutaneously.
- When giving injections or performing venous or arterial punctures, use the smallest gauge needle possible and apply gentle, prolonged pressure to the site after the needle is removed.
- Caution client to avoid activities that increase the risk for trauma (e.g., shaving with a straight-edge razor, using stiff bristle toothbrush or dental floss).

Cuts or mucous membrane irritation may cause excessive bleeding.

- Whenever possible, avoid intubations (e.g., nasogastric) and procedures that can cause injury to the rectal mucosa (e.g., taking temperature rectally, inserting a rectal suppository, administering an enema).

Decreases bleeding associated with trauma.

- Pad side rails if client is confused or restless.

These actions decreases risk for client injury.

- Perform actions to prevent injury (e.g., keep bed in low position; keep needed items within easy reach; assist with ambulation; keep floor clear of clutter; provide ambulatory aids).
- Instruct client to avoid blowing nose forcefully or straining to have a bowel movement; consult physician about an order for a decongestant and/or laxative if indicated.

Reduces pressure in esophageal vessels.

- Administer the following if ordered:
  - Vitamin K (e.g., phytonadione) injections
  - Platelets
  - Fresh frozen plasma
  - Cryoprecipitate

Administration of these medications improves clotting ability.

If bleeding occurs and does not subside spontaneously:

- Apply firm, prolonged pressure to bleeding area(s) if possible.

Each action enhances the body's clotting ability.

- If epistaxis occurs, place client in a high-Fowler's position and apply pressure and ice pack to nasal area.
- Maintain oxygen therapy as ordered.
- Administer vitamin K (e.g., phytonadione) injections, whole blood, or blood products (e.g., fresh frozen plasma, platelets) as ordered.
- Assess for and report signs and symptoms of hypovolemic shock (e.g., restlessness; confusion; significant decrease in B/P; rapid, weak pulse; rapid respirations; cool skin; urine output <30 mL/h).

Notifying the physician allows for prompt modification of the treatment plan.

Collaborative Diagnosis **RISK FOR ASCITES**

Definition: An accumulation of fluid in the peritoneal cavity

Related to:
- Low plasma colloid osmotic pressure associated with hypoalbuminemia (a result of decreased hepatic synthesis of albumin and prolonged inadequate nutrition)
- Increased pressure in the portal system and hepatic lymph system associated with blood flow backup resulting from structural changes in the liver
- A generalized increase in hydrostatic pressure associated with excess fluid volume

CLINICAL MANIFESTATIONS

Subjective	Objective
Verbalization of abdominal discomfort	Increasing abdominal girth; dull percussion note over the abdomen; abdominal fluid wave; protruding umbilicus; bulging flanks; dyspnea

RISK FACTORS
- Poor nutritional status
- Chronic illness
- Impaired synthesis of proteins
- Hyperaldosteronism

DESIRED OUTCOMES

The client will have decreased ascites if present as evidenced by:
   a. Decrease in abdominal girth
   b. Abdominal percussion note more tympanic

NURSING ASSESSMENT

Assess for signs and symptoms of ascites:
- Increase in abdominal girth (abdominal girth should be measured daily at the same time and in the same location on the abdomen with client in the same position)
- Dull percussion note over abdomen with finding of shifting dullness
- Presence of abdominal fluid wave
- Protruding umbilicus and bulging flanks.

RATIONALE

Early recognition of the signs and symptoms of ascites allows for prompt treatment.

THERAPEUTIC INTERVENTIONS

Dependent/Collaborative Actions
Implement measures to reduce excess fluid volume, promote mobilization of fluid back into the vascular space, and prevent further third-spacing:
- Restrict sodium intake as ordered.
- Maintain fluid restrictions if ordered.
- Encourage client to rest periodically in a recumbent position. **D** ✦

- Administer diuretics if ordered (e.g., potassium-sparing diuretics such as spironolactone and amiloride are often used initially). **D** ✦
If signs and symptoms of ascites are present and persist or worsen:
- Consult physician.

- Assist with paracentesis and administer albumin infusions if ordered.

- Prepare client for a portal systemic shunt procedure (e.g., transjugular intrahepatic portosystemic shunt [TIPS]) if planned.

RATIONALE

These actions decrease fluid retention.

Lying down reduces peripheral pooling of blood, which increases effective circulating volume and renal blood flow and subsequently promotes diuresis.
Diuretics reduce fluid volume by increasing urinary output, and improve renal blood flow, which increases water excretion and reduces activation of the renin-angiotensin-aldosterone mechanism.

Notification of the physician allows for prompt modification of treatment plan.
Paracentesis removes fluid from abdomen.
Albumin increases colloid osmotic pressure and pulls fluid back into the vascular system.
This procedure treats portal hypertension and subsequently reduces ascites.

NDx = NANDA-I Diagnosis   **D** = Delegatable Action   ● = UAP   ✦ = LVN/LPN   ⊖▶ = Go to ⊖volve for animation

Collaborative Diagnosis   **RISK FOR HEPATORENAL SYNDROME**

Definition: Acute renal failure associated with cirrhosis

Related to:
- Decreased renal blood flow possibly associated with:
  - A decrease in intravascular volume resulting from:
    (1) Third-spacing and sequestration of fluid in the splanchnic system
    (2) Treatment-induced fluid loss (e.g., paracentesis, diuretic therapy)
  - Intrarenal vasoconstriction that may result from increased levels of certain renal arteriolar vasoconstrictors (e.g., angiotensin, endothelin), increased sympathetic nervous system activity, and impaired synthesis of renal vasodilators such as prostaglandin E_2

CLINICAL MANIFESTATIONS

Subjective	Objective
N/A	Increases serum creatinine levels; decreased creatinine clearance; urine output <30 mL/hr; peripheral edema

RISK FACTORS
- Edema
- Medication regimen
- Impairment of vascular regulatory mechanisms

DESIRED OUTCOMES

The client will maintain adequate renal function as evidenced by:
  a. Serum creatinine level within normal range
  b. Creatinine clearance and urine sodium within normal range
  c. Urine output at least 30 mL/h

NURSING ASSESSMENT	RATIONALE
Assess for and report signs and symptoms of hepatorenal syndrome (e.g., increased serum creatinine level, decreased creatinine clearance, low urine sodium level, urine output <30 mL/h).	*Early recognition of signs and symptoms of hepatorenal syndrome allows for prompt intervention.*

THERAPEUTIC INTERVENTIONS	RATIONALE

Dependent/Collaborative Actions
Implement measures to reduce the risk for hepatorenal syndrome:
- Perform actions to maintain adequate renal blood flow:
  - Maintain an adequate fluid intake; if client is on a fluid restriction, maintain the maximum fluid intake allowed. **D** ✦

    Maintenance of adequate vascular fluid volume maintains cardiac output/renal blood flow.
  - Administer albumin infusions if ordered.

    Albumin increases intravascular volume and via osmotic pressure pulls that fluid into the vascular system.
  - Consult physician about reducing the dose of diuretic ordered if client loses more than 1 kg of weight per day.

    Vigorous diuresis can reduce the intravascular volume enough to decrease renal blood flow and precipitate the hepatorenal syndrome.
- Consult physician regarding discontinuation of prescribed medications that can be nephrotoxic (e.g., nonsteroidal anti-inflammatory agents, aminoglycosides).

  These medications can cause nephrotoxicity decreases renal functioning and blood flow.

If signs and symptoms of the hepatorenal syndrome occur:
- Administer intravenous infusions of dopamine, argipressin, and/or albumin if ordered.

  These medications increase renal blood flow and help to maintain blood pressure.
- Prepare client for dialysis if indicated.

  Decreases client's fear and anxiety.

Collaborative Diagnosis **RISK FOR BLEEDING ESOPHAGEAL VARICES**

Definition: A life-threatening complication associated with cirrhosis and portal hypertension

Related to:
* Tortuosity and increased fragility of small vessels in the esophagus
* Increased bleeding tendency

CLINICAL MANIFESTATIONS

Subjective	**Objective**
Verbalization of feeling light headed, dizziness; confusion	Hematemesis; blood in stools; hypotension; tachycardia; diminished RBC count, Hct and Hgb levels

RISK FACTORS
* Alcohol ingestion
* Chronic illness
* Portal hypertension
* Poor mastication of food
* Esophageal reflux

DESIRED OUTCOMES

The client will not experience bleeding of esophageal varices as evidenced by:
   a. Absence of hematemesis and melena
   b. B/P and pulse rate within normal range for client
   c. Stable or improved RBC count, Hct and Hgb levels

NURSING ASSESSMENT	**RATIONALE**
Assess for and report signs and symptoms of bleeding esophageal varices:	*Early recognition of signs and symptoms of bleeding esophageal varices allows for prompt intervention.*
• Hematemesis	
• Blood in stools	
• Hypotension	
• Tachycardia	
• Diminished RBC count, Hct and Hgb levels	

THERAPEUTIC INTERVENTIONS	**RATIONALE**

Dependent/Collaborative Actions
Implement measures to reduce risk of bleeding from esophageal varices:
* Perform actions to reduce excess fluid volume.
  * Restrict sodium intake as ordered.
  * Maintain fluid restrictions if ordered. **D** ✦
  * Encourage client to rest periodically in a recumbent position. **D** ✦

  * Administer diuretics if ordered (e.g., potassium-sparing diuretics such as spironolactone and amiloride are often used initially). **D** ✦

* Instruct client to avoid activities such as straining to have a bowel movement, coughing, sneezing, and lifting heavy objects.
* Consult physician about an order for a laxative, antitussive, and/or decongestant if indicated.
* Instruct client to avoid eating foods that might cause mechanical trauma to the esophageal varices (e.g., chips).
* Administer a nonselective beta-adrenergic blocker (e.g., propranolol, nadolol) (a nitrate such as isosorbide may be given with the beta-adrenergic blocker).
* Administer vitamin K and blood products if ordered.

These actions decrease fluid retention and pressure on the esophageal varices.

Lying down reduces peripheral pooling of blood, which increases effective circulating volume and renal blood flow and subsequently promotes diuresis.
Diuretics reduce fluid volume by increasing urinary output and improve renal blood flow, which increases water excretion and reduces activation of the renin-angiotensin-aldosterone mechanism.
Avoiding these activities prevents sudden increases in intra-abdominal pressure that increases pressure in the esophageal vessels.
Straining with bowel movements and coughing increase intra-thoracic pressure, which may increase bleeding from varices.
Prevents unnecessary trauma to the esophageal varices.

Beta blockers reduces portal pressure, which reduces pressure in the esophageal vessels.

Vitamin K and blood products improve the body's clotting ability.

Continued...

THERAPEUTIC INTERVENTIONS	RATIONALE
If signs and symptoms of bleeding esophageal varices occur:	
• Turn client on side and suction as necessary.	*Reduces risk of aspiration.*
• Maintain oxygen therapy as ordered.	*Improves cellular oxygenation.*
• Assist with administration of octreotide (Sandostatin) or vasopressin if ordered (nitroglycerin is often given with vasopressin).	*Octreotide and vasopressin cause constriction of the splanchnic vessels and reduce blood flow to the portal vein.* *Nitroglycerin lowers portal pressure and reduces vasoconstrictor side effects of vasopressin.*
• Prepare client for endoscopic sclerotherapy or ligation of varices if planned.	*Reduces fear and anxiety.*
• Assist with insertion of a gastroesophageal balloon tube (e.g., Sengstaken-Blakemore tube, Minnesota tube); maintain balloon pressure and suction and perform lavage as ordered.	*A gastroesophageal balloon tube places pressure on the esophageal varices to decrease bleeding and increase clotting.*
• Administer vitamin K (e.g., phytonadione) injections, whole blood, or blood products (e.g., fresh frozen plasma, platelets) as ordered.	*Vitamin K, blood, and blood products increase the body's clotting ability.*
• Prepare client for a transjugular intrahepatic porto-systemic shunt (TIPS) or surgery (e.g., esophageal trans-ection with reanastomosis, distal splenorenal shunt) if planned.	*Reduces client's fear and anxiety.*

Collaborative Diagnosis   RISK FOR HEPATIC (PORTAL-SYSTEMIC) ENCEPHALOPATHY (HEPATIC COMA)

Definition: Central nervous system damage associated with liver disease

Related to:
• Altered brain function associated with:
  • The effect of toxic end products of intestinal protein digestion (e.g., ammonia) on the brain
  • Replacement of true neurotransmitters by false neurotransmitters
  • Increased brain sensitivity to certain substances (e.g., benzodiazepines, gamma-aminobutyric acid [GABA])
  • Decreased activity of urea cycle enzymes if zinc deficiency is present

CLINICAL MANIFESTATIONS

Subjective	Objective
Verbalization of weakness and lethargy	Changes in fine motor movements such as handwriting and drawing; asterixis; slowed or slurred speech; emotional liability; agitation; belligerence; disorientation; fetor hepaticus; unresponsiveness; increased serum ammonia level

RISK FACTORS
• Inability of body to remove toxins
• Hypokalemia
• Medication regimen

DESIRED OUTCOMES

The client will not develop hepatic encephalopathy as evidenced by:
  a. Usual speech and handwriting
  b. Usual mental status
  c. Absence of asterixis and fetor hepaticus
  d. Serum ammonia level within normal range

NURSING ASSESSMENT	RATIONALE
Assess for and report signs and symptoms of hepatic encephalopathy (e.g., change in handwriting, inability to draw simple figures or numbers, asterixis, slow or slurred speech, inability to concentrate, emotional lability, disordered sleep, agitation, belligerence, disorientation, lethargy, fetor hepaticus [musty or fruity odor on breath], unresponsiveness).	*Early recognition of signs and symptoms of hepatic encephalopathy allows for prompt intervention.*
Monitor serum ammonia levels; report elevated values.	

THERAPEUTIC INTERVENTIONS	RATIONALE

Dependent/Collaborative Actions

Implement measures to reduce the risk for hepatic coma:

- Perform actions to eliminate or control the following conditions that increase levels of ammonia and other nitrogenous substances:
  - Constipation — *Results in increased formation and absorption of ammonia and mercaptans from the gut.*
  - Gastrointestinal hemorrhage — *Intestinal bacteria convert the protein in blood to ammonia and other nitrogenous substances.*
  - Hypokalemia and/or metabolic alkalosis — *These conditions contribute to increased levels of ammonia.*
  - Renal failure — *Decreases excretion of ammonia.*
  - Excessive protein intake — *Intestinal bacteria convert protein to ammonia and other nitrogenous substances.*
  - Infection — *Bacteria that produce urease break urea into ammonia.*
  - Dehydration/hypovolemia — *Reduced blood flow to the liver results in decreased detoxification of ammonia and other toxins.*
  - If client is to receive blood transfusions, request fresh rather than stored blood. — *Stored blood contains more ammonia and citrate.*
- Consult physician about discontinuation of prescribed medications that are potential hepatotoxins (e.g., isoniazid, amiodarone, 6-mercaptopurine, erythromycin, phenytoin). — *Discontinuation of hepatotoxic medications prevent further liver damage.*
- Administer central nervous system depressants such as narcotics, sedative-hypnotics, and antianxiety agents with extreme caution. — *Many of these agents are metabolized in the liver and may precipitate nonnitrogenous coma.*

If signs and symptoms of hepatic encephalopathy occur:

- Maintain client on strict bedrest. — *Rest reduces metabolic demands on the liver.*
- Maintain dietary protein restrictions as ordered; increase protein intake slowly as encephalopathy resolves and encourage intake of vegetable proteins rather than animal proteins. — *Vegetable proteins are less ammoniagenic.*
- Ensure a high carbohydrate intake or administer intravenous glucose or tube feedings as ordered. — *A high CHO intake or IV glucose provides a rapid energy source and decreases metabolism of endogenous proteins.*
- Administer enemas and/or cathartics as ordered. — *Enemas and/or cathartics hastens expulsion of intestinal contents so that bacteria have less time to convert proteins to ammonia and other nitrogenous substances.*
- Administer the following medications if ordered:
  - Antimicrobials that suppress activity of the intestinal flora (e.g., neomycin, metronidazole) — *Antimicrobials suppress activity of intestinal flora, which decreases protein breakdown in the intestine and subsequently reduces the formation of nitrogenous substance.*
  - Lactulose — *Stimulates catharsis and creates an acidic medium in the intestine (the acidity reduces bacterial growth and the resultant formation of nitrogenous substances and also traps ammonia in the colon by promoting the conversion of NH_3 to the poorly absorbed NH_4).*
  - Benzodiazepine receptor antagonists (e.g., flumazenil) — *Blocks benzodiazepine uptake in the brain and may improves cognition in clients with hepatic encephalopathy.*
  - Zinc supplements — *Stimulates ureagenesis (several enzymes in the urea cycle are zinc dependent).*
- Institute general safety precautions. — *Prevents client injury.*

Nursing Diagnosis INEFFECTIVE FAMILY THERAPEUTIC REGIMEN MANAGEMENT NDx

Definition: Pattern of regulating and integrating into family processes a program for treatment of illness and the sequelae of illness that is unsatisfactory for meeting specific health goals

CLINICAL MANIFESTATIONS

Subjective	Objective
Verbalizes inability to manage illness; verbalizes inability to follow prescribed regimen	Inaccurate follow-through with instructions; inappropriate behaviors

RISK FACTORS

- Ineffective family process
- Change in lifestyle
- Chronic illness

DESIRED OUTCOMES

The client will demonstrate the probability of effective therapeutic regimen management as evidenced by:
  a. Willingness to learn about and participate in treatment plan and care
  b. Statements reflecting ways to modify personal habits and integrate treatments into lifestyle
  c. Statements reflecting an understanding of the implications of not following the prescribed treatment plan

NOC OUTCOMES

Compliance behavior; treatment behavior: illness or injury; knowledge: treatment regimen; health beliefs: perceived resources; health beliefs: perceived ability to perform

NIC INTERVENTIONS

Self-modification assistance; values clarification; substance use treatment; teaching: prescribed diet; financial resource assistance; support system enhancement

NURSING ASSESSMENT

Assess for indications that the client may be unable to manage the therapeutic regimen effectively:
- Statements reflecting inability to manage care at home
- Failure to adhere to treatment plan (e.g., not adhering to dietary modifications and fluid restrictions, refusing medications)
- Statements reflecting a lack of understanding of the factors that will cause further progression of liver failure
- Statements reflecting an unwillingness or inability to modify personal habits and integrate necessary treatments into lifestyle
- Statements reflecting the view that cirrhosis has resolved once he/she is feeling better, or that there is no way to control the disease and efforts to comply with treatments are useless

RATIONALE

Allows the nurse to tailor the client's education based on client's abilities and concerns.

THERAPEUTIC INTERVENTIONS

RATIONALE

Independent Actions

Implement measures to promote effective therapeutic regimen management:
- Explain cirrhosis in terms the client can understand; stress that cirrhosis is a chronic disease and adherence to the treatment plan is necessary in order to delay and/or prevent complications.
- Encourage questions and clarify misconceptions client has about cirrhosis and its effects.

Increased client knowledge about the disease process and self-care will improve adherence.

THERAPEUTIC INTERVENTIONS	RATIONALE
• Encourage client to participate in the treatment plan.	*Improves client's sense of control and ability to care for self once discharged*
• Provide instructions on weighing self and calculating dietary sodium and protein content; allow time for return demonstration.	*Important to know whether a significant weight gain is occurring, which can represent increased fluid retention.*
• Determine areas of difficulty and misunderstanding and reinforce teaching as necessary.	*Increased client knowledge about the disease process and self-care will improve adherence.*
• Provide client with written instructions about scheduled appointments with health care provider, medications, signs and symptoms to report, weighing self, and dietary modifications.	*Provides information resource for client and significant others to refer to as needed after discharge*
• Assist client to identify ways treatments can be incorporated into lifestyle; focus on modifications of lifestyle rather than complete change.	*Improves client's adherence to treatment regimen if client determines how lifestyle can be modified.*
• Encourage client to discuss concerns about the cost of hospitalization, medications, and lifelong follow-up care; obtain a social service consult to assist with financial planning and to obtain financial aid if indicated.	*Allows client to clarify issues and support in dealing with his/her illness.*
• Provide information about and encourage utilization of community resources that can assist client to make necessary lifestyle changes (e.g., drug and alcohol rehabilitation programs).	*Provides ongoing assistance once client is discharged.*
• Reinforce behaviors suggesting future compliance with the therapeutic regimen (e.g., statements reflecting plans for integrating treatments into lifestyle, participation in diet planning, statements reflecting an understanding of the importance of eliminating alcohol intake).	*Enhances client's self-confidence for self-care and adherence to treatment regimen.*
• Include significant others in explanations and teaching sessions and encourage their support; reinforce the need for client to assume responsibility for managing as much of care as possible.	*Enhances client's potential for adherence to the treatment regimen.*
Consult appropriate health care provider (e.g., social worker, physician) about referrals to community agencies if continued instruction, support, or supervision is needed.	*Provides a multidisciplinary approach to care after client is discharged.*

DISCHARGE TEACHING/CONTINUED CARE

Nursing Diagnosis # DEFICIENT KNOWLEDGE NDx; INEFFECTIVE SELF-HEALTH MANAGEMENT NDx*

Definition: Absence or deficiency of cognitive information related to specific topic (lack of specific information necessary for clients/significant others) to make informed choices regarding condition/treatment/lifestyle changes; pattern of regulating and integrating into daily living a therapeutic regimen for treatment of illness and the sequelae of illness that is unsatisfactory for meeting specific health goals

CLINICAL MANIFESTATIONS

Subjective	Objective
Verbalizes inability to manage illness; verbalizes inability to follow prescribed regimen	Inaccurate follow through with instructions; inappropriate behaviors; experience of manageable complications of cirrhosis

*The nurse should select the diagnostic label that is most appropriate for the client's discharge teaching needs.

NDx = NANDA-I Diagnosis **D** = Delegatable Action ● = UAP ✦ = LVN/LPN ⊖▶ = Go to ⊖volve for animation

Continued...

RISK FACTORS

* Cognitive deficit
* Financial concerns
* Failure to take action to reduce risk factors for complications of cirrhosis
* Inability to care for oneself
* Difficulty in modifying personal habits and integrating treatments into lifestyle

NOC OUTCOMES	NIC INTERVENTIONS
Knowledge: diet; knowledge: disease process; knowledge: treatment regimen	Health system guidance; teaching: individual; teaching: disease process; teaching: prescribed diet; teaching: prescribed activity/exercise substance abuse treatment

NURSING ASSESSMENT	RATIONALE
Assess the client's ability to learn and readiness to learn. Assess the client's understanding of teaching.	*Learning is more effective when the client is motivated and understands the importance of what is to be learned. Readiness to learn changes based on situations, physical and emotional challenges.*

THERAPEUTIC INTERVENTIONS	RATIONALE

Desired Outcome: The client will identify ways to prevent further liver damage

Independent Actions
Provide the following instructions regarding ways to prevent further liver damage:

* Avoid the following hepatotoxic agents: *Hepatotoxic substances increase liver problems in processing proteins and medications.*
  * Alcohol
  * Cleaning agents containing carbon tetrachloride and solvents (these are toxic even when inhaled)
  * Industrial chemicals such as nitrobenzene, disulfide, and tetrachloroethane
* Take acetaminophen (e.g., Tylenol) only when necessary and do not exceed the recommended dose.
* Adhere to the following precautions to prevent hepatitis:
  * Eat only in restaurants that have been inspected and approved by health authorities.   *Foods must be appropriately prepared and under the appropriate hygienic conditions.*
  * If blood transfusions are anticipated, arrange to donate and receive autologous blood rather than commercially obtained blood if possible.   *Prevents exposure to blood products that may carry hepatitis.*
  * Avoid sharing food or eating utensils and handling toiletry items of others.   *These actions prevent sharing of body fluids, which increases potential for exposure to hepatitis A and/or B.*
  * Practice safe sex (e.g., condom use for intercourse).
  * Avoid anal sex.
  * Do not share drug paraphernalia (e.g., needles, syringes, cookers, rinse water, straws for intranasal inhalation).
  * Get vaccinations for hepatitis A and B if recommended by health care provider.   *Decreases risk if exposed to hepatitis A and/or B.*
  * If traveling to a developing country:
    (1) Receive immune globulin and vaccines for hepatitis (e.g., hepatitis B vaccine, hepatitis A vaccine) as recommended by health care provider.
    (2) Drink only bottled water and avoid eating raw fruits and vegetables washed or prepared with local water when in the country.

THERAPEUTIC INTERVENTIONS	RATIONALE

Desired Outcome: The client will verbalize an understanding of the rationale for and components of the recommended diet

Independent Actions

Explain the rationale for a diet low in sodium and provide information about decreasing sodium intake:

- Read food labels and calculate sodium content of items; avoid those products that tend to have a high sodium content (e.g., canned soups and vegetables, tomato juice, commercial baked goods, commercially prepared frozen or canned entrees and sauces).
- Do not add salt when cooking foods or to prepared foods; use low-sodium herbs and spices if desired.
- Avoid cured and smoked foods.
- Avoid salty snack foods.
- Avoid commercially prepared fast foods.
- Avoid routine use of over-the-counter medications with a high sodium content (e.g., some antacids, Alka-Seltzer).

Obtain a dietary consult to assist client in planning meals that will meet prescribed dietary modifications.

Increased sodium intake leads to retention of fluid, which may increase the incidence of ascites and lower extremity edema.

Provides multidisciplinary approach to client care.

THERAPEUTIC INTERVENTIONS	RATIONALE

Desired Outcome: The client will identify ways to reduce stress on or trauma to the esophageal blood vessels

Independent Actions

Provide the following instructions about ways to reduce stress on or trauma to the esophageal blood vessels:

Adhere to prescribed measures to reduce fluid retention (e.g., fluid restriction, low-sodium diet, diuretics).

Avoid activities that increase intra-abdominal pressure (e.g., straining to have a bowel movement, coughing, sneezing, lifting heavy objects).

Avoid eating foods that might cause mechanical trauma to the esophageal varices (e.g., chips).

Prevents increased fluid volume which puts increased pressure on the esophageal vessels.

These activities increase intrathoracic pressure, which places additional pressure on the esophageal vessels.

May cause tearing of the esophageal vessels.

THERAPEUTIC INTERVENTIONS	RATIONALE

Desired Outcome: The client will identify ways to prevent bleeding

Independent Actions

Instruct client about ways to minimize risk of bleeding:

- Avoid taking aspirin and other nonsteroidal anti-inflammatory agents (e.g., ibuprofen) on a regular basis.
- Use an electric rather than a straight-edge razor.
- Floss and brush teeth gently.
- Cut nails carefully.
- Avoid situations that could result in injury (e.g., contact sports).
- Avoid putting sharp objects (e.g., toothpicks) in mouth.
- Do not walk barefoot.
- Avoid blowing nose forcefully.
- Avoid straining to have a bowel movement.

Instruct client to control any bleeding by applying firm, prolonged pressure to the area if possible.

Aspirin blocks platelet adherence, which is necessary for clotting, and will increase bleeding.

These actions decrease the risk of injury.

Avoiding these actions decreases pressure on esophageal vessels.

Improves body's blood clotting ability.

NDx = NANDA-I Diagnosis   **D** = Delegatable Action   ● = UAP   ✦ = LVN/LPN   ⊖▶ = Go to ⊖volve for animation

Continued...

THERAPEUTIC INTERVENTIONS	RATIONALE

Desired Outcome: The client will identify ways to reduce the risk of infection

Independent Actions

Instruct client in ways to reduce risk of infection:

• Continue with coughing and deep breathing or use of incentive spirometer every 2 hours while awake as long as activity is limited.	*Improves lung expansion and decreases stasis of secretions.*
• Increase activity as tolerated.	
• Avoid contact with persons who have an infection.	*Decreases risk for exposure to infection.*
• Avoid crowds, especially during flu and cold seasons.	
• Decrease or stop smoking.	*Smoking decreases ciliary activity and the ability to expel infectious agents with coughing.*
• Drink at least 10 glasses of liquid per day unless on a fluid restriction.	*Maintains adequate hydration and vascular fluid volume.*
• Adhere to recommended diet.	*Malnutrition decreases the client's ability to fight off infection.*
• Take supplemental vitamins and minerals as prescribed.	
• Maintain good personal hygiene.	*Prevents cross-contamination.*
• Receive immunizations (e.g., influenza vaccine, pneumococcal vaccine, hepatitis vaccines) if approved by health care provider.	*Enhances body's immune system and resistance to infection.*

THERAPEUTIC INTERVENTIONS	RATIONALE

Desired Outcome: The client will identify ways to relieve pruritus

Independent Actions

Instruct client in and/or implement measures to relieve pruritus:

• Apply cool, moist compresses to pruritic areas.	*Cool/cold compresses provide a counter sensation that decreases the urge to rub or scratch the area.*
• Apply emollient creams or ointments frequently.	*Creams and ointments prevent dryness and subsequent itchy skin.*
• Add emollients, cornstarch, or baking soda to bath water.	*Adding these products to bath water decreases skin dryness and provides a protective barrier.*
• Use tepid water and mild soaps for bathing.	*Use of tepid water and mild soaps decreases skin dryness.*
• Pat skin dry after bathing, making sure to dry thoroughly.	*Rubbing of the skin with a towel after a bath can stimulate itching.*
• Maintain a cool environment.	*A cool environment provides a counter sensation that decreases urge to rub or scratch.*
• Encourage participation in diversional activity.	*Distracts client from focusing on the itch.*
• Use relaxation techniques.	
• Use cutaneous stimulation techniques (e.g., massage, pressure, vibration, stroking with soft brush) at sites of itching or acupressure points.	*Cutaneous stimulation decreases itching sensations by blocking neurotransmission of the sensation.*
• Encourage client to wear loose cotton garments and avoid clothes or blankets made from wool.	*Decreases skin irritation.*
• Take medications as prescribed:	
• Antihistamines (e.g., diphenhydramine, hydroxyzine [Atarax])	*Antihistamines block histamine, which stimulates itchy sensations.*
• Bile acid–sequestering agents (e.g., cholestyramine)	*Bile acid–sequestering agents bind with the bile acids in the intestines, prevents absorption and enhances elimination, thereby decreasing itch sensations.*

THERAPEUTIC INTERVENTIONS	RATIONALE

Desired Outcome: The client will state signs and symptoms to report to the health care provider

Independent Actions

Stress the importance of reporting the following signs and symptoms:

• Rapid weight gain or loss	*Indicates changes in protein levels and retention of fluid volume.*
• Increasing size of abdomen	*Indicates ascites.*

THERAPEUTIC INTERVENTIONS	RATIONALE
• Increased swelling of lower extremities	
• Increasing shortness of breath	*May indicate heart failure.*
• Increased itchiness or yellowing of skin	*Indicates jaundice or increasing retention of bile acids.*
• Temperature elevation lasting more than 2 days	*Indicates infection.*
• Red, rust-colored, or smoky urine; bloody or tarry stools; blood in sputum or vomitus; persistent bleeding from nose, mouth, or skin; prolonged or excessive menses; excessive bruising; severe or persistent headache; or sudden abdominal or back pain	*Indicates inability of the body's clotting factors to control bleeding.*
• Tremors or changes in behavior, speech, or handwriting	*Indicates changes in neurological status.*

THERAPEUTIC INTERVENTIONS	RATIONALE
Desired Outcome: The client will identify community resources that can assist with home management and adjustment to lifestyle changes necessary for effective management of cirrhosis	
Independent Actions	
Provide information regarding community resources that can assist client and significant others with home management and adjustment to changes necessary for effective management of cirrhosis (e.g., Meals on Wheels, home health agencies, transportation services, drug and alcohol rehabilitation programs, counseling services).	*Provides for continuation of care after discharge from the acute care facility.*

THERAPEUTIC INTERVENTIONS	RATIONALE
Desired Outcome: The client will verbalize an understanding of a plan for adhering to recommended follow-up care including future appointment with health care provider, medications prescribed, and activity level	
Independent Actions	
Reinforce the importance of keeping follow-up appointments with health care provider.	*Cirrhosis is a chronic illness, and follow-up appointments are important to maintain health status.*
Explain the rationale for, side effects of, and food and drug interactions and importance of taking medications prescribed.	*Knowledge of medications and how they impact the system improves client adherence to treatment regimen and understanding of the importance of adhering to the prescribed medication regimen. The client must be able to recognize alterations in functioning related to medication administration and what clinical manifestations that should be reported to the health care provider.*
Reinforce physician's instructions regarding activity level. Stress the importance of rest.	*Important in maintaining health status and ability to maintain activities of daily living.*

ADDITIONAL NURSING DIAGNOSES

RISK FOR IMPAIRED TISSUE INTEGRITY NDx
Related to:
• Damage to the skin and/or subcutaneous tissue associated with prolonged pressure on the tissues, friction, and/or shearing if mobility is decreased
• Increased fragility of the skin associated with edema and malnutrition
• Excessive scratching associated with pruritus

RISK FOR INFECTION NDx
Related to:
• Lowered resistance to infection associated with:
  • Diminished function of the Kupffer cells in the liver (these cells normally phagocytize bacteria)

• Malnutrition
• Leukopenia resulting from hypersplenism (if venous congestion has resulted in splenomegaly, the spleen will destroy leukocytes faster than usual)
• Serum complement deficiency resulting from decreased production of complement proteins by the liver
• Colonization of bacteria in the ascitic fluid (spontaneous bacterial peritonitis)
• Stasis of secretions in the lungs and urinary stasis if mobility is decreased

RISK FOR INJURY NDx
Falls related to:
• Weakness
• Dizziness (can result from anemia and the postural hypotension that occurs with third-spacing)

Continued...

- Balance and gait disturbances that can occur with deficiencies of thiamine and/or vitamin B_{12}
- Disturbed thought processes (e.g., agitation, confusion) Burns and lacerations related to:
- Paresthesias that can occur with deficiencies of thiamine and vitamin B_{12}
- Tremors and jerky, restless movements associated with delirium tremens ("DTs") if present

INEFFECTIVE COPING NDx
Related to:
- Changes in appearance (e.g., edema, ascites, jaundice, spider angiomas, gynecomastia)
- Alterations in sexual functioning (e.g., impotence, decreased libido)
- Dependence on others to meet self-care needs
- Disturbed thought processes
- Stigma of having a chronic illness
- Possible changes in lifestyle and roles

DISTURBED SLEEP PATTERN NDx
Related to: Unfamiliar environment, frequent assessments and treatments, decreased physical activity, discomfort, fear, anxiety, and inability to assume usual sleep position because of orthopnea

FEAR AND ANXIETY NDx
Related to:
- Difficulty breathing
- Unfamiliar environment and separation from significant others
- Lack of understanding of the diagnosis, diagnostic tests, and treatments
- Uncertainty of prognosis
- Financial concerns
- Possibility of changes in lifestyle and roles

HEPATITIS

Hepatitis is widespread inflammation of the liver. It is most commonly caused by a virus but can also be caused by bacteria, an autoimmune reaction, or toxic injury to the liver by drugs, alcohol, industrial chemicals, or plant poisons. The five major viruses that cause hepatitis are the hepatitis A virus (HAV), hepatitis B virus (HBV), hepatitis C virus (HCV), hepatitis E virus (HEV), and the delta virus or hepatitis D virus (HDV). Several other viruses (e.g., hepatitis G virus) have been identified but occur rarely and do not appear to cause significant liver disease.

Hepatitis A and E are both spread by the fecal-oral route. Hepatitis A is the most common cause of acute hepatitis in the United States. Hepatitis E is similar in many respects to hepatitis A but is seen predominantly in persons who live in or have traveled to developing countries. Hepatitis B is transmitted sexually, perinatally, and parenterally (primarily in intravenous drug users who share needles). In the United States and many developed countries, sexual transmission is now the prevalent mode of transmission of hepatitis B. Hepatitis C is the most common blood-borne disease in the United States and the cause of chronic hepatitis in the majority of cases. End-stage liver disease associated with chronic hepatitis C is now the leading indication for liver transplants in the United States. Hepatitis C is transmitted predominantly by the parenteral route, with intravenous drug use and sharing of drug paraphernalia being the most common risk factors. The risk for perinatal and sexual transmission is relatively low. Hepatitis D appears to require the presence of the HBV for its replication and is therefore only seen in HBV-infected persons.

The various forms of hepatitis have similar clinical manifestations. Signs and symptoms vary in severity, and many cases (particularly of hepatitis C) go undetected because the person either has very mild symptoms or is asymptomatic. Elevated serum aminotransferases (alanine aminotransferase [ALT] and aspartate aminotransferase [AST]) are hallmarks of acute hepatitis. Other signs and symptoms include flulike symptoms, mild-to-moderate right upper quadrant pain, and symptoms of bile flow obstruction (e.g., jaundice, pruritus, dark amber urine, light-colored stools). The only definitive way to distinguish the various forms of viral hepatitis is by the presence of antigens and antigenic subtypes and the subsequent development of antibodies to these antigens.

Hospitalization of persons with hepatitis is usually not indicated except for certain high-risk persons (e.g., the elderly, immunocompromised persons, persons with other disease conditions that may be difficult to manage with hepatitis) and persons with severe disease. Signs and symptoms of severe disease include a marked prolongation of prothrombin time, a serum bilirubin level more than 10 times normal, symptoms of encephalopathy, the presence of edema and/or ascites, or an inability to maintain adequate hydration.

Acute viral hepatitis is a major public health problem because it is highly communicable and because there is currently no effective treatment. Most cases are self-limited and resolve completely without complications, but a small percentage of cases of hepatitis B and as many as 70% to 85% of cases of hepatitis C do progress to a chronic state, which can then progress to cirrhosis or hepatocellular carcinoma. The treatment of acute hepatitis is primarily supportive and directed toward reducing the metabolic demands on the liver and promoting cell regeneration. If the client has hepatitis B, C, or D, close follow-up should be encouraged to determine whether medication therapy (e.g., interferon, ribavirin, adefovir) is indicated to prevent and treat chronic hepatitis.

This care plan focuses on the adult client with acute viral hepatitis hospitalized because of persistent nausea, worsening of liver function test results, and a prolonged prothrombin time. Much of the information is applicable to clients receiving follow-up care in an extended care facility or home setting.

OUTCOME/DISCHARGE CRITERIA

The client will:
1. Have resolution of nausea
2. Have no evidence of bleeding or progressive liver degeneration
3. Have an adequate nutritional intake
4. Perform activities of daily living without fatigue
5. Identify ways to prevent the spread of hepatitis to others
6. Identify ways to prevent further liver damage
7. Verbalize an understanding of the rationale for and components of the recommended diet
8. State signs and symptoms to report to the health care provider
9. Verbalize an understanding of and a plan for adhering to recommended follow-up care including activity level, medications prescribed, and future appointments with health care provider and for laboratory studies

---

Nursing Diagnosis   # RISK FOR DEFICIENT FLUID VOLUME NDx

Definition: Decreased intravascular volume, interstitial and/or intracellular fluid

Related to:
- Decreased oral intake associated with anorexia and nausea
- Excessive loss of fluid if diaphoresis and/or persistent vomiting is present

CLINICAL MANIFESTATIONS

Subjective	Objective
Verbalization of thirst; feeling weak	Decreased urine output; increased urine concentration; weakness; sudden weight loss (except in third-spacing); decreased venous filling; increased body temperature; decreased pulse volume/pressure; change in mental status; elevated Hct; decreased skin/tongue turgor; dry skin/mucus membranes; increased pulse rate; decreased B/P

RISK FACTORS
- Inadequate intake
- Exposure to pathogens
- Medication regimen

DESIRED OUTCOMES

The client will not experience a deficient fluid volume as evidenced by:
  a. Normal skin turgor
  b. Moist mucous membrane
  c. Stable weight
  d. B/P and pulse rate within normal range for client and stable with position change
  e. Capillary refill time less than 2 to 3 seconds
  f. Usual mental status
  g. BUN and Hct within normal range
  h. Balanced intake and output

NOC OUTCOMES

Fluid balance; hydration

NIC INTERVENTIONS

Fluid monitoring; fluid management; intravenous (IV) therapy; nausea management

NURSING ASSESSMENT	RATIONALE
Assess for and report signs and symptoms of deficient fluid volume: - Decreased skin turgor, dry mucous membranes, thirst - Weight loss of 2% or greater over a short period - Postural hypotension and/or low B/P - Weak, rapid pulse	*Early recognition of signs and symptoms of fluid volume deficit allows for prompt intervention.*

NDx = NANDA-I Diagnosis   **D** = Delegatable Action   ● = UAP   ✦ = LVN/LPN   ⊝▶ = Go to ⊝volve for animation

Continued...

NURSING ASSESSMENT	RATIONALE

- Capillary refill time greater than 2 to 3 seconds
- Flat neck veins when supine
- Decreased urine output with increased specific gravity (reflects an actual rather than potential fluid deficit)
- Change in mental status
- Increased BUN and Hct values

THERAPEUTIC INTERVENTIONS	RATIONALE

Independent Actions

Implement measures to prevent deficient fluid volume:

- Perform actions to reduce nausea and prevent vomiting:
  - Instruct client to ingest food/fluid slowly.
  - Eliminate noxious sights and odors. **D** ● ✦

- Perform actions to improve oral intake:
  - Encourage rest before meals.
  - Provide oral hygiene before meals. **D** ● ✦
  - Allow adequate time for meals; reheat foods and fluids as needed. **D** ● ✦

- Perform actions to reduce fever if present (administer tepid sponge bath, administer antipyretics if ordered).

- Maintain fluid intake of at least 2300 mL/day unless contraindicated; if oral intake is inadequate or contraindicated, maintain intravenous and/or enteral fluid therapy as ordered.

Nausea often causes the client to have decreased fluid intake. Persistent vomiting results in excessive loss of fluid. These actions help prevent the experience of nausea.

Minimizes fatigue.

Removes unpleasant tastes, which often improves the taste of foods/fluids.

Reduction of fever decreases fluid loss from diaphoresis.

Adequate fluid intake needs to be provided in order to ensure adequate hydration.

Nursing Diagnosis   IMBALANCED NUTRITION: LESS THAN BODY REQUIREMENTS NDx

Definition: Inadequate intake or insufficient nutrition to meet the body's metabolic needs

Related to:

- Decreased oral intake associated with anorexia and nausea
- Loss of nutrients associated with persistent vomiting if present
- Reduced metabolism and storage of nutrients by the liver associated with an alteration in normal liver function as a result of inflammation
- Malabsorption of fats and fat-soluble vitamins associated with impaired bile flow resulting from inflammation of the liver
- Increased utilization of nutrients associated with the increased metabolic rate that is present with infection

CLINICAL MANIFESTATIONS

Subjective	Objective
Report of lack of appetite; fatigue; irritability; poor self-esteem	Loss of weight with adequate food intake; body weight 20% or more under ideal weight; sore, inflamed buccal cavity; capillary fragility; pale conjunctiva and mucous membranes; poor muscle tone; excessive hair loss; amenorrhea

RISK FACTORS

- Chronic illness
- Change in normal digestive process
- Treatment regimen
- Exposure to pathogens

DESIRED OUTCOMES

The client will maintain an adequate nutritional status as evidenced by:
  a. Weight within normal range for the client
  b. Normal BUN and serum albumin, prealbumin, Hct, and Hgb levels and normal lymphocyte count
  c. Improved strength and activity tolerance
  d. Healthy oral mucous membrane

NOC OUTCOMES

Nutritional status

NIC INTERVENTIONS

Nutritional monitoring; nutrition management; nutrition therapy; nutritional counseling; nausea management

NURSING ASSESSMENT

Assess for and report signs and symptoms of malnutrition:
- Weight significantly below client's usual weight or below normal for client's age, height, and body frame
- Abnormal BUN and low serum albumin, prealbumin, Hct, Hgb, and ammonia levels and low lymphocyte count
- Weakness and fatigue
- Sore, inflamed oral mucous membrane
- Pale conjunctiva

Monitor percentage of meals and snacks client consumes. Report a pattern of inadequate intake.

RATIONALE

Early recognition and reporting of signs and symptoms of malnutrition allow for prompt intervention.

An awareness of the amount of food/fluid the client consumes alerts the nurse to deficits in nutritional intake. Reporting an inadequate intake allows for prompt intervention.

THERAPEUTIC INTERVENTIONS

Independent Actions

Implement measures to maintain an adequate nutritional status:
- Perform actions to improve oral intake:
  - Implement measures to prevent vomiting if indicated (e.g., eliminate noxious sights and odors). **D** ● ✦
  - Implement measures to control diarrhea if present (e.g., discourage intake of spicy foods and foods high in fiber or lactose).
  - Maintain a clean environment and a relaxed, pleasant atmosphere. **D** ● ✦

  - Encourage a rest period before meals.

  - Provide oral hygiene before meals. **D** ● ✦

  - Serve foods/fluids that are appealing to the client and adhere to personal and cultural (e.g., religious, ethnic) preferences whenever possible.

  - Serve frequent, small meals rather than large ones if client is weak, fatigues easily, and/or has a poor appetite.
  - Allow adequate time for meals; reheat foods and fluids as needed. **D** ● ✦

  - Limit fluid intake with meals unless the fluid has high nutritional value.
  - Increase activity as allowed and tolerated. **D** ● ✦

RATIONALE

Vomiting results in actual loss of nutrients and fluid volume.

Increased intestinal motility that occurs with or causes diarrhea results in a decreased absorption of nutrients in the bowel.

Noxious sights and odors can inhibit the feeding center in the hypothalamus. Maintaining a clean environment helps prevent this from occurring, which may improve appetite and oral intake.

Minimizes fatigue which decreases client's ability to complete a meal.

Removes unpleasant tastes, which often improves the taste of foods/fluids.

Foods/fluids that appeal to the client's senses (especially sight and smell) and are in accordance with personal and cultural preferences are most likely to stimulate appetite and promote interest in eating.

Providing small rather than large meals can enable a client who is weak or fatigues easily to finish a meal.

Clients who feel rushed during meals tend to become anxious, lose their appetite, and stop eating. Appetite is also suppressed if foods/fluids normally served hot or warm become cold and do not appeal to the client.

Limiting fluid intake with meals reduces early satiety and subsequent decreased food intake.

Activity promotes a sense of well-being, which can improve appetite.

NDx = NANDA-I Diagnosis   **D** = Delegatable Action   ● = UAP   ✦ = LVN/LPN   ⊖▶ = Go to ⊖volve for animation

Continued...

THERAPEUTIC INTERVENTIONS	RATIONALE
• Encourage client to consume meals that are well balanced and high in essential nutrients; offer dietary supplements if client's caloric intake is inadequate.	*The client must consume a diet that is well balanced and high in essential nutrients in order to meet nutritional needs. Dietary supplements are often needed to help accomplish this.*
• Assist and instruct client to adhere to the following dietary recommendations:	
• Avoid skipping meals.	*Skipping meals may decrease caloric and nutritional intake.*
• Consume a diet high in calories (2000-3000 calories/day) and carbohydrates; if unable to tolerate food, suck on hard candy and drink fruit juices and regular soft drinks.	
• Maintain a moderate to high protein intake (unless serum ammonia level is high or clinical evidence of encephalopathy is present).	*Adequate protein intake promotes healing of the liver.*

Dependent/Collaborative Actions

Implement measures to maintain an adequate nutritional status:

• Administer medications that may be ordered to improve client's nutritional status (e.g., antiemetics, antidiarrheals, vitamins and minerals). **D** ✦	*These medications decrease incidence of nausea, vomiting, and diarrhea. Vitamin and minerals may be required to maintain adequate nutritional status*
• Obtain a dietary consult if necessary.	*A dietitian is best able to evaluate whether the foods/fluids selected will meet the client's nutritional needs.*
• Perform a calorie count if ordered. Report information to the dietitian and physician.	*A calorie count provides information about the caloric and nutritional value of the foods/fluids the client consumes. The information obtained helps the dietitian and physician determine whether an alternative method of nutritional support is needed.*
Consult the physician about an alternative method of providing nutrition (e.g., parenteral nutrition, tube feeding) if client does not consume enough food or fluids to meet nutritional needs.	*If the client's oral intake is inadequate, an alternative method of providing nutrients needs to be implemented.*

Nursing Diagnosis **IMPAIRED COMFORT** NDx **(PRURITUS)**

Definition: Perceived lack of ease, relief and transcendence in physical, psychospiritual, environmental and social dimensions

Related to: Stimulation of itch receptors in the skin by bile acid metabolites that accumulate in the blood as a result of bile flow obstruction

CLINICAL MANIFESTATIONS

Subjective	Objective
Complaint of skin itching	Persistent scratching or rubbing of skin

RISK FACTORS
• Chronic illness
• Increased toxins in the blood

DESIRED OUTCOMES

The client will experience relief of pruritus as evidenced by:
  a. Verbalization of same
  b. No scratching or rubbing of skin

NOC OUTCOMES

Comfort level; symptom control

NIC INTERVENTIONS

Pruritus management

NURSING ASSESSMENT	RATIONALE
Assess for the following: • Reports of itchiness • Persistent scratching or rubbing of skin	Early recognition of signs and symptoms of pruritus allows for prompt intervention.

THERAPEUTIC INTERVENTIONS	RATIONALE

Independent Actions

Instruct client in and/or implement measures to relieve pruritus:

• Apply cool, moist compresses to pruritic areas. **D** ● ✦	A cool/cold compress provides a counter sensation that decreases the urge to rub or scratch the area.
• Apply emollient creams or ointments frequently. **D** ● ✦	Application of creams and emollients prevents skin dryness.
• Add emollients, cornstarch, or baking soda to bath water. **D** ● ✦	Addition of these products to bath water decreases skin dryness and provides a protective barrier.
• Use tepid water and mild soaps for bathing. **D** ● ✦	Tepid water and mild soaps for bathing decreases incidence of skin dryness.
• Pat skin dry after bathing, making sure to dry thoroughly. **D** ● ✦	Rubbing of the skin after a bath with a towel can stimulate itching.
• Maintain a cool environment. **D** ● ✦	A cool environment provides a counter sensation that decreases urge to rub or scratch.
• Encourage participation in diversional activity.	Distracts client from focusing on the itch.
• Use relaxation techniques.	
• Use cutaneous stimulation techniques (e.g., massage, pressure, vibration, stroking with soft brush) at sites of itching or acupressure points.	Cutaneous stimulation blocks the neurotransmission of the itch sensation.
• Encourage client to wear loose cotton garments and avoid clothes or blankets made from wool.	Wearing loose clothing and non-wool blankets decrease skin irritation.

Dependent/Collaborative Actions

Instruct client in and/or implement measures *to relieve pruritus:*

• Administer the following medications if ordered:	
• Antihistamines (e.g., diphenhydramine, hydroxyzine [Atarax]) **D** ✦	Antihistamines block histamine, which stimulates itchy sensations.
• Bile acid–sequestering agents (e.g., cholestyramine)	Bile acid–sequestering agents bind with the bile acids in the intestines, prevents absorption and enhances elimination, thereby decreasing itch sensations.
Consult appropriate health care provider (e.g., clinical nurse specialist, physician) if above measures fail to alleviate pruritus or if the skin becomes excoriated.	Notification of the appropriate health care provider allows for prompt alterations in treatment plan.

Nursing Diagnosis ## NAUSEA NDx

Definition: A subjective, unpleasant wavelike sensation in the back of the throat, epigastrium, or abdomen that may lead to the urge or need to vomit

Related to: Stimulation of the vomiting center associated with stimulation of the visceral afferent pathways as a result of:
• Inflammation of the gastrointestinal tract resulting from immune complex–mediated tissue responses to the viral infection
• Gaseous distention resulting from impaired fat digestion if bile flow is obstructed
• Venous congestion in the gastrointestinal tract if portal hypertension has developed

CLINICAL MANIFESTATIONS

Subjective	Objective
Complaint of nausea	N/A

Continued...

RISK FACTORS	DESIRED OUTCOME

- Chronic illness
- Treatment regimen
- Exposure to pathogens/toxins

The client will experience relief of nausea as evidenced by verbalization of same.

NOC OUTCOMES	NIC INTERVENTIONS

Nausea and vomiting severity

Nausea management; environmental management: comfort

NURSING ASSESSMENT	RATIONALE

Assess for complaints of nausea.

Early recognition of nausea allows for prompt treatment.

THERAPEUTIC INTERVENTIONS	RATIONALE

Independent Actions

Implement measures to reduce nausea and prevent vomiting:

- Eliminate noxious sights and odors from the environment. **D** ● ✦

  Noxious stimuli can cause stimulation of the vomiting center.

- Instruct client to change positions slowly.

  Rapid movement can result in stimulation of the chemoreceptor trigger zone and subsequent excitation of the vomiting center.

- Encourage client to take deep, slow breaths when nauseated. **D** ✦

  Provides relaxation and helps to decrease nausea.

- Encourage client to avoid intake of foods/fluids high in fat (e.g., butter, cream, whole milk, ice cream, fried foods, gravies, nuts).

  Avoiding foods/fluids high in fat prevents a delay in gastric emptying and reduces nausea associated with impaired fat digestion.

- Avoid serving foods with an overpowering aroma; remove lids from hot foods before entering room. **D** ● ✦

  Noxious stimuli can cause stimulation of the vomiting center.

- Instruct client to eat dry foods (e.g., toast, crackers) and avoid drinking liquids with meals if nauseated.

  Eating dry foods and avoidance of drinking liquids with meals decreases the incidence of nausea.

- Provide small, frequent meals; instruct client to ingest foods and fluids slowly.

  Eating small frequent meals and eating slowly prevents overdistention of the stomach and stimulation of the chemoreceptor trigger zone and subsequent excitation of the vomiting center.

- Instruct client to avoid foods/fluids that irritate the gastric mucosa (e.g., spicy foods; caffeine-containing beverages such as tea, coffee, and colas).

  Avoidance of foods that irritate the gastric mucosa decreases the incidence of nausea.

Dependent/Collaborative Actions

Implement measures to reduce nausea and prevent vomiting:

- Administer antiemetics if ordered (phenothiazines are contraindicated because of their potential cholestatic effects).

  Antiemetics decrease nausea and/or vomiting.

Consult physician if above measures fail to control nausea.

Notification of the physician allows for prompt alterations in treatment plan.

Nursing Diagnosis   # RISK FOR BLEEDING NDx

Definition: At risk for a decrease in blood volume that may compromise health

Related to:

- Decreased production of clotting factors associated with impaired liver function and impaired vitamin K absorption if bile flow is obstructed (normal bile flow is necessary for absorption of vitamin K)
- Thrombocytopenia associated with hypersplenism (if venous congestion has resulted in splenomegaly, the spleen will destroy platelets faster than usual)

DESIRED OUTCOMES

The client will not experience unusual bleeding as evidenced by:
  a. Skin and mucous membranes free of petechiae, purpura, ecchymoses, and active bleeding
  b. Absence of unusual joint pain
  c. No increase in abdominal girth
  d. Absence of frank and occult blood in stool, urine, and vomitus
  e. Usual menstrual flow
  f. Vital signs within normal range for client
  g. Stable or improved Hct and Hgb values

NURSING ASSESSMENT	RATIONALE
Assess client for and report signs and symptoms of unusual bleeding: • Petechiae, purpura, ecchymoses • Gingival bleeding • Prolonged bleeding from puncture sites, epistaxis, hemoptysis • Unusual joint pain • Increase in abdominal girth • Frank or occult blood in stool, urine, or vomitus • Menorrhagia • Restlessness, confusion	*Early recognition of signs and symptoms of bleeding and progressive liver degeneration allows for prompt intervention.*

THERAPEUTIC INTERVENTIONS	RATIONALE

Dependent/Collaborative Actions

Implement measures to prevent bleeding:

- Avoid giving injections whenever possible; consult physician about prescribing an alternative route for medications ordered to be given intramuscularly or subcutaneously.

  Giving the client injections increases risk of bleeding when clotting factors are diminished.

- When giving injections or performing venous or arterial punctures, use the smallest gauge needle possible and apply gentle, prolonged pressure to the site after the needle is removed.

  These actions help to decrease bruising and improve clotting at the injection site.

- Caution client to avoid activities that increase the risk for trauma (e.g., shaving with a straight-edge razor, using stiff bristle toothbrush or dental floss).

  Trauma increases the risk of bleeding when clotting factors are diminished.

- Pad side rails if client is confused or restless. **D** ● ✦

  Decreases potential for client injury.

- Whenever possible, avoid intubations (e.g., nasogastric) and procedures that can cause injury to the rectal mucosa (e.g., inserting a rectal suppository or tube, administering an enema).

  Trauma during procedures increases the risk of bleeding when clotting factors are diminished.

- Perform actions to reduce the risk for falls (e.g., avoid unnecessary clutter in room, instruct client to wear shoes/slippers with nonslip soles when ambulating). **D** ● ✦

  Placing client on risk for falls protocol decreases risk for injury.

- Instruct client to avoid blowing nose forcefully or straining to have a bowel movement; consult physician about an order for a decongestant and/or laxative if indicated.

  These actions may rupture small blood vessels and increase the incidence of bleeding.

- Administer the following if ordered to improve clotting ability:
  - Vitamin K (e.g., phytonadione) injections **D** ✦
  - Platelets
  - Fresh frozen plasma (FFP)

  Administration of Vitamin K, platelets and FFP replaces deficient clotting factors.

If bleeding occurs and does not subside spontaneously:

- Apply firm, prolonged pressure to bleeding area(s) if possible.

  Application of pressure to the bleeding site improves clotting ability.

- If epistasis occurs, place client in a high-Fowler's position, have client lean forward and apply pressure and/or ice pack to nasal area. **D** ● ✦

  Proper positioning helps to prevent aspiration of blood from the nasal cavity. Application of pressure or ice to the nasal area improves clotting.

- Maintain oxygen therapy as ordered. **D** ✦

  Provides supplemental oxygenation to the tissues.

- If esophageal bleeding occurs:
  - Turn client on side and suction as necessary. **D** ✦

    These actions reduce the risk for aspiration.

  - Assist with administration of octreotide (Sandostatin) or vasopressin if ordered.

    Octreotide/vasopressin constricts splanchnic vessels and reduces blood flow to the portal vein, decreasing pressure on esophageal varices.

  - Prepare client for endoscopic sclerotherapy or ligation of varices if planned.

    Decreases client's fear and anxiety.

NDx = NANDA-I Diagnosis   **D** = Delegatable Action   ● = UAP   ✦ = LVN/LPN   ⊖▶ = Go to ⊖volve for animation

Continued...

THERAPEUTIC INTERVENTIONS	RATIONALE
• Assist with insertion of a gastroesophageal balloon tube (e.g., Sengstaken-Blakemore tube, Minnesota tube); maintain balloon pressure, suction client, and perform lavage if ordered.	*The gastroesophageal balloon tube places pressure on bleeding varices, which improves clotting.*
• Administer vitamin K (e.g., phytonadione) injections, whole blood, or blood products (e.g., FFP, platelets) as ordered.	*Administration of vitamin K, blood, FFP, and platelets replace deficient clotting factors.*
• Assess for and report signs and symptoms of hypovolemic shock (e.g., restlessness; confusion; significant decrease in B/P; rapid, weak pulse; rapid respirations; cool skin; urine output <30 mL/h).	*Allows for prompt alteration in treatment plan.*

Collaborative Diagnosis   RISK FOR PROGRESSIVE LIVER DEGENERATION (E.G., FULMINANT HEPATITIS, CHRONIC ACTIVE HEPATITIS)

Definition: Degradation of the liver

Related to: Continued degeneration/necrosis of liver cells

CLINICAL MANIFESTATIONS

Subjective	Objective
Reports of weakness, itching	Increased jaundice, weakness, and pruritus Edema, ascites, bleeding Encephalopathy (e.g., change in handwriting, slow or slurred speech, emotional lability, agitation, asterixis, disorientation, lethargy) Further increase in prothrombin time Further elevation of serum AST, ALT, alkaline phosphatase, and bilirubin; low serum albumin

RISK FACTORS
• Chronic illness
• Inadequate/ineffective treatment regimen
• Non-adherence to treatment regimen

DESIRED OUTCOMES

The client will not experience progressive liver degeneration as evidenced by:
  a. Resolutions of signs and symptoms of hepatitis
  b. Absence of edema, ascites, and bleeding
  c. Usual mental status
  d. Coagulation test results and serum AST, ALT, alkaline phosphatase, bilirubin, and albumin levels within or returning toward normal limits

NURSING ASSESSMENT	RATIONALE
Assess for signs and symptoms of progressive liver degeneration: • Worsening of signs and symptoms (e.g., increased jaundice, weakness, and pruritus) • Edema, ascites • Bleeding • Encephalopathy (e.g., change in handwriting, slow or slurred speech, emotional lability, agitation, asterixis, disorientation, lethargy) • Further increase in prothrombin time • Further elevation of serum AST, ALT, alkaline phosphatase, and bilirubin levels • Low serum albumin level	*Early recognition of signs and symptoms of progressive liver degeneration allows for prompt intervention.*

THERAPEUTIC INTERVENTIONS	RATIONALE
Dependent/Collaborative Actions	
If signs and symptoms of progressive liver degeneration occur:	
• Implement measures to prevent an increase in levels of ammonia and other nitrogenous substances (e.g., administer neomycin if ordered, administer lactulose if ordered, maintain prescribed dietary protein restriction). **D ✦**	*Neomycin attacks the ammonia forming bacteria in the gastrointestinal tract. Lactulose draws ammonia from the blood stream into the colon for excretion. A low protein diet reduces the buildup of nitrogen metabolites and ammonia in the blood stream.*
• Implement measures to reduce the risk for injury (e.g., keep side rails up, maintain seizure precautions). **D ● ✦**	*Implement hospital protocols to reduce risk for injury.*
• Prepare client for liver transplant if planned.	*Decreases client's fear and anxiety and improves client understanding of procedure.*

DISCHARGE TEACHING/CONTINUED CARE

Nursing Diagnosis **DEFICIENT KNOWLEDGE** NDx**; INEFFECTIVE FAMILY THERAPEUTIC REGIMEN MANAGEMENT** NDx**; OR INEFFECTIVE SELF-HEALTH MANAGEMENT* NDx**

Definition: Absence or deficiency of cognitive information related to specific topic (lack of specific information necessary for clients/significant others) to make informed choices regarding condition/treatment/lifestyle changes; pattern of regulating and integrating into daily living and family processes a therapeutic regimen for treatment of illness and the sequelae that are unsatisfactory for meeting specific health goals

CLINICAL MANIFESTATIONS

Subjective	Objective
Verbalizes inability to manage illness; verbalizes inability to follow prescribed regimen	Inaccurate follow through with instructions; inappropriate behaviors; experience of preventable complications of hepatitis

RISK FACTORS

• Cognitive deficit
• Financial concerns
• Failure to take action to reduce risk factors for complications of hepatitis
• Inability to care for oneself
• Difficulty in modifying personal habits and integrating treatments into lifestyle

NOC OUTCOMES	NIC INTERVENTIONS
Knowledge: disease process; knowledge: treatment regimen; knowledge: health behavior; knowledge: infection control	Health system guidance; teaching: disease process; teaching: prescribed diet; teaching: prescribed medication; communicable disease management; teaching: individual

NURSING ASSESSMENT	RATIONALE
Assess client's knowledge base related to the disease process.	*The client's knowledge base provides the basis for education.*
Assess for indications that the client may be unable to effectively manage the therapeutic regimen:	*Early recognition of inability to understand disease process or self-care allows for change in teaching modality.*
• Statements reflecting inability to manage care at home	
• Failure to adhere to treatment plan (e.g., refusing medications)	

*The nurse should select the diagnostic label that is most appropriate for the client's discharge teaching needs.

Continued...

NURSING ASSESSMENT	RATIONALE

- Statements reflecting a lack of understanding of factors that may cause further progression hepatitis
- Statements reflecting an unwillingness or inability to modify personal habits and integrate necessary treatments into lifestyle
- Statements reflecting view that there is not cure for most forms of hepatitis or that the situation is hopeless, and efforts to comply with the treatment plan are useless

THERAPEUTIC INTERVENTIONS	RATIONALE

Desired Outcome: The client will identify ways to prevent the spread of hepatitis to others

Independent Actions

Provide the following instructions on ways to prevent the spread of hepatitis to others:

- If client has hepatitis A, instruct him/her to adhere to the following precautions for 1 to 2 weeks after the onset of jaundice:
  - Wash hands thoroughly after having a bowel movement.
  - Use separate toilet facilities if possible; if separate toilet facilities are not available, clean toilet seat with a chlorine solution after use.
  - Wash bedding, towels, and underwear in hot, soapy water; wash them separately from other articles.
  - Do not donate blood or work in food services until approved by physician.
- If client has hepatitis B, C, or D, instruct him/her to adhere to the following precautions until health care provider states that transmitting hepatitis to others is no longer a risk:
  - Wash hands thoroughly after urinating and having a bowel movement.
  - Do not share personal articles (e.g., toothbrush, straight-edge razor, thermometer, washcloth).
  - Do not share food, cigarettes, or eating utensils.
  - If any injections (e.g., insulin, vitamin B_{12}) are given at home, use disposable equipment and dispose of it properly to reduce the risk of others coming in contact with contaminated needles.
  - Do not share drug paraphernalia (e.g., needles, straws for intranasal inhalation).
  - Use disposable eating utensils or wash utensils separately in hot, soapy water.
  - Avoid intimate sexual contact; once sexual activity is resumed, avoid intercourse during menstruation and intermenstrual bleeding and make sure that a condom is used during intercourse.
  - Do not donate blood.

These actions by the client prevent exposure of others to the client's blood and/or body fluids.

Instruct client to inform household and sexual contacts to see health care provider for appropriate immunization and testing for early detection of hepatitis.

Allows for testing and appropriate treatment of individuals who have been exposed to the individual with hepatitis

THERAPEUTIC INTERVENTIONS	RATIONALE

Desired Outcome: The client will identify ways to prevent further liver damage

Independent Actions

Provide the following instructions regarding ways to prevent further liver damage:

- Avoid alcohol intake for a minimum of 6 months (many sources recommend a year).
- Avoid contact with substances known to be injurious to the liver (e.g., cleaning agents containing carbon tetrachloride, solvents, industrial chemicals such as nitrobenzene, disulfide, and tetrachloroethane).
- Take acetaminophen (e.g., Tylenol) only when necessary and do not exceed the recommended dose or take it after drinking alcohol because of its potential toxic effect.
- Take precautions to prevent recurrent hepatitis (client is immune only to the viral type he/she has had):
  - Avoid unnecessary transfusions; if transfusions are necessary, arrange to donate and receive autologous blood rather than commercially obtained blood if possible.
  - Practice safe sex (e.g., condom use during intercourse); if sexual partner is a carrier, consult health care provider about receiving a hepatitis B vaccination.
  - Avoid sharing food, eating utensils, and toiletry items.
  - Avoid sharing drug paraphernalia (e.g., needles, syringes, cookers, rinse water, straws for intranasal inhalation).
  - Eat only in restaurants that have been inspected and approved by health authorities.
  - Get vaccinations for hepatitis A and B if recommended by health care provider.
  - Avoid anal sex.
  - If traveling to a developing country:
    (1) Receive immune globulin and vaccines for hepatitis (e.g., hepatitis B vaccine, hepatitis A vaccine) as recommended by health care provider.
    (2) Drink only bottled water and avoid eating raw fruits and vegetables washed or prepared with local water when in the country.
- Inform all health care providers of history of hepatitis because a number of medications (e.g., chlorpromazine, acetaminophen, allopurinol, amiodarone, erythromycin, 6-mercaptopurine, phenytoin) can be hepatotoxic and should not be prescribed if alternatives are available.

Alcohol is hepatotoxic and will exacerbate the clinical manifestations of hepatitis.

These agents are hepatotoxic and should be avoided.

Acetaminophen at high doses is hepatotoxic and when combined with alcohol the two substances compete for the substrates of metabolism.

These actions decrease the client's exposure to other viral types of hepatitis or individuals with other viral infections.

Informing all health care providers of history of hepatitis prevents unintended prescription of medications that may be hepatotoxic.

Desired Outcome: The client will verbalize an understanding of the rationale for and components of the recommended diet

Independent Actions

Explain to client that adherence to the recommended diet will promote healing of the liver and reduce the risk of further liver damage.

Knowledge of the required diet and the impact of this diet on the system allows the client some mechanism of control of his/her disease and the ability to have an active part in treatment and care.

Continued...

THERAPEUTIC INTERVENTIONS	RATIONALE

Desired Outcome: The client will state signs and symptoms to report to the health care provider

Independent Actions

Stress the importance of reporting the following signs and symptoms:

- Persistent or recurrent loss of appetite, nausea, fatigue, or weight loss
- Vomiting
- Increased itchiness or yellowing of skin
- Swelling of lower extremities, rapid weight gain, or increased size of abdomen
- Red, rust-colored, or smoky urine; bloody or tarry stools; blood in sputum or vomitus; prolonged or excessive bleeding from nose, mouth, or skin; prolonged or excessive menses; excessive bruising; severe or persistent headache; or sudden abdominal or back pain
- Changes in behavior, speech, or handwriting

These are signs and symptoms of progression of liver disease and the client's health care professional should be notified to initiate prompt interventions.

THERAPEUTIC INTERVENTIONS	RATIONALE

Desired Outcome: The client will verbalize an understanding of and a plan for adhering to recommended follow-up care including activity level, medications prescribed, and future appointments with health care provider and for laboratory studies

Independent Actions

Reinforce physician's instructions regarding activity level. Stress the importance of rest during convalescent phase (from 6 weeks to 6 months).

Rest is critical for client healing and prevention of further liver damage.

Reinforce the importance of keeping follow-up appointments with health care provider and for laboratory studies (liver enzyme levels and serological markers provide information about immunity, presence of a carrier state, and chronicity, which helps determine the need for additional treatment [e.g., interferon, ribavirin, adefovir] and teaching).

Follow-up is critical because this is a long-term illness that requires various tests and evaluations to be treated properly.

If medication is prescribed to prevent/treat chronic hepatitis, explain the rationale for, side effects of, and importance of taking the medications prescribed (e.g., interferon, ribavirin, adefovir). If client is to administer own interferon, provide instructions on subcutaneous injection technique.

Knowledge of the medication regimen and the impact of these medications on the system, as well as how the medication regimen can be incorporated into the client's lifestyle, allows the client some mechanism of control of his/her disease and the ability to have an active part in treatment and care.
Encourages adherence with treatment regimen.

Provide client with information about and encourage participation in drug and alcohol rehabilitation programs if indicated.

Reduces further liver damage and potential infections.

Implement measures to improve client's compliance:

- Include significant others in teaching if possible.

Involvement of the client's significant others helps them to support the client and improves client's adherence to the treatment regimen.

- Encourage questions and allow time for reinforcement and clarification of information provided.

Improves client understanding of treatment regimen and reinforces self-reliance and confidence in ability to care for self.

- Provide written instructions regarding scheduled appointments with health care provider and for laboratory studies, medications prescribed, activity restrictions, and signs and symptoms to report.

Provides the client and significant others a resource of information following discharge from the acute care facility.

ADDITIONAL NURSING DIAGNOSES

ACUTE PAIN NDx

- **Right upper quadrant** related to inflammation of the liver
- **Myalgias/arthralgias** related to the presence of circulating immune complexes and activation of the complement system associated with viral infection

RISK FOR ACTIVITY INTOLERANCE NDx

Related to:
- Inadequate nutritional status
- Increased energy utilization associated with the increased metabolic rate present in an infectious process
- Difficulty resting and sleeping associated with frequent assessments and treatments, discomfort, anxiety, and unfamiliar environment

FEAR AND ANXIETY NDx

Related to:
- Unfamiliar environment and lack of understanding of diagnosis and diagnostic tests
- Lack of definitive treatment for hepatitis and the possibility of serious complications
- Discomfort associated with nausea, pain, and pruritus
- Possible transmission of disease to others and rejection by others because of their fear of contracting hepatitis
- Temporary restrictions of some usual activities (e.g., vigorous exercise, contact sports, sexual activity, alcohol consumption)

PANCREATITIS, ACUTE

Acute pancreatitis is an inflammation of the pancreas that occurs when the enzymes it produces become activated in the pancreas rather than in the duodenum. The subsequent autodigestion causes pathological changes that range from a mild local inflammatory response to extensive tissue and vascular damage that can result in life-threatening complications such as shock and multiple organ failure. After an episode of mild to moderate acute pancreatitis, the structure and function of the pancreas often return to normal. However, with more severe and/or recurrent episodes of acute pancreatitis, irreversible changes can occur and chronic pancreatitis can develop.

It is theorized that pancreatic duct obstruction, pancreatic ischemia, direct injury to the acinar cells, and reflux of bile into the pancreatic duct are among the mechanisms that trigger the activation of enzymes in the pancreas. The most common causes of acute pancreatitis are biliary tract disease and heavy alcohol intake. Some less frequent causes include external trauma to the abdomen, trauma to the pancreas during pancreatic endoscopy or abdominal surgery, infections, drugs (e.g., azathioprine, mercaptopurine, didanosine, pentamidine, estrogen, thiazides, valproic acid), and metabolic disorders such as chronic hypercalcemia and genetic hyperlipidemia.

Signs and symptoms of acute pancreatitis usually include severe, continuous epigastric pain that radiates to the back, nausea, vomiting, fever (usually low-grade), and abdominal tenderness and distention. The focus of medical treatment is to prevent further autodigestion of the pancreas and prevent systemic complications by decreasing stimulation of the pancreatic enzymes until normal outflow resumes. If the cause of the pancreatitis is biliary tract disease, surgery (e.g., removal of gallstones that may be blocking the pancreatic duct) is usually performed after pancreatic inflammation has subsided and the client is in stable condition.

This care plan focuses on the adult client hospitalized with acute pancreatitis. Some of the information is applicable to clients receiving follow-up care in an extended care facility or home setting.

OUTCOME/DISCHARGE CRITERIA

The client will:
1. Have no signs and symptoms of complications
2. Have relief of severe pain
3. Have an adequate nutritional intake
4. Identify ways to prevent overstimulation of and further trauma to the pancreas
5. Verbalize an understanding of recommended dietary modifications
6. State signs and symptoms to report to the health care provider
7. Verbalize an understanding of and a plan for adhering to recommended follow-up care including future appointments with health care provider and medications prescribed.

Nursing Diagnosis **INEFFECTIVE BREATHING PATTERN** NDx

Definition: Inspiration and/or expiration that does not provide adequate ventilation

Related to:
- Increased rate of respirations associated with fear and anxiety
- Decreased rate of respirations associated with the depressant effect of some medications (e.g., narcotic [opioid] analgesics, some antiemetics)
- Decreased depth of respirations associated with:
  - Depressant effects of some medications (e.g., narcotic [opioid] analgesics, some antiemetics)
  - Fear, anxiety, decreased activity, and reluctance to breathe deeply because of pain
  - Restricted chest expansion resulting from positioning (client often positions self on side with knees and trunk flexed to reduce pain) and pressure on the diaphragm (can occur as a result of accumulation of gastrointestinal gas and fluid and ascites if present)
  - Decreased lung compliance (distensibility) if pleural effusion is present

CLINICAL MANIFESTATIONS

Subjective	Objective
Complaints of shortness of breath	Dyspnea; orthopnea; increased respiratory rate; decreased depth of breathing; decreased inspiratory/expiratory pressure; decreased minute ventilation; decreased vital capacity; nasal flaring; use of accessory muscles to breathe; assumption of three-point position; altered chest excursion; pursed-lip breathing; prolonged expiration phases; increased anterior-posterior diameter

RISK FACTORS
- Treatment regimen
- Biliary tract disorder
- Autoimmune disorder

DESIRED OUTCOMES

The client will have an improved breathing pattern as evidenced by:
  a. Normal rate and depth of respirations
  b. Decreased dyspnea
  c. Symmetrical chest excursion

NOC OUTCOMES

Respiratory status: ventilation

NIC INTERVENTIONS

Ventilation assistance; respiratory monitoring

NURSING ASSESSMENT	RATIONALE
Assess for signs and symptoms of an ineffective breathing pattern: • Shallow or slow respirations • Limited chest excursion • Tachypnea or dyspnea • Use of accessory muscles when breathing	*Early recognition of signs and symptoms of an ineffective breathing pattern allows for prompt intervention.*
Assess/monitor pulse oximetry (arterial oxygen saturation [Sao$_2$]), arterial blood gas (ABG) values as indicated.	*Monitoring continuous Sao$_2$ readings allows for the early detection of hypoxia.* *Assessment of ABG values provides a more direct measurement of both the partial pressure of oxygen in arterial blood (Pao$_2$) and the partial pressure of carbon dioxide in arterial blood (Paco$_2$), both of which reflect the adequacy of ventilation.*

THERAPEUTIC INTERVENTIONS	RATIONALE
Independent Actions Implement measures to improve breathing pattern: • Perform actions to reduce fear and anxiety (e.g., assure client that staff is nearby; provide a calm, restful environment; explain all tests and procedures). **D** ✦	*Prevents the shallow and/or rapid breathing that can occur with fear and anxiety*

THERAPEUTIC INTERVENTIONS	RATIONALE
• Perform actions to reduce pressure on the diaphragm:	
• Implement measures to reduce the accumulation of gas and fluid in the gastrointestinal tract (avoid carbonated beverages and chewing gum; avoid gas-producing foods). **D** ✦	*These actions decrease incidence of abdominal distention and pressure on the diaphragm.*
• When severe pain has subsided, place client in a semi- to high-Fowler's position unless contraindicated; position with pillows. **D** ✦	*Prevents slumping and decreases pressure on the diaphragm preventing adequate lung expansion.*
• If client must remain flat in bed, assist with position change at least every 2 hours. **D** ● ✦	*Changing position while on bed rest prevents skin breakdown and stasis of lung secretions.*
• Instruct client to deep breathe or use incentive spirometer every 1 to 2 hours.	*Deep breathing and use of incentive spirometry improves lung expansion.*
Dependent/Collaborative Actions	
• Implement measures to prevent further third-spacing and/or promote mobilization of fluid back into vascular space (administer albumin infusions, withhold fluid and food as ordered).	*Reduces ascites and pressure on the diaphragm, which blocks adequate lung expansion.*
• Perform actions to prevent and treat pleural effusion (reduce oral fluid intake, insert nasogastric tube and maintain suction as ordered).	*Reduces stimulation of the pancreas and removes hydrochloric acid from the stomach*
• Increase activity as allowed and tolerated. **D** ✦	*Increases client's willingness and ability to move*
• Administer central nervous system depressants judiciously; hold medication and consult physician if respiratory rate is less than 12 breaths/min.	*Central nervous system depressants can significantly reduce respiratory rate and subsequently cause a significant decrease in oxygenation.*
Consult appropriate health care provider (e.g., respiratory therapist, physician) if:	*Notifying the appropriate health care provider allows for prompt modification of treatment plan.*
• Ineffective breathing pattern continues.	
• Signs and symptoms of atelectasis (e.g., diminished or absent breath sounds, dull percussion note over affected area, increased respiratory rate, dyspnea, tachycardia, elevated temperature) develop.	
• Signs and symptoms of impaired gas exchange (e.g., restlessness, irritability, confusion, significant decrease in oximetry results, decreased PaO_2 and increased $PaCO_2$ levels) are present.	

Nursing/Collaborative Diagnosis **IMBALANCED FLUID AND ELECTROLYTES**

Definition: Risk for developing an imbalance of electrolytes and fluids in the intracellular and extracellular compartments of the body

Related to:
- **Deficient fluid volume NDx** related to:
  - Decreased oral intake
  - Excessive loss of fluid associated with vomiting and nasogastric tube drainage
  - Third-spacing of intravascular fluid
- **Hypokalemia, hypochloremia, and metabolic alkalosis** related to loss of electrolytes and hydrochloric acid associated with vomiting and nasogastric tube drainage
- **Hypocalcemia** related to:
  - Binding of calcium to the undigested fats in the intestine (enzymes such as lipase and phospholipase A are not released into the intestinal tract to digest fats so calcium binds with the free fats and is excreted in the stool)
  - Hypoalbuminemia associated with increased vascular permeability that occurs with inflammation (albumin is needed to transport nonionized calcium in the blood)
  - Binding of calcium to free fatty acids in areas of tissue necrosis
- **Third-spacing** related to increased vascular permeability associated with the inflammatory response and activation of kinin peptides such as bradykinin and kallidin (occurs when the pancreatic enzyme trypsin enters systemic circulation)

NDx = NANDA-I Diagnosis   **D** = Delegatable Action   ● = UAP   ✦ = LVN/LPN   ⊖▶ = Go to ⊖volve for animation

Continued...

CLINICAL MANIFESTATIONS

Subjective	Objective
Complaints of fatigue and weakness; complaints of dizziness; anxiousness; irritability; complaints of numbness and tingling of fingers, toes, or circumoral area	Decreased skin turgor; dry mucous membranes; weight loss of 2% or greater over a short period; postural hypotension; weak rapid pulse; flat neck veins when supine; changes in mental status; capillary refill greater than 2 to 3 seconds; decreased urine output with increased specific gravity; cardiac dysrhythmias; vomiting; hypoactive or absent bowel sounds; muscle twitching; positive Chvostek's and Trousseau's sign; hyperactive reflex

RISK FACTORS

- Failure of regulatory mechanisms
- Chronic illness
- Inadequate intake
- Exposure to pathogens

DESIRED OUTCOMES

The client will not experience deficient fluid volume, hypokalemia, hypochloremia, hypocalcemia, or metabolic alkalosis as evidenced by:

  a. Normal skin turgor
  b. Moist mucous membranes
  c. Stable weight
  d. B/P and pulse rate within normal range for client and stable with position change
  e. Capillary refill time less than 2 to 3 seconds
  f. Usual mental status
  g. Balanced intake and output
  h. Urine specific gravity within normal range
  i. Soft, nondistended abdomen with normal bowel sounds
  j. Absence of cardiac dysrhythmias, muscle weakness, paresthesias, muscle twitching or spasms, dizziness, tetany, and seizure activity
  k. Negative Chvostek's and Trousseau's signs
  l. BUN, Hct, serum electrolyte, and arterial blood gas values within normal range

NOC OUTCOMES

Fluid balance; electrolyte and acid-base balance

NIC INTERVENTIONS

Fluid monitoring; fluid/electrolyte management; electrolyte management: hypokalemia; electrolyte management: hypocalcemia; acid-base monitoring; acid-base management: metabolic alkalosis

NURSING ASSESSMENT

Assess for and report signs and symptoms of:
- Deficient fluid volume:
- Decreased skin turgor, dry mucous membranes, thirst
- Weight loss of 2% or greater over a short period
- Postural hypotension and/or low B/P
- Weak, rapid pulse
- Capillary refill time greater than 2 to 3 seconds
- Flat neck veins when supine
- Change in mental status
- Decreased urine output with increased specific gravity (reflects an actual rather than potential fluid volume deficit)
- Increased BUN and Hct values

RATIONALE

Early recognition of signs and symptoms of imbalanced fluid and electrolytes allows for prompt intervention.

NURSING ASSESSMENT

RATIONALE

- Hypokalemia (e.g., cardiac dysrhythmias, postural hypotension, muscle weakness, nausea and vomiting, abdominal distention, hypoactive or absent bowel sounds)
- Hypochloremia and metabolic alkalosis (e.g., dizziness, paresthesias, muscle twitching or spasms, hypoventilation, elevated pH and total carbon dioxide content [TCO_2])
- Hypocalcemia (e.g., anxiousness; irritability; numbness or tingling of fingers, toes, or circumoral area; positive Chvostek's and Trousseau's signs; hyperactive reflexes; tetany; seizures).

THERAPEUTIC INTERVENTIONS

RATIONALE

Dependent/Collaborative Actions

Implement measures to prevent or treat deficient fluid volume, hypokalemia, hypochloremia, hypocalcemia, and metabolic alkalosis:

- Perform actions to reduce nausea and vomiting (maintain fluid and food restrictions as ordered; reduce pain, eliminate noxious sights and odors from the environment). **D** ● ✦

These actions prevent loss of fluid and electrolytes and alterations in metabolic status.

- If a nasogastric tube is present and needs to be irrigated frequently and/or with large volumes of solution, irrigate it with normal saline rather than water.

Maintains patency.

- Administer fluid and electrolyte replacements as ordered.

Replaces lost fluid and electrolytes to normalize values.

- Maintain a fluid intake of at least 2500 mL/day unless contraindicated. **D** ● ✦

Adequate fluid intake is required to maintain adequate circulatory volume.

- When oral intake is allowed:
  - Assist client to select the following foods/fluids:
    (1) Those high in potassium (e.g., bananas, potatoes, cantaloupe, avocados, raisins)

    Maintains adequate level of potassium.

    (2) Those high in calcium such as milk and milk products (if client is on a low-fat diet, items such as ice cream, whole milk, butter, and cream should be omitted)

    Maintains adequate level of calcium.

- Administer pancreatic enzymes (e.g., pancreatin, pancrelipase) if ordered.

Promotes fat digestion so that there is less fat available to bind with calcium.

Consult physician if signs and symptoms of deficient fluid volume and electrolyte imbalances persist or worsen.

Notification of the physician allows for prompt alterations in treatment plan.

Monitor serum albumin levels. Report below-normal levels.

Low serum albumin levels result in fluid shifting out of the vascular space because albumin normally maintains plasma colloid osmotic pressure.

Implement measures to prevent further third-spacing and/or promote mobilization of fluid back into vascular space:

- Administer albumin infusions if ordered.

Albumin increases colloid osmotic pressure which pulls fluid into the vascular compartment.

- Perform actions to decrease pancreatic stimulation; withhold all food and oral fluid as ordered. **D** ✦

Food and fluid, especially those that are acidic or have a high protein or fat content, upon entering the duodenum cause the release of secretin and/or cholecystokinin, which stimulate the output of pancreatic secretions.

Implement measures to reduce hydrochloric acid in the stomach.

As hydrochloric acid enters the duodenum, it stimulates the release of secretin, which is believed to stimulate a significant output of pancreatic secretions.

Continued...

THERAPEUTIC INTERVENTIONS	RATIONALE
• Insert a nasogastric tube and maintain suction as ordered.	*Placing a nasogastric tube to suction removes the acid from the stomach.*
• Administer histamine receptor antagonists (e.g., famotidine, ranitidine, nizatidine) if ordered.	*Histamine receptor antagonists inhibit the action of histamine on the parietal cells, which blocks gastric acid secretion.*
• Minimize client's exposure to odor and sight of food until oral intake is allowed.	*Decreasing the client's exposure to the sight and odor of food prevents stimulation of gastric secretions and the subsequent output of pancreatic secretions.*
Consult physician if signs and symptoms of third-spacing persist or worsen.	*Notification of the physician allows for prompt alterations in treatment plan.*

Nursing Diagnosis IMBALANCED NUTRITION: LESS THAN BODY REQUIREMENTS NDx

Definition: Inadequate intake or insufficient nutrition to meet the body's metabolic needs

Related to:
• Decreased oral intake associated with nausea, pain, prescribed dietary restrictions, and feeling of fullness resulting from abdominal distention
• Loss of nutrients associated with vomiting
• Decreased utilization of nutrients associated with impaired digestion of fats, proteins, and carbohydrates resulting from loss of normal outflow of pancreatic enzymes
• Increased nutritional needs associated with the increased metabolic rate that occurs with pancreatitis

CLINICAL MANIFESTATIONS

Subjective	Objective
Verbalization of lack of appetite; fatigue; irritability; poor self-esteem	Loss of weight with adequate food intake; body weight 20% or more under ideal weight; sore, inflamed buccal cavity; capillary fragility; pale conjunctiva and mucous membranes; poor muscle tone; excessive hair loss; amenorrhea

RISK FACTORS
• Impaired digestion
• Poor diet
• Treatment regimen

DESIRED OUTCOMES

The client will maintain an adequate nutritional status as evidenced by:
  a. Weight within normal range for the client
  b. Normal BUN and serum albumin, prealbumin, Hct, and Hgb levels and normal lymphocyte count
  c. Usual strength and activity tolerance
  d. Healthy oral mucous membrane

NOC OUTCOMES

Nutritional status

NIC INTERVENTIONS

Nutritional monitoring; nutrition management; nutrition therapy; nausea management; pain management; total parenteral nutrition (TPN) administration

NURSING ASSESSMENT	RATIONALE
Assess for and report signs and symptoms of malnutrition: • Weight significantly below client's usual weight or below normal for client's age, height, and body frame • Abnormal BUN and low serum albumin, prealbumin, Hct, and Hgb levels and low lymphocyte count	*Early recognition and reporting of signs and symptoms of malnutrition allows for prompt intervention.*

NURSING ASSESSMENT

- Weakness and fatigue
- Sore, inflamed oral mucous membrane
- Pale conjunctiva

Monitor percentage of meals and snacks client consumes. Report a pattern or inadequate intake.

RATIONALE

An awareness of the amount of foods/fluids the client consumes alerts the nurse to deficits in nutritional intake. Reporting an inadequate intake allows for prompt intervention.

THERAPEUTIC INTERVENTIONS

Independent Actions

Implement measures to maintain an adequate nutritional status:

- Limit activity as ordered.
- When food or oral fluids are allowed:
- Perform actions to improve oral intake:
  - Implement measures to reduce ascites and the accumulation of gas and fluid in the gastrointestinal tract (e.g., proper positioning, encourage client not to eat or drink foods that cause gas production [caffeine, beans, drinking with a straw, chewing gum]).
  - Implement measures to reduce nausea and vomiting (maintain fluid and food restrictions as ordered, reduce pain, eliminate noxious sights and odors from the environment).
  - Increase activity as allowed and tolerated. **D** ● ✦

  - Maintain a clean environment and a relaxed, pleasant atmosphere. **D** ● ✦

  - Allow adequate time for meals; reheat foods/fluids if necessary. **D** ● ✦

  - Limit fluid intake with meals (unless the fluids have high nutritional value). **D** ✦
  - Ensure that meals are well balanced and high in essential nutrients.

RATIONALE

Limiting activity decreases energy utilization and metabolic rate.

These actions reduce abdominal distention and the subsequent feeling of fullness and early satiety.

These actions prevent loss of fluid and electrolytes.

Activity usually promotes a sense of well-being, which can improve appetite.

Noxious sites and odors can inhibit the feeding center in the hypothalamus. Maintaining a clean environment helps prevent this from occurring. In addition, maintaining a relaxed, pleasant atmosphere can help reduce the client's stress and promote a feeling of well-being, which tends to improve appetite and oral intake.

Clients who feels rushed during meals tend to become anxious, lose their appetite, and stop eating. Appetite is also suppressed if foods/fluids normally served hot or warm become cold and do not appeal to the client.

Drinking liquids with meals distends the stomach and may cause satiety before an adequate amount of food is consumed.

Maintenance of nutritional status

Dependent/Collaborative Actions

Implement measures to maintain an adequate nutritional status:

Administer TPN if ordered.

- Administer vitamins and minerals.

- Administer pancreatic enzymes (e.g., pancreatin, pancrelipase)
- Administer albumin

Implement measures to reduce pain (position properly, administer pain meds as ordered). **D** ✦

- Perform a calorie count if ordered. Report information to dietitian and physician.

Reassess nutritional status on a regular basis and report decline.

Provides nutrition if client is unable to tolerate oral intake.

Vitamins, minerals, and supplements are needed to maintain metabolic functioning.

Supplemental pancreatic enzymes aid in the digestion of foods.

Albumin increases osmotic pressure and pulls fluid into the vascular compartment.

Pain reduction increases a client's appetite and ability to tolerate diet.

A dietitian is best able to evaluate whether the foods/fluids selected will meet the client's nutritional needs.

Allows for prompt alterations in treatment plan.

NDx = NANDA-I Diagnosis   **D** = Delegatable Action   ● = UAP   ✦ = LVN/LPN   ⊜▶ = Go to ⊜volve for animation

Nursing Diagnosis ACUTE PAIN NDx (EPIGASTRIC WITH RADIATION TO THE BACK)

Definition: Unpleasant sensory and emotional experience arising from actual or potential tissue damage or described in terms of such damage (International Association for the Study of Pain); sudden or slow onset of any intensity from mild to severe with an anticipated or predictable end and a duration of less than 6 months

Related to:
• Distention of the pancreas associated with inflammation and obstruction of pancreatic ducts
• Peritoneal irritation associated with escape of activated pancreatic enzymes into the peritoneum

CLINICAL MANIFESTATIONS

Subjective	Objective
Verbal or coded report of pain; difficulty sleeping due to experience of pain	Autonomic responses (e.g., diaphoresis; changes in B/P, respiration, pulse; pupillary dilatation); expressive behavior (e.g., restlessness, moaning, crying, vigilance, irritability, sighing); changes in appetite and eating; protective gestures; guarding behavior; facial mask; evidence of sleep disturbance (eyes lack luster, fixed or scattered movement, beaten look, grimace); self-focus; narrowed focus (altered time perception, impaired thought processes, reduced interaction with people and environment); distraction behavior (e.g., pacing, seeking out other people and/or activities, repetitive activities)

RISK FACTORS	DESIRED OUTCOMES

• Exposure to pathogens
• Acute/chronic illness
	The client will experience diminished pain as evidenced by:
	    a. Verbalization of a decrease in or absence of pain
	    b. Relaxed facial expression and body positioning
	    c. Increased participation in activities
	    d. Stable vital signs

NOC OUTCOMES	NIC INTERVENTIONS
Pain control; comfort level	Pain management; analgesic administration; patient-controlled analgesia (PCA) assistance

NURSING ASSESSMENT	RATIONALE
Assess for signs and symptoms of pain (e.g., verbalization of pain, grimacing, reluctance to move, restlessness, diaphoresis, increased B/P, tachycardia).	*Early recognition of signs and symptoms of pain allows for prompt intervention and improved pain control.*
Assess client's perception of the severity of pain using a pain intensity rating scale.	*An awareness of the severity of pain being experienced helps determine the most appropriate interventions for pain management. Use of a pain intensity rating scale gives the nurse a clearer understanding of the pain being experienced and promotes consistency when communicating with others about the client's pain experience.*
Assess the client's pain pattern (e.g., location, quality, onset, duration, precipitating factors, aggravating factors, alleviating factors).	*Knowledge of the client's pain pattern assists in the identification of effective pain management interventions.*
Ask the client to describe previous pain experiences and methods used to manage pain effectively.	*Many variables affect a client's response to pain (e.g., age, sex, coping style, previous experience with pain, culture, cause of pain). Knowledge of the client's usual response to pain and methods previously used to manage pain effectively enables the nurse to evaluate the client's pain more accurately and facilitates the identification of effective strategies for pain management.*

THERAPEUTIC INTERVENTIONS	RATIONALE

Independent Actions

Implement measures to reduce pain:

- Implement measures to reduce fear and anxiety (e.g., assure client that the need for pain relief is understood, plan methods for achieving pain control with client, provide a calm, restful environment). **D** ✦

Promotes relaxation and subsequently increases the client's threshold and tolerance for pain.

- Perform actions to promote rest (e.g., minimize environmental activity and noise). **D** ● ✦

These actions reduce fatigue and subsequently increases the client's threshold and tolerance for pain.

Dependent/Collaborative Actions

Implement measures to reduce pain:

- Administer analgesics before activities and procedures that can cause pain and before pain becomes severe.

Improves ability to perform activities of daily living without discomfort.

- Perform actions to reduce pancreatic stimulation:
  - Withhold all food and oral fluid as ordered. **D** ✦

Food and fluid, especially those that are acidic or have a high protein or fat content, upon entering the duodenum cause the release of secretin and/or cholecystokinin, which stimulate the output of pancreatic secretions.

  - Implement measures to reduce the amount of hydrochloric acid in the stomach:

As hydrochloric acid enters the duodenum, it stimulates the release of secretin; some physicians believe that the secretin released stimulates a significant output of pancreatic enzymes secretion.

  (1) Insert a nasogastric tube and maintain suction if ordered.

Removes fluid and hydrochloric acid from the stomach.

  (2) Administer histamine₂-receptor antagonists (e.g., famotidine, ranitidine, nizatidine) if ordered.

Histamine receptor antagonists and proton-pump inhibitors suppress secretion of gastric acid.

  - Minimize client's exposure to odor and sight of food until oral intake is allowed.

Prevents stimulation of gastric secretions and the subsequent output of pancreatic secretions.

  - When oral intake is allowed:
  (1) Advance diet slowly.

Slow advancement increases tolerance to oral intake.

  (2) Provide small, frequent meals rather than three large ones. **D** ✦

Small frequent meals decreases stretch of the stomach and subsequent discomfort.

  (3) Avoid foods/fluids high in fat (e.g., butter, cream, whole milk, ice cream, fried foods, gravies, nuts), spicy foods, and caffeine-containing beverages (e.g., coffee, tea, colas) if ordered.

These foods cause release of pancreatic enzymes, which causes pain.

- Allow client to sit or lie with knees and trunk flexed. **D** ● ✦

This position relieves pressure on the inflamed pancreas.

- Provide or assist with additional nonpharmacological measures for pain relief (e.g., massage; position change; progressive relaxation exercises; restful environment; diversional activities such as watching television, reading, or conversing).

Nonpharmacological pain management includes a variety of interventions. It is believed that most of these are effective because they stimulate closure of the gating mechanism in the spinal cord and subsequently block the transmission of pain impulses. In addition, some interventions are thought to stimulate the release of endogenous analgesics (e.g., endorphins) that inhibit the transmission of pain impulses and/or alter the client's perception of pain. Many of the nonpharmacological interventions also help decrease pain by promoting relaxation.

- Administer analgesics as ordered and encourage client to use PCA device as instructed.

Analgesics reduce pain; use of a PCA device allows client control over pain regulation.

- If client is receiving epidural analgesia, perform actions to maintain patency of the system (e.g., keep tubing free of kinks, tape catheter securely, use caution when moving client to avoid dislodging catheter).

Use of epidural analgesia helps to decrease pain without causing increased sedation.

- Assist with peritoneal lavage if performed.

May be done to remove some of the activated pancreatic enzymes and debris that cause peritoneal irritation and subsequent pain

Consult appropriate health care provider (e.g., pharmacist, pain management specialist, physician) if above measures fail to provide adequate pain relief.

Allows for prompt alterations in the treatment plan.

NDx = NANDA-I Diagnosis **D** = Delegatable Action ● = UAP ✦ = LVN/LPN ⊖▶ = Go to ⊖volve for animation

Nursing Diagnosis **NAUSEA** NDx

Definition: An unpleasant, wavelike sensation in the back of the throat, epigastrium, or throughout the abdomen that may or may not lead to vomiting

Related to:
- Stimulation of the vomiting center associated with:
  - Stimulation of the visceral afferent pathways from abdominal distention and inflammation of the pancreas
  - Stimulation of the cerebral cortex resulting from pain and stress

CLINICAL MANIFESTATIONS

Subjective	Objective
Complaints of nausea	N/A

RISK FACTORS
- Exposure to pathogens
- Acute/chronic illness
- Inadequate pain relief

DESIRED OUTCOMES
The client will experience relief of nausea and vomiting as evidenced by:
  a. Verbalization of relief of nausea
  b. Absence of vomiting

NOC OUTCOMES
Nausea and vomiting severity

NIC INTERVENTIONS
Nausea management; vomiting management; environmental management: comfort

NURSING ASSESSMENT	RATIONALE
Assess for nausea and vomiting. Determine: • Duration • Frequency • Severity	*Identification of the signs and symptoms of nausea and vomiting allows for prompt intervention.*

THERAPEUTIC INTERVENTIONS	RATIONALE

Independent Actions
Implement measures to reduce nausea and vomiting:

- Maintain NPO restrictions as ordered. **D** ● ✦

  Prevents accumulation of fluid in the stomach and decreases the experience of vomiting.

- Eliminate noxious sights and odors from the environment. **D** ● ✦

  Noxious stimuli can cause stimulation of the vomiting center.

- Instruct client to change positions slowly. **D** ● ✦

  Rapid movements can result in chemoreceptor trigger zone stimulation and subsequent excitation of the vomiting center.

- Provide oral hygiene after each emesis. **D** ● ✦

  Removes the taste of emesis from the mouth and helps to decrease subsequent nausea.

- Reduce pain via positioning or distractions. **D** ✦

  Pain may stimulate chemoreceptor trigger zone and produce nausea.

- Perform actions to reduce fear and anxiety (e.g., assure client that staff are nearby, provide a calm, restful environment, explain all tests and procedures).

  Fear and anxiety may produce nausea.

- Encourage client to take deep, slow breaths when nauseated. **D** ● ✦

  Helps to relax the client and reduce stress.

Dependent/Collaborative Actions
Implement measures to reduce nausea and vomiting:

- Administer antiemetics as ordered. **D** ✦

  Raises the threshold of the chemoreceptor trigger zone, thus decreasing nausea.
  Administer phenothiazines cautiously because of their potential cholestatic effect.

- Administer analgesics as ordered.

  The client may experience nausea as a result of pain.

THERAPEUTIC INTERVENTIONS	RATIONALE
• Insert nasogastric tube and maintain suction as ordered.	*This reduces stomach contents and decreases the incidence of nausea and vomiting.*
• When oral intake is allowed:	*Oral intake helps to maintain nutritional status and should be advanced slowly so that the incidence of nausea is decreased.*
• Advance diet as tolerated.	
• Avoid serving foods with an overpowering aroma; remove lids from hot foods before entering room. **D ● ✦**	*Noxious stimuli stimulate the vomiting center.*
• Provide small, frequent meals; instruct client to ingest foods and fluids slowly.	*Provides adequate nutrition and small, frequent meals don't over stimulate the stomach. Large meals may increase nausea.*
• Instruct client to eat dry foods (e.g., toast, crackers) and avoid drinking liquids with meals if nauseated.	*Decreases nausea before arising from bed.*
• Instruct client to avoid the following:	
(1) Foods/fluids high in fat (e.g., butter, cream, whole milk, ice cream, fried foods, gravies, nuts)	*Stimulates secretion of pancreatic enzymes, which increase pain and nausea.*
(2) Foods/fluids that irritate the gastric mucosa (e.g., spicy foods; caffeine-containing beverages such as tea, coffee, and colas)	*Decreases gastric irritation and possible subsequent nausea.*
Consult a physician or a pharmacist if nausea continues.	*Allows for changes in intervention to decrease/eliminate nausea.*

Nursing Diagnosis IMPAIRED COMFORT NDx (ABDOMINAL DISTENTION AND GAS PAIN)

Definition: Perceived lack of ease, relief and transcendence in physical psychospiritual, environmental and social dimensions

Related to: Abdominal distention

CLINICAL MANIFESTATIONS

Subjective	Objective
Verbal reports of abdominal fullness or gas pain	Clutching or guarding of the abdomen; restlessness; reluctance to move; grimacing; increasing abdominal girth

RISK FACTORS
- Decreased peristalsis
- Immobility

DESIRED OUTCOMES

The client will experience diminished abdominal distention and gas pain as evidenced by:
  a. Verbalization of decreased abdominal fullness and pain
  b. Relaxed facial expression and body positioning
  c. Decrease in abdominal girth

NOC OUTCOMES

Comfort level; symptom control

NIC INTERVENTIONS

Flatulence reduction

NURSING ASSESSMENT	RATIONALE
Assess for and report signs and symptoms of abdominal distention or gas pain.	*Early recognition of signs and symptoms of abdominal distention or gas pain allows for prompt intervention.*

Continued...

THERAPEUTIC INTERVENTIONS	RATIONALE

Independent Actions

Implement measures to reduce the accumulation of gas and fluid in the gastrointestinal tract:

- Encourage and assist client with frequent position changes and ambulation as soon as allowed and tolerated. **D** ●

- Instruct the client to avoid activities such as chewing gum, drinking through a straw, and smoking.

- Maintain patency of nasogastric, gastric, or intestinal tube if present. **D** ✦

- When oral intake is allowed, instruct client to avoid intake of carbonated beverages and gas-producing foods (e.g., cabbage, onions, beans).

- Encourage client to eructate and expel flatus whenever the urge is felt. **D** ✦

Activity stimulates peristalsis and expulsion of flatus.

Avoiding these activities reduces air swallowing and subsequent abdominal distention.

Maintaining the patency of tubes designed to decompress the abdomen ensures adequate evacuation of gas, reducing distention.

Intake of this type of fluids/foods increases abdominal distention.

Relieves abdominal distention.

Dependent/Collaborative Actions

Implement measures to reduce the accumulation of gas and fluid in the gastrointestinal tract:

- Maintain food and oral fluid restrictions as ordered. **D** ✦

- Consult physician regarding insertion of a rectal tube or administration of a return-flow enema if indicated.

- Encourage use of nonnarcotic analgesics once the period of severe pain has subsided. **D** ✦

- Administer gastrointestinal stimulants (e.g., metoclopramide, bisacodyl) if ordered. **D** ✦

- Administer antiflatulents (e.g., simethicone).

- Administer pancreatic enzymes (e.g., pancreatin, pancrelipase).

Consult physician if signs and symptoms of abdominal distention and gas pain persist or worsen.

Prevents abdominal distention, especially if there is reduced or absent peristalsis.

Notifying the appropriate health care provider allows for modification of the treatment plan.

Narcotic [opioid] analgesics depress gastrointestinal activity, contributing further to gas and the risk of constipation.

Gastrointestinal stimulants increase gastrointestinal motility.

Antiflatulents reduce gas accumulation in the gastrointestinal tract.

Pancreatic enzymes aid in digestion.

Notifying the appropriate health care provider allows for modification of the treatment plan.

Nursing Diagnosis   RISK FOR INFECTION NDx (SEPSIS)

Definition: An increased risk for being invaded by pathogenic organisms

Related to:
- Release of bacteria into the blood associated with:
  - Presence of infected necrotic areas or leakage of infected pseudocysts or abscesses (necrotic areas, pseudocysts, and abscesses can develop as a result of destruction of pancreatic and surrounding tissue by the activated proteolytic enzymes)
  - Peritonitis (if it occurs)
- Decreased resistance to infection associated with decreased nutritional status
- Break in skin integrity associated with frequent venipunctures or presence of invasive lines (e.g., intravenous catheter, hemodynamic monitoring devices)

CLINICAL MANIFESTATIONS

Subjective	Objective
Report of chills/lethargy; loss of appetite	Elevated temperature; diaphoresis; tachypnea; tachycardia; confusion increase in WBC count above previous levels and/or significant change in differential; positive blood cultures

RISK FACTORS
- Exposure to pathogens
- Failure of immune response
- Poor nutritional status

DESIRED OUTCOMES

The client will not experience sepsis as evidenced by:
   a. No further increase in temperature
   b. Absence of chills and diaphoresis
   c. Pulse and respiratory rate within normal range for client
   d. WBC and differential counts returning to normal
   e. Negative blood culture results

NOC OUTCOMES

Immune status; infection severity

NIC INTERVENTIONS

Infection protection; infection control

NURSING ASSESSMENT	**RATIONALE**
Assess for and report signs and symptoms of sepsis (e.g., increase in temperature, chills, diaphoresis, tachypnea, tachycardia, increase in WBC count above previous levels and/or significant change in differential, positive blood cultures).	Early recognition of signs and symptoms of sepsis allows for prompt intervention.

THERAPEUTIC INTERVENTIONS	**RATIONALE**

Dependent/Collaborative Actions

Implement measures to prevent sepsis:

- Perform actions to decrease pancreatic stimulation (e.g., keep client NPO; maintain nasogastric tube to suction).

  These actions reduce destruction of pancreatic and peripancreatic tissue and subsequent development of necrotic areas, pseudocysts, and abscesses.

- Perform actions to prevent and treat peritonitis (e.g., keep client NPO, place client in semi-Fowler's position, administer antimicrobials).

  Prevents and decreases incidence of peritonitis.

- Prepare client for drainage of an abscess or pseudocyst or surgical resection of necrotic tissue if planned.

  Prevents spread of infection and decreases incidence of sepsis.

- Maintain sterile technique during all invasive procedures (e.g., venous and arterial punctures).

  Decreases incidence of bacteria being introduced in the system.

- Perform actions to maintain an adequate nutritional status (e.g., increase activity as tolerated; maintain a clean environment and a relaxed, pleasant atmosphere; serve several small meals rather than three large ones).

  Adequate nutrition is necessary for cellular development and to fight off infection.

- Perform actions to reduce stress (e.g., reduce pain and nausea; provide a calm, restful environment; explain diagnostic tests and treatment plan).

  Stress reduction prevents an increase in secretion of cortisol, which interferes with some immune responses.

- Change intravenous line sites, tubing, and solutions according to hospital policy and maintain a closed system for intravenous infusions whenever possible.

  Decreases potential for the introduction of foreign bacteria into the system.

- Anchor catheters/tubings (e.g., intravenous) securely.

  Reduces trauma to the tissues and the risk for introduction of pathogens associated with in-and-out movement of the tubing.

- Administer antimicrobials as ordered.

  Antimicrobials prevent and/or treat infections.

- If signs and symptoms of sepsis occur, assess for and immediately report signs and symptoms of septic shock (e.g., systolic B/P <90 mm Hg; rapid, weak pulse; restlessness; agitation; confusion; urine output <30 mL/h; cool, pale, mottled, and/or cyanotic extremities; capillary refill time >3 seconds; diminished or absent peripheral pulses).

  Allows for prompt alterations in treatment plan.

NDx = NANDA-I Diagnosis   **D** = Delegatable Action   ● = UAP   ✦ = LVN/LPN   ⊝▶ = Go to ⊝volve for animation

Collaborative Diagnosis   RISK FOR HYPOVOLEMIC SHOCK

Definition: A form of shock in which the blood volume is so significantly decreased that the heart is unable to supply blood to the body

Related to:

- Deficient fluid volume associated with restricted oral intake and fluid loss resulting from vomiting and nasogastric tube drainage
- Peripheral vasodilation and increased vascular permeability with subsequent third-spacing associated with activation of kinin peptides such as bradykinin and kallidin (occurs when the pancreatic enzyme trypsin enters systemic circulation)
- Hemorrhage associated with destruction of elastic fibers of the blood vessels by the proteolytic enzyme elastase (elastase is activated in the pancreas by trypsin and causes localized vessel damage in addition to the vessel wall destruction that occurs when it enters the systemic circulation)

CLINICAL MANIFESTATIONS

Subjective	Objective
Report of feeling agitated; anxiety	Changes in mental status; agitation; confusion; hypotension; tachycardia; cool skin; restlessness; rapid respirations; pallor and cyanosis; oliguria

RISK FACTORS

- Inadequate fluid intake
- Increased toxins in the blood
- Failure of regulatory mechanisms

DESIRED OUTCOMES

The client will not develop hypovolemic shock as evidenced by:
  a. Usual mental status
  b. Stable vital signs
  c. Skin warm and usual color
  d. Palpable peripheral pulses
  e. Urine output at least 30 mL/h

NURSING ASSESSMENT

Assess for and report signs and symptoms of:
- Deficient fluid volume and third-spacing:
  - Decreased skin turgor, dry mucous membranes, thirst
  - Weight loss of 2% or greater over a short period
  - Postural hypotension and/or low B/P
  - Weak, rapid pulse
  - Capillary refill time greater than 2 to 3 seconds
  - Flat neck veins when supine
  - Change in mental status
  - Decreased urine output with increased specific gravity (reflects an actual rather than potential fluid volume deficit)
  - Increased BUN and Hct
- Bleeding (e.g., gray-blue discoloration around umbilicus [Cullen's sign], green-blue or purple-blue discoloration of flanks [Grey Turner's sign], increased abdominal or back pain, increased abdominal girth, decreasing B/P and increased pulse rate, decreased Hct and Hgb levels)
- Hypovolemic shock:
  - Restlessness, agitation, confusion, or other change in mental status
  - Significant decrease in B/P
  - Postural hypotension
  - Rapid, weak pulse
  - Rapid respirations
  - Cool skin
  - Pallor, cyanosis
  - Diminished or absent peripheral pulses
  - Urine output less than 30 mL/h

RATIONALE

Early recognition of signs and symptoms of hypovolemic shock allows for prompt intervention.

THERAPEUTIC INTERVENTIONS	RATIONALE

Dependent/Collaborative Actions

Implement measures to prevent hypovolemic shock:

- Perform actions to prevent or treat imbalanced fluid and electrolytes.
- Perform actions to reduce pancreatic stimulation (e.g., withhold all food and oral fluid intake as ordered; insert a nasogastric tube and maintain to suction as ordered; administer histamine receptor antagonists).

Actions that decrease the amount of elastase that is activated and released into the tissue and systemic circulation and thereby decreases the risk for bleeding and loss of vascular fluid volume.

If signs and symptoms of hypovolemic shock occur:

- Place client flat in bed with legs elevated unless contraindicated.

  Placing the client in this position increases B/P and blood flow to the vital organs.
- Monitor vital signs frequently.

  Monitors changes in client's status.
- Administer oxygen as ordered.

  Maintains tissue oxygenation.
- Administer whole blood, blood products, and/or volume expanders if ordered.

  Administration of blood and blood products increases vascular fluid volume and B/P.
- Prepare client for transfer to the critical care unit and insertion of hemodynamic monitoring devices (e.g., central venous catheter, intra-arterial catheter) if indicated.

  Central monitoring of hemodynamic status can be done in the critical care unit.

⊖▶ Collaborative Diagnosis   RISK FOR PERITONITIS

Definition: Inflammation of the peritoneum

Related to:

- Escape of activated pancreatic enzymes from the pancreas into the peritoneum
- Leakage of necrotic substances into the peritoneum associated with rupture of an infected pancreatic or peripancreatic abscess or pseudocyst
- Suppuration in areas of pancreatic and peripancreatic necrosis

CLINICAL MANIFESTATIONS

Subjective	Objective
Verbalization of increasing abdominal pain; rebound tenderness; nausea	Temperature above 38°C; rigid abdomen; diminished or absent bowel sounds; tachycardia; hypotension; tachypnea; elevated WBC count

RISK FACTOR

- Exposure to pathogens

DESIRED OUTCOMES

The client will not develop peritonitis as evidenced by:
  a. Gradual resolution of abdominal pain
  b. Soft, nondistended abdomen
  c. Temperature declining toward normal
  d. Stable vital signs
  e. Decreased nausea and vomiting
  f. Gradual return of normal bowel sounds
  g. WBC count declining toward normal

NURSING ASSESSMENT	RATIONALE

Assess for and report signs and symptoms of peritonitis (e.g., increase in severity of abdominal pain; generalized abdominal pain; rebound tenderness; distended, rigid abdomen; further increase in temperature; tachycardia; tachypnea; hypotension; increased nausea and vomiting; diminished or absent bowel sounds; WBC count that increases or fails to decline toward normal).

Early recognition of signs and symptoms of peritonitis allows for prompt intervention.

Continued...

THERAPEUTIC INTERVENTIONS	RATIONALE
Dependent/Collaborative Actions Implement measures to prevent peritonitis: • Perform actions to reduce pancreatic stimulation (e.g., maintain food and oral fluid restrictions if ordered, place client in semi-Fowler's position,). **D** ✦ • Administer antimicrobials if ordered. • Prepare client for drainage or removal of infected pseudocysts and abscesses and resection of necrotic tissue if planned. If signs and symptoms of peritonitis occur: • Withhold oral intake as ordered. • Place client on bedrest in a semi-Fowler's position. • Prepare client for diagnostic tests (e.g., abdominal radiograph, computed tomography, ultrasonography) if planned. • Insert a nasogastric tube and maintain suction as ordered. • Administer antimicrobials as ordered. • Administer intravenous fluids and/or blood volume expanders if ordered to prevent or treat shock. • Prepare client for and assist with peritoneal lavage if performed.	*These actions decrease activation of the pancreatic enzymes within the pancreas and reduce the risk for their escape into the peritoneum.* *Antimicrobials treat and/or prevent infections.* *Decreases client's fear and anxiety.* *Proper positioning assists in pooling or localizing gastrointestinal contents in the pelvis rather than under the diaphragm.* *Decreases client's fear and anxiety.* *Removal of the gastric contents decreases activation of the pancreatic enzymes within the pancreas and reduces the risk for their escape into the peritoneum.* *Antimicrobials prevent and/or treat infection.* *Administration of IV fluids or blood expanders increase vascular fluid volume.* *Peritoneal lavage removes toxins from the peritoneal cavity.*

Collaborative Diagnosis   RISK FOR HYPERGLYCEMIA

Definition: Elevated serum glucose levels

Related to:
• Increased glucagon and decreased insulin output associated with damage to the pancreatic islet cells resulting from activation of pancreatic enzymes in the pancreas
• The increased glucagon, cortisol, and catecholamine output that occurs with stress

CLINICAL MANIFESTATIONS

Subjective	Objective
Verbalization of feeling hungry and tired	Polydipsia; polyuria; polyphagia; change in mental status; blood glucose level greater than 200 mg/dL

RISK FACTORS

• Failure of regulatory mechanisms
• Inadequate treatment regimen

DESIRED OUTCOMES

The client will maintain a safe blood glucose level as evidenced by:
   a. Absence of polydipsia, polyuria, and polyphagia
   b. Usual mental status
   c. Serum glucose between 60 and 200 mg/dL

NURSING ASSESSMENT	RATIONALE
Assess for and report signs and symptoms of hyperglycemia (e.g., polydipsia, polyuria, polyphagia, change in mental status, blood glucose levels >200 mg/dL or greater than the parameter specified by physician).	*Early recognition of signs and symptoms of hyperglycemia allows for prompt intervention.*

THERAPEUTIC INTERVENTIONS	RATIONALE

Dependent/Collaborative Actions

Implement measures to prevent hyperglycemia:

- Perform actions to reduce pancreatic stimulation (e.g., maintain food and oral fluid restrictions if ordered, place client in semi-Fowler's position, administer antimicrobials).

- Perform actions such as relieving discomfort, explaining all tests and procedures, and providing a restful environment in order to reduce stress.

If signs and symptoms of hyperglycemia occur:

- Administer insulin or oral hypoglycemic agents if ordered.
- Assess for and report signs and symptoms of ketoacidosis (e.g., warm, flushed skin; thirst; weakness; lethargy; hypotension; increased abdominal pain; fruity odor on breath; Kussmaul respirations; blood glucose >250 mg/dL; ketones in blood and urine; low serum pH and CO_2 content).

- If client does not have a history of diabetes or chronic pancreatitis, offer assurance that the hyperglycemia is expected to resolve as the pancreatitis does.

Decreases activation of the pancreatic enzymes within the pancreas and prevents further damage to the pancreatic islet cells.

Stress causes an increased output of epinephrine, norepinephrine, glucagon, and cortisol that results in a further increase in blood glucose levels.

Insulin and oral hypoglycemic decreases blood glucose levels.
Notification of the physician of signs and symptoms of ketoacidosis allow for modification of the treatment plan.

Collaborative Diagnosis ## RISK FOR PLEURAL EFFUSION

Definition: Accumulation of fluids within the pleural cavity

Related to:

- Increased capillary permeability of and damage to the pleural vessels associated with the escape of activated pancreatic enzymes into systemic circulation
- Passage of exudate from the peritoneal cavity to the pleural cavity through the transdiaphragmatic lymph channels

CLINICAL MANIFESTATIONS

Subjective	Objective
Verbalization of shortness of breath	Dyspnea; tachypnea; asymmetrical chest excursion; dull percussion note; diminished or absent breath sounds over the affected area; chest radiograph showing pleural effusion

RISK FACTOR

- Increased toxins in the blood

DESIRED OUTCOMES

The client will not experience pleural effusion as evidenced by:
  a. Unlabored respirations at 12 to 20 breaths/min
  b. Symmetrical chest excursion
  c. Resonant percussion note throughout lung fields
  d. Normal breath sounds

NURSING ASSESSMENT	RATIONALE

Assess for and report signs and symptoms of pleural effusion (e.g., dyspnea, chest pain, decreased chest excursion on affected side, dull percussion note and diminished or absent breath sounds over the affected area, chest radiograph showing pleural effusion).

Early recognition of signs and symptoms of pleural effusion allows for prompt intervention.

Continued...

THERAPEUTIC INTERVENTIONS	RATIONALE
Dependent/Collaborative Actions	
Implement measures to reduce pancreatic stimulation (e.g., maintain food and oral fluid restrictions if ordered, place client in semi-Fowler's position, administer antimicrobials).	*These actions reduce the release of activated pancreatic enzymes into the systemic circulation and transdiaphragmatic lymph channels.*
If signs and symptoms of pleural effusion occur, prepare client for thoracentesis if planned.	*Removes fluid from the lungs, which increases client's ability to breathe.*

Collaborative Diagnosis RISK FOR ORGAN ISCHEMIA/DYSFUNCTION (MULTIPLE ORGAN DYSFUNCTION SYNDROME [MODS])

Definition: A life-threatening syndrome in which the body is unable to maintain homeostasis without intervention

Related to:

* Hypoperfusion of major organs associated with hypovolemic and/or septic shock if present and decreased myocardial contractility (can occur as a result of the release of myocardial depressant factor in response to the inflammatory process that occurs in pancreatitis)
* Microvascular thrombosis associated with disseminated intravascular coagulation (DIC) if it occurs (activation of clotting mechanisms can occur in response to the presence of activated proteolytic enzymes in the blood vessels and/or the procoagulant effects of some inflammatory mediators)

CLINICAL MANIFESTATIONS

Subjective	Objective
N/A	Severe hypotension; tachycardia; urine output less than 30 mL/h; dyspnea, tachypnea; altered arterial blood gas values with low PaO_2; elevated serum BUN and creatinine levels; crackles throughout lungs; changes in mental status

RISK FACTORS

* Failure of regulatory mechanisms
* Exposure to pathogens

DESIRED OUTCOMES

The client will not develop organ ischemia/dysfunction as evidenced by:
  a. Usual mental status
  b. Urine output at least 30 mL/h
  c. Unlabored respirations at 12 to 20 breaths/min
  d. Audible breath sounds without an increase in adventitious sounds
  e. Absence of new or increased abdominal pain, distention, nausea, vomiting, and diarrhea
  f. BUN and serum creatinine, aspartate aminotransferase (AST), alanine aminotransferase (ALT), and lactate dehydrogenase (LDH) levels within normal range

NURSING ASSESSMENT	RATIONALE
Assess for and report signs and symptoms of organ ischemia/dysfunction:	*Early recognition of organ ischemia/dysfunction allows for prompt intervention.*
• Cerebral ischemia (e.g., change in mental status)	
• Renal insufficiency (e.g., urine output <30 mL/h, elevated BUN and serum creatinine levels)	
• Acute respiratory distress syndrome (e.g., dyspnea, increase in respiratory rate, low SaO_2, crackles)	
• Gastrointestinal ischemia (e.g., increased abdominal pain, nausea, and abdominal distention; continued hypoactive or absent bowel sounds; development of or increased episodes of vomiting; diarrhea; hematemesis; blood in stool)	
• Liver dysfunction (e.g., increased serum AST, ALT, and LDH levels)	

THERAPEUTIC INTERVENTIONS	RATIONALE

Dependent/Collaborative Actions

Implement measures to reduce the risk for organ ischemia/dysfunction:

- Perform actions to prevent hypovolemic shock (administer fluids and electrolytes as ordered; maintain fluid intake of at least 2500 mL/day).

- Perform actions to prevent sepsis (administer antimicrobials as ordered; maintain sterile technique on all procedures; maintain adequate nutrition status).

- Perform actions to treat DIC if it occurs (e.g., implement safety precautions to prevent further bleeding; administer fresh frozen plasma, platelets, and/or cryoprecipitate if ordered; administer medications such as heparin and antithrombin III if ordered to interrupt clotting).

- Maintain intravenous therapy as ordered.
- Maintain oxygen therapy as ordered.
- Administer vasopressors (e.g., dopamine, norepinephrine) and/or positive inotropic agents (e.g., dobutamine) as ordered.

If signs and symptoms of organ ischemia/MODS occur, prepare client for transfer to critical care unit.

When pancreatic tissue dies, pancreatic enzymes and blood may escape into the abdomen causing sepsis, which subsequently leads to systemic hypoperfusion.

These actions prevent introduction of bacteria into the system; nutrition is important for the body's ability to fight off infections.

Actions maintain fluid volume, replace utilized clotting factors, and prevent injury to client.

Maintains adequate vascular fluid volume.
Maintains adequate oxygenation of tissues.
Vasopressors and positive inotropic agents cause vasoconstriction and increase the force of cardiac contractions to maintain adequate tissue perfusion and cardiac output.
Client requires intensive monitoring and care that will be received in the intensive care unit.

DISCHARGE CARE/CONTINUED CARE

Nursing Diagnosis ## DEFICIENT KNOWLEDGE NDx; INEFFECTIVE FAMILY THERAPEUTIC REGIMEN MANAGEMENT NDx; or INEFFECTIVE SELF HEALTH MANAGEMENT NDx*

Definition: Absence or deficiency of cognitive information related to specific topic (lack of specific information necessary for clients/significant others) to make informed choices regarding condition/treatment/lifestyle changes; pattern of regulating and integrating into daily living and family processes a therapeutic regimen for treatment of illness and the sequelae that are unsatisfactory for meeting specific health goals

Related to:

- Specific topic (lack of specific information necessary for clients/significant others) to make informed choices regarding condition/treatment/lifestyle changes
- Pattern of regulating and integrating into daily living and family processes a therapeutic regimen for treatment of illness and the sequelae of illness that is unsatisfactory for meeting specific health goals

CLINICAL MANIFESTATIONS

Subjective	Objective
Verbalizes inability to manage illness; verbalizes inability to follow prescribed regimen	Inaccurate follow through with instructions; inappropriate behaviors; experience of preventable complications of pancreatitis

---

*The nurse should select the diagnostic label that is most appropriate for the client's discharge teaching needs.

Continued...

RISK FACTORS

- Cognitive deficit
- Financial concerns
- Failure to take action to reduce risk factors for complications of pancreatitis
- Inability to care for oneself
- Difficulty in modifying personal habits and integrating treatments into lifestyle

DESIRED OUTCOMES

The client will:
  a. Identify ways to prevent overstimulation of and further trauma to the pancreas
  b. Verbalize an understanding of recommended dietary modifications
  c. State signs and symptoms to report to the health care provider
  d. Verbalize an understanding of and a plan for adhering in recommended follow-up care including future appointments with heath care provider and medications prescribed

NOC OUTCOMES

Knowledge: treatment regimen; knowledge: diet; knowledge: disease process

NIC INTERVENTIONS

Health system guidance; teaching: individual; teaching: disease process; teaching: prescribed diet; teaching: prescribed medication

NURSING ASSESSMENT

Assess client's knowledge base related to the disease process.
Assess for indications that the client may be unable to effectively manage the therapeutic regimen:
- Statements reflecting inability to manage care at home
- Failure to adhere to treatment plan (e.g., refusing medications)
- Statements reflecting a lack of understanding of factors that may cause further progression of pancreatitis
- Statements reflecting an unwillingness or inability to modify personal habits and integrate necessary treatments into lifestyle

RATIONALE

The client's knowledge base provides the basis for education.
Early recognition of inability to understand disease process or self-care allows for change in teaching modality.

THERAPEUTIC INTERVENTIONS

Desired Outcome: The client will identify ways to prevent overstimulation of and further trauma to the pancreas

Independent Actions
Instruct client in importance of avoiding overstimulation of the pancreas for the length of time specified by the physician (may be for a few months or for life depending on the cause of the pancreatitis and if permanent pancreatic damage has occurred).
Instruct client in ways to prevent overstimulation of and further trauma to the pancreas:
- Maintain a balanced program of rest and exercise.
- Avoid drinking alcohol.

- Adhere to recommended dietary modifications.
If indicated, provide information about and encourage use of community resources that can assist client to make necessary lifestyle changes (e.g., alcohol rehabilitation program).

Desired Outcome: The client will verbalize an understanding of recommended dietary modifications

RATIONALE

Decreases stimulation of the pancreas.
Alcohol can cause blockage of pancreatic ducts that drain into the pancreatic duct.
Prevents overstimulation of the pancreas.
Provides continuum of care postdischarge from the acute care facility.

THERAPEUTIC INTERVENTIONS	RATIONALE

Independent Actions
Instruct client regarding dietary modifications necessary to prevent overstimulation of the pancreas during the recovery period:
* Eat small, frequent meals rather than three large ones.
* Avoid foods/fluids high in fat (e.g., butter, cream, whole milk, ice cream, fried foods, gravies, nuts).
* Avoid spicy foods and caffeine-containing beverages (e.g., coffee, tea, colas).

Obtain a dietary consult if client needs assistance in planning meals that incorporate dietary modifications.

Enhances client's knowledge of foods that the client likes to eat and can tolerate.

Smaller meals require less pancreatic enzymes.
Foods/fluids high in fat increase the release of pancreatic enzymes.

Spicy foods can simulate increased release of pancreatic enzymes.

THERAPEUTIC INTERVENTIONS	RATIONALE

Desired Outcome: The client will state signs and symptoms to report to the health care provider

Independent Actions
Instruct client to report:
* Stools that float and are grayish, greasy, and foul-smelling
* Persistent or recurrent abdominal or back pain
* Nausea or vomiting
* Abdominal distention or increasing feeling of fullness
* Excessive thirst or excessive urination
* Irritability or confusion
* Continued or unexplained weight loss
* Bluish areas on the back or abdomen
* Persistent or recurrent temperature elevation
* Fever, chills
* Difficulty breathing
* Reddened, tender nodules on skin

Indicates a very high fat content resulting from impaired flow of the pancreatic enzyme lipase into the intestinal tract.
May indicate recurrence of pancreatitis as well as the complications of bleeding and infection.
These symptoms may indicate decreased insulin production and increased serum glucose levels.

May indicate bleeding within the abdomen.
These symptoms may indicate an infection.

This could be indicative of destruction of superficial tissue by activated pancreatic enzymes such as lipase and phospholipase A that have entered the systemic circulation of tissues; if this relatively rare condition occurs, it is usually weeks to months after the episode of acute pancreatitis.

THERAPEUTIC INTERVENTIONS	RATIONALE

Desired Outcome: The client will verbalize an understanding of and a plan for adhering in recommended follow-up care including future appointments with heath care provider and medications prescribed

Independent Actions
Reinforce the importance of keeping follow-up appointments with health care provider.

Explain the rationale for, side effects of, and importance of taking medications prescribed (e.g., vitamins, antimicrobials, pancreatic enzymes). Inform client of pertinent food and drug interactions.

Implement measures to improve client's compliance:
* Include significant others in teaching sessions if possible.
* Encourage questions and allow time for reinforcement and clarification of information provided.

* Provide written instructions on scheduled appointments with health care provider, medications prescribed, and signs and symptoms to report.

Allows the health care provider to monitor client's health status.

Knowledge of medications and how they impact the system improves client adherence to treatment regimen and understanding of the importance of adhering to the prescribed medication regimen. The client must be able to recognize alterations in functioning related to medication administration and know what clinical manifestations should be reported to the health care provider.

Allows for others to support client as needed.
Allows for a more complete understanding of the client's condition by client and significant others and for the nurse to evaluate client's knowledge of the treatment regimen.
Written instructions provide an information resource following discharge from the acute care facility.

NDx = NANDA-I Diagnosis   **D** = Delegatable Action   ● = UAP   ✦ = LVN/LPN   ⊖▶ = Go to ⊖volve for animation

ADDITIONAL DIAGNOSES

IMPAIRED ORAL MUCOUS MEMBRANE: DRYNESS NDx

Related to:

- Deficient fluid volume associated with restricted oral intake and fluid loss resulting from vomiting and nasogastric tube drainage
- Decreased salivation associated with deficient fluid volume, restricted oral intake, and the side effect of some medications (e.g., narcotic [opioid] analgesics, some antiemetics)
- Mouth breathing if nasogastric tube is in place

FEAR AND ANXIETY NDx

Related to:

- Severe pain
- Unfamiliar environment
- Lack of understanding of diagnostic tests, treatment plan, and prognosis

11 The Client with Alterations in the Kidney and Urinary Tract

BLADDER NECK SUSPENSION (VESICOURETHRAL SUSPENSION)

A bladder neck suspension is a surgical procedure performed to restore the bladder neck and proximal urethra to a well-supported retropubic position. It is performed to correct anatomical urinary stress incontinence associated with excessive mobility of the urethra and/or lowering of the position of the bladder neck (vesicourethral segment) resulting from pelvic floor weakness. The surgery is indicated when conservative measures for treating stress incontinence (e.g., pelvic floor exercises, biofeedback, estrogen therapy, sympathomimetic agents, periurethral bulking) have failed to produce significant improvement.

A number of techniques can be used to suspend the bladder neck and proximal urethra to their proper retropubic position. Most of these techniques involve placement of sutures in the periurethral and/or vaginal fascia and anchoring the sutures to the underside of the pubic symphysis or to an endopelvic ligament or muscle. Another procedure, considered by some authorities to be a bladder neck suspension technique, is called a pubovaginal or suburethral sling and involves the creation of a sling using a ribbon of fascia or synthetic material. This sling is then passed below the urethra and anchored to the urethropelvic ligament and/or vesicopelvic fascia. The approaches that are used for bladder suspension surgery include an abdominal approach (e.g., Marshall-Marchetti-Krantz, Burch), a vaginal approach in combination with suprapubic laparoscopy (e.g., Stamey, Raz), or a "no incision" laparoscopic approach (e.g., Gittes). The particular surgery and the approach selected depend on the physiological condition of the client, the type of incontinence present, previous pelvic surgeries the client has had,

the presence of associated pelvic floor abnormalities (e.g., uterine prolapse, cystocele, rectocele), and the need for additional abdominal surgery.

This care plan focuses on the adult client having bladder neck suspension surgery. If repair of a cystocele and/or rectocele is planned concurrently, use this care plan in conjunction with the Care Plan on Colporrhaphy.

OUTCOME/DISCHARGE CRITERIA

The client will:
1. Have evidence of normal healing of surgical wound(s)
2. Have adequate urine output
3. Have no evidence of wound or urinary tract infection
4. Have no signs and symptoms of postoperative complications
5. Demonstrate care of suprapubic catheter if present
6. Demonstrate the ability to measure residual urine
7. State signs and symptoms to report to the health care provider
8. Verbalize an understanding of and a plan for adhering to recommended follow-up care including future appointments with health care provider, medications prescribed, activity restrictions, and measures to prevent constipation

Preoperative—Refer to Standardized Preoperative Care Plan.
Postoperative—Use in conjunction with the Standardized Postoperative Care Plan.

Nursing Diagnosis **URINARY RETENTION** NDx

Definition: Incomplete emptying of the bladder

Related to:
- Obstruction of the urethral and/or suprapubic catheters if present
- Impaired urination after removal of the catheter(s) associated with:
  - Edema of the bladder neck and urethra resulting from surgical trauma
  - Increased tone of the urinary sphincters resulting from sympathetic nervous system stimulation (can result from pain, fear, and anxiety)

NDx = NANDA-I Diagnosis   **D** = Delegatable Action   ● = UAP   ✦ = LVN/LPN   ⊖▶ = Go to ⊖volve for animation   709

Continued...
- Decreased perception of bladder fullness resulting from the depressant effect of anesthesia and some medications (e.g., narcotic [opioid] analgesics)
- Relaxation of the bladder muscle resulting from the depressant effect of anesthesia and some medications (e.g., narcotic [opioid] analgesics) and stimulation of the sympathetic nervous system (can result from pain, fear, and anxiety)
- Urethral obstruction resulting from excessive elevation of the bladder neck

CLINICAL MANIFESTATIONS

Subjective	Objective
Verbalization of sensation of bladder fullness	Bladder distention; small, frequent voiding or absence of urine output; dysuria; dribbling of urine; residual urine; overflow incontinence

RISK FACTORS
- Surgery
- Preoperative poor bladder tone

DESIRED OUTCOMES

The client will not experience urinary retention as evidenced by:
  a. No reports of bladder fullness and suprapubic discomfort
  b. Absence of bladder distention and dribbling of urine
  c. Balanced intake and output 48 hours after surgery
  d. Voiding adequate amounts at expected intervals after removal of the catheter(s)

NOC OUTCOMES

Urinary elimination

NIC INTERVENTIONS

Urinary retention care; tube care: urinary; urinary catheterization: intermittent

NURSING ASSESSMENT

Assess for and report the following:
- Urinary retention when suprapubic and/or urethral catheters are present (e.g., reports of bladder fullness or suprapubic discomfort, bladder distention, absence of fluid in urinary drainage tubing, output that continues to be less than intake 48 hours after surgery)
- Urinary retention after catheter removal (e.g., reports of bladder fullness or suprapubic discomfort, bladder distention, output that continues to be less than intake 48 hours after surgery, frequent voiding of small amounts [25-60 mL] of urine).

RATIONALE

Early recognition of the signs and symptoms of urinary retention allows for prompt intervention.

THERAPEUTIC INTERVENTIONS

Independent Actions
Implement measures to prevent urinary retention:
- Perform actions to maintain patency of urinary catheter(s):
  - Keep drainage tubing free of kinks. **D** ● ✦
  - Keep collection container below level of bladder. **D** ● ✦
  - Tape catheter tubing securely (suprapubic catheter tubing to abdomen, urethral catheter tubing to thigh).
  - Irrigate catheter if ordered. **D** ✦
- After urethral catheter is removed, open suprapubic catheter as scheduled or if client is unable to void voluntarily.

RATIONALE

Kink free tubing prevents backup of urine within the catheter(s).

Securely taping the catheter tubing prevents inadvertent removal.

Prevents blockage of catheter.
If the client feels the urge to urinate but suppresses it by contracting the external urinary sphincter, the urge will subside and not recur until the bladder fills more. If the client repeatedly suppresses the urge to urinate and the bladder fills too much or is chronically distended, the micturition reflex becomes less sensitive and does not effectively stimulate urination when the bladder fills.

THERAPEUTIC INTERVENTIONS	RATIONALE
• When both urethral and suprapubic catheters have been removed: • Instruct client to urinate when the urge is first felt. Implement measures to promote relaxation during voiding attempts (e.g., provide privacy, hold a warm blanket against abdomen, administer prescribed analgesic if client has pain, encourage client to read).	*A client who is relaxed when trying to urinate is better able to relax the pelvic floor muscles and external urinary sphincter and allow voiding to occur.*
If the client is having difficulty voiding, run water, place hands in warm water, and/or pour warm water over perineum unless contraindicated. **D** ● ✦	*These measures have been found to trigger the micturition reflex and thereby promote voiding. They also promote a sense of relaxation, which facilitates voiding.*
Allow client to assume a normal position for voiding (usually sitting for females and standing for males) unless contraindicated. **D** ● ✦	*A sitting or standing position uses gravity to facilitate bladder emptying. Allowing the client to assume a normal voiding position also promotes relaxation, which facilitates voiding.*
• Perform intermittent catheterization as ordered if post-voiding residual urine exceeds the established parameter (usually 50-100 mL). **D** ✦	*Intermittent catheterization as indicated prevents bladder distention.*

Nursing Diagnosis   RISK FOR CONSTIPATION NDx

Definition: A decrease in normal frequency of defecation accompanied by difficult or incomplete passage of stool and/or passage of excessively hard, dry stool.

Related to:
• Decreased gastrointestinal motility associated with manipulation of the bowel (if an abdominal approach was used), decreased activity, and the depressant effect of the anesthetic and narcotic (opioid) analgesics
• Reluctance to defecate associated with fear of pain and possible disruption of sutures

CLINICAL MANIFESTATIONS

Subjective	Objective
Verbalization of straining with defecation; feeling of rectal fullness or pressure; abdominal pain inability to pass stool; headache; indigestion nausea; abdominal tenderness	Change in bowel pattern; bright red blood with stool; presence of soft, pastelike stool in rectum; distended abdomen; dark, black, or tarry stool; increased abdominal pressure; percussed abdominal dullness; pain with defecation; decreased volume of stool; decreased frequency; dry, hard, formed stool; palpable rectal mass; anorexia; change in abdominal growling (borborygmi); atypical presentation in older adults (e.g., change in mental status, urinary incontinence, unexplained falls, elevated body temperature); severe flatus hypoactive or hyperactive bowel sounds; palpable abdominal mass; abdominal tenderness with or without palpable muscle resistance; vomiting; oozing liquid stool

RISK FACTORS
• Immobility
• Lack of fiber in pre-operative diet
• Inadequate fluid replacement

DESIRED OUTCOMES

The client will maintain usual bowel elimination pattern as evidenced by:
 a. Usual frequency of bowel movements
 b. Passage of soft, formed stool
 c. Absence of abdominal distention and pain, feeling of rectal fullness or pressure, and straining during defecation

Continued...

NOC OUTCOMES	NIC INTERVENTIONS
Bowel elimination; gastrointestinal function; hydration; symptom control	Constipation/impaction management

NURSING ASSESSMENT	RATIONALE
Ascertain client's usual bowel elimination habits.	*Knowledge of the client's usual bowel elimination habits is essential in determining whether constipation is present because the frequency of defecation varies among individuals.*
Assess for signs and symptoms of constipation: • Decrease in frequency of bowel movements • Passage of hard, formed stools • Anorexia • Abdominal distention and pain • Feeling of fullness or pressure in rectum • Straining during defecation	*Early recognition of signs and symptoms of constipation allows for prompt intervention.*
Assess bowel sounds. Report a pattern of decreasing bowel sounds.	*Bowel sounds are produced by peristaltic activity. A pattern of decreasing bowel sounds indicates a decrease in bowel motility, which can lead to and be present with constipation.*

THERAPEUTIC INTERVENTIONS	RATIONALE

Independent Actions

Encourage client to defecate whenever the urge is felt. **D** ✦	*If the client feels the urge to defecate but suppresses it by contracting the external anal sphincter, the defecation reflex will subside after a few minutes and not recur for several hours or until additional feces enters the rectum. Repeated inhibition of the defecation reflex results in progressive weakening of the reflex. In addition, when the defecation reflex is inhibited, feces remain in the colon longer and water continues to be absorbed from the feces, making the stool drier, harder, and subsequently more difficult to evacuate.*
Assist client to toilet or bedside commode or place in high-Fowler's position on bedpan for bowel movements unless contraindicated. **D** ● ✦	*A sitting position aids in the expulsion of stool by taking advantage of gravity. This position also enhances the client's ability to perform the Valsalva maneuver, which increased intra-abdominal pressure and forces the fecal contents downward and into the rectum where the defecation reflex is then elicited.*
Encourage client to relax, provide privacy, and have call signal within reach during attempts to defecate. **D** ● ✦	*Measures that promote relaxation enable the client to relax the levator ani muscle and external anal sphincter, which facilitates evacuation of stool.*
Instruct client to increase intake of foods high in fiber (e.g., bran, whole-grain breads and cereals, fresh fruits and vegetables) unless contraindicated.	*Foods high in fiber provide bulk to the fecal mass and keep the stool soft because of the ability of fiber to absorb water. This stimulates peristalsis, which promotes more rapid movement of stool through the colon.*
Encourage client to drink hot liquids (e.g., coffee, tea) upon arising in the morning.	*Ingestion of hot fluids can stimulate peristalsis.*

Dependent/Collaborative Actions

Instruct client to maintain a minimal fluid intake of 2500 mL/day unless contraindicated.	*Inadequate fluid intake reduces the water content of feces which results in a hard, dry stool that is difficult to evacuate.*
Increase activity as allowed and tolerated.	*Ambulation stimulates peristalsis, which promotes the passage of stool through the intestines.*
Instruct client to request an analgesic before attempting to defecate.	*This eases the surgical site pain associated with increased intra-abdominal perineal pressure that occurs with defecation.*
Consult physician about an order for a stool softener if one has not been ordered.	*Makes passage of stool easier after surgery.*

Collaborative Diagnosis   RISK FOR BLADDER, URETHRAL, OR URETERAL INJURY

Definition: Surgery-related bladder injury

Related to: Accidental tear or ligation during the surgical procedure

CLINICAL MANIFESTATIONS

Subjective	Objective
Verbalization of back pain	Hematuria; significantly increased urine output

RISK FACTOR	DESIRED OUTCOMES
• Surgical procedure	The client will experience healing of bladder, urethral, or ureteral injury if it occurs as evidenced by: a. Gradual resolution of hematuria and backache b. Urine output greater than 200 mL within 6 to 8 hours after surgery

NURSING ASSESSMENT	RATIONALE
Assess for and report signs and symptoms of bladder, urethral, or ureteral injury (e.g., persistent or increasing hematuria or backache, urine output less than 200 mL in first 6-8 hours after surgery).	*Early recognition of signs and symptoms of urinary tract injury allows for prompt intervention.*

THERAPEUTIC INTERVENTIONS	RATIONALE
Independent Actions If signs and symptoms of bladder, urethral, or ureteral injury are present: • Continue to monitor output carefully. • Prepare client for surgical repair if indicated.	*Changes in output may indicate an injury to the urinary tract.* *Decreases fear and anxiety*

Collaborative Diagnosis   RISK FOR URINARY TRACT INFECTION; WOUND INFECTION

Definition: At risk for invasion of the body by pathogenic organisms

Urinary tract infection
Related to:

- Increased growth and colonization of microorganisms associated with urinary stasis
- Introduction of pathogens associated with the presence of urethral and/or suprapubic catheters and performance of intermittent catheterizations if being done

Wound infection
Related to:

- Wound contamination associated with introduction of pathogens during or after surgery (particularly high risk with a vaginal approach because of the proximity of the incision to the perianal area)
- Decreased resistance to infection associated with factors such as diminished blood flow to wound area or an inadequate nutritional status

CLINICAL MANIFESTATIONS

Subjective	Objective
Verbalization of frequency, urgency, and burning upon urination; chills	Elevated temperature; urinalysis—increased white blood cells (WBCs) and presence of bacteria; positive urine cultures

Continued...

RISK FACTORS

- Poor surgical hygiene
- Surgical procedure

DESIRED OUTCOMES

The client will remain free of urinary tract and/or infection as evidenced by:
   a. Clear urine
   b. Absence of frequency, urgency, and burning on urination
   c. Absence of chills and fever
   d. Urinalysis slowing fewer than 5 WBCs, negative leukocyte esterase and nitrates, and absence of bacteria
   e. No redness, swelling or drainage from surgical site
   f. Negative urine cultures

NURSING ASSESSMENT

Assess for and report signs and symptoms of urinary tract infection:
- Cloudy urine
- Reports of frequency or urgency, or burning on urination
- Chills
- Elevated temperature
- Urinalysis showing greater than 5 WBCs per high-power field, positive leukocyte esterase or nitrates, or presence of bacteria
- Positive urine culture

RATIONALE

Early recognition of signs and symptoms of urinary tract infection allows for prompt intervention.

THERAPEUTIC INTERVENTIONS

Independent Actions
Implement measures to prevent urinary tract infection:
- Perform actions to prevent urinary retention (e.g., instruct client to urinate when the urge is first felt, provide privacy for urination, hold a warm blanket against the abdomen, encourage client to relax if possible, run warm water, pour warm water over perineal area). **D** ✦
- Instruct female client to wipe from front to back after urinating or defecating. **D** ✦
- Assist client with perineal care routinely and after each bowel movement. **D** ● ✦

RATIONALE

These actions reduce the risk of urinary stasis and subsequent urinary tract infection.

Personal hygiene performed in this manner reduces the risk for wound infection if a vaginal incision is present.
Proper perineal care removes pathogens from the perineal area.

DISCHARGE TEACHING/CONTINUED CARE

Nursing Diagnosis

DEFICIENT KNOWLEDGE NDx; INEFFECTIVE FAMILY THERAPEUTIC REGIMEN MAINTENANCE NDx; OR INEFFECTIVE SELF-HEALTH MANAGEMENT* NDx

Definition: Absence or deficiency of cognitive information related to specific topic (lack of specific information necessary for clients/significant others) to make informed choices regarding condition/treatment/lifestyle changes; Pattern of regulating and integrating into daily living and family processes a therapeutic regimen for treatment of illness and the sequelae of illness that is unsatisfactory for meeting specific health goals

*The nurse should select the diagnostic label that is most appropriate for the client's discharge teaching needs.

CLINICAL MANIFESTATIONS

Subjective	Objective
Verbalizes inability to manage illness; verbalizes inability to follow prescribed regimen	Inaccurate follow through with instructions; inappropriate behaviors; experience of preventable complications of following surgery.

RISK FACTORS

- Cognitive deficit
- Financial concerns
- Failure to take action to reduce risk factors for posts operative complications
- Inability to care for oneself
- Difficulty in modifying personal habits and integrating treatments into lifestyle

NOC OUTCOMES	NIC INTERVENTIONS
Knowledge: treatment regimen	Health system guidance; teaching: individual; teaching: psychomotor skill; teaching: disease process

NURSING ASSESSMENT	RATIONALE
Assess the client's ability to learn and readiness to learn Assess the client's understanding of teaching	*Learning is more effective when the client is motivated and understands the importance of what is to be learned. Readiness to learn changes based on situations, physical and emotional challenges.*

THERAPEUTIC INTERVENTIONS	RATIONALE

Desired Outcome: The client will demonstrate care of suprapubic catheter if present.

Independent Actions
Provide the following instructions about care of suprapubic catheter if client is discharged with one in place:
- Tape catheter securely to abdomen.
- Keep skin around catheter insertion site clean and dry.
- Keep drainage tubing free of kinks.
- Keep collection bag below level of bladder.

Allow time for questions, clarification, and return demonstration.

The client needs to know how to appropriately care for the suprapubic catheter to prevent it from becoming dislodged, to promote drainage, and to prevent insertion site or urinary tract infection.

Improves client's understanding of treatment regimen and confidence in ability to care for self.

THERAPEUTIC INTERVENTIONS	RATIONALE

Desired Outcome: The client will demonstrate the ability to measure residual urine.

Independent Actions
Provide the following instructions about how to measure residual urine (the client who needs to measure residual urine and does not have a suprapubic catheter will need to be instructed on how to perform self-catheterization):
- Unclamp the suprapubic catheter after urinating or at prescribed intervals (usually every 4 hours if unable to urinate).
- Leave the suprapubic catheter unclamped for 10 minutes, reclamp the catheter, and then empty the bag and measure the amount of urine.
- Measure and record the amount of urine voided and the amount of residual urine.

The client measures residual urine to determine when the catheter may be removed. The client should be given step-by-step instructions on how to measure residual urine.

Continued...

THERAPEUTIC INTERVENTIONS	RATIONALE
Instruct client to contact physician's office once the residual urine amounts are consistently less than 100 mL for 2 consecutive days.	*Residual urine less that 100 mL for 2 consecutive days indicates that the suprapubic catheter is ready to be removed.*
Allow time for questions, clarification, and return demonstration.	*Improves client's understanding of treatment regimen and confidence in ability to care for self.*

THERAPEUTIC INTERVENTIONS	RATIONALE

Desired Outcome: The client will state signs and symptoms to report to the health care provider.

Independent Actions

Instruct client to report these additional signs and symptoms:	*These clinical manifestations should be reported to the health care provider because they indicate a potential surgical complication.*
• Difficulty breathing	*Indicates a possible pulmonary embolism.*
• Productive cough of discolored sputum	*Indicates a possible infection.*
• Unusual or excessive drainage from the wound site	
• Pain or swelling in the calf of one or both legs	*Indicates a deep vein thrombosis.*
• Stress incontinence	*Indicates possible urinary retention.*
• Unusual and continuous abdominal or pelvic pain	*May indicate an infection.*
• Temperature above 38° C (100.4° F)	*Indicates a possible infection.*
• Persistent bright red vaginal bleeding or clots	*Indicates possible rupture of vaginal sutures if sutures were used.*
• Persistent inability to void voluntarily	*Indicates possible infection and lack of nervous stimulation to void.*
• Persistent residual urine amounts in excess of 100 mL	*Indicates inability of the client to completely empty the bladder.*

THERAPEUTIC INTERVENTIONS	RATIONALE

Desired Outcome: The client will verbalize an understanding of and a plan for adhering to recommended follow-up care including future appointments with health care provider, medications prescribed, activity restrictions, and measures to prevent constipation.

Independent Actions

Instruct client to avoid vigorous exercise and lifting objects over 15 lb until healing is complete (about 6 weeks).	*Vigorous exercise and lifting more than 15 lb creates increased pressure on the abdominal muscles and may cause dehiscence of the suture line.*
If client has a vaginal incision, instruct her to:	*These actions help prevent infection.*
• Perform good perineal hygiene, particularly after defecation.	
• Avoid inserting anything into vagina (e.g., tampons, douches) or having sexual intercourse until advised by physician (usually for 6 weeks).	
• Reinforce measures to prevent constipation:	*These actions decrease incidence of constipation.*
• Drink 8 to 10 glasses of water a day unless contraindicated.	
• Eat foods that are high in fiber (e.g., fresh fruits and vegetables, whole-grain cereals).	
• Take 1 to 2 stool softeners (e.g., Dialose) a day.	
Instruct client to contact physician's office or follow physician's instructions regarding the appropriate measures to take if there is a 2-day span without a bowel movement.	*The physician may recommend that the client self-administer a small-volume enema or laxative suppository.*

CYSTECTOMY WITH URINARY DIVERSION

Cystectomy is the removal of the bladder and is accompanied by a procedure to divert urinary flow. It may be performed to treat a malignancy of the bladder, congenital bladder anomalies, neurogenic bladder, and irreparable bladder trauma. A cystectomy may also be performed to prevent further deterioration of renal function associated with chronic bladder infection. In some cases, the surgery includes removal of just the bladder (simple cystectomy), but when there is an invasive malignancy, a more radical procedure is performed. In men, a radical cystectomy usually includes removal of the bladder, prostate, seminal vesicles, a portion of the vas deferens, and some or all of the pelvic lymph nodes. In women, a radical cystectomy usually includes removal of the bladder, urethra, uterus, fallopian tubes, ovaries, a portion of the anterior vaginal wall, and some or all of the pelvic lymph nodes.

There are several ways to accomplish urinary diversion. The most common surgical method is the conventional conduit (incontinent urinary diversion). In this procedure, the ureters are implanted in a portion of a resected segment of intestine and then the end of the segment is brought through the abdominal wall to create a stoma. Because no valves are incorporated into the construction of the conventional conduit, drops of urine usually flow from the stoma every few seconds, resulting in the client's need to wear a urinary collection appliance at all times.

The second most common surgical method to accomplish urinary diversion is the continent internal reservoir (e.g., Kock pouch, Mainz pouch, Indiana pouch). In this method, the ureters are implanted in a resected portion of intestine that has been remodeled to create a reservoir. Another segment of the reservoir is used to create the stoma that is brought out through the abdominal wall. The reflux of urine from the reservoir back through the ureters and the uncontrolled flow of urine from the reservoir through the stoma are prevented by the surgical positioning of the ureters, reservoir, and stoma or by the construction of one-way valves at these sites. After healing occurs, a catheter is inserted into the stoma at regularly scheduled intervals (usually every 4-6 hours once the reservoir stretches to its full capacity) to drain the reservoir. If the system functions properly, the client does not need to wear a urinary collection appliance over the stoma.

Two less commonly used methods of urinary diversion are cutaneous ureterostomy (direct implantation of the ureters into the abdominal wall) and nephrostomy (insertion of catheters into the kidneys via flank incisions). These methods are usually reserved for clients who cannot tolerate lengthy surgery and/or have a short life expectancy.

The type of urinary diversion selected depends on many factors including the client's preference, age, body build, ability to learn about and participate in care of the urinary diversion, prognosis, and ability to tolerate lengthy surgery; the integrity of the client's ureters, kidneys, and intestinal tract; the advice of the enterostomal therapy nurse; and the expertise of the surgeon.

This care plan focuses on the adult client hospitalized for a cystectomy with urinary diversion by means of a conventional conduit. Some additional nursing interventions are also included for the client with a continent internal reservoir. Much of the postoperative information is applicable to clients receiving follow-up care in an extended care facility or home setting.

OUTCOME/DISCHARGE CRITERIA

The client will:
1. Maintain an adequate urine output via the urinary diversion
2. Have surgical pain controlled
3. Have evidence of normal healing of surgical wound
4. Have a medium pink to red, moist stoma and intact peristomal skin
5. Have no signs and symptoms of postoperative complications
6. Verbalize a basic understanding of the anatomical changes that have occurred as a result of the surgery
7. Demonstrate the ability to change the urostomy appliance and maintain stomal and peristomal skin integrity
8. Demonstrate the ability to properly clean reusable urostomy equipment
9. Demonstrate the ability to drain and irrigate a continent internal reservoir if present
10. Identify ways to control odor of the urostomy drainage and appliance
11. Identify ways to prevent urinary tract infection
12. State signs and symptoms to report to the health care provider
13. Share thoughts and feelings about altered urinary elimination and its effect on body image and lifestyle
14. Identify appropriate community resources that can assist with home management and adjustment to changes resulting from the urinary diversion
15. Verbalize an understanding of and a plan for adhering to recommended follow-up care including future appointments with health care provider, wound care, activity level, and medications prescribed

For a full, detailed care plan on this topic, go to http://evolve.elsevier.com/Haugen/careplanning/.

NEPHRECTOMY

Nephrectomy is the surgical removal of the kidney. Conditions that are commonly treated by nephrectomy include renal carcinoma, massive traumatic injury to the kidney, polycystic kidney disease (especially if the kidney is bleeding or severely infected), calculi, renal tuberculosis, pyelonephritis, glomerulonephritis, and renal sclerosis resulting from hypertension. The kidney may also be removed for the purpose of donation.

The surgical approach used to perform a nephrectomy depends on the extensiveness of the planned surgery; the client's age, body build, and physiological status; the underlying pathology; and prior surgical incisions. The approach commonly used for a simple nephrectomy (removal of just the kidney) is the subcostal flank approach. Other approaches (e.g., thoracoabdominal, transabdominal, dorsolumbar) may be necessary when greater visualization, improved access, or

Continued...

a radical nephrectomy (removal of the kidney, renal artery and vein, adrenal gland, proximal ureter, regional lymph nodes, and surrounding fat and fascia) is necessary. Although it is most often necessary to remove the entire kidney, advances in renal imaging, earlier diagnosis of renal disease, and improved surgical techniques have provided surgeons with an option of performing a partial nephrectomy (nephron-sparing nephrectomy) in some instances. In these situations, a laparoscopic rather than an open approach is often feasible.

This care plan focuses on the adult client hospitalized for a simple unilateral nephrectomy. Much of the postoperative information is applicable to clients receiving follow-up care in an extended care facility or home setting. The care plan will need to be individualized according to the client's diagnosis, prognosis, and plans for subsequent treatment.

OUTCOME/DISCHARGE CRITERIA

The client will:
1. Have evidence of normal healing of the surgical wound
2. Have adequate functioning of the remaining kidney
3. Have clear, audible breath sounds throughout lungs
4. Have no signs and symptoms of postoperative complications
5. Verbalize ways to maintain health of the remaining kidney
6. State signs and symptoms to report to the health care provider
7. Share thoughts and feelings about the loss of the kidney
8. Verbalize an understanding of and a plan for adhering to recommended follow-up care including future appointments with health care provider, medications prescribed, activity level, wound care, and plans for subsequent treatment of the underlying disorder.

See Standardized Preoperative and Postoperative Care Plans for additional diagnoses.

Nursing Diagnosis **INEFFECTIVE BREATHING PATTERN** NDx

Definition: Inspiration and/or expiration that does not provide adequate ventilation

Related to:
- Increased rate of respirations associated with fear and anxiety
- Decreased rate of respirations associated with the depressant effect of anesthesia and some medications (e.g., narcotic [opioid] analgesics, some antiemetics)
- Decreased depth of respirations associated with:
  - Depressant effect of anesthesia and some medications (e.g., narcotic [opioid] analgesics, some antiemetics)
  - Reluctance to breathe deeply resulting from incisional pain and fear of dislodging chest tube if present (a chest tube is usually inserted after a thoracoabdominal approach and may be needed after a flank approach)
  - Positioning, weakness, fatigue, and elevation of the diaphragm (can occur if abdominal distention is present)

CLINICAL MANIFESTATIONS

Subjective	Objective
Verbal report of shortness of breath and difficulty breathing	Alterations in depth of breathing; altered chest excursion; bradypnea; decreased minute ventilation; use of accessory muscles to breathe

RISK FACTORS	DESIRED OUTCOMES

• Surgery
• Obesity
• Immobility
	The client will maintain an effective breathing pattern as evidenced by:
	  a. Normal rate and depth of respirations
	  b. Absence of dyspnea

NOC OUTCOMES	NIC INTERVENTIONS
Respiratory status: ventilation	Respiratory monitoring; ventilation assistance

NURSING ASSESSMENT	RATIONALE
Assess for signs and symptoms of the following: • Ineffective breathing pattern • Shallow or slow respirations • Limited chest excursion • Tachypnea or dyspnea • Use of accessory muscles when breathing	*Early recognition of signs and symptoms of an ineffective breathing pattern allows for prompt intervention.*

NURSING ASSESSMENT	RATIONALE
Assess/monitor pulse oximetry (arterial oxygen saturation [SaO$_2$]), arterial blood gas (ABG) values as indicated.	Monitoring continuous SaO$_2$ readings allows for the early detection of hypoxia. Assessment of ABG values allows for a more direct measurement of both the partial pressure of oxygen in arterial blood (PaO$_2$) and the partial pressure of carbon dioxide in arterial blood (PcCO$_2$), both of which reflect the adequacy of ventilation.

THERAPEUTIC INTERVENTIONS	RATIONALE

Independent Actions

Implement measures to improve breathing pattern:

- Perform actions to reduce fear and anxiety:
  - Promote a calm, restful environment. **D** ● ✦
  - Assure client that deep breathing will not dislodge chest tube if present. **D** ✦

  Reducing fear and anxiety helps prevent shallow and/or rapid breathing.

- Perform actions to reduce pain:
  - Reposition client for comfort. **D** ● ✦
  - Instruct and assist client to support incision when moving or coughing.

  Reducing pain helps increase the client's willingness to move and breathe more deeply.

- Perform actions to reduce the accumulation of gas and fluid in the gastrointestinal tract:
  - Maintain patency of nasogastric, gastric, or intestinal tubes if present. **D** ✦

  Reducing the accumulation of gas in the gastrointestinal tract decreases pressure on the diaphragm, facilitating more effective ventilation.

- Perform actions to increase strength and improve activity tolerance:
  - Implement measures to conserve energy. **D** ● ✦

  Increasing activity tolerance enables the client to breathe more deeply and participate in activities to improve breathing pattern.

- Assist client to deep breathe or use incentive spirometer every 1 to 2 hours. **D** ✦

  Deep breathing and use of an incentive spirometer promote maximal inhalation and lung expansion.

- Instruct client to breathe slowly if hyperventilating.

  Hyperventilation is an ineffective breathing pattern that can lead to respiratory alkalosis. A client can often slow breathing rate by concentrating on doing so.

- Place client in a semi- to high-Fowler's position unless contraindicated. **D** ● ✦

  A semi- to high-Fowler's position allows for maximal diaphragmatic excursion and lung expansion.

- If client must remain flat in bed, assist with position change at least every 2 hours. **D** ● ✦

  Compression of the thorax and subsequent limited chest wall expansion occur when the client lies in one position. Frequent repositioning promotes maximal chest wall and lung expansion.

- Provide pillow support between lower costal margin and iliac crest when client is lying on operative side. **D** ● ✦

  Decreases strain on flank incision and subsequently increases the ease of deep breathing

Dependent/Collaborative Actions

Implement measures to improve breathing pattern:

- Increase activity as allowed and tolerated. **D** ● ✦

  During activity, especially ambulation, the client usually takes deeper breaths, thus increasing lung expansion.

- Assist with positive airway pressure techniques if ordered:
  - Continuous positive airway pressure (CPAP)
  - Bilevel positive airway pressure (BiPAP)
  - Flutter/positive expiratory pressure (PEP) device

  Positive airway pressure techniques increase intrapulmonary (alveolar) pressure, which helps reexpand collapsed alveoli and prevent further alveoli collapse.

- Administer central nervous system depressants judiciously:
  - Hold medication and consult physician if respiratory rate is less than 12 breaths/min. **D** ✦

  Central nervous system depressants cause depression of the respiratory center in the brainstem, which can result in a decreased rate and depth of respiration.

- Perform actions to reduce pain:
  - Administer analgesics before activities and procedures that can cause pain and before pain becomes severe. **D** ✦

  Reducing pain helps increase the client's willingness to move and breathe more deeply.

NDx = NANDA-I Diagnosis   **D** = Delegatable Action   ● = UAP   ✦ = LVN/LPN   ⊖▶ = Go to ⊖volve for animation

Continued...

THERAPEUTIC INTERVENTIONS	RATIONALE
Consult appropriate health care provider if: • Ineffective breathing pattern continues. • Client develops signs and symptoms of impaired gas exchange such as restlessness, irritability, confusion, significant decrease in oximetry results, decreased PaO$_2$ and increased PaCO$_2$ levels.	*Notifying the appropriate health care provider allows for modification of treatment plan.*

Collaborative Diagnosis   RISK FOR HYPOVOLEMIC SHOCK

Definition: A form of shock in which the blood volume is so significantly decreased that the heart is unable to supply blood to the body

Related to: Excessive blood loss during surgery (the renal area is highly vascular) and hemorrhage after surgery

CLINICAL MANIFESTATIONS

Subjective	Objective
Report of feeling lightheaded or dizzy	Confusion; agitation; restlessness; hypotension; tachycardia; urine output less than 30 mL/h; cool skin; diminished or absent peripheral pulses; pallor; cyanosis

RISK FACTORS
• Failure of regulatory mechanisms
• Inadequate fluid volume replacement

DESIRED OUTCOMES

The client will not develop hypovolemic shock as evidenced by:
a. Usual mental status
b. Stable vital signs
c. Skin warm and usual color
d. Palpable peripheral pulses
e. Urine output at least 30 mL/h

NURSING ASSESSMENT	RATIONALE
Assess for and report signs and symptoms of hypovolemic shock: • Restlessness, agitation, confusion, or other change in mental status • Significant decrease in blood pressure (B/P) • Postural hypotension • Rapid, weak pulse • Rapid respirations • Cool skin • Pallor, cyanosis • Diminished or absent peripheral pulses • Urine output less than 30 mL/h	*Early recognition of signs and symptoms of hypovolemic shock allows for prompt of intervention.*
Monitor hemoglobin (Hgb), hematocrit (Hct), and prothrombin time (PT)/partial thromboplastin time (PTT) values.	*Elevated clotting times may contribute to postoperative hemorrhage and hypovolemic shock. Monitoring Hgb/Hct and PT/PTT will allow for implementation of the appropriate interventions.*
Monitory hemodynamic values if present: • Central venous pressure (CVP)	*If present, hemodynamic values are beneficial in guiding fluid resuscitation and preventing fluid volume overload.*

THERAPEUTIC INTERVENTIONS	RATIONALE
Dependent/Collaborative Actions Implement measures to prevent hypovolemic shock: • If bleeding occurs, apply firm, prolonged pressure to area if possible.	*These actions prevent further loss of blood or volume, which may contribute to hypovolemic shock.* *Promotes clotting.*

THERAPEUTIC INTERVENTIONS	RATIONALE
• Perform actions to prevent deficient fluid volume.	
• Instruct client to splint incisional area with hands or pillow when turning and coughing.	*Splinting the incision area when turning and coughing reduces stress on the surgical wound to reduce risk for hemorrhage.*
• Implement measures to reduce nausea and vomiting (e.g., administer medications for pain, eliminate noxious sights and odors, reduce fear and anxiety, instruct to change position slowly).	*Retching action with vomiting places stress on the surgical wound. Preventing nausea and vomiting reduces this.*
If signs and symptoms of hypovolemic shock occur:	
• Place client flat in bed with legs elevated unless contraindicated.	*Elevation of legs facilitates the return of blood pooled in the extremities to the central circulation, improving blood flow to the vital organs.*
• Monitor vital signs frequently.	
If signs and symptoms of hypovolemic shock occur:	
• Administer oxygen as ordered.	*Supplemental oxygen is beneficial because oxygen delivery to the tissues is compromised in shock states.*
• Administer blood and/or volume expanders if ordered.	*Blood and/or fluid volume expanders will help restore circulating volume. The agent of choice is driven by laboratory values.*

• Prepare client for insertion of hemodynamic monitoring devices:
  • Central venous catheter
  • Intra-arterial catheter
	Hemodynamic monitoring devices can measure preload/filling pressures, which are low in hypovolemic shock states.

***It is not appropriate to delegate nursing actions for a client in hypovolemic shock because continuous assessment and evaluation of interventions is necessary.**	

Collaborative Diagnosis RISK FOR PARALYTIC ILEUS

Definition: Paralysis of the intestines resulting in blockage of the intestines

Related to:
- Manipulation of the bowel during surgery
- Depressant effect of anesthesia and some medications (e.g., narcotic [opioid] analgesics, some antiemetics) on bowel motility
- Hypovolemia if it occurs (can cause decreased blood supply to the intestine)

CLINICAL MANIFESTATIONS

Subjective	Objective
Verbal reports of persistent abdominal pain and cramping	Firm, distended abdomen; absent bowel sounds; failure to pass flatus; abdominal radiograph showing distended bowel

RISK FACTORS
- Surgery
- Inadequate fluid volume replacement
- Immobility

DESIRED OUTCOMES

The client will not develop a paralytic ileus as evidenced by:
  a. Absence or resolution of abdominal pain and cramping
  b. Soft, nondistended abdomen
  c. Gradual return of bowel sounds
  d. Passage of flatus

NURSING ASSESSMENT	RATIONALE
Assess for and report signs and symptoms of paralytic ileus: • Development of or persistent abdominal pain and cramping	*Early recognition of signs and symptoms allows for prompt intervention.*

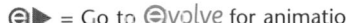

Continued...

NURSING ASSESSMENT	RATIONALE
• Firm, distended abdomen • Absent bowel sounds • Failure to pass flatus • Abdominal radiograph showing distended bowel	

THERAPEUTIC INTERVENTIONS	RATIONALE

Dependent/Collaborative Actions

Implement measures to prevent paralytic ileus:

• Increase activity as soon as allowed and tolerated.	*Activity increases peristalsis.*
• Perform actions to prevent hypokalemia (e.g., prevent nausea and vomiting, administer fluid and electrolytes as ordered, when oral intake is allowed help client to select foods high in potassium).	*Prevention of hypokalemia is important because it prevents resultant decrease in peristalsis.*
• Perform actions to maintain adequate tissue perfusion (e.g., maintain fluid intake of 2500 mL/day unless contraindicated, administer blood and blood products as ordered, instruct and assist client to perform active foot and leg exercises every 1-2 hours while awake).	*Maintains adequate blood supply to the bowel.*
• Administer gastrointestinal stimulants (e.g., metoclopramide) if ordered.	*Gastrointestinal stimulants stimulate peristalsis.*

If signs and symptoms of paralytic ileus occur:

• Withhold all oral intake.	*Decreases potential for a bowel obstruction.*
• Insert nasogastric tube and maintain suction as ordered.	*Placement of an NG tube to facilitate suction helps remove fluid and gastric secretions from the stomach and decreases potential for a bowel obstruction.*

Collaborative Diagnosis **RISK FOR PNEUMOTHORAX**

Definition: An accumulation of air in the pleural space that compromises lung expansion

Related to: An accumulation of air in the pleural space associated with surgical opening of the pleura (occurs most frequently with thoracoabdominal and flank approaches) and/or malfunction of chest tube if present

CLINICAL MANIFESTATIONS

Subjective	**Objective**
Verbalization of shortness of breath	Absent breath sounds; hyperresonant percussion; rapid, shallow, and/or labored respirations; restlessness; agitation; confusion; arterial blood gas values that have worsened; chest radiograph showing a lung collapse

RISK FACTORS	**DESIRED OUTCOMES**

• Surgery
• Immobility
• Ineffective cough effort
	The client will experience normal lung reexpansion if pneumothorax occurs as evidenced by:
	  a. Audible breath sounds and resonant percussion note by the third to fourth postoperative day
	  b. Unlabored respirations at 12 to 20 breaths/min
	  c. Arterial blood gas values returning toward normal
	  d. Chest radiograph showing lung reexpansion

NURSING ASSESSMENT	RATIONALE
Assess for and immediately report signs and symptoms of: • Malfunction of the chest drainage system (e.g., respiratory distress, lack of fluctuation in water seal chamber without evidence of lung reexpansion, excessive bubbling in water seal chamber, significant increase in subcutaneous emphysema)	*Early recognition of the signs and symptoms of pneumothorax allows for prompt intervention.*

NURSING ASSESSMENT	RATIONALE
• Further lung collapse (e.g., extended area of absent breath sounds with hyperresonant percussion note; rapid, shallow, and/or labored respirations; tachycardia; increased chest pain; restlessness; confusion; arterial blood gas results that have worsened; significant decrease in oximetry results) Monitor chest radiograph results. Report findings of delayed lung reexpansion or further lung collapse.	

THERAPEUTIC INTERVENTIONS	RATIONALE

Independent Actions

Implement measures to promote lung reexpansion and prevent further lung collapse:
- Perform actions to maintain patency and integrity of chest drainage system:
  - Maintain fluid levels in the water seal and suction chambers as ordered. — *Maintains negative pressure within the lungs*
  - Maintain occlusive dressing over chest tube insertion site. — *An occlusive dressing over the chest tube insertion site maintains negative pressure seal.*
  - Tape all connections securely. — *Securely taping the tubings/connections prevents tubing from being disconnected and maintains a closed drainage system*
  - Tape the tubing to the chest wall close to insertion site. — *Taping the tubing to the chest wall reduces the risk of inadvertent removal of the chest tube.*
  - Position tubing to promote optimum drainage (e.g., coil excess tubing on bed rather than allowing it to hang down below the collection device, keep tubing free of kinks). — *These actions promote chest tube drainage.*
  - Drain fluid that accumulates in tubing into the collection chamber. — *Maintains patency of the drainage system.*
  - Avoid stripping of chest tubes. If ordered, milk tubing using a hand-over-hand method while moving along the drainage tube. — *Chest tube stripping increases high negative pressures in the pleural space and may damage lung tissues.*
  - Keep drainage collection device below level of client's chest at all times. — *Maintaining the drainage device below the level of the client's chest prevents backflow of drainage into the lungs.*
- Perform actions to facilitate the escape of air from the pleural space (e.g., maintain suction as ordered, ensure that the air vent is open on the drainage collection device if system is to water seal only).
- Perform actions to improve breathing pattern and facilitate airway clearance (e.g., encourage client to cough and deep breathe every 1 to 2 hours; use incentive spirometry every 2 hours; ambulate as ordered and as tolerated). — *These actions improve lung expansion and removal of secretions.*

If signs and symptoms of further lung collapse occur:
- Maintain client on bedrest in a semi- to high-Fowler's position. — *Positioning the client in a semi- to high-Fowler's position improves the client's ability to expand the lungs.*
- Maintain oxygen therapy as ordered. — *Supplemental oxygen helps maintain tissue oxygenation.*
- Assess for and immediately report signs and symptoms of tension pneumothorax (e.g., severe dyspnea, increased restlessness and agitation, rapid and/or irregular pulse rate, hypotension, neck vein distention, shift in trachea from midline). — *Emergency treatment is required to prevent further respiratory difficulty.*
- Assist with clearing of existing chest tube and/or insertion of a new tube. — *Reestablishes a closed drainage system.*

DISCHARGE TEACHING/CONTINUED CARE

Nursing Diagnosis **DEFICIENT KNOWLEDGE NDx; INEFFECTIVE FAMILY THERAPEUTIC REGIMEN MANAGEMENT NDx; OR INEFFECTIVE HEALTH MAINTENANCE* NDx**

Definition: Absence or deficiency of cognitive information related to specific topic (lack of specific information necessary for client/significant others) to make informed choices regarding condition/treatment/lifestyle changes; pattern of regulating and integrating into daily living and family processes a therapeutic regimen for treatment of illnesses and the sequelae of illness that is unsatisfactory for meeting specific health goals.

CLINICAL MANIFESTATIONS

Subjective	Objective
Verbalizes inability to manage illness; verbalizes inability to follow prescribed regimen	Inaccurate follow through with instructions; inappropriate behaviors; experience of preventable complications of surgery and living with one kidney.

RISK FACTORS

- Cognitive deficit
- Financial concerns
- Failure to take action to reduce risk factors for complications of surgery
- Inability to care for oneself
- Difficulty in modifying personal habits and integrating treatments into lifestyle

NOC OUTCOMES

Knowledge: treatment regimen; knowledge: cardiac disease management

NIC INTERVENTIONS

Teaching: individual; teaching: disease process; teaching: prescribed activity/exercise; teaching: prescribed medication; health system guidance

NURSING ASSESSMENT	**RATIONALE**
Assess client's readiness and ability to learn. Assess meaning of illness to client.	*Early recognition of readiness to learn and meaning of illness to client allows for implementation of the appropriate teaching interventions.*

THERAPEUTIC INTERVENTIONS	**RATIONALE**

Desired Outcome: The client will verbalize ways to maintain health of the remaining kidney.

Independent Actions
Instruct client regarding ways to maintain health of the remaining kidney:

- Adhere to precautions to prevent a urinary tract infection:
  - Perform actions to prevent urinary stasis:
    - (1) Drink at least 10 glasses of liquid per day unless contraindicated.   *Hydration is required to maintain vascular fluid volume and adequate blood flow to the kidneys.*
    - (2) Urinate whenever the urge is felt.   *Prevents stasis of urine in the bladder.*
    - (3) Avoid long periods of inactivity (if unable to maintain a program of moderate activity, be sure to change positions frequently).

*The nurse should select the diagnostic label that is most appropriate for the client's needs.

THERAPEUTIC INTERVENTIONS	RATIONALE
• Wipe from front to back after urinating and defecating (if female).	*Appropriate perineal hygiene prevents urinary tract exposure to vaginal or rectal bacteria.*
• Keep perineal area clean and dry.	
• Immediately report signs and symptoms of a urinary tract infection (e.g., chills; fever; urgency, frequency, or burning on urination; cloudy or foul-smelling urine).	*Urinary tract infections require prompt treatment.*
• Notify physician if a cold or other infection persists for more than 2 to 3 days or if unable to maintain an adequate fluid intake.	*Hydration is important to maintain fluid volume and adequate blood flow to the kidneys.*
• Inform other health care providers about the nephrectomy so that prophylactic antimicrobials may be initiated before dental work and invasive procedures such as cystoscopy and minor surgeries.	*Helps prevent infections.*
• Avoid activities that might cause trauma to the remaining kidney (e.g., contact sports, horseback riding).	*Prevents injury.*
• Inform physician of all prescription and nonprescription medications being taken and before taking any new medications since they might cause damage to the remaining kidney (e.g., ibuprofen, ciprofloxacin, captopril, quinine, naproxen, lithium, neomycin, gentamicin, pentamidine, vancomycin, cyclosporine).	*Many medications are nephrotoxic and should not be taken.*
• Consult health care provider before undergoing any diagnostic test involving the use of contrast media.	*Some agents used during these procedures can damage the remaining kidney.*
• If nephrectomy was performed because of renal calculi, reinforce physicians' instructions about diet, drug therapy, and daily fluid requirements.	*Prevents formation of stones in the remaining kidney.*
• If surgery was necessary because of renal hypertension, reinforce the physician's instructions about methods of controlling B/P (e.g., dietary modification, medication, physical exercise on regular basis, weight loss if overweight).	*Client needs to control B/P to prevent destruction of the nephrons on the remaining kidney.*

THERAPEUTIC INTERVENTIONS	RATIONALE

Desired Outcome: The client will state signs and symptoms to report to the health care provider.

Independent Actions

Instruct client to report signs and symptoms to their health care provider:	*These clinical manifestations should be reported to the health care provider because they require prompt intervention.*
• Difficulty breathing	*May indicate a pulmonary embolism.*
• Productive cough of discolored sputum	
• Unusual or excessive drainage from the wound site	*May indicate an infection.*
• Pain or swelling in the calf of one or both legs	*May indicate a deep vein thrombosis.*
• Unusual and continuous abdominal or pelvic pain	*May indicate an infection.*
• Temperature above 38° C (100.4° F)	
• Unexplained weight gain	*May indicate loss of or changes in kidney function.*
• Decreased urine output	
• Flank pain on the unoperative side	
• Blood in the urine	

THERAPEUTIC INTERVENTIONS	RATIONALE

Desired Outcome: The client will verbalize an understanding of and a plan for adhering to recommended follow-up care including future appointments with health care provider, medications prescribed, activity level, wound care, and plans for subsequent treatment of the underlying disorder.

NDx = NANDA-I Diagnosis   **D** = Delegatable Action   ● = UAP   ✦ = LVN/LPN   ⊖▶ = Go to ⊖volve for animation

Continued...

THERAPEUTIC INTERVENTIONS	RATIONALE

Independent Actions

Reinforce physician's instructions regarding activity:

* Gauge activity according to tolerance and allow adequate rest periods.
* Avoid lifting objects over 7 to 10 lb, pushing heavy objects, and exercising strenuously for specified length of time (usually 4-8 weeks).

These actions prevent unnecessary stress on the suture line.

Clarify plans for follow-up visits and subsequent treatment of the underlying disorder (e.g., chemotherapy, radiation therapy) if appropriate.

Clarity of information improves client's understanding of long-term care and adherence to treatment regimen.

RENAL FAILURE: ACUTE AND CHRONIC

Renal failure can be classified as acute or chronic. Acute renal failure (ARF) is an abrupt loss of kidney function that can lead to chronic renal failure (CRF) if the conditions that led to acute failure are not corrected. ARF may be classified as prerenal, intrarenal, and postrenal failure. Prerenal failure is a condition in which blood flow to the kidneys has been significantly decreased so the kidneys are no longer able to concentrate urine. The loss of renal blood flow is caused by conditions such as hypovolemia due to blood loss from trauma, severe hypotension from sepsis, cardiac failure, massive pulmonary embolism, and renal artery clamping or stenosis. Intrarenal failure results from an injury to the kidney itself. Potential causes of intrarenal failure include acute tubular necrosis, glomerulopathies, malignant hypertension, bilateral acute pyelonephritis, and injury to the glomerulus from medications and dye used during procedures. Postrenal failure results from a blockage of urine outflow from the kidneys. Causes of postrenal failure include kidney stones, tumors, injury and/or edema that blocks the ureters, and an enlarged prostate.

Diagnosis and treatment of ARF focuses on the cause of the failure. The challenge in diagnosing ARF is to differentiate between the types of renal failure. A thorough client history, which includes surgeries, cardiac disorders, and trauma, will help identify the underlying cause of renal failure. Other important diagnostic studies include urinalysis, blood urea nitrogen (BUN) and serum creatinine levels and ratio, and the fractional excretion of sodium. The results of these studies vary depending upon the type of ARF present.

ARF and recovery of renal function progress in phases: initiation, oliguric, diuretic, and recovery. The initiation phase begins with the insult to the kidneys and occurs until signs and symptoms are identifiable. This phase can last from hours to days. Prevention of permanent injury may be possible within this phase. The oliguric phase begins when the urine output is decreased to approximately 50 to 400 mL/day. This phase can resolve within hours or can last for up to 3 weeks. Typical signs and symptoms of this phase include hypotension, nausea and vomiting, anorexia, diarrhea, constipation, bleeding, anemia, lethargy, memory impairment,

and seizures. Electrolyte changes are also seen in this phase and include decreased serum sodium and calcium levels and increased serum potassium and phosphate levels. The neurological changes noted above occur with increased nitrogenous waste products that accumulate in the brain and other areas of the nervous system. The diuretic phase begins with a gradual increase in daily urine output of at least 1 to 3 L/day. In this phase, the kidneys are beginning to recover waste excretion processes but cannot concentrate urine. The client may experience hypovolemia and hypotension related to the excessive fluid loss. In the recovery phase, the BUN and serum creatinine levels begin to decline and glomerular filtration rates (GFRs) increase. This phase may take 1 to 2 weeks; however, it can take up to 1 year for renal function to stabilize.

ARF is reversible in most individuals, but it can lead to CRF. CRF is a progressive, irreversible loss of kidney function that usually develops gradually over many years. The leading causes of CRF are diabetes mellitus, hypertension, and glomerulonephritis. Other causes include pyelonephritis/interstitial nephritis, obstruction of the urinary tract by conditions such as benign prostatic hypertrophy, and hereditary conditions such as polycystic kidney disease. CRF can also develop after ARF that has resulted in irreversible renal damage.

Creatinine clearance is the measurement that is used to determine the effectiveness of renal function. As renal failure progresses, creatinine clearance declines, reflecting a decrease in the GFR and the percentage of functioning nephrons. The severity of CRF can be classified by the proportion of renal function that has been lost and is often divided into stages. In the first stage, diminished renal reserve, the GFR can be as low as 30% of normal, but the renal dysfunction usually goes undiagnosed because homeostatic mechanisms are able to maintain fluid balance and keep serum electrolyte, urea nitrogen, and creatinine levels within normal ranges.

Renal insufficiency, the middle stage, begins when the GFR is about 25% of normal. At this point in the disease process, creatinine clearance continues to decline and azotemia (the retention of nitrogenous substances in the blood) begins. The BUN and serum creatinine levels are elevated but are not high enough to cause symptoms that are problematic for the client. During this stage, the client progresses from a nonoliguric phase, in which the kidneys are unable to concentrate the urine, to a state of oliguria. When this occurs, symptoms become evident and result mainly from a decreased ability of the kidneys to excrete fluid and electrolytes.

The last stage of CRF is end-stage renal disease (ESRD). It occurs when the GFR is less than about 10% of normal and nitrogenous substances (e.g., urea, creatinine) accumulate to levels high enough to cause toxic effects on other body systems. Typical signs and symptoms of ESRD can include lethargy, irritability, extreme fatigue and weakness, pruritus, nausea and vomiting, muscle cramping, and stomatitis. Fluid, electrolyte, and acid-base imbalances also worsen and, in this stage, dialysis or kidney transplantation is necessary for survival.

This care plan focuses on the adult client with renal insufficiency who has progressed from the nonoliguric to the oliguric phase and is hospitalized for treatment and further evaluation of renal function. Much of the information is also applicable to clients in an extended care facility or home setting.

3. Have fluid, electrolyte, and acid-base balance stabilized within a safe range
4. Tolerate expected level of activity
5. Have no evidence of infection
6. Have an adequate nutritional status
7. Verbalize a basic understanding of CRF
8. Identify ways to slow the progression of kidney damage
9. Verbalize an understanding of fluid restrictions and dietary modifications
10. Demonstrate the ability to accurately weigh self, measure fluid intake and output, and monitor own B/P
11. Identify ways to reduce the risk of infection
12. Identify ways to manage signs and symptoms that often occur as a result of CRF
13. Share feelings and concerns about the effects of renal failure on lifestyle and roles
14. State signs and symptoms to report to the health care provider
15. Identify community resources that can assist with adjustment to changes resulting from CRF
16. Verbalize an understanding of and a plan for adhering to recommended follow-up care including future appointments with health care provider and medications prescribed

OUTCOME/DISCHARGE CRITERIA

The client will:
1. Not have signs and symptoms of uremic syndrome
2. Have B/P within a safe range

Nursing Diagnosis # RISK FOR EXCESS FLUID VOLUME NDx

Definition: Increased isotonic fluid retention

Related to:
- Retention of sodium and water associated with a decreased glomerular filtration rate (occurs as a result of the decrease in the number of functioning nephrons) and activation of the renin-angiotensin-aldosterone mechanism (can occur if renal blood flow is decreased as a result of the underlying disease process)
- Fluid intake in excess of prescribed restrictions

CLINICAL MANIFESTATIONS

Subjective	Objective
Verbalization of shortness of breath	Weight gain of 2% or greater over a short period; hypertension; presence of an S_3 heart sound; tachycardia; intake greater than output; changes in mental status; crackles (rales) and diminished or absent breath sounds; dyspnea, orthopnea; peripheral edema; distended neck veins; chest radiograph showing pulmonary vascular congestion, pleural effusion, or pulmonary edema

---

NDx = NANDA-I Diagnosis   **D** = Delegatable Action   ● = UAP   ✦ = LVN/LPN   ⊜▶ = Go to ⊜volve for animation

Continued...

RISK FACTOR

- Failure of regulatory mechanisms

DESIRED OUTCOMES

> The client will experience resolution of excess fluid volume as evidenced by:
> a. Decline in weight toward client's normal
> b. B/P within normal range for client
> c. Absence of an S_3 heart sound
> d. Normal pulse volume
> e. Balanced intake and output
> f. Usual mental status
> g. Normal breath sounds
> h. Absence of dyspnea, orthopnea, peripheral edema, and distended neck veins

NOC OUTCOMES

Fluid balance; electrolyte and acid-base balance; fluid overload severity

NIC INTERVENTIONS

Fluid/electrolyte monitoring; fluid management

NURSING ASSESSMENT	**RATIONALE**
Assess for and report signs and symptoms of excess fluid volume: • Weight gain of 2% or greater over a short period • Elevated B/P (B/P may not be elevated if fluid has shifted out of vascular space) • Presence of an S_3 heart sound • Bounding pulse • Intake greater than output • Changes in mental status • Crackles (rales) and diminished or absent breath sounds • Dyspnea, orthopnea • Peripheral edema • Distended neck veins • Chest radiograph showing pulmonary vascular congestion, pleural effusion, or pulmonary edema	*Early recognition of signs and symptoms of excess fluid volume allows for prompt intervention.*

THERAPEUTIC INTERVENTIONS	**RATIONALE**
Dependent/Collaborative Actions Implement measures to reduce excess fluid volume: • Maintain fluid restrictions as ordered (intake allowed is usually 500-700 mL plus the amount of urine output in the previous 24 hours). **D** ✦	*Reduction of excess fluid volume reduces stress on the heart and vascular system.*
• Instruct client in ways to alleviate thirst and/or keep oral mucous membranes moist (e.g., space fluid intake evenly throughout the hours client is awake, rinse mouth frequently with water, breathe through nose rather than mouth).	*Ability to alleviate thirst and keep oral mucous membranes moist promotes compliance with oral fluid restrictions.*
• Weigh client daily at the same time of day using the same scale and with similar weight of clothing. **D** ✦	*Daily weights are important for comparisons. A sudden weight gain may be an indication of fluid volume excess.*
• If client is receiving numerous and/or a large volume of intravenous medications, consult the pharmacist to prevent excessive fluid administration (e.g., stop primary infusion during administration of intravenous medications, dilute medication in the minimum amount of solution).	*Prevents fluid volume excess.*
• Restrict sodium intake as ordered. **D** ✦	*Reducing sodium intake decreases fluid retention.*
• Administer diuretic if ordered. **D** ✦	*Diuretics increases excretion of water.*
Consult physician if signs and symptoms of excess fluid volume persist or worsen.	*Notification of the physician allows for prompt alterations in treatment plan.*

Collaborative Diagnosis **RISK FOR SODIUM IMBALANCE**

Definition: Sodium levels higher or lower than normal

Hyponatremia related to excessive fluid intake in relation to output (causes a dilutional hyponatremia) and loss of sodium associated with diuretic therapy

Hypernatremia related to:
- Decreased ability of the kidneys to excrete sodium
- Increased aldosterone output associated with activation of the renin-angiotensin-aldosterone mechanism if decreased renal blood flow has occurred as a result of the underlying disease process
- Dietary sodium intake in excess of prescribed restrictions

CLINICAL MANIFESTATIONS

Subjective	Objective
Hyponatremia: Verbalization of nausea; abdominal cramps; weakness	**Hyponatremia:** Vomiting; confusion; seizures; low serum sodium level
Hypernatremia: Verbalization of thirst; weakness	**Hypernatremia:** Dry, sticky mucous membranes; restlessness; elevated temperature; seizures; elevated serum sodium level

RISK FACTORS

- Poor adherence to dietary regimen
- Changes in regulatory mechanisms

DESIRED OUTCOMES

The client will maintain a safe serum sodium level as evidenced by:
  a. Absence of nausea, vomiting, abdominal cramps, and thirst
  b. Moist mucous membranes
  c. Usual mental status
  d. Usual muscle strength
  e. Absence of seizure activity
  f. Serum sodium level within a safe range for client

NOC OUTCOMES

Fluid balance; electrolyte balance

NIC INTERVENTIONS

Fluid/electrolyte monitoring; electrolyte management: hyponatremia; electrolyte management: hypernatremia

NURSING ASSESSMENT	**RATIONALE**
Assess for and report signs and symptoms of: • Hyponatremia (e.g., nausea, vomiting, abdominal cramps, lethargy, confusion, weakness, seizures, and low serum sodium level) • Hypernatremia (e.g., thirst; dry, sticky mucous membranes; restlessness; lethargy; weakness; elevated temperature; seizures; elevated serum sodium level)	*Early recognition of signs and symptoms of sodium imbalance allows for prompt intervention.*

THERAPEUTIC INTERVENTIONS	**RATIONALE**
Dependent/Collaborative Actions Implement measures to prevent or treat hyponatremia: • Maintain fluid restrictions as ordered. • Increase dietary allotment of sodium if ordered. **D ● ✦** • Administer loop diuretics. **D ● ✦** Implement measures to prevent or treat hypernatremia: • Maintain maximum fluid intake allowed. • Maintain dietary sodium restrictions if ordered.	 *Maintenance of fluid restrictions prevents dilutional hyponatremia.* *Increased intake of sodium decreases the dilutional effects of fluid retention.* *Loop diuretics promotes excretion of water.* *Maintains appropriate balance between vascular fluid volume and sodium volume.*

 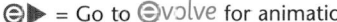

Continued...

THERAPEUTIC INTERVENTIONS	RATIONALE
• Administer thiazide diuretics if ordered. **D** ✦ Consult a physician if unsafe serum sodium levels persist.	*Thiazide diuretics increase excretion of sodium and water. Notification of the physician allows for prompt alternation in treatment plan.*

Collaborative Diagnosis ## RISK FOR HYPERKALEMIA

Definition: Serum potassium levels above normal limits

Related to:
- Decreased ability of the kidneys to excrete potassium
- Increased cellular release of potassium associated with progressive renal tissue damage and metabolic acidosis
- Dietary potassium intake in excess of prescribed restrictions
- Use of potassium-sparing diuretics or medications and salt substitutes containing potassium

CLINICAL MANIFESTATIONS

Subjective	Objective
Verbalization of muscle weakness	Bradycardia with irregular pulse; diarrhea and intestinal colic; electrocardiogram (ECG) showing peaked T wave, prolonged PR interval, and/or widened QRS; elevated serum potassium level

RISK FACTORS
- Poor adherence to dietary regimen
- Medication regimen
- Changes in regulatory mechanisms

DESIRED OUTCOMES

The client will maintain a safe serum potassium level as evidenced by:
  a. Regular pulse at 60 to 80 beats/min
  b. Absence of paresthesias
  c. Usual muscle tone and strength
  d. Absence of diarrhea and intestinal colic
  e. Normal ECG
  f. Serum potassium level within a safe range for client

NOC OUTCOMES

Fluid balance; electrolyte fluid overload severity; kidney function

NIC INTERVENTIONS

Fluid/electrolyte monitoring; fluid management; electrolyte management: hyperkalemia

NURSING ASSESSMENT	RATIONALE
Assess for and report signs and symptoms of hyperkalemia (e.g., slow or irregular pulse; paresthesias; muscle weakness and flaccidity; diarrhea and intestinal colic; ECG showing peaked T wave, prolonged PR interval, and/or widened QRS; elevated serum potassium level).	*Early recognition of the signs and symptoms of hyperkalemia allows for prompt intervention.*

THERAPEUTIC INTERVENTIONS	RATIONALE
Dependent/Collaborative Actions Implement measures to prevent or treat hyperkalemia: • Maintain dietary restrictions of potassium by limiting intake of foods/fluid such as bananas, potatoes, raisins, avocados, and orange juice. **D** ● ✦	*Restricting intake of potassium-rich foods helps maintain a normal level of potassium for the client.*

THERAPEUTIC INTERVENTIONS	RATIONALE
• Instruct client to consult physician or dietitian about which salt substitute can safely be used.	*Most salt substitutes contain potassium.*
• Perform actions to reduce the cellular release of potassium:	
• Implement measures to spare body proteins and prevent tissue breakdown:	
(1) Encourage client to consume the amount of dietary protein allotted. **D** ✦	*During the breakdown of proteins, potassium is released.*
(2) Provide allotted amount of carbohydrates.	*Ingestion of carbohydrates spares protein by providing a quick energy source.*
(3) Perform actions to prevent infection (use sterile technique when doing invasive procedures, use good hand washing and encourage client to do the same, rotate intravenous line sites according to hospital policy). **D** ✦	*Prevention of an infection prevents an increase in the metabolic rate and a subsequent increase in protein catabolism.*
• Implement measure to prevent or treat metabolic acidosis (e.g., administer sodium bicarbonate).	*In metabolic acidosis, potassium is moved out of the cell in exchange for hydrogen, thus increasing the extracellular potassium level.*
• If signs and symptoms of hyperkalemia are present, consult physician before administering prescribed potassium supplements and other medications that can increase potassium levels (e.g., potassium penicillin G, potassium-sparing diuretics, some beta-blockers and angiotensin-converting enzyme [ACE] inhibitors).	*Prevents increased potassium levels.*
• Administer the following medications if ordered:	
• Loop diuretics **D** ✦	*Increases renal excretion of potassium.*
• Cation-exchange resins (e.g., sodium polystyrene sulfonate [Kayexalate] **D** ✦	*Administration of sodium polystyrene sulfonate increases potassium excretion via the intestines (action by exchanging sodium for potassium).*
• Intravenous insulin and hypertonic glucose solutions	*Infusion of hypertonic glucose solutions and insulin enhances transport of potassium back into cells.*
If signs and symptoms of hyperkalemia persist or worsen:	
• Consult physician.	*Notification of the physician allows for prompt alterations in treatment plan.*
• Have intravenous calcium preparation (e.g., calcium gluconate) readily available.	*Administration of calcium gluconate counteracts the effect of a high potassium level on the heart.*

Collaborative Diagnosis # RISK FOR HYPOCALCEMIA

Definition: Serum calcium levels below normal range

Related to:
• Decreased intestinal absorption of calcium associated with inability of the kidneys to activate vitamin D (the active metabolite of vitamin D is needed to stimulate calcium absorption from the small intestine)
• Hyperphosphatemia (causes a reciprocal drop in calcium)

CLINICAL MANIFESTATIONS

Subjective	Objective
Verbalization of feeling anxious; verbalization of numbness or tingling in fingers, toes, or circumoral area	Irritability; positive Chvostek's and Trousseau's signs; hyperactive reflexes; tetany; seizures; serum calcium level that is lower than normal

Continued...

RISK FACTORS

- Decreased levels of vitamin D
- Failure of regulatory mechanisms

DESIRED OUTCOMES

The client will maintain a safe serum calcium level as evidenced by:
  a. Usual mental status
  b. Negative Chvostek's and Trousseau's signs
  c. Absence of numbness and tingling in fingers, toes, and circumoral area; hyperreflexia; tetany; and seizure activity
  d. Serum calcium level within a safe range for client

NOC OUTCOMES

Fluid balance; electrolyte balance

NIC INTERVENTIONS

Fluid/electrolyte monitoring; fluid management; electrolyte management: hypocalcemia

NURSING ASSESSMENT

Assess for and report signs and symptoms of hypocalcemia (e.g., anxiousness, irritability, positive Chvostek's and Trousseau's signs, numbness or tingling of fingers, toes, or circumoral area; hyperactive reflexes; tetany; seizures; serum calcium level that is lower than normal for client).

RATIONALE

Early recognition of signs and symptoms of hypocalcemia allows for prompt intervention.

THERAPEUTIC INTERVENTIONS

Dependent/Collaborative Actions
Implement measures to prevent or treat hypocalcemia:
- Provide sources of calcium (e.g., milk and milk products). **D ● ✦**

- Administer activated vitamin D (e.g., paricalcitol, calcitriol) and calcium supplements if ordered. **D ● ✦**

- Perform measures to prevent or treat hyperphosphatemia (e.g., restrict phosphorus intake).

- Avoid rapid or aggressive treatment of acidosis.

If signs and symptoms of hypocalcemia occur:
- Institute seizure precautions.
- Administer calcium preparations (e.g., calcium gluconate, calcium carbonate) as ordered.

RATIONALE

Ensures that calcium is present in client's diet.

Vitamin D is required for the absorption of calcium.

Calcium and phosphate have an inverse relationship, and a high phosphate level leads to hypocalcemia.

Rapidly reversing acidosis can result in decreased ionization of calcium.

Prevents client injury.

Increases calcium levels.

Collaborative Diagnosis   # HYPERPHOSPHATEMIA

Definition: Serum phosphate levels above normal range

Related to: Hypocalcemia (an inverse relationship exists between phosphorus and calcium) and decreased ability of the kidneys to excrete phosphorus

CLINICAL MANIFESTATIONS

Subjective	Objective
Verbalization of numbness or tingling in hands and feet	Tetany; seizures; elevated serum phosphorus level

RISK FACTOR

- Failure of regulatory mechanisms

DESIRED OUTCOMES

The client will maintain a safe serum phosphorus level as evidenced by:
  a. Absence of paresthesias, tetany, and seizure activity.
  b. Serum phosphorus level within a safe range for client.

NOC OUTCOMES	NIC INTERVENTIONS
Fluid balance; electrolyte balance	Fluid/electrolyte monitoring; fluid management; electrolyte management: hyperphosphatemia

NURSING ASSESSMENT	RATIONALE
Assess for and report signs and symptoms of hyperphosphatemia (e.g., paresthesias, tetany, seizures, higher than normal serum phosphorus level for client).	*Early recognition of signs and symptoms of hyperphosphatemia allows for prompt treatment.*

THERAPEUTIC INTERVENTIONS	RATIONALE

Dependent/Collaborative Actions

Implement measures to prevent or treat hyperphosphatemia:

• Restrict dietary intake of phosphorus if ordered by limiting intake of foods/fluids such as poultry, nuts, milk, milk products, eggs, legumes, and some cola beverages. **D** ● ✦	*These foods contain phosphate and will increase blood phosphate levels.*
• Administer phosphate-binding medications such as sevelamar (e.g., Renagel), aluminum-containing agents (e.g., Amphojel, Basaljel), calcium acetate (e.g., PhosLo), and calcium carbonate (e.g., Tums) if ordered. **D** ● ✦	*Administration of phosphate-binding medications binds with phosphate and decreases the free phosphate levels available in the body.*
• Consult physician if signs and symptoms of hyperphosphatemia persist or worsen.	*Notification of the physician allows for prompt alterations in treatment plan.*

Collaborative Diagnosis **RISK FOR HYPERMAGNESEMIA**

Definition: Serum magnesium level above normal range

Related to:

- Decreased ability of the kidneys to excrete magnesium
- Excessive intake of magnesium-containing antacids, laxatives, or foods

CLINICAL MANIFESTATIONS

Subjective	Objective
Verbalization of nausea; weakness	Flushed, warm skin; vomiting; drowsiness; hypotension; bradypnea; bradycardia; higher than normal serum magnesium level

RISK FACTORS	DESIRED OUTCOMES

• Poor adherence to dietary regimen
• Use of certain OTC medications
• Failure of the regulatory mechanisms
	The client will maintain a safe serum magnesium level as evidenced by:
	  a. Absence of flushing, nausea, vomiting, and muscle weakness
	  b. Usual mental status
	  c. Vital signs within normal range for client
	  d. Serum magnesium level within a safe range for client

NOC OUTCOMES	NIC INTERVENTIONS
Fluid balance; electrolyte balance	Fluid/electrolyte monitoring; fluid management; electrolyte management: hypermagnesemia

---

NDx = NANDA-I Diagnosis   **D** = Delegatable Action   ● = UAP   ✦ = LVN/LPN   ⊖▶ = Go to ⊖volve for animation

Continued...

NURSING ASSESSMENT	RATIONALE
Assess for and report signs and symptoms of hypermagnesemia (e.g., flushed, warm skin; nausea; vomiting; muscle weakness; drowsiness; lethargy; hypotension; bradypnea; bradycardia; higher than normal serum magnesium level for client).	*Early recognition of signs and symptoms of hypermagnesemia allows for prompt intervention.*

THERAPEUTIC INTERVENTIONS	RATIONALE
Dependent/Collaborative Actions Implement measures to prevent or treat hypermagnesemia:	
• Avoid giving laxatives and antacids that contain magnesium (e.g., Milk of Magnesia, Gelusil, Mylanta, Maalox). **D** ✦	*Magnesium is absorbed from these agents.*
• Maintain dietary restrictions of magnesium if ordered by limiting intake of foods/fluids such as seafood, green leafy vegetables, and legumes. **D** ✦	*Because the kidneys are unable to regulate the electrolytes, decreasing intake of magnesium is the most appropriate way to maintain decreased level.*
Consult physician if signs and symptoms of hypermagnesemia persist or worsen.	*Notification of the physician allows for prompt alterations of interventions.*

Collaborative Diagnosis   RISK FOR METABOLIC ACIDOSIS

Definition: Elevated level of serum acidity

Related to:
• Decreased ability of the kidneys to excrete hydrogen ions and reabsorb bicarbonate
• Hyperkalemia (the body attempts to compensate for high serum potassium levels by shifting hydrogen ions into the vascular space in exchange for potassium ions)

CLINICAL MANIFESTATIONS

Subjective	Objective
Verbalization of a headache and nausea	Drowsiness; disorientation; stupor; rapid, deep respirations; vomiting; cardiac dysrhythmias; lower than usual pH; increased anion gap

RISK FACTOR	DESIRED OUTCOMES
• Changes in regulatory mechanisms	The client will not experience metabolic acidosis as evidenced by: a. Usual mental status b. Unlabored respirations at 12 to 20 breaths/min c. Absence of headache, nausea, vomiting, and cardiac dysrhythmias d. Arterial blood gas values within a safe range for client e. Anion gap within a normal range

NOC OUTCOMES	NIC INTERVENTIONS
Fluid balance; acid-base balance; kidney function	Fluid/electrolyte monitoring; acid-base monitoring; acid-base management: metabolic acidosis

NURSING ASSESSMENT	RATIONALE
Assess for and report signs and symptoms of metabolic acidosis (e.g., drowsiness; disorientation; stupor; rapid, deep respirations; headache; nausea; vomiting; cardiac dysrhythmias; lower than usual pH and CO_2 content; increased anion gap).	*Early recognition of signs and symptoms of metabolic acidosis allows for prompt intervention.*

THERAPEUTIC INTERVENTIONS	RATIONALE

Dependent/Collaborative Actions

Implement measures to prevent or treat metabolic acidosis:

- Perform actions to prevent or treat hyperkalemia (e.g., maintain dietary restrictions of potassium, limit use of salt substitutes, limit intake of dietary protein). **D** ✦

- Administer sodium bicarbonate if ordered.

Consult physician if signs and symptoms of acidosis persist or worsen.

Decreases potassium levels in the system or prevents elevated potassium levels from occurring.

Administration of bicarbonate decreases acidosis of the blood. Notification of the physician allows for prompt alterations in treatment plan.

Nursing Diagnosis

IMBALANCED NUTRITION: LESS THAN BODY REQUIREMENTS NDx

Definition: Inadequate intake or insufficient nutrition to meet the body's metabolic needs

Related to:

- Decreased oral intake associated with fatigue and dislike of prescribed diet
- Prescribed dietary modifications (especially protein restrictions that are necessary in order to control the serum levels of nitrogenous substances)

CLINICAL MANIFESTATIONS

Subjective	Objective
Verbalization of lack of appetite, fatigue, poor self-esteem	Loss of weight with adequate food intake; body weight 20% or more under ideal weight; sore, inflamed buccal cavity; capillary fragility; irritability; pale conjunctiva and mucous membranes; poor muscle tone; excessive hair loss; amenorrhea

RISK FACTORS

- Poor adherence to dietary regimen
- Chronic illness

DESIRED OUTCOMES

The client will maintain an adequate nutritional status as evidenced by:
   a. Weight within normal range for the client
   b. Serum albumin, prealbumin, Hct, and Hgb levels and lymphocyte count within normal range
   c. Usual or improved strength and activity tolerance
   d. Healthy oral mucous membrane

NOC OUTCOMES

Appropriate appetite; positive body image; bowel elimination; compliance with prescribed diet; adequate hydration; weight maintenance behavior

NIC INTERVENTIONS

Nutritional monitoring; nutritional counseling; nutritional management; nutrition therapy; weight gain assistance; weight management

NURSING ASSESSMENT	RATIONALE

Assess for and report signs and symptoms of malnutrition:

- Weight significantly below client's usual weight or below normal for client's age, height, and body frame
- Low serum albumin, prealbumin, Hct, and Hgb levels and low lymphocyte count
- Weakness and fatigue (may also reflect decreasing renal function)
- Sore, inflamed oral mucous membrane
- Pale conjunctiva

Monitor percentage of meals and snacks client consumes. Report a pattern or inadequate intake.

Early recognition and reporting of signs and symptoms of malnutrition allow for prompt intervention.

An awareness of the amount of foods/fluids the client consumes alerts the nurse to deficits in nutritional intake. Reporting an inadequate intake allows for prompt intervention.

NDx = NANDA-I Diagnosis   **D** = Delegatable Action   ● = UAP   ✦ = LVN/LPN   ⊖▶ = Go to ⊖volve for animation

Continued...

THERAPEUTIC INTERVENTIONS	RATIONALE

Independent Actions

Implement measures to improve oral intake:

- Increase activity as allowed and tolerated. **D** ● ✦

  Activity usually promotes a general feeling of well-being, which can result in improved appetite.

- Maintain a clean environment and a relaxed, pleasant atmosphere. **D** ● ✦

  Noxious sites and odors can inhibit the feeding center in the hypothalamus. Maintaining a clean environment helps prevent this from occurring. In addition, maintaining a relaxed, pleasant atmosphere can help reduce the client's stress and promote a feeling of well-being, which tends to improve appetite and oral intake.

- Encourage a rest period before meals if indicated.

  The physical activity of eating requires some expenditure of energy. Fatigue can reduce the client's desire and ability to eat.

- Provide oral hygiene before meals. **D** ● ✦

  Oral hygiene moistens the oral mucous membrane, which may make it easier to chew and swallow. It also freshens the mouth and removes unpleasant tastes. This can improve the taste of foods/fluids, which helps stimulate appetite and increase oral intake.

- Serve foods/fluids that are appealing to the client and adhere to personal and cultural (e.g., religious, ethnic) preferences whenever possible.

  Foods/fluids that appeal to the client's senses (especially sight and smell) and are in accordance with personal and cultural preferences are most likely to stimulate appetite and promote interest in eating.

- Serve frequent, small meals rather than large ones if client is weak, fatigues easily, and/or has a poor appetite. **D** ✦

  Providing small rather than large meals can enable a client who is weak or fatigues easily to finish a meal.

- Allow adequate time for meals; reheat foods/fluids if necessary. **D** ● ✦

  Clients who feel rushed during meals tend to become anxious, lose their appetite, and stop eating.

- Encourage client to eat the maximum amount of protein allowed; instruct client to satisfy protein requirements with foods/fluids that are complete proteins and contain essential amino acids (e.g., eggs, milk, meat, poultry) if serum phosphorus level is not too high.

  Client needs to have protein to maintain normal body functions.

Dependent/Collaborative Actions

Perform a calorie count if ordered. Report information to the dietitian and physician.

The client must consume a diet that is well balanced and high in essential nutrients in order to meet nutritional needs. Dietary supplements are often needed to help accomplish this.

Consult the physician about an alternative method of providing nutrition (e.g., parenteral nutrition, tube feeding) if client does not consume enough food or fluids to meet nutritional needs.

Notification of the physician allows for prompt alteration in the treatment plan.

Collaborative Diagnosis   RISK FOR UREMIA SYNDROME

Definition: A syndrome associated with progressive renal failure

Related to: Accumulations of serum nitrogenous substances (e.g., creatinine, urea) associated with extensive loss of renal function (signs and symptoms usually occur when the glomerular filtration rate falls to <10% of normal)

CLINICAL MANIFESTATIONS

Subjective	Objective
Reports of inability to concentrate; increasing weakness and fatigue; hallucinations; nausea; itching; muscle cramps; restless feelings in the legs during rest; joint pain; metallic or bitter taste in mouth	Increasing serum BUN and creatinine levels; cardiac dysrhythmias; confusion; sallow or grayish bronze skin; stomatitis; vomiting; unusual bleeding; pericarditis; fever; asterixis; seizures

RISK FACTOR

- Failure of regulatory mechanisms

DESIRED OUTCOMES

The client will not experience uremic syndrome as evidenced by:
  a. Pulse regular at 60 to 100 beats/min
  b. Usual mental status
  c. Usual skin color
  d. Improved strength and activity tolerance
  e. No reports of nausea, insomnia, itching, muscle cramping, joint pain, paresthesias, and taste alterations
  f. Intact oral mucous membrane
  g. Absence of vomiting, unusual bleeding, pericarditis, asterixis, and seizure activity

NURSING ASSESSMENT

Assess for and report the following:
- Increasing BUN and serum creatinine levels
- Decreasing creatinine clearance levels
- Signs and symptoms of uremic syndrome:
  - Cardiac dysrhythmias
  - Difficulty concentrating, lethargy, confusion, or hallucinations
  - Sallow or grayish bronze skin
  - Increased weakness or fatigue
  - Reports of nausea, insomnia, itching, muscle cramps, joint pain, paresthesias, restless feeling in legs during periods of inactivity, or metallic or bitter taste in mouth
  - Stomatitis
  - Vomiting
  - Unusual bleeding (e.g., ecchymoses; prolonged bleeding from puncture sites; gingival bleeding; frank or occult blood in stool, urine, or vomitus)
  - Pericarditis (e.g., chest pain that frequently radiates to shoulder, neck, back, and arm [usually left]; pericardial friction rub; elevated temperature)
  - Asterixis, seizures

RATIONALE

Early recognition of signs and symptoms of uremic syndrome allows for prompt intervention.

THERAPEUTIC INTERVENTIONS

Independent Actions

Implement measures to reduce the levels of serum nitrogenous substances to prevent uremic syndrome:
- Perform actions to maintain an adequate nutritional status (e.g., serve small, frequent meals; allow adequate time to complete meals; eat the appropriate amount of proteins; take dietary supplements if indicated). **D** ● ✦
- Maintain dietary protein restrictions.
- Perform actions to prevent infection (e.g., maintain adequate fluid intake, use sterile technique during all invasive procedures, promote good hand washing, change peripheral intravenous line sites according to hospital policy).
- Implement measures as ordered to control disease conditions such as diabetes that have caused or contributed to renal failure.

Dependent/Collaborative Actions

- Consult the physician before administering medications that are known to be nephrotoxic (e.g., nonsteroidal anti-inflammatory drugs [NSAIDs], aminoglycosides).

RATIONALE

These actions assist the client in maintenance of an adequate nutritional status while reducing catabolism of body proteins, which contribute to uremic syndrome.

Prevention of infection prevents an increase in the metabolic rate and subsequent cellular catabolism.

Prevents further renal damage.

Client should be informed of medications that are nephrotoxic and should not take any over-the-counter medications without consulting his/her health care provider.

NDx = NANDA-I Diagnosis   **D** = Delegatable Action   ● = UAP   ✦ = LVN/LPN   ⊖▶ = Go to ⊖volve for animation

Continued...

THERAPEUTIC INTERVENTIONS	RATIONALE
If signs and symptoms of uremic syndrome occur:	
• Prepare client for dialysis if planned.	*Dialysis removes toxins from the blood.*
• Maintain a safe environment for client (e.g., side rails up while in bed, assistance with ambulation as needed, constant supervision if indicated, seizure precautions).	*Implementation of hospital policy related to falls and other precautions decreases potential for client injury.*
• Administer antidysrhythmics as ordered; restrict activity if indicated. **D** ✦	*Treats cardiac dysrhythmias.*
• Administer antiemetics as ordered. **D** ✦	*Antiemetics decrease the incidence of nausea.*
• Provide small, frequent meals; instruct client to ingest foods/fluids slowly.	
• Use tepid water and mild soap for bathing; apply emollient creams or ointments frequently. **D** ● ✦	*Use of tepid water for bathing and creams and ointments reduces the incidence of pruritus.*
• Administer antihistamines if ordered. **D** ✦	*Antihistamines block the release of histamines, which stimulate itchy sensations.*
• Instruct client to push feet against a hard surface when leg cramps occur; apply warm packs to affected areas.	*These actions help control muscle cramps.*
• Instruct client to avoid substances such as extremely hot, spicy, or acidic foods/fluids; assist with frequent oral hygiene; apply oral protective pastes as ordered.	*Avoidance of hot, spicy, and/or acidic foods reduces the severity of stomatitis.*
• Apply gentle, prolonged pressure after injections and venous and arterial punctures; instruct client to use an electric rather than a straight-edge razor and to use a soft bristle toothbrush for oral hygiene.	*These actions prevent and/or decrease incidence of bleeding.*
• Apply firm, prolonged pressure to bleeding area if possible; administer clotting factors or vitamin K if ordered.	*Administration of clotting factors and/or vitamin K helps improve body's clotting ability and control bleeding.*
• Maintain activity restrictions as ordered; administer an anti-inflammatory agent and analgesics if ordered. **D** ✦	*Anti-inflammatory agents treat pericarditis. Analgesics decrease sensation of pain.*

Collaborative Diagnosis RISK FOR HYPERTENSION

Definition: Increased B/P of greater than 120 mm Hg systolic and 80 mm Hg diastolic

Related to:
• Excess fluid volume
• Peripheral vasoconstriction associated with increased stimulation of the renin-angiotensin mechanism (possibly in response to diminished renal blood flow)
• Cardiovascular changes resulting from the underlying disease processes (e.g., diabetes)
• Effect of some medications (e.g., erythropoietin)

CLINICAL MANIFESTATIONS

Subjective	Objective
Reports of headache and dizziness	Blood pressure greater than 120/80 mm Hg

RISK FACTORS
• Medication regimen
• Poor adherence to fluid restrictions
• Chronic illness

DESIRED OUTCOMES

The client will not experience hypertension as evidenced by:
   a. B/P within a safe range for client
   b. No reports of headache and dizziness

NURSING ASSESSMENT	RATIONALE
Assess for and report signs and symptoms of hypertension (e.g., B/P greater than client's usual level [a B/P > 140/90 mm Hg is usually considered to be significant], headache, dizziness).	*Early recognition of signs and symptoms of hypertension allows for prompt intervention.*

THERAPEUTIC INTERVENTIONS	RATIONALE

Dependent/Collaborative Actions

Implement measures to prevent or control hypertension:

- Perform actions to reduce excess fluid volume.
  - Maintain fluid restrictions as ordered (usually 500-700 mL plus amount of urine output). **D** ● ✦
  - Instruct client to spread fluid intake throughout the day.

- Administer antihypertensives. **D** ✦
- Perform actions to prevent or treat hypernatremia:
  - Maintain maximum fluid intake allowed.
  - Maintain dietary sodium restrictions if ordered.
  - Administer thiazide diuretics if ordered. **D** ✦

Consult physician if hypertension persists or worsens.

Fluid restrictions help maintain appropriate vascular fluid volume.

Distributing fluid intake throughout the day helps moisten oral mucous membranes and improves compliance with oral fluid restrictions.
Antihypertensive medications decrease B/P.

Maintains appropriate sodium and fluid ratios.
Restricts increase in sodium levels.
Thiazide diuretics stimulate functioning nephrons to excrete sodium.
Notification of the physician allows for prompt alterations in treatment plan.

DISCHARGE TEACHING/CONTINUED CARE

Nursing Diagnosis | # DEFICIENT KNOWLEDGE NDx; INEFFECTIVE FAMILY THERAPEUTIC REGIMEN MANAGEMENT NDx; OR INEFFECTIVE SELF-HEALTH MANAGEMENT⁼ NDx

Definition: Absence or deficiency of cognitive information related to specific topic (lack of specific information) necessary for client/significant others to make informed choices regarding condition/treatment/lifestyle changes; pattern of regulating and integrating into daily living and family processes a therapeutic regimen for treatment of illnesses and the sequelae of illness that is unsatisfactory for meeting specific health goals.

Related to:

- Specific topic (lack of specific information necessary for clients/significant others) to make informed choices regarding condition/treatment/lifestyle changes
- Pattern of regulating and integrating into daily living and family processes a therapeutic regimen for treatment of illness and the sequelae of illness that is unsatisfactory for meeting specific health goals

CLINICAL MANIFESTATIONS

Subjective	Objective
Verbalizes inability to manage illness; verbalizes inability to follow prescribed regimen	Inaccurate follow through with instructions; inappropriate behaviors; experience of preventable complications of renal failure

RISK FACTORS

- Cognitive deficit
- Financial concerns
- Failure to take action to reduce risk factors for complications of renal failure
- Inability to care for oneself
- Difficulty in modifying personal habits and integrating treatments into lifestyle

---

*The nurse should select the diagnostic label that is most appropriate for the client's discharge teaching needs.

NDx = NANDA-I Diagnosis   **D** = Delegatable Action   ● = UAP   ✦ = LVN/LPN   ⊖▶ = Go to ⊖volve for animation

Continued...

NOC OUTCOMES	NIC INTERVENTIONS
Knowledge: treatment regimen; knowledge: diet; knowledge: infection control; knowledge: cardiac medication	Health system guidance; teaching: individual; teaching: disease process; teaching: prescribed activity/exercise; teaching: prescribed medication

NURSING ASSESSMENT	RATIONALE
Assess client's readiness and ability to learn. Assess meaning of illness to client.	*Early recognition of readiness to learn and meaning of illness to client allows for implementation of the appropriate teaching interventions.*

THERAPEUTIC INTERVENTIONS	RATIONALE

Desired Outcome: The client will verbalize a basic understanding of renal failure.

Independent Actions

Explain renal failure in terms that client can understand. Use appropriate teaching aids (e.g., pictures, videotapes, kidney models).	*Client's understanding of the disease process will increase adherence with treatment regimen.*

THERAPEUTIC INTERVENTIONS	RATIONALE

Desired Outcome: The client will identify ways to slow the progression of kidney damage.

Independent Actions
Provide instructions regarding ways to slow the progression of kidney damage:

• Control hypertension by adhering to dietary modifications and taking medications as prescribed.	*Prevents further damage to the kidneys.*
• Reduce the risk of urinary tract infection by:	
• Cleaning perianal area thoroughly after each bowel movement	*Proper perineal hygiene prevents urinary tract exposure to vaginal or rectal bacteria.*
• Wiping from front to back after urination and defecation (if female)	
• Consuming the maximum amount of fluids allowed	*Maintenance of appropriate fluid intake maintains vascular fluid volume.*
• Reduce the risk of nephrotoxic reactions by:	
• Consulting the appropriate health care provider before:	
(1) Taking any additional prescription and nonprescription drugs	*Many over-the-counter and prescription medications are nephrotoxic.*
(2) Undergoing diagnostic testing that requires use of a contrast medium	*Inform health care provider of renal failure as dyes used in diagnostic testing can be nephrotoxic.*
(3) Resuming any occupation or hobby involving exposure to chemicals or fumes	*Fumes may be nephrotoxic.*
• Avoiding contact with products such as antifreeze, pesticides, carbon tetrachloride, mercuric chloride, lead, arsenic, and creosote.	*Free radicals associated with these materials increase destruction of renal tissue.*
Assist client and significant others to identify ways in which the above-described health care measures can be incorporated into lifestyle.	*Allows client control of how he/she will be able to care for self postdischarge. It will also provide confidence in his/her ability to care for self.*

THERAPEUTIC INTERVENTIONS	RATIONALE

Desired Outcome: The client will verbalize an understanding of fluid restrictions and dietary modifications.

Independent Actions

Reinforce the importance of adhering to and following physician's instructions about fluid restrictions and dietary modifications.	*The client should understand the impact of following prescribed fluid restrictions and dietary modification as well as the impact on the system when the restrictions and modifications are not followed.*

THERAPEUTIC INTERVENTIONS	RATIONALE
Reinforce dietitian's instructions on how to calculate and measure dietary allotments. Have client develop sample menus.	*Allows client to determine appropriate meals based on treatment regimen.*
If client is on a protein- and sodium-restricted diet, inform him/her that numerous salt-free and protein-free products are available. Provide names of local stores that carry these products.	*Provides client with options for diet and flavoring of foods.*
If client is on a fluid restriction, instruct to:	
• Take oral medications with soft foods (e.g., applesauce, pudding).	*This allows client to take medications without using liquids.*
• Reduce thirst by:	
• Sucking on hard candy, popsicles, or ice cubes made with favorite juices	*Maintains moist oral mucous membranes without fluid volume excess and decreases thirst. Be sure to caution client that the fluid volume of the popsicle and ice cubes must be considered as oral fluid intake.*
• Spacing fluids evenly throughout the hours client is awake	*Spacing fluid intake throughout the day helps maintain moist oral mucous membranes and improves client adherence to fluid restrictions.*
• Set out the 24-hour allotment of liquids in the morning in order to visualize the amount allowed for the day.	*Helps client determine when are the best times to drink fluid allotment.*

THERAPEUTIC INTERVENTIONS	RATIONALE

Desired Outcome: The client will demonstrate the ability to accurately weigh self, measure fluid intake and output, and monitor own B/P.

Independent Actions

If client needs to monitor weight, instruct client to weigh at the same time, on the same scale, and with similar amounts of clothing on.	*Weight measurements should be performed daily at the same time and under the same conditions for more precise measurements.*
Demonstrate how to measure and record fluid intake and urinary output if indicated. Stress that any substance that is liquid at room temperature is counted as fluid intake.	*Accurate documentation and monitoring are important to determine appropriate amount of fluid intake.*
If client needs to monitor B/P, provide instructions on how to take, read, and record it.	*Regular monitoring of blood pressure helps prevent hypertension and its deleterious effects on the kidneys.*
Allow time for questions, clarification, practice, and return demonstration. Instruct client to take record of weights, fluid intake, urinary output, and B/P readings to appointments with health care provider.	*Allowing time for questions, clarification, and return demonstrations allows the nurse to evaluate the effectiveness of teaching and make the appropriate adjustments to the teaching plan. It also improves client's self-confidence in his/her ability to care for self and manage disease process.*

THERAPEUTIC INTERVENTIONS	RATIONALE

Desired Outcome: The client will identify ways to reduce the risk of infection.

Independent Actions

Instruct client in ways to reduce the risk of infection:	
• Avoid contact with persons who have an infection.	*These actions prevent exposure to individuals who may have an infection or improve the client's ability to fight infections.*
• Avoid crowds during the flu or cold season.	
• Decrease or stop smoking.	
• Drink allotted amounts of liquids.	
• Maintain good personal hygiene.	
• Maintain a good nutritional status.	
• Maintain an adequate balance between activity and rest.	
• Take antimicrobials as prescribed before scheduled dental work, invasive diagnostic procedures, or surgery.	*Prevents infection from normal body flora.*

Continued...

THERAPEUTIC INTERVENTIONS	RATIONALE

Desired Outcome: The client will identify ways to manage signs and symptoms that often occur as a result of chronic renal failure.

Independent Actions

Provide instructions regarding ways to manage the following signs and symptoms that often occur as a result of chronic renal failure:

- Weakness and fatigue
  - Schedule frequent rest periods throughout the day.
  - Maintain a good nutritional status.
- Dry mouth
  - Space fluid allotments evenly throughout waking hours.
  - Perform oral hygiene frequently.
- Decreased libido (can occur as a result of weakness, fatigue, depression, and side effects of some medications)
  - Schedule rest periods before and after sexual activity.
  - Explore creative ways of expressing sexuality (e.g., massage, fantasies, cuddling).

Knowledge of disease process and how to decrease the impact of risk factors and disease progression helps the client and family understand why lifestyle changes are required to maintain health status. This improves client's adherence to treatment regimen and allows client to maintain a level of independence for as long as possible.

THERAPEUTIC INTERVENTIONS	RATIONALE

Desired Outcome: The client will state signs and symptoms to report to the health care provider.

Independent Actions

Instruct client to report the following:

- Weight gain of more than 0.5 kg (1 lb) per day or a continued weight loss
- Persistent nausea or vomiting

- Increasing fatigue or weakness
- Difficulty concentrating and making decisions
- Confusion
- Persistent or severe headache
- Palpitations or chest pain
- Red, rust-colored, or smoky urine; bloody or tarry stools; blood in sputum or vomitus; persistent bleeding from nose, mouth, or any cut; prolonged or excessive menses; excessive bruising; or sudden abdominal or back pain
- Fever or chills
- Numbness or tingling in extremities, persistent restless feeling in legs during periods of inactivity
- Change in skin color (e.g., bronze, yellow-gray, brownish gray, increased pallor)
- Impotence, infertility, or amenorrhea

- Increasing B/P

- Swelling of feet, ankles, or hands
- Shortness of breath
- Diarrhea or constipation

- Persistent itching
- Oral pain or breakdown of oral mucous membrane

These clinical manifestations should be reported to the health care provider and require prompt attention.
This level of weight gain indicates fluid volume excess.

Persistent nausea and vomiting may indicate changes in serum electrolyte levels.
These clinical manifestations indicate a decreased ability of the kidneys to remove toxins from the body.

Indicates increased B/P or vascular fluid volume.

May indicate infection, anemia, or decreased level of clotting factors.

Indicates an infection.
May indicate anemia and/or changes in electrolyte levels.

May indicate anemia or dialysis-related hemochromatosis.

Could indicate hormonal imbalances caused by increasing serum levels of nitrogenous substances.
Increasing blood pressure may indicate excess vascular fluid volume and/or increased sodium levels.

Diarrhea and/or constipation can occur as a side effect of antacid therapy; physicians generally recommend alternating antacids containing magnesium with those containing aluminum or calcium to prevent these bowel problems.
May indicate high plasma calcium levels.
Increased uremia.

THERAPEUTIC INTERVENTIONS	RATIONALE
• Muscle pain or cramping • Twitching or seizures • Joint or bone pain	*Decreased serum potassium/magnesium.* *May indicate uremic encephalopathy.* *Could indicate renal osteodystrophy resulting from effects of hypo-calcemia and hyperphosphatemia.*

THERAPEUTIC INTERVENTIONS	RATIONALE

Desired Outcome: The client will identify community resources that can assist with adjustment to changes resulting from chronic renal failure.

Independent Actions

Provide information about community resources that can assist the client and significant others to adjust to changes resulting from chronic renal failure (e.g., local chapter of the American Kidney Association, vocational rehabilitation, social services, counseling services).

Provides for continuum of care and support of the client after discharge from the acute care facility.

Initiate a referral if indicated.

May be required for client to receive service or coverage by health care insurance/Medicare/Medicaid.

THERAPEUTIC INTERVENTIONS	RATIONALE

Desired Outcome: The client will verbalize an understanding of and a plan for adhering to recommended follow-up care including future appointments with health care provider and medications prescribed.

Independent Actions

Reinforce the importance of keeping follow-up appointments with health care provider.

Client should understand that he/she has a chronic illness and should be monitored by a health care professional to maintain level of health as long as possible.

Explain the rationale for, side effects of, and importance of taking prescribed medications. Inform client of pertinent food and drug interactions.

Reinforce the importance of consulting the appropriate health care provider (e.g., pharmacist, nurse practitioner, physician) before taking any prescription and nonprescription drugs. Explain that:

• Some drugs such as ibuprofen, neomycin, and naproxen are nephrotoxic and can hasten the progression of renal failure.

Knowledge of medications and how they impact the system improves client adherence to treatment regimen and understanding of the importance of adhering to the prescribed medication regimen. The client must be able to recognize alterations in functioning related to medication administration and what clinical manifestations should be reported to the health care provider.

Nephrotoxic medications hasten the progression of renal failure.

• Some drugs such as aspirin and digoxin are excreted by the kidneys and can rapidly build to toxic levels in the body (usual dosages may need to be reduced or a different medication may need to be taken).

Some drugs quickly build up to toxic levels because they are excreted by the kidneys.

• Some drugs contain ingredients that affect electrolyte balance and elevate B/P (e.g., many cold remedies).

Include significant others in explanations and teaching sessions, and encourage their support.

Including significant others in teaching helps them understand how to appropriately support the client and improves adherence to the treatment regimen.

Reinforce the need to the client to assume responsibility for managing as much of care as possible.

Improves client's confidence in ability to care for self and maintain independence as long as possible.

ADDITIONAL NURSING DIAGNOSES

ACTIVITY INTOLERANCE NDx
Related to:
- Inadequate tissue oxygenation associated with anemia resulting from:
  - Decreased secretion of erythropoietin as a result of impaired renal function (erythropoietin stimulates the bone marrow to produce red blood cells [RBCs])
  - Shortened survival time of RBCs (as renal failure progresses, the nitrogenous substances in the blood increase and cause increased hemolysis of RBCs)
- Inadequate nutritional status

RISK FOR CONSTIPATION NDx
Related to:
- Decreased intake of foods high in fiber and fluids associated with prescribed restrictions
- Decreased gastrointestinal motility associated with decreased activity and the effect of some medications (e.g., those containing aluminum or calcium, iron preparations)

RISK FOR INFECTION NDx
Related to:
- Lowered natural resistance associated with:
  - Changes in leukocyte function and a depressed immune response resulting from the effects of increasing levels of serum nitrogenous substances
  - Inadequate nutritional status

- Stasis of respiratory secretions and urinary stasis if mobility is decreased

IMPAIRED ORAL MUCOUS MEMBRANE NDx
Related to: Prescribed fluid restrictions

FEAR AND ANXIETY NDx
Related to:
- Prescribed fluid restriction
- Lack of understanding of diagnosis, diagnostic tests, and treatment plan
- Uncertainty as to extensiveness of loss of renal function
- Anticipated change in health status, lifestyle, and roles as a result of progressive loss of renal function
- Awareness of probable future need for dialysis or renal transplantation
- Financial concerns

GRIEVING NDx
Related to: Progressive loss of kidney function and the effects of this on lifestyle and roles

12 The Client with Alterations in Musculoskeletal Function

AMPUTATION

An amputation is the removal of all or part of a limb. Amputation of an upper or lower extremity may be performed to treat conditions such as tumors, uncontrollable infection, or gangrene and may be indicated in situations involving tissue destruction resulting from trauma or thermal injury (e.g., frostbite, electrocution, burns). Most amputations, however, are performed on the lower extremities of persons with severe peripheral vascular disease. In these instances, the ischemic limb is removed to prevent life-threatening infection and/or relieve severe, persistent discomfort. The level of amputation (e.g., above the knee, below the knee) is determined by factors such as the adequacy of circulation in the involved extremity; the client's age, general health, and anticipated mobility; and the requirements for proper fit and optimal function of the prosthetic device.

The two types of surgical amputations are open and closed. The open type is performed if the client has an infected limb. The wound is left open, treated until the infection resolves, and then closed during a second surgical procedure. An open amputation may also be done if the client has a very high risk for developing a wound or bone infection postoperatively. A closed amputation, which consists of soft tissue flaps sutured over the bone, is the type of amputation that is more frequently performed. The basic techniques for postoperative management of the residual limb after a closed amputation include use of a soft compression dressing or use of a rigid dressing. The technique selected depends on the client's underlying disease process and physiological status and whether the prosthetic fitting will be immediate, early (usually within 10-30 days), or delayed or is not expected to occur (unplanned).

This care plan focuses on the adult client hospitalized for a planned below-the-knee, closed amputation.* Much of the postoperative information is applicable to clients receiving follow-up care in an extended care facility or home setting.

OUTCOME/DISCHARGE CRITERIA

The client will:
1. Have pain controlled
2. Have evidence of normal healing of the surgical wound
3. Achieve expected level of mobility
4. Have no signs and symptoms of postoperative complications
5. Demonstrate appropriate ways to prevent contractures, increase strength, and improve mobility
6. Demonstrate correct transfer and ambulation techniques and proper use of ambulatory aids
7. Identify ways to maintain health of the remaining lower extremity
8. Demonstrate the ability to care for the residual limb
9. Verbalize how to care for the prosthesis and residual limb if a permanent prosthesis is planned
10. Identify ways to manage phantom limb pain if it occurs
11. State signs and symptoms to report to the health care provider
12. Share feelings and thoughts about the change in body image and effects of the amputation on lifestyle and roles
13. Identify community resources that can assist with home management and adjustment to changes resulting from the amputation
14. Verbalize an understanding of and a plan for adhering to recommended follow-up care including future appointments with health care provider, prosthetist, and physical therapist; medications prescribed; and activity level

For a full, detailed care plan on this topic, go to http://evolve.elsevier.com/Haugen/careplanning/.

---

*If an above-the-knee amputation is planned, refer to medical-surgical nursing texts for additional nursing diagnoses and related actions that might be appropriate.

NDx = NANDA-I Diagnosis   **D** = Delegatable Action   ● = UAP   ✦ = LVN/LPN   ⊝▶ = Go to ⊝volve for animation

FRACTURED HIP WITH INTERNAL FIXATION OR PROSTHESIS INSERTION

A fractured hip is the term used to describe a fracture of the proximal end of the femur. Hip fractures are classified according to the specific location of the fracture. A common classification system divides hip fractures into three types: femoral neck fractures (also referred to as intracapsular fractures), intertrochanteric fractures, and subtrochanteric fractures (the latter two types are sometimes referred to as extracapsular fractures).

A fractured hip is one of the most common orthopedic injuries in the elderly because of the increased incidence of osteoporosis and falls in the elderly population. Although a fractured hip can be treated by traction, the preferred treatment is surgery because it allows earlier mobility.

Surgery involves insertion of a femoral head prosthesis or reduction and internal fixation of the fracture with an intramedullary fixation device, cannulated screws, or a dynamic compression hip screw with a plate assembly. Internal fixation with preservation of the femoral head is the preferred treatment for hip fractures, but the femoral head and neck can be replaced with a prosthetic device (e.g., Austin Moore prosthesis) if an intracapsular fracture has occurred and factors are present that increase the risk for avascular necrosis and/or nonunion. Ideally, surgery is performed within 12 to 24 hours after the injury, especially if the client has a displaced femoral neck. During the preoperative period, traction is usually applied to stabilize and reduce the fracture and reduce muscle spasms and pain.

This care plan focuses on the elderly adult client who is hospitalized for surgical repair of a hip fracture. Much of the postoperative information is applicable to clients receiving follow-up care in an extended care facility or home setting.

OUTCOME/DISCHARGE CRITERIA

The client will:
1. Have evidence of normal healing of the surgical wound
2. Have clear, audible breath sounds throughout lungs
3. Have expected level of mobility
4. Have adequate fracture reduction and healing
5. Have hip pain controlled
6. Have no signs and symptoms of infection or postoperative complications
7. Demonstrate correct transfer and ambulation techniques and proper use of ambulatory aids
8. Demonstrate the ability to correctly perform the prescribed exercises
9. Verbalize an understanding of activity and position restrictions necessary to prevent dislocation of the prosthesis or internal fixation device
10. Identify ways to reduce the risk of falls in the home environment
11. Share thoughts and feelings about the need to transfer to or remain in an extended care or assisted living facility
12. State signs and symptoms to report to the health care provider
13. Identify community resources that can assist with home management and provide transportation
14. Verbalize an understanding of and a plan for adhering to recommended follow-up care including future appointments with health care provider and physical therapist, medications prescribed, activity level, and wound care.

PREOPERATIVE: USE IN CONJUNCTION WITH THE STANDARDIZED PREOPERATIVE CARE PLAN

RELATED PREOPERATIVE NURSING/COLLABORATIVE DIAGNOSES

FEAR/ANXIETY

Related to:
- Severe pain
- Lack of understanding of traction device and planned surgical procedure
- Unfamiliar environment and separation from significant others
- Anticipated postoperative discomfort and loss of control associated with the effects of anesthesia
- Financial concerns associated with hospitalization
- Potential embarrassment or loss of dignity associated with body exposure
- Possibility of changes in usual lifestyle, permanent disability, or death

PREOPERATIVE: USE IN CONJUNCTION WITH THE STANDARDIZED PREOPERATIVE CARE PLAN

Nursing Diagnosis   ## ACUTE PAIN NDx (HIP)

Definition: Unpleasant sensory and emotional experience arising from actual or potential tissue damage

Related to: fracture of the bone, tissue trauma, and muscle spasms

CLINICAL MANIFESTATIONS

Subjective	Objective
Verbalization of pain	Grimacing; reluctance to move; clutching hip/thigh; restlessness; diaphoresis; increased B/P; tachycardia

RISK FACTORS

- Trauma
- Dislocation
- Fractures

DESIRED OUTCOMES

The client will experience diminished hip pain as evidenced by:
   a. Verbalization of a reduction in pain
   b. Relaxed facial expression and body positioning
   c. Stable vital signs

NOC OUTCOMES

Comfort level; pain control

NIC INTERVENTIONS

Analgesic administration; pain management; environmental management: comfort

NURSING ASSESSMENT	RATIONALE

Assess for and report signs and symptoms of pain
- Verbalization of pain
- Grimacing, clutching hip, diaphoresis, increased B/P, tachycardia

Assess client's perception of the severity of pain using a pain intensity rating scale.

Assess the client's pain pattern:
- Location, quality, onset, duration, precipitating factors, aggravating factors, alleviating factors

Early recognition of signs and symptoms of acute hip pain allows for prompt intervention.

THERAPEUTIC INTERVENTIONS	RATIONALE

Independent Actions

Implement measures to reduce pain:
- Perform actions to reduce fear and anxiety about the pain experience:
  - Assure client that the need for pain relief is understood; plan methods for achieving pain control with client.
- Perform actions to reduce fear and anxiety:
  - Reduce environmental stimulation.
  - Provide explanation prior to procedures.
- Perform actions to promote rest:
  - Minimize environmental activity and noise.
  - Limit the number of visitors and their length of stay.
- Provide or assist with additional nonpharmacological measures for pain relief.
  - Relaxation exercises
  - Diversional activities such as watching television, reading, or conversing

Promotes relaxation and subsequently increases the client's threshold and tolerance for pain.

Actions help to reduce fatigue and subsequently increase the client's threshold and tolerance for pain.

Dependent/Collaborative Actions

Implement measures to reduce pain:
- Administer analgesics and muscle relaxants if ordered.

- Perform actions to maintain effective traction on the injured extremity.
  - Ensure that weights are hanging freely.
  - Do not allow footplate or ropes to rest on end of bed.
  - Keep affected heel off bed.
  - Keep knots away from pulley device.
  - Do not remove traction unless specifically ordered.

Administering analgesics before activities and procedures that can cause pain and before pain becomes severe improves mobility.
Client is usually placed in Buck's traction preoperatively to stabilize and reduce the fracture and reduce muscle spasms and pain.

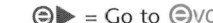 **NDx** = NANDA-I Diagnosis   **D** = Delegatable Action   ● = UAP   ✦ = LVN/_PN   ⊖▶ = Go to ⊖volve for animation

Continued...

THERAPEUTIC INTERVENTIONS	RATIONALE
• Do not lift the weights in order to facilitate moving the client or performing other care.	*This reduces traction pull and can cause severe muscle spasm.*
• Limit head of bed elevation to 20 degrees to 25 degrees except for meals and toileting.	*Actions help to maintain the prescribed traction force.*
• Place a trochanter roll or sandbag firmly against the lateral aspect of injured hip and upper thigh (should extend from iliac crest to midthigh).	*Trochanter rolls/sandbags help to maintain leg in proper alignment.*
• Consult physician if extremity appears out of alignment; do not attempt to realign extremity.	*An attempt to realign the extremity may cause further tissue trauma.*
• Move client carefully, keeping injured extremity well supported.	
If turning is allowed, place pillow between legs before turning.	*In order to prevent adduction and further strain on the fracture site*
Consult appropriate health care provider if above measures fail to provide adequate pain relief:	*Notifying the appropriate health care provider allows for modification of the treatment plan.*
• Physician, pharmacist	
• Pain management specialist	

Nursing Diagnosis ## RISK FOR PERIPHERAL NEUROVASCULAR DYSFUNCTION NDx (FRACTURED EXTREMITY)

Definition: At risk for disruption in circulation, sensation, or motion of an extremity

Related to:
• Trauma to or excessive pressure on the nerves or blood vessels as a result of the injury
• Displaced bone fragments
• Blood accumulation and edema at fracture site
• Improper alignment, application of skin traction device, or traction on the injured extremity

CLINICAL MANIFESTATIONS

Subjective	Objective
Verbalization of numbness or tingling in leg or foot; increased pain in extremity or buttock (new or increased pain that occurs during passive movement is a symptom of compartment syndrome)	Diminished or absent pedal pulses; capillary refill time in toes greater than 2 to 3 seconds; pallor, cyanosis, or coolness of the extremity; inability to flex or extend knee, foot, or toes

RISK FACTORS
• Immobilization
• Mechanical compression
• Vascular obstruction

DESIRED OUTCOMES

The client will maintain normal neurovascular function in the injured extremity as evidenced by:
  a. Palpable pedal pulses
  b. Capillary refill time in toes less than 2 to 3 seconds
  c. Extremity warm and usual color
  d. Ability to flex and extend knee, foot, and toes
  e. Absence of numbness and tingling in leg and foot
  f. No increase in pain in extremity or buttock

NOC OUTCOMES

Tissue perfusion: peripheral

NIC INTERVENTIONS

Circulatory care: arterial insufficiency; circulatory care: venous insufficiency; positioning; lower extremity monitoring; pressure management; heat/cold application

NURSING ASSESSMENT	RATIONALE
Assess for and report signs and symptoms of neurovascular dysfunction in the injured extremity: • Numbness or tingling in leg or foot • Increased pain in extremity or buttock • Diminished or absent pedal pulses • Capillary refill time in toes greater than 2 to 3 seconds • Pallor, cyanosis, or coolness of the extremity • Inability to flex or extend knee, foot, or toes	*Early recognition of signs and symptoms of neurovascular dysfunction allows for prompt intervention.*

THERAPEUTIC INTERVENTIONS	RATIONALE
Independent Actions Implement measures to prevent neurovascular dysfunction in injured extremity: • Place a trochanter roll or sandbag firmly against lateral aspect of injured hip and upper thigh (should extend from the iliac crest to midthigh). **D** ✦ • Make sure skin traction device (e.g., elastic wraps, foam boot with Velcro strap) is applied properly (if necessary to reapply, obtain assistance so that one person can maintain traction on the leg during the reapplication process). **D** ✦ • Make sure that excessive or prolonged pressure is not exerted on Achilles tendon and medial and lateral aspects of knee and ankle. **D** ✦	*Actions help to maintain proper alignment, preventing undue pressure on nerves.*
If signs and symptoms of neurovascular dysfunction occur: • Assess for and correct improper positioning of the injured extremity and traction device and external cause of excessive pressure.	*Correcting improper positioning of extremity and traction devices can prevent nerve damage by preventing stretching/inflammation of associated nerves.*
Dependent/Collaborative Actions Implement measures to prevent neurovascular dysfunction in injured extremity: • Maintain traction as ordered. **D** ✦ • Do not attempt to realign injured leg unless specifically ordered. **D** ✦ • Do not turn client on injured side unless specifically ordered. **D** ✦	*An attempt to align extremity may cause further trauma to the nerves and blood vessels.* *May cause further displacement of fracture and decrease blood flow to area.*
If signs and symptoms of neurovascular dysfunction occur: • Notify physician if the signs and symptoms persist or worsen. • Prepare client for surgical intervention (e.g., internal fixation, insertion of hip prosthesis).	*Notifying the appropriate health care provider allows for modification of the treatment plan.*

POSTOPERATIVE: USE IN CONJUNCTION WITH THE STANDARDIZED POSTOPERATIVE CARE PLAN

Nursing Diagnosis **RISK FOR PERIPHERAL NEUROVASCULAR DYSFUNCTION** NDx **(OPERATIVE EXTREMITY)**

Definition: At risk for disruption in circulation, sensation, or motion of an extremity

Related to:
• Trauma to or excessive pressure on the nerves or blood vessels as a result of surgery and the initial injury
• Blood accumulation and edema in the surgical area
• Improper alignment of operative extremity
• Tight or improperly positioned abductor device straps
• Dislocation of prosthesis or internal fixation device

NDx = NANDA-I Diagnosis   **D** = Delegatable Action   ● = UAP   ✦ = LVN/LPN   ⊖▶ = Go to ⊖volve for animation

Continued...

CLINICAL MANIFESTATIONS

Subjective	Objective
Verbalization of numbness or tingling in leg or foot; increased pain in extremity or buttock (new or increased pain that occurs during passive movement is a symptom of compartment syndrome)	Diminished or absent pedal pulses; capillary refill time in toes greater than 2 to 3 seconds; pallor, cyanosis, or coolness of the extremity; inability to flex or extend knee, foot, or toes

RISK FACTORS
- Mechanical compression
- Vascular obstruction
- Immobilization

DESIRED OUTCOMES
The client will maintain normal neurovascular function in the operative extremity.

NOC OUTCOMES
Tissue perfusion: peripheral

NIC INTERVENTIONS
Circulatory care: arterial insufficiency; circulatory care: venous insufficiency; positioning; lower extremity monitoring; pressure management; heat/cold application

---

NURSING ASSESSMENT	RATIONALE
Assess for and report signs and symptoms of neurovascular dysfunction in the operative extremity: • Numbness or tingling in leg or foot • Increased pain in extremity or buttock • Diminished or absent pedal pulses • Capillary refill time in toes greater than 2 to 3 seconds • Pallor, cyanosis, or coolness of the extremity • Inability to flex or extend knee, foot, or toes	*Early recognition of signs and symptoms of neurovascular dysfunction allows for prompt intervention.*

THERAPEUTIC INTERVENTIONS	RATIONALE

Independent Actions
Implement measures to prevent neurovascular dysfunction in the operative extremity:
• Maintain extremity in proper alignment. **D** ✦
• Perform actions to prevent dislocation of prosthesis or internal fixation device: **D** ●
  • Perform actions to prevent adduction of the operative extremity: **D** ●
    (1) Keep two or three pillows or abductor device between legs at all times.
    (2) Do not move operative extremity past midline.
• Make sure that straps on abductor device are not too tight and are not exerting pressure on the popliteal space, lateral calf immediately below the knee, and lateral malleolus. **D** ✦
• Apply ice pack or cooling pad to operative hip if ordered to reduce edema; remove ice if signs and symptoms of compartment syndrome (e.g., deep, throbbing, unrelenting pain; pain in buttock or thigh with passive movement of the hip or knee) are present. **D** ✦
If signs and symptoms of neurovascular dysfunction occur:
• Assess for and correct improperly applied or tight straps on abductor device and improper positioning of operative extremity; do not attempt to realign extremity if extreme rotation has occurred.
	Maintaining proper alignment of affected limb prevents stretching/inflammation of associated nerves, reducing pain and muscle spasms.
	If a prosthesis has been inserted, the patient is at increased risk for dislocation.
	
	Reducing edema alleviates pressure on surrounding nerves, decreasing the risk for nerve dysfunction.

THERAPEUTIC INTERVENTIONS	RATIONALE

Dependent/Collaborative Actions

If signs and symptoms of neurovascular dysfunction occur:

- Notify physician if the signs and symptoms persist or worsen.
- Prepare client for closed reduction or return to surgery if planned.

Notifying the appropriate health care provider allows for modification of the treatment plan.

Collaborative Diagnosis | # RISK FOR HYPOVOLEMIC SHOCK

Definition: Low blood flow shock due to loss of intravascular fluid volume

Related to: Excessive bleeding associated with fracture of the proximal femur (bones are quite vascular) and intraoperative and postoperative blood loss

CLINICAL MANIFESTATIONS

Subjective	Objective
N/A	Restlessness; agitation; confusion; significant decrease in B/P; postural hypotension; rapid, weak pulse; tachypnea; cool skin; pallor; cyanosis; diminished or absent pulses; urine output less than 30 mL/h

RISK FACTORS

- Long bone fractures
- Coagulopathy
- Inadequate fluid/blood replacement

DESIRED OUTCOMES

The client will not develop hypovolemic shock.

NURSING ASSESSMENT	RATIONALE

Assess for and report signs and symptoms of hypovolemic shock in the operative extremity:

- Restlessness
- Agitation
- Confusion
- Significant decrease in B/P
- Postural hypotension
- Rapid, weak pulse
- Tachypnea
- Cool skin
- Pallor, cyanosis
- Diminished or absent pulses
- Urine output less than 30 mL/h

Early recognition of signs and symptoms of hypovolemic shock allows for prompt intervention.

THERAPEUTIC INTERVENTIONS	RATIONALE

Dependent/Collaborative Actions

Implement measures to prevent hypovolemic shock:

- If bleeding occurs, apply firm, prolonged pressure to the area if possible.
- Carefully measure wound drainage and administer replacement fluids as ordered. **D** ✦

If signs and symptoms of hypovolemic shock occur:

- Place client flat in bed with legs elevated unless contraindicated.
- Monitor vital signs frequently.
- Administer oxygen as ordered.
- Administer blood and/or volume expanders.

Absolute hypovolemia, when fluid is lost through hemorrhage, requires fluid resuscitation with the appropriate replacement: normal saline, colloids, or blood products. Careful measurement of wound drainage and adequate volume replacement can help to prevent hypovolemic shock.

NDx = NANDA-I Diagnosis   **D** = Delegatable Action   ● = UAP   ✦ = LVN/LPN   ⊖▶ = Go to ⊖volve for animation

RISK FOR DISLOCATION OF PROSTHESIS OR INTERNAL FIXATION DEVICE

Definition: Temporary displacement of one or more bones in a joint in which opposing bone surfaces lose contact

Related to:
• Improper movement or positioning of operative extremity
• Noncompliance with weight-bearing limitations
• Delayed healing of the fracture
• Infection of the bone or surrounding tissue

CLINICAL MANIFESTATIONS

Subjective	**Objective**
Reports of sudden, severe pain in operative hip; sudden inability to participate in usual exercise and ambulation regimen	Significant (>10 degrees) external rotation of the operative leg; operative leg more than 2.5 cm (1 inch) shorter than unoperative leg; decline in neurovascular status in operative leg

RISK FACTORS
• Fractures
• Congenital disorders

DESIRED OUTCOMES

The client will not experience dislocation of the prosthesis or internal fixation device as evidenced by:
  a. Continued resolution of hip pain
  b. Ability to maintain operative leg in proper alignment
  c. Length of operative leg equal to unoperative leg
  d. Ability to adhere to exercise and ambulation regimen
  e. Normal neurovascular status in operative leg

NURSING ASSESSMENT	**RATIONALE**
Assess for and report signs and symptoms of dislocation of the hip or external fixation device: • Sudden, severe pain in operative hip • Sudden inability to participate in usual exercise and ambulation regimen • Significant (>10 degrees) external rotation of the operative leg • Operative leg more than 2.5 cm (1 inch) shorter than unoperative leg • Decline in neurovascular status in operative leg	*Early recognition of signs and symptoms of a dislocated hip allows for prompt intervention.*

THERAPEUTIC INTERVENTIONS	**RATIONALE**

Independent Actions
Implement measures to reduce the risk for dislocation of the prosthesis or internal fixation device:
• Perform actions to prevent adduction of the operative extremity:
  • Keep two or three pillows or abductor device between legs at all times. **D** ✦ ●
  • Remind client not to cross legs. **D** ✦
  • Do not move operative extremity past midline. **D** ✦
• Maintain the operative extremity in proper alignment. **D** ✦
• Maintain restrictions on head-of-bed elevation if ordered (some physicians order a 45 degree to 60 degree maximum elevation for the first few days after surgery). **D** ✦
	Actions help to prevent adduction of the operative extremity, which may increase the risk of dislocation.
	
	Incorrect alignment of the affected extremity can result in increased pain and nonunion/malunion.
	Restricting head-of-bed elevation helps to reduce hip flexion and the risk for dislocation.

THERAPEUTIC INTERVENTIONS	RATIONALE
• Perform actions to prevent extreme (beyond 90 degree) hip flexion:	
• Instruct client not to lean forward to reach objects on end of bed or on floor or to put on slippers, socks, or shoes.	
• Raise the entire bed to client's midthigh level before client gets in or out of bed. **D ✦**	*Action helps to reduce the degree of hip flexion that occurs when client sits on edge of bed.*
• Provide a high, firm chair (or elevate sitting surface with pillows) and an elevated toilet seat for client's use. **D ✦ ●**	*Action helps to reduce degree of hip flexion when client sits down.*
• Do not elevate operative leg when sitting in chair. **D ✦ ●**	
• Maintain restrictions on turning (usually allowed to turn on unoperative side only) and always turn client with pillows between legs. **D ✦**	*Actions help to maintain proper body alignment, reducing the risk of dislocation.*
• Reinforce weight-bearing limitations ordered (partial weight-bearing is usually allowed as soon as ambulation is started after prosthesis insertion; weight-bearing restrictions vary after internal fixation depending on the stability of the fracture reduction and fixation).	
• Perform actions to prevent and treat wound infection and osteomyelitis.	*Osteomyelitis ultimately deprives bone of its underlying blood supply, leading to necrosis and death of bone, which may weaken the joint, resulting in displacement.*
• Use good hand hygiene and encourage client to do the same.	
• Instruct client to avoid touching wound.	
If signs and symptoms of dislocation of prosthesis or internal fixation device occur:	
• Maintain client on bedrest.	
• Prepare client for radiographs of surgical area.	
• Prepare client for closed reduction or surgical repair of the dislocation if planned.	

Collaborative Diagnosis ## RISK FOR THROMBOEMBOLISM

Definition: Formation in a blood vessel of a clot (thrombus) that breaks loose and is carried by the bloodstream to plug another vessel

Related to:
- Venous stasis associated with increased blood viscosity (can result from deficient fluid volume), decreased mobility, and pressure exerted on blood vessels by abductor device
- Hypercoagulability associated with increased release of tissue thromboplastin into the blood (occurs as a result of surgical trauma) and hemoconcentration and increased blood viscosity (can occur as a result of deficient fluid volume)
- Trauma to vein walls during surgery

CLINICAL MANIFESTATIONS

Subjective	Objective
Deep vein thrombosis: verbalization of pain or tenderness in an extremity	Increased circumference of an extremity; unusual warmth of an extremity; positive Homans' sign; distention of superficial vessels in an extremity
Pulmonary embolism: verbalization of acute onset of chest pain; apprehension	Tachypnea; dyspnea; tachycardia

RISK FACTORS
- Virchow's triad
- Orthopedic surgery
- Inadequate hydration

DESIRED OUTCOMES

The client will not develop a deep vein thrombus or pulmonary embolism.

NDx = NANDA-I Diagnosis   **D** = Delegatable Action   **●** = UAP   **✦** = LVN/LPN   ⊖▶ = Go to ⊖volve for animation

Continued...

NURSING ASSESSMENT	RATIONALE
Assess for and report signs and symptoms of thromboembolism:	*Early recognition of signs and symptoms of a thromboembolism allows for prompt intervention.*
• Deep vein thrombosis: pain or tenderness in an extremity; increased circumference of an extremity; unusual warmth of an extremity; positive Homans' sign; distention of superficial vessels in an extremity	
• Pulmonary embolism: acute onset of chest pain; apprehension; tachypnea; dyspnea; tachycardia	

THERAPEUTIC INTERVENTIONS	RATIONALE
Dependent/Collaborative Actions	
Implement additional measures to prevent thrombus formation:	
• Make sure that straps on abductor device do not exert excessive pressure on any area. **D** ✦	*Excessive pressure obstructs venous blood flow, increasing venous stasis and the risk for thromboembolism.*
• Make sure that antiembolism stockings are applied correctly and that intermittent pneumatic compression device is correctly applied and functioning properly. **D** ✦	
• Encourage client to perform active foot exercises every 1 to 2 hours while awake; provide adequate analgesia to promote client compliance.	*Ensuring adequate pain relief enhances the client's ability to perform actions that promote mobility and reduce venous stasis.*
• Administer anticoagulants if ordered.	*Anticoagulants are routinely ordered for the prevention and treatment of deep vein thrombosis.*
• Assist client with ambulation as soon as allowed.	*Anticoagulation does not dissolve the clot, but it prevents clot propagation, the development of any new thrombi, and embolization.*

Collaborative Diagnosis   RISK FOR FAT EMBOLISM SYNDROME (FES)

Definition: Systemic fat globules from fractures that are distributed into tissues and organs after a traumatic skeletal injury

Related to: Release of fat globules from the bone marrow and injured surrounding tissue into the bloodstream associated with fracture of a long bone and subsequent surgery on the bone

CLINICAL MANIFESTATIONS

Subjective	Objective
N/A	Restlessness, apprehension, confusion; sudden onset of dyspnea; tachypnea; elevated pulse rate and temperature; petechiae on the chest, neck, or axilla; low partial pressure of oxygen in arterial blood (Pao_2) level; unexpected decrease in hematocrit (Hct) and hemoglobin (Hgb) levels; thrombocytopenia

RISK FACTORS
• Traumatic skeletal injury

DESIRED OUTCOMES

The client will not experience FES as evidenced by:
a. Usual mental status
b. Unlabored respirations at 12 to 20 breaths/min
c. Absence of petechiae
d. Pao_2 within normal limits

NURSING ASSESSMENT	RATIONALE
Assess for and report signs and symptoms of FES: • Restlessness • Apprehension • Confusion • Sudden onset of dyspnea • Tachypnea • Elevated pulse rate and temperature • Petechiae on the chest, neck, or axilla	*Early recognition of signs and symptoms of FES allows for prompt intervention.*
Assess pulse oximetry/arterial blood gas values for hypoxia/low Pao₂ level.	*Lungs are usually impacted by fat emboli obstructing vessels that supply blood to lung tissue, resulting in ischemia and infarction.*
Assess hemogram for unexpected decrease in Hct and Hgb levels; thrombocytopenia	*Two of several minor criteria associated with FES.*

THERAPEUTIC INTERVENTIONS	RATIONALE
Dependent/Collaborative Actions	
Minimize movement of the fractured extremity during the first few days after the injury. **D ✦ ●**	*Initially, limited mobility after a hip fracture helps to reduce the risk for fat emboli.*
If signs and symptoms of FES occur:	
• Maintain client on bedrest and move fractured extremity as little as possible to prevent further emboli. **D ✦ ●**	
• Administer oxygen and assist with positive airway pressure techniques (e.g., positive end expiratory pressure) if ordered. **D ✦**	*Improves oxygenation in the presence of hypoxia.*
• Prepare client for chest radiograph or lung scan.	
• Administer intravenous fluids as ordered. **D ✦**	*Intravenous fluid administration helps to maintain adequate perfusion to vital organs and prevent shock.*
• Administer corticosteroids if ordered. **D ✦**	*Corticosteroids help to reduce cerebral edema and pulmonary inflammation.*

Collaborative Diagnosis RISK FOR AVASCULAR NECROSIS/DELAYED HEALING OF FRACTURED BONE

Definition: A condition in which poor blood supply to an area of the bone leads to bone death (avascular necrosis) or delayed healing of fractured bone

Related to:
• Avascular necrosis related to an inadequate blood supply to the bone (occurs primarily after intracapsular fractures)
• Delayed healing of fractured bone related to:
• Inadequate reduction and internal fixation of fracture
• Diminished blood supply to fracture site
• Thin or absent periosteum in neck of femur (decreases the healing potential)
• Inadequate nutritional status
• Preexisting osteoporosis
• Development of infection in the fractured bone and/or surrounding tissue

CLINICAL MANIFESTATIONS

Subjective	Objective
Reports of persistent hip pain; inability to make expected progress in physical therapy program	Limited range of motion of operative leg; radiology reports showing delayed healing of fracture

Continued...

RISK FACTORS	DESIRED OUTCOMES

• Dislocation injuries
• Subluxation injuries
	The client will not experience avascular necrosis or delayed healing of the fracture as evidenced by:
	  a. Resolution of hip pain
	  b. Expected progression in prescribed physical therapy program
	  c. Radiology reports showing evidence of normal stages of bone healing

NURSING ASSESSMENT	RATIONALE
Assess for and report signs and symptoms of avascular necrosis and/or delayed healing of the fracture: • Persistent hip pain • Limited range of motion of operative leg Assess radiology results for delayed healing of fractures.	*Early recognition of signs and symptoms of avascular necrosis or delayed healing of a fracture allows for prompt intervention.*

THERAPEUTIC INTERVENTIONS	RATIONALE

Dependent/Collaborative Actions
Implement measures to promote healing of the fracture:
• Maintain operative leg in proper alignment. **D** ✦
• Maintain restrictions on weight-bearing as ordered.
• Maintain an adequate nutritional status. **D** ✦ ●
• Encourage client to consume foods/fluids high in calcium and vitamin D.
• Perform actions to prevent and treat wound infection and osteomyelitis.
  • Use proper hand hygiene.
  • Encourage patient not to touch wounds.
• Discourage smoking.
• Administer the following if ordered: **D** ✦
  • Calcium preparations
  • Vitamin D
  • Medications to inhibit bone resorption
If signs and symptoms of avascular necrosis or delayed healing of the fracture occur:
• Prepare client for diagnostic tests (e.g., radiographs, computed tomography [CT] scan, bone scan, magnetic resonance imaging) if planned.
• Prepare client for surgical intervention if planned.
	
	Immobility and callus formation increase calcium needs.
	
	Infection reduces blood supply to the bone, leading to necrosis and death of the bone.
	
	Evidence strongly suggests that smoking decreases tissue perfusion and may delay bone union.
	The growth of bone tissue requires adequate supplies of calcium.

DISCHARGE TEACHING/CONTINUED CARE

Nursing Diagnosis | # DEFICIENT KNOWLEDGE NDx, INEFFECTIVE SELF-HEALTH MANAGEMENT NDx, OR INEFFECTIVE HEALTH MAINTENANCE*

Definition: Absence or deficiency of cognitive information related to specific topic; pattern of regulating and integrating into daily living a therapeutic regimen for treatment of illness and the sequelae of illness that is unsatisfactory for meeting specific health goals; inability to identify, manage; and/or seek out help to manage health

---

*The nurse should select the nursing diagnostic label that is most appropriate for the client's discharge teaching needs.

CLINICAL MANIFESTATIONS

Subjective	Objective
Verbalization of lack of knowledge about health practices	Lack of expressed interest in improving behavior; exaggerated behavior; inaccurate follow-through of instructions

RISK FACTORS
- Cognitive limitation
- Unfamiliarity with resources
- Complex therapeutic regimen
- Insufficient resources

NOC OUTCOMES

Knowledge: fall prevention; knowledge: prescribed activity; knowledge: treatment regimen

NIC INTERVENTIONS

Health system guidance; teaching: individual; teaching: prescribed activity/exercise

NURSING ASSESSMENT

Assess client's readiness and ability to learn.
Assess meaning of illness to client.

RATIONALE

Early recognition of readiness to learn and meaning of illness to client allows for implementation of the appropriate teaching interventions.

THERAPEUTIC INTERVENTIONS

RATIONALE

Desired Outcome: The client will demonstrate correct transfer and ambulation techniques and proper use of ambulatory aids.

Independent Actions
Reinforce instructions about correct transfer and ambulation techniques, amount of weight-bearing allowed, and proper use of ambulatory aids (a walker is preferable for most elderly clients because it provides the greatest stability).

Allow time for questions, clarification, and practice of transfer and ambulation techniques.

Performing transfer techniques and using assistive devices correctly reduce the risk of injury.

Allows the nurse to reinforce patient education and to evaluate the need for further instruction.

THERAPEUTIC INTERVENTIONS

RATIONALE

Desired Outcome: The client will demonstrate the ability to correctly perform the prescribed exercises.

Independent Actions
Reinforce instructions on muscle strengthening and range-of-motion exercises.

Explain importance of performing muscle strengthening and range-of-motion exercises 3 to 4 times a day.

Allow time for questions, clarification, and return demonstration of prescribed exercises.

Improves mobility, flexibility, and reduces the risk of muscle atrophy.
Builds muscle mass, increasing strength and support to joint.

Allows the nurse to reinforce patient education and to evaluate the need for further instruction.

THERAPEUTIC INTERVENTIONS

RATIONALE

Desired Outcome: The client will verbalize an understanding of activity and position restrictions necessary to prevent dislocation of the prosthesis or internal fixation device.

Continued...

THERAPEUTIC INTERVENTIONS	RATIONALE

Independent Actions

Instruct client to adhere to the following activity and position restrictions for at least 2 months (time may vary depending on physician preference) in order to prevent dislocation of prosthesis or internal fixation device:

- Turn only as directed by physician (many physicians allow turning to unoperative side only).
- Keep pillows between legs when lying on back or side and when turning.
- Never cross legs.
- Do not sit on low chairs, stools, or toilets; place a cushion on low chairs; rent or purchase an elevated toilet seat for home use; and use the high toilets designed for the handicapped when in public facilities.
- Do not elevate operative leg higher than hip when sitting.
- Sit in chairs with arms and use the arms to raise self off chair.
- Support weight on unoperative leg when raising self from a sitting position.
- Use assistive devices (e.g., long-handled shoe horn, long-handled grabber) to assist with activities that require flexing hip beyond 90 degrees (e.g., putting on shoes and socks, reaching objects on the floor or in low cupboards or drawers, pulling bed covers up from end of bed).
- Keep operative leg in proper alignment and avoid extreme internal and external rotation of leg.
- Do not drive until approved by physician (usually about 6 weeks after surgery).
- When riding in a car:
  - Sit on a firm pillow or cushion to prevent hip flexion of more than 90 degrees.
  - Keep operative leg extended (a sudden impact of the knee against the dashboard can dislodge the prosthesis).
- Do not resume sexual activity until approved by physician; when sexual activity is resumed, avoid positions that involve extreme rotation of the operative leg, flexing hip beyond 90 degrees, and moving operative leg past the midline.
- Avoid lifting heavy objects, excessive twisting and turning of body, walking on uneven surfaces, and activities that place excessive strain on hip (e.g., jogging).

Actions help to reduce pain that can result from poor body alignment and helps to prevent dislocation.

Crossing the legs increases the risk of venous thromboembolism.

Sitting on a low chair can force the hip into greater than 90 degrees flexion, which can predispose the client to dislocation.

THERAPEUTIC INTERVENTIONS	RATIONALE

Desired Outcome: The client will identify ways to reduce the risk of falls in the home environment.

Independent Actions

If client is to return home, provide the following instructions on how to reduce the risk for falls at home:

- Keep electrical cords out of pathways.
- Remove unnecessary furniture and provide wide pathways for ambulation.
- Remove scatter rugs.
- Provide adequate lighting at all times.
- Do not climb stairs until permission is given by physician.

Actions reduce potential causes of in-home falls.

THERAPEUTIC INTERVENTIONS	RATIONALE

Desired Outcome: The client will state signs and symptoms to report to the health care provider.

Independent Actions
Instruct client to report these additional signs and symptoms:
- Persistent or increased pain or spasms in operative extremity
- Loss of sensation or movement in operative extremity
- Inability to maintain operative extremity in a neutral position
- Inability to bear weight on operative extremity once weight-bearing is allowed
- Shortening of operative extremity (will probably be noticed as a limp once full weight-bearing is resumed)

Educating the client regarding signs and symptoms to report to the health care provider allows for implementing appropriate interventions, altering the plan of care, and reducing the risk of potential complications.

THERAPEUTIC INTERVENTIONS	RATIONALE

Desired Outcome: The client will identify community resources that can assist with home management and provide transportation.

Independent Actions
Provide information about community resources that can assist the client and significant others with home management and provide transportation.

Social support can aid the client in obtaining necessary resources to adapt to physical changes and obtain the necessary long-term assistance to maintain independence.

THERAPEUTIC INTERVENTIONS	RATIONALE

Desired Outcome: The client will verbalize an understanding of and a plan for adhering to recommended follow-up care including future appointments with health care provider and physical therapist, medications prescribed, activity level, and wound care.

Independent Actions
Reinforce the importance of keeping appointments with physical therapist.
If a hip prosthesis was inserted, instruct client to inform other health care providers about the hip prosthesis so that prophylactic antimicrobials can be started before any dental work, invasive diagnostic procedures, or surgery is performed.
Inform client that the hip prosthesis or fixation device may activate metal detector alarms. Recommend carrying an identification/information card if available.

Adherence to a plan of care reduces the risk of complications and improves patient outcomes.

RELATED CARE PLANS

Preoperative
Postoperative

ADDITIONAL NURSING DIAGNOSES

ACUTE PAIN NDx (HIP)
Related to tissue trauma and reflex muscle spasms associated with the initial injury, surgery, and strain on the area postoperatively

IMPAIRED PHYSICAL MOBILITY NDx
Related to:
- Pain and weakness in weight-bearing extremity associated with the fracture and subsequent surgical repair
- Prescribed activity and weight-bearing restrictions after internal fixation or prosthesis insertion
- Generalized weakness associated with surgery
- Depressant effect of anesthesia and some medications (e.g., narcotic [opioid] analgesics, centrally acting muscle relaxants, some antiemetics)
- Fear of falling, moving operative hip improperly, and compromising surgical wound

NDx = NANDA-I Diagnosis   **D** = Delegatable Action   ● = UAP   ✦ = LVN/LPN   ⊖▶ = Go to ⊖volve for animation

Continued...

RISK FOR INFECTION NDx
Related to:

- Stasis of pulmonary secretions associated with decreased mobility and weak cough effort (an increased risk with elderly clients)
- Wound contamination associated with introduction of pathogens during or after surgery (risk is increased because of close proximity of wound to perineal area)
- Decreased resistance to infection associated with factors such as an inadequate nutritional status and decreased effectiveness of immune system if client is elderly
- Increased growth and colonization of microorganisms in the urine associated with urinary stasis if mobility is decreased and introduction of pathogens if indwelling catheter is present

RISK FOR FALLS NDx
Related to:

- Weakness, fatigue, and postural hypotension associated with the effects of major surgery and physiological changes that may have occurred if client is elderly

- Central nervous system depressant effect of some medications (e.g., narcotic [opioid] analgesics, centrally acting muscle relaxants, some antiemetics)
- Weakness and pain in weight-bearing extremity associated with the initial injury and surgery on the hip
- Difficulty with transfer and ambulation techniques

GRIEVING NDx
Related to:

- Physical limitations imposed by the hip fracture and surgery
- Need for assistance with activities of daily living
- Possible change in roles and future living situation
- Possible permanent disability and death

LAMINECTOMY/DISKECTOMY WITH OR WITHOUT FUSION

A laminectomy is the surgical removal of the lamina of a vertebra. It may be performed to allow for removal of a neoplasm or bone fragments that are putting pressure on nerve roots or the spinal cord or to enable a rhizotomy or cordotomy to be performed to treat intractable pain. Most commonly, a laminectomy is performed to gain access to a herniated nucleus pulposus (HNP, "ruptured disk") so that a diskectomy (removal of the herniated portion of the disk) can be accomplished.

Disk herniation is usually the result of trauma (e.g., falls, vehicular accidents) or strain caused by factors such as improper or repeated lifting of heavy objects, twisting, sneezing, or coughing. Age-related degenerative changes in the disks, supporting ligaments, and vertebrae make the disks more prone to rupture. The most common sites of disk herniation are C5-6, C6-7, L4-5, and L5-S1. These areas of the spine are the most flexible and therefore are subjected to a greater amount of movement and strain. Signs and symptoms of lumbar disk herniation can include low back pain that radiates down the buttock, thigh, calf, and ankle on the affected side; muscle spasms in the lower back; muscle weakness, diminished knee and ankle reflexes, numbness, or tingling in the affected lower extremity; constipation; and/or urinary retention. Clinical manifestations of cervical disk herniation can include neck pain that radiates to the shoulder, arm, and fingers on the affected side; stiff neck; muscle spasms in the neck; and/or muscle weakness, diminished biceps and triceps reflexes, numbness, or tingling in the affected upper extremity.

A diskectomy is usually indicated if conservative measures such as rest, heat or cold applications, anti-inflammatory

medications, analgesics, muscle relaxants, and local steroid injections fail to control pain or if neurological deficits persist or worsen. Disk removal is usually accomplished by a microdiskectomy or laminectomy and can be performed using an anterior and/or posterior approach. The surgical procedure performed depends on the location and size of the herniated disk and physician preference. If the vertebral column in the surgical area is unstable, a spinal fusion may be performed along with a laminectomy. The surgical immobilization of the unstable area is accomplished using a bone graft (autograft [usually from the iliac crest], allograft, or bone substitute) or implanted fixation devices such as cages, plates, screws, and rods.

This care plan focuses on the adult client admitted for a laminectomy that is being performed to remove an HNP. The care of a client hospitalized for a laminectomy with spinal fusion is also discussed. Much of the postoperative information is applicable to clients receiving follow-up care in an extended care facility or home setting.

OUTCOME/DISCHARGE CRITERIA

The client will:
1. Have improved neurological function
2. Have evidence of normal healing of the surgical wound
3. Have intact skin under the stabilization device if one is present
4. Have pain controlled

5. Have no signs and symptoms of postoperative complications
6. Identify ways to prevent recurrent disk herniation
7. Demonstrate the ability to correctly apply and remove the stabilization device if one is required
8. Verbalize an understanding of ways to maintain skin integrity when wearing a stabilization device
9. State signs and symptoms to report to the health care provider
10. Verbalize an understanding of and a plan for adhering to recommended follow-up care including future appointments with health care provider, medications prescribed, activity level, and wound care

PREOPERATIVE: USE IN CONJUNCTION WITH THE STANDARDIZED PREOPERATIVE CARE PLAN

RELATED PREOPERATIVE NURSING/COLLABORATIVE DIAGNOSES

DEFICIENT KNOWLEDGE NDx

Related to: the surgical procedure, routines associated with surgery, physical preparation for laminectomy and spinal fusion (if planned), sensations that normally occur after surgery and anesthesia, and postoperative care.

POSTOPERATIVE: USE IN CONJUNCTION WITH THE STANDARDIZED POSTOPERATIVE CARE PLAN

Nursing Diagnosis # RISK FOR PERIPHERAL NEUROVASCULAR DYSFUNCTION NDx

Definition: At risk for disruption in circulation, sensation, or motion of an extremity

Related to:
- Trauma to the nerves or blood vessels during surgery
- Blood accumulation and inflammation in the surgical area
- Dislocation of the bone graft or implanted fixation devices (if a fusion was performed)
- Excessive external pressure on the nerves or blood vessels associated with improper fit or application of the stabilization device (e.g., cervical collar, back brace, corset)

CLINICAL MANIFESTATIONS

Subjective	Objective
Reports of numbness or tingling in extremities; development of or increase in pain in extremities	Diminished or absent peripheral pulses; capillary refill time greater than 2 to 3 seconds; pallor, cyanosis, or coolness of extremities; inability to flex or extend feet, toes, hands, or fingers; diminished or absent reflexes in extremities; development of or increase in muscle weakness

RISK FACTORS
- Mechanical compression
- Vascular obstruction
- Immobilization

DESIRED OUTCOMES

The client will have usual or improved peripheral neurovascular function as evidenced by:
  a. Palpable peripheral pulses
  b. Capillary refill time less than 2 to 3 seconds
  c. Extremities warm and usual color
  d. Ability to flex and extend feet, toes, hands, and fingers
  e. Usual or improved reflexes, muscle tone, and sensation in extremities
  f. No new or increased pain in extremities

NDx = NANDA-I Diagnosis   **D** = Delegatable Action   ● = UAP   ✦ = LVN/LPN   ⊖▶ = Go to ⊖volve for animation

Continued...

NOC OUTCOMES	NIC INTERVENTIONS
Neurological status: spinal sensory/motor function; tissue perfusion: peripheral	Neurological monitoring; positioning: neurological; circulatory care: arterial insufficiency; circulatory care: venous insufficiency

NURSING ASSESSMENT	RATIONALE
Assess for and report signs and symptoms of peripheral neurovascular dysfunction (check upper extremities after surgery on the cervical area and lower extremities after surgery on the lumbar area • Numbness or tingling in extremities • Development of or increase in pain in extremities • Diminished or absent peripheral pulses • Capillary refill time greater than 2 to 3 seconds • Pallor, cyanosis, or coolness of extremities • Inability to flex or extend feet, toes, hands, or fingers • Diminished or absent reflexes in extremities • Development of or increase in muscle weakness	*Early recognition of signs and symptoms of peripheral neurovascular dysfunction allows for prompt intervention.*

THERAPEUTIC INTERVENTIONS	RATIONALE

Independent Actions

Implement measures to reduce the risk for peripheral neurovascular dysfunction:
*   Perform actions to reduce strain on the surgical area: **D** ✦
    *   Keep spine in proper alignment.
    *   Prevent hyperextension, extreme flexion, or twisting of spine.
    *   Position to maintain flattening of lumbosacral spine:
        (1) Side lying with knees flexed
        (2) Supine with slight knee flexion
*   Maintain wound suction and patency of wound drain.

Reducing strain on the surgical area helps to prevent bleeding and subsequent hematoma formation in the surgical area and to reduce the risk for dislocation of the bone graft or implanted fixation devices (if fusion was performed).

Reduces the accumulation of blood in the surgical area and subsequently prevents increased pressure on nerves and blood vessels.

*   Apply stabilization device properly; notify orthotist if it appears to create excessive pressure on any area.

Dependent/Collaborative Actions

Implement measures to reduce the risk for peripheral neurovascular dysfunction:
*   Perform actions to reduce strain on the surgical area.
    *   Ensure client is always positioned with spine in proper alignment
    *   Apply stabilization device
*   Administer corticosteroids if ordered.

Actions help to stabilize surgical area.

Corticosteroids help to reduce inflammation in the surgical area.

If signs and symptoms of peripheral neurovascular dysfunction occur:
*   Assess for and correct improper body alignment and external cause of excessive pressure (e.g., tight or improperly applied stabilization device).
*   Notify physician if signs and symptoms persist or worsen.
*   Prepare client for surgical intervention (e.g., evacuation of hematoma, repositioning of dislocated bone graft or implanted fixation devices) if planned.

Allows for prompt intervention to reduce complications resulting in permanent nerve dysfunction (e.g., hematoma, dislocated bone graft).

Nursing Diagnosis **ACUTE PAIN** NDx

Definition: Unpleasant sensory and emotional experience arising from actual or potential tissue damage.

Related to:

- Tissue trauma and reflex muscle spasms associated with the surgery
- Removal of bone if an autograft was used to achieve spinal fusion (the bone is usually taken from the client's iliac crest)
- Stretching and compression of sensory nerves associated with blood accumulation and inflammation in the surgical area
- Irritation from drainage tube (wound drain may be present, especially after a spinal fusion)
- Stress on surgical area associated with movement
- Release of pressure on compressed spinal nerve root after removal of the herniated nucleus pulposus (improved sensory nerve function can cause a temporary increase in pain in area[s] of previously diminished sensation).

CLINICAL MANIFESTATIONS

Subjective	Objective
Verbalization of pain; reluctance to move	Grimacing; restlessness; diaphoresis; increased B/P; tachycardia

RISK FACTORS

- Altered limited mobility
- Inadequate pain relief

DESIRED OUTCOMES

The client will experience diminished pain.

NOC OUTCOMES

Pain control; comfort level

NIC INTERVENTIONS

Pain management; analgesic administration

NURSING ASSESSMENT	RATIONALE
Assess the patient for signs and symptoms of pain: - Verbalization of pain - Reluctance to move - Grimacing - Restlessness - Diaphoresis - Increased B/P - Tachycardia	*Early recognition of signs and symptoms of pain allows for prompt intervention.*

THERAPEUTIC INTERVENTIONS	RATIONALE

Independent Actions

Implement additional measures to reduce pain:

- Perform actions to reduce strain on the surgical area: **D** ✦
  - Ensure that client is always positioned with spine in proper alignment. **D** ✦

  - Apply stabilization device if ordered.
  - If stabilization device loosens, reapply it or tighten straps or screws if allowed, or consult orthotist about adjustment of the device.
  - Implement measures to prevent hyperextension, extreme flexion, and/or twisting of spine (e.g., instruct and assist client to logroll when turning; put needed items within easy reach; if a cervical laminectomy was performed, place a small pillow or folded pad under client's head rather than a full-size pillow; assist with bathing and dressing as needed). **D** ✦ ●

Reducing strain on the surgical area helps to prevent bleeding and subsequent hematoma formation in the surgical area and to reduce the risk for dislocation of the bone graft or implanted fixation devices (if fusion was performed).
Stabilization helps to provide additional support to surgical area.

Continued...

THERAPEUTIC INTERVENTIONS	RATIONALE
• If lumbar laminectomy was performed, assist client to maintain a position that results in flattening of the lumbosacral spine (e.g., slight knee flexion when supine, knees flexed while in side-lying position, feet elevated on footstool when sitting in chair). **D** ✦ ●	*Interventions help to reduce stretching of the nerves and muscles in the lower back.*
• Instruct client to avoid sitting or standing for longer than 20- to 30-minute intervals (some physicians instruct clients to sit only during meals and ambulate only short distances when progressive activity begins).	
• Instruct client to avoid straining to have a bowel movement (especially after lumbar laminectomy) and vigorous coughing; consult physician about an order for a laxative and antitussive if indicated.	*Helps to reduce tension on incision lines.*
• If appropriate, perform actions to reduce pressure on bone graft donor site (e.g., position client so he/she is not lying on site, protect the site with padding if stabilization device is worn over it).	

Dependent/Collaborative Actions

Implement additional measures to reduce pain:
• Administer corticosteroids if ordered.   *Steroids help to reduce inflammation in the surgical area.*

Nursing Diagnosis   **ACTUAL/RISK FOR IMPAIRED SKIN INTEGRITY** NDx

Definition: Risk for altered epidermis and/or dermis

Related to:
• Disruption of tissue associated with the surgical procedure
• Irritation of skin associated with contact with wound drainage, use of tape, and pressure from tubes and/or stabilization device if present

CLINICAL MANIFESTATIONS

Subjective	Objective
Verbal reports of pain	Color changes, redness, swelling, warmth (signs of infection); surgical incisions; abrasions/tears

RISK FACTORS
• Physical immobility
• Shearing forces
• Pressure

DESIRED OUTCOMES

The client will:
  a. Experience normal healing of the surgical wound
  b. Maintain tissue integrity in areas in contact with wound drainage, tape, tubings, and stabilization device as evidenced by absence of redness and irritation, and no skin breakdown

NOC OUTCOMES

Wound healing: primary intention; tissue integrity: skin and mucous membranes

NIC INTERVENTIONS

Skin surveillance; positioning; wound care; pressure management

NURSING ASSESSMENT	RATIONALE
Assess the patient for signs and symptoms of skin irritation and breakdown: • Areas in contact with wound drainage, tape, and tubings • Area under stabilization device	*Early recognition of signs and symptoms of actual or impaired skin integrity allows for prompt intervention.*

NURSING ASSESSMENT	RATIONALE

- Color changes, redness, swelling, warmth (signs of infection)
- Surgical incisions
- Abrasions/tears

Assess the site of impaired tissue integrity and determine the cause.

THERAPEUTIC INTERVENTIONS	RATIONALE

Independent Actions

Implement measures to prevent skin irritation and breakdown under stabilization device:

- Apply stabilization device securely enough to keep it from rubbing and irritating the skin but not too tightly. **D** ✦
- Position client so that stabilization device is not causing excessive pressure on any area. **D** ✦
- Assist client to put a cotton T-shirt on under back brace or corset and ensure that the shirt is dry and wrinkle-free. **D** ✦ ●
- Apply a thin layer of a dry lubricant such as powder or cornstarch to skin under stabilization device in order to reduce friction. **D** ✦ ●
- Pad areas over bony prominences before applying stabilization device.
- Instruct client to refrain from inserting anything under the stabilization device.
- Consult physician or orthotist if stabilization device is putting excessive pressure on the skin.

If tissue breakdown occurs:

- Notify appropriate health care provider (e.g., physician, wound care specialist).
- Perform care of involved area(s) as ordered or per standard hospital procedure.

Constant pressure applied to the skin reduces blood flow to the tissues.

Notifying the physician allows for modification of the treatment plan.

Collaborative Diagnosis **RISK FOR RESPIRATORY DISTRESS**

Definition: Severe difficulty breathing

Related to:

- Trauma to the phrenic nerve during surgery and/or compression of the phrenic nerve after surgery associated with inflammation or accumulation of blood in the surgical area (can occur with a cervical laminectomy because the phrenic nerve arises at the C3-5 level)
- Tracheal compression associated with inflammation or accumulation of blood in the surgical area after a cervical laminectomy (particularly if the anterior approach was used)
- Closure of the glottis associated with paralysis of the vocal cords (can occur as a result of injury to the bilateral recurrent laryngeal nerves during an anterior cervical laminectomy)

CLINICAL MANIFESTATIONS

Subjective	Objective
Cervical laminectomy: statements of difficulty swallowing or choking sensation	Cervical laminectomy: increased swelling in the neck or bulging of the wound; rapid and/or labored respirations, stridor, sternocleidomastoid muscle retraction, restlessness, agitation; abnormal arterial blood gas values; decrease in pulse oximetry values

---

Continued...

RISK FACTORS

* Coagulopathy
* Elevated blood pressure
* Third spacing of fluid

DESIRED OUTCOMES

The client will not experience respiratory distress as evidenced by:
  a. Unlabored respirations at 12 to 20 breaths/min
  b. Absence of stridor and sternocleidomastoid muscle retraction
  c. Usual mental status
  d. Oximetry results within normal range
  e. Arterial blood gas values within normal range

NURSING ASSESSMENT

Assess client for signs and symptoms of respiratory distress:
* Verbalization of difficulty swallowing
* Swelling in neck; rapid, labored respiration, stridor, retractions, agitation

Monitor pulse oximetry and arterial blood gas values for abnormalities.

RATIONALE

Early recognition of signs and symptoms of respiratory distress allows for prompt intervention.

THERAPEUTIC INTERVENTIONS

RATIONALE

Independent Actions

Have tracheostomy and suction equipment readily available after cervical laminectomy.

Implement measures to prevent respiratory distress after a cervical laminectomy:

* Implement measures to reduce strain on the surgical area:
  * Keep neck in proper alignment. **D** ✦
  * Ensure that cervical collar is applied correctly.
  * Instruct and assist client to support neck when moving.
* Elevate head of bed 30 degrees to 45 degrees unless contraindicated.
* Apply ice pack to incisional area as ordered. **D** ✦ ●
* Administer corticosteroids if ordered. **D** ✦
* Maintain wound suction and patency of wound drain. **D** ✦

If signs and symptoms of respiratory distress occur:
* Place client in a high-Fowler's position unless contraindicated.
* Loosen neck dressing or cervical collar if it appears tight.
* Administer oxygen as ordered.
* Assist with intubation or emergency tracheostomy if performed.
* Prepare client for surgical evacuation of hematoma or repair of the bleeding vessel(s) if planned.

Actions help to reduce inflammation and/or prevent bleeding and subsequent hematoma formation in the surgical area.

Application of ice reduces postsurgical swelling along incision site. Patent drains help to prevent the accumulation of blood in the surgical area.

Collaborative Diagnosis **RISK FOR CEREBROSPINAL FLUID LEAK**

Definition: Leakage of the cerebrospinal fluid into the tissues and out of the CNS compartment

Related to: Inadvertent damage to and/or incomplete closure of the dura (care is taken during surgery to keep the dura intact; however, it is sometimes necessary to incise dura that extends along the involved nerve)

CLINICAL MANIFESTATIONS

Subjective	Objective
Reports of headache	Clear drainage from the incision; presence of glucose in wound drainage as shown by positive results on a glucose reagent strip (be aware, blood will test positive for glucose); yellowish ring ("halo") around bloody or serosanguineous drainage on lower back or neck dressing, sheet, or pillowcase *(cerebrospinal fluid [CSF] dries in concentric circles)*

RISK FACTORS
- Surgical Damage
- Injury

DESIRED OUTCOMES

The client will have resolution of CSF leak if it occurs as evidenced by:
  a. Absence of CSF drainage from lower back or neck incision
  b. No reports of headache

NURSING ASSESSMENT

Assess for and report signs and symptoms of a CSF leak:
- Reports of headache
- Clear drainage from incision
- Presence of glucose in wound drainage

RATIONALE

Early recognition of signs and symptoms of CSF leak allows for prompt intervention.

THERAPEUTIC INTERVENTIONS

Dependent/Collaborative Actions
Implement measures to reduce strain on the surgical area.
- Keep neck in proper alignment
- Instruct and assist client when moving

If signs and symptoms of CSF leak occur:
- Maintain activity restrictions as ordered to reduce stress on the dural tear. **D ✦ ●**
- Change dressing as soon as it becomes damp; maintain meticulous sterile technique when changing dressing. **D ✦**
- Administer antimicrobials if ordered. **D ✦**
- Assess for and report signs and symptoms of meningitis (e.g., fever; chills; new, increasing, or persistent headache; nuchal rigidity; photophobia; positive Kernig's and Brudzinski's signs).
- Prepare client for surgical repair of the torn dura if planned (usually the torn dura heals spontaneously within a few days).

RATIONALE

Actions help to promote healing of the dura and subsequent resolution of CSF leak.

Collaborative Diagnosis # RISK FOR LARYNGEAL NERVE DAMAGE

Definition: Injury to one or both of the nerves that are attached to the voice box

Related to: Surgical trauma or pressure on the nerve(s) associated with inflammation or accumulation of blood in the surgical area (can occur with an anterior cervical laminectomy)

CLINICAL MANIFESTATIONS

Subjective	Objective
Reports of voice changes (hoarseness; weak, whispery voice; inability to speak)	Respiratory distress (rapid and/or labored respirations, stridor, sternocleidomastoid muscle retraction, restlessness, agitation; abnormal arterial blood gas values; decrease in pulse oximetry values)

RISK FACTORS
- Hematoma at surgical site
- Edema/swelling at surgical site

DESIRED OUTCOMES

The client will experience resolution of laryngeal nerve damage if it occurs as evidenced by:
  a. Improved voice tone and quality
  b. Gradual resolution of hoarseness
  c. Absence of respiratory distress

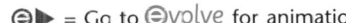

Continued...

NURSING ASSESSMENT	RATIONALE
Assess for the following indications of laryngeal nerve damage: • Hoarseness • Weak, whispery voice • Respiratory distress • Stridor • Retractions • Restlessness • Agitation	*Early recognition of signs and symptoms of laryngeal nerve damage allows for prompt intervention.*

THERAPEUTIC INTERVENTIONS	RATIONALE

Independent Actions

Implement measures to reduce pressure on the laryngeal nerves (e.g., elevated head of bed, ice to surgical site, monitor for swelling).

Assess arterial blood gases for abnormal values and pulse oximetry.

• Encourage client to avoid unnecessary talking. **D** ✦ ●   *Action helps to rest the vocal cords.*

• Implement measures to facilitate communication (e.g., provide pad and pencil, flash cards, or Magic Slate; ask questions that require a short answer or nod of head). **D** ✦ ●

Reinforce physician's explanation regarding the permanence of voice changes (voice tone and quality usually return to normal as inflammation subsides).

If signs and symptoms of laryngeal nerve damage occur:

• Notify physician immediately if signs and symptoms of respiratory distress occur, client is unable to speak, or hoarseness or voice changes worsen.   *Notifying the physician allows for modification of the treatment plan.*

Collaborative Diagnosis # RISK FOR PARALYTIC ILEUS

Definition: Paralysis of the intestinal musculature caused by trauma, peritonitis, electrolyte imbalance, or spasmolytic agents

Related to:
• Impaired innervation of the intestinal tract after a lumbar laminectomy associated with stimulation of sympathetic nerves and/or loss of parasympathetic nerve function in the operative area
• Depressant effect of anesthesia and some medications (e.g., centrally acting muscle relaxants, narcotic [opioid] analgesics, some antiemetics)

CLINICAL MANIFESTATIONS

Subjective	Objective
Reports of persistent abdominal pain and cramping	Firm, distended abdomen; absent bowel sounds; failure to pass flatus

RISK FACTORS
• Immobility
• Narcotic administration

DESIRED OUTCOMES

The client will not develop a paralytic ileus as evidenced by:
  a. Absence or resolution of abdominal pain and cramping
  b. Soft, nondistended abdomen
  c. Gradual return of bowel sounds
  d. Passage of flatus

NURSING ASSESSMENT	RATIONALE
Assess for and report signs and symptoms of paralytic ileus: • Abdominal pain • Cramping • Distended abdomen • Absent bowel sounds • Failure to pass stool Monitor results of abdominal radiographs for abnormalities (distended bowel).	*Early recognition of signs and symptoms of paralytic ileus allows for prompt intervention.*

THERAPEUTIC INTERVENTIONS	RATIONALE
Dependent/Collaborative Actions Implement measures to prevent paralytic ileus: • Increase activity as soon as allowed and tolerated. • Administer gastrointestinal stimulants.	*Ambulation helps to stimulate motility of the gastrointestinal tract.*

DISCHARGE TEACHING/CONTINUED CARE

Nursing Diagnosis | # DEFICIENT KNOWLEDGE NDx, INEFFECTIVE FAMILY THERAPEUTIC REGIMEN MANAGEMENT NDx, OR INEFFECTIVE HEALTH MAINTENANCE NDx*

Definition: Absence or deficiency of cognitive information related to a specific topic; pattern of regulating and integrating into family processes a program for treatment of illness and its sequelae that is unsatisfactory for meeting specific health goals; inability to identify, manage, and/or seek out help to maintain health.

CLINICAL MANIFESTATIONS

Subjective	Objective
Verbalization of the problem	Demonstrated lack of knowledge about basic health practices; demonstrated lack of adaptive behaviors; impaired personal support systems; inaccurate follow through of instructions

RISK FACTORS
• Cognitive deficit
• Financial concerns
• Inability to care for oneself

NOC OUTCOMES	NIC INTERVENTIONS
Knowledge: treatment regimen	Health system guidance; teaching: individual; teaching: prescribed activity/exercise

NURSING ASSESSMENT	RATIONALE
Assess client's readiness and ability to learn. Assess meaning of illness to client.	*Early recognition of readiness to learn and meaning of illness to client allows for implementation of the appropriate teaching interventions.*

THERAPEUTIC INTERVENTIONS	RATIONALE
Desired Outcome: The client will identify ways to prevent recurrent disk herniation.	

*The nurse should select the nursing diagnostic label that is most appropriate for the client's discharge teaching needs.

NDx = NANDA-I Diagnosis   **D** = Delegatable Action   ● = UAP   ✦ = LVN/LPN   ⊖▶ = Go to ⊖volve for animation

Continued...

THERAPEUTIC INTERVENTIONS	RATIONALE

Independent Actions

Inform client about ways to reduce back and/or neck strain and subsequently reduce the risk of recurrent disk herniation:

• Lose weight if overweight.

Maintaining a normal body weight reduces stress/strain on the back.

• Support the spine adequately (e.g., sleep on a firm mattress; sit on firm, straight-backed or contoured chairs; wear stabilization device as prescribed).

• Use proper body mechanics (e.g., bend at the knees rather than waist, push rather than pull heavy objects, carry items close to body).

Use of proper body mechanics reduces the risk of injury.

• Keep spine in good alignment (e.g., avoid excessive bending or twisting, maintain good posture).

Reduces stress on back, reducing the risk of injury.

• Wear flat or low-heeled shoes; avoid wearing high heels.

Helps to maintain proper posture.

• Adhere to prescribed, progressive exercise program to strengthen back, neck, shoulders, arms, legs, and abdominal muscles.

Stronger, well-developed muscles provide better support to bony spine.

Provide a dietary consult regarding a weight reduction program if indicated.

Refer client to an occupational therapist and/or vocational rehabilitation specialist for assistance in modifying daily routines or pursuing different job opportunities if indicated.

Allow time for client to practice proper body alignment when sitting, standing, and walking; proper positioning when resting; and any exercises allowed in immediate postoperative period. Encourage client to think about and plan movements before doing them.

Ensuring client's understanding of proper body mechanics reduces the risk of additional injury. Allow time for questions and return demonstration to assess the need for further instruction.

THERAPEUTIC INTERVENTIONS	RATIONALE

Desired Outcome: The client will demonstrate the ability to correctly apply and remove stabilization device if one is required.

Independent Actions

Reinforce instructions on the correct way to apply and remove stabilization device (e.g., cervical collar, back brace, corset) if client needs to wear one after discharge.

Reduces the risk of injury associated with improper use of stabilization devices.

THERAPEUTIC INTERVENTIONS	RATIONALE

Desired Outcome: The client will verbalize an understanding of ways to maintain skin integrity when wearing a stabilization device.

Independent Actions

If client is to be discharged with a stabilization device, instruct client to examine skin daily when device is off (if device should not be removed, demonstrate how to examine underneath it using a mirror and flashlight).

Early, prompt recognition of potential areas of skin breakdown allows for prompt intervention.

Instruct client in ways to maintain skin integrity if a stabilization device needs to be worn:

• Apply device properly and maintain spine in good alignment to avoid undue pressure in any area.

• Wear a cotton T-shirt under back brace or corset and keep shirt dry and wrinkle-free.

THERAPEUTIC INTERVENTIONS	RATIONALE

- Apply a thin layer of powder or cornstarch to skin under stabilization device to reduce irritation caused by friction.
- Avoid inserting anything under the device.
- Place padding between stabilization device and bony prominences.

THERAPEUTIC INTERVENTIONS	RATIONALE

Desired Outcome: The client will state signs and symptoms to report to the health care provider.

Independent Actions

Instruct client to report these additional signs and symptoms:

- Decreased movement or sensation in extremities
- Coolness or bluish color of extremities
- Increasing or recurrent numbness, tingling, or pain in surgical area or extremities
- Difficulty standing up straight (after lumbar surgery) or keeping neck straight (after cervical surgery)
- Persistent and/or severe headache
- Drainage of clear or bloody fluid from incision
- Persistent hoarseness or difficulty swallowing (after cervical laminectomy)
- Reddened or irritated area on skin underneath stabilization device

Educating the client regarding signs and symptoms to report to the health care provider allows for implementing appropriate interventions, altering the plan of care, and reducing the risk of potential complications.

THERAPEUTIC INTERVENTIONS	RATIONALE

Desired Outcome: The client will verbalize an understanding of and a plan for adhering to recommended follow-up care including future appointments with health care provider, medications prescribed, activity level, and wound care.

Independent Actions

Reinforce physician's instructions regarding activity (the restrictions will vary depending on extensiveness of surgery, client's condition, and physician preference):

- Avoid lifting objects weighing more than 5 to 10 lb.
- Progress through exercise program as prescribed.
- Avoid sitting or standing for longer than 30 minutes at a time (especially after surgery on lumbar area).
- Schedule adequate rest periods.
- Avoid driving a car (causes increased flexion of the spine) and taking long car rides (the vibrations can jar the spine and long periods without significant changes in position can increase stiffness and discomfort) until allowed.
- Do not participate in contact sports.

Following activity restrictions allows for healing of surgical site and building up increased tolerance for activity.

RELATED CARE PLANS

Preoperative
Postoperative
Urinary retention

TOTAL JOINT ARTHROPLASTY (HIP/KNEE)

A total hip replacement (arthroplasty) is a surgical procedure in which the ball and socket components of the hip joint are replaced with prosthetic devices. There are a variety of prosthetic devices available. The prostheses are either cemented in place using an agent called polymethylmethacrylate or are uncemented (cementless). Uncemented prostheses have porous surfaces that permit bone ingrowth to occur and provide biological fixation. A total hip replacement is performed to relieve joint pain that has been resistant to conservative management and/or improve joint mobility in persons with severe arthritis. It may also be performed to treat avascular necrosis of the femoral head, congenital hip deformity, and failure of previous reconstructive hip surgery.

A total knee replacement (arthroplasty) is a surgical procedure in which the articular surfaces of the tibia, femur, and patella are replaced with prosthetic devices. It is performed to relieve joint pain that has not been controlled by conservative management and/or to improve joint mobility in persons with severe arthritis, congenital knee deformity, hemophilic arthropathy, or severe intra-articular injury.

There are a variety of prostheses available. The type most frequently used is the tricompartmental prosthesis that has separate femoral, tibial, and patellar components. Fixation of the prosthesis is accomplished by using a cement-like agent called polymethylmethacrylate or, if left uncemented, by bone ingrowth into the porous outer surface on the prostheses.

This care plan focuses on the adult client hospitalized for a total hip/knee replacement. Much of the postoperative information is applicable to clients receiving follow-up care in an extended care facility or home setting.

OUTCOME/DISCHARGE CRITERIA

The client will:
1. Have evidence of normal healing of the surgical wound
2. Have clear, audible breath sounds throughout lungs
3. Have reduced hip/knee pain
4. Have expected degree of mobility of hip/knee joint
5. Have no signs and symptoms of infection or postoperative complications
6. Demonstrate correct transfer and ambulation techniques and proper use of ambulatory aids
7. Demonstrate the ability to correctly perform the prescribed exercises
8. Verbalize an understanding of activity and position restrictions necessary to prevent dislocation of the hip prosthesis
9. Identify ways to reduce the risk of loosening of the knee prosthesis(es)
10. Identify ways to reduce the risk of falls in the home environment
11. State signs and symptoms to report to the health care provider
12. Identify community resources that can assist with home management and provide transportation
13. Verbalize an understanding of and a plan for adhering to recommended follow-up care including future appointments with health care provider and physical therapist, medications prescribed, activity level, and wound care

PREOPERATIVE: USE IN CONJUNCTION WITH THE STANDARDIZED PREOPERATIVE CARE PLAN

RELATED PREOPERATIVE NURSING/COLLABORATIVE DIAGNOSES

Deficient Knowledge: Regarding the surgical procedure, hospital routines associated with surgery, physical preparation for total knee replacement, sensations that normally occur after surgery and anesthesia, and postoperative care

POSTOPERATIVE: USE IN CONJUNCTION WITH THE STANDARDIZED POSTOPERATIVE CARE PLAN

Nursing Diagnosis | # RISK FOR PERIPHERAL NEUROVASCULAR DYSFUNCTION NDx (OPERATIVE EXTREMITY)

Definition: At risk for disruption in circulation sensation or motion of an extremity

Related to:
Hip
- Trauma to or excessive pressure on the nerves or blood vessels during surgery
- Blood accumulation and edema in the surgical area
- Improper alignment of operative extremity

- Pressure exerted by balanced suspension device or straps on abductor wedge
- Dislocation of the prosthesis(es)

Related to:
Knee
- Trauma to or excessive pressure on the nerves or blood vessels during surgery
- Blood accumulation and edema in the surgical area
- Improper alignment of operative extremity
- Pressure exerted by the dressing, knee immobilizer, or continuous passive motion (CPM) machine
- Dislocation of the prosthesis(es)

CLINICAL MANIFESTATIONS

Subjective	Objective
Reports of increased pain in the extremity; numbness or tingling in the foot or toes (knee); pain in the foot during passive motion of toes or foot; numbness or tingling in the leg or foot (hip)	Diminished or absent pedal pulses; capillary refill time in toes greater than 2 to 3 seconds; pallor, cyanosis, or coolness of the extremity; inability to flex or extend knee, foot, or toes (knee)

RISK FACTORS

- Fracture
- Immobilization
- Mechanical compression (brace)
- Vascular obstruction

DESIRED OUTCOMES

The client will maintain normal neurovascular function in the operative extremity as evidenced by:
  a. Palpable pedal pulses
  b. Capillary refill time in toes less than 2 to 3 seconds
  c. Extremity warm and usual color
  d. No increase in pain in extremity
  e. Ability to flex and extend foot and toes **(knee)**
  f. Absence of numbness and tingling in foot and toes **(knee)**
  g. Absence of foot pain during passive movement of toes and foot **(knee)**
  h. Ability to flex and extend knee, foot, and toes **(hip)**
  i. Absence of numbness and tingling in leg or foot **(hip)**

NOC OUTCOMES

Tissue perfusion: peripheral

NIC INTERVENTIONS

Circulatory care: arterial insufficiency; circulatory care: venous insufficiency; lower extremity monitoring; positioning; pressure management; heat/cold application

NURSING ASSESSMENT

Assess for and report signs of neurovascular dysfunction in the operative extremity:
- Increased pain in the extremity
- Numbness or tingling in the foot or toes (knee)
- Pain in the foot during passive motion of toes or foot
- Numbness or tingling in the leg or foot (hip)
- Diminished or absent pedal pulses
- Capillary refill time in toes greater than 2 to 3 seconds
- Pallor, cyanosis, or coolness of the extremity
- Inability to flex or extend knee, foot, or toes (knee)

RATIONALE

Early recognition of signs and symptoms of neurovascular dysfunction allows for prompt intervention.

THERAPEUTIC INTERVENTIONS

RATIONALE

Independent Actions
Implement measures to reduce the risk for peripheral neurovascular dysfunction:
- Perform actions to reduce or prevent hematoma formation:

NDx = NANDA-I Diagnosis **D** = Delegatable Action ● = UAP ✦ = LVN/LPN ⊝▶ = Go to ⊝volve for animation

Continued...

THERAPEUTIC INTERVENTIONS	RATIONALE
• Maintain patency of wound drainage system (e.g., prevent kinking of tubing, empty collection device as needed, keep collection device below the level of surgical site, maintain suction as ordered). **D** ✦	*Maintaining patency of a drainage system if used helps to reduce the accumulation of fluid in the surgical area, decreasing pressure on surrounding nerves.*
Knee arthroplasty specific	
• Elevate operative leg on pillow (when not in CPM machine) for the first 48 hours after surgery; place pillows so knee flexion is avoided. **D** ✦ ●	*Elevation of the affected limb helps to reduce edema in the surgical area. Limiting knee flexion helps to reduce pressure on peroneal nerve.*
• Position leg so that knee immobilizer and CPM machine are not causing excessive pressure on any area. **D** ✦	
• Loosen straps of knee immobilizer if it appears to be too tight. **D** ✦	
• Notify physician if dressing appears to be too tight.	
Hip arthroplasty specific	
• Make sure that balanced suspension device and straps on abductor wedge are not exerting pressure on the popliteal space, Achilles tendon, and lateral and medial aspects of the knee and ankle.	*Excessive pressure on the popliteal space compresses arteries, nerves, and veins, decreasing perfusion and increasing the risk for nerve damage. In addition, the risk for deep vein thrombosis increases because of altered perfusion.*
• Perform actions to prevent dislocation of prosthesis:	*Provides appropriate support, preventing further injury.*
• Maintain extremity in proper alignment (e.g., external rotation of hip). **D** ✦	*Maintaining the affected extremity in proper alignment reduces the risk of dislocation.*
• Immobilize the knee in an extended position after surgery. **D** ✦	
• Assist with full weight-bearing after surgery. **D** ✦ ●	
If signs and symptoms of neurovascular dysfunction occur:	
• Assess for and correct causes of excessive pressure on operative leg (e.g., tight straps immobilizing devices, improper positioning).	*Excessive pressure/compression of operative leg may result in nerve dysfunction. Search for correctable causes if the client is displaying symptoms of the problem.*
Dependent/Collaborative Actions	
Implement measures to reduce the risk for peripheral neurovascular dysfunction: **D** ●	
• Apply ice pack or cooling pad to operative hip if ordered.	*Cold therapy is most appropriate immediately after surgery because it facilitates vasoconstriction, thereby reducing bleeding, swelling, congestion, and pain at the surgical site.*
• Obtain and review postoperative radiographs.	*Radiographs will confirm the presence of fractures.*
If signs and symptoms of neurovascular dysfunction occur:	
• Notify physician.	*Notifying the physician allows for modification of the treatment plan.*
• Prepare client for closed reduction and/or surgical intervention.	

Nursing Diagnosis ## ACTUAL/RISK FOR IMPAIRED TISSUE INTEGRITY NDx

Definition: Damage to mucous membrane, corneal, integumentary, or subcutaneous tissues

Related to:
• Disruption of tissue associated with the surgical procedure
• Delayed wound healing associated with factors such as decreased nutritional status and inadequate blood supply to wound area
• Irritation of skin associated with contact with wound drainage, pressure from tubes, and use of tape
• Excessive or prolonged pressure on tissues from balanced suspension device, straps on abductor wedge, and elastic wraps or stockings
• Damage to the skin and/or subcutaneous tissue associated with prolonged pressure on tissues, friction, and shearing while mobility is decreased

CLINICAL MANIFESTATIONS

Subjective	Objective
N/A	Pallor and/or redness of skin in the following areas: skin in contact with wound drainage, tape, or tubing; back, coccyx, and buttocks; elbows and/or heels; skin in areas at edges of compression dressing or joint immobilizer; areas in contact with CPM machine; areas under elastic wraps or compression stockings

RISK FACTORS

- Imbalanced nutrition
- Immobility
- Mechanical pressure

DESIRED OUTCOMES

The client will:
  a. Experience normal healing of the surgical wound
  b. Maintain tissue integrity as evidenced by absence of redness and irritation, and no skin breakdown

NOC OUTCOMES

Tissue integrity: skin and mucous membranes; wound healing: primary intention

NIC INTERVENTIONS

Incision site care; skin surveillance; positioning; pressure ulcer prevention; pressure management; skin care: topical treatments

NURSING ASSESSMENT

Assess for and report signs and symptoms of skin breakdown:
- Pallor and/or redness of skin in the following areas:
  - Skin in contact with wound drainage, tape, or tubing
  - Back, coccyx, and buttocks
  - Elbows and/or heels
  - Skin in areas at edges of compression dressing or joint immobilizer
  - Areas in contact with CPM machine
  - Areas under elastic wraps or compression stockings

RATIONALE

Early recognition of signs and symptoms of actual or impaired skin integrity allows for prompt intervention.

THERAPEUTIC INTERVENTIONS

RATIONALE

Independent Actions

Implement measures to prevent tissue irritation and breakdown in areas in contact with wound drainage, tape, and tubings:
- Maintain patency of drainage tubes. **D** ✦

- Apply collection device over drains and incisions that are draining continuously. **D** ✦
- Ensure client is not lying on drainage tubes. **D** ✦ ●
- Perform actions to decrease skin irritation from tape:
  - Use only the necessary amount of tape. **D** ✦
  - Use hypoallergenic tape.
  - Use Montgomery straps or tubular netting.

Implement measures to prevent tissue breakdown associated with decreased mobility:
- Position client properly; use pressure-reducing or pressure-relieving devices (e.g., pillows, alternating pressure mattress) if indicated. **D** ✦ ●
- Instruct client to use overhead trapeze to lift self and shift weight at least every 30 minutes.
- Gently massage around reddened areas at least every 2 hours. **D** ✦

Maintaining patency of drainage tubes helps to prevent the possibility of leakages around tubes.

Pressure on the skin may compromise circulation to that area.

Decreases incident of allergic reactions.
Decreases exposure of the skin to avoid repeated application and removal of tape.

Actions help to reduce constant pressure on skin and bony prominences, improving circulation to skin.

Actions prevent shearing of client's skin.

Actions stimulate circulation to the skin.

Continued...

THERAPEUTIC INTERVENTIONS	RATIONALE
• Apply a thin layer of a dry lubricant such as powder or cornstarch to bottom sheet or skin and to opposing skin surfaces (e.g., axillae) if indicated. **D** ✦ ●	*Actions help to reduce friction.*
• Lift and move client carefully using a turn sheet and adequate assistance. **D** ●	*Prevents shearing forces against client's skin.*
• Perform actions to keep client from sliding down in bed (e.g., limit length of time client is in semi-Fowler's position to 30-minute intervals). **D** ●	
• If turning is allowed, turn client every 2 hours, maintaining proper alignment. **D** ●	*Turning from side to side decreases constant pressure on bony prominences.*
Implement measures to prevent irritation and breakdown on elbows and heels:	*Actions help to reduce the risk of skin surface abrasion and shearing.*
• Massage elbows and heels with lotion frequently. **D** ✦ ●	
• Encourage client to use overhead trapeze to move self rather than pushing up with heel and elbows.	
• Provide elbow and heel protectors if indicated. **D** ●	
Implement measures to prevent tissue breakdown under elastic wraps or stockings:	*Moisture facilitates skin breakdown.*
• Remove elastic wraps or stockings at least twice daily, bathe and thoroughly dry skin, and reapply smoothly. **D** ✦ ●	
• Check wraps or stockings frequently and reapply if they have slipped or become wrinkled. **D** ✦	
• If areas of redness develop under wraps or stockings, consult physician before reapplying.	
Implement measures to prevent tissue breakdown associated with excessive pressure caused by balanced suspension device or abductor wedge **(hip arthroplasty):**	*Balanced suspension devices or abductor wedges may promote tissue breakdown during the healing process.*
• Make sure metal parts on suspension device are not resting on any area of extremity.	
• Maintain proper alignment of extremity in suspension device. **D** ✦	
• Make sure that straps holding abductor wedge in place are not too tight. **D** ✦	
Implement measures to prevent tissue breakdown in areas in contact with the compression dressing, knee immobilizer, and CPM machine **(knee arthroplasty):**	
• Loosen straps on knee immobilizer if it appears to be too tight. **D** ✦	
• Apply cornstarch to skin under immobilizer to reduce friction and irritation. **D** ●	
• Keep dressing dry.	
• Position the operative extremity so the knee immobilizer and CPM machine are not causing excessive pressure on any area. **D** ✦	
• Ensure CPM machine is padded appropriately. **D** ✦	

Dependent/Collaborative Actions

If tissue breakdown occurs:

• Notify appropriate health care provider (e.g., physician, wound care specialist).	*Notifying the physician allows for modification of the treatment plan.*
• Perform care of involved areas as ordered or per standard hospital procedure.	

Nursing Diagnosis # IMPAIRED PHYSICAL MOBILITY NDx

Definition: Limitation in independent, purposeful, physical movement of the body or of one or more extremities

Related to:
- Pain and weakness in weight-bearing extremity associated with surgery on the hip/knee
- Prescribed activity and weight-bearing restrictions after total hip replacement
- Generalized weakness associated with surgery
- Depressant effect of anesthesia and some medications (e.g., narcotic [opioid] analgesics, centrally acting muscle relaxants, some antiemetics)
- Fear of falling, dislodging drainage tube, dislocating prostheses, and compromising surgical wound

CLINICAL MANIFESTATIONS

Subjective	Objective
N/A	Decreased reaction time; difficulty turning; limited ability to perform gross motor skills; limited range of motion; postural instability; slowed movements; uncoordinated movements

RISK FACTORS
- Malnutrition
- Musculoskeletal impairment
- Pain

DESIRED OUTCOMES

The client will maintain maximum physical mobility within prescribed activity and weight-bearing restrictions.

NOC OUTCOMES

Mobility

NIC INTERVENTIONS

Exercise therapy: joint mobility; exercise therapy: muscle control; exercise therapy: ambulation

NURSING ASSESSMENT	**RATIONALE**

Assess for and report signs and symptoms of impaired physical mobility:
- Decreased reaction time
- Difficulty turning
- Limited ability to perform gross motor skills
- Limited range of motion
- Postural instability
- Slowed movements
- Uncoordinated movements

Early recognition of signs and symptoms of impaired physical mobility allows for prompt intervention.

THERAPEUTIC INTERVENTIONS	**RATIONALE**

Independent Actions
Implement measures to increase client's mobility:
- Perform actions to reduce pain.
  - Keep operative extremity in proper alignment.
  - Move operative extremity gently. **D** ✦
- Encourage client to use overhead trapeze to move self.
- Reinforce physical therapist's instructions regarding additional muscle strengthening exercises, transfer and ambulation techniques, and use of ambulatory aids.
- Perform actions to prevent falls:
  - Keep bed in low position with side rails up. **D** ●
  - Keep items within easy reach. **D** ●
- Assist client with ambulation as soon as allowed (usually by postoperative day 2). **D** ●

Actions help to strengthen arm and shoulder muscles needed for proper use of ambulatory aids.

NDx = NANDA-I Diagnosis   **D** = Delegatable Action   ● = UAP   ✦ = LVN/LPN   ⊖▶ = Go to ⊖volve for animation

Continued...

THERAPEUTIC INTERVENTIONS	RATIONALE

Dependent/Collaborative Actions

Consult appropriate health care provider (e.g., physician, physical therapist) if client is unable to achieve expected level of mobility.

Notifying the physician allows for modification of the treatment plan.

Collaborative Diagnosis

RISK FOR HEMORRHAGE AND/OR HEMATOMA FORMATION

Definition: Severe bleeding that is difficult to control

Related to:
- Surgical trauma to blood vessels
- Use of anticoagulants or antiplatelet agents before and after surgery

CLINICAL MANIFESTATIONS

Subjective	Objective
N/A	Hemorrhage; excessive wound drainage (expected loss is 200-500 mL in the first 24 hours, diminishing to less than 100 mL/24 hours by 48 hours after surgery); significant decrease in red blood cell (RBC) count, Hct, and Hgb levels; signs and symptoms of hematoma formation (e.g., increased pain and tense swelling in buttock and/or thigh)

RISK FACTORS

- Anticoagulation therapy
- Disruption of surgical site

DESIRED OUTCOMES

The client will not experience hemorrhage or hematoma formation as evidenced by:
   a. Expected amount of wound drainage
   b. No further decrease in RBC count, Hct, and Hgb levels
   c. No significant increase in hip pain
   d. Absence of tense swelling in surgical area

NURSING ASSESSMENT	RATIONALE

Assess client for and report signs and symptoms of hemorrhage and/or hematoma formation:

Hemorrhage
- Excessive wound drainage (expected loss is 200-500 mL in the first 24 hours, diminishing to less than 100 m/24 hours by 48 hours after surgery)
- Significant decrease in RBC count, Hct, and Hgb levels

Hematoma formation
- Signs and symptoms of hematoma formation (e.g., increased pain and tense swelling in buttock and/or thigh)

Early recognition of signs and symptoms of hemorrhage or hematoma formation allows for prompt intervention.

THERAPEUTIC INTERVENTIONS	RATIONALE

Independent Actions

Maintain pressure dressing over operative site as ordered.

Keep trochanter roll or sandbag placed firmly against operative site for the first 24 to 48 hours after surgery to provide additional pressure on surgical site.

Actions help to reduce operative site bleeding and/or prevent hematoma formation.

Apply ice pack or cooling pad to operative hip if ordered.

Promotes vasoconstriction, which decreases edema.

THERAPEUTIC INTERVENTIONS	RATIONALE
Maintain patency of wound drainage system if present.	*Prevents stasis of secretions, which may contribute to infection.*
If signs and symptoms of excessive bleeding or hematoma formation occur, prepare client for return to surgery to ligate bleeding vessels and/or drain hematoma if planned.	*Notifying the physician allows for modification of the treatment plan.*

Collaborative Diagnosis # RISK FOR DISLOCATION OF HIP PROSTHESIS(ES)

Definition: A severe injury of the ligamentous structures that surround a joint

Related to:
- Weakness of the hip muscles
- Improper positioning or movement of the operative extremity
- Noncompliance with weight-bearing limitations

CLINICAL MANIFESTATIONS

Subjective	Objective
Reports of sudden, severe hip pain followed by continuous pain and muscle spasms with movement	Abnormal rotation of operative leg; inability to move or bear weight on operative leg; shortening of operative leg; decline in neurovascular status in operative leg

RISK FACTOR
- Malposition of operative limb

DESIRED OUTCOMES

The client will not experience dislocation of the hip prosthesis(es) as evidenced by:
  a. Continued resolution of hip pain
  b. Ability to maintain operative leg in proper alignment
  c. Ability to adhere to expected exercise and ambulation regimen
  d. Usual length of operative extremity
  e. Normal neurovascular status in operative leg

NURSING ASSESSMENT	RATIONALE
Assess client for signs and symptoms of dislocation of the hip prosthesis(es): • Sudden, severe hip pain followed by continuous pain and muscle spasms with movement • Abnormal rotation of operative leg • Inability to move or bear weight on operative leg • Shortening of operative leg • Decline in neurovascular status in operative leg	*Early recognition of signs and symptoms of hip prosthesis(es) dislocation allows for prompt intervention.*

THERAPEUTIC INTERVENTIONS	RATIONALE
Independent Actions Maintain bedrest as ordered (may be on bedrest for first 24 hours after surgery). Perform actions to prevent adduction of the operative extremity (if a posterolateral approach was used): • Maintain extremity in abducted position using balanced suspension device, an abduction wedge, or two or three pillows between legs. **D** ✦ ● • Remind client to avoid crossing legs. • Do not move operative extremity past midline. **D** ✦ ● • Turn client only as ordered and always with pillows between legs. **D** ✦ ●	*Actions help to prevent dislocation of hip prosthesis(es).*

NDx = NANDA-I Diagnosis   **D** = Delegatable Action   ● = UAP   ✦ = LVN/LPN   ⊝▶ = Go to ⊝volve for animation

Continued...

THERAPEUTIC INTERVENTIONS	RATIONALE
If client had an anterolateral approach, maintain restrictions on abduction.	
Maintain operative extremity in proper alignment; instruct client to avoid extreme internal and external rotation of operative leg. **D** ✦ ●	
Maintain restrictions on head-of-bed elevation if ordered (some physicians order a 45-60 degrees maximum for first 2 to 3 days after surgery) to reduce hip flexion. **D** ✦ ●	*Actions help to reduce hip flexion.*
Perform actions to prevent extreme (beyond 90 degrees) hip flexion:	
• Instruct client not to lean forward to reach objects on end of bed or on floor or to put on slippers, socks, or shoes.	
• Raise the entire bed to client's midthigh level before client gets in or out of bed in order to reduce the degree of hip flexion that occurs when client sits on edge of bed. **D** ✦ ●	
• Provide a high, firm chair (or elevate sitting surface with pillows) and an elevated toilet seat for client's use to reduce degree of hip flexion when client sits down. **D** ✦ ●	
• Do not elevate operative leg when client is sitting in chair.	
Reinforce importance of adhering to recommended weight-bearing restrictions (the amount of weight-bearing allowed is based on the type of prostheses inserted; partial weight-bearing is usually allowed as soon as ambulation is started).	
Instruct and assist client to pivot and bear weight on the unoperative leg when transferring from bed to chair and raising self out of chair.	
If signs and symptoms of dislocation of the prosthesis(es) occur:	
• Maintain client on bedrest.	
• Prepare client for radiographs of the surgical area.	
• Prepare client for closed reduction (e.g., traction) or surgical relocation of the prosthesis(es) if planned.	

Collaborative Diagnosis   RISK FOR DISLOCATION OF KNEE PROSTHESIS(ES)

Definition: A severe injury of the ligamentous structures that surround a joint

Related to: Rotation of or excessive pressure on the knee

CLINICAL MANIFESTATIONS

Subjective	Objective
Sudden, severe knee pain followed by continuous pain and muscle spasms with movement	Abnormal rotation of lower portion of the operative leg; inability to move or bear weight on operative leg; decline in neurovascular status in operative leg

RISK FACTORS

• Improper alignment of extremities
• Inappropriate weight bearing

DESIRED OUTCOMES

The client will not experience dislocation of the hip prosthesis(es) as evidenced by:
  a. Continued resolution of knee pain
  b. Ability to maintain operative leg in proper alignment
  c. Ability to adhere to expected exercise and ambulation regimen
  d. Usual length of operative extremity
  e. Normal neurovascular status in operative leg

NURSING ASSESSMENT	RATIONALE
Assess client for signs and symptoms of dislocation of the knee prosthesis(es): • Sudden, severe knee pain followed by continuous pain and muscle spasms with movement • Abnormal rotation of lower portion of the operative leg • Inability to move or bear weight on operative leg • Decline in neurovascular status in operative leg	*Early recognition of signs and symptoms of knee prosthesis(es) dislocation allows for prompt intervention.*

THERAPEUTIC INTERVENTIONS	RATIONALE
Independent Actions Instruct client to avoid hyperextension, rotation, and acute flexion of the knee. Reinforce physician's instructions regarding the amount of weight-bearing allowed (usual order is partial weight-bearing initially with progressive weight-bearing as tolerated). Reinforce instructions and assist client with gait training and proper use of ambulatory aids. Reinforce the importance of wearing knee immobilizer when ambulating. If signs and symptoms of prosthesis(es) dislocation or stress fracture occur: • Maintain client on bedrest. **D** ✦ ● • Prepare client for radiographs of operative leg. • Prepare client for closed reduction or surgical intervention (e.g., realignment of prosthesis, internal fixation of fracture) if planned.	*Actions help to prevent dislocation of hip prosthesis(es).*

Collaborative Diagnosis ## RISK FOR THROMBOEMBOLISM

Definition: Formation in a blood vessel of a clot (thrombus) that breaks loose and is carried by the bloodstream to plug another vessel

Related to:
• Trauma to vein walls during surgery
• Hypercoagulability associated with increased release of tissue thromboplastin into the blood (occurs as a result of surgical trauma) and hemoconcentration and increased blood viscosity (can occur as a result of deficient fluid volume)
• Venous stasis associated with decreased mobility, increased blood viscosity (can result from deficient fluid volume), and pressure exerted on veins by balanced suspension device or abductor wedge **(hip)**
• Venous stasis associated with use of a tourniquet on operative leg during surgery; pressure exerted on the veins by the dressing, knee immobilizer, or CPM machine; decreased mobility; and increased blood viscosity (can result from deficient fluid volume) **(knee)**

CLINICAL MANIFESTATIONS

Subjective	Objective
Deep vein thrombosis: reports of pain or tenderness in an extremity	Increased circumference of an extremity; unusual warmth of an extremity; positive Homans' sign; distention of superficial vessels in an extremity
Pulmonary embolism: reports of acute onset of chest pain; apprehension	Tachypnea; dyspnea; tachycardia

RISK FACTORS
• Immobility
• Inadequate hydration
• Orthopedic surgery

DESIRED OUTCOMES
The client will not develop a deep vein thrombus or pulmonary embolism.

NDx = NANDA-I Diagnosis   **D** = Delegatable Action   ● = UAP   ✦ = LVN/LPN   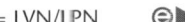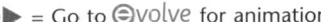 = Go to Ⓔvolve for animation

Continued...

NURSING ASSESSMENT	RATIONALE
Assess for and report signs and symptoms of thromboembolism: • **Deep vein thrombosis:** pain or tenderness in an extremity; increased circumference of an extremity; unusual warmth of an extremity; positive Homans' sign; distention of superficial vessels in an extremity • **Pulmonary embolism:** acute onset of chest pain; apprehension; tachypnea; dyspnea; tachycardia	*Early recognition of signs and symptoms of a thromboembolism allows for prompt intervention.*

THERAPEUTIC INTERVENTIONS	RATIONALE
Dependent/Collaborative Actions Assist client to perform leg exercises and ambulate as soon as allowed. **D ✦ ●** Make sure that antiembolism stockings are applied correctly and that intermittent pneumatic compression device is correctly applied and functioning properly. **D ✦** Perform actions to reduce risk of compromising venous return: • Ensure elastic wraps, stockings, or dressings are not too tight. **D ✦** • Avoid use of knee gatch or pillows under knees. **D ✦** • Discourage prolonged sitting or standing. • Make sure that balanced suspension device or straps on abductor wedge do not exert excessive pressure on any area **(hip). D ✦** • Make sure exercise sling is not exerting pressure on the popliteal space **(knee). D ✦** • Loosen knee immobilizer if too tight. **D ✦** Administer anticoagulants or antiplatelet agents if ordered.	*Actions help to prevent thrombus formation.* *Anticoagulants are routinely ordered for the prevention and treatment of deep vein thrombosis.* *Anticoagulation does not dissolve the clot, but it prevents clot propagation, the development of any new thrombi, and embolization.*

Collaborative Diagnosis   RISK FOR FAT EMBOLISM SYNDROME (FES)

Definition: Systemic fat globules from fractures that are distributed into tissues and organs after a traumatic skeletal injury

Related to: Release of fat from the bone marrow into the blood associated with trauma to the bone during preparation for and implantation of the hip or knee prosthesis

CLINICAL MANIFESTATIONS

Subjective	Objective
N/A	Restlessness, apprehension, confusion; sudden onset of dyspnea; tachypnea; elevated pulse rate and temperature; petechiae on the chest, neck, or axilla; low Pao_2 level; unexpected decrease in Hct and Hgb levels; thrombocytopenia

RISK FACTOR
- Fracture of long bones

DESIRED OUTCOMES

The client will not experience fat embolism syndrome as evidenced by:
a. Usual mental status
b. Unlabored respirations at 12 to 20 breaths/min
c. Absence of petechiae
d. Pao_2 within normal limits

NURSING ASSESSMENT

Assess for and report signs and symptoms of FES:
- Restlessness, apprehension, confusion
- Sudden onset of dyspnea
- Tachypnea
- Elevated pulse rate and temperature
- Petechiae on the chest, neck, or axilla
- Low Pao_2 level
- Unexpected decrease in Hct and Hgb levels
- Thrombocytopenia

RATIONALE

Early recognition of signs and symptoms of FES allows for prompt intervention.

THERAPEUTIC INTERVENTIONS

Dependent/Collaborative Actions
Move operative extremity gently and avoid excessive movement of the extremity during the first few days after surgery to reduce the risk for fat emboli. **D** ✦ ●

If signs and symptoms of FES occur:
- Maintain client on bedrest and move fractured extremity as little as possible to prevent further emboli. **D** ✦ ●
- Administer oxygen and assist with positive airway pressure techniques (e.g., positive end-expiratory pressure) if ordered. **D** ✦
- Prepare client for chest radiograph or lung scan.
- Administer intravenous fluids as ordered.

- Administer corticosteroids if ordered.

RATIONALE

Initially, limited mobility after a hip fracture helps to reduce the risk for fat emboli.

Intravenous fluid administration helps to maintain adequate perfusion to vital organs and prevent shock.
Corticosteroids help to reduce cerebral edema and pulmonary inflammation.

DISCHARGE TEACHING/CONTINUED CARE

Nursing Diagnosis
DEFICIENT KNOWLEDGE NDx, INEFFECTIVE FAMILY THERAPEUTIC REGIMEN MANAGEMENT NDx, OR INEFFECTIVE SELF-HEALTH MAINTENANCE NDx*

Definition: Absence or deficiency of cognitive information related to specific topic; pattern of regulating and integrating into family processes and daily living a program for treatment of illness and the sequelae of illness that is unsatisfactory for meeting specific health goals

CLINICAL MANIFESTATIONS

Subjective	Objective
Verbalization of the problem	Demonstrated lack of knowledge about basic health practices; demonstrated lack of adaptive behaviors; impaired personal support systems; inaccurate follow-through of instructions

*The nurse should select the nursing diagnostic label that is most appropriate for the client's discharge teaching needs.

NDx = NANDA-I Diagnosis   **D** = Delegatable Action   ● = UAP   ✦ = LVN/LPN   ⊖▶ = Go to ⊖volve for animation

Continued...

RISK FACTORS

- Cognitive limitations
- Financial concerns
- Inadequate support system

NOC OUTCOMES	NIC INTERVENTIONS
Knowledge: fall prevention; knowledge: prescribed activity; knowledge: treatment regimen	Health system guidance; teaching: individual; teaching: prescribed activity/exercise

NURSING ASSESSMENT	RATIONALE
Assess client's readiness and ability to learn. Assess meaning of illness to client.	*Early recognition of readiness to learn and meaning of illness to client allows for implementation of the appropriate teaching interventions.*

THERAPEUTIC INTERVENTIONS	RATIONALE

Desired Outcome: The client will demonstrate correct transfer and ambulation techniques and proper use of ambulatory aids.

Independent Actions	
Reinforce instructions about correct transfer and ambulation techniques and proper use of walker, quad cane, or crutches.	*Performing transfer techniques and using assistive devices correctly reduces the risk of injury.*
Reinforce physician's instructions about amount of weight-bearing on operative extremity.	
Allow time for questions, clarification, and practice of transfer and ambulation techniques.	*Allows the nurse to reinforce patient education and to evaluate the need for further instruction.*

THERAPEUTIC INTERVENTIONS	RATIONALE

Desired Outcome: The client will demonstrate the ability to correctly perform the prescribed exercises.

Independent Actions	
Reinforce the physical therapist's instructions on prescribed exercises and the importance of continuing the exercises for the prescribed length of time.	*Regular physical activity helps to maintain bone mass, increase lean muscle mass, and increase muscular strength, improving overall function and range of motion.*
Inform client that walking and swimming are good aerobic exercises.	*Lower impact exercises such as walking and swimming reduce the risk of loosening the implant.*
Allow time for questions, clarification, and return demonstration of prescribed exercises.	*Allows the nurse to reinforce patient education and to evaluate the need for further instruction.*

Desired Outcome: The client will identify ways to reduce the risk of loosening of the prosthesis(es).

THERAPEUTIC INTERVENTIONS	RATIONALE

Independent Actions

Hip arthroplasty

Instruct client to adhere to the following activity and position restrictions (length of time the restrictions are necessary varies but ranges from 2-6 months):

These actions are important for the client to adhere to to prevent dislocation of the prosthesis.
Anything that requires joint flexion beyond 90 degrees should be avoided.

- Turn only as directed by physician (many physicians allow client to turn to unoperative side only).
- Instruct client to keep pillow between legs when lying on back or side and when turning.
- Never cross legs.
- Do not sit on low chairs, stools, or toilets; place a cushion on low chairs, rent or purchase an elevated toilet seat for home use, and use the high toilets designated for the handicapped when in public facilities.
- Do not elevate operative leg higher than hip when sitting.
- Sit in chairs with arms and use the arms to raise self off chair.
- Support weight on unoperative leg when raising self from a sitting position.
- Use assistive devices (e.g., long-handled shoe horn, long-handled grabber) to assist with activities that require flexing hip beyond 90 degrees (e.g., putting on shoes and socks, reaching objects on the floor or in low cupboards or drawers, pulling bed covers up from end of bed).
- Keep operative leg in proper alignment and avoid extreme internal and external rotation of leg.
- Do not drive until approved by physician (usually about 6 weeks after surgery).
- When riding in a car:
  - Sit on a firm pillow or cushion to prevent hip flexion of more than 90 degrees.
  - Keep operative leg extended (a sudden impact of the knee against the dashboard can dislodge the prostheses).
- When sexual activity is resumed, avoid positions that involve extreme rotation of the operative leg, flexing hip beyond 90 degrees, and moving operative leg past the midline.
- Avoid lifting heavy objects, excessive twisting and turning of body, and activities that place excessive strain on hip (e.g., jogging, jumping).

Knee arthroplasty

Inform client of the possibility of loosening of the prosthesis (usually does not occur until 2 to 3 years after surgery).

Instruct client to report increasing pain or instability of operative knee (may indicate loosening of the prosthesis).

Instruct client regarding ways to minimize risk of loosening of the prosthesis(es):

- Adhere to weight-bearing restrictions if prescribed.
- Avoid unusual twisting of knee.
- Avoid contact sports.
- Do not force knee beyond comfortable degree of flexion and avoid kneeling.
- Avoid placing undue stress on knees (e.g., do not lift and carry heavy objects, maintain ideal body weight, avoid activities such as jogging).

Continued...

THERAPEUTIC INTERVENTIONS	RATIONALE

Desired Outcome: The client will identify ways to reduce the risk of falls in the home environment.

Independent Actions

Provide the following instructions on ways to reduce risk of falls at home:

- Keep electrical cords out of pathways.
- Remove unnecessary furniture and provide wide pathways for ambulation.
- Remove scatter rugs.
- Provide adequate lighting at all times.
- Avoid unnecessary stair climbing.

Actions reduce potential causes of in-home falls.

THERAPEUTIC INTERVENTIONS	RATIONALE

Desired Outcome: The client will state signs and symptoms to report to the health care provider.

Independent Actions

Instruct client to report these additional signs and symptoms:

- Persistent or increased pain or spasms in operative extremity
- Loss of sensation or movement in operative extremity
- Inability to bear expected amount of weight on operative extremity
- Inability to maintain operative extremity in a neutral position
- Instability of operative extremity (feeling of knee "giving out") or shortening of the operative extremity (noticed as a limp in a hip client)

Educating the client regarding signs and symptoms to report to the health care provider allows for implementing appropriate interventions, altering the plan of care, and reducing the risk of potential complications.

THERAPEUTIC INTERVENTIONS	RATIONALE

Desired Outcome: The client will identify community resources that can assist with home management and provide transportation.

Independent Actions

Provide information about community resources that can assist client and significant others with home management and provide transportation (e.g., home health agencies, Meals on Wheels, church groups, transportation services). Initiate a referral if indicated.

Social support can aid the client in obtaining necessary resources to adapt to physical changes and obtain the necessary long-term assistance to maintain independence.

THERAPEUTIC INTERVENTIONS	RATIONALE

Desired Outcome: The client will verbalize an understanding of and a plan for adhering to recommended follow-up care including future appointments with health care provider and physical therapist, medications prescribed, activity level, and wound care.

Independent Actions

Reinforce the importance of keeping appointments with physical therapist.

Teach client the rationale for, side effects of, schedule for taking, and importance of taking prescribed medications.

Adherence to a plan of care reduces the risk of complications and improves patient outcomes.

THERAPEUTIC INTERVENTIONS	RATIONALE

Instruct client to inform other health care providers of history of total joint arthroplasty so prophylactic antimicrobials can be started before any dental work, invasive diagnostic procedures, or surgery is performed.

Inform client that the prosthetic device may activate metal detector alarms. Recommend carrying an identification/information card verifying presence of the device.

RELATED CARE PLANS

Preoperative
Postoperative

ADDITIONAL NURSING DIAGNOSES

ACUTE PAIN NDx

Related to tissue trauma and reflex muscle spasms associated with the surgery, blood accumulation and edema in surgical area, and improper positioning of the operative extremity

ACTIVITY INTOLERANCE NDx

Related to:
- Tissue hypoxia associated with anemia (there can be significant blood loss because the hip is a very vascular area)
- Difficulty resting and sleeping associated with discomfort, position restrictions, fear, and anxiety

RISK FOR INFECTION NDx

Related to:
- Introduction of pathogens into the wound during or after surgery
- Hematoma formation (increases the likelihood of infection by providing a good medium for growth of pathogens and compromising blood flow to the area)
- Increased susceptibility to infection associated with decreased effectiveness of immune system if client is elderly and immunosuppression if client has been taking corticosteroids to treat the joint disorder necessitating the surgery (e.g., rheumatoid arthritis)
- Hematogenous seeding of wound from distant sites (e.g., urinary tract)

RISK FOR FALLS NDx

Related to:
- Weakness, fatigue, and postural hypotension associated with the effects of major surgery and physiological changes that may have occurred if client is elderly
- Central nervous system depressant effect of some medications (e.g., narcotic [opioid] analgesics, centrally acting muscle relaxants, some antiemetics)
- Weakness and pain in weight-bearing extremity associated with surgery on the hip
- Difficulty with transfer and ambulation techniques

13

The Client with Alterations in the Breast and Reproductive System

COLPORRHAPHY (ANTERIOR AND POSTERIOR REPAIR)

Colporrhaphy is the surgical tightening of the vaginal wall and relaxed pelvic muscles. An anterior colporrhaphy is performed to correct a cystocele, which is a herniation of the bladder through weakened supportive fascia of the anterior vaginal compartment. Urethral hypermotility is often present with a cystocele and various techniques for providing urethrovesical angle support during an anterior colporrhaphy can be used to correct this problem. A posterior colporrhaphy is performed if weakening of the supporting fascia has resulted in a rectocele (herniation of the rectum into the posterior vaginal wall). If both an anterior and posterior colporrhaphy are done at the same time, the surgery is referred to as an anteroposterior (AP) repair. Colporrhaphy is usually performed transvaginally through an incision in the vaginal wall (an incision in the perineum also may be made during a posterior colporrhaphy). An abdominal approach is sometimes used to perform a colporrhaphy depending on the client's diagnosis and need for additional abdominal surgery.

Cystoceles and rectoceles are caused by relaxation of the pelvic floor support system, which is usually associated with changes that occur with childbirth and are exacerbated by aging, loss of estrogen stimulation, and factors such as obesity and chronic abdominal straining (e.g., chronic cough, chronic constipation). Signs and symptoms of a cystocele may include stress incontinence, a feeling of incomplete emptying of the bladder after voiding, and a sensation of fullness or pressure in the pelvic area and/or a feeling that organs are "falling out." Indications that a rectocele may be present are difficult or incomplete emptying of the rectum, constipation, and a heavy or "falling out" feeling in the vagina. Colporrhaphy is indicated when conservative management (e.g., perineal exercises, insertion of a pessary) no longer controls signs and symptoms.

This care plan focuses on the adult client having a transvaginal anterior and posterior repair. The information is applicable to clients having surgery in a hospital or outpatient (e.g., surgical care center) setting.

OUTCOME/DISCHARGE CRITERIA

The client will:
1. Have evidence of normal healing of surgical wound
2. Have adequate urine output
3. Have surgical pain controlled
4. Have no signs and symptoms of infection or postoperative complications
5. Identify ways to decrease the risk of reherniation of the bladder and rectum
6. Identify ways to relieve surgical site discomfort
7. State signs and symptoms to report to the health care provider
8. Verbalize an understanding of and a plan for adhering to recommended follow-up care including future appointments with health care provider, medications prescribed, and limitations on sexual activity.

PREOPERATIVE: REFER TO THE STANDARDIZED PREOPERATIVE CARE PLAN

POSTOPERATIVE: USE IN CONJUNCTION WITH THE STANDARDIZED POSTOPERATIVE CARE PLAN

Nursing Diagnosis ## URINARY RETENTION NDx

Definition: Incomplete emptying of the bladder

Related to: Obstruction of the urethral and/or suprapubic catheter(s); impaired urination after removal of catheter(s) associated with:
- Edema of the bladder neck and urethra resulting from surgical trauma
- Increased tone of the urinary sphincters resulting from sympathetic nervous system stimulation (can result from pain, fear, and anxiety)
- Decreased perception of bladder fullness resulting from the depressant effect of anesthesia and some medications (e.g., narcotic [opioid] analgesics)
- Relaxation of the bladder muscle resulting from the depressant effect of anesthesia and some medications (e.g., narcotic [opioid] analgesics) and stimulation of the sympathetic nervous system (can result from pain, fear, and anxiety)

CLINICAL MANIFESTATIONS

Subjective	Objective
Verbal reports of bladder fullness or suprapubic discomfort	Urinary retention when suprapubic and/or urethral catheter(s) are present: bladder distention; absence of fluid in urinary drainage tubing; output that continues to be less than intake 48 hours after surgery Urinary retention after catheter removal: bladder distention, output that continues to be less than intake 48 hours after surgery, frequent voiding of small amounts 25-60 mL of urine.

RISK FACTORS
- Surgery
- Medication regimen

DESIRED OUTCOMES

The client will not experience urinary retention as evidenced by:
- a. No reports of bladder fullness and suprapubic discomfort
- b. Absence of bladder distention
- c. Balanced intake and output within 48 hours after surgery
- d. Voiding adequate amounts at expected intervals after removal of the catheter(s)

NOC OUTCOMES

Urinary elimination

NIC INTERVENTIONS

Urinary retention care; tube care: urinary

NURSING ASSESSMENT

Assess for and report signs and symptoms of urinary retention:
- Bladder fullness
- Suprapubic discomfort
- Bladder distention
- Absence of fluid in urinary drainage tubing

RATIONALE

Early recognition of signs and symptoms of urinary retention allows for prompt intervention.

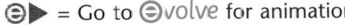

Continued...

THERAPEUTIC INTERVENTIONS	RATIONALE

Independent Actions

Implement measures to prevent urinary retention:
- Keep drainage tubing free of kinks. **D** ● ✦
- Keep collection container below level of bladder. **D** ● ✦
- Anchor catheter tubing securely to prevent inadvertent removal. **D** ● ✦

Actions help prevent urinary retention by maintaining patency of urinary catheter.

After removal of catheter:
- Instruct client to urinate when the urge is first felt. **D** ● ✦
- Promote actions that facilitate relaxation during voiding attempts:
  - Provide privacy. **D** ● ✦
  - Hold a warm blanket against abdomen. **D** ● ✦
- Perform actions that may help trigger the micturition reflex and promote relaxation:
  - Run water. **D** ● ✦
  - Pour warm water over perineum. **D** ● ✦
- Allow client to assume a normal position for voiding if allowed.

Prevents stasis

Helps to initiate urine stream

Dependent/Collaborative Actions

Implement measures to prevent urinary retention:
- After urethral catheter is removed, open suprapubic catheter (if one is present) as scheduled and/or if client is unable to void voluntarily.
- Consult physician if urinary retention persists or if actions fail to alleviate urinary retention.

Notifying the physician allows for modification of the treatment plan.

Nursing Diagnosis **RISK FOR CONSTIPATION** NDx

Definition: Decrease in normal frequency of defecation, accompanied by difficult or incomplete passage of stool and/or passage of excessively dry stool

Related to: Decreased gastrointestinal motility associated with decreased activity and the depressant effect of the anesthetic and narcotic (opioid) analgesics; reluctance to defecate associated with fear of pain and reherniation of the bladder and rectum; decreased intake of fluids and foods high in fiber

CLINICAL MANIFESTATIONS

Subjective	Objective
Increasing abdominal pain; feeling of fullness or pressure in rectum	Decrease in frequency of bowel movements; passage of hard, formed stools; anorexia; abdominal distention; straining during defecation

RISK FACTORS
- Immobility
- Poor preoperative intake of food and fiber
- Medication regimen

DESIRED OUTCOMES

The client will not experience constipation as evidenced by:
   a. Usual frequency of bowel movements about 2 days after usual oral intake is resumed
   b. Passage of soft, formed stool
   c. Absence of increasing abdominal distention and pain, feeling of rectal fullness or pressure, and straining during defecation

NOC OUTCOMES	NIC INTERVENTIONS
Bowel elimination	Constipation/Impaction management; pain management

NURSING ASSESSMENT	RATIONALE
Assess for and report signs and symptoms of constipation: • Increasing abdominal pain • Feeling of fullness or pressure in rectum • Decrease in frequency of bowel movements • Passage of hard, formed stools • Anorexia • Abdominal distention • Straining during defecation	*Early recognition of signs and symptoms of constipation allows for prompt intervention.*

THERAPEUTIC INTERVENTIONS	RATIONALE

Independent Actions
Implement additional measures to prevent constipation:
* Encourage client to defecate when urge is felt. **D** ✦

  If client suppresses the urge to defecate by contracting the anal sphincters, the defecation reflex will subside after a few minutes and not occur again for several hours.
* Instruct client to request an analgesic prior to attempting to defecate.

  An analgesic will help ease the surgical site pain associated with the increased intra-abdominal and perineal pressure that occur with defecation.

Dependent/Collaborative Actions
Implement additional measures to prevent constipation:
* Increase activity as allowed. **D** ● ✦

  Ambulation stimulates peristalsis, which promotes passage of stool through the intestines.
* Maintain minimum fluid intake of 2500 mL unless contra-indicated. **D** ✦

  Inadequate fluid intake reduces the water content of feces, which results in dry, hard stool.
* When diet advances, encourage client to increase intake of foods high in fiber.

  Foods high in fiber provide bulk to the fecal mass and keep the stool soft because of the ability of fiber to absorb water.

Nursing Diagnosis **RISK FOR INFECTION** NDx

Definition: At risk for being invaded by pathogenic organisms

Related to:
a. **Vaginal/perineal wound infection** related to:
   * Wound contamination associated with introduction of pathogens during or after surgery (a high risk with this surgery because of the close proximity of the incisions to the perianal area)
   * Decreased resistance to infection associated with factors such as age and an inadequate nutritional status
b. **Urinary tract infection** related to:
   * Increased growth and colonization of microorganisms associated with urinary stasis
   * Introduction of pathogens associated with the presence of an indwelling catheter

CLINICAL MANIFESTATIONS

Subjective	Objective
Vaginal/perineal wound infection: increased pain in wound area **Urinary tract infection:** verbal reports of frequency, urgency, and burning on urination	**Vaginal/perineal wound infection:** chills; fever; redness, heat, swelling in wound area; unusual wound drainage; foul smelling odor from wound area; persistent elevation in WBC count; change in differential count; positive wound cultures **Urinary tract infection:** cloudy urine; positive urine culture; abnormal urinalysis

Continued...

RISK FACTORS

- Inadequate immune response
- Surgery

DESIRED OUTCOMES

The client will remain free of wound infection as evidenced by:
   a. Absence of chills/fever
   b. Absence of redness, heat, swelling, and increased pain in wound area
   c. Usual drainage from wounds
   d. White blood cell (WBC) and differential counts returning toward normal
   e. Negative cultures of wound drainage
   f. Clear urine
   g. Absence of frequency, urgency, and burning on urination
   h. Negative urine culture

NOC OUTCOMES

Infection severity; immune status; wound healing: primary intention

NIC INTERVENTIONS

Infection control; infection protection; perineal care; urinary retention care

NURSING ASSESSMENT

Assess for and report signs and symptoms of vaginal perineal wound or urinary tract infection:
- Chills
- Fever
- Redness, heat, swelling in wound area
- Unusual wound drainage
- Foul smelling odor from wound area

Assess results of urinalysis, urine, and/or wound cultures reporting abnormalities.

RATIONALE

Early recognition of signs and symptoms of infection allows for prompt intervention.

THERAPEUTIC INTERVENTIONS

Independent Actions

Use good hand hygiene and encourage client to do the same.

Implement measures to reduce the risk of wound infection:
- Instruct client to avoid touching incisions, dressings, and/ or drainage tubings.
- Use sterile technique during all dressing changes and wound care. **D** ✦
- Assist client with perineal care every shift and after each bowel movement. **D** ● ✦

Implement measures to reduce the risk of urinary tract infection:
- Instruct client to wipe from front to back after urination and defecation.
- If catheter is present, perform catheter care at least twice a day. **D** ● ✦

Implement measures to prevent urinary retention when urinary catheter is present (e.g. keep drainage tubing free of kinks, keep collection container below bladder).

Dependent/Collaborative Actions

Administer antimicrobials as ordered.
Obtain urine/wound cultures as ordered.

Consult appropriate health care provider if signs and symptoms of a wound infection or urinary tract infection is present.

RATIONALE

Good hand hygiene removes transient flora, which reduces the risk of transmission of pathogens.

Use of sterile technique reduces the risk of introducing pathogens into the body.

The perineal area contains a large number of organisms. Routine cleansing reduces the risk of colonization of organisms.

Normal unobstructed voiding flushes microorganisms from the mucosal lining of the urethra. Urine that accumulates in the bladder creates an environment conducive to colonization of bacteria.

Notifying the appropriate health care provider allows for modification of the treatment plan.

Collaborative Diagnosis   RISK FOR REHERNIATION OF THE BLADDER OR RECTUM

Definition: Protrusion of the bladder or rectum into the vaginal canal

Related to: Stress on internal sutures associated with increased intra-abdominal, bladder, rectal, or vaginal pressure

CLINICAL MANIFESTATIONS

Subjective	Objective
Difficulty evacuating stool, or pelvic pressure	Persistent or increasing stress incontinence

RISK FACTORS

- Poor abdominal muscle tone
- Surgery
- Distended abdomen

DESIRED OUTCOMES

The client will not experience reherniation of the bladder and rectum as evidenced by:
   a. Absence of stress incontinence
   b. No difficulty with evacuation of stool
   c. Gradual resolution of pelvic pressure

NURSING ASSESSMENT	RATIONALE
Assess for and report signs and symptoms of reherniation of the bladder or rectum: • Difficulty evacuating stool, or pelvic pressure • Persistent or increasing stress incontinence	*Early recognition of signs and symptoms of reherniation of bladder or rectum allows for prompt intervention.*

THERAPEUTIC INTERVENTIONS	RATIONALE
Independent Actions Perform actions to prevent urinary retention (instruct client to urinate when urge is first felt, provide privacy, hold warm blanket against abdomen, run water pour warm water over perineum). **D ● ✦**	*These actions reduce pressure on the suture line.*
Perform actions to prevent constipation (e.g. encourage client to defecate when urge is first felt, encourage client to relax, provide privacy, increase intake of liquids and fiber). **D ● ✦**	
Perform actions to prevent increased intra-abdominal pressure: • Instruct client to remain in a flat or semi-Fowler's position rather than a high Fowler's position while in bed. • Instruct client to avoid any activities that may create a Valsalva response (e.g., straining to have a bowel movement, lifting or carrying a heavy object, holding breath while moving in bed, coughing).	*Actions help prevent stress on the internal sutures and reduce the risk for reherniation of the bladder and rectum.*
Administer a laxative, antiemetic, and antitussive if ordered. **D ● ✦**	*Medications help prevent straining to have a bowel movement and control nausea, vomiting, and persistent cough.*
Caution client to avoid prolonged standing and sitting. If reherniation occurs: • Maintain client on bed rest. **D ● ✦** • Prepare client for surgical repair if planned.	

Collaborative Diagnosis   RISK FOR BLADDER, URETHRAL, OR URETERAL INJURY

Definition: Inadvertent injury to the bladder, urethra, or ureters during surgery

Related to: Accidental tear or ligation during the surgical procedure

CLINICAL MANIFESTATIONS

Subjective	Objective
Reports of persistent or increasing complaints of a backache	Persistent or increasing hematuria; urine output <200 mL in the first 6 to 8 hours after surgery

NDx = NANDA-I Diagnosis   **D** = Delegatable Action   ● = UAP   ✦ = LVN/LPN   ⊖▶ = Go to ⊖volve for animation

Continued...

RISK FACTOR	DESIRED OUTCOMES
• Surgery	The client will experience healing of bladder, urethral, or ureteral injury if it occurs as evidenced by: a. Gradual resolution of hematuria and backache b. Urine output >200 mL within 6 to 8 hours after surgery

NURSING ASSESSMENT	RATIONALE
Assess for and report signs and symptoms of bladder, urethral, or ureteral injury—persistent or increasing hematuria: • Persistent or increasing complaints of a backache	*Early recognition of signs and symptoms of bladder or urethral injury allows for prompt intervention.*

THERAPEUTIC INTERVENTIONS	RATIONALE
Independent Actions If signs and symptoms of bladder, urethral, or ureteral injury are present: • Continue to monitor output carefully. **D** ● ✦ • Notify the physician/surgeon. • Prepare client for surgical repair if indicated.	*Notifying the appropriate health care provider allows for modification of the treatment plan.*

DISCHARGE TEACHING/CONTINUED CARE

Nursing Diagnosis
DEFICIENT KNOWLEDGE NDx, INEFFECTIVE FAMILY THERAPEUTIC REGIMEN NDx, OR INEFFECTIVE SELF-HEALTH MANAGEMENT* NDx

Definition: Absence or deficiency of cognitive information related to specific topic (lack of specific information) necessary for client/significant others to make informed choices regarding condition/treatment/lifestyle changes; pattern of regulating and integrating into daily living and family processes a therapeutic regimen for treatment of illnesses and the sequelae of illness that is unsatisfactory for meeting specific health goals.

CLINICAL MANIFESTATIONS

Subjective	Objective
Verbalizes inability to manage illness and inability to follow prescribed regimen	Inaccurate follow through with instructions; inappropriate behavior; refusal to participate in care

RISK FACTORS
• Cognitive deficit
• Inability to care for self
• Difficulty in integrating changes into lifestyle

NOC OUTCOMES	NIC INTERVENTIONS
Knowledge: disease process; knowledge: treatment regimen; knowledge: prescribed activity	Health system guidance; teaching: individual; teaching: disease process; pelvic muscle exercise; teaching: prescribed activity/exercise

NURSING ASSESSMENT	RATIONALE
Assess client's readiness and ability to learn. Assess meaning of illness to client.	*Early recognition of readiness to learn and meaning of illness to client allows for implementation of the appropriate teaching interventions.*

*The nurse should select the nursing diagnostic label that is most appropriate for the client's discharge teaching needs.

THERAPEUTIC INTERVENTIONS	RATIONALE

Desired Outcomes: The client will identify ways to decrease the risk of reherniation of the bladder and rectum.

Independent Actions

Provide the following instructions:

- Reinforce instructions about avoiding prolonged sitting and standing and any activity that may create a Valsalva response (e.g., straining to have a bowel movement, lifting or carrying heavy objects, coughing) for at least 6 weeks.
- Instruct client to urinate whenever the urge is felt or at least every 4 hours.
- Reinforce instructions about how to prevent constipation (e.g., drink at least 8 glasses of water daily, increase intake of foods high in fiber, take stool softeners as prescribed).

Instruct client in additional ways to reduce the risk of reherniation of the bladder and rectum:

- Do perineal exercises (e.g., stopping and starting urinary stream, alternately contracting and relaxing the gluteal muscles) when healing is complete (usually in 6 weeks) to help maintain tone of the pelvic muscles.
- Adhere to a weight reduction diet and exercise program if overweight.

Actions help minimize pressure on the internal suture lines and decrease the risk of reherniation of the bladder and/or rectum.

Actions help strengthen the pelvic floor muscles.

THERAPEUTIC INTERVENTIONS	RATIONALE

Desired Outcomes: The client will identify ways to relieve surgical site discomfort.

Independent Actions

Provide the following instructions regarding ways to relieve discomfort in the surgical area:

- Take a sitz bath 2 to 3 times/day.

- Avoid prolonged sitting and standing.
- Sit on a foam pad or pillow.
- Take analgesics as prescribed.

Warm water is soothing to suture line and promotes blood flow and healing.
Actions increase pressure on surgical site causing pain.
Provides support to surgical site
Analgesics decrease discomfort.

THERAPEUTIC INTERVENTIONS	RATIONALE

Desired Outcomes: The client will state signs and symptoms to report to the health care provider.

Independent Actions

Instruct the client to report these additional signs and symptoms to the health care provider:

- Foul-smelling vaginal discharge
- Heavy, bright-red vaginal bleeding or the passage of clots that are thumb-size or larger
- Persistent or recurrent stress incontinence, difficulty evacuating stool, or feeling of pressure in pelvic area (may indicate reherniation of bladder or rectum)
- Persistent painful intercourse (client should avoid intercourse for approximately 6 weeks)
- Presence of urine or stool in vaginal drainage (indicative of fistula formation)
- Excessive swelling or pain in perineal area

These clinical manifestations are an indication of complications including infection, bleeding, possible nerve damage, or fistula formation. These should be reported to the health care provider for treatment.

Continued...

THERAPEUTIC INTERVENTIONS	RATIONALE

Desired Outcomes: The client will verbalize an understanding of and a plan for adhering to recommended follow-up care including future appointments with health care provider, medications prescribed, and limitations on sexual activity.

Independent Actions

Instruct client not to have sexual intercourse until permitted by physician (usually 6 weeks).

Inform client that loss of vaginal sensation is usually temporary but may persist for several months.

Reinforce importance of keeping follow-up appointments with the health care provider.

Implement measures to improve client adherence:
- Include significant others in teaching sessions if possible.
- Encourage questions and allow time for reinforcement and clarification of information.
- Provide written instructions.

Adhering to a prescribed treatment plan is important to prevent the development of complications and to promote adequate wound healing.

ADDITIONAL CARE PLANS

ACUTE PAIN NDx

Related to: Tissue trauma and reflex muscle spasms associated with the surgical procedure

HYSTERECTOMY WITH SALPINGECTOMY AND OOPHORECTOMY

Hysterectomy is the surgical removal of the uterus. It is performed to treat conditions such as malignant and non-malignant growths in the uterus and cervix, symptomatic endometriosis, uterine prolapse, intractable pelvic infection, irreparable rupture of the uterus, and dysfunctional or life-threatening uterine bleeding. Both the uterus and cervix are removed in a total hysterectomy. A panhysterectomy is the removal of the uterus, cervix, fallopian tubes, and ovaries and is often referred to as a total abdominal hysterectomy with bilateral salpingectomy and oophorectomy (TAH-BSO). A radical hysterectomy also includes a partial vaginectomy and dissection of the pelvic lymph nodes.

A vaginal or abdominal approach can be used to perform a hysterectomy. The approach used depends on factors such as the woman's pelvic anatomy and size of the uterus, whether repairs to the vaginal wall or pelvic floor are needed, the presence of other medical conditions, previous abdominal surgeries, and the diagnosis.

This care plan focuses on the adult client hospitalized for a total abdominal hysterectomy with salpingectomy and oophorectomy.

OUTCOME/DISCHARGE CRITERIA

The client will:
1. Have evidence of normal healing of surgical wound
2. Have clear, audible breath sounds throughout lungs
3. Have adequate urine output
4. Have surgical pain controlled
5. Have no signs and symptoms of postoperative complications
6. Verbalize an understanding of the effects of surgical menopause
7. Identify ways to achieve sexual satisfaction
8. Verbalize an understanding of medications ordered including the rationale for the prescription, food and drug interactions, side effects, schedule for taking, and importance of taking as prescribed
9. State signs and symptoms to report to the health care provider
10. Share feelings about the loss of reproductive ability
11. Verbalize an understanding of and a plan for adhering to recommended follow-up care including future appointments with health care provider, activity limitations, and wound care.

PREOPERATIVE: USE IN CONJUNCTION WITH THE STANDARDIZED PREOPERATIVE CARE PLAN

RELATED PREOPERATIVE NURSING DIAGNOSES

FEAR/ANXIETY
Related to:

- Anticipated loss of control associated with the effects of anesthesia
- Anticipated effects of surgery on femininity and reproductive ability
- Fear of rejection by partner
- Unfamiliar environment and separation from significant others

- Potential embarrassment or loss of dignity associated with body exposure during preoperative care, surgery, and postoperative care
- Lack of understanding of the surgical procedure and postoperative expectations and care
- Anticipated surgical findings and postoperative discomfort
- Financial concerns associated with hospitalization
- Diagnosis of cancer (if present) and prognosis.

POSTOPERATIVE: USE IN CONJUNCTION WITH THE STANDARDIZED POSTOPERATIVE CARE PLAN

Nursing Diagnosis | ## URINARY RETENTION NDx

Definition: Incomplete emptying of the bladder

Related to:
a. Obstruction of the urinary catheter
b. Impaired urination after removal of catheter associated with:

- Decreased perception of bladder fullness associated with the depressant effect of anesthesia and some medications (e.g., narcotic [opioid] analgesics)
- Increased tone of the urinary sphincters associated with sympathetic nervous system stimulation resulting from pain, fear, and anxiety
- Relaxation of the bladder muscle associated with nerve trauma and/or edema in the bladder area resulting from surgical manipulation; the depressant effect of anesthesia and some medications (e.g., narcotic [opioid] analgesics); stimulation of the sympathetic nervous system (can result from pain, fear, and anxiety)

CLINICAL MANIFESTATIONS

Subjective	Objective
Verbal reports of bladder fullness or suprapubic discomfort	Bladder distention, absence of fluid in urinary drainage tubing, output that continues to be < intake 48 hours after surgery; frequent voiding of small amounts [25-60 mL] of urine.

RISK FACTORS

- Surgery
- Medication regimen

DESIRED OUTCOMES

The client will not experience urinary retention as evidenced by:
  a No reports of bladder fullness and suprapubic discomfort
  b Absence of bladder distention
  c Balanced intake and output within 48 hours after surgery
  d Voiding adequate amounts at expected intervals after removal of the catheter

NOC OUTCOMES

Urinary elimination

NIC INTERVENTIONS

Urinary retention care; tube care: urinary

NDx = NANDA-I Diagnosis   **D** = Delegatable Action   ● = UAP   ✦ = LVN/LPN   ⊖▶ = Go to ⊖volve for animation

Continued...

NURSING ASSESSMENT	RATIONALE
Assess for and report signs and symptoms of urinary retention: • Verbal reports of bladder fullness or suprapubic discomfort • Bladder distention • Absence of fluid in urinary drainage tubing • Output that continues to be < intake 48 hours after surgery • Frequent voiding of small amounts [25-60 mL] of urine	*Early recognition of signs and symptoms of urinary retention allows for prompt intervention.*

THERAPEUTIC INTERVENTIONS	RATIONALE
Independent Actions Implement measures to prevent urinary retention: • Keep drainage tubing free of kinks. **D** ● ✦ • Keep collection container below level of bladder. **D** ● ✦ • Anchor catheter tubing securely to prevent inadvertent removal. **D** ● ✦	*Actions help prevent urinary retention by maintaining patency of urinary catheter.*

After removal of catheter:
• Instruct client to urinate when the urge is first felt.
• Promote actions that facilitate relaxation during voiding attempts.
  • Provide privacy. **D** ● ✦
  • Hold a warm blanket against abdomen. **D** ● ✦
Perform actions that may help trigger the micturition reflex and promote relaxation:
• Run water. **D** ● ✦
• Pour warm water over perineum. **D** ● ✦
• Allow client to assume a normal position for voiding if allowed. **D** ● ✦
	Actions help prevent urinary retention after removal of urinary catheter.

Consult physician if urinary retention persists or if actions fail to alleviate urinary retention.	*Notifying the physician allows for modification of the treatment plan.*

Collaborative Diagnosis **RISK FOR BLADDER OR URETERAL INJURY**

Definition: Inadvertant injury to the bladder or ureters during surgery.

Related to: Accidental tear or ligation during the surgical procedure

CLINICAL MANIFESTATIONS

Subjective	Objective
Verbalizes persistent or increasing complaints of a backache	Persistent or increasing hematuria; urine output <200 mL in the first 6 to 8 hours after surgery

RISK FACTORS
• Surgery

DESIRED OUTCOMES

The client will experience healing of bladder, urethral, or ureteral injury if it occurs as evidenced by:
  a. Gradual resolution of hematuria and backache
  b. Urine output >200 mL within 6 to 8 hours after surgery

NURSING ASSESSMENT	RATIONALE
Assess for and report signs and symptoms of bladder or ureteral injury: • Persistent or increasing complaints of a backache • Persistent or increasing hematuria • Urine output <200 mL in the first 6 to 8 hours after surgery	*Early recognition of signs and symptoms of bladder or ureteral injury allows for prompt intervention.*

THERAPEUTIC INTERVENTIONS	RATIONALE
Independent Actions If signs and symptoms of bladder, urethral, or ureteral injury are present: • Continue to monitor output carefully. **D** ● ✦ • Notify the physician/surgeon. • Prepare client for surgical repair if indicated.	*Notifying the appropriate health care provider allows for modification of the treatment plan.*

Collaborative Diagnosis ⬛ RISK FOR THROMBOEMBOLISM

Definition: A clot attached to a vessel wall that detaches and circulates within the blood

Related to:
a. Trauma to the pelvic veins during surgery
b. Venous stasis associated with:
   • Decreased activity
   • Increased blood viscosity (can result from deficient fluid volume)
   • Pelvic congestion resulting from inflammation in the surgical area
   • Abdominal distention (the distended intestine may put pressure on the abdominal vessels)
   • Pressure on the pelvic and calf vessels during surgery if a vaginal approach was used (client is placed in lithotomy position for this approach)
c. Hypercoagulability associated with increased release of tissue thromboplastin into the blood (occurs as a result of surgical trauma) and hemoconcentration and increased blood viscosity (can result from deficient fluid volume)

CLINICAL MANIFESTATIONS

Subjective	Objective
Reports deep vein thrombus: reports of pain, tenderness	**Deep vein thrombus:** swelling, unusual warmth, and/or positive Homans' sign in extremity
Reports arterial thrombus: reports of numbness, and/or pain in extremity	**Arterial thrombus:** diminished or absent peripheral pulses; pallor, coolness
Reports cerebral ischemia: N/A	**Cerebral ischemia:** decreased level of consciousness, alteration in usual sensory and motor function
Reports pulmonary embolism: reports of sudden onset of chest pain, increased dyspnea	**Pulmonary embolism:** increased restlessness and apprehension, significant decrease in SaO_2

RISK FACTORS
• Immobility
• Inadequate fluid volume
• Surgery
• Decreased venous return

DESIRED OUTCOMES

The client will not develop a thromboembolism as evidenced by:
   a. Absence of pain, tenderness, swelling, and numbness in extremities
   b. Usual temperature and color of extremities
   c. Palpable and equal peripheral pulses
   d. Usual mental status
   e. Usual sensory and motor function
   f. Absence of sudden chest pain and dyspnea

Continued...

NURSING ASSESSMENT	RATIONALE
Assess for signs and symptoms of thromboebolism	
DVT: Pain, tenderness, Swelling, unusual warmth, or positive humans' sign in extremity	*Early recognition of signs and symptoms of thromboembolism allows prompt intervention.*
Arterial thrombus: Numbness and/or pain in the extremity, diminished or absent pulses, pallor, coolness	
Pulmonary embolism: Sudden onset of chest pain, increased dyspnea, increased restlessness, apprehension, significant decrease in SaO$_2$	

THERAPEUTIC INTERVENTIONS	RATIONALE
Collaborative Actions	
Implement measures to prevent thrombus formation:	*Actions help prevent pooling of blood in lower extremities.*
• Avoid having client in a high Fowler's position **D** ● ✦	
• Encourage client to lie flat for short periods at least every 4 hours. **D** ● ✦	*Increases blood return to the legs.*
• Assist client with ambulation as soon as allowed. **D** ● ✦	
• Consult physician about an order for antiembolism stockings or pneumatic compression devices if the patient remains inactive.	
• Maintain adequate fluid intake of at least 2500 mL/day unless contraindicated. **D** ✦	*Adequate hydration helps thin circulating blood volume reducing the risk of embolism formation.*
• Administer anticoagulants as ordered. **D** ✦	*Anticoagulants*

DISCHARGE TEACHING/CONTINUED CARE

Nursing Diagnosis

DEFICIENT KNOWLEDGE NDx, INEFFECTIVE FAMILY THERAPEUTIC REGIMEN NDx OR INEFFECTIVE SELF-HEALTH MANAGEMENT* NDx

Definition: Absence or deficiency of cognitive information related to specific topic (lack of specific information necessary) for client/significant others to make informed choices regarding condition/treatment/lifestyle changes; pattern of regulating and integrating into daily living and family processes a therapeutic regimen for treatment of illnesses and the sequelae of illness that is unsatisfactory for meeting specific health goals.

CLINICAL MANIFESTATIONS

Subjective	Objective
Verbalizes inability to manage illness and inability to follow prescribed regimen	Inaccurate follow through with instructions; inappropriate behavior; refusal to participate in care

RISK FACTORS
• Cognitive deficit
• Inability to care for self

NOC OUTCOMES	NIC INTERVENTIONS
Knowledge: treatment regimen; knowledge: prescribed activity	Health system guidance; teaching: individual; teaching: prescribed medication; teaching: prescribed activity/exercise

NURSING ASSESSMENT	RATIONALE
Assess client's readiness and ability to learn. Assess meaning of illness to client.	*Early recognition of readiness to learn and meaning of illness to client allows for implementation of the appropriate teaching interventions.*

*The nurse should select the nursing diagnostic label that is most appropriate for the client's discharge teaching needs.

THERAPEUTIC INTERVENTIONS	RATIONALE

Desired Outcomes: The client will verbalize an understanding of the effects of surgical menopause.

Independent Actions

Reinforce the physician's explanation of surgical menopause and its possible effects (e.g., hot flashes, facial hair growth, decrease in vaginal lubrication, insomnia, fatigue, nervousness, palpitations, depression).

Explain the probable effects of the surgery on sexual functioning (e.g., decreased libido, vaginal dryness, painful intercourse).

Having a greater understanding of the physiological effects of surgery will aid the client in understanding potential effects of surgery and allow for time to grieve, develop effective coping skills, and seek out the social support necessary to adjust to the effects of surgery.

THERAPEUTIC INTERVENTIONS	RATIONALE

Desired Outcomes: The client will identify ways to achieve sexual satisfaction.

Independent Actions

Instruct client in ways to promote sexual satisfaction:
- Use a water-soluble lubricant in the vagina to prevent pain during intercourse.
- Take hormone replacements (e.g., estrogen) as prescribed.
- Try different positions for intercourse to determine whether some positions are more comfortable than others.

Reinforce physician's instructions regarding when client can resume sexual intercourse (usually 4 to 6 weeks).

The amount of vaginal lubrication decreases as a result of the effects of surgically induced menopause.

Waiting to resume sexual intercourse provides time for appropriate healing.

THERAPEUTIC INTERVENTIONS	RATIONALE

Desired Outcomes: The client will verbalize an understanding of medications ordered including rationale for prescription, food and drug interactions, side effects, schedule for taking, and importance of taking as prescribed.

Independent Actions

Explain the rationale for, side effects of, schedule for taking, and importance of taking hormone replacement therapy as prescribed.

Inform client of pertinent interactions between estrogen and other medications she is taking.

Instruct client to inform physician of any other prescription and nonprescription medications she is taking and to inform all health care providers of medications being taken.

Taking medications as prescribed is important to achieve maximum benefits of therapy and prevent adverse effects. Understanding the purpose and side effects of medications improves adherence.

Decreases potential for adverse drug effects.

THERAPEUTIC INTERVENTIONS	RATIONALE

Desired Outcomes: The client will state signs and symptoms to report to the health care provider.

Independent Actions

Instruct the client to report these additional signs and symptoms:
- Foul-smelling vaginal discharge (it is normal to have an increased amount of discharge about 2 weeks postoperatively when internal sutures are absorbed)
- Heavy, bright-red vaginal bleeding or the passage of clots that are thumb-size or larger
- Excessive depression or difficulty dealing with changes in body image

These clinical manifestations are indications of infection, trauma, and other complications. These should be reported to the health care provider for modification of the treatment plan.

Continued...

THERAPEUTIC INTERVENTIONS	RATIONALE

- Excessive discomfort associated with effects of surgical menopause
- Adverse reactions to estrogen replacement therapy

THERAPEUTIC INTERVENTIONS	RATIONALE

Desired Outcomes: The client will verbalize an understanding of and a plan for adhering to recommended follow-up care including future appointments with health care provider, activity limitations, and wound care.

Independent Actions

Reinforce the physician's instructions regarding the need to:

Adhering to a prescribed treatment plan helps promote positive outcomes and prevents complications.
Avoiding heavy lifting allows for appropriate physical healing.

- Avoid lifting objects over 10 pounds, sitting for long periods, stair climbing, and strenuous physical activity (e.g., vacuuming, aerobics) for 6 to 8 weeks postoperatively.
- Avoid driving for at least a week after surgery.
- Avoid douching, using tampons, and having sexual intercourse for 4 to 6 weeks postoperatively.

Reinforce importance of keeping follow-up appointments with the health care provider.

Follow-up appointments are important to monitor progress. Involving the client's significant other improves client adherence to treatment regimen.

Implement measures to improve client adherence:

- Include significant others in teaching sessions if possible.
- Encourage questions and allow time for reinforcement and clarification of information.
- Provide written instructions.

ADDITIONAL CARE PLANS

ACUTE PAIN NDx
Related to:

- Tissue trauma and reflex muscle spasms associated with the surgical procedure

DISTURBED SELF-CONCEPT*
Related to:

- Loss of reproductive organs with subsequent inability to bear children
- Feeling of loss of femininity and sexuality

GRIEVING† NDx
Related to:

- Loss of reproductive ability, early menopause, diagnosis of cancer (if present), and the possibility of premature death

RISK FOR INFECTION NDx
Related to:

- Wound contamination associated with introduction of pathogens during or following surgery
- Decreased resistance to infection associated with factors such as age and an inadequate nutritional status
- Increased growth and colonization of microorganisms associated with urinary stasis
- Introduction of pathogens associated with the presence of an indwelling catheter

MASTECTOMY

A mastectomy is the surgical removal of all or part of the breast and is usually performed to treat breast cancer. The type of mastectomy is based on factors such as the location, type, and size of the tumor; the number of tumors; breast size; axillary lymph node status; whether the client has received prior irradiation of the breast; and client preference. The two major types of surgeries performed to treat resectable breast cancer are a modified radical mastectomy and breast-conserv-

---

*This diagnostic label includes the nursing diagnoses of Disturbed body image, Low self-esteem, and Ineffective role performance.
†This diagnostic label includes Anticipatory grieving and Grieving following the actual losses.

ing surgery (e.g., lumpectomy, quadrantectomy, partial or segmental mastectomy).

A modified radical mastectomy includes removal of the breast and an axillary node dissection. The pectoral muscles and surrounding nerves are left intact, which allows the client to retain the shape of her breast and avoid the shoulder and arm limitations and skin graft requirements that accompany a radical mastectomy. Leaving the muscles and nerves intact facilitates reconstructive surgery, which may be performed at the time of the mastectomy or delayed for several months depending on physician and client preference and additional treatment planned.

The additional treatment (e.g., chemotherapy, hormone therapy, external radiation therapy) that may be considered after a modified radical mastectomy depends on factors such as the immunological and menopausal status of the client, tumor type and size, and amount of lymph node involvement. Breast-conserving surgery is an option for many women with stage I or stage II breast cancer. It involves excision of the tumor, a surrounding margin of normal tissue, and an axillary lymph node dissection. It is followed by a course of radiation therapy to eradicate any residual tumor and reduce the risk for tumor recurrence.

Axillary node dissection has traditionally been performed with all invasive breast cancer to stage the tumor. Sentinel node biopsy (lymphatic mapping) is a procedure currently being used to help identify axillary node involvement and avoid unnecessary lymph node dissection. This procedure can be done the day of surgery. If the sentinel node is negative for cancer cells, an axillary dissection is not necessary, which eliminates the need for axillary drains and reduces the risk for lymphedema.

This care plan focuses on the female adult client hospitalized for a modified radical mastectomy. Much of the postoperative information is applicable to clients receiving follow-up care in a home setting.

OUTCOME/DISCHARGE CRITERIA

The client will:
1. Have evidence of normal healing of surgical wounds
2. Have clear, audible breath sounds throughout lungs
3. Have surgical pain controlled
4. Have no signs and symptoms of postoperative complications
5. Identify ways to reduce the risk of trauma to and infection in the arm on the operative side
6. Identify ways to prevent and treat lymphedema of the arm on the operative side
7. Demonstrate the ability to care for wound drainage device if present
8. Demonstrate the ability to perform the prescribed exercises and verbalize an understanding of additional exercises to be done once the incision has healed
9. Verbalize the importance of and demonstrate the ability to perform a breast self-examination (BSE) on the remaining breast and operative site
10. State the factors to consider in selecting a breast prosthesis
11. State signs and symptoms to report to the health care provider
12. Share thoughts and feelings about the change in body image
13. Identify community resources that can assist with adjustment to the diagnosis of cancer and the loss of a breast
14. Verbalize an understanding of and a plan for adhering to recommended follow-up care including future appointments with health care provider, medications prescribed, activity level, wound care, and plans for subsequent treatment.

PREOPERATIVE: USE IN CONJUNCTION WITH THE STANDARDIZED PREOPERATIVE CARE PLAN

RELATED PREOPERATIVE NURSING DIAGNOSES

FEAR/ANXIETY NDx
Related to:
- Diagnosis of cancer, treatment plan, and prognosis
- Anticipated loss of control associated with the effects of anesthesia
- Anticipated loss of femininity and physical attractiveness and possible change in relationship with significant other associated with the disfiguring effect of the mastectomy
- Unfamiliar environment and separation from significant others

- Anticipated surgical findings and postoperative pain
- Lack of understanding of the surgical procedure and postoperative expectations and care
- Potential embarrassment or loss of dignity associated with body exposure during preoperative care, surgery, and postoperative assessments and treatments
- Financial concerns associated with hospitalization and subsequent treatment (if planned)

Nursing Diagnosis	**DEFICIENT KNOWLEDGE** NDx

Definition: Absence or deficiency of cognitive information related to a specific topic

CLINICAL MANIFESTATIONS

Subjective	Objective
Verbalization of the problem	Exaggerated behaviors

RISK FACTORS

- Unfamiliar environment
- Anxiety about the future

DESIRED OUTCOMES

The client will:
- Verbalize an understanding of the surgical procedure, preoperative care, and postoperative sensations and care
- Demonstrate the ability to perform activities designed to prevent postoperative complications

NOC OUTCOMES	NIC INTERVENTIONS
Knowledge: disease process; knowledge: treatment regimen	Teaching: preoperative; teaching: individual; teaching: prescribed activity/exercise

NURSING ASSESSMENT	RATIONALE
Assess client's readiness and ability to learn. Assess meaning of illness to client.	*Early recognition of readiness to learn and meaning of illness to client allows for implementation of the appropriate teaching interventions.*

THERAPEUTIC INTERVENTIONS	RATIONALE

Independent Actions

Provide the following information about sensations that may occur after a mastectomy:

- Explain to client that it is common to have sensations of pain, numbness, and tingling in the operative area (these sensations usually subside within a year).
- Assure client that the sense that both breasts are present (phantom breast sensation) is common.
- Explain to client that she may feel a change in balance at first, particularly if breasts are large.

Provide additional instructions regarding ways to prevent complications after a mastectomy:

- Inform the client that she must keep upper arm on operative side close to her body for a few days after surgery (length of time will vary according to physician preference).
- Explain that exercise of the hand, arm, and shoulder on the operative side.
- Demonstrate recommended postmastectomy exercises (e.g., squeezing a ball, flexion and extension of the fingers and wrist, wall climbing, rope pulley exercises, arm swings, rope turning); inform client that hand and wrist exercises are usually begun the day after surgery with gradual progression to full range-of-motion exercises of arm and shoulder on operative side when incision has healed.

Instruct client on ways to minimize or prevent lymphedema of the arm on operative side:

- Keep arm on operative side elevated on pillows with elbow above heart level and hand higher than elbow in the early postoperative period.

Clients vary in physical and cognitive ability to learn. When educating clients, nurses need to determine a client's ability to read and understand written materials. If literacy barriers are present, alternative educational materials should be provided. Allow time for questions, clarification, and return demonstration of any learned actions.

Prevents tension on the suture lines and subsequent hematoma formation and seroma formation.

These are essential to facilitate and improve lymphatic and blood circulation, maintain muscle tone, and prevent contractures.

These exercises improve circulation and lymphatic return from the upper extremities.

Supports lymphatic drainage

THERAPEUTIC INTERVENTIONS	RATIONALE
• Perform recommended postmastectomy exercises as soon as allowed.	
• Avoid having BP measurements, injections, blood draws, and intravenous infusions in arm on operative side.	*These procedures increase the risk of infection or traum and subsequent lymphedema.*

POSTOPERATIVE: USE IN CONJUNCTION WITH THE STANDARDIZED POSTOPERATIVE CARE PLAN

Nursing Diagnosis ## ACUTE PAIN NDx (CHEST AND ARM ON OPERATIVE SIDE)

Definition: Unpleasant sensory and emotional experience arising from actual or potential tissue damage or described in terms of such damage (International Association for the Study of Pain); sudden or slow onset of any intensity from mild to severe with an anticipated or predictable end and a duration of <6 months.

Related to: Tissue trauma and reflex muscle spasms associated with surgery, irritation from drainage tubes, and strain on the surgical area postoperatively

CLINICAL MANIFESTATIONS

Subjective	Objective
Verbalization of pain	Grimacing; reluctance to move; restlessness; diaphoresis; increased BP; tachycardia

RISK FACTORS
• Surgical procedure

DESIRED OUTCOMES
The client will experience diminished pain in the chest and arm on the operative side as evidenced by:
a. Verbalization of a decrease in or absence of pain
b. Relaxed facial expression and body positioning
c. Increased participation in activities
d. Stable vital signs

NOC OUTCOMES
Pain control; comfort level; pain: adverse psychological reaction

NIC INTERVENTIONS
Pain management; analgesic administration

NURSING ASSESSMENT	RATIONALE
Assess for and report signs and symptoms of pain: • Verbalization of pain • Grimacing • Reluctance to move • Restlessness • Diaphoresis • Increased BP • Tachycardia	*Early recognition of signs and symptoms of pain allows for prompt intervention.*

THERAPEUTIC INTERVENTIONS	RATIONALE
Independent Actions Perform actions that will help prevent or alleviate pain: • Place client in a semi-Fowler's position during the immediate postoperative period. • Elevate the arm on the operative side on pillows, keeping elbow above the level of the heart and hand higher than the elbow. **D ✦**	*Actions help reduce pain in the chest and arm on the operative side.* *Improves vascular and lymph return and swelling*

NDx = NANDA-I Diagnosis **D** = Delegatable Action ● = UAP ✦ = LVN/LPN ⊖▶ = Go to ⊖volve for animation

Continued...

THERAPEUTIC INTERVENTIONS	RATIONALE
• Do not use arm on the operative side for intravenous therapy, blood draws, injections, and BP measurements. **D** ● ✦	*Actions help decrease tension on the incision, promote circulation, and prevent venous congestion in affected arm.*
• Move the operative extremity gently. **D** ● ✦	
• Reinforce the importance of adhering to arm and shoulder movement restrictions.	
• Maintain patency of wound drainage system (e.g., prevent kinking of tubing, empty collection device as needed, maintain suction as ordered, keep collection device below surgical wound). **D** ● ✦	*Actions help prevent fluid accumulation in the operative site, thereby reducing pain.*
• Securely anchor drainage tubes and collection device.	
• If a sling is ordered, apply it to the client's arm before client gets out of bed.	*Action reduces pain by supporting the affected arm and reducing strain on the surgical site.*
• Instruct client to get out of bed on the unaffected side (promotes the use of the unaffected arm rather than the arm on the operative side when getting up).	*Action helps reduce pain by reducing strain on the surgical site*
• Place needed items within easy reach.	
Dependent/Collaborative Actions	
Administer analgesics as ordered:	*Narcotics, non-narcotic analgesics, and NSAIDs are used for pain relief.*
• Narcotics	
• Nonnarcotic analgesics	
• Nonsteroidal anti-inflammatory agents	
Consult appropriate health care provider if above measures fail to provide adequate pain relief.	*Notifying the appropriate health care provider allows for modification of the treatment plan.*

Collaborative Diagnosis ## RISK FOR LYMPHEDEMA OF ARM ON OPERATIVE SIDE

Definition: Chronic swelling or feeling of tightness in the arm or hand due to an accumulation of lymphatic fluid in the soft tissue of the arm

Related to: Interruption in usual lymph flow associated with surgical removal of axillary lymph nodes and channels, edema in the operative area, and infection of or trauma to operative arm

CLINICAL MANIFESTATIONS

Subjective	Objective
Verbal reports of numbness, tingling, pain, sensation of heaviness or tightness or weakness in affected arm	Edema (measure arm on operative side at points 5-10 cm above and below elbow)

RISK FACTORS

- Surgical procedure
- Exposure to pathogens

DESIRED OUTCOMES

The client will not develop lymphedema of the arm on the operative side as evidenced by:
  a. Absence or gradual resolution of numbness, tingling, and weakness of the arm
  b. Absence of pain and feeling of heaviness and tightness in the arm
  c. Absence of edema in the arm

NURSING ASSESSMENT	RATIONALE
Assess for and report signs and symptoms of lymphedema of the arm on the operative side:	*Early recognition of signs and symptoms of lymphedema allows for prompt intervention.*
• Verbal reports of numbness, tingling, pain, sensation of heaviness or tightness or weakness in affected arm	
• Edema (measure arm on operative side at points 5-10 cm above and below elbow)	

THERAPEUTIC INTERVENTIONS	RATIONALE
Independent Actions	
Perform actions to prevent lymphedema:	*Measures help prevent lymphedema of arm on operative side.*
• Place client in a semi-Fowler's position during the immediate postoperative period.	
• Elevate arm on the operative side on pillows, keeping elbow above the level of the heart and hand higher than elbow. **D** ✦	
• Place a sign above bed to remind personnel not to use arm on operative side for intravenous therapy, blood draws, injections, and BP measurements. **D** ● ✦	*Actions help decrease risk of infection or trauma and subsequent lymphedema.*
Perform actions to prevent wound infection:	
• Instruct and assist client to perform postmastectomy exercises as soon as allowed.	*Actions help promote lymphatic drainage.*
Dependent/Collaborative Actions	
If signs and symptoms of lymphedema occur:	
• Notify the appropriate health care provider.	*Notifying the appropriate health care provider allows for modification of the treatment plan.*
• Apply an elastic pressure gradient sleeve to the affected arm if ordered to reduce edema.	
• Assist and instruct client in manual massage of the affected arm and/or use of sequential compression device on affected arm if ordered.	
• Administer antimicrobial agents if ordered.	*Medications help prevent or treat cellulitis and lymphangitis.*

Collaborative Diagnosis **RISK FOR MOTOR AND SENSORY IMPAIRMENT OF THE ARM AND/OR SHOULDER ON THE OPERATIVE SIDE**

Definition: Change in function and sensation of an extremity

Related to: Transection of or trauma to the nerves during surgery; pressure on nerves associated with lymphedema if it occurs; nonadherence with prescribed exercise program

CLINICAL MANIFESTATIONS

Subjective	Objective
Reports of new or increased numbness, tingling, or weakness in arm	Inability to move joints through expected range of motion

RISK FACTORS
• Surgery
• Fatigue

DESIRED OUTCOMES

The client will have expected motor and sensory function of the arm and shoulder on the operative side as evidenced by:
  a. Ability to put hand, arm, and shoulder through expected range of motion
  b. No reports of new or increased numbness, tingling, or weakness in arm

NURSING ASSESSMENT	RATIONALE
Assess for and report signs and symptoms of motor and/or sensory impairment of the arm and shoulder on operative side:	*Early recognition of signs and symptoms of fat embolism syndrome allows for prompt intervention.*
• Reports of new or increased numbness, tingling, or weakness in arm	
• Inability to move joints through expected range of motion	

 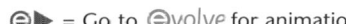

Continued...

THERAPEUTIC INTERVENTIONS	RATIONALE

Independent Actions

Perform actions to prevent lymphedema:
* Initiate postmastectomy exercises as soon as allowed.
* Encourage use of arm on operative side to perform activities of daily living as soon as allowed.

If signs and symptoms of impaired arm or shoulder function occur, assist with prescribed physical therapy.

Measures help prevent arm and shoulder dysfunction. Interventions aimed at prevention of lymphedema reduce pressure on surrounding nerves.

Collaborative Diagnosis   # RISK FOR SEROMA FORMATION

Definition: A collection of serous fluid at the site of surgery, armpit, or shoulder blade

Related to: Delayed or impaired flap adherence associated with irregular shape of chest wall, impaired wound drainage, and excessive movement of operative area with arm and shoulder use

CLINICAL MANIFESTATIONS

Subjective	**Objective**
N/A	Unusual swelling around incision site, less than expected amount of drainage in collection device, continued drainage from incision

RISK FACTORS
* Ineffective therapeutic regime
* Excessive movement of upper extremities

DESIRED OUTCOMES

The client will not develop a seroma at the surgical site as evidenced by:
 a. No unusual swelling around incision
 b. Expected amount of wound drainage in collection device
 c. Absence of continued drainage from incision

NURSING ASSESSMENT	RATIONALE

Assess for and report signs and symptoms of seroma formation:
* Unusual swelling around incision site
* Less than expected amount of drainage in collection device
* Continued drainage from incision

Early recognition of signs and symptoms of seroma formation allows for prompt intervention.

THERAPEUTIC INTERVENTIONS	RATIONALE

Independent Actions

Implement measures to prevent seroma formation:
* Maintain compression dressing over operative site if one is in place. **D** ✦
* Maintain patency of wound drainage system (e.g., prevent kinking of tubing, empty collection device as needed, keep collection device below surgical wound, maintain suction as ordered). **D** ✦

Action helps promote skin flap adherence so that fluid cannot accumulate in any dead space beneath the flap.

* Place needed items within easy reach to prevent excessive arm and shoulder movement.

Decreases stretching of arms, which decreases wound healing.

* If a sling is ordered, apply it to client's arm before client gets out of bed.

Supports the arm and reduces strain on the surgical site.

* Reinforce importance of adhering to arm and shoulder movement restrictions.

Decreases strain/pulling at the surgical site.

If seroma formation occurs:
* Notify the appropriate health care provider.
* Prepare client for needle aspiration of fluid if planned.

Notifying the appropriate health care provider allows for modification of the treatment plan.

THERAPEUTIC INTERVENTIONS	RATIONALE
• Assist with application of compression dressing if not already present.	
• Administer antimicrobials if ordered.	*Treatment of infections.*

Collaborative Diagnosis RISK FOR HEMATOMA FORMATION

Definition: Localized collection of partially clotted or clotted blood

Related to: Inadequate hemostasis during surgery, stress on vessels in operative area, and impaired drainage from the operative area

CLINICAL MANIFESTATIONS

Subjective	Objective
Verbalizes increased pain at surgical site	Swelling, and discoloration of operative site; less than expected amount of wound drainage in collection device

RISK FACTORS
- Surgery
- Inadequate drainage of surgical site or lymph system

DESIRED OUTCOMES

The client will not develop a hematoma at the surgical site as evidenced by:
  a. No unusual increase in pain, swelling, and skin discoloration in operative area
  b. Expected amount of wound drainage in collection device

NURSING ASSESSMENT	RATIONALE
Assess for and report signs and symptoms of hematoma formation:	*Early recognition of signs and symptoms of hematoma formation allows for prompt intervention.*
• Increased pain at surgical site	
• Swelling and discoloration of operative site	
• Less than expected amount of wound drainage in collection device	

THERAPEUTIC INTERVENTIONS	RATIONALE
Independent Actions Implement measures to prevent hematoma formation:	*Action helps prevent strain on the surgical site and subsequent bleeding.*
• Caution client to adhere to arm and shoulder movement restrictions.	
• Maintain compression dressing over operative site if one is in place. **D** ✦	
• Maintain patency of wound drainage system (e.g., prevent kinking of tubing, empty collection device as needed, keep collection device below surgical wound, maintain suction as ordered).	*Prevents accumulation of fluid at the surgical site.*
If signs and symptoms of hematoma formation occur, prepare client for evacuation of hematoma and repair of bleeding vessels if planned.	

Collaborative Diagnosis RISK FOR NECROSIS OF SKIN FLAP

Definition: Localized death of living tissue

Related to: Inadequate blood supply in flap or infection of surgical wound

NDx = NANDA-I Diagnosis   **D** = Delegatable Action   ● = UAP   ✦ = LVN/LPN   ⊖▶ = Go to ⊖volve for animation

Continued...

CLINICAL MANIFESTATIONS

Subjective	Objective
N/A	Decreased warmth of skin flap, pallor or cyanosis of skin flap, capillary refill time greater than 2 to 3 seconds; pale, cool, darkened tissue; separation of wound edges; foul odor from flap area.

RISK FACTORS

- Surgery
- Poor circulation

DESIRED OUTCOMES

The client will not experience necrosis of the skin flap as evidenced by:
  a. Skin flap warm and expected color
  b. Approximated wound edges
  c. Absence of foul odor from flap area

NURSING ASSESSMENT	RATIONALE
Assess for and report signs and symptoms of impaired blood flow to skin flap and/or skin flap necrosis: • Decreased warmth of skin flap, pallor or cyanosis of skin flap • Capillary refill time greater than 2 to 3 seconds • Pale, cool, darkened tissue; separation of wound edges • Foul odor from flap area	*Early recognition of signs and symptoms of flap necrosis allows for prompt intervention.*

THERAPEUTIC INTERVENTIONS	RATIONALE
Independent Actions Perform actions to maintain adequate circulation to wound area:	*Interventions help prevent skin flap necrosis.*
• Implement measures to prevent and treat seroma and hematoma formation (maintain patency of drains, maintain compression dressing).	*Prevents accumulation of fluid at the surgical site, which can impair healing.*
• Consult physician about reapplying or loosening the dressing if client reports increased tightness of dressing or if dressing appears too tight.	
• Position client on unoperative side or back. • Encourage client not to smoke.	*Improved drainage of fluid out of surgical site.* *Smoking causes vasoconstriction.*
Perform actions to promote healing of surgical incision and prevent wound infection (e.g., Change dressings as ordered; promote proper nutrition; support client in performing exercises).	
If signs and symptoms of skin flap necrosis occur, notify appropriate health care provider and, prepare client for surgical revision of flap.	

Nursing Diagnosis   ## DISTURBED SELF-CONCEPT*

Definitions: **Disturbed body image NDx:** Confusion in mental picture of one's physical self

        Situational low self-esteem NDx: Development of a negative perception of self-worth in response to a current situation

Related to: Loss of a breast; temporary dependence on others for assistance with self-care associated with restricted arm movement; possible altered sexuality patterns associated with decreased libido, perceived loss of femininity, and fear of rejection by partner

---

*This diagnostic label includes the nursing diagnoses of Disturbed body image, Low self-esteem.

CLINICAL MANIFESTATIONS

Subjective	Objective
Verbalization of negative feelings about self	Lack of participation in activities of daily living, refusal to look at mastectomy site, withdrawal from significant others

RISK FACTORS

- Surgical procedure
- Loss of image of self

DESIRED OUTCOMES

The client will demonstrate beginning adaptation to the loss of her breast and integration of the change in body image as evidenced by:
  a. Verbalization of feelings of self-worth and sexual adequacy
  b. Active participation in activities of daily living
  c. Willingness to look at surgical site
  d. Maintenance of relationships with significant others

NOC OUTCOMES

Body image; self-esteem; psychosocial adjustment: life change

NIC INTERVENTIONS

Body image enhancement; grief work facilitation; self-esteem enhancement; role enhancement; counseling: emotional support; support system enhancement

NURSING ASSESSMENT

Assess for signs and symptoms of a disturbed self-concept:
- Verbalization of negative feelings about self
- Lack of participation in activities of daily living
- Refusal to look at mastectomy site
- Withdrawal from significant others

RATIONALE

Early recognition of signs and symptoms of disturbed self-concept allows for prompt intervention.

THERAPEUTIC INTERVENTIONS

RATIONALE

Independent Actions
Implement measures to facilitate the grieving process:
Assist the client to identify and use coping techniques that have been helpful in the past.
Implement measures to facilitate client's adjustment to the effects of the loss of a breast on her sexuality:
- Facilitate communication between client and partner; focus on feelings the couple share and assist them to identify factors that may affect their sexual relationship.
- Arrange for uninterrupted privacy during hospital stay if desired by the couple.
- Assist client with usual grooming and makeup habits.
- Demonstrate acceptance of client using techniques such as touch and frequent visits.
- Encourage significant others to do the same.
- Stay with client during first dressing change and encourage her to express feelings about appearance of incision and change in body. If the client is reluctant to look at the surgical site, provide support and encouragement to do so before discharge.
- Encourage client's participation in activities that can assist her to integrate the physical change that has occurred (e.g., exercise, grooming, bathing, wound care).
If breast reconstruction has not been performed:
- Encourage client to discuss possibilities for future reconstruction of breast with physician if desired.

A change in body appearance can initiate a grieving response. Resolution of grief assists the client to accept changes experienced and integrate the changes into self-concept.

Involving partner in care of the client can help facilitate partner's adjustment to the change in client's appearance and subsequently decrease the possibility of partner's rejection of client.

Allows client to visualize a more "normal" future.

Continued...

THERAPEUTIC INTERVENTIONS	RATIONALE
• Discuss the variety of prostheses available and ways to obtain one.	
• Assist client's and significant others' adjustment by listening, facilitating communication, and providing information.	
• Support behaviors suggesting positive adaptation to the loss of a breast (e.g., willingness to look at and care for wound, compliance with exercise program, maintenance of relationships with significant others).	
• Reinforce the temporary nature of operative side arm movement restrictions.	
• Encourage client contact with others so that she can test and establish a new self-image.	
• Encourage visits and support from significant others.	
• Encourage client to pursue usual roles and interests and to continue involvement in social activities.	
• Provide information about and encourage use of community agencies and support groups (e.g., Reach to Recovery; sexual, family, and individual counseling services).	*Provides client/family support following discharge from acute care facility.*
Dependent/Collaborative Actions	
Consult appropriate health care provider (e.g., psychiatric nurse clinician, physician) if client seems unwilling or unable to adapt to the loss of her breast.	*Notifying the appropriate health care provider allows for modification of the treatment plan.*

DISCHARGE TEACHING/CONTINUED CARE

Nursing Diagnosis **DEFICIENT KNOWLEDGE NDx, INEFFECTIVE FAMILY THERAPEUTIC REGIMEN NDx, OR INEFFECTIVE SELF-HEALTH MANAGEMENT NDx***

Definition: Absence or deficiency of cognitive information related to specific topic (lack of specific information) necessary for client/significant others to make informed choices regarding condition/treatment/lifestyle changes; Pattern of regulating and integrating into daily living and family processes a therapeutic regimen for treatment of illnesses and the sequelae of illness that is unsatisfactory for meeting specific health goals.

CLINICAL MANIFESTATIONS

Subjective	**Objective**
Verbalizes inability to manage illness and inability to follow prescribed regimen	Inaccurate follow-through with instructions; inappropriate behavior; refusal to participate in care

RISK FACTORS
• Cognitive deficit
• Failure to take action to reduce risk factors
• Inability to care for self

NOC OUTCOMES	**NIC INTERVENTIONS**
Knowledge: disease process; knowledge: treatment regimen; knowledge: treatment procedure(s); knowledge: health resources	Health system guidance; teaching: individual; teaching: disease process; teaching: prescribed activity/exercise; teaching: psychomotor skill

*The nurse should select the nursing diagnostic label that is most appropriate for the client's discharge teaching needs.

NURSING ASSESSMENT	RATIONALE
Assess client's readiness and ability to learn. Assess meaning of illness to client.	*Early recognition of readiness to learn and meaning of illness to client allows for implementation of the appropriate teaching interventions.*

THERAPEUTIC INTERVENTIONS	RATIONALE

Desired Outcomes: The client will identify ways to reduce the risk of trauma to and infection in the arm on the operative side.

Independent Actions
Provide the following instructions:
- Avoid cuts by pushing cuticles back instead of cutting them and trimming fingernails carefully.
- Wear heavy work gloves when gardening and rubber gloves when in contact with steel wool, harsh chemicals, abrasive compounds, or water for prolonged periods.
- Wear insulated gloves when reaching into a hot oven or handling hot items.
- Use a thimble when sewing to avoid pinpricks.
- Keep pressure off the affected arm (e.g., avoid wearing tight jewelry and clothes with constricting bands, carry heavy objects such as purse or packages with the unaffected arm).
- Offer only the unaffected arm for blood pressure readings, injections, blood drawing, and intravenous therapy.
- Wash any break in the skin on the affected arm with soap and water and cover the area with a protective dressing.
- Use an electric rather than a straight-edge razor when shaving underarm area.
- Apply a lanolin hand cream several times/day to prevent drying and cracking of the skin.
- Use insect repellant when in an area where stinging or biting insects may be located.
- Avoid prolonged exposure to the sun to prevent burns.

Actions help reduce the risk of trauma to and infection in the arm on operative side:

THERAPEUTIC INTERVENTIONS	RATIONALE

Desired Outcome: The client will identify ways to prevent and treat lymphedema of the arm on the operative side.

Independent Actions
Instruct client in ways to prevent lymphedema of the arm on operative side:
- Elevate the affected arm on pillows for 30 to 45 minutes at least 3 times a day for the prescribed length of time (usually 6-12 weeks).
- Sleep on unaffected side or back with affected arm elevated for the prescribed length of time (usually 6-12 weeks).
- Avoid placing the affected extremity in a dependent position for extended periods.

Reinforce physician's instructions regarding ways to treat lymphedema if present:
- Perform manual massage of the affected arm if prescribed.
- Wear an elastic pressure gradient sleeve as recommended.

These actions help facilitate lymph drainage by gravity.

These actions decrease lymphedema.

THERAPEUTIC INTERVENTIONS	RATIONALE

Desired Outcomes: The client will demonstrate the ability to care for wound drainage device if present.

NDx = NANDA-I Diagnosis   **D** = Delegatable Action   ● = UAP   ✦ = LVN/LPN   ⊖▶ = Go to ⊖volve for animation

Continued...

THERAPEUTIC INTERVENTIONS	RATIONALE
Independent Actions If the client is to be discharged with wound drain(s) and a suction device, demonstrate how to empty and establish negative pressure in the collection device and provide these additional instructions: • Keep the collection device positioned below the insertion site. • Keep the tubing pinned to the dressing and avoid kinks and strain on the tubing. • Empty the collection device at least twice daily or more often if needed. • Keep a record of the amount of drainage (drains will typically be removed once the drainage is <20-30 mL in 24 hours).	*Proper wound care is necessary to prevent infection and promote optimum wound healing. Allow time for return demonstration to assess client understanding of instructions and the need for further education.*

THERAPEUTIC INTERVENTIONS	RATIONALE
Desired Outcomes: The client will demonstrate the ability to perform the prescribed exercises and verbalize an understanding of additional exercises to be done once the incision has healed. **Independent Actions** Reinforce teaching about postmastectomy exercises: • Emphasize the need to perform hand and elbow exercises regularly and begin full range-of-motion exercises of the arm and shoulder once the incision has healed.	*Postoperative exercises are necessary to prevent contraction and promote return of optimum range of motion.*

THERAPEUTIC INTERVENTIONS	RATIONALE
Desired Outcomes: The client will verbalize the importance of and demonstrate the ability to perform a breast self-examination (BSE) on the remaining breast and operative site. **Independent Actions** Explain the reasons for monthly BSE of the remaining breast and operative site. • Explore with client ways to remember to carry out BSE. The examination should be done a week after conclusion of menses or on a specific date if postmenopausal. • Demonstrate, using a model, film, or chart, how to do a BSE.	*Performance of preventative screening measures at regular intervals can alert clients to findings that require further evaluation by a health care provider.*

THERAPEUTIC INTERVENTIONS	RATIONALE
Desired Outcomes: The client will state the factors to consider in selecting a breast prosthesis. **Independent Actions** If acceptable to client, invite a Reach to Recovery volunteer or prosthetist to share information about the various prostheses available. Suggest that client wear a soft, temporary prosthesis until complete healing of the incision has occurred. Encourage the client to take significant other or a close friend with her for the initial fitting of the prosthesis in order to provide emotional support. Emphasize that it is important to select or make a prosthesis that will balance the chest to avoid difficulties with posture and subsequent back, shoulder, and neck discomfort.	*Selection of a prosthetic will be a very personal choice by the client, and including members of a social support network may facilitate appropriate selection.*

THERAPEUTIC INTERVENTIONS	RATIONALE

Desired Outcomes: The client will state signs and symptoms to report to the health care provider.

Independent Actions

Instruct client to report these additional signs and symptoms:

- New or increased sensations of numbness, tingling, heaviness, or tightness in hand, arm, or shoulder on operative side
- Increasing weakness of the affected arm
- Decreased ability to move shoulder or arm on operative side (full range of motion should be regained within 3-6 months)
- Warmth or redness of the affected arm
- Increase in size of arm on affected side (client may be instructed to measure arm circumference weekly at points about 2-4 inches above and below elbow and compare with unaffected arm); inform client that transient edema may occur as she increases use of the affected arm and that this should subside as collateral lymphatic circulation develops
- Increased swelling around incision(s)
- Purulent, foul-smelling drainage from incision site(s) or wound drain insertion site
- Dressings that become saturated with drainage more than once a day
- Unexpected increase in or absence of drainage in collection device

Educating the client regarding signs and symptoms requiring evaluation by a health care provider can help to reduce the occurrence of complications and improve health outcomes.

THERAPEUTIC INTERVENTIONS	RATIONALE

Desired Outcomes: The client will identify community resources that can assist with adjustment to the diagnosis of cancer and the loss of a breast.

Independent Actions

Provide information about community resources that can assist the client and significant others with adjustment to the diagnosis of cancer and the mastectomy (e.g., American Cancer Society, Reach to Recovery, National Lymphedema Network, National Breast Cancer Coalition, home health agencies, individual and family counselors).

- Initiate a referral if appropriate.

Identification of a social support network can assist the client in selection of the appropriate type of support system to meet the adjustment needs of the individual.

THERAPEUTIC INTERVENTIONS	RATIONALE

Desired Outcomes: The client will verbalize an understanding of and a plan for adhering to recommended follow-up care including future appointments with health care provider, medications prescribed, activity limitations, exercises, wound care, and plans for subsequent treatment.

Independent Actions

Reinforce physician's explanations and instructions regarding future treatment (e.g., chemotherapy, radiation therapy, hormone therapy such as tamoxifen, breast reconstruction) if planned.

- Explain the importance of having follow-up breast exams and mammography as prescribed.

Ensuring the client understands the importance of adhering to a treatment plan may reduce the occurrence of adverse outcomes. The client should be given time to clarify and answer questions as appropriate.

Continued...

THERAPEUTIC INTERVENTIONS	RATIONALE
Reinforce the physician's instructions regarding activity limitations. Instruct client to:	

- Avoid lifting heavy objects (over 5-10 pounds) until wound has healed (usually about 4-6 weeks).
- Avoid driving until approved by physician (usually about 2 weeks).

Review physician's instructions regarding exercises (e.g., squeezing a ball, bending and flexing wrist and elbow, hand wall climbing, pulley exercises, rope turning, arm swings, elbow pull-in, scissors). Instructions should include when to start exercises, frequency, and a written description and/or pictures of how to perform them.

ADDITIONAL CARE PLANS

GRIEVING NDx
Related to:

- Loss of a breast and subsequent change in body image
- Potential for premature death associated with the diagnosis of cancer

SELF-CARE DEFICIT NDx
Related to:

- Impaired physical mobility associated with pain, the depressant effect of anesthesia and some medications (e.g., narcotic [opioid] analgesics, some antiemetics), fear of dislodging tubes and compromising surgical wound, and prescribed arm movement restrictions on the operative side

INEFFECTIVE COPING NDx
Related to:

- Perceived loss of femininity and embarrassment associated with loss of a breast
- Fear of rejection by significant others
- Fear, anxiety, and feelings of loss of control associated with the diagnosis of cancer, subsequent treatment (e.g., external radiation therapy, chemotherapy, hormone therapy) if planned, and possibility of disease recurrence

⊖▶ RADICAL PROSTATECTOMY

A radical prostatectomy is performed to treat cancer of the prostate. The surgery includes removal of the prostate gland, prostatic capsule, seminal vesicles, and part of the vas deferens. In addition, a portion of the bladder neck is sometimes removed before the anastomosis of the remaining urethra to the bladder neck. A pelvic lymphadenectomy is usually performed concurrently if the cancer has spread into the pelvic lymph nodes. A radical prostatectomy is accomplished via a retropubic or perineal approach depending on the size and position of the prostate, the anticipated extensiveness of surgery, and physician preference. Occasionally, the client will receive external radiation therapy before surgery to reduce the tumor size. If there is evidence of lymph node involvement, a course of external radiation therapy may be done after the client recovers from the surgery.

This care plan focuses on the adult client with cancer of the prostate who is admitted for a radical prostatectomy. Much of the postoperative information is applicable to clients receiving follow-up care in an extended care facility or home setting.

OUTCOME/DISCHARGE CRITERIA

The client will:
1. Have adequate urine output
2. Have normal healing of the surgical wound
3. Have surgical pain controlled
4. Have no signs and symptoms of infection or postoperative complications
5. Demonstrate the ability to perform care related to the urinary catheter and drainage system
6. Identify ways to manage urinary incontinence if it occurs after catheter removal
7. Identify ways to manage bowel incontinence if present
8. Share feelings and concerns about the diagnosis of cancer, the prognosis, and changes in body functioning that may occur as a result of a radical prostatectomy
9. State signs and symptoms to report to the health care provider
10. Verbalize an understanding of and a plan for adhering to recommended follow-up care including future appointments with health care provider, medications prescribed, activity level, wound care, and plans for subsequent treatment.

PREOPERATIVE: USE IN CONJUNCTION WITH THE STANDARDIZED PREOPERATIVE CARE PLAN

RELATED PREOPERATIVE NURSING DIAGNOSIS

FEAR/ANXIETY NDx

Related to:

- Diagnosis of cancer, treatment plan, and prognosis
- Potential embarrassment or loss of dignity associated with body exposure during preoperative care, surgery, and postoperative assessments and treatments
- Anticipated loss of control associated with effects of anesthesia

- Lack of understanding of the surgical procedure and postoperative expectations and care
- Anticipated surgical findings, postoperative pain, and changes in body functioning
- Unfamiliar environment and separation from significant others
- Financial concerns associated with hospitalization

POSTOPERATIVE: USE IN CONJUNCTION WITH THE STANDARDIZED POSTOPERATIVE CARE PLAN

For a full, detailed care plan on this topic, go to http://evolve.elsevier.com/Haugen/careplanning/.

TRANSURETHRAL RESECTION OF THE PROSTATE

Transurethral resection of the prostate (TURP) is the surgical removal of a prostatic adenoma through the urethra, while leaving the true prostate and its fibrous capsule intact. It may be performed to remove a small cancerous prostatic tumor but most frequently is done to remove a benign prostatic neoplasm that has enlarged enough to block the bladder neck or urethra. The most common cause of a benign neoplasm is benign prostatic hyperplasia (BPH).

BPH is common in men over 50 years of age and results from age-associated changes in androgen levels. Hyperplasia usually occurs gradually and involves the medial portion of the prostate gland, which surrounds the urethra. Treatment is indicated when signs and symptoms of prostatism (e.g., urgency, frequency, hesitancy, decreased force of urinary stream, nocturia, post-void dribbling) become problematic or when complications such as recurrent urinary tract infection, urinary retention, hematuria, renal calculi, or hydronephrosis occur.

TURP is the most common surgical method for treating BPH. If the prostate gland is quite large, an open prostatectomy using a suprapubic or retropubic approach may be necessary. Methods such as medication therapy (e.g., doxazosin, tamsulosin, terazosin, finasteride), balloon urethroplasty, laser incision or removal of prostatic tissue, placement of a stent or coil in the prostatic urethra, and thermal therapy also may be used to treat symptomatic BPH. Factors influencing

the treatment method selected include the client's age and health status, size of the enlarged prostate, presence of complications, and physician preference and expertise.

This care plan focuses on the adult client with BPH who is undergoing a transurethral resection of the prostate. The information is applicable to client's having surgery in a hospital or outpatient (e.g., surgical care center) setting.

OUTCOME/DISCHARGE CRITERIA

The client will:

1. Have adequate urine output
2. Have bladder spasms controlled
3. Have no signs and symptoms of infection or postoperative complications
4. Identify ways to prevent bleeding in the surgical area
5. Identify ways to regain or maintain control of bladder emptying
6. State signs and symptoms to report to the health care provider
7. Verbalize an understanding of and a plan for adhering to recommended follow-up care including future appointments with health care provider, medications prescribed, and activity level

PREOPERATIVE: USE IN CONJUNCTION WITH THE STANDARDIZED PREOPERATIVE CARE PLAN

Nursing Diagnosis **URINARY RETENTION**

Definition: Incomplete emptying of the bladder

Related to: Obstruction of the urethra and/or bladder neck by the enlarged prostate; loss of bladder muscle tone associated with hypertrophy of the bladder wall (as BPH develops, the detrusor muscle hypertrophies in an attempt to increase its ability to push urine past the bladder neck or urethral obstruction; this hypertrophied muscle has poor contractility)

NDx = NANDA-I Diagnosis   **D** = Delegatable Action   ● = UAP   ✦ = LVN/LPN   ⊖▶ = Go to ⊖volve for animation

Continued...

CLINICAL MANIFESTATIONS

Subjective	Objective
Reports of bladder fullness or suprapubic discomfort	Bladder distention, output less than intake

RISK FACTOR

- Decreased function of the genitourinary system

DESIRED OUTCOMES

The client will experience resolution of urinary retention if it occurs as evidenced by:
   a. No reports of bladder fullness and suprapubic discomfort
   b. Absence of bladder distention
   c. Balanced intake and output

NOC OUTCOMES	NIC INTERVENTIONS
Urinary elimination	Urinary catheterization; tube care: urinary

NURSING ASSESSMENT	RATIONALE
Assess for and report signs and symptoms of urinary retention: • Reports of bladder fullness or suprapubic discomfort • Bladder distention, output less than intake	*Early recognition of signs and symptoms of urinary retention allow for prompt intervention.*

THERAPEUTIC INTERVENTIONS	RATIONALE
Independent Actions If urinary catheter is present: • Keep drainage tubing free of kinks. **D** ● ✦ • Keep collection container below level of bladder. **D** ● ✦ • Tape catheter securely to abdomen or thigh.	*Maintaining patency of indwelling urinary catheter prevents urinary retention.* *Prevents inadvertent removal*
Dependent/Collaborative Actions Insert or assist with insertion of a urethral catheter as ordered (if insertion is difficult because of obstruction of the prostatic urethra or bladder neck, it may be necessary to use a stylet or a firm, specially angled catheter). Assist with insertion of a suprapubic catheter if unable to insert a urethral catheter because of obstruction. Consult physician if signs and symptoms of urinary retention persist despite implementation of above actions.	*Actions help treat urinary retention if present.* *Notifying the appropriate health care provider allows for modification of the treatment plan.*

Nursing Diagnosis DEFICIENT KNOWLEDGE NDx

Definition: Absence or deficiency of cognitive information related to specific topic (lack of specific information) necessary for client/significant others to make informed choices regarding condition/treatment/lifestyle changes

CLINICAL MANIFESTATIONS

Subjective	Objective
Verbalizes inability to manage illness	Inaccurate follow through with instructions; inappropriate behavior; refusal to participate in care

RISK FACTOR

- Unknown environment, routines associated with surgery

NOC OUTCOMES

Knowledge: treatment regimen; knowledge: treatment procedure(s)

NIC INTERVENTIONS

Health system guidance; teaching: preoperative; teaching: individual; teaching: procedure/treatment

NURSING ASSESSMENT

Assess client's readiness and ability to learn
Assess meaning of illness to client

RATIONALE

Early recognition of readiness to learn and meaning of illness to client allows for implementation of the appropriate teaching interventions

THERAPEUTIC INTERVENTIONS

RATIONALE

Desired Outcomes: The client will:

a. Verbalize an understanding of the surgical procedure, preoperative care, and postoperative sensations and care
b. Demonstrate the ability to perform activities designed to prevent postoperative complications

Independent Actions

Provide information about usual preoperative routines for surgery to be performed.

Provide additional information regarding care after a TURP:

- Explain that bed rest is usually ordered for 6 to 18 hours after surgery; activity is then increased gradually (the level of activity allowed depends on physician preference, extensiveness of the resection, and the amount of postoperative bleeding client experiences).
- Explain that a urinary catheter will be in place for 24 to 48 hours after surgery.
- Describe the procedure and rationale for intermittent and continuous bladder irrigations.
- Explain that traction may be applied to the catheter for 4 to 5 hours postoperatively and again as needed (traction is accomplished by pulling down on the urethral catheter and anchoring it securely to the client's leg so that tension is maintained).

Explain that the following can be expected:

- Red urine that gradually lightens in color (urine color usually goes from bright red to pink within 24-36 hours and to light pink or dark amber within 72 hours) but often temporarily becomes more red when activity increases
- Some blood clots in urine
- Some bloody drainage from urethra Describe signs and symptoms that can be indicative of bladder spasms (e.g., leakage of urine around catheter, feeling of an urgent need to urinate or defecate, pressure in bladder); stress that these signs and symptoms should be reported to the nurse so that catheter patency can be checked and medication can be given as needed to reduce discomfort.

Explain that after the catheter is removed:

- A mild to moderate burning sensation may be experienced when urinating and that this is expected to decrease with each voiding and resolve within 1 to 2 days.
- Urinary symptoms experienced preoperatively (e.g., urgency, frequency, hesitancy, postvoid dribbling) may still be present or may even increase temporarily postoperatively due to poor bladder muscle tone and/or tissue trauma from the surgery and catheter (these symptoms usually resolve within 2-3 weeks).

Clients vary in physical and cognitive ability to learn. When educating clients, nurses need to determine a client's ability to read and understand written materials. If literacy barriers are present, alternative educational materials should be provided. Allow time for questions, clarification, and return demonstration of any learned actions.

A urethral catheter with three lumens is usually inserted to allow drainage of bladder and simultaneous infusion of irrigation solution if needed.

The catheter balloon puts pressure on the surgical site to control bleeding.

Helps client to understand what to expect postoperatively.

Continued...

THERAPEUTIC INTERVENTIONS	RATIONALE
Reinforce physician's explanation regarding effects of TURP on sexual functioning (after surgery, the client usually experiences retrograde ejaculation as a result of direct trauma to the internal urinary sphincter and/or widening of the bladder neck; normal ejaculatory function usually returns within weeks or months).	

POSTOPERATIVE: USE IN CONJUNCTION WITH THE STANDARDIZED POSTOPERATIVE CARE PLAN

Nursing Diagnosis RISK FOR EXCESS FLUID VOLUME NDx OR WATER INTOXICATION ("TUR Syndrome")

Definition: "TUR syndrome" results from the absorption of large volumes of bladder irrigation fluid during the procedure

Related to: Vigorous fluid therapy during and immediately after surgery; increased secretion of antidiuretic hormone (output of antidiuretic hormone [ADH] is stimulated by trauma, pain, and anesthetic agents); excessive absorption of irrigation solution via the prostatic veins during and after surgery

CLINICAL MANIFESTATIONS

Subjective	Objective
Reports of dyspnea; orthopnea	Elevated BP; presence of S_3 heart sound; bounding pulse, change in mental status; intake greater than output; low serum sodium and osmolality; decreased BUN, Hct, serum sodium and osmolality; chest radiograph results demonstrating pulmonary congestion

RISK FACTORS

- Surgery
- Excessive bladder irrigation
- Endocrine response to trauma

DESIRED OUTCOMES

The client will not experience excess fluid volume or water intoxication as evidenced by:
  a. Stable weight
  b. Stable BP
  c. Absence of S_3 heart sound
  d. Normal pulse volume
  e. Balanced intake and output within 48 hours after surgery
  f. Usual mental status
  g. BUN, Hct, serum sodium and osmolality within normal range
  h. Absence of dyspnea, orthopnea, edema, and distended neck veins

NOC OUTCOMES

Fluid overload severity; fluid balance

NIC INTERVENTIONS

Fluid monitoring; fluid management

NURSING ASSESSMENT	RATIONALE
Assess for and report signs and symptoms of fluid volume excess: • Dyspnea, Orthopnea • Increased blood pressure	*Early recognition of signs and symptoms of fluid volume excess allow for prompt intervention.*

NURSING ASSESSMENT	RATIONALE

- S_1 heart sound: bounding pulse, change in mental status
- Intake greater than output

Assess serum electrolytes, BUN, Hct, serum sodium and osmolality, reporting any abnormal values.

Assess chest radiograph results, reporting any abnormalities.

THERAPEUTIC INTERVENTIONS	RATIONALE

Dependent/Collaborative Actions

Use normal saline rather than hypotonic solutions for bladder irrigations.

Do not increase frequency of bladder irrigations or speed up continuous irrigation unless indicated.

Actions help reduce absorption of fluid via the prostatic veins to further reduce the risk for excess fluid volume and/or water intoxication.

Notify physician if signs and symptoms of fluid overload develop.

Notifying the appropriate health care provider allows for modification of the treatment plan.

Nursing Diagnosis IMPAIRED COMFORT NDx (BLADDER SPASMS)

Definition: Perceived lack of ease, relief, and transcendence in physical, psychospiritual environmental, and social dimensions

Related to: Irritation of the bladder wall associated with tissue trauma during surgery, presence of urinary catheter, rapid infusion of irrigation solution, and distention of the bladder (can occur if urine flow becomes obstructed); increased pressure on the bladder neck and prostatic fossa if traction is applied to the urethral catheter (traction may be applied to pull the catheter balloon into the prostatic fossa to put pressure on bleeding vessels)

CLINICAL MANIFESTATIONS

Subjective	Objective
Reports of suprapubic discomfort; urgent need to urinate or defecate	Leakage of urine around the urinary catheter; intermittent periods of increase in bloody urine/bladder irrigation

RISK FACTORS

- Surgery
- 3-way urinary catheterization
- Bladder irrigation

DESIRED OUTCOMES

The client will experience relief of bladder spasms as evidenced by:
  a. Verbalization of relief of suprapubic discomfort
  b. No reports of an urgent need to urinate or defecate
  c. No leakage of urine around the urinary catheter

NOC OUTCOMES

Comfort level; symptom control

NIC INTERVENTIONS

Medication administration; tube care: urinary

NURSING ASSESSMENT	RATIONALE

Assess for and report signs and symptoms of altered comfort: bladder spasms:
- Suprapubic discomfort
- Urgent need to urinate or defecate
- Leakage of urine around the urinary catheter
- Intermittent periods of increase in bloody urine/bladder irrigation

Early recognition of signs and symptoms of altered comfort: bladder spasms allow for prompt intervention.

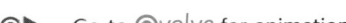

Continued...

THERAPEUTIC INTERVENTIONS	RATIONALE

Independent Actions

Maintain patency of the urinary catheter (e.g., irrigate as needed, keep tubing free of kinks).

Perform actions to reduce movement of the catheter:
* Anchor catheter securely to client's abdomen or thigh.
* Instruct client to avoid pulling on and twisting the catheter.

Release traction on the catheter as soon as ordered. **D** ✦

Do not increase frequency of bladder irrigations or speed up continuous irrigation unless bleeding is noted or blood clots or tissue debris are present. **D** ✦

Instruct client to avoid attempting to urinate around the catheter and straining to urinate after catheter is removed.

Perform actions to prevent urinary retention.

If bladder spasms occur:
* Encourage client to take short, frequent walks unless contraindicated. **D** ✦
* Decrease the rate of continuous bladder irrigation if urine is not red and blood clots and tissue debris are not present.

Actions help decrease the risk of bladder spasms and prevent bladder distention.

Reduces pressure on the bladder neck and fossa.

Excessive or rapid bladder irrigation can irritate the bladder mucosa.

Attempts to forcefully contract bladder can stimulate bladder spasms.

Walking seems to reduce spasms.

Dependent/Collaborative Actions

If bladder spasms occur:
* Administer belladonna and opium (B&O) rectal suppositories if ordered (this is combination of an antimuscarinic and narcotic analgesic).

Consult physician if above measures fail to control bladder spasms.

Reduces spasm of the bladder muscle and the client's perception of discomfort; it is only prescribed when the urinary catheter is present because it can cause urinary retention.

Notifying the appropriate health care provider allows for modification of the treatment plan.

Nursing Diagnosis   # IMPAIRED URINARY ELIMINATION NDx

Definition: Disturbance in urine elimination

Related to:

Retention related to:
a. Obstruction of the urinary catheter
b. Difficulty urinating after removal of the catheter associated with:
  * Loss of bladder muscle tone resulting from hypertrophy of the detrusor muscle as BPH developed, overdistention of the bladder preoperatively, and/or decompression of the bladder when the catheter was present
  * Relaxation of the bladder muscle resulting from stimulation of the sympathetic nervous system (can result from surgical site discomfort, fear, and anxiety) and the depressant effect of some medications (e.g., narcotic [opioid] analgesics)
  * Decreased perception of bladder fullness resulting from the depressant effect of some medications (e.g., narcotic [opioid] analgesics)
  * Obstruction of the urethra and bladder neck by blood clots, tissue debris, and/or edema (can occur as a result of surgical instrumentation, irritation from the urethral catheter, and/or pressure from the catheter balloon if traction was applied postoperatively)

Incontinence after catheter removal related to: Trauma to the urinary sphincter(s) associated with surgical instrumentation, irritation from the urethral catheter, and/or pressure from the catheter balloon if traction was applied postoperatively

CLINICAL MANIFESTATIONS

Subjective	Objective
Reports of bladder fullness; increasing need to strain to empty bladder; increasing urgency	Bladder distention; absence of urine in urinary drainage bag; output that continues to be less than intake 48 hours after surgery; voiding frequent small amounts of urine (after removal of catheter).

RISK FACTORS
- Surgical procedure
- Preoperative urinary retention
- Medication regimen

DESIRED OUTCOMES

The client will:
a. Not experience urinary retention as evidenced by:
   - No reports of bladder fullness and suprapubic discomfort
   - Absence of bladder distention
   - Balanced intake and output within 48 hours after surgery
   - Voiding adequate amounts at expected intervals after removal of catheter
b. Experience urinary continence

NOC OUTCOMES

Urinary continence; urinary elimination

NIC INTERVENTIONS

Urinary incontinence care; urinary retention care; bladder irrigation; tube care: urinary; pelvic muscle exercise

---

NURSING ASSESSMENT	RATIONALE
Assess for and report signs of impaired urinary elimination: • Reports of bladder fullness • Increasing need to strain to empty bladder • Increasing urgency • Bladder distention • Absence of urine in urinary drainage bag • Output that continues to be less than intake 48 hours after surgery • Voiding frequent small amounts of urine (after removal of catheter)	*Early recognition of signs and symptoms of impaired urinary elimination allow for prompt intervention.*

THERAPEUTIC INTERVENTIONS	RATIONALE

Independent Actions

Implement measures to maintain patency of the urinary catheter:
- Keep drainage tubing free of kinks. **D** ● ✦
- Keep collection container below level of bladder.
- Tape catheter securely to abdomen or thigh. **D** ● ✦
- Perform bladder irrigations as ordered to flush out blood clots and tissue debris if present.

After removal of the catheter, implement measures to prevent urinary retention:
- Offer urinal or assist client to bathroom every 2 to 4 hours if indicated. **D** ● ✦
- Instruct client to urinate when the urge is first felt.
- Perform actions to promote relaxation during voiding attempts (e.g., provide privacy, have client sit to void, hold a warm blanket against abdomen).
- Perform actions that may help trigger the micturition reflex and promote a sense of relaxation during voiding attempts (e.g., run water, place client's hands in warm water, encourage client to urinate when in shower). **D** ● ✦
- Allow client to assume a normal position for voiding unless contraindicated. **D** ● ✦

Implement measures to prevent trauma to the urinary sphincter(s) while the catheter is in place to reduce the risk of urinary incontinence after removal of the catheter:
- Anchor catheter securely to client's abdomen or thigh. **D** ✦

Maintaining patency of urinary catheter helps prevent urinary retention.

Prevents inadvertent removal of the catheter

A hypotonic bladder can be easily distended.

Improves ability to urinate.

Prevents excessive movement of the catheter.

NDx = NANDA-I Diagnosis   **D** = Delegatable Action   ● = UAP   ✦ = LVN/LPN   ⊜▶ = Go to ⊜volve for animation

Continued...

THERAPEUTIC INTERVENTIONS	RATIONALE
After removal of the catheter, implement measures to reduce the risk of urinary incontinence:	
• Keep urinal within client's reach and provide easy access to bathroom. **D ● ✦**	*Reduces delay in toileting.*
• Allow client to assume a normal position for voiding unless contraindicated to promote complete bladder emptying. **D ✦**	
• Instruct client to perform perineal exercises (e.g., stopping and starting stream during voiding; squeezing buttocks together, then relaxing the muscles) regularly.	*Actions help strengthen pelvic floor muscles and improve tone of the external urinary sphincter.*
• Limit oral fluid intake in the evening. **D ✦**	*Actions help decrease the possibility of nighttime incontinence.*
• Instruct client to limit intake of alcohol and beverages containing caffeine.	*Alcohol and caffeine have a mild diuretic effect and act as irritants to the bladder; these factors may make urinary control more difficult.*
• Instruct client to space fluids evenly throughout the day rather than drinking a large quantity at one time.	*Rapid filling of bladder can result in increased incontinence.*
Dependent/Collaborative Actions	
Implement measures to prevent trauma to the urinary sphincter(s) while the catheter is in place to reduce the risk of urinary incontinence after removal of the catheter:	*Reduces pressure on and possible damage to the internal urinary sphincter.*
• If urethral catheter traction is ordered to control bleeding, release it as soon as allowed (traction should not be maintained for longer than 4 to 5 hours without being released).	
If signs and symptoms of urinary retention occur after removal of the catheter, consult physician about intermittent catheterization or reinsertion of an indwelling catheter.	*Notifying the appropriate health care provider allows for modification of the treatment plan.*
If urinary incontinence persists, consult physician regarding intermittent catheterization, reinsertion of an indwelling catheter, or use of external collection device (e.g., condom catheter).	

Collaborative Diagnosis   **RISK FOR HYPOVOLEMIC SHOCK**

Definition: A type of low blood flow shock that occurs when there is a loss of intravascular fluid volume; loss of fluid volume may be absolute resulting from fluid lost from hemorrhage, dieresis, or gastrointestinal losses

Related to: Hemorrhage (the prostate gland is very vascular)

CLINICAL MANIFESTATIONS

Subjective	Objective
N/A	Bright red drainage (could indicate arterial bleeding) or persistent darker drainage (venous bleeding) and blood clots in urinary catheter; persistent redness of and blood clots in urine after removal of the catheter; significant decrease in RBC, Hct, and Hgb levels; tachypnea; hypotension; decreased urine output; pallor; cool, clammy skin; anxiety; confusion; agitation

RISK FACTOR
• Inadequate fluid volume replacement

DESIRED OUTCOMES

The client will not develop hypovolemic shock as evidenced by:
  a. Usual mental status
  b. Stable vital signs
  c. Skin warm and usual color
  d. Palpable peripheral pulses
  e. Urine output at least 30 mL/hr

NURSING ASSESSMENT	RATIONALE
Assess for and report signs and symptoms of hypovolemic shock: • Bright red drainage (could indicate arterial bleeding) or persistent darker drainage (venous bleeding) and blood clots in urine • After removal of the catheter; significant decrease in RBC, Hct, and Hgb levels • Tachypnea; hypotension; decreased urine output; pallor; cool, clammy skin; anxiety; confusion and agitation Assess serum Hgb/Hct and report any abnormalities.	*Early recognition of signs and symptoms of hypovolemic shock allow for prompt intervention.*

THERAPEUTIC INTERVENTIONS	RATIONALE
Independent Actions Maintain traction on the urethral catheter as ordered (provides direct pressure on the bleeding vessels). • Anchor catheter tubing securely to client's abdomen or thigh to minimize movement of catheter. • Caution client to avoid pulling on the catheter. • Instruct client to take short rather than long walks and to avoid sitting for long periods. • Instruct client to avoid straining to have a bowel movement; consult physician regarding an order for a laxative if indicated. Implement measures to prevent urinary retention. • Instruct client to return to bed and limit activity for a few hours if urine becomes more red when ambulating or sitting in chair.	*Measures help to prevent or control hemorrhage to prevent hypovolemic shock.* *Actions help to prevent trauma to and/or unnecessary pressure on the prostatic area thereby reducing the risk of hemorrhage.* *Actions help prevent distention of the bladder and subsequent pressure on the newly coagulated blood vessels in the operative area.*

Collaborative Diagnosis RISK FOR THROMBOEMBOLISM

Definition: A clot attached to a vessel wall that detaches and circulates within the blood

Related to: Venous stasis associated with pressure on the pelvic and calf vessels during surgery (the client is usually in lithotomy position) and decreased activity

CLINICAL MANIFESTATIONS

Subjective	Objective
Deep vein thrombus: report of pain, tenderness	**Deep vein thrombus:** swelling, unusual warmth, and/or positive Homans' sign in extremity
Arterial thrombus: report of numbness, and/or pain in extremity	**Arterial thrombus:** diminished or absent peripheral pulses; pallor, coolness
Cerebral ischemia: N/A	**Cerebral ischemia:** decreased level of consciousness, alteration in usual sensory and motor function
Pulmonary embolism: report of sudden onset of chest pain, increased dyspnea	**Pulmonary embolism:** increased restlessness and apprehension, significant decrease in SaO_2

RISK FACTORS
• Immobility
• Inadequate fluid replacement

DESIRED OUTCOMES

The client will not develop a thromboembolism as evidenced by:
a. Absence of pain, tenderness, swelling, and numbness in extremities
b. Usual temperature and color of extremities
c. Palpable and equal peripheral pulses
d. Usual mental status
e. Usual sensory and motor function
f. Absence of sudden chest pain and dyspnea

Continued...

NURSING ASSESSMENT	RATIONALE
Assess for and report signs and symptoms of deep vein thrombus; arterial embolus in an extremity; cerebral ischemia; or pulmonary embolism.	*Early recognition of signs and symptoms of thromboembolism allow prompt intervention.*

- Deep vein thrombosis: pain, tenderness, swelling, unusual warmth, and/or positive Homans' sign in extremity
- Arterial thrombus: numbness and/or pain in exteremity; diminished or absent peripheral pulses; pallor, coolness
- Cerebral ischemia: decreased level of consciousness; alteration in usual sensory and motor function
- Pulmonary embolism: sudden onset of chest pain; increased dyspnea; increased restlessness and apprehension; significant decrease in saO_2

THERAPEUTIC INTERVENTIONS	RATIONALE

Independent Actions

Implement measures to prevent thrombus formation: *These actions improve circulation to the lower extremities*
- Perform actions to prevent pooling of blood in extremities.
- Promote active foot and leg exercises. **D** ✦
- Encourage and assist with ambulation. **D** ✦
- Discourage positions that compromise blood flow in lower extremities (e.g., don't use knee gatch on the bed, don't put pillows beneath the knees, remind patient not to cross legs while seated). **D** ✦
- Be aware that prophylactic anticoagulant and antiplatelet medications may be contraindicated because of the high risk of hemorrhage during and after surgery on the prostate gland.

DISCHARGE TEACHING/CONTINUED CARE

Nursing Diagnosis   **DEFICIENT KNOWLEDGE NDx, INEFFECTIVE FAMILY THERAPEUTIC REGIMEN NDx, OR INEFFECTIVE HEALTH MAINTENANCE* NDx**

Definition: Absence or deficiency of cognitive information related to specific topic (lack of specific information) necessary for client/significant others to make informed choices regarding condition/treatment/lifestyle changes; pattern of regulating and integrating into daily living and family processes a therapeutic regimen for treatment of illnesses and the sequelae of illness that is unsatisfactory for meeting specific health goals. Inability to identify, manage, or seek out help to maintain health

CLINICAL MANIFESTATIONS

Subjective	Objective
Verbalizes inability to manage illness and inability to follow prescribed regimen	Inaccurate follow-through with instructions; inappropriate behavior; refusal to participate in care

RISK FACTORS
- Cognitive Deficit
- Failure to take action to reduce risk factors
- Inability to care for oneself
- Difficulty in modifying personal habits and integrating treatments into lifestyle

NOC OUTCOMES	NIC INTERVENTIONS
Knowledge: disease process; knowledge: treatment regimen	Health system guidance; teaching: individual; teaching: disease process; teaching: prescribed activity/exercise; pelvic muscle exercise

*The nurse should select the nursing diagnostic label that is most appropriate for the client's discharge teaching needs.

NURSING ASSESSMENT	RATIONALE
Assess client's ability to learn and readiness to learn Assess understanding of patient teaching	*Learning is more effective when the client is motivated and understands the importance of what is to be learned. Readiness to learn is based on situations, physical, and emotional challenges.*

THERAPEUTIC INTERVENTIONS	RATIONALE

Desired Outcomes: The client will identify ways to prevent bleeding in the surgical area.

Independent Actions

Instruct client in ways to prevent bleeding in the surgical area: • Avoid straining during defecation (provide instructions about increasing fluid intake and intake of foods high in fiber if client tends to be constipated). • Avoid long walks, prolonged sitting, long car rides, running, climbing stairs quickly, strenuous exercise, sexual intercourse, and lifting objects over 10 pounds for as long as recommended by physician (usually for 2-6 weeks after discharge). • Consult physician before resuming preoperative medications such as aspirin and other NSAIDs, warfarin, and clopidogrel (physicians often recommend waiting 1-2 weeks after surgery if possible before resuming these medications).	*Decreased bleeding promotes improvement in healing.*

THERAPEUTIC INTERVENTIONS	RATIONALE

Desired Outcomes: The client will identify ways to regain or maintain control of bladder emptying.

Independent Actions

Instruct client in ways to regain or maintain control of bladder emptying: • Try to urinate every 2 to 3 hours and whenever the urge is felt. • Urinate in a standing or sitting position to facilitate bladder emptying. • Avoid drinking large quantities of liquids over a short period. • Limit intake of alcohol and caffeine-containing beverages. • Avoid activities that make it difficult to empty bladder as soon as the urge is felt (e.g., long car rides, lengthy meetings) to prevent retention and the subsequent risk for incontinence. • Perform perineal exercises (e.g., stopping and starting stream during voiding; squeezing buttocks together, then relaxing the muscles) 10 to 20 times/hour while awake until urinary control is regained. If client is experiencing urinary incontinence, instruct to: • Wear disposable underwear liners or absorbent undergarments such as Attends if necessary.	*Alcohol and caffeine have a mild diuretic effect and act as irritants to the bladder; these factors may make urinary control more difficult.* *Stop drinking liquids a few hours before bedtime (reduces risk of urine retention and nighttime incontinence).* *Improves bladder control*

THERAPEUTIC INTERVENTIONS	RATIONALE

Desired Outcomes: The client will state signs and symptoms to report to the health care provider.

Continued...

THERAPEUTIC INTERVENTIONS	RATIONALE

Independent Actions

Instruct client to report these additional signs and symptoms:

- Persistent burgundy colored or bright red urine (inform client that some blood is expected intermittently for 2-3 weeks after surgery but that urine should become pink to amber after he rests and increases fluid intake for a couple of hours)
- Presence of large blood clots or continued passage of smaller clots
- Development of or increase in frequency, burning, or pain when urinating
- Decrease in urine output or force and caliber of urinary stream
- Bladder distention
- Unexpected loss of bladder control
- Cloudy urine unrelated to orgasm
- Persistent or increased bladder spasms

Consult physician if urinary incontinence persists, worsens, or interferes with daily life so that various options (e.g., biofeedback, insertion of artificial urinary sphincter) can be discussed.

Educating the client regarding signs and symptoms requiring evaluation by a health care provider can help reduce the occurrence of complications and improve health outcomes.

It is expected that urine will be cloudy after orgasm if client is experiencing retrograde ejaculation.

THERAPEUTIC INTERVENTIONS	RATIONALE

Desired Outcomes: The client will verbalize an understanding of and a plan for adhering to recommended follow-up care including future appointments with health care provider, medications prescribed, and activity level.

Independent Actions

Reinforce the physician's instructions regarding the importance of lying down and increasing fluid intake for a few hours if amount of blood or number of blood clots in the urine increases.

Explain the importance of having a digital rectal examination and a blood test for prostate-specific antigen (PSA) done each year (cancer of the prostate and recurrent BPH can develop because the entire prostate gland is not removed during a TURP).

Ensuring the client understands the importance of adhering to a treatment plan may reduce the occurrence of adverse outcomes. The client should be given time to clarify and answer questions as appropriate.

ADDITIONAL NURSING DIAGNOSES

RISK FOR INFECTION: URINARY TRACT
Related to:

- Introduction of pathogens associated with instrumentation of urinary tract during surgery, presence of indwelling catheter, and frequent bladder irrigations

- Increased growth and colonization of microorganisms associated with urinary stasis resulting from decreased activity and urinary retention if it occurs

14

The Client Receiving Treatment for Neoplastic Disorders

CHEMOTHERAPY

This care plan focuses on the use of cytotoxic drugs (chemotherapeutic agents) in the treatment of cancer. Chemotherapy is used alone or in combination with radiation therapy, surgery, and/or biotherapy to achieve a cure, control tumor growth, or provide relief of symptoms associated with advanced disease (palliation). Success of the therapy depends on the size, type, and location of the tumor in addition to the client's physiological and psychological condition.

Cytotoxic drugs are classified according to chemical structure (e.g., antimetabolites, mitotic inhibitors [vinca alkaloids, plant alkaloids], alkylating agents), primary mode of action (e.g., interfere with folic acid synthesis, produce cross-links of DNA strands), or effect on the cell life cycle. Some drugs are more effective during a specific phase of the cell cycle and are referred to as cell cycle phase-specific or cell cycle-specific (e.g., mitotic inhibitors, antimetabolites). The cytotoxic agents that interrupt the cell replication process without regard to the phase of the cell cycle are classified as cell cycle phase-nonspecific or cell cycle-nonspecific (e.g., alkylating agents, antitumor antibiotics).

The primary effect of cytotoxic drugs is to interrupt cell replication. It is believed that cytotoxic drugs kill a fixed percentage, rather than a specific number, of tumor cells with each dose and that tumors with a large percentage of growing cells will experience greater cell death than tumors with a smaller percentage of growing cells. Cells in the resting phase are less responsive to chemotherapeutic agents and are better able to repair themselves if damaged during treatment.

The finding that tumor cells may develop resistance to chemotherapeutic agents has resulted in the development of multiple drug protocols in which a combination of drugs is given simultaneously or in a particular sequence. The additive and sometimes synergistic effects that occur when drugs are used together allow an increased percentage of tumor cell kill without a concomitant increase in drug-induced toxicities. The dose, combination, and treatment schedule for the drugs are determined by factors such as the physiological status of the client and the drug's action on the cell cycle, metabolism, toxic effects, and nadir. Cytotoxic agents are most frequently given intravenously, but routes such as oral, subcutaneous, topical, and direct instillation into the target area (e.g.,

peritoneum, bladder, cerebrospinal fluid) are used when appropriate.

Cytotoxic drugs do not discriminate between the normal and the cancerous cell and, as a result, the client may experience certain side effects and/or toxic effects after their administration. The drugs have the greatest effect on rapidly dividing cancerous and normal cells (e.g., bone marrow, skin, hair follicles, lining of the gastrointestinal tract). Because of this lack of selectivity between the cancerous and the normal cell, nursing care of the recipient of the drugs is indeed a challenge.

This care plan focuses on the adult client hospitalized for an initial or subsequent cycle of chemotherapy and/or management of side effects of treatment with cytotoxic agents. Much of the information is applicable to clients receiving chemotherapy and/or follow-up care in an outpatient facility or home setting.

OUTCOME/DISCHARGE CRITERIA

The client will:
1 Have no signs and symptoms of toxic effects of cytotoxic agents
2 Have side effects of cytotoxic agents under control
3 Have fatigue at a manageable level
4 Have an adequate or improved nutritional status
5 Identify ways to prevent infection during periods of lowered immunity
6 Demonstrate appropriate oral hygiene techniques
7 Identify techniques to control nausea and vomiting
8 Verbalize ways to improve appetite and nutritional status
9 Verbalize ways to manage and cope with persistent fatigue
10 Verbalize ways to prevent bleeding when platelet counts are low
11 Verbalize ways to adjust to alterations in reproductive and sexual functioning
12 Verbalize ways to promote independence and prevent injury if neuropathies are present

Continued...

13. Demonstrate the ability to care for a central venous catheter, a peritoneal catheter, or an implanted infusion device if in place
14. Verbalize an understanding of the care and precautions necessary if an Ommaya reservoir is in place
15. Verbalize an understanding of an implanted infusion pump and precautions necessary if one is in place
16. State signs and symptoms to report to the health care provider
17. Share thoughts and feelings about changes in body image resulting from chemotherapy

18. Identify community resources that can assist with home management and adjustment to the diagnosis of cancer and chemotherapy and its effects
19. Verbalize an understanding of and a plan for adhering to recommended follow-up care including medications prescribed and schedule for chemotherapy, laboratory studies, and future appointments with health care provider

---

Nursing Diagnosis **IMBALANCED NUTRITION: LESS THAN BODY REQUIREMENTS** NDx

Definition: Intake of nutrients insufficient to meet metabolic needs

Related to:
- Decreased oral intake associated with:
  - Oral, pharyngeal, and esophageal pain and difficulty swallowing resulting from mucositis if it has developed
  - Anorexia resulting from factors such as depression, fear, anxiety, fatigue, discomfort, early satiety, altered sense of taste and smell, and increased levels of certain cytokines that depress appetite (e.g., interleukin-1, tumor necrosis factor)
  - Altered mental status (can result from fluid and electrolyte imbalances, hypoxia, or tumor involvement of the brain)
- Loss of nutrients associated with vomiting and diarrhea if present
- Impaired utilization of nutrients associated with:
  - Accelerated and inefficient metabolism of proteins, carbohydrates, and/or fats resulting from factors such as increased levels of cortisol, glucagon, and certain cytokines (e.g., tumor necrosis factor, interleukin-1)
  - Decreased absorption of nutrients resulting from loss of intestinal absorptive surface if mucositis has developed
- Utilization of available nutrients by the malignant cells rather than the host

CLINICAL MANIFESTATIONS

Subjective	Objective
Verbal reports of weakness and fatigue	Significant weight loss; abnormal blood urea nitrogen (BUN) and low serum prealbumin, albumin, and transferrin levels; sore, inflamed oral mucous membrane; pale conjunctiva

RISK FACTORS
- Inability to ingest foods
- Inability to absorb nutrients
- Inability to digest foods

DESIRED OUTCOMES

The client will have or attain an adequate nutritional status as evidenced by:
  a. Weight within or returning toward normal range for client
  b. Normal BUN and serum prealbumin, albumin, and transferrin levels
  c. Usual strength and activity tolerance
  d. Healthy oral mucous membrane

NOC OUTCOMES

Nutritional status; appetite

NIC INTERVENTIONS

Nutritional monitoring; nutrition management; nutrition therapy; nausea management; pain management

NURSING ASSESSMENT	RATIONALE
Assess for and report signs and symptoms of malnutrition: • Weakness • Fatigue • Significant weight loss • Sore, inflamed oral mucous membrane • Pale conjunctiva Monitor percentage of meals and snacks client consumes. Report a pattern of inadequate intake. Monitor serum BUN and serum prealbumin, albumin, and transferrin levels.	*Early recognition of signs and symptoms of malnutrition allows for prompt intervention.*

THERAPEUTIC INTERVENTIONS	RATIONALE

Independent Actions
  • Implement measures to maintain or promote an adequate nutritional status.
  • Implement measures to reduce nausea and vomiting (e.g., provide mints or sour candy for client to suck on to eliminate noxious odors).

  Vomiting results in loss of nutrients.

  • Implement measures to reduce oral, pharyngeal, esophageal, and abdominal pain (e.g., encourage client to suck on ice during infusion).

  Pain can decrease client's appetite and result in decreased oral intake.

• Implement measures to assist client to adjust psychologically to the diagnosis of cancer and treatment with chemotherapy (e.g., reassure client hair loss is temporary; encourage client to wear wig).

  Improves self-esteem and decreases depression, which may impact a clients desire to eat.

• Implement measures to compensate for taste alterations that might be present:

  Enhancing the taste of foods/fluids and providing nutritious alternatives to those that taste unpleasant to the client help to stimulate appetite and improve oral intake.

  • Encourage client to select mild-tasting fish, cold chicken or turkey, eggs, and cheese as protein sources if beef or pork tastes bitter or rancid.
  • Provide meat for breakfast if aversion to meat tends to increase as day progresses.
  • Marinate meats in red wine or sweet and sour sauce.
  • Add extra sweeteners to foods if acceptable to client.
  • Experiment with different flavorings, seasonings, and textures.
  • Serve food cold or at room temperature (can decrease some peculiar tastes).
  • Provide client with plastic rather than metal eating utensils if metallic taste is present. **D ●**
• If client is having difficulty swallowing:
  • Implement measures to reduce the severity of stomatitis and/or relieve dryness of the oral mucous membrane (e.g., encourage client to suck on sugarless candy).

  Action helps to stimulate salivation.

  • Assist client to select foods that require little or no chewing and are easily swallowed (e.g., custard, eggs, canned fruit, mashed potatoes).
  • Avoid serving foods that are sticky (e.g., peanut butter, soft bread, honey).
  • Moisten dry foods with gravy or sauces.
• Serve food warm if indicated. **D ● ✦**

  Warm food can stimulate sense of smell and subsequent appeal of certain foods.

• Increase activity as tolerated. **D ● ✦**

  Activity usually promotes a sense of well-being, which can improve appetite.

• Obtain a dietary consult if necessary to assist client in selecting foods/fluids that are appealing and adhere to personal and cultural preferences.

  Foods/fluids that appeal to the client's senses and are in accordance with personal and cultural preferences are most likely to stimulate appetite and promote interest in eating.

NDx = NANDA-I Diagnosis **D** = Delegatable Action **●** = UAP **✦** = LVN/LPN **⊖▶** = Go to ⊖volve for animation

Continued...

THERAPEUTIC INTERVENTIONS	RATIONALE
• Encourage a rest period before meals. **D** ●	*The physical activity of eating requires some expenditure of energy. Fatigue can reduce the client's desire and ability to eat.*
• Maintain a clean environment and a relaxed, pleasant atmosphere. **D** ● ✦	*Noxious sites and odors can inhibit the feeding center in the hypothalamus.*
	Maintaining a clean environment helps prevent this from occurring. In addition, maintaining a relaxed, pleasant atmosphere can help reduce the client's stress and promote a feeling of well-being, which tends to improve appetite and well-being.
• Provide oral hygiene before meals. **D** ● ✦	*Oral hygiene moistens the mouth, which makes it easier to chew and swallow; it also removes unpleasant tastes, which often improves the taste of foods/fluids.*
• Provide largest amount of calories and protein when appetite is the best (usually at breakfast).	
• Serve frequent, small meals rather than large ones if client is weak, fatigues easily, and/or has a poor appetite.	*Small rather than large meals can enable a client who is weak or fatigues easily to finish a meal. Smaller meals also seem less overwhelming.*
• Encourage significant others to bring in client's favorite foods and eat with him/her.	*Favorite foods eaten along with family members help to make eating more of a familiar social experience.*
• Limit fluid intake with meals (unless the fluid has high nutritional value).	*Limiting fluids helps to reduce early satiety and subsequent decreased food intake.*
• Allow adequate time for meals; reheat foods/fluids if necessary.	*Clients who feel rushed during meals tend to become anxious, lose their appetite, and stop eating.*
• Ensure that meals are well balanced and high in essential nutrients; offer high-calorie, high-protein dietary supplements (e.g., milk shakes, puddings, or eggnog made with cream or powdered milk reconstituted with whole milk; commercially prepared dietary supplements) if indicated.	*Clients must consume a diet that is well balanced and high in essential nutrients in order to meet their nutritional needs. Dietary supplements are often needed to help accomplish this.*
• Perform actions to control diarrhea (e.g., avoid foods high in fiber, coffee, alcohol, spicy or fatty foods).	*Foods may irritate bowel or cause the stool to be more liquid.*

Dependent/Collaborative Actions

Implement measures to maintain or promote an adequate nutritional status:	
• Administer appetite stimulants (e.g., megestrol acetate, dronabinol) if ordered.	
• Administer vitamins and minerals if ordered. **D** ✦	*Vitamins and minerals are needed to maintain metabolic functioning.*
• Perform a calorie count if ordered. Report information to dietitian and physician.	*A calorie count provides information about the caloric intake and nutritional value of the foods/fluids the client consumes. The information helps the dietician and physician determine whether an alternative method of nutritional support is needed.*
Consult physician regarding an alternative method of providing nutrition (e.g., parenteral nutrition, tube feedings) if client does not consume enough food or fluids to meet nutritional needs.	*Notification of the appropriate health care provider allows for modification of the treatment plan.*

Nursing Diagnosis   ACUTE/CHRONIC PAIN NDx

Definition: Pain is an unpleasant sensory and emotional experience arising from actual or potential tissue damage, or described in terms of such damage.

Acute: sudden or slow onset of pain in any intensity from mild to severe with anticipated or predictable end and a duration of less than 6 months

Chronic: sudden or slow onset of pain of any intensity from mild to severe, constant or recurring without anticipated or predictable end and a duration of greater than 6 months

Related to:

• **Oral, pharyngeal, esophageal, and/or abdominal pain** related to mucositis associated with the effects of cytotoxic drugs on the rapidly dividing cells of the gastrointestinal mucosa

• **Muscle and bone pain** (the cause is not known but it sometimes occurs in persons receiving paclitaxel and high doses of vinblastine or etoposide)

- **Neuropathic pain** related to the effects of some cytotoxic drugs (e.g., paclitaxel, cisplatin, vinca alkaloids) on the peripheral nerves

CLINICAL MANIFESTATIONS

Subjective	**Objective**
Verbal reports of oral, pharyngeal, esophageal, and/or abdominal pain; statements of painful swallowing; reports of gastric pain induced by spicy or acidic foods; reports of achiness (usually in lower extremities); reports of numbness, tingling, burning, or shooting pain in extremity(ies)	Grimacing; reluctance to move; clutching abdomen; restlessness

RISK FACTORS

- Chronic disability
- Injury agents (chemical)

DESIRED OUTCOMES

The client will experience diminished pain as evidenced by:
    a. Verbalization of a decrease in or absence of pain
    b. Relaxed facial expression and body positioning
    c. Increased participation in activities

NOC OUTCOMES

Pain control; comfort level

NIC INTERVENTIONS

Pain management; environmental management: comfort; analgesic administration; oral health restoration

NURSING ASSESSMENT	RATIONALE
Assess for and report signs and symptoms of acute/chronic pain. Assess client's perception of the severity of pain using a pain intensity rating scale. Assess the client's pain pattern (e.g., location, quality, onset, duration, precipitating factors, alleviating factors).	*Early recognition of signs and symptoms of acute/chronic pain allows for prompt intervention.*

THERAPEUTIC INTERVENTIONS	RATIONALE

Independent Actions
Implement measures to reduce pain:

- Perform actions to reduce fatigue (e.g., schedule frequent rest periods; minimize environmental noise). **D** ● ✦

  Reducing fatigue helps to increase the client's threshold and tolerance for pain.

- Perform actions to reduce fear and anxiety in order to promote relaxation and subsequently increase the client's threshold and tolerance for pain (e.g., maintain calm, supportive, confident manner).

  Fear and anxiety can decrease the client's threshold for pain and thereby heighten the perception of pain.

- Provide or assist with nonpharmacological methods for pain relief (e.g., massage; position change; progressive relaxation exercises; guided imagery; restful environment; diversional activities such as watching television, reading, or conversing). **D** ● ✦

  Nonpharmacological interventions are believed to be effective because they stimulate closure of the gating mechanism in the spinal cord and block the transmission of pain impulses.

- If client has oral, pharyngeal, esophageal, or abdominal pain:
  - Perform actions to reduce the severity of stomatitis (e.g., encourage client to perform oral hygiene frequently using soft bristle toothbrush or soft tip swab).

    Actions help to reduce irritation to dry, inflamed oral mucosa.

  - Instruct client to avoid substances that might further irritate the gastrointestinal mucosa (e.g., extremely hot, spicy, or acidic foods/fluids; dry or hard foods; raw vegetables).
  - Offer cool, soothing liquids such as nonacidic juices and ices. **D** ● ✦

Continued...

THERAPEUTIC INTERVENTIONS	RATIONALE

Dependent/Collaborative Actions

Implement measures to reduce pain:

*   If client has oral, pharyngeal, esophageal, or abdominal pain:
    *   Instruct client to gargle with a saline solution every 2 hours or spray mouth with a solution containing diphenhydramine and water (1 oz diphenhydramine and 1 qt water) if ordered.
    *   Administer topical anesthetics/analgesics and oral protective agents (e.g., mixture of diphenhydramine, antacid, and Xylocaine Viscous; sucralfate oral suspension) if ordered. **D** ✦
*   Administer the following medications if ordered to manage pain: **D** ✦
    *   Nonopioid (nonnarcotic) analgesics
    *   Skeletal muscle relaxants

    *   Antidepressants
    *   Opioid (narcotic) analgesics or opioid analgesics combined with *N*-methyl-D-aspartate (NMDA) receptor antagonists
    *   Corticosteroids
*   Apply a cooling pad or ice pack to painful extremity unless contraindicated. **D** ● ✦

Consult appropriate health care provider (e.g., pharmacist, physician, pain management specialist) if pain persists or worsens.

Actions help to soothe the oral mucous membrane.

Pharmacological therapy is an effective method of relieving pain.

Muscle relaxants help to reduce pain associated with muscle spasms.
Antidepressants are often used to treat neuropathic pain.

Steroids help to reduce inflammation, which may cause gain.
Action may help reduce mild neuropathic pain.

Notifying the appropriate health care provider allows for modification of the treatment plan.

Nursing Diagnosis IMPAIRED ORAL MUCOUS MEMBRANE NDx

Definition: Disruption of lips and soft tissue of the oral cavity

Related to:

Dryness related to reduced oral intake
Stomatitis related to:
*   Malnutrition and inadequate oral hygiene
*   Disruption in the renewal process of mucosal epithelial cells associated with toxic effects of cytotoxic drugs (particularly antimetabolites, antitumor antibiotics, mitotic inhibitors, and taxanes)
*   Infection, particularly gingival, during the period of myelosuppression

CLINICAL MANIFESTATIONS

Subjective	Objective
Reports of burning pain in mouth; difficulty swallowing; taste changes	Dryness of the oral mucosa; inflamed and/or ulcerated oral mucosa; viscous saliva; positive results of cultured specimens from oral lesions

RISK FACTORS

*   Chemical irritants
*   Decreased salivation
*   Barriers to oral self-care
*   Malnutrition
*   Medication side effects

DESIRED OUTCOMES

The client will maintain a healthy oral cavity as evidenced by:
  a. Absence of inflammation
  b. Pink, moist, intact mucosa
  c. No reports of oral dryness and burning
  d. Ability to swallow without discomfort

NOC OUTCOMES	NIC INTERVENTIONS
Oral hygiene	Oral health maintenance; oral health restoration

NURSING ASSESSMENT	RATIONALE

Assess client for dryness of the oral mucosa and signs and symptoms of stomatitis:
- Reports of burning pain in mouth
- Difficulty swallowing
- Taste changes
- Dryness of the oral mucosa
- Inflamed and/or ulcerated oral mucosa
- Viscous saliva
- Positive results of cultured specimens from oral lesions

Early recognition of signs and symptoms of impaired oral mucosa allows for prompt intervention.

THERAPEUTIC INTERVENTIONS	RATIONALE

Independent Actions

Implement measures to prevent or reduce the severity of stomatitis and/or relieve dryness of the oral mucous membrane:
- Encourage client to chew on ice during chemotherapy infusion, especially if receiving 5-fluorouracil.
- Reinforce importance of and assist client with oral hygiene after meals and snacks; avoid use of products that contain lemon and glycerin and mouthwashes containing alcohol.
- Instruct and assist client to perform oral hygiene using a soft bristle toothbrush or sponge-tipped swab and to floss teeth gently.
- Have client rinse mouth frequently with warm saline solution, baking soda and warm water, or chlorhexidine gluconate (Peridex), or mist oral cavity frequently using a spray bottle. **D** ● ✦
- Lubricate client's lips frequently. **D** ● ✦
- Encourage client to suck on sugarless candy or chew sugarless gum. **D** ● ✦
- Encourage client not to smoke or chew tobacco.
- Encourage client to use a saliva substitute such as Salivart if indicated.
- Instruct client to avoid substances that might further irritate the oral mucosa (e.g., hot, spicy, or acidic foods/fluids).
- Perform actions to promote an adequate nutritional status (e.g., serve food cold or at room temperature; experiment with different seasonings, textures).

If stomatitis is not controlled:
- Increase frequency of oral hygiene. **D** ● ✦
- If client has dentures, remove and replace only for meals. **D** ●

Lemon glycerin or alcohol-containing products have a drying and irritating effect on the oral mucous membrane.

Use of appropriate oral hygiene devices and techniques helps to effectively remove food particles and debris from client's mouth without causing trauma to the oral mucous membrane.

Lubricating lips helps prevent drying and cracking.
Sucking on candy stimulates saliva secretion.

Smoking dries the oral mucous membrane.

Irritation and subsequent inflammation can occur when tobacco is in contact with the oral mucosa.

Actions help to compensate for taste alterations that the client may be experiencing.

Dependent/Collaborative Actions

Implement measures to prevent or reduce the severity of stomatitis and/or relieve dryness of the oral mucous membrane:
- Encourage a fluid intake of at least 2500 mL/day unless contraindicated.
- Provide client with a prophylactic antifungal oral suspension or lozenge (e.g., nystatin) if ordered. **D** ✦

Consult appropriate health care provider (e.g., oncology nurse specialist, physician) if signs and symptoms of dryness and stomatitis persist or worsen.

Adequate hydration helps keep the oral mucosa moist, which reduces the risk of cracking and breakdown.

Notifying the appropriate health care provider allows for modification of the treatment plan.

NDx = NANDA-I Diagnosis   **D** = Delegatable Action   ● = UAP   ✦ = LVN/LPN   ⊝▶ = Go to ⊝volve for animation

Collaborative Diagnosis **RISK FOR BLEEDING**

Definition: Escape of blood from an injured vessel.
Related to: Thrombocytopenia associated with chemotherapy-induced bone marrow suppression

CLINICAL MANIFESTATIONS

Subjective	Objective
N/A	Petechiae, purpura, or ecchymoses; gingival bleeding; prolonged bleeding from puncture sites; epistaxis, hemoptysis; unusual joint pain; frank or occult blood in stool, urine, or vomitus; increase in abdominal girth; menorrhagia; restlessness, confusion; decreasing blood pressure (B/P) and increased pulse rate; decrease in hematocrit (Hct) and hemoglobin (Hgb) levels

RISK FACTORS

- Trauma

DESIRED OUTCOMES

The client will not experience unusual bleeding as evidenced by:
   a. Skin and mucous membranes free of petechiae, purpura, ecchymoses, and active bleeding
   b. Absence of unusual joint pain
   c. Absence of frank and occult blood in stool, urine, and vomitus
   d. No increase in abdominal girth
   e. Usual menstrual flow
   f. Usual mental status
   g. Vital signs within normal range for client
   h. Stable or improved Hct and Hgb levels

NURSING ASSESSMENT

Assess client for and report signs and symptoms of unusual bleeding:
- Petechiae
- Purpura
- Ecchymoses
- Gingival bleeding
- Prolonged bleeding from puncture sites
- Epistaxis
- Hemoptysis
- Unusual joint pain
- Frank or occult blood in stool, urine, or vomitus
- Increase in abdominal girth
- Menorrhagia
- Restlessness
- Confusion
- Decreasing B/P and increased pulse rate
- Decrease in Hct and Hgb levels

Monitor platelet count and coagulation test results (e.g., bleeding time). Report significant worsening of values.

If platelet count is low, coagulation test results are abnormal, or Hct and Hgb levels decrease, test all stools, urine, and vomitus for occult blood. Report positive results.

RATIONALE

Early recognition of signs and symptoms of bleeding allows for prompt intervention.

THERAPEUTIC INTERVENTIONS	RATIONALE

Dependent/Collaborative Actions

Implement measures to prevent bleeding:

- Avoid giving injections whenever possible; consult physician about prescribing an alternative route for medications ordered to be given intramuscularly or subcutaneously.
- When giving injections or performing venous and arterial punctures, use the smallest gauge needle possible.
- Apply gentle, prolonged pressure to puncture sites after injections, venous and arterial punctures, and diagnostic tests such as bone marrow aspiration.
- Take B/P only when necessary and avoid overinflating the cuff.
- Caution client to avoid activities that increase the risk for trauma (e.g., shaving with a straight-edge razor, using stiff bristle toothbrush or dental floss).
- Whenever possible, avoid intubations (e.g., nasogastric) and procedures that can cause injury to rectal mucosa (e.g., taking temperatures rectally, inserting a rectal suppository or tube, administering an enema).
- Pad side rails if client is confused or restless.
- Perform actions to reduce the risk for falls (e.g., keep bed in low position with side rails up when client is in bed, avoid unnecessary clutter in room, instruct client to wear slippers/shoes with nonslip soles when ambulating).
- Instruct client to avoid blowing nose forcefully or straining to have a bowel movement; consult physician about an order for a decongestant and/or laxative if indicated.
- Administer the following if ordered:
  - Platelet-stimulating factor
  - Estrogen-progestin preparations to suppress menses
  - Platelets

If bleeding occurs and does not subside spontaneously:

- Apply firm, prolonged pressure to bleeding area(s) if possible.
- If epistaxis occurs, place client in high-Fowler's position and apply pressure and ice pack to nasal area.
- Maintain oxygen therapy as ordered.
- Administer whole blood or blood products (e.g., platelets) as ordered.

Thrombocytopenia predisposes patients to bleeding. Actions that increase the risk for bleeding should be avoided in clients with thrombocytopenia.

Actions help to decrease bleeding temporarily, support adequate oxygenation in the presence of loss of RBCs, and replace deficient blood components.

Collaborative Diagnosis # RISK FOR IMPAIRED RENAL FUNCTION

Definition: Inability of the kidney to appropriately concentrate urine and excrete waste products

Related to:

- Direct toxic effects of some cytotoxic agents (e.g., cisplatin, high doses of methotrexate, streptozocin) on renal cells
- Nephropathy associated with:
  - Excessive uric acid accumulation resulting from the rapid lysis of large numbers of tumor cells
  - Precipitation of certain drugs (e.g., high doses of methotrexate) in the renal tubules and collecting ducts as a result of low urinary pH and inadequate hydration before, during, and after drug administration

CLINICAL MANIFESTATIONS

Subjective	Objective
N/A	Urine output less than 30 mL/h; urine specific gravity fixed at or less than 1.010; elevated BUN and serum creatinine levels; decreased creatinine clearance

---

Continued...

RISK FACTORS

- Chemotherapeutic agents
- Impaired volume status

DESIRED OUTCOMES

The client will maintain adequate renal function as evidenced by:
  a. Urine output at least 30 mL/h
  b. BUN and serum creatinine levels and creatinine clearance within normal range

NURSING ASSESSMENT

Assess for and report signs and symptoms of impaired renal function:

- Urine output less than 30 mL/h
- Urine specific gravity fixed at or less than 1.010
- Elevated BUN and serum creatinine levels
- Decreased creatinine clearance

Assess for and report a urine output below 100 mL/h during and for 24 hours after administration of nephrotoxic drugs.

RATIONALE

Early recognition of signs and symptoms of impaired renal function allows for prompt intervention.

THERAPEUTIC INTERVENTIONS

Dependent/Collaborative Actions

- Implement measures to maintain adequate renal function:

  - Hydrate client with at least 150 mL/h of fluid, unless contraindicated, for 6 to 24 hours before administration of drugs known to be nephrotoxic (e.g., cisplatin, high doses of methotrexate, streptozocin).
  - Administer intravenous fluids as ordered during administration of nephrotoxic drugs and for 24 hours after. **D** ✦

- Administer the following medications as ordered:
  - Diuretics (e.g., furosemide, mannitol)

  - Xanthine oxidase inhibitor (e.g., allopurinol)

  - Sodium bicarbonate

  - Leucovorin calcium (e.g., folinic acid)

  - Chemoprotectant agent (e.g., amifostine)

If signs and symptoms of impaired renal function occur:

- Assess for and report signs of acute renal failure (e.g., oliguria or anuria; weight gain of 2% or greater over a short time; edema; elevated B/P; lethargy and confusion; increasing BUN and serum creatinine, phosphorus, and potassium levels).
- Prepare client for dialysis if indicated.

RATIONALE

Adequate hydration ensures optimum perfusion of the kidney, which is necessary for the health of the functional nephron units.

Adequate hydration helps to maintain a high rate of glomerular blood flow.

Diuretics help to promote more rapid plasma clearance of the cytotoxic agent.

Xanthine oxidase inhibitors help to decrease the formation of uric acid.

Sodium bicarbonate helps to alkalinize the urine and subsequently increase the solubility of uric acid in the urine and prevent the precipitation of methotrexate in renal tubules and collecting ducts.

Folic acid helps to diminish the toxic effects of cytotoxic agents such as methotrexate on the renal cells.

Chemoprotective agents help to protect the renal cells against toxicity from some cytotoxic agents (e.g., cisplatin).

Recognition of signs and symptoms of impaired renal function allows for prompt intervention.

Collaborative Diagnosis   **RISK FOR HEMORRHAGIC CYSTITIS**

Definition: Inflammation of the bladder resulting in bleeding

Related to: Irritation and ulceration of the bladder mucosa by toxic metabolites of certain cytotoxic agents, particularly cyclophosphamide and ifosfamide

CLINICAL MANIFESTATIONS

Subjective	Objective
Reports of dysuria; suprapubic pain	Frank or occult blood in urine; urinary frequency/urgency

RISK FACTORS

- Chemotherapy

DESIRED OUTCOMES

The client will not develop hemorrhagic cystitis as evidenced by absence of dysuria, urinary frequency and urgency, suprapubic pain, and hematuria.

NURSING ASSESSMENT

Assess for and report signs and symptoms of hemorrhagic cystitis:
- Dysuria
- Suprapubic pain
- Frank or occult blood in urine
- Urinary frequency/urgency

RATIONALE

Early recognition of signs and symptoms of hemorrhagic cystitis allows for prompt intervention.

THERAPEUTIC INTERVENTIONS

RATIONALE

Dependent/Collaborative Actions

Implement measures to prevent hemorrhagic cystitis:
- Ensure that client is vigorously hydrated; maintain intravenous fluids at the rate ordered (often as high as 200 mL/h during chemotherapy). **D** ✦
- Administer cyclophosphamide early in the day and encourage client to void at least every 4 hours, before going to bed, and at least once during the night.
- Administer mesna (Mesnex) if ordered.

- Maintain continuous bladder irrigation before and after administration of cyclophosphamide or ifosfamide if ordered.

If signs and symptoms of hemorrhagic cystitis occur:
- Discontinue cytotoxic drug administration and notify physician.
- Continue with fluid administration as ordered. **D** ✦
- Administer diuretics as ordered. **D** ✦

- Assist with or perform bladder irrigations as ordered.
- Maintain continuous bladder irrigation with silver nitrate or alum (potassium aluminum sulfate) solution if ordered to stop bleeding.
- Prepare client for the following if planned:
  - Cystoscopy to cauterize bleeding vessels
  - Intravesical instillation of formalin to control persistent, severe bleeding

Adequate hydration ensures ability to reduce the concentration of toxic drug metabolites in the bladder.

Actions help to prevent stasis of toxic drug metabolites in the bladder.

Mesna helps to interact with and inactivate the toxic drug metabolites of ifosfamide.
Continuous bladder irrigation helps flush metabolites from the bladder and prevent the formation of obstructive clots should bleeding occur.

To increase urine output and thereby decrease the concentration of toxic drug metabolites in the urine.

Bladder irrigations help to facilitate removal of drug metabolites and flush clots from the bladder.

Collaborative Diagnosis ## RISK FOR DRUG EXTRAVASATION

Definition: Infiltration of drugs into soft tissues leading to local tissue irritation and sloughing

Related to: Extravasation of vesicant drugs (e.g., most antitumor antibiotics, teniposide, vinblastine, vincristine, paclitaxel)

Continued...

CLINICAL MANIFESTATIONS

Subjective	Objective
Reports of stinging or burning pain at infusion site or along vein	Swelling, blanching, or coolness of skin around infusion site

RISK FACTORS

- Infiltration of intravenous lines
- Multiple punctures in the same vein

DESIRED OUTCOMES

The client will not experience drug extravasation as evidenced by:
  a. Absence of swelling, blanching, and coolness of skin around infusion site
  b. No reports of stinging or burning pain at infusion site or along the vein

NURSING ASSESSMENT

Assess for signs and symptoms of drug extravasation:
- Reports of stinging or burning pain at infusion site or along vein
- Swelling, blanching, or coolness of skin around infusion site

Ensure that infusion site and surrounding tissue are visible at all times.

RATIONALE

Early recognition of signs and symptoms of drug extravasation allows for prompt intervention.

THERAPEUTIC INTERVENTIONS

Dependent/Collaborative Actions
Implement measures to prevent drug extravasation:
- Select the best vein possible for vesicant drug administration:
  - Do not use a vein that has been previously used for vesicant agents.
  - Use a large vein in forearm if possible; avoid the antecubital fossa and small veins in the hand.
  - Do not use an existing peripheral intravenous catheter that is more than 24 hours old.
  - Avoid extremities with compromised circulation.
  - Consult physician about insertion of a central venous catheter if large and/or frequent doses of a vesicant are planned.
- Do not perform multiple punctures in the same vein.
- Tape intravenous catheter securely, but not too tight.
- Do not irrigate catheter forcefully or use a high pressure setting on infusion device.
- Perform actions to ensure that the drug is infusing into the vein:
  - Test patency of vein before administration of cytotoxic drug.
  - Stay with client while a vesicant drug is infusing; check site every 2 to 3 minutes.
- Perform actions to prevent increased irritation of the vein:
  - Dilute drug according to manufacturer's recommendations.
  - Administer drug at recommended rate of infusion.
- Stop infusion if there is any indication that the drug is not infusing properly.
- When the drug infusion is complete, flush intravenous catheter with a minimum of 30 mL of normal saline; apply pressure to site for at least 4 minutes after catheter removal to minimize oozing.

RATIONALE

This vein is more fragile and previous use increases the risk for extravasation.
Extravasation in these areas can destroy nerves and tendons.

This prevents excessive damage to the vein and decreases the risk of extravasation.

Prevents leakage from the vessel after infusion has begun.

Irrigating forcefully may disrupt the integrity of the vessel, resulting in infiltration.

Ensuring adequate blood return prior to the administration of cytotoxic agents reduces the risk of extravasation.

THERAPEUTIC INTERVENTIONS	RATIONALE
If signs and symptoms of drug extravasation occur: • Stop infusion immediately. • Treat area of extravasation as ordered (treatment varies depending on drug used) or per standard hospital procedure. • Assess the site frequently for signs of increased inflammation, blistering, and necrosis. • Administer analgesics as ordered (severe pain is common after extravasation).	*Infusion must be discontinued immediately and area treated per hospital protocol to avoid extensive tissue damage.*

Collaborative Diagnosis | RISK FOR CARDIAC DYSRHYTHMIAS

Definition: Disturbance of the heart rhythm

Related to: Cardiotoxic effects of certain cytotoxic drugs (e.g., cyclophosphamide, high doses of ifosfamide, doxorubicin, daunorubicin, paclitaxel)

CLINICAL MANIFESTATIONS

Subjective	Objective
Reports of lightheadedness; palpitations	Irregular apical pulse; pulse rate below 60 or above 100 beats/min; apical-radial pulse deficit; syncope; palpitations; abnormal rate, rhythm, or configurations on electrocardiogram (ECG)

RISK FACTORS

• Electrolyte imbalance

DESIRED OUTCOMES

The client will experience resolution of cardiac dysrhythmias if they occur as evidenced by:
   a. Regular apical pulse at 60 to 100 beats/min
   b. Equal apical and radial pulse rates
   c. Absence of syncope and palpitations
   d. ECG reading showing normal sinus rhythm

NURSING ASSESSMENT	RATIONALE
Assess for and report signs and symptoms of cardiac dysrhythmias: • Reports of lightheadedness, palpitations • Irregular apical pulse • Pulse rate below 60 or above 100 beats/min • Apical-radial pulse deficit • Syncope • Abnormal rate, rhythm, or configurations on ECG	*Early recognition of signs and symptoms of cardiac dysrhythmias allows for prompt intervention.*
Monitor liver and kidney function studies and report abnormal results.	*Cardiotoxicity can result from delayed metabolism or excretion of cytotoxic drugs by the liver or kidneys.*

THERAPEUTIC INTERVENTIONS	RATIONALE
Dependent/Collaborative Actions Administer a cardioprotectant agent (e.g., dexrazoxane) if ordered.	*Cardioprotective agents help to reduce the risk of anthracycline-induced cardiac damage.*
If cardiac dysrhythmias occur: • Initiate cardiac monitoring and prepare client for an ECG if ordered.	*Allows for proper identification of dysrhythmias and the implementation of the appropriate interventions.*
• Administer antidysrhythmic agents (e.g., Lidocaine, digoxin, diltiazem, esmolol, amiodarone, atropine) if ordered.	

NDx = NANDA-I Diagnosis   **D** = Delegatable Action   ● = UAP   ✦ = LVN/LPN   ⊝▶ = Go to ⊝volve for animation

Continued...

THERAPEUTIC INTERVENTIONS	RATIONALE
• Restrict client's activity based on his/her tolerance and severity of the dysrhythmia. • Maintain oxygen therapy as ordered. • Assess cardiovascular status frequently and report signs and symptoms of inadequate tissue perfusion (e.g., decrease in B/P, cool skin, cyanosis, diminished peripheral pulses, declining urine output, restlessness and agitation, shortness of breath). • Have emergency cart readily available for defibrillation, cardioversion, or cardiopulmonary resuscitation.	*Life threatening dysrhythmias such as ventricular fibrillation require use of equipment maintuined on emergency carts.*

Collaborative Diagnosis | **RISK FOR INFLAMMATION AND FIBROSIS OF LUNG TISSUE**

Related to: Toxic effects of some cytotoxic agents on the lung (e.g., busulfan, bleomycin, carmustine, mitomycin)

CLINICAL MANIFESTATIONS

Subjective	Objective
Verbal reports of shortness of breath	Dry, hacking, persistent cough; fever; tachypnea; dyspnea on exertion; wheezing; crackles

RISK FACTORS
• Chemotherapeutic agents
• Radiation therapy

DESIRED OUTCOMES

The client will experience decreased signs and symptoms of pulmonary inflammation and fibrosis if they occur as evidenced by:
  a. Decreased coughing
  b. Afebrile status
  c. Decreased dyspnea
  d. Improved breath sounds

NURSING ASSESSMENT	RATIONALE
Assess for and report signs and symptoms of pulmonary inflammation and fibrosis, particularly if client is reaching total allowable cumulative dose of cytotoxic agent(s) known to cause pulmonary toxicity: • Verbal reports of shortness of breath • Dry, hacking, persistent cough • Fever • Tachypnea • Dyspnea on exertion • Wheezing • Crackles	*Early recognition of signs and symptoms of pulmonary inflammation/fibrosis allows for prompt intervention.*

THERAPEUTIC INTERVENTIONS	RATIONALE

Dependent/Collaborative Actions
If signs and symptoms of pulmonary inflammation and fibrosis occur:
• Discontinue infusion of cytotoxic agent as ordered.
• Prepare client for diagnostic studies (e.g., chest radiograph, pulmonary function studies, computed tomography (CT) or gallium scan, fiberoptic bronchoscopy) if planned.
• Maintain oxygen therapy as ordered.
• Administer the following medications if ordered:
  • Corticosteroids
  • Bronchodilators
	Discontinuing of the medication prevents further exposure to the toxic agents.
	
	Maintain's supplemental tissue oxygenation.
	
	Corticosteroids reduce the inflammatory response.
	Bronchodilators dilate the bronchi and bronchioles, decrease airway resistance, and improve airflow.

Collaborative Diagnosis **RISK FOR NEUROTOXICITY**

Definition: Destructive or poisonous effect upon nerve tissue

Related to: The toxic effects of certain cytotoxic agents (e.g., vincristine, vinblastine, cisplatin, ifosfamide, etoposide, high doses of methotrexate or cytarabine) on the nerves

CLINICAL MANIFESTATIONS

Subjective	Objective
Reports of numbness and tingling of extremities; burning pain in extremity; unusual muscle weakness; blurred vision	Constipation; ataxia; gait disturbances; difficulty with fine motor movements; foot drop or wrist drop; hearing loss; nystagmus; memory loss; confusion; expressive aphasia; seizures

RISK FACTORS

- Chemotherapeutic agents

DESIRED OUTCOMES

The client will adapt to the signs and symptoms of neurotoxicity if it occurs and not experience injury associated with those signs and symptoms.

NURSING ASSESSMENT

Assess for and report signs and symptoms of neurotoxicity:
- Numbness and tingling of extremities
- Burning pain in extremity
- Unusual muscle weakness
- Blurred vision
- Constipation
- Ataxia, gait disturbances
- Difficulty with fine motor movements
- Foot drop or wrist drop
- Hearing loss
- Nystagmus
- Memory loss
- Confusion
- Expressive aphasia
- Seizures

RATIONALE

Early recognition of signs and symptoms of neurotoxicity allows for prompt intervention.

THERAPEUTIC INTERVENTIONS

Dependent/Collaborative Actions

Assure client that most changes in neurological function may be reversible if reported immediately and the neurotoxic drug is discontinued.

If signs and symptoms of neurotoxicity occur:
- Implement measures to prevent falls:
  - Keep bed in low position. **D** ●
  - Avoid unnecessary clutter in the room. **D** ●

- Implement measures to prevent burns and cuts:
  - Let hot foods/fluids cool slightly before serving.
  - Assess temperature of bath water before bathing.
- Institute seizure precautions if indicated.
- Implement measures to assist client to adapt to the following if present:
  - Constipation
    (1) Encourage fluid intake. **D** ✦
    (2) Increase fiber intake.

RATIONALE

Recognition of signs and symptoms of neurotoxicity allows for implementation of the appropriate interventions and modification of the treatment plan.

Neurotoxicity can result in ataxia, which may predispose the client to falls.

Common clinical manifestations associated with neoplastic drugs include numbness in extremities (polyneuropathy), which may interfere with normal response to hot foods, water.

NDx = NANDA-I Diagnosis   **D** = Delegatable Action   ● = UAP   ✦ = LVN/LPN   ⊖▶ = Go to ⊖volve for animation

Continued...

THERAPEUTIC INTERVENTIONS	RATIONALE

• Pain in extremities
  (1) Assist with position changes. **D** ●
  (2) Assist with guided imagery. **D** ● ✦	

• Foot drop (1) Instruct client to perform active foot exercises every 1 to 2 hours while awake. **D** ● ✦	*Musculoskeletal effects associated with neurotoxicity include myalgia, joint stiffness, and muscle weakness.*
• Wrist drop (1) Instruct client to perform active wrist exercises every 1 to 2 hours while awake. **D** ● ✦	

• Impaired hearing
  (1) Face client when speaking.
  (2) Use gestures.
	Improves ability to communicate with client.

• Memory loss
  (1) Assist to make lists. **D** ● ✦
  (2) Repeat information as needed.
	Actions assist clients with memory loss, visual or auditory hallacinations, and confusion that can result from neurotoxicity.

• Confusion
  (1) Decrease environmental stimuli. **D** ● ✦
  (2) Keep daily routines consistent. **D** ● ✦	

• Expressive aphasia
  (1) Encourage client to use short words.
  (2) Encourage client to use gestures.	

Consult physician if signs and symptoms of neurotoxicity persist or worsen.	

Collaborative Diagnosis   RISK FOR ANAPHYLAXIS

Definition: A rapid and severe hypersensitivity reaction occurring within minutes of exposure to an antigen

Related to: A hypersensitivity response to a cytotoxic drug (e.g., cyclophosphamide, cisplatin, L-asparaginase, teniposide, paclitaxel).

CLINICAL MANIFESTATIONS

Subjective	Objective
Reports of anxiety; generalized urticaria and pruritus; reports of abdominal cramps, tightness in throat, ringing in ears, or numbness	Agitation; flushing of the skin; dyspnea; wheezing; stridor; irregular and/or increased pulse rate; decline in B/P; edema (particularly common in face, hands, and feet)

RISK FACTORS

• Incomplete immune systems

DESIRED OUTCOMES

The client will not develop an anaphylactic reaction as evidenced by:
  a. Usual mental status
  b. Usual skin color
  c. Absence of urticaria and pruritus
  d. No reports of abdominal cramps, tightness in throat, ringing in ears, and numbness
  e. Absence of dyspnea, wheezing, and stridor
  f. Stable vital signs
  g. Absence of edema

NURSING ASSESSMENT	RATIONALE
Assess for and report signs and symptoms of an anaphylactic reaction: • Anxiety/agitation • Generalized urticaria and pruritus	*Early recognition of signs and symptoms of anaphylaxis allows for prompt intervention.*

NURSING ASSESSMENT	RATIONALE

- Reports of abdominal cramps, tightness in throat, ringing in ears, or numbness
- Flushing of the skin
- Dyspnea, wheezing, stridor
- Irregular and/or increased pulse rate
- Decline in B/P
- Edema (particularly common in face, hands, and feet)

THERAPEUTIC INTERVENTIONS	RATIONALE

Dependent/Collaborative Actions

Implement measures to prevent an anaphylactic reaction:

- Consult physician before giving any drug that is the same as or similar to one the client has reacted to previously.
- Administer a test dose before giving drug if appropriate.
- Administer the following medications if ordered:
  - Corticosteroids **D** ✦
  - Histamine$_1$ receptor antagonists **D** ✦

If signs and symptoms of an anaphylactic reaction occur:

- Discontinue the cytotoxic drug but keep intravenous line open with a normal saline solution.
- Administer oxygen as ordered.
- Administer the following medications if ordered:
  - Sympathomimetics such as epinephrine or dopamine

  - Antihistamines (e.g., diphenhydramine)

  - Bronchodilators (e.g., theophylline)
  - Corticosteroids

- Assess for and report signs and symptoms of anaphylactic shock (e.g., increased restlessness; significant decrease in B/P; rapid, weak pulse; increased dyspnea; cool, pale skin).

Administration of corticosteroids and/or histamine$_1$ receptor antagonists helps to reduce sensitivity to the cytotoxic agent.

Prevents further reaction to the drug and maintains an access line for IV medication administration if needed.

Sympathomimetics help to relieve bronchospasm and stimulate peripheral vasoconstriction, while dopamine helps maintain B/P and organ perfusion.

Antihistamines help to reduce the sensitivity reaction and control pruritus and urticaria.

Bronchodilators alleviate bronchospasm.

Corticosteroids reduce the allergic response and maintain usual vascular wall permeability.

Reporting signs and symptoms of shock allows for modification of the treatment plan.

Nursing Diagnosis RISK FOR DISTURBED SELF-CONCEPT* NDx

Definition: **Disturbed body image NDx:** comfusion in mental picture of one's physical self.
Situational low self-esteem NDx: Development of negative perception of self-worth in response to a current situation.

Related to:

- Changes in appearance associated with the side effects of chemotherapy (e.g., alopecia, excessive weight loss, skin and nail changes) and external drug infusion catheter if present
- Possible alteration in usual sexual activities associated with weakness, fatigue, reduced levels of testosterone (can occur with chemotherapy for prostate or testicular cancer or lymphoma), psychological factors, and vaginal discomfort (may result from mucositis and premature menopause if ovarian failure occurs)
- Possible temporary or permanent infertility associated with gonadal dysfunction resulting from extensive therapy with some cytotoxic drugs (e.g., some alkylating agents)
- Increased dependence on others to meet self-care needs
- Changes in lifestyle and roles associated with effects of the disease process and its treatment

CLINICAL MANIFESTATIONS

Subjective	Objective
Verbalization of negative feelings about self; lack of a plan for adapting to necessary changes in lifestyle	Withdrawal from significant others; lack of participation in activities of daily living

*This diagnostic lable includes the nursing diagnoses of disturbed body image and situational low self-esteem.

NDx = NANDA-I Diagnosis   **D** = Delegatable Action   ● = UAP   ✦ = LVN/LPN   ⊝▶ = Go to ⊝volve for animation

Continued...

RISK FACTORS

- Illness treatment
- Altered body image

DESIRED OUTCOMES

The client will demonstrate beginning adaptation to changes in appearance, body functioning, lifestyle, and roles as evidenced by:

    a. Verbalization of feelings of self-worth and sexual adequacy

    b. Maintenance of relationships with significant others

    c. Active participation in activities of daily living

    d. Verbalization of a beginning plan for adapting lifestyle to changes resulting from the disease process and residual effects of chemotherapy

NOC OUTCOMES

Self-esteem; personal autonomy; psychosocial adjustment: life change; body image

NIC INTERVENTIONS

Body image enhancement; self-esteem enhancement; role enhancement; emotional support; support system enhancement

NURSING ASSESSMENT

Assess for signs and symptoms of a disturbed self-concept
- Subjective
- Objective

RATIONALE

Early recognition of signs and symptoms of disturbed self-concept allows for prompt intervention.

THERAPEUTIC INTERVENTIONS

RATIONALE

Independent Actions

Implement measures to facilitate the grieving process.

Discuss with client improvements in appearance and functioning that can realistically be expected.

Implement measures for the following changes in body functioning and appearance if appropriate:

- Alopecia
  - Inform client that hair loss can be expected approximately 2 weeks after initiation of chemotherapy; may be sudden, gradual, partial, or complete; and can include scalp hair, pubic hair, beard, eyebrows, and eyelashes.
  - Reassure client that hair loss is temporary (regrowth sometimes occurs before cessation of treatment but usually occurs 2-3 months after it).
  - Inform client that hair regrowth may be a different color, texture, and consistency.
  - Encourage client to cut hair very short.
  - Inform client that the rate of scalp hair loss can be reduced by:
    - (1) Brushing hair gently using a soft bristle brush
    - (2) Shampooing hair only once or twice a week and using a gentle shampoo and lukewarm water
    - (3) Avoiding use of equipment/products that dry hair (e.g., hot rollers, hair dryers, curling iron, dyes)
    - (4) Avoiding hair styles that create tension on hair (e.g., ponytails, braids)
  - Encourage client to wear a wig, scarf, hat, false eyelashes, or makeup if desired to camouflage hair loss.
  - Inform client of community resources that can provide information and assistance with ways to facilitate adjustment to changes in appearance (e.g., American Cancer Society, Look Good-Feel Better Program).

Actions help to assist client to adapt to changes in body functioning and appearance.

Clients may exhibit a range of emotional responses at the prospect of losing hair, including anger, grief, embarrassment, and fear. Educating the client regarding hair loss may alleviate anxiety and allow the client to explore feelings associated with this side effect.

Cutting the hair very short helps to decrease the anxiety related to seeing large quantities of hair fall out.

Provides client ways to control hair loss.

Helps to improve client's self esteem.

THERAPEUTIC INTERVENTIONS	RATIONALE

• Skin changes (e.g., redness, rashes, peeling, increased sensitivity to sun, acne, darkening along the vein used for cytotoxic drug administration)
    • Inform client that skin and vein hyperpigmentation may occur if cytotoxic drugs such as bleomycin, busulfan, methotrexate, and fluorouracil are being administered.
    • Inform client that skin and vein discoloration is usually temporary.
    • Instruct client to avoid exposure to sunlight and to use sunscreen to prevent an increase in photosensitivity reactions.
    • Assist client to identify types of clothing that can be worn to camouflage skin changes.
	Educating the client about skin changes associated with chemotherapy may help alleviate anxiety and allow the client to explore feelings associated with this side effect.

• Nail changes
    • Inform client that nails may thicken and stop growing, develop ridges, darken, and detach from nail bed during treatment with certain cytotoxic drugs (e.g., cyclophosphamide, doxorubicin, bleomycin, fluorouracil).
    • Reassure client that normal nail growth will resume when chemotherapy is completed.
	Educating the client about nail changes associated with chemotherapy may help alleviate anxiety.

• Infertility
    • Clarify physician's explanation that infertility is a possible permanent effect of chemotherapy.
    • Discuss alternative methods of becoming a parent (e.g., artificial insemination, adoption) if of concern to client.
	Educating the client about infertility may help alleviate anxiety and allow the client to explore alternative treatments.

• Impotence
    • Encourage client to discuss it with physician (impotence usually resolves after cessation of therapy).
    • Suggest alternative methods of sexual gratification if appropriate.
    • Discuss ways to be creative in expressing sexuality (e.g., massage, fantasies, cuddling).
	Educating the client about impotence may help alleviate anxiety and allow the client to explore alternative treatments.

Assist client with usual grooming and makeup habits if necessary. **D** ●	
Support behaviors suggesting positive adaptation to changes that have occurred (e.g., interest in personal appearance, maintenance of relationships with significant others).	*These actions promote positive self-esteem and clients ability to maintain supportive relationships.*
Assist client's and significant others' adjustment to changes by listening, facilitating communication, and providing information.	
Encourage significant others to allow client to do what he/she is able.	*Actions help encourage the client to be independent and/or develop self-esteem.*
Encourage client contact with others.	*Contact with others helps the client to test and establish a new self-image.*
Encourage visits and support from significant others.	
Consult appropriate health care provider (e.g., psychiatric nurse clinician, physician) if client seems unwilling or unable to adapt to changes that have occurred as a result of cancer and its treatment.	

DISCHARGE TEACHING/CONTINUED CARE

Nursing Diagnosis   **DEFICIENT KNOWLEDGE** NDx**; INEFFECTIVE THERAPEUTIC REGIMEN MANAGEMENT** NDx**; OR INEFFECTIVE HEALTH MAINTENANCE***

Definition: Absence of deficiency of cognitive information related to a specific, topic; pattern of regulating and integrating into family processes a program for treatment of illness and its sequelae that is unsatisfactory in meeting specific health goals; inability to identify, manage, and/or seek out help to maintain health.

RISK FACTORS
- Cognitive limitations
- Lack of recall
- Diminished fine/gross motor skills

NOC OUTCOMES	NIC INTERVENTIONS
Knowledge: disease process; knowledge: treatment regimen; knowledge: energy conservation; knowledge: treatment procedure(s)	Health system guidance; teaching: disease process; teaching: prescribed medication; teaching: prescribed activity/exercise; teaching: procedure/treatment; nutrition management

CLINICAL MANIFESTATIONS

Subjective	Objective
Verbalization of interest in learning; verbalization of the problem	Exaggerated behaviors; inaccurate follow-through of instructions

NURSING ASSESSMENT	RATIONALE
• Assess client's willingness to learn and knowledge related to the disease and treatment process • Assess for indications that the client may be unable to effectively management the therapeutic regimen	*The client's willingness to learn and knowledge base provides the foundation for education.* *Early recognition of inability to understand disease process or provide self-care allows for changes in the teaching plan.*

THERAPEUTIC INTERVENTIONS	RATIONALE

Desired Outcome: The client will identify ways to prevent infection during periods of lowered immunity.

Independent Actions

Explain to client that his/her resistance to infection is reduced when white blood cell (WBC) counts are low. Emphasize need to adhere closely to recommended techniques to prevent infection.

Instruct the client in ways to prevent infection:

- Avoid crowds, persons with any sign of infection, and persons who have recently been vaccinated.
- Use good hand hygiene (e.g., wash hands using an anti-bacterial soap, use an alcohol-base hand rub).

  Good hand hygiene is paramount in preventing infection.

- Wear gloves to protect hands during activities such as cleaning and gardening.

  Animal feces are often present in garden soil and, if ingested, can lead to infection in an immunocompromised client.

- Take axillary rather than oral temperature if stomatitis is present.

  Axillary temperature assessment is more comfortable for a client with stomatitis.

- Lubricate skin frequently to prevent dryness and subsequent cracking.
- Maintain sterile technique when caring for a central venous or peritoneal catheter, an Ommaya reservoir, or an implanted infusion device (e.g., MediPort) if in place.

  Sterile technique is paramount when dealing with indwelling catheters to prevent catheter line sepsis.

- Avoid unnecessary rectal invasion (e.g., temperature taking, enemas, suppositories, sexual activity) to prevent rectal trauma.

  Damage or perforation of the bowel can lead to sepsis in an immunocompromised client.

- Avoid constipation to prevent damage to the bowel mucosa from hard or impacted stool.

  Adequate hydration prevents constipation.

---

*The nurse should select the nursing diagnostic label that is most appropriate for the client's discharge teaching needs.

THERAPEUTIC INTERVENTIONS	RATIONALE
• Wash perianal area thoroughly with soap and water after each bowel movement and after sexual activity; instruct female client to always wipe from front to back after urination and defecation.	*Prevents cross contamination between the vagina and the rectum. Actions prevent urinary tract contamination from faecal bacteria.*
• Drink at least 10 glasses of liquid a day unless contraindicated.	*Maintains adequate hydration.*
• Cough and deep breathe or use incentive spirometer every 2 hours until usual activity is resumed.	*Supports lung expansion and movement of secretions if present* *Coughing and deep breathing keep alveoli expanded, improve gas exchange, and facilitate expectoration of secretions, preventing pneumonia.*
• Stop smoking.	*Smoking damages the mucociliary system, which helps facilitate the expectoration of secretions.* *Prevents chronic lung irritation and paralyzing of cilia.*
• Perform meticulous oral hygiene after meals and at bedtime, change denture care solution daily, and replace toothbrush routinely.	*Maintains oral hydration and prevents oral infections.*
• Avoid douching unless ordered.	*Douching disturbs normal vaginal flora and may cause trauma to the vaginal mucosa.* *Prevents loss of normal flora.*
• Maintain an optimal nutritional status (e.g., diet high in protein, calories, vitamins, and minerals).	*Maintains wellness and body's ability to fight infection.*
• Avoid sharing eating utensils.	*Prevents infection.*
• Maintain an adequate balance between activity and rest.	
• Cleanse respiratory equipment as instructed; change water in humidifiers daily.	*Prevents infection.*
• Decrease risk of food-borne illness:	*Prevents infection or illness from food sources.*
• Avoid intake of foods with a high microorganism content (e.g., unwashed fruits and vegetables; undercooked eggs, meat, poultry, and seafood).	
• Be sure that juices and ciders are pasteurized or processed and that milk and cheese are pasteurized.	
• Thoroughly wash hands and food preparation items and surfaces (e.g., knives, cutting board, countertop) before and after cooking, especially when working with raw meat, poultry, and fish.	
• Thaw food items in the refrigerator rather than on kitchen counter.	
• Avoid picking up animal waste or cleaning animal litter boxes and bird cages.	
• Avoid elective surgery and dental work.	
• Reinforce the importance of taking prescribed medications such as colony-stimulating factors and prophylactic antimicrobial agents.	

THERAPEUTIC INTERVENTIONS	RATIONALE

Desired Outcome: The client will demonstrate appropriate oral hygiene techniques.

Independent Actions

Explain the rationale for and importance of frequent oral hygiene.	*Frequent oral hygiene is necessary in the neutropenic client to keep the oral cavity clean, moist, and free of bacterial infection so adequate nutritional intake can occur.*
Provide instructions regarding oral hygiene techniques:	
• Cleanse mouth after eating and at bedtime; increase frequency to every 2 hours if stomatitis is present.	
• Use a soft bristle toothbrush.	*Prevents trauma to fragile mucous membranes*
• Rinse mouth with the following solutions as prescribed:	*Reduces oral dryness*
• Salt or baking soda and warm water	
• Chlorhexidine gluconate (Peridex)	

Continued...

THERAPEUTIC INTERVENTIONS	RATIONALE
• Mist oral cavity frequently using a spray bottle and/or take sips of water frequently.	
• Avoid commercial mouthwashes that have an alcohol base.	*These are drying to the oral mucosa.*

THERAPEUTIC INTERVENTIONS	RATIONALE

Desired Outcome: The client will verbalize ways to improve appetite and nutritional status.

Independent Actions

Instruct client in methods to control nausea and vomiting:

• Eat foods that are cool or room temperature (hot foods frequently have an overpowering aroma that stimulates nausea).

• Eat dry foods (e.g., toast, crackers) or sip cold carbonated beverages if nausea is present.

• Eat several small meals per day instead of three large ones.

• Avoid drinking liquids with meals.

• Select bland foods (e.g., mashed potatoes, cottage cheese) rather than fatty, spicy foods.

• Rest after eating.

• If feasible, have someone else prepare the food.

• Avoid offensive odors and sights.

• Cleanse mouth frequently.

• Take deep, slow breaths when nauseated.

• Take antiemetics on a regular basis for prescribed length of time and if nausea is persistent.

Instruct client in ways to improve appetite and maintain an adequate nutritional status:

• Try fish, cheese, chicken, and eggs as protein sources instead of beef and pork if taste distortion is a problem.

• Increase amount of sugar or sweeteners and seasonings usually used in foods and beverages.

• Use plastic utensils and cook food in glass or plastic containers if metallic taste is present.

• Eat in a pleasant environment with company if possible.

• Perform frequent, meticulous oral hygiene to eliminate unpleasant tastes in mouth.

• Try recommended methods of controlling nausea.

• Eat several high-calorie, high-protein, nutritious small meals each day rather than three large ones; use nutritional supplements if needed to maintain an adequate caloric intake.

• Plan ahead for low-energy days (e.g., have some prepared meals available; maintain an ample supply of nutritious, minimal preparation foods such as eggs, tuna fish, cheese, peanut butter, and yogurt; keep nutritious snacks and beverages within easy reach).

• Take vitamins, minerals, and appetite stimulants (e.g., megestrol acetate, dronabinol) as prescribed.

Nausea and vomiting commonly occur after chemotherapy and/or radiation. Prevention and control of nausea and vomiting are necessary to ensure adequate nutrition.

Cells of the mucosal lining of the stomach are highly proliferative. Intestinal mucosa is very sensitive to radiation and chemotherapy. Nausea, vomiting, diarrhea, mucositis, and anorexia are all gastrointestinal effects that can affect a client's nutritional status. Actions help facilitate optimum nutritional status for clients undergoing chemotherapy.

THERAPEUTIC INTERVENTIONS	RATIONALE

Desired Outcome: The client will verbalize ways to manage and cope with persistent fatigue.

THERAPEUTIC INTERVENTIONS	RATIONALE

Independent Actions

Instruct client in ways to manage and cope with persistent fatigue:

- View fatigue as a protective mechanism rather than a problematic limitation.
- Determine ways in which daily patterns of activity can be modified to conserve energy and prevent excessive fatigue (e.g., spread light and heavy tasks throughout the day, take short rests during an activity whenever possible, sit during an activity whenever possible, take several short rest periods during the day instead of one long one).
- Determine whether life demands are realistic in light of physical state and adjust short- and long-term goals accordingly.
- Avoid situations that are particularly fatiguing such as those that are boring, frustrating, or require prolonged or strenuous physical activity.
- Participate in a moderate exercise program (e.g., walking or bicycling 20-30 minutes 3-4 times/wk).
- Participate in "attention-restoring" activities (e.g., walking outside, gardening).

Fatigue affects most all clients undergoing chemotherapy and/or radiation. Fatigue may be related to anemia or side effects of therapy.

THERAPEUTIC INTERVENTIONS	RATIONALE

Desired Outcome: The client will verbalize ways to prevent bleeding when platelet counts are low.

Independent Actions

Instruct client in ways to minimize risk of bleeding:

- Avoid taking aspirin and other nonsteroidal anti-inflammatory agents (e.g., ibuprofen).
- Consult health care provider before routinely taking herbs that can increase the risk of bleeding (e.g., ginkgo, arnica, chamomile).
- Brush teeth gently using a soft bristle toothbrush; do not use dental floss or put sharp objects (e.g., toothpicks) in mouth.
- Use an electric rather than a straight-edge razor.
- Cut nails and cuticles carefully.
- Use caution when ambulating to prevent falls or bumps and do not walk barefoot.
- Be attentive when using scissors, knives, and tools to reduce the risk of cuts.
- Avoid contact sports and other activities that could result in injury.
- Avoid straining to have a bowel movement.
- Avoid blowing nose forcefully.
- Avoid wearing constrictive clothing (e.g., garters, knee-high stockings).
- Use an ample amount of water-soluble lubricant before sexual intercourse and avoid anal sexual activity, douching, use of rectal suppositories, and enemas in order to prevent trauma to the vaginal and rectal mucosa.
- Avoid heavy lifting.

Instruct client to control any bleeding by applying firm, prolonged pressure to the area if possible.

A client who is thrombocytopenic is at risk for increased bleeding and should be instructed on actions to prevent and/or control bleeding.

Continued...

THERAPEUTIC INTERVENTIONS	RATIONALE

Desired Outcome: The client will verbalize ways to adjust to alterations in reproductive and sexual functioning.

Independent Actions

Assure client that many of the side effects of chemotherapy (e.g., decreased libido, impotence) are temporary or can be treated.

Explain to the female client that ovarian failure during chemotherapy may result in irritability, hot flashes, and other symptoms of premature menopause.

Instruct client in the childbearing years to use contraception during chemotherapy and for at least 2 years after completion of chemotherapy (many cytotoxic drugs cause genetic abnormalities in the developing fetus).

Encourage client to rest before sexual activity if fatigue is a problem.

Instruct client in measures to decrease discomfort associated with decreased vaginal secretions and mucositis:

* Use an ample amount of water-soluble lubricant before intercourse.
* Use vaginal steroid cream if prescribed to ease dryness and inflammation if present.
* Take a sitz bath 2 to 3 times a day.
* Avoid intercourse until mucositis of the vaginal canal resolves.

Instruct client to take hormone replacements (e.g., estrogen, testosterone) as prescribed.

Reproductive and sexual dysfunction vary depending upon treatment protocol. Clients should be educated as to appropriate alternatives to reproductive and sexual dysfunction.

THERAPEUTIC INTERVENTIONS	RATIONALE

Desired Outcome: The client will verbalize ways to promote independence and prevent injury if neuropathies are present.

Independent Actions

Instruct client in measures to promote independence and prevent injury if neuropathies are present:

* Use adaptive devices to facilitate performance of activities of daily living (e.g., zipper pulls; buttoners; molded sock aids; elastic shoe laces or Velcro straps; special pens, pencils, or utensils that are easy to grasp).
* Take extra precautions to prevent falls (e.g., have handrails in hallways and tubs and showers, avoid unnecessary clutter in pathways, wear shoes/slippers with nonskid soles, secure all carpets/rugs).
* Adhere to precautions to prevent burns (e.g., check temperature of bath water [should be <110°F], wear mitts when handling hot items) and cuts (e.g., shield fingers when using a sharp knife, avoid the use of motorized tools such as lawnmowers and saws, use adapted nail clippers).

Helps client to maintain independence as much as possible and prevent injury.

THERAPEUTIC INTERVENTIONS	RATIONALE

Desired Outcome: The client will demonstrate the ability to care for a central venous catheter, a peritoneal catheter, or an implanted infusion device if in place.

Independent Actions

Provide instructions related to care of a central venous catheter (e.g., Groshong) if appropriate:

* Change dressing if present according to protocol using aseptic technique.

Clients should be instructed on the proper care of indwelling catheters to avoid catheter-related sepsis.

THERAPEUTIC INTERVENTIONS	RATIONALE

• Observe exit site for changes in appearance, redness, swelling, and unusual drainage.
• Flush catheter according to protocol to maintain patency.
• Replace injection cap as directed.
• Tape catheter securely to the chest wall to prevent accidental dislodgment.
• Notify physician if unable to flush catheter, if signs and symptoms of infection occur at exit site, or if catheter appears to be leaking.
Provide instructions related to care of a peritoneal catheter if in place:
• Change dressing according to protocol using aseptic technique.
• Keep catheter capped between treatments.
• Keep water below the level of the catheter when taking a tub bath (a tub bath may be taken 7-10 days after catheter insertion).
• Observe for and notify physician if any of the following occur:
    • Redness, swelling, or change in appearance of insertion site
    • Unusual drainage from exit site
    • Increasing abdominal pain
    • Chills or fever
    • Increased abdominal distention between treatments
    • Persistent nausea or vomiting
    • Dyspnea
Provide instructions related to care of an implanted infusion device (e.g., MediPort, Port-a-Cath) if in place:
• Keep appointment to have device flushed or flush as instructed.
• Avoid trauma to insertion site.
• Notify physician if area around infusion device becomes reddened or painful.
	Clients should be instructed on the proper maintenance of implanted infusion devices to ensure catheter patency and prevent infection.

THERAPEUTIC INTERVENTIONS	RATIONALE
Desired Outcome: The client will verbalize an understanding of the care and precautions necessary if an Ommaya reservoir is in place. **Independent Actions** Provide instructions related to care and precautions necessary if an Ommaya reservoir is in place: • Wash site daily with soap and water. • Observe for and report redness, drainage, or discomfort at insertion site; stiff neck; persistent headache; or persistent nausea and vomiting. • Avoid activities that could result in trauma to the head and damage to the reservoir (e.g., contact sports).	*Clients should be instructed on the proper care of the reservoir site to prevent both infection and device damage.*

THERAPEUTIC INTERVENTIONS	RATIONALE
Desired Outcome: The client will verbalize an understanding of an implanted infusion pump and precautions necessary if one is in place. **Independent Actions** Reinforce physician's explanation about the purpose of the infusion pump and how it works.	*Allows for client understanding and ability to care for self, while maintaining some degree of independence.*

NDx = NANDA-I Diagnosis **D** = Delegatable Action ● = UAP ✦ = LVN/LPN ⊜▶ = Go to ⊜volve for animation

Continued...

THERAPEUTIC INTERVENTIONS	RATIONALE

Instruct client to avoid activities that could result in abdominal trauma and dislodgment of pump.

Caution client to notify physician if:

- Air travel is planned (client should carry an explanatory letter since pump may trigger airport weapon security devices; flow rate of pump may also need to be adjusted if the flight time is lengthy).
- Body temperature is elevated more than 2°F for more than 24 hours (an increase in vapor pressure in the pump can increase flow rate).
- Client plans to move to an area of greater or lesser altitude (alterations in the pump's flow rate may need to be made).
- Redness, swelling, or drainage occurs at incisional or refilling site.

Emphasize importance of keeping appointments to have pump refilled (permanent blockage of the catheter can occur if pump is allowed to empty completely).

THERAPEUTIC INTERVENTIONS	RATIONALE

Desired Outcome: The client will state signs and symptoms to report to the health care provider.

Independent Actions

Instruct client to observe for and report the following:

- Signs and symptoms of infection (stress that usual signs of infection are diminished in people with altered bone marrow function and/or a suppressed immune system and that it is necessary to monitor closely for the following signs and symptoms):
  - Temperature above 38°C (100.4°F)
  - Changes in odor, color, or consistency of urine or pain with urination
  - White patches in mouth
  - Crusted ulcerations around or in oral cavity
  - Swollen, reddened, coated tongue
  - Painful rectal or vaginal area
  - Unusual vaginal drainage
  - Changes in the appearance or temperature of skin, particularly around puncture sites
  - Persistent productive or nonproductive cough
- Signs and symptoms of bleeding (e.g., excessive bruising, black stools, persistent nosebleeds or bleeding from gums, sudden swelling in joints, red or smoke-colored urine, blood in vomitus)
- Signs and symptoms of hemorrhagic cystitis (e.g., blood in urine, pain on urination, urinary frequency or urgency)
- Signs and symptoms of extravasation (e.g., coolness, pain, swelling, and/or skin changes at infusion site)
- Signs and symptoms of pulmonary dysfunction (e.g., shortness of breath; persistent, dry, hacking cough; fever)
- Signs and symptoms of dehydration (e.g., dry mouth, significant weight loss, concentrated urine, lightheadedness)
- Signs and symptoms of cardiotoxicity (e.g., irregular or rapid heart rate, increased weakness and fatigue, shortness of breath, unexplained weight gain, swelling of extremities); emphasize that cardiotoxicity can occur several days to months after administration of drugs known to cause it.

Prompt reporting of adverse signs and symptoms allows for modification of the treatment plan and may reduce the risk of complications.

THERAPEUTIC INTERVENTIONS	RATIONALE
• New or increased signs and symptoms of neurotoxicity (e.g., numbness and tingling of extremities, change in hearing acuity, blurred vision, constipation, change in motor function and coordination, burning pain in extremity, impaired memory or ability to communicate)	
• Persistent diarrhea, nausea, vomiting, and/or decreased oral intake	
• Significant weight loss	
• Inability to cope with the effects of the diagnosis and treatment	
Instruct client to keep a record of signs and symptoms, activities at the time the symptoms occur, measures taken to achieve relief, and the effect of the measures taken.	*Detailed accounts of signs and symptoms can aid practitioners in the formulation of appropriate interventions.*
Instruct client to take the information to each appointment with the health care provider.	

THERAPEUTIC INTERVENTIONS	RATIONALE

Desired Outcome: The client will identify community resources that can assist with home management and adjustment to the diagnosis of cancer and chemotherapy and its effects.

Independent Actions

Provide information about and encourage use of community resources that can assist client and significant others with home management and adjustment to diagnosis of cancer and chemotherapy and its effects (e.g., American Cancer Society, counselors, social service agencies, Meals on Wheels, Make Today Count, Look Good-Feel Better Program, hospice, community support groups).	*Actions can assist clients in coping with the psychoemotional issues associated with chemotherapy. Actions can help clients manage their illness and normalize their experiences.*

THERAPEUTIC INTERVENTIONS	RATIONALE

Desired Outcome: The client will verbalize an understanding of and a plan for adhering to recommended follow-up care including medications prescribed and schedule for chemotherapy, laboratory studies, and future appointments with health care provider.

Independent Actions

Thoroughly explain rationale for, side effects of, and importance of taking medications prescribed. Inform client of pertinent food and drug interactions.	*Improves client's adherence to treatment regimen.*

Reinforce physician's explanation of planned chemotherapy schedule.

Discuss with client any difficulties with adhering to the schedule and assist in planning ways to overcome these.

Reinforce importance of keeping appointments for chemotherapy and laboratory studies.

Reinforce importance of keeping follow-up appointments with health care provider.

Implement measures to improve client compliance:

- Include significant others in teaching sessions.
- Encourage questions and allow time for reinforcement and clarification of information provided.
- Provide written instructions regarding ways to maintain nutritional status, future appointments with health care provider and laboratory, medications prescribed, and signs and symptoms to report.

NDx = NANDA-I Diagnosis   **D** = Delegatable Action   ● = UAP   ◆ = LVN/LPN   ⊖▶ = Go to ⊖volve for animation

ADDITIONAL NURSING DIAGNOSES

FEAR/ANXIETY NDx
Related to:
- Unfamiliar environment
- Lack of knowledge about chemotherapy including administration procedure, expected side effects, and impact on usual lifestyle and roles if admitted for chemotherapy
- Need for hospitalization to manage current side effects and/or toxic effects of chemotherapy and possibility of additional untoward effects with a subsequent cycle of chemotherapy
- Financial concerns
- Diagnosis of cancer with potential for premature death

NAUSEA NDx
Related to: Stimulation of the vomiting center associated with:
- The effect of some cytotoxic drugs (those with a high emetic potential include carboplatin, cisplatin, dacarbazine, mechlorethamine, streptozocin, and carmustine), the by-products of cellular destruction, and the foul taste created by some cytotoxic agents
- Stimulation of the visceral afferent pathways resulting from inflammation of the gastrointestinal mucosa if mucositis is present
- Stimulation of the cerebral cortex resulting from stress and a conditioned response to previous experience with nausea and vomiting after the administration of cytotoxic drugs

FATIGUE NDx
Related to:
- A buildup of cellular waste products associated with rapid lysis of cancerous and normal cells exposed to cytotoxic drugs
- Difficulty resting and sleeping associated with fear, anxiety, and discomfort
- Tissue hypoxia associated with anemia (a result of malnutrition and chemotherapy-induced bone marrow suppression)
- Overwhelming emotional demands associated with the diagnosis of cancer and treatment with chemotherapy
- Increased energy expenditure associated with an increase in the metabolic rate resulting from continuous, active tumor growth and increased levels of certain cytokines (e.g., tumor necrosis factor, interleukin-1)
- Malnutrition
- Side effects of other medications client may be receiving (e.g., narcotic [opioid] analgesics, antiemetics, antianxiety agents, biotherapy agents such as interferons and interleukins)

DIARRHEA NDx
Related to: Increased peristalsis and disorders of intestinal secretion and absorption associated with inflammation and ulceration of the gastrointestinal mucosa resulting from effects of cytotoxic drugs (particularly many of the antimetabolites, topoisomerase-1 inhibitors, and antitumor antibiotics) on the rapidly dividing epithelial cells in the intestine

RISK FOR INFECTION NDx
Related to: Lowered natural resistance associated with:
- Malnutrition
- Chemotherapy-induced bone marrow suppression
- Long-term treatment with corticosteroids (may be used in treatment of certain types of cancer)
- Disruption in normal, endogenous microbial flora resulting from antimicrobial therapy
- Impaired immune system functioning resulting from certain malignancies (e.g., Hodgkin's disease, lymphoma, multiple myeloma, leukemia)
- Break in mucosal surfaces
- Break in skin integrity
- Stasis of secretions in lungs

GRIEVING NDx
Related to:
- Changes in body image and usual roles and lifestyle
- Diagnosis of cancer with potential for premature death

RISK FOR IMPAIRED SKIN INTEGRITY NDx
Related to:
- Increased skin fragility associated with malnutrition and dryness (a result of the effects of cytotoxic drugs on sebaceous and sweat glands)
- Frequent contact of the skin with irritants associated with diarrhea if present
- Damage to the skin and/or subcutaneous tissue associated with prolonged pressure on tissues, friction, or shearing if mobility is decreased

RISK FOR CONSTIPATION NDx
Related to: Decreased gastrointestinal motility associated with:
- Autonomic neuropathy resulting from some cytotoxic drugs (e.g., vinblastine, teniposide, vindesine, vinorelbine)
- Depressant effect of medications administered to control symptoms such as pain, nausea, and vomiting (e.g., narcotic [opioid] analgesics, some antiemetics)
- Decreased activity
- Increased sympathetic nervous system activity resulting from anxiety
- Decreased intake of fiber and fluids

SELF-CARE DEFICIT NDx
Related to:
- Fatigue, weakness, and discomfort
- Sedation associated with the effects of some medications administered to control pain, anxiety, nausea, and vomiting
- Tactile and proprioceptive impairments associated with the neurotoxic effects of some cytotoxic agents (particularly platinum, procarbazine, paclitaxel, or etoposide)

DISTURBED SLEEP PATTERN NDx
Related to:
- Nausea, vomiting, and pain
- Anxiety, fear, and grief
- Frequent need to defecate associated with diarrhea if present

INEFFECTIVE COPING/IMPAIRED ADJUSTMENT

Related to: Persistent discomfort associated with the side effects of chemotherapy, fear, anxiety, chronic fatigue, feeling of powerlessness, and uncertainty of prognosis

RISK FOR POWERLESSNESS NDx

Related to:
- The possibility of disease progression and death despite treatment

- Dependence on others to assist with basic needs as a result of fatigue, weakness, and discomfort
- Possible alterations in roles, relationships, and future plans associated with changes that occur as a result of the cancer and the side effects/toxic effects of the cytotoxic drugs

⊖▶ EXTERNAL RADIATION THERAPY (TELETHERAPY)

Radiation therapy is one of the four major modes of treatment for cancer. It can be either external (teletherapy) or internal (brachytherapy) and is a local treatment in which cellular destruction occurs only at the treatment site. It is most effective on well-oxygenated tumors with a high growth fraction. Unfortunately, radiation therapy is not a selective process, and changes in cellular structure and function occur in both cancerous and normal cells within the treatment field. The normal cells, however, have a greater capacity for self-repair.

The effect of radiation therapy on the cell begins immediately and continues through several reproductive cycles of the cell. The time of cellular death and the side effects experienced by the client depend on the number of grays (Gy) or centigrays (cGy) received, the volume of tissue irradiated, whether or not both strands of DNA are broken, the extent of the damage to the cell's reproductive abilities, and the cell's ability to repair damage. The side effects that most clients receiving external radiation experience are a skin reaction at the radiation treatment site, fatigue, malaise, and anorexia. Other side effects experienced depend on the anatomic site being radiated, the mitotic rate of the cells within the treatment field, fractionation of the dose, total dose delivered, and the general condition of the client.

Although it may be used alone, radiation therapy is increasingly being used in combination with surgery, chemotherapy, and/or biotherapy to achieve palliation, control, or cure of cancer. External radiation is also used with brachytherapy to treat certain cancers (e.g., prostate, endometrial) more effectively. Radiation therapy in combination with surgical treatment of some cancers has resulted in the need for less extensive surgery.

Minimization of damage to normal tissue with maximum tumor kill is a primary goal of radiation therapy. This goal is being accomplished more frequently as a result of advances in technology and techniques. Computerized three-dimensional treatment planning provides more accurate targeting of tumor tissue, and the use of equipment that contains multiple computer-operated shields results in preservation of a greater amount of the normal tissue surrounding the tumor. Radiosensitizers that increase the sensitivity of tumor cells to radiation, and radioprotectants that help protect normal cells from radiation damage may be used during teletherapy for some clients to achieve this same goal. In addition, changes in standard radiation protocols (e.g., more frequent, smaller doses of radiation) are being made in some instances to increase tumor cell kill and decrease damage to normal cells.

This care plan focuses on the adult client hospitalized for initiation of external radiation therapy or
for management of side effects associated with radiation therapy. Much of the information is applicable to the client undergoing treatment on an outpatient basis.

OUTCOME/DISCHARGE CRITERIA

The client will:
1. Have an adequate or improved nutritional status
2. Have fatigue at a manageable level
3. Have evidence of normal healing of skin at site of irradiation
4. Have no signs and symptoms of complications of radiation therapy
5. Verbalize an understanding of appropriate skin care for site of irradiation
6. Identify techniques to control nausea and vomiting
7. Verbalize ways to improve appetite and nutritional status
8. Identify ways to reduce the risk of dental caries and periodontal disease and manage stomatitis if present
9. Identify ways to prevent bleeding if platelet counts are low
10. Identify ways to prevent infection if WBC counts are low
11. Verbalize an understanding of and ways to manage the effects of radiation therapy on sexual and reproductive functioning
12. Verbalize ways to manage and cope with persistent fatigue
13. Verbalize an understanding of the signs and symptoms of lymphedema and ways to manage it if it occurs
14. State signs and symptoms to report to the health care provider
15. Share feelings and thoughts about the diagnosis of cancer and the effects of radiation therapy on body image
16. Identify community resources that can assist with home management and adjustment to the diagnosis of cancer and radiation therapy and its effects
17. Verbalize an understanding of and a plan for adhering to recommended follow-up care including medications prescribed and future appointments with health care provider, radiation department, and laboratory

For a full, detailed care plan on this topic, go to http://evolve.elsevier.com/Haugen/careplanning/.

NDx = NANDA-I Diagnosis   **D** = Delegatable Action   ● = UAP   ✦ = LVN/LPN   ⊖▶ = Go to ⊖volve for animation

⊖▶ INTERNAL RADIATION THERAPY (BRACHYTHERAPY)

Internal radiation therapy (brachytherapy) involves either permanent or temporary placement of a radioactive isotope directly into a tumor (interstitial) or near a tumor (intracavity or intraluminal). Brachytherapy can be used alone or as part of a multimodal treatment approach for the purpose of controlling local disease, treating areas at high risk for disease reoccurrence, preserving vital organ function, and sparing damage to normal tissue. Brachytherapy is used for a variety of gynecological, breast, head, neck, lung, liver, colon, bladder, and prostate cancers.

Brachytherapy is classified according to the location of the implant (intracavity, interstitial, surface [mold/plaques]), type of loading (hot, manual afterload, remote afterload), dose rate (low, medium, high), duration of treatment (permanent, temporary), or type of emission (gamma, beta, neutron). Brachytherapy is indicated for the following uses: (1) alone in the treatment of small localized tumors; (2) alone or in combination with chemotherapy, surgery, or hyperthermia; (3) for the purpose of shrinking more bulky tumors; and (4) in palliative cases to reduce overall treatment time.

Nurses providing direct care to patients undergoing internal radiation therapy must adhere to safety precautions designed to keep occupational exposure to radiation at the lowest possible level. Safety precautions are based on the key principles of time, distance, and shielding. To reduce occupational exposure, nurses should limit the time in direct contact to 30 minutes per 8-hour shift. The intensity of the radiation decreases as the distance from the source of the radiation increases. Finally, whenever possible, nurses should stay behind a lead shield device when handling radioactive sources or interacting with patients. Lead shielding can be very cumbersome in practice and provide a false sense of security to the nurse. Maximizing distance and efficient time management often provide nurses with adequate protection. Nurses caring for radioactive patients should wear some type of personal monitoring device to monitor and track exposure. It is recommended that nurses providing care for these patients should be rotated to prevent constant exposure.

This care plan focuses on the adult client hospitalized for initiation of internal radiation therapy or for management of side effects associated with radiation therapy. Much of the information is applicable to the client undergoing treatment on an outpatient basis.

OUTCOME/DISCHARGE CRITERIA

The client will:
1. Have an adequate or improved nutritional status
2. Have fatigue at a manageable level
3. Have evidence of normal healing of skin at the site of irradiation
4. Have no signs and symptoms of complications of radiation therapy
5. Verbalize an understanding of appropriate skin care for the site of irradiation
6. Verbalize ways to improve appetite and nutritional status
7. Verbalize an understanding of and ways to manage the effects of radiation therapy on sexual and reproductive functioning
8. Verbalize ways to manage and cope with persistent fatigue
9. Verbalize an understanding of the signs and symptoms of lymphedema and ways to manage it if it occurs
10. State signs and symptoms to report to the health care provider
11. Share feelings and thoughts about the diagnosis of cancer and the effects of radiation therapy on body image
12. Identify community resources that can assist with home management and adjustment to the diagnosis of cancer and radiation therapy and its effects
13. Verbalize an understanding of and a plan for adhering to recommended follow-up care including medications prescribed and future appointments with health care provider, radiation department, and laboratory.

Go to *http://evolve.elsevier.com/Haugen/careplanning/* for the full, detailed care plan.

15 Nursing Care of the Elderly Client

Persons who are 65 and older are the fastest growing segment of the population, making the elderly a major portion of the health care consumer population. Older persons are in the final stage of development during which many adaptations need to be made by the client because of the physiological changes that occur with aging. The extent or degree of the changes that take place depends on genetic and environmental factors as well as on the client's previous attention to health maintenance. As a client reaches old age, there may also be many changes in roles, relationships, and ability to maintain his/her usual lifestyle. These factors create psychosocial concerns that need to be addressed.

This care plan focuses on the elderly client needing health care. It includes the nursing diagnoses that reflect the biopsychosocial changes that commonly occur with old age and are intensified with the stressors of illness. This care plan can be used in conjunction with the care plans in this text that are appropriate to the client's specific medical diagnosis(es) or surgery and is intended for use in an acute or extended care facility or in a home setting.

Nursing Diagnosis **INEFFECTIVE TISSUE PERFUSION** NDx

Definition: Decrease in oxygen resulting in the failure to nourish the tissues at the capillary level

Related to:
- Decreased cardiac output associated with:
  - Impaired relaxation and contractility of the heart associated with stiffening of the ventricular walls
  - Increased cardiac workload resulting from an increase in vascular resistance, thickened and rigid cardiac valves, and stress of current illness
- Increased vascular resistance associated with decreased elasticity and increased rigidity of the arterial vessels associated with changes in the proportion of elastin and collagen in the vessel walls and accumulation of substances such as calcium and lipids
- Decrease in baroreceptor sensitivity
- Peripheral pooling of blood associated with loss of muscle tone in extremities, decreased competency of venous valves, and venous dilation (results from loss of vascular elasticity)

CLINICAL MANIFESTATIONS

Subjective	Objective
Reports of increased fatigue and weakness; confusion; reports dizziness or lightheadedness and syncopal episodes	Variations in blood pressure (B/P); irregular, rapid, or slow pulse; increase in loudness of existing murmurs; dyspnea; increased crackles; edema; jugular vein distention (JVD); changes in electrocardiogram (ECG); restlessness; cool, pale skin; decreased or absent peripheral pulses; capillary refill >2 to 3 seconds; elevated blood urea nitrogen (BUN) and serum creatinine levels; oliguria; claudication; angina

---

Continued...

RISK FACTORS

- Immobility
- Inadequate fluid intake
- Vascular changes

DESIRED OUTCOMES

The client will maintain adequate tissue perfusion as evidenced by:
a. B/P within normal range for client
b. Usual mental status
c. Absence of dizziness or lightheadedness and syncope
d. Extremities warm with absence of pallor and cyanosis
e. Palpable peripheral pulses
f. Capillary refill time <2 to 3 seconds
g. Absence of edema
h. BUN and serum creatinine levels within normal limits for an elderly client
i. Urine output ≥20 mL/h
j. Absence of exercise-induced pain

NOC OUTCOMES

Circulation status; cardiac pump effectiveness

NIC INTERVENTIONS

Circulatory care: arterial insufficiency; circulatory care: venous insufficiency; cardiac precautions

NURSING ASSESSMENT

Assess for and report signs and symptoms of:
- Decreased cardiac output (can lead to diminished tissue perfusion):
  - Variations in B/P

  - Irregular, rapid, or slow pulse

  - Increase in loudness of existing systolic murmurs or presence of diastolic murmur
  - Development of or an increase in loudness of S_3 and/or S_4 gallop rhythm
  - Development of or increase in fatigue and weakness
  - Development of or increase in dyspnea
  - New finding of or increased crackles
  - Edema
  - JVD
  - Abnormal ECG readings
  - Chest radiograph showing pleural effusion or pulmonary edema
- Diminished tissue perfusion:
  - Significant decrease in B/P

  - Decline in systolic B/P of >20 mm Hg when client changes from a lying to sitting or standing position
  - Restlessness, confusion, or other change in mental status
  - Reports of dizziness or lightheadedness or occurrence of syncopal episodes
  - Cool, pale, or cyanotic skin
  - Diminished or absent peripheral pulses
  - Capillary refill time >2 to 3 seconds
  - Edema
  - Elevated BUN and serum creatinine levels
  - Oliguria
  - Claudication
  - Angina

RATIONALE

Early recognition of signs and symptoms of decreased cardiac output allows for prompt intervention.

May be increased because of compensatory vasoconstriction and may be decreased when compensatory mechanisms and pump fail

The incidence of dysrhythmias increases with age and is of concern because of the coexisting decrease in cardiac reserve.

Soft systolic murmurs are often present in elderly clients because of sclerosed valves.

An S_4 can be present in healthy adult clients.

Crackles in the morning are a common finding in an elderly adult client.

Expected age-related changes include left axis deviation and some prolongation of the PR and QT intervals.

Elevated systolic B/P is often present in elderly clients because of the age-related stiffening of the arteries and impaired baroreceptor function.

In an elderly client, there is often a decline in systolic B/P of 12 to 20 mm Hg with this position change because of a decrease in baroreceptor sensitivity and vasomotor responsiveness.

The BUN and serum creatinine levels tend to be slightly elevated because of the age-related decline in renal function.

THERAPEUTIC INTERVENTIONS	RATIONALE

Independent Actions

Implement measures to maintain adequate tissue perfusion:

- Perform actions to reduce cardiac workload and help maintain an adequate cardiac output:
  - Place client in a semi- to high-Fowler's position whenever possible. **D** ● ✦ — *Prevents slumping*
  - Instruct client to avoid activities that create a Valsalva response (e.g., straining to have a bowel movement, holding breath while moving up in bed). — *These activities decrease the heart rate and subsequently cardiac output.*
  - Implement measures to promote rest and conserve energy (e.g., maintain activity restrictions, minimize environmental noise, limit number of visitors and length of stay). **D** ● ✦ — *Decreases stress on the heart and body's oxygenation demands*
  - Implement measures to maintain an adequate respiratory status (place in high Fowler's position, change position every 2 hours, instruct client in deep breathing exercises every 2 hours). **D** ● ✦ — *Promotes adequate tissue oxygenation*
  - Discourage smoking. — *Nicotine has a cardiostimulatory effect and causes vasoconstriction; the carbon monoxide in smoke reduces oxygen availability.*
  - Discourage excessive intake of beverages high in caffeine such as coffee, tea, and colas. **D** ✦ — *Caffeine is a myocardial stimulant and can increase myocardial oxygen consumption.*
  - Provide small meals rather than large ones. **D** ✦ — *Large meals can increase cardiac workload because they require an increase in blood supply to the gastrointestinal tract to aid digestion.*
  - Increase activity gradually as allowed and tolerated. **D** ✦ — *Improves stamina and cardiac functioning*
- Perform actions to reduce peripheral pooling of blood and increase venous return: — *Improves venous return to the heart*
  - Instruct client in and assist with active foot and leg exercises every 1 to 2 hours during periods of decreased activity.
  - Encourage and assist client with ambulation as allowed and tolerated. **D** ● ✦
- Instruct and assist client to change from a supine to an upright position slowly. **D** ● ✦ — *Allows time for autoregulatory mechanisms to adjust to the change in the distribution of blood associated with an upright position*
- Discourage positions that compromise blood flow in lower extremities (e.g., crossing legs, pillow under knees, use of knee gatch, sitting for long periods, prolonged standing). **D** ● ✦ — *These positions increase pooling of blood in the feet and leg, decreasing venous return to the heart.*
- Maintain a comfortable room temperature and provide client with adequate clothing and blankets. **D** ● ✦ — *Exposure to cold causes generalized vasoconstriction.*

Dependent/Collaborative Actions

Implement measures to maintain adequate tissue perfusion:

- Maintain a fluid intake of 1500 to 2000 mL/day unless contraindicated; if oral intake is inadequate or contraindicated, maintain intravenous and/or enteral fluid therapy as ordered. — *There is a greater risk for fluid overload in the elderly client because of the age-related decline in the kidney's ability to excrete a large volume of water in response to sudden volume excess.*

Consult appropriate health care provider if signs and symptoms of diminished tissue perfusion persist or worsen. — *Allows for prompt alterations in treatment plan.*

IMPAIRED RESPIRATORY FUNCTION*

Definition: Inability of an individual to maintain adequate ventilation of the respiratory tract and perfusion of oxygen (O_2) and carbon dioxide (CO_2) between the lungs and vascular system to maintain adequate tissue oxygenation

Ineffective breathing pattern (NDx)
Related to:
- Loss of alveolar elasticity (results in reduced efficiency of air expulsion)
- Decreased chest expansion associated with calcification of costal cartilage and weakened respiratory muscles
- Decreased responsiveness of chemoreceptors to hypoxia and hypercapnia

Ineffective airway clearance (NDx) Related to stasis of secretions associated with decreased activity during illness and an age-related decrease in ciliary activity and cough effectiveness
Impaired gas exchange (NDx)
Related to:
- Loss of effective lung surface associated with a reduced number of alveoli, changes in the alveolar walls, and accumulation of secretions in the bronchioles and alveoli (can result from ineffective airway clearance)
- Reduced airflow associated with loss of alveolar elasticity, restricted chest expansion, and premature closure of small airways
- Decreased pulmonary blood flow associated with a decrease in the number of capillaries surrounding the alveoli, fibrosis of the pulmonary vessels, and a generalized decrease in tissue perfusion

CLINICAL MANIFESTATIONS

Subjective	Objective
Reports of shortness of breath	Irritability, confusion, somnolence Dyspnea; orthopnea; use of accessory muscles when breathing; asymmetrical chest excursion; adventitious breath sounds; diminished or absent breath sounds; abnormal breath sounds; decreased oximetry results; abnormal chest radiograph

RISK FACTORS
- Sedentary lifestyle
- Chronic illness
- Respiratory system changes

DESIRED OUTCOMES

The client will experience adequate respiratory function as evidenced by:
- a. Normal rate and depth of respirations
- b. Absence of dyspnea
- c. Symmetrical chest excursion
- d. Usual or improved breath sounds
- e. Usual mental status
- f. Oximetry results within normal range for an elderly client
- g. Arterial blood gas values within normal range for an elderly client

NOC OUTCOMES

Respiratory status: ventilation; respiratory status: airway patency; respiratory status: gas exchange

NIC INTERVENTIONS

Respiratory monitoring; airway management; chest physiotherapy; oxygen therapy; cough enhancement

NURSING ASSESSMENT	RATIONALE
Assess for and report signs and symptoms of impaired respiratory function:	*Early recognition of signs and symptoms of impaired respiratory function allows for prompt intervention.*
• Rapid, shallow, or slow respirations	*Decreased oxygenation to the tissues*
• Dyspnea, orthopnea	*Results from alveolar collapse associated with age-related hypoven-*
• Use of accessory muscles when breathing	*tilation and decreased activity*
• Asymmetrical chest excursion	

*This diagnostic label includes the following nursing diagnoses: ineffective breathing pattern, ineffective airway clearance, and impaired gas exchange.

NURSING ASSESSMENT	RATIONALE
• Adventitious breath sounds (e.g., crackles [rales], rhonchi); crackles may be heard, especially on initial morning assessment	*Diminished sounds are often present in the elderly client because of reduced airflow.*
• Diminished or absent breath sounds	
• Cough	
• Restlessness, irritability	
• Confusion, somnolence	
• Abnormal arterial blood gas values (partial pressure of oxygen in arterial blood [PaO_2] is normally lower in the elderly client)	
• Significant decrease in oximetry results	*Oxygen saturation is normally lower in the elderly client.*
• Abnormal chest radiograph results	

THERAPEUTIC INTERVENTIONS	RATIONALE

Independent Actions

Implement measures to maintain an adequate respiratory status:

• Place client in a semi- to high-Fowler's position unless contraindicated; position with pillows. **D** ● ✦	*Prevents slumping and improves lung expansion*
• If client must remain flat in bed, assist with position change at least every 2 hours. **D** ● ✦	*Improves lung expansion and decreases stasis of lung secretions*
• Instruct client to deep breathe or use incentive spirometer every 1 to 2 hours.	*These actions improve lung expansion of mobilization of secretions.*
• Perform actions to decrease pain if present (e.g., splint/protect painful area during movement, administer prescribed analgesics before planned activity). **D** ● ✦	*Client will be hesitant to take deep breaths if pain is present.*
• Perform actions to decrease fear and anxiety (e.g., explain procedures, provide a calm environment). **D** ● ✦	*Fear and anxiety can cause the client to breathe in shallow and/or rapid breaths.*
• Instruct client in and assist with diaphragmatic and pursed-lip breathing techniques if indicated.	*Improves oxygenation*
• Instruct and assist client to cough or "huff" every 1 to 2 hours. **D** ✦	*Improves lung expansion and oxygenation*
• Discourage smoking.	*Irritants in smoke increase mucus production, further impair ciliary function, and can damage the bronchial and alveolar walls; the carbon monoxide decreases oxygen availability*
• Instruct client to avoid intake of gas-forming foods (e.g., beans, cabbage, cauliflower, onions), carbonated beverages, and large meals.	*Prevents gastric distention and pressure on the diaphragm*
• Maintain activity restrictions as ordered; increase activity gradually as allowed and tolerated. **D** ● ✦	*Improves cardiac output and exercise stamina*

Dependent/Collaborative Actions

Implement measures to maintain an adequate respiratory status:

• Implement measures to thin tenacious secretions and reduce dryness of the respiratory mucous membrane:	
• Maintain a fluid intake of 1500 to 2000 mL/day unless contraindicated. **D** ● ✦	*Maintains adequate vascular fluid volume*
• Humidify inspired air if ordered. **D** ✦	*Moisturizes air and helps to thin secretions*
• If client has difficulty mobilizing secretions:	
• Assist with or perform postural drainage therapy (PDT) if ordered.	*Helps to mobilize and excrete secretions*
• Consult physician about use of a mucolytic (e.g., acetylcysteine) or diluent or hydrating agent (e.g., water, saline) via nebulizer.	*These medications improve client's ability to expectorate secretions*
• Suction as needed.	

NDx = NANDA-I Diagnosis   **D** = Delegatable Action   ● = UAP   ✦ = LVN/LPN   ⊖▶ = Go to ⊖volve for animation

Continued...

THERAPEUTIC INTERVENTIONS	RATIONALE
• Assist with positive airway pressure techniques (e.g., continuous positive airway pressure [CPAP], bilevel positive airway pressure [BiPAP], flutter/positive expiratory pressure [PEP] device) if ordered.	*Manually removes secretions*
• Maintain oxygen therapy if ordered. **D** ✦	*Provides supplemental oxygenation to support tissue requirements*
• Administer central nervous system depressants judiciously because of their respiratory depressant effect; hold medication and consult physician if respiratory rate is <12 breaths/min.	*The possibility of respiratory depression is increased in the elderly because of their altered metabolism, distribution and excretion of drugs, and decreased responsiveness of chemoreceptors to hypoxia and hypercapnia.*
Consult appropriate health care provider (e.g., physician, respiratory therapist) if signs and symptoms of impaired respiratory function persist or worsen.	*Allows for prompt alteration in treatment plan*

Nursing Diagnosis **RISK FOR DEFICIENT FLUID VOLUME** NDx

Definition: Decreased intravascular, interstitial, and/or intracellular fluid. This refers to dehydration, water loss alone without change in sodium.

Related to:
• Age-related decrease in total body water
• Decreased fluid intake associated with:
  • Restrictions imposed by current illness and/or treatment plan
  • Diminished thirst sensation
  • Desire to avoid nocturia and/or urinary incontinence
• Age-related decline in kidney's ability to conserve water when a deficit is caused by disease or environmental factors

CLINICAL MANIFESTATIONS

Subjective	Objective
Report of dry mouth, report of confusion	Decreased skin turgor; dry skin and mucous membranes; weight loss of 2% or greater over a short period; hypotension; weak, rapid pulse; capillary refill time >2 to 3 seconds; flat neck veins when lying flat; elevated BUN, serum creatinine, and hematocrit (Hct) levels; oliguria; change in mental status; decreased urine output

RISK FACTORS
• Changes in regulatory systems
• Inadequate fluid intake
• Medication regimen

DESIRED OUTCOMES

The client will not experience deficient fluid volume as evidenced by:
  a. Normal skin and tongue turgor for client
  b. Moist mucous membranes
  c. Stable weight
  d. B/P and pulse within normal range for client with no further increase in postural hypotension
  e. Capillary refill time <2 to 3 seconds
  f. BUN and Hct levels within normal range for age
  g. Usual mental status
  h. Balanced intake and output

NOC OUTCOMES

Fluid balance

NIC INTERVENTIONS

Fluid monitoring; fluid management; hypovolemia management; intravenous (IV) therapy

NURSING ASSESSMENT	RATIONALE
Assess for and report signs and symptoms of deficient fluid volume:	*Early recognition of signs and symptoms of deficient fluid volume allows for prompt intervention.*
• Decreased skin turgor	*Not always a reliable indicator because decreased skin turgor is a normal age-related change; turgor is best assessed over the forehead or sternum in an elderly client.*
• Decreased tongue turgor	*The tongue will be smaller than usual and have more than one longitudinal furrow.*
• Dry mucous membranes, thirst	*Thirst may not be a reliable indicator because saliva production and sensation of thirst are diminished in elderly clients.*
• Weight loss of 2% or greater over a short period	*May indicate fluid loss*
• Low B/P and/or decline in systolic B/P of >20 mm Hg when client sits up	*A drop of 15 to 20 mm Hg is not unusual in elderly clients because of decreased baroreceptor sensitivity and vasomotor responsiveness.*
• Weak, rapid pulse	*Indicates decreased vascular volume*
• Capillary refill time >2 to 3 seconds	
• Neck veins flat when client is supine	
• Elevated BUN and Hct levels	
• Change in mental status (e.g., confusion)	*Indicates decreased volume to maintain cerebral perfusion pressure*
• Decreased urine output	*Indicates an actual rather than potential fluid volume deficit*

THERAPEUTIC INTERVENTIONS	RATIONALE
Independent Actions	
Implement measures to prevent deficient fluid volume:	*Maintains adequate vascular volume*
• Maintain a fluid intake of 1200 to 2500 mL/day and instruct client to continue this regimen after discharge unless contraindicated. **D** ● ✦	
Dependent /Collaborative Actions	
Implement measures to prevent deficient fluid volume:	
• Maintain IV and/or enteral fluid therapy if ordered.	*Administer IV fluids cautiously because the elderly client is also at risk for fluid overload.*

Nursing Diagnosis IMBALANCED NUTRITION: LESS THAN BODY REQUIREMENTS NDx

Definition: Intake of nutrients insufficient to meet metabolic needs

Related to:
- Decreased oral intake associated with:
  - Anorexia resulting from factors such as depression, loneliness, diminished sense of smell and/or taste, early satiety, and dyspepsia
  - Difficulty chewing and swallowing food resulting from poor dentition, a decreased amount of saliva, and weakened chewing and swallowing muscles
  - Decreased ability to purchase and/or prepare healthy foods
- Decreased utilization of nutrients associated with impaired digestion resulting from:
  - Decreased ability to chew foods thoroughly
  - Reduced secretion of digestive enzymes (e.g., salivary ptyalin, hydrochloric acid, pepsin, lipase)
- Reduced absorption of nutrients associated with hypochlorhydria, decreased intestinal blood flow, and atrophy of the absorptive surface of the intestine

CLINICAL MANIFESTATIONS

Subjective	Objective
Reports of abdominal pain and cramping; sore buccal cavity	Aversion to eating; body weight 20% or more under ideal; capillary fragility; hair loss; lack of food; lack of interest in food; pale mucous membranes; low serum albumin, prealbumin, Hct, and hemoglobin (Hgb) levels; and low lymphocyte count

NDx = NANDA-I Diagnosis   **D** = Delegatable Action   ● = UAP   ✦ = LVN/LPN   ⊖▶ = Go to ⊖volve for animation

Continued...

RISK FACTORS

- Living on a fixed income
- Changes in taste sensation
- Medication regimen

DESIRED OUTCOMES

The client will maintain an adequate nutritional status as evidenced by:
- a. Weight within normal range for client
- b. Normal serum albumin, prealbumin, Hct, and Hgb levels and normal lymphocyte count for client's age
- c. Usual strength and activity tolerance
- d. Healthy oral mucous membrane

NOC OUTCOMES

Nutritional status

NIC INTERVENTIONS

Nutritional monitoring; appetite; nutrition management; nutrition therapy; nutritional counseling

NURSING ASSESSMENT	RATIONALE
Assess for and report signs and symptoms of malnutrition:	*Early recognition of signs and symptoms of malnutrition allows for prompt intervention.*
• Weight significantly below client's usual weight or below normal for client's age, height, and body frame	*Indicates that client has not maintained a proper diet. When using height and weight charts, be aware that weight is expected to decline gradually with age.*
• Low serum albumin, prealbumin, Hct, and Hgb levels and low lymphocyte count	*These indicate protein depletion. Low Hct and Hgb levels and low white blood cell (WBC) count lead to anemia and potential infections.*
• Weakness and fatigue	
• Sore, inflamed oral mucous membrane	
• Pale conjunctiva	
• Lower-than-normal anthropometric measurements such as skinfold thickness, body circumferences (e.g., hip, waist, mid-upper arm), and bioelectrical impedance analysis	
Monitor percentage of meals and snacks client consumes. Report a pattern of inadequate intake.	

THERAPEUTIC INTERVENTIONS	RATIONALE
Independent Actions	
Implement measures to maintain an adequate nutritional status:	
• Perform actions to improve oral intake:	
• Implement measures to relieve dyspepsia, gastric fullness, and gas pain. **D** ● ✦	*Decreases pressure in the abdomen which helps to improve appetite*
• Increase activity as allowed and tolerated. **D** ● ✦	*Activity usually promotes a sense of well-being, which can improve appetite; it also promotes gastric emptying, which reduces feeling of gastric fullness.*
• Maintain a clean environment and a relaxed, pleasant atmosphere. **D** ● ✦	*Helps improve appetite*
• Implement measures to decrease sense of isolation and aloneness (e.g., use touch to demonstrate acceptance; encourage significant others to visit; schedule time to sit and speak with the client each day).	*Promotes a sense of well-being, which can improve appetite*
• Encourage a rest period before meals if client is weak or fatigues easily. **D** ● ✦	*Fatigue can reduce the client's desire and ability to eat.*
• Provide frequent, small meals rather than large ones if client is weak, fatigues easily, and/or has a poor appetite. **D** ● ✦	
• Provide oral hygiene before eating. **D** ● ✦	*Oral hygiene moistens the mouth, which may make it easier to chew and swallow; it also removes unpleasant tastes, which often improves the taste of foods/fluids.*
• Serve foods/fluids that are appealing to client. **D** ● ✦	*Visual appeal is especially important if sense of smell is diminished.*

THERAPEUTIC INTERVENTIONS	RATIONALE
• Encourage significant others to bring in client's favorite foods unless contraindicated and eat with client to make eating more of a familiar social experience. **D** ✦	*Clients may be more inclined to eat food they like.*
• Provide a soft, ground, or pureed diet if client has difficulty chewing.	*Easier for client to chew and swallow*
• Implement measures to compensate for taste alterations and/or dislike of prescribed diet:	
(1) Serve foods warm to stimulate sense of smell. **D** ● ✦	*Improves taste of foods that should be served warm and can improve intake*
(2) Encourage client to experiment with different flavorings and seasonings. **D** ● ✦	*Adds different flavors*
(3) Instruct client to use salt substitutes and salt-free herbs and spices if receiving a low-sodium diet.	*Decreases salt intake and subsequent fluid retention*
(4) Encourage client to add extra sweeteners to foods unless contraindicated.	*Helps improve taste of foods*
(5) Provide alternative sources of protein if meats such as beef or pork taste bitter or rancid.	*Improves nutritional status*
• Limit fluid intake with meals. **D** ✦	*Unless the fluid has high nutritional value, the fluid should be avoided as it may cause early satiety and subsequent decreased food intake.*
• Allow adequate time for meals; reheat foods/fluids if necessary. **D** ● ✦	*Improves intake of nutrients*
• Ensure that meals are well balanced and high in essential nutrients; offer high-protein supplements if client is having difficulty maintaining an adequate caloric intake.	*Ensures adequate nutrition is maintained*

Dependent/Collaborative Actions

Implement measures to maintain an adequate nutritional status:

• Administer vitamins and minerals if ordered. **D** ✦	*Supplements regular diet*
• Perform a calorie count if ordered. Report information to dietitian and physician.	*It is important to know how many calories and what type client is eating.*
• Consult physician regarding an alternative method of providing nutrition (e.g., parenteral nutrition, tube feedings) if client does not consume enough food or fluids to meet nutritional needs.	*Allows for alteration in treatment plan*
• If indicated, obtain a social service consult to assist client in arranging for services such as Meals on Wheels and home health aides for feeding assistance at home.	*Provides for continuum of care*
• Obtain a dietary consult if necessary to assist client in selecting foods/fluids that meet nutritional needs as well as personal and cultural preferences whenever possible.	*Provides a multidisciplinary approach to care*
• If client has dentures, assist with putting them in before meals; if dentures do not fit properly, obtain a dental consult.	*Improves client's ability to macerate foods*

Nursing Diagnosis

IMPAIRED COMFORT NDx (DYSPEPSIA, GASTRIC FULLNESS, AND/OR GAS PAIN)

Definition: Perceived lack of ease, relief, and transcendence in the physical, psychospiritual, environmental, and social dimensions

Related to:

- Increased gastroesophageal sensitivity to irritants associated with thinning of the esophageal and gastric mucosa
- Gastroesophageal reflux associated with decreased tone of the lower esophageal sphincter
- Impaired digestion of many foods associated with reduced secretion of digestive enzymes (e.g., hydrochloric acid, pepsin, lipase)
- Delayed esophageal and gastric emptying associated with decreased gastroesophageal motility
- Accumulation of intestinal gas associated with decreased peristalsis

NDx = NANDA-I Diagnosis　　**D** = Delegatable Action　　● = UAP　　✦ = LVN/LPN　　⊖▶ = Go to ⊖volve for animation

Continued...

CLINICAL MANIFESTATIONS

Subjective	Objective
Reports of indigestion, feeling of fullness; reports of gas pain; reluctance to eat; reluctance to move	Grimacing; clutching at the abdomen; frequent eructation

RISK FACTORS	DESIRED OUTCOMES

• Medication regimen
• Sedentary lifestyle
• Changes in GI system functioning
	The client will experience diminished dyspepsia, gastric fullness, and gas pain as evidenced by:
	  a. Verbalization of same
	  b. Relaxed facial expression and body positioning
	  c. Diminished eructations

NOC OUTCOMES	NIC INTERVENTIONS
Comfort level	Flatulence reduction

NURSING ASSESSMENT	RATIONALE
Assess for signs and symptoms of dyspepsia, gastric fullness, or gas pain (e.g., verbal reports of indigestion, fullness, or gas pain; grimacing; clutching and guarding of abdomen; rubbing epigastric area; restlessness; reluctance to move; frequent eructation; reluctance to eat).	*Early recognition of signs and symptoms of dyspepsia, gastric fullness, or gas pain allows for prompt intervention.*

THERAPEUTIC INTERVENTIONS	RATIONALE

Independent Actions

Implement measures to reduce dyspepsia, gastric fullness, and gas pain:

• Provide small, frequent meals rather than three large ones. **D** ✦	*Reduces gastrointestinal (GI) reflux and GI fullness*
• Instruct client to ingest foods and fluids slowly. **D** ✦	
• Maintain client in high-Fowler's position during and for ≥30 minutes after meals and snacks unless contraindicated. **D** ● ✦	*Uses gravity to help move food through the GI tract*
• Instruct client to avoid spicy foods; alcohol; caffeine-containing beverages such as coffee, tea, and colas; and fried foods.	*Spicy foods, alcohol, and caffeine-containing beverages cause irritation to the GI mucosa, and fried foods are hard to digest.*
• Encourage and assist client with frequent position changes and ambulation as allowed and tolerated. **D** ● ✦	*Activity stimulates peristalsis and expulsion of flatus.*
• Instruct client to avoid activities such as gum-chewing and drinking through a straw.	*Reduces air swallowing*
• Instruct client to avoid intake of carbonated beverages and gas-producing foods (e.g., cabbage, onions, beans).	*Reduces gas in the abdomen*
• Encourage client to eructate and expel flatus whenever the urge is felt. **D** ✦	*Releases gas from the system*
• Encourage client to quit smoking.	*Smoking increases gastric acid production, alters the tone of the lower esophageal sphincter, and causes air swallowing.*

Dependent/Collaborative Actions

Implement measures to reduce dyspepsia, gastric fullness, and gas pain:

• Administer the following medications if ordered: • Antacids and cytoprotective agents (e.g., sucralfate, misoprostol) **D** ✦	*Antacids and cytoprotective agents protect the gastroesophageal mucosa*
• Antiflatulents (e.g., simethicone) **D** ✦	*Antiflatulents reduce gas accumulation.*
• GI stimulants (e.g., metoclopramide) **D** ✦	*GI stimulants promote gastric emptying.*
Consult appropriate health care provider if signs and symptoms of dyspepsia, gastric fullness, or gas pain persist or worsen.	*Allows for alterations in treatment plan*

Nursing Diagnosis | DISTURBED SENSORY PERCEPTION NDx

Definition: Change in the amount of patterning of incoming stimuli accompanied by a diminished, exaggerated, distorted, or impaired response to such stimuli

Visual Related to: the lens becoming more opaque, losing elasticity, and yellowing; loss of ciliary muscle tone; decreased pupil size; and changes in the cornea, retina, macula, and vitreous humor.

Auditory Related to: degenerative changes in the inner ear and eardrum and cerumen accumulation

Gustatory Related to: a diminished sense of smell and atrophy of the taste buds (there is usually only a modest, quality-specific loss of taste in healthy elderly clients)

Olfactory Related to: a decreased number of sensory cells in the nasal lining and atrophy of the olfactory bulb at the base of the brain

Kinesthetic Related to: a decrease in vestibular sensitivity and ability to perceive movement

Tactile Related to: a decreased number of sensory receptors in the skin

CLINICAL MANIFESTATIONS

Subjective	Objective
Reports of difficulties with vision, hearing, smell, and taste; reports of difficulty moving	Overreaching or underreaching for objects; high volume on radio or television; heavy use of spices on foods, lack of coordination; unsteady when on feet; use of heating pad at higher-than-expected temperatures

RISK FACTOR

• Changes in ability to receive and perceive stimuli

DESIRED OUTCOMES

The client will demonstrate adaptation to disturbed sensory perception as evidenced by:
   a. Appropriate verbal and nonverbal responses
   b. Expected level of participation in self-care activities and treatment plan
   c. Safe responses to environmental stimuli

NOC OUTCOMES

Hearing compensation behavior; sensory function: cutaneous; sensory function: hearing; sensory function: proprioception; sensory function: taste and smell; sensory function: vision

NIC INTERVENTIONS

Communication enhancement: visual deficit; communication enhancement: hearing deficit; environmental management; peripheral sensation management

NURSING ASSESSMENT

Assess client for the following:
• Vision changes (e.g., statements of decreased visual acuity, altered depth perception, inability to adjust to changes in lighting, increased sensitivity to glare, or altered color perception; overreaching or underreaching for objects)
• Decreased auditory ability (e.g., statements of not being able to hear or understand what others are saying, inappropriate responses to auditory stimuli, irritability, increased volume of speech, not speaking when spoken to, increased volume of radio and television)
• Altered sense of taste and smell (e.g., statements of same, decreased food intake, heavy use of sugar or seasonings)
• Diminished kinesthetic sense (e.g., unsteadiness on feet, swaying, lack of coordination)
• Diminished tactile sensation (e.g., statements of diminished feeling in extremities, holding or touching very hot objects, use of heating pad at higher-than-expected temperatures)

RATIONALE

Early recognition of changes in sensory functioning allows for prompt intervention.

Continued...

THERAPEUTIC INTERVENTIONS	RATIONALE

Independent Actions

If client's vision is impaired:

- Ensure that lighting is adequate but not too bright. **D ● ✦**

  Elderly individuals have increased sensitivity to glare.

- Avoid sudden changes in light intensity. **D ● ✦**

  Elderly clients often adjust more slowly to changes in lighting.

- Reduce the glare from windows by partially closing blinds or curtains. **D ● ✦**

  Increased sensitivity to glare makes it more difficult to see.

- Provide a night-light. **D ● ✦**

  Facilitates adaptation to a darkened environment and improves night vision

- Provide large-print reading material if available. **D ● ✦**

  Easier for client to read with reading glasses.

- Keep frequently used items within the visual range. **D ● ✦**

  The visual field narrows with aging and keeping things within the visual range decreases risk of falls.

- Encourage client to wear his/her glasses; make sure glasses are clean. **D ● ✦**

  Improves visual acuity and ability to see through lenses

- Provide auditory rather than visual diversionary activities if indicated. **D ● ✦**

  Relieves boredom

- Inform client of resources available if additional information about visual aids is desired (e.g., American Foundation for the Blind).

  Provides for continuum of care once discharged from the acute care facility

- Assist with activities such as filling out menus and reading mail and legal documents as needed.

  Assists the client in making decisions

If client's hearing is impaired:

- Consult appropriate health care provider about removal of ear wax if there is excessive cerumen accumulation in the ear.

  Cerumen blocks vibratory action of sound waves on the eardrum and diminishes hearing.

- Provide adequate lighting in room so client can read lips and see facial expressions and gestures. **D ● ✦**

  Facilitates communication

- Reduce environmental noise. **D ● ✦**

  Background noise can make it difficult for the client to hear during conversations and other interactions.

- Get client's attention (e.g., touch client's shoulder, stand within visual field) before beginning conversation. **D ● ✦**

  Assures client involvement even with a hearing deficit

- Remind client to use hearing aid; ensure that it is functioning well, positioned correctly, and free of cerumen.

  Facilitates communication

- Face client and stay within 3 to 6 feet of client while speaking. **D ● ✦**

  Too much distance between individuals will impact how well the client hears a conversation.

- Lower tone of voice, speak slightly louder than usual, and avoid talking rapidly. **D ● ✦**

  Facilitates communication

- Avoid lowering voice at end of sentences. **D ● ✦**

  This action makes it more difficult for client to follow conversation.

- Use simple sentence. **D ● ✦**

  Facilitates communication

- Articulate clearly but avoid overenunciation of words. **D ● ✦**

- Rephrase sentences if client does not understand what is being said. **D ● ✦**

- Employ related nonverbal cues such as gestures when appropriate. **D ● ✦**

- Use alternative forms of communication (e.g., word cards, paper and pencil, Magic Slate) if indicated. **D ● ✦**

- Respond to client's call signal in person rather than over intercommunication system. **D ● ✦**

  Client may not understand what is spoken via the call-signal system.

- Encourage client to have an audiometric examination if indicated.

  Determines level of hearing loss and proper intervention

- Provide client and significant others with information about available resources that can assist with recommendations about hearing aids and assisted listening devices (e.g., amplifiers for the telephone and television, lighted rather than sound-producing smoke alarms).

  Provides for continuum of care postdischarge from an acute care facility

THERAPEUTIC INTERVENTIONS	RATIONALE
Implement measures to compensate for taste alterations if present:	
• Serve foods warm.	*These actions stimulate sense of smell and taste, which improves*
• Encourage client to experiment with different flavorings and seasoning.	*appetite and thus nutritional status.*
• Encourage client to add extra sweeteners to foods unless contraindicated.* **D** ● ✦	
Implement measures to prevent burns if client has decreased tactile sensation:	*These safety measures help prevent burns.*
• Let hot foods and fluids cool slightly before serving. **D** ● ✦	
• Supervise client while smoking if indicated. **D** ● ✦	
• Assess temperature of bath water and direct heat application (e.g., heating pad, warm compress) before and during use. **D** ● ✦	
Implement measures to reduce the risk for falls if client's vision and/or sense of position or balance seems impaired:	
• Keep bed in low position. **D** ● ✦	*Prevents potential for client falling when getting out of bed*
• Keep needed items within easy reach and assist client to identify their location. **D** ● ✦	*Prevents stretching to reach objects and possible loss of balance or falling out of bed*
• Encourage client to request assistance whenever needed; have call signal within easy reach. **D** ● ✦	*Assures client that someone is available to help them*
• Use lap belt when client is in chair if indicated. **D** ● ✦	*Prevents client from sliding out of the chair*
• Keep floor free of clutter and wipe up spills. **D** ● ✦	*Improves client safety*
• Instruct and assist client to get out of bed slowly and change position slowly.	*Reduces dizziness associated with postural hypotension*
• Provide ambulatory aids (e.g., walker, cane) if appropriate. **D** ● ✦	*Improves balance when walking*
Instruct client and significant others in above methods of adapting to disturbed sensory perceptions.	*Provides for continuum of care*
Dependent/Collaborative Actions	
Consult appropriate health care provider if disturbed sensory perceptions worsen.	*Allows prompt alteration in intervention*

Nursing Diagnosis RISK FOR IMPAIRED SKIN INTEGRITY NDx

Definition: At risk for skin being adversely altered

Related to:
• Increased fragility of the skin associated with decreased nutritional status and age-related dryness, loss of elasticity, and thinning of skin
• Frequent contact with irritants if urinary incontinence is present
• Accumulation of waste products and decreased oxygen and nutrient supply to the skin and subcutaneous tissue associated with decreased blood flow to the skin resulting from:
  • An age-related decrease in dermal vascularity
  • Prolonged pressure on the tissues if mobility is decreased

NOC OUTCOMES	NIC INTERVENTIONS
Tissue integrity: skin and mucous membrane	Skin surveillance; positioning; skin care: topical treatments; pressure ulcer prevention

RISK FACTORS	DESIRED OUTCOMES
• Poor nutritional status	The client will maintain skin integrity as evidenced by:
• Chronic illness	a. Absence of redness and irritation
• Sedentary lifestyle	b. No skin breakdown
• Inadequate fluid intake	

 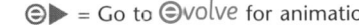

Continued...

NURSING ASSESSMENT	RATIONALE
Determine client's risk for skin breakdown using a risk assessment tool (e.g., Norton Scale, Braden Scale, Gosnell Scale).	*Early recognition of signs and symptoms of skin breakdown allows for prompt intervention.* *Use of a scale provides for standardized assessment.*
Inspect the skin (especially bony prominences, dependent areas, perineum, and areas of decreased sensation and/or edema) for pallor, redness, and breakdown.	

THERAPEUTIC INTERVENTIONS	RATIONALE

Independent Actions

Implement measures to prevent skin breakdown:

• Assist client to turn at least every 2 hours. **D** ● ✦	*Elderly clients may require more frequent position changes because of decreased blood flow to the skin, reduced amounts of protective subcutaneous fat, and a decreased ability to sense pressure and discomfort.*
Position client properly; use pressure-reducing or pressure-relieving devices (e.g., pillows, gel or foam cushions, alternating pressure mattress, air-fluidized bed) if indicated. **D** ● ✦	*Decreases the amount of pressure placed on the skin*
• Gently massage around reddened areas at least every 2 hours. **D** ● ✦	*Improves circulation, which increases supply of oxygen and nutrients*
• Apply a thin layer of a dry lubricant such as powder or cornstarch to bottom sheet or skin and to opposing skin surfaces (e.g., axillae, beneath breasts) if indicated. **D** ● ✦	*Reduces friction between client's skin and the bed linens*
• Lift and move client carefully using a turn sheet and adequate assistance. **D** ● ✦	*Prevents accidental skin tears*
• Perform actions to keep client from sliding down in bed (e.g., gatch knees slightly when head of bed is elevated 30 degrees or higher, limit length of time client is in a semi-Fowler's position to 30-minute intervals). **D** ● ✦	*Reduces the risk of skin surface abrasion and shearing*
• Instruct or assist client to shift weight at least every 30 minutes. **D** ● ✦	*Changes area of pressure on the skin and decreases incidence of skin breakdown*
• Keep client's skin clean. **D** ● ✦	*Removes surface microorganisms, which if allowed to accumulate increase the risk of irritation and infection*
• Keep bed linens dry and wrinkle free. **D** ● ✦	*Moisture harbors microorganisms that can cause irritation and/or infection. Keeping linens wrinkle free decreases the possibility of friction.*
• Thoroughly dry skin after bathing and as often as needed, paying special attention to skin folds and opposing skin surfaces (e.g., axillae, perineum, beneath breasts); pat skin dry rather than rub. **D** ● ✦	*Excessive moisture or prolonged skin exposure softens the epidermal cells and makes them less resistant to damage.*
• Ensure that external devices such as braces, casts, and restraints are applied properly.	*Prevents accidental skin tears and allows for adequate circulation*
• Provide elbow and heel protectors if indicated. **D** ● ✦	*Reduces pressure on these areas*
• Encourage client to wear socks while in bed. **D** ● ✦	*Helps reduce friction on heels and decreases incidence of skin breakdown.*
• Increase activity as allowed and tolerated.	*Improves circulation*
• Avoid use of harsh soaps and hot water; use a mild soap and tepid water for bathing. **D** ● ✦	*Reduces dryness of the skin*
• Apply moisturizing lotion and/or emollient to skin at least once a day.	*Reduces friction and helps prevent skin surface irritation and abrasion*
• Assist client with total bath or shower every other day rather than daily. **D** ● ✦	*Reduces drying of the skin*
• Encourage a fluid intake of 1500 to 2000 mL/day unless contraindicated.	*Ensures skin is well hydrated*
• Protect skin from wound drainage and urinary incontinence (e.g., change dressing when damp, apply drainage collection device; take client regularly to the bathroom, encourage client to urinate when urge is felt, allow client to assume normal position for voiding). **D** ✦	*Prevents skin irritation resulting from exposure to wound drainage or urine*

THERAPEUTIC INTERVENTIONS	RATIONALE
• Assist client to thoroughly cleanse and dry perineal area with soft tissue or cloth after each episode of incontinence; apply a protective ointment or cream. **D ● ✦**	*Excessive exposure of skin to urine increases the potential for skin breakdown.*
• If use of absorbent products such as pads or undergarments is necessary, select those that effectively absorb moisture and keep it away from the skin. **D ● ✦**	*Decreases skin exposure to moisture and potential for irritation and breakdown*
• Apply a protective covering such as a hydrocolloid or transparent membrane dressing to areas of the skin susceptible to breakdown (e.g., coccyx, elbows, heels).	*Decreases friction between skin and bed linens or clothing*
• Use caution with application of heat or cold to areas of decreased sensation or circulatory impairment. **D ✦**	*Prevents potential burn to the skin*
• Maintain optimal nutritional status. **D ✦**	*Proper nutrition is required to maintain the appropriate amount of subcutaneous tissue and prevent skin from becoming thin and losing its elasticity.*

Dependent/Collaborative Actions

If skin breakdown occurs:

• Notify appropriate health care provider (e.g., physician, wound care specialist).	*Allows for alteration in treatment plan*
• Perform care of involved area(s) as ordered or per standard hospital procedure. **D ✦**	*Provides standardized care for skin breakdown*

Nursing Diagnosis ## IMPAIRED ORAL MUCOUS MEMBRANE NDx

Definition: Disruption of the lips and soft tissue of the oral cavity

Dryness Related to decreased saliva production associated with a gradual decline in salivary gland activity

Irritation and breakdown Related to dryness and thinning of the oral mucosa

CLINICAL MANIFESTATIONS

Subjective	**Objective**
Reports of dryness, irritation	Breakdown of oral mucosa

RISK FACTORS	DESIRED OUTCOMES
• Chronic changes • Inadequate fluid intake • Medication regimen	The client will maintain a moist, intact oral mucous membrane.

NOC OUTCOMES	NIC INTERVENTIONS
Oral hygiene	Oral health maintenance; oral health restoration; oral health promotion

NURSING ASSESSMENT	RATIONALE
Assess client for dryness, irritation, and breakdown of the oral mucosa.	*Early recognition of signs and symptoms of impaired mucous membranes allows for prompt intervention.*

THERAPEUTIC INTERVENTIONS	RATIONALE

Independent Actions

Implement measures to decrease dryness and irritation of the oral mucous membrane:

• Instruct and assist client to perform oral hygiene as often as needed; avoid products that contain lemon and glycerin and mouthwashes containing alcohol. **D ✦**	*These products have a drying and irritating effect on the oral mucous membrane.*
• Instruct and assist client to perform oral hygiene using a soft bristle toothbrush or sponge-tipped swab and to floss teeth gently. **D ✦**	*A soft bristle toothbrush or sponge-tipped swab decreases potential for mucous membrane irritation.*

NDx = NANDA-I Diagnosis   **D** = Delegatable Action   ● = UAP   ✦ = LVN/LPN   ⊖▶ = Go to ⊖volve for animation

Continued...

THERAPEUTIC INTERVENTIONS	RATIONALE
• Encourage client to rinse mouth frequently with water. **D ● ✦**	*Helps to keep mucous membranes moist*
• Lubricate client's lips frequently. **D ● ✦**	*Helps prevents lips from chafing*
• Encourage client to breathe through nose rather than mouth.	*Breathing through the nose prevents air from drying out the oral mucous membranes.*
• Encourage client not to smoke or chew tobacco. **D ✦**	*Smoking dries the mucosa; tobacco acts as an irritant to the oral mucosa.*
• Encourage a fluid intake of 1500 to 2000 mL/day unless contraindicated. **D ✦**	*Maintains adequate vascular fluid volume*
• Encourage client to chew sugarless gum or suck on sugarless hard candy. **D ✦**	*Stimulates salivation and helps to maintain moist mucous membranes*
• Encourage client to use artificial saliva. **D ✦**	*Lubricates the mucous membranes and prevents dryness or irritation*
If mucosa is irritated or cracked:	
• Assist client to select soft, bland foods.	
• Instruct client to avoid foods/fluids that are extremely hot.	
• If client has dentures, remove and replace only for meals **D ✦**	*Relieves discomfort, prevents further irritation and breakdown and promotes healing.*
Dependent/Collaborative Actions	
Implement measures to decrease dryness and irritation of the oral mucous membrane:	
• Inspect client's dentures; obtain a dental consult if dentures are rough, cracked, or ill-fitting.	*Improves client's ability to eat without discomfort*
If mucosa is irritated or cracked:	
• Administer topical anesthetics, oral protective agents, and analgesics as ordered.	*These medications protect oral mucosa from further breakdown, decrease pini, and promote healing*
Consult appropriate health care provider (i.e., dentist) if dryness, irritation, breakdown, or discomfort persists.	*Allows for multidisciplinary care*

Nursing Diagnosis **RISK FOR ACTIVITY INTOLERANCE** NDx

Definition: Verbal report of fatigue or weakness; abnormal heart rate or B/P response to activity; exertional discomfort or dyspnea, ECG changes reflecting dysrhythmias or ischemia

Related to:
• Decreased tissue oxygenation associated with diminished functional reserve capacity of the respiratory and cardiac systems during stress/illness
• Decrease in strength and endurance associated with the loss of muscle mass that occurs with aging
• Inadequate nutritional status
• Inadequate rest and sleep associated with age-related changes in sleep pattern and effects of current illness and hospitalization on sleep pattern

CLINICAL MANIFESTATIONS

Subjective	Objective
Report of weakness or fatigue; report of exertional chest pain and/or dizziness	Exertional dyspnea; exertional changes in heart rate and B/P

RISK FACTORS
• Medication regimen
• Poor dietary intake
• Changes in the musculoskeletal system
• Sedentary lifestyle

DESIRED OUTCOMES

The client will not experience activity intolerance as evidenced by:
   a. No reports of fatigue and weakness
   b. Ability to perform activities of daily living without exertional dyspnea, chest pain, diaphoresis, dizziness, and a significant change in vital signs

NOC OUTCOMES	NIC INTERVENTIONS
Activity tolerance; energy conservation; self-care: activities of daily living; self-care status	Energy management; nutrition management; sleep enhancement

NURSING ASSESSMENT	RATIONALE
Assess for signs and symptoms of activity intolerance: • Statements of fatigue or weakness • Exertional dyspnea, chest pain, diaphoresis, or dizziness • Abnormal heart rate response to activity (e.g., increase in rate of 20 beats/min above resting rate, rate not returning to preactivity level within 10 minutes after stopping activity, change from regular to irregular rate); be aware that the pulse rate increases only slightly with activity and returns to preactivity level slowly in an elderly client • A significant change (15-20 mm Hg) in B/P with activity	*Early recognition of activity intolerance allows for prompt intervention.*

THERAPEUTIC INTERVENTIONS / RATIONALE

Independent Actions

Implement measures to maintain adequate activity tolerance:

• Maintain activity restrictions as ordered. **D** ● ✦ — *Promotes rest and/or conserves energy*

• Minimize environmental activity and noise. **D** ● ✦

• Group nursing interventions. **D** ● ✦ — *Allows for periods of uninterrupted rest*

• Limit the number of visitors and their length of stay. **D** ● ✦ — *Reduces client fatigue*

• Assist client with self-care activities as needed. **D** ● ✦ — *Conserves client energy*

• Keep supplies and personal articles within easy reach. **D** ● ✦ — *Prevents client from having to get up to obtain supplies and personal articles.*

• Assist client in using energy-saving techniques (e.g., using shower chair when showering, sitting to brush teeth or comb hair). **D** ● ✦ — *Conserves energy*

• Discourage smoking and excessive intake of beverages high in caffeine such as coffee, tea, and colas. **D** ✦ — *Both nicotine and excessive caffeine intake can increase cardiac workload and myocardial oxygen utilization.*

• Perform actions to maintain an adequate respiratory status (e.g., encourage use of incentive spirometer; elevate head of bed; assist with turning, coughing, and deep breathing). **D** ✦ — *Maintaining or improving respiratory status increases the amount of oxygen available for energy production.*

• Maintain adequate nutritional status. — *Provides energy for activities*

• Increase client's activity gradually as allowed and tolerated; periods of activity should be short, frequent, and interspersed with rest periods. — *Improves stamina for increasing activity*

• Instruct client to report a decreased tolerance for activity; caution client that tolerance for vigorous activity may be diminished. — *This is due to age-related changes in thermoregulatory mechanisms and sympathetic nervous system response.*

• Instruct client to stop any activity that causes chest pain, shortness of breath, dizziness, or extreme fatigue or weakness. — *These symptoms indicate that insufficient oxygen is reaching the tissues and that activity has been increased beyond a therapeutic level.*

Dependent/Collaborative Actions

Implement measures to maintain adequate activity tolerance:

• Implement measures to increase cardiac output (e.g., administer positive inotropic agents, vasodilators, or antidysrhythmics as ordered; elevate the head of the bed) if decreased cardiac output is contributing to the client's activity intolerance. — *Sufficient cardiac output is necessary to maintain an adequate blood flow and oxygen supply to the tissues. Adequate tissue oxygenation promotes more efficient energy production, which subsequently improves client's activity tolerance.*

• Consult physician if signs and symptoms of activity intolerance develop and persist or worsen. — *Allows for prompt alteration in treatment plan.*

Nursing Diagnosis IMPAIRED PHYSICAL MOBILITY NDx

Definition: Limitation in independent, purposeful physical movement of the body or of one or more extremities

Related to:
- Decreased muscle strength associated with the loss of muscle mass that occurs with aging
- Weakness and fatigue associated with decreased functional reserve capacity of the respiratory and cardiac systems during stress and illness, inadequate nutritional status, and difficulty resting and sleeping
- Joint aching and stiffness that may be present as a result of degenerative changes in the joints
- Fear of falling
- Physical limitations/activity restrictions associated with current diagnosis and/or treatment plan

CLINICAL MANIFESTATIONS

Subjective	Objective
Report of pain, discomfort, or fatigue with activities	Decreased reaction time; difficulty moving; engages in substitution for movement; supporting the affected limb; exertional dyspnea; contractures; limited ability to perform gross and fine motor skills; limited range of motion; intentional movement-induced tremor; postural instability; uncoordinated movements

RISK FACTORS
- Pain
- Chronic illness
- Decreased muscle mass
- Sedentary lifestyle

DESIRED OUTCOME

The client will maintain an optimal level of physical mobility within prescribed activity restrictions.

NOC OUTCOMES

Mobility; ambulation: balance

NIC INTERVENTIONS

Exercise therapy: joint mobility; exercise therapy: ambulation; exercise promotion

NURSING ASSESSMENT	RATIONALE
Assess client's movement ability and activity tolerance. Use a tool such as the Assessment Tool for Safe Patient Handling and Movement or the Functional Independence Measures (FIM)	*Assessment of mobility is used to best determine how to facilitate movement. Assessment of activity tolerance provides a baseline for patient strength and endurance with movement.*
Assess for cause of immobility.	*It is important to determine whether the cause of immobility is physical or psychological, and to plan interventions to improve mobility.*
Assess circulation, motion, and feeling in digits.	*Circulation may be compromised by edema of extremities, which can lead to tissue necrosis and/or contractures.*
Assess skin integrity.	*Routine examination of the skin provides for early detection and intervention of pressure sores. Pressure sores develop quickly in patients who are immobile.*
Assess need for assist devices.	*Determine client's need for assistive devices as well as proper use of wheelchairs, walkers, canes, etc., to reduce incidence of falls.*

THERAPEUTIC INTERVENTIONS	RATIONALE
Independent Actions Encourage and implement strength training activities: • Active and/or passive range of motion **D** ● ✦ • Ambulation **D** ● ✦ • Use of trapeze for pull-ups • Allow client to perform as many activities of daily living as they are able **D** ● ✦	*Inactivity contributes to muscle weakening. Contractures can develop as early as 8 hours after a client becomes immobile. These activities maintain and increase client's strength and ability to move.*

THERAPEUTIC INTERVENTIONS	RATIONALE
Use assistive devices to help client with movement: • Crutches • Gait belt **D** ● ✦ • Walker **D** ● ✦	*Use of assistive devices help the caregivers decrease the potential for falls and/or injuries.*
Encourage patient with positive reinforcement during activities. **D** ● ✦	*A positive approach to activities supports the client's accomplishment and engagement in new activities, and improves self-esteem.*
If client complains of joint aching or stiffness: • Encourage client to perform mild exercise of affected joint(s) upon awakening in the morning. **D** ✦	*Reduces stiffness and improves mobility*
Encourage activity and participation in self-care as allowed and tolerated. **D** ● ✦	*Client should be as active as possible to prevent potential loss of mobility.*
Encourage client to continue a regular exercise program after discharge.	*Improves strength and stamina for activities. Client needs to understand the importance of continuing an exercise program post-discharge to maintain mobility.*
Encourage the support of significant others.	*Involves significant others in client care*
Allow them to assist with range-of-motion exercises, positioning, and activity unless contraindicated. **D** ✦	*Exercises improve stamina for activities and improve muscle strength. Allowing significant others to engage in care of the client helps them to understand what is required to assist the client in maintaining mobility.*

Dependent/Collaborative Actions

If client complains of joint aching or stiffness: • Consult physician regarding application of heat to affected joint(s).	*Application of heat helps to relax joints and relieve stiffness.*
• Administer analgesics (e.g., nonsteroidal anti-inflammatories) if ordered.	*Analgesics reduce joint pain.*
Consult appropriate health care provider if client is unable to achieve expected level of mobility or if range of motion becomes more restricted.	*Allows for prompt alteration in treatment plan*

Nursing Diagnosis ## SELF-CARE DEFICIT NDx (BATHING, DRESSING, FEEDING, AND/OR TOILETING)

Definition: Impaired ability to perform or complete activities of daily living (ADLs), such as feeding, dressing, bathing and toileting

Related to:
• Impaired physical mobility
• Weakness and fatigue
• Lack of motivation and/or presence of cognitive impairments that result in the elderly client attaching less importance to or forgetting usual grooming and hygiene practices

RISK FACTORS
• Sedentary lifestyle
• Lack of interest in self-appearance

DESIRED OUTCOMES

The client will perform self-care activities within physical limitations and activity restrictions imposed by the treatment plan.

CLINICAL MANIFESTATIONS

Subjective	**Objective**
Verbal reports of inability to care for self	Refusal to care for self unbrushed hair, mismatched outfits, body odo

NOC OUTCOMES

Self-care: ADLs

NIC INTERVENTIONS

Self-care assistance

NDx = NANDA-I Diagnosis   **D** = Delegatable Action   ● = UAP   ✦ = LVN/LPN   ⊖▶ = Go to ⊖volve for animation

Continued...

NURSING ASSESSMENT	RATIONALE
Assess client's ability to perform ADLs including feeding, dressing, bathing, and toileting.	*Early recognition of client's inability to perform ADLs allows for prompt intervention.*
Assess client's need to use assistive devices.	

THERAPEUTIC INTERVENTIONS	RATIONALE

Independent Actions

With client, develop a realistic plan for meeting daily physical needs.	*Client involvement in developing outcomes improves adherence to treatment regimen.*
Implement measures to facilitate client's ability to perform self-care activities:	
• Schedule care at a time when client is most likely to be able to participate (e.g., after rest periods, not immediately after meals or treatments).	*Clients are more likely to be willing to participate if they feel rested.*
• Keep needed objects within easy reach. **D ● ✦**	*Allows client to care for self without asking for assistance*
• Consult occupational therapist about assistive devices available (e.g., long-handled hairbrush and shoehorn) if indicated.	*May improve clients ability to care for self*
• Allow adequate time for the accomplishment of self-care activities. **D ● ✦**	*Elderly clients tend to be slower in reacting to stimuli and in moving.*
• Maintain a daily exercise routine at the level the client is capable of. **D ● ✦**	*Maintains mobility and improves stamina to perform ADLs*
• Maintain adequate nutritional status.	*Provides energy to perform ADLs*
Encourage maximum independence within physical limitations and prescribed activity restrictions.	*Improves client's confidence that he/she can care for self*
Assist the client with activities he/she is unable to perform independently.	*Conserves energy and decreases frustration with completion of ADLs*
Inform significant others of client's abilities to perform own care. Explain the importance of encouraging and allowing client to maintain an optimal level of independence and allowing client to complete activities at his/her own pace.	*Elderly clients make take longer to complete ADLs. Hurrying clients may cause accidents and will increase their level of frustration in performance of ADLs. Performing ADLs for clients may decrease their level of independent functioning.*

Nursing Diagnosis IMPAIRED URINARY ELIMINATION* NDx

Definitions:
  Urge incontinence NDx: Dysfunction in urine elimination
  Stress incontinence NDx: Loss of <50 mL of urine occurring with increased abdominal pressure
  Reflex incontinence NDx: Involuntary loss of urine at somewhat predictable intervals when a specific bladder volume is reached
  Functional incontinence NDx: Inability of usually continent person to reach toilet in time to avoid unintentional loss of urine
  Total incontinence Continuous and unpredictable loss of urine (**NDx**)
Frequency and urgency Related to: incomplete bladder emptying, decrease in bladder capacity, and uninhibited bladder contractions in response to small volumes of urine (bladder detrusor muscle hyperactivity or instability)
Retention Related to:
• Decrease in bladder muscle tone
• Obstruction of the bladder outlet by an enlarged prostate or fecal impaction
• Decreased attention to the urge to urinate
• Difficulty urinating associated with anxiety about a lack of privacy and possibly having to use a bedpan or urinal
• The effect of some medications (e.g., sedatives, narcotic [opioid] analgesics, anticholinergics)
Incontinence (stress, urge, functional) Related to:
• Decreased tone of the external urinary sphincter and an incompetent bladder outlet (a result of lessening of the urethrovesical junction angle in women) associated with degenerative changes in the urethra and pelvic floor muscles and structural supports of the bladder (occurs more in women as a result of childbearing and estrogen deficiency)
• Decreased bladder capacity and an increase in uninhibited bladder contractions in response to small volumes of urine (bladder detrusor muscle hyperactivity or instability)

*The nurse should select the appropriate nursing diagnosis that is most appropriate based on the nursing assessment.

- Overflow of urine associated with overdistention of the bladder if urinary retention is present
- Delays in toileting associated with:
  - Inability to get to the toilet in time to urinate resulting from unfamiliar environment and impaired physical mobility
  - Difficulty removing clothing in a timely manner when needing to urinate resulting from reduced manual dexterity

CLINICAL MANIFESTATIONS

Subjective	Objective
Urge Incontinence: Reports of involuntary loss of urine	**Urge Incontinence:** Observed inability to reach commode in time to avoid urine loss
Stress Incontinence: Reports of leakage of small amounts of urine on exertion, with coughing, sneezing, and/or laughing	**Stress Incontinence:** Observe leakage of urine during exertion, coughing, sneezing, and/or laughing
Reflex Incontinence: Reports of inability to inhibit or initiate voiding or sensation of bladder fullness	**Reflex Incontinence:** N/A
Functional Incontinence: Reports loss of urine prior to getting to the commode; amount of time to reach commode exceeds length of time between sensing the urge to void and uncontrolled voiding; report of being incontinent only in the morning	**Functional Incontinence:** N/A

RISK FACTORS

- Medication regimen
- Changes in urinary system functioning
- Childbearing

DESIRED OUTCOMES

The client will maintain or regain optimal urinary elimination as evidenced by:
a. Voiding at normal intervals
b. No reports of urgency, frequency, bladder fullness, and suprapubic discomfort
c. Absence of bladder distention
d. Absence of incontinence
e. Balanced intake and output

NOC OUTCOMES

Urinary continence; urinary elimination

NIC INTERVENTIONS

Urinary incontinence care; urinary retention care; urinary habit training; urinary bladder training; pelvic muscle exercise

NURSING ASSESSMENT	RATIONALE
Assess for signs and symptoms of impaired urinary elimination:	*Early recognition of signs and symptoms of impaired urinary elimination allows for prompt intervention.*
• Frequent voiding of small amounts (25-60 mL) of urine	
• Nocturia	
• Reports of urgency, frequency, bladder fullness, or suprapubic discomfort	
• Bladder distention	
• Incontinence	
• Output less than intake	
Monitor client's pattern of fluid intake and urination (e.g., times and amounts of fluid intake, types of fluids consumed, times and amounts of voluntary and involuntary voiding, reports of sensation of need to void, activities preceding incontinence).	*Knowledge of the client's fluid intake and urination pattern assists in the identification of factors that may be causing urinary incontinence. This information helps the nurse plan individualized interventions that promote urinary continence.*
Catheterize client if ordered.	*Determination of the amount of residual urine*
Assist with urodynamic studies (e.g., urethral pressure profile, uroflowmetry, cystometrogram) if ordered.	*Determines cause of altered urinary elimination*

Continued...

THERAPEUTIC INTERVENTIONS	RATIONALE

Independent Actions

Implement measures to promote optimal urinary elimination:

- Offer bedpan or urinal or assist client to bedside commode or bathroom every 2 to 4 hours if indicated. **D** ● ✦

- Instruct client to urinate when the urge is first felt. **D** ✦

- Implement measures to promote relaxation during voiding attempts (e.g., provide privacy, encourage client to read). **D** ● ✦

- Implement measures involving use of water and warmth to promote voiding (e.g., run water, place client's hands in warm water, pour warm water over perineum). **D** ● ✦

- Allow client to assume a normal position for voiding unless contraindicated. **D** ● ✦

- Instruct client to lean upper body forward and/or gently press downward on lower abdomen during voiding attempts unless contraindicated.

- Maintain normal bowel function measures.

- Implement measures to reduce delays in toileting (e.g., have call signal within client's reach and respond promptly to requests for assistance; have bedpan, urinal, or bedside commode readily available to client; provide easy access to bathroom; provide client with easy-to-remove clothing such as pajamas with Velcro closures or an elastic waistband). **D** ● ✦

- Instruct client to perform pelvic floor muscle exercises (e.g., stopping and starting stream during voiding; squeezing buttocks together, then relaxing the muscles) several times a day if appropriate.

- Instruct client to continue these exercises after discharge, emphasizing that it will take several weeks of exercise before improvement may be noted.

- Instruct client to space fluids evenly throughout the day rather than drinking a large quantity at one time.

- Limit oral fluid intake in the evening. **D** ● ✦

- Instruct client to avoid drinking alcohol and beverages containing caffeine.

Urinary incontinence occurs when the pressure in the bladder becomes greater than the pressure exerted by the urinary sphincters.

Emptying the bladder before the pressure becomes too great reduces the risk of incontinence.

Improves the client's ability to completely empty the bladder

Triggers the micturition reflex and promotes relaxation, which improves client's ability to empty the bladder

A sitting or standing position uses gravity to facilitate bladder emptying. The more completely the bladder is emptied, the less risk there is of incontinence.

This puts pressure on the bladder, which helps create a sensation of bladder fullness, which stimulates the micturition reflex.

Constipation increases pressure on the bladder outlet causing increased urinary retention.

Delays in toileting increase the chance of urinary incontinence.

Strengthens pelvic floor muscles and improves tone of the external urinary sphincter

Provides for continuum of care once discharged from the acute care facility

Decreases frustration in knowing that improvement will not be seen for several weeks

Rapid filling of the bladder can result in incontinence if client has decreased urinary sphincter control.

Decreases the possibility of nighttime incontinence

Alcohol and caffeine have a mild diuretic effect and act as irritants to the bladder; both factors may make urinary control more difficult.

Dependent/Collaborative Actions

Implement measures to promote optimal urinary elimination:

- Administer the following medications if ordered:
  - Cholinergic (parasympathomimetic) agents (e.g., bethanechol) **D** ✦

  - Estrogen preparations **D** ✦
  - Anticholinergics (e.g., oxybutynin, tolterodine) **D** ✦

  - Sympathomimetic agents (e.g., ephedrine) **D** ✦
- If urinary incontinence persists:
  - Use biofeedback techniques if appropriate.

  - Instruct and assist client with bladder retraining program if appropriate.

Cholinergics stimulate bladder contractions and promote complete bladder emptying if incontinence is associated with overflow resulting from urinary retention.

May be used to treat stress incontinence in postmenopausal women

Anticholinergics decrease bladder detrusor muscle hyperactivity and reduce episodes of urge incontinence.

Sympathomimetics increase urethral sphincter tone.

Assists client in regaining control over the pelvic floor muscles and external urinary sphincter

Establishes a schedule of when client should empty his/her bladder with the goal of decreasing urinary elimination problems

THERAPEUTIC INTERVENTIONS	RATIONALE
• Consult physician regarding intermittent catheterization, insertion of an indwelling catheter, or use of an external collection device (e.g., condom catheter).	*Allows for alteration in treatment plan*

Nursing Diagnosis **RISK FOR CONSTIPATION** NDx

Definition: Decrease in normal frequency of defecation accompanied by difficult or incomplete passage of stool and/or passage of excessively hard, dry stool

Related to:
• Decreased gastrointestinal motility associated with age and exacerbated by decreased activity and anxiety during illness
• Failure to respond to the urge to defecate associated with dulling of the impulses that sense the signal to defecate, inability to get to the toilet independently, and/or reluctance to use a bedpan or bedside commode
• Difficulty evacuating stool associated with weakened abdominal muscles and decreased lubrication of stools (a result of diminished intestinal mucus production)
• Decreased intake of fiber and fluids
• Possible chronic laxative use

CLINICAL MANIFESTATIONS

Subjective	Objective
Reports of pain on defecation	Infrequent bowel movements; hard, dry stool; chronic laxative use

RISK FACTORS	DESIRED OUTCOMES
• Poor muscle tone • Inadequate fluid/fiber intake • Medication regimen • Sedentary lifestyle	The client will not experience constipation as evidenced by: a. Usual frequency of bowel movements b. Passage of soft, formed stool c. Absence of abdominal distention and pain, feeling of rectal fullness or pressure, and straining during defecation

NOC OUTCOMES	NIC INTERVENTIONS
Bowel elimination; symptom control	Constipation/impaction management

NURSING ASSESSMENT	RATIONALE
Assess for signs and symptoms of constipation (e.g., decrease in frequency of bowel movements; passage of hard, formed stools; anorexia; abdominal distention and pain; feeling of fullness or pressure in rectum; straining during defecation). Assess bowel sounds. Report a pattern of decreasing bowel sounds.	*Early recognition of signs and symptoms of constipation allows for prompt intervention.*

THERAPEUTIC INTERVENTIONS	RATIONALE
Independent Actions Implement measures to prevent constipation: • Encourage client to defecate whenever the urge is felt. **D** ✦	*Prevents stool from remaining too long in the bowel and becoming hard*
• Encourage client to relax, provide privacy, and have call signal within reach during attempts to defecate. **D** ● ✦	*Measures that promote relaxation enable the client to relax the levator ani muscle and external anal sphincter, which facilitates evacuation of stool.*
• Encourage client to establish a regular time for defecation, preferably within an hour after a meal.	*Promotes routine defecation*

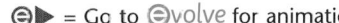

NDx = NANDA-I Diagnosis   **D** = Delegatable Action   ● = UAP   ✦ = LVN/LPN   ⊖▶ = Go to ⊖volve for animation

Continued...

THERAPEUTIC INTERVENTIONS	RATIONALE
• Instruct client to increase intake of foods high in fiber (e.g., bran, whole-grain breads and cereals, fresh fruits and vegetables) unless contraindicated.	*Fiber adds bulk to the intestinal contents.*
• Instruct client to maintain a minimum fluid intake of 1500 to 2000 mL/day unless contraindicated.	*Adequate hydration is important in having a soft stool.*
• Encourage client to drink hot liquids (e.g., tea) upon arising in the morning. **D** ● ✦	*Stimulates peristalsis*
• Increase activity as allowed and tolerated. **D** ● ✦	*Activity improves peristalsis and strengthens the abdominal muscles.*
• Encourage client to perform isometric abdominal strengthening exercises unless contraindicated.	*This type of exercise strengthens the abdominal muscles and stimulates peristalsis.*
• Perform actions to reduce fear and anxiety (e.g., explain procedures, provide care in a confident manner). **D** ✦	*Promotes relaxation*
• If client is taking analgesics for pain management, encourage the use of nonnarcotic rather than narcotic (opioid) analgesics when appropriate. **D** = ✦	*Analgesics decrease peristalsis and promote constipation.*
• Instruct client to continue with actions to promote regular bowel function after discharge (e.g., maintain a fluid intake of ≥6 to 8 glasses per day, increase intake of foods high in fiber, participate in regular exercise program).	*Provides for continuum of care postdischarge from the acute care facility*

Dependent/Collaborative Actions
Implement measures to prevent constipation:

• Administer laxatives or cathartics and/or enemas if ordered. **D** ● ✦	*These medications promote evacuation of the bowel.*
Consult physician about checking for an impaction and digitally removing stool if client has not had a bowel movement in 3 days, if client is passing liquid stool, or if other signs and symptoms of constipation are present.	
Consult appropriate health care provider if signs and symptoms of constipation persist and appear to be an ongoing problem.	*Allows for prompt alterations in treatment plan*

Nursing Diagnosis DISTURBED SLEEP PATTERN NDx

Definition: Time-limited disruption of sleep (natural, periodic suspension of consciousness) amount and quality

Related to:
• Fear, anxiety, change in environment if in hospital or extended care facility, and discomfort associated with present illness
• Age-related nocturia
• Age-related changes in the stages of sleep resulting in frequent awakenings and less deep restorative sleep

CLINICAL MANIFESTATIONS

Subjective	**Objective**
Statements of difficulty falling asleep; statements of not feeling well rested	Frequent awakenings

RISK FACTORS
• Sedentary lifestyle
• Chronic illness
• Medication regimen
• Daytime napping

DESIRED OUTCOMES

The client will attain optimal amount of sleep as evidenced by statements of feeling well rested.

NOC OUTCOMES	NIC INTERVENTIONS
Sleep	Sleep enhancement

NURSING ASSESSMENT	RATIONALE
Assess for signs and symptoms of a disturbed sleep pattern (e.g., statements of difficulty falling asleep, frequent awakenings, or not feeling well rested). Assess client's regular sleep patterns (e.g., hour of bedtime, frequency and length of naps).	*Early recognition of signs and symptoms of disrupted sleep patterns allows for prompt intervention.*

THERAPEUTIC INTERVENTIONS	RATIONALE

Independent Actions
Implement measures to promote sleep:

- Discourage excessive napping during the day unless signs and symptoms of sleep deprivation exist. **D** ✦

- Perform actions to reduce fear and anxiety (e.g., explain procedures, provide care in a confident manner). **D** ● ✦
- Perform actions to reduce dyspepsia, gastric fullness, and gas pain if present (don't eat foods that promote gas; avoid sodas) and discomfort associated with client's diagnosis and treatment.
- Inform client of normal changes in sleep pattern that occur with aging.
- Encourage participation in relaxing diversional activities during the evening. **D** ● ✦
- Discourage intake of foods and fluids high in caffeine (e.g., chocolate, coffee, tea, colas) in the evening. **D** ● ✦
- Offer client an evening snack that includes milk unless contraindicated. **D** ● ✦
- Allow client to continue usual sleep practices (e.g., position; time; presleep routines such as reading, watching television, and listening to music) whenever possible. **D** ● ✦
- Satisfy basic needs such as comfort and warmth before sleep. **D** ● ✦
- Encourage client to limit intake of fluids in the evening and urinate just before bedtime. **D** ✦
- Encourage client to avoid drinking alcohol in the evening.
- Encourage client to avoid smoking before bedtime. **D** ● ✦
- Reduce environmental distractions (e.g., close door to client's room; use night-light rather than overhead light whenever possible; lower volume of paging system; keep staff conversations at a low level and away from client's room; close curtains between clients in a semiprivate room or ward; keep beepers and alarms on low volume; have earplugs available for client if needed). **D** ✦
- Perform actions to reduce interruptions during sleep (70-100 minutes of uninterrupted sleep is usually needed to complete one sleep cycle):
  - Restrict visitors.
  - Group care (e.g., medications, treatments, physical care, assessments) whenever possible

Client will have more hours of sleep if they don't nap during the day. Elderly clients may have short naps during the day because of shorter nighttime sleep time.
Promotes relaxation and rest

Causes discomfort and interferes with sleep

Reduces concerns about quality and amount of sleep necessary to maintain health
Decreases stress and promotes rest

Caffeine is a stimulant and will make it difficult for the client to rest.
Milk contains L-tryptophan, which is believed to help induce and maintain sleep.
Allowing client normal sleep practices will decrease disruption of sleep patterns while in the acute care facility.

Promotes relaxation

Reduces nocturia

Alcohol interferes with rapid eye movement (REM) sleep.
Nicotine is a stimulant.
Most individuals sleep in a dark, quiet environment.

Interruptions decrease REM sleep, causing disruption of sleep patterns.

NDx = NANDA-I Diagnosis   **D** = Delegatable Action   ● = UAP   ✦ = LVN/LPN   ⊜▶ = Go to ⊜volve for animation

Continued...

THERAPEUTIC INTERVENTIONS	RATIONALE

Dependent/Collaborative Actions

Implement measures to promote sleep:

- Review medications that client takes with pharmacist or physician and identify those that can interfere with sleep (e.g., nicotine transdermal systems, theophylline, corticosteroids, diuretics, diphenhydramine or other over-the-counter sleep aids, some antidepressants); if possible, administer medications such as corticosteroids and diuretics early in the day rather than late afternoon or evening and encourage client to continue this schedule for these medications at home.
- Administer prescribed sedative-hypnotic only if indicated; administer these agents cautiously; inform client that over-the-counter sleep aids (e.g., diphenhydramine) can interfere with the quality of sleep and daytime functioning and should not be taken on a regular basis. **D** ✦

Consult appropriate health care provider if signs and symptoms of sleep deprivation (e.g., irritability, lethargy, agitation, inability to concentrate) occur and persist or worsen.

Medications that may interfere with sleep should be given as early in the day as possible.

The metabolism, distribution, and excretion of drugs are often altered in the elderly client.

Allows for prompt alterations in treatment plan

Nursing Diagnosis   RISK FOR INFECTION NDx

Definition: At increased risk for being invaded by pathogenic organisms

Related to:

- Stasis of respiratory secretions associated with decreased activity during illness and age-related decrease in ciliary activity and cough effectiveness
- Decrease in immunity associated with:
  - An age-related decline in T-cell and B-cell function and the number of functional macrophages in the skin and alveoli
  - An inadequate nutritional status (if present)
- Decrease in effectiveness of the body's physical barriers associated with changes in the skin and mucous membranes
- Urinary stasis associated with decreased activity during illness and the urinary retention that can result from a decrease in bladder muscle tone, the effect of certain medications, an enlarged prostate, and difficulty urinating in a new environment
- Favorable environment for growth of pathogens in vagina associated with an increase in the pH of vaginal secretions

CLINICAL MANIFESTATIONS

Subjective	Objective
Reports of fatigue and lack of appetite Reports of frequency, urgency, or burning when urinating	• Elevated temperature • Chills • Increased pulse rate • Malaise, lethargy, acute confusion • Abnormal breath sounds • Productive cough of purulent, green, or rust-colored sputum • Cloudy urine • Urinalysis showing a WBC count greater than 5, positive leukocyte esterase or nitrites, or presence of bacteria • Heat, pain, redness, swelling, or unusual drainage in any area • Elevated WBC count and/or significant change in differential

RISK FACTORS

- Chronic illness
- Injury
- Inadequate immune system response
- Increased susceptibility to pathogens

DESIRED OUTCOMES

The client will remain free of infection as evidenced by:
a. Absence of fever and chills
b. Pulse rate within normal limits
c. Normal breath sounds
d. Cough productive of clear mucus only
e. Voiding clear urine without reports of burning and increased frequency and urgency
f. Absence of heat, pain, redness, swelling, and unusual drainage in any area
g. Usual mental status
h. WBC and differential counts within normal range for elderly client
i. Negative results of cultured specimens

NOC OUTCOMES

Immune status; infection severity

NIC INTERVENTIONS

Infection protection; infection control; incision site care; tube care; wound care

NURSING ASSESSMENT

Assess for and report signs and symptoms of infection:

- Increase in temperature above client's usual level (be aware that normal temperature in the elderly client may be <37°C)
- Chills
- Increased pulse rate
- Abnormal breath sounds
- Cough productive of purulent, green, or rust-colored sputum
- Loss of appetite
- Cloudy urine
- Reports of burning when urinating
- Reports of increased urinary frequency or urgency
- Urinalysis showing a WBC count >5 per high-power field, positive leukocyte esterase or nitrites, or the presence of bacteria
- Heat, pain, redness, swelling, or unusual drainage in any area
- Malaise, lethargy, acute confusion
- Increase in WBC count and/or significant change in differential
- Positive results of cultured specimens (e.g., urine, vaginal drainage, wound drainage, sputum, blood)

RATIONALE

Early recognition of signs and symptoms of infection allows for prompt intervention.
Be aware that some signs and symptoms vary because of an age-related decline in thermoregulatory, immune, and sympathetic nervous system responses.
As the elderly have a diminished shivering reflex
The elderly client may not demonstrate the classic elevation in pulse rate that occurs with infection because of a decreased sympathetic nervous system response.

THERAPEUTIC INTERVENTIONS

Independent Actions
Implement measures to prevent infection:
- Maintain a fluid intake of ≥1500 to 2000 mL/day unless contraindicated.
- Use good hand hygiene and encourage client to do the same. **D** ● ✦
- Adhere to the appropriate precautions established to prevent transmission of infection to the client (standard precautions, transmission-based precautions on other clients, neutropenic precautions). **D** ● ✦

RATIONALE

Maintains adequate hydration and vascular fluid volume

Hand hygiene removes transient flora, which reduces the risk of transmission of pathogens.
Helps prevent the transmission of microorganisms and reduces the client's risk of infection

Continued...

THERAPEUTIC INTERVENTIONS	RATIONALE
• Use sterile technique during invasive procedures (e.g., urinary catheterizations, venous and arterial punctures, injections, wound care) and dressing changes. **D** ✦	*Reduces the possibility of introducing pathogens into the body*
• Anchor catheters/tubings (e.g., urinary, intravenous, wound drainage) securely. **D** ● ✦	*Reduces the risk for trauma to the tissues and the risk for introduction of pathogens associated with in-and-out movement of the tubing*
• Change equipment, tubings, and solutions used for treatments such as intravenous infusions, respiratory care, irrigations, and enteral feedings according to hospital policy.	*The longer that equipment, tubings, and solutions are in use, the greater the chance of colonization of microorganisms, which can then be introduced into the body.*
• Change peripheral intravenous line sites according to hospital policy.	*Peripheral intravenous line sites are changed routinely to reduce persistent irritation of one area of a vein wall and the resultant colonization of microorganisms at that site.*
• Maintain a closed system for drains (e.g., wound, chest tube, urinary catheter) and intravenous infusions whenever possible.	*Prevents introduction of pathogens into the body*
• Protect client from others with infections and instruct client to continue this after discharge. **D** ● ✦	*Protecting the client from others with infections reduces the client's risk of exposure to pathogens.*
• Maintain adequate nutritional status. **D** ✦	*Adequate nutrition is needed to maintain normal function of the immune system.*
• Perform actions to prevent and treat irritation and breakdown of the oral mucous membrane (e.g., maintain oral hydration, use a soft tooth brush, don't use glycerine swabs for mouth care). **D** ● ✦	*Frequent oral hygiene helps prevent infection by removing most of the food, debris, and many of the microorganisms that are present in the mouth. It also helps maintain the integrity of the oral mucosa, which provides a physical and chemical barrier to pathogens.*
• Instruct and assist client to perform good perineal care routinely and after each bowel movement. **D** ● ✦	*The perineal area contains a large number of organisms. Routine cleansing of the area reduces the risk of colonization of organisms and subsequent perineal, urinary tract, and/or vaginal infection.*
• Perform actions to maintain an adequate respiratory status (e.g., use incentive spirometry every 2 hours, change position every 2 hours, ambulate as able).	*Reduces stasis of respiratory secretions and the risk of a respiratory tract infection*
• Perform actions to prevent or treat urinary retention (e.g., encourage clients to void when they experience the urge, maintain adequate fluid volume). **D** ● ✦	*Prevents urine accumulation in the bladder, which creates an environment conducive to the growth and colonization of microorganisms, and reduces the risk of urinary tract infection*
• Perform actions to prevent skin breakdown (promote ambulation, change positions of bed-ridden clients every 2 hours, maintain adequate hydration). **D** ● ✦	*Skin breakdown removes one of the physical barriers to the body.*
• If client has a wound, provide appropriate wound care (e.g., use dressing materials that maintain a moist wound surface, assist with debridement of necrotic tissue, use dressing materials that absorb excess exudate, maintain patency of wound drains). **D** ✦	*Facilitates wound healing and reduces the number of pathogens that enter or are present in the wound*
• Perform actions to reduce stress (e.g., reduce fear, anxiety, and pain; help client identify and use effective coping mechanisms). **D** ● ✦	*Prevents an increase in cortisol secretion, which is important because cortisol interferes with some immune responses*

Dependent/Collaborative Actions
Implement measures to prevent infection:

• Instruct client to receive vaccinations (e.g., pneumococcal pneumonia, tetanus, influenza) at recommended intervals if appropriate.	*Immunizations are often recommended to reduce the possibility of some infections in high-risk clients (e.g., those clients who are immunosuppressed, elderly, or have a chronic disease).*
• Consult appropriate health care provider regarding:	
• Initiation of antimicrobial therapy if indicated **D** ✦	*Prevents and/or treats infection*
• Antimicrobial orders that do not seem appropriate (e.g., prolonged use of antimicrobials, excessively high doses of an antimicrobial, unnecessary use of broad-spectrum or multiple antimicrobials) **D** ✦	*Reduces the risk of elimination of the client's natural flora and/or the development of drug-resistant microorganisms*

| Nursing Diagnosis | **RISK FOR FALLS** NDx |

Definition: Increased susceptibility to falling that may cause physical harm

Related to:
- Dizziness or syncope associated with decreased cerebral tissue perfusion that can result from certain medications (e.g., antihypertensive agents) and from age-related vascular changes, decrease in cardiac output, and postural hypotension
- Loss of balance associated with the effect of certain medications (e.g., sedatives, narcotic [opioid] analgesics) and the changes in posture, reduced coordination, delayed reaction time, and impaired proprioception that can occur with aging
- Tripping associated with age-related gait abnormalities (e.g., decreased step height and length) and impaired vision
- Weakness associated with an age-related decrease in muscle strength and the general deconditioning that can occur with reduced physical activity

CLINICAL MANIFESTATIONS

Subjective	Objective
Expressed concern for safety during ambulation; stated history of previous falls	Unsteadiness when ambulating; use of ambulation aids; visual field deficits; confusion; orthostatic hypotension; medication therapy (e.g., antihypertensives, diuretics, hypnotics, antianxiety agents, narcotics, tranquilizers, antidepressants); anemias, arthritis

RISK FACTORS
- Medication
- Sedentary lifestyle
- Safety hazards in the home
- Weakness

DESIRED OUTCOMES

The client will not experience falls.

NOC OUTCOMES

Fall prevention behavior; knowledge: fall prevention

NIC INTERVENTIONS

Fall prevention; environmental management: safety

NURSING ASSESSMENT	RATIONALE
Assess client's risk for falls using standardized assessment tool (e.g., Fall Risk Assessment).	*A client's risk for falls increases with the number of risk factors. Determining the client's risk for falls allows implementation of the appropriate preventive measures.*
Assess client's balance and mobility skills.	*Determining the client's baseline status allows for the implementation of the appropriate preventive measures*
Evaluate client's medications to determine whether they place the client at increased risk for falls.	*Some medications may cause excessive drowsiness, altered mental states, or physiological changes such as orthostatic hypotension that can increase the risk of falls in clients. Early identification of such medications allows for implementation of appropriate preventive measures.*

THERAPEUTIC INTERVENTIONS	RATIONALE

Independent Actions
Implement measures to reduce the risk for falls:
- Keep bed in low position with side rails up when client is in bed. **D** ● ✦   *Prevents client from falling when getting out of bed*
- Keep needed items within easy reach and assist client to identify their location. **D** ● ✦   *Prevents clients from stretching to obtain items and losing their balance and falling*
- Encourage client to request assistance whenever needed; have call signal within easy reach. **D** ● ✦   *Provides assurance to clients that someone will assist them as needed and that they can remain in bed till assistance arrives*
- Use lap belt when client is in chair if indicated. **D** ● ✦   *Prevents sliding out of a chair*
- Instruct client to wear well-fitting slippers/shoes with nonslip soles and low heels when ambulating.   *Decreases potential for falls and improves ambulation*
- Keep floor free of clutter and wipe up spills promptly. **D** ● ✦   *Prevents tripping over clutter or slipping on wet floors*

NDx = NANDA-I Diagnosis   **D** = Delegatable Action   ● = UAP   ✦ = LVN/LPN   ⊖▶ = Go to ⊖volve for animation

Continued...

THERAPEUTIC INTERVENTIONS	RATIONALE
• Instruct and assist client to get out of bed slowly.	*Reduces dizziness associated with postural hypotension*
• Carefully position tubings and equipment. **D** ● ✦	*Prevents tripping over equipment*
• Accompany client during ambulation and use a transfer safety belt if client is weak or dizzy. **D** ● ✦	*Provides stability when ambulating and helps prevent falls*
• Provide ambulatory aids (e.g., walker, cane) if client is weak or unsteady on feet. **D** ● ✦	*Provides stability when ambulating*
• Reinforce instructions from physical therapist on correct ambulation and transfer techniques.	*Improves client adherence and improves safety*
• If vision is impaired, orient client to surroundings, room, and arrangement of furniture and identify obstacles during ambulation.	*Ensures that client is able to see obstacles in pathway when ambulating*
• Instruct client to move slowly, use wider stance when ambulating, and avoid rapidly turning head or body.	*Prevents loss of balance when ambulating*
• Instruct client to ambulate in well-lit areas and to use handrails if needed.	*Allows client to see obstacles that may be in pathway when ambulating*
• Do not rush client; allow adequate time for ambulation to the bathroom and in hallway. **D** ● ✦	*Elderly clients move more slowly; allowing them adequate time for ambulation decreases their frustration and risk for falls.*
• Make sure that shower has a nonslip bottom surface and that shower chair; secure bath mat, call signal, grab bars, and adequate lighting are present.	*Decreases risk for slipping and falling while on wet surfaces*
• Maintain adequate strength and activity tolerance and an optimal level of physical mobility.	*Provides for client stamina while performing activities of daily living*
• If client is at high risk for falls and gets up without assistance despite reminders to request assistance:	*Institute facility's falls protocol.*
• Attach an alarm device to bed or chair. **D** ● ✦	*Notifies health care personnel if client leaves the chair or bed*
Include client and significant others in planning and implementing measures to prevent falls. **D** ● ✦	*Helps family understand what they can do to assist client and reduce risk for falls*
Discuss:	
• The need to evaluate living environment for hazards (e.g., thick or loose carpets, inadequate or loose railings, insufficient lighting) and make necessary modifications	*Improves safety*
• The importance of participating in a regular exercise program for conditioning and muscle strengthening and continuing with therapy for gait and balance training if needed	*Provides conditioning and muscle strengthening and improves balance*
• The importance of continuing appropriate safety precautions after discharge	*Prevents falls*
If falls occur, initiate appropriate first aid and notify physician.	*Allows for prompt intervention*

Dependent/Collaborative Actions

Implement measures to reduce the risk for falls:

• If client is at high risk for falls and gets up without assistance despite reminders to request assistance:	
• Consult physician about the temporary use of jacket or wrist restraints.	*Helps prevent falls of clients who won't remain in the bed or chair to protect them from falling*
• Administer central nervous system depressants judiciously. **D** ✦	*Central nervous system depressants decrease client's level of consciousness and increase risk for falls.*

Nursing Diagnosis   # RISK FOR ASPIRATION NDx

Definition: At risk for entry of gastrointestinal secretions, oropharyngeal secretions, solids, or fluids into tracheobronchial passages

Related to: Diminished gag reflex and the gastroesophageal reflux that can occur as a result of decreased tone of the lower esophageal sphincter

CLINICAL MANIFESTATIONS

Subjective	Objective
Not applicable	Rhonchi, dull percussion note over affected lung area, cough, tachypnea, dyspnea, tachycardia, presence of tube feeding in tracheal aspirate, chest radiograph showing pulmonary infiltrate

RISK FACTORS

- Changes in esophageal sphincter tone
- Medication regimen

DESIRED OUTCOMES

The client will not aspirate secretions or foods/fluids as evidenced by:
  a. Clear breath sounds
  b. Resonant percussion note over lungs
  c. Absence of cough, tachypnea, and dyspnea

NOC OUTCOMES

Aspiration prevention

NIC INTERVENTIONS

Aspiration precautions

NURSING ASSESSMENT	RATIONALE
Assess for and report signs and symptoms of aspiration of secretions or foods/fluids (e.g., rhonchi, dull percussion note over affected lung area, cough, tachypnea, dyspnea, tachycardia, presence of tube feeding in tracheal aspirate, chest radiograph showing pulmonary infiltrate).	*Early recognition of signs and symptoms of aspiration of secretions or foods/fluids allows for prompt intervention.*

THERAPEUTIC INTERVENTIONS	RATIONALE

Independent Actions
Implement measures to reduce the risk for aspiration:

- Perform actions to reduce gastroesophageal reflux (e.g., provide small frequent meals rather than three large ones; instruct client to ingest food slowly; maintain client in high-Fowler's position during and for ≥30 minutes after ingestion of foods and fluids). **D ● ✦**

  Prevents stomach from becoming too full and incidence gastric fluid reflux into the oropharynx

- Instruct client to avoid laughing and talking while eating and drinking.

  Prevents food/fluids from moving into the trachea rather than the esophagus

- Encourage client to concentrate on eating and drinking and allow ample time for meals and snack. **D ● ✦**

  Allows client to fully chew foods, which makes them easier to swallow and reduces the risk of aspiration

- Instruct and assist client to perform oral hygiene after meals. **D ● ✦**

  Ensures that food particles do not remain in the mouth

- If client is receiving tube feedings, check tube placement before each feeding or on a routine basis if tube feeding is continuous, and do not administer tube feeding if the residual exceeds a specified amount (usually 75-100 mL). **D ✦**

  Prevents overdistention of the stomach and subsequent increased pressure, which can force gastric contents into the oropharynx and increase the risk for aspiration

Dependent/Collaborative Actions
If signs and symptoms of aspiration occur:

- Perform tracheal suctioning.

  Manually removes contents from the trachea

- Withhold oral intake.

  Prevents further aspiration

- Prepare client for chest radiograph.

Nursing Diagnosis ## RISK FOR INJURY NDx **(BURNS)**

Definition: At risk for injury as a result of environmental conditions interacting with the individual's adaptive and defensive resources

Related to: Age-related decrease in tactile sensation

NDx = NANDA-I Diagnosis   **D** = Delegatable Action   **●** = UAP   **✦** = LVN/LPN   ⊖▶ = Go to ⊖volve for animation

Continued...

RISK FACTORS

• Changes in sensations

DESIRED OUTCOMES

The client will not experience burns.

CLINICAL MANIFESTATIONS

Subjective	Objective
Burn patterns on body	Not applicable

NOC OUTCOMES

Knowledge: personal safety; knowledge: medication

NIC INTERVENTIONS

Environmental management: safety; medication management

THERAPEUTIC INTERVENTIONS	RATIONALE

Independent Actions

Implement measures to prevent burns:

• Let hot foods and fluids cool slightly before serving. **D ● ✦**

Prevents accidental burns

• Supervise client while smoking if indicated. **D ● ✦**

Provides safety to client; decreases potential for accidental fire and subsequent burns

• Assess temperature of bath water and direct heat application (e.g., heating pad, warm compress) before and during use. **D ● ✦**

Client may have decreased feeling; this action provides a safety measure to prevent injury.

If burns occur, initiate appropriate first aid and notify physician.

Allows for prompt intervention should a burn occur

Nursing Diagnosis RISK FOR INJURY NDx (PATHOLOGICAL FRACTURES)

Definition: At risk for injury as a result of environmental conditions interacting with the individual's adaptive and defensive resources.

Pathological fractures Related to: osteoporosis associated with an imbalance between bone resorption and bone formation resulting from decreased estrogen levels in women, calcium deficiency (results from decreased dietary intake and decreased absorption due to vitamin D deficiency), and decreased activity

CLINICAL MANIFESTATIONS

Subjective	Objective
Report of pain in joints and/or bones	Decrease in mobility; decrease in range of motion of extremities; abnormal joint positioning; swelling over skeletal structures; radiographs showing pathologic fractures

RISK FACTORS

• Decreased calcium absorption
• Sedentary lifestyle
• Medication regimen
• Chronic illness
• Poor diet

DESIRED OUTCOMES

The client will not experience pathological fractures as evidenced by:
  a. Usual mobility and range of motion
  b. Absence of unusual motion, abnormal joint position, and obvious deformity of any body part
  c. Absence of pain and swelling over skeletal structures
  d. Radiographs showing absence of fractures

NOC OUTCOMES

Knowledge: personal safety; knowledge: medication

NIC INTERVENTIONS

Environmental management: safety; medication management

NURSING ASSESSMENT	RATIONALE
Assess for and report signs and symptoms of pathological fractures (e.g., decrease in mobility or range of motion, motion at site where motion does not usually occur, abnormal joint position or obvious deformity, pain or swelling over skeletal structures, radiographs showing pathological fracture).	*Early recognition of signs and symptoms of fractures allows for prompt interventions.*

THERAPEUTIC INTERVENTIONS	RATIONALE

Independent Actions

Implement measures to prevent pathological fractures:

- Move client carefully; obtain adequate assistance as needed. **D** ● ✦ — *Prevents potential falls and fractures*
- When turning client, logroll and support all extremities. **D** ● ✦ — *Prevents dangling of extremities during turning and decreases the potential for injury*
- Use smooth movements when moving client; avoid pulling or pushing on body parts. **D** ● ✦ — *Prevents sharp, jerking movements, which may cause fractures*
- Initiate and follow facility safety protocol. **D** ● ✦ — *Provides standardized care to prevent accidental falls and bone injury.*
- Assist client to maintain maximum mobility. **D** ● ✦ — *Weight-bearing exercises reduce bone breakdown.*
- Discourage smoking and excessive caffeine and alcohol intake. **D** ✦
- Encourage client to consume a diet that has adequate amounts of protein, vitamins, and calcium. — *Ensures an adequate amount of nutrients required for healthy bones*
- Emphasize need for client to follow a regular exercise program after discharge. — *Provides for continuum of care once client is discharged from the acute care facility*

Dependent/Collaborative Actions

Implement measures to prevent pathological fractures:

- Consult physician about use of a tilt table if client is immobile. — *Facilitates weight-bearing*
- Administer calcium preparations, vitamin D, and medications that inhibit bone resorption (e.g., calcitonin, alendronate) if ordered. **D** ● ✦ — *These preparations improve potential for bone health and decrease in pathological fractures*

If fractures occur:

- Maintain activity restrictions if ordered. **D** ● ✦ — *Prevents further bone injury*
- Apply external stabilization device (e.g., cervical collar, brace, splint, sling) if ordered. — *Stabilizes bone for healing*
- Prepare client for surgery (e.g., internal fixation) if planned. — *Decreases client's fear and anxiety*
- Administer analgesics and/or muscle relaxants if ordered. **D** ✦ — *Controls pain associated with pathological fractures*

Nursing Diagnosis | DRUG TOXICITY

Definition: An accumulation drug(s) in the bloodstream that may lead to severe side effects

Related to:

- An increase in cell receptor sensitivity to some drugs
- Changes in the usual distribution of drugs associated with factors such as a decrease in total body water, a decrease in lean body mass, an increase in total body fat, and a decrease in serum albumin
- Impaired metabolism and excretion of drugs associated with diminished liver and kidney function
- Synergistic effect that occurs with some combinations of medications (elderly clients are often taking a number of medications)

CLINICAL MANIFESTATIONS

Subjective	Objective
Report of confusion; blurred vision; anorexia; nausea; dizziness; itchy skin	Ataxia; vomiting; diarrhea; dysrhythmias; postural hypotension; stridor; rash; urticaria; agitation; elevated BUN, serum creatinine, and serum transaminase levels

---

NDx = NANDA-I Diagnosis **D** = Delegatable Action ● = UAP ✦ = LVN/LPN ⊖▶ = Go to ⊖volve for animation

Continued...

RISK FACTORS

- Polypharmacy
- Changes in distribution
- Inadequate fluid intake
- Poor diet

DESIRED OUTCOMES

The client will not develop drug toxicity as evidenced by absence of signs and symptoms commonly associated with drug toxicity such as:

a. Ataxia, agitation, confusion, and blurred vision
b. Anorexia, nausea, vomiting, and diarrhea
c. Dizziness, dysrhythmias, and postural hypotension
d. Dyspnea and stridor
e. Rash and urticaria
f. Elevated BUN, serum creatinine, and serum transaminase levels

NOC OUTCOMES

Knowledge: personal safety; knowledge: medication

NIC INTERVENTIONS

Environmental management: safety; medication management

NURSING ASSESSMENT

Assess client for signs and symptoms that might be indicative of drug toxicity (e.g., ataxia, agitation, confusion, blurred vision, anorexia, nausea, vomiting, diarrhea, dizziness, dysrhythmias, postural hypotension, dyspnea, stridor, rash, urticaria, elevated BUN, serum creatinine, and serum transaminase levels). Be aware that the signs and symptoms will vary depending on drugs being taken.

RATIONALE

Early recognition of signs and symptoms of drug toxicity allows for prompt intervention.

THERAPEUTIC INTERVENTIONS

Independent Actions

Implement measures to prevent drug toxicity:

- Educate client about common adverse effects of drugs being taken and ways to avoid toxicity; encourage client to report adverse effects or any other unusual symptoms immediately.

- Obtain baseline vital signs and results of laboratory studies indicative of renal and hepatic function.

- Monitor blood levels (e.g., peak, trough) of drugs as ordered and report results to physician; be aware that the elderly client may experience toxic effects when drug levels are within the "normal" therapeutic range.

- Before discharge:
  - Provide client and family members with clear, simple, written instructions for taking medications prescribed; include drug name, dose, schedule, route of administration, special precautions such as incompatible foods or drugs, and adverse reactions to observe for.

  - Assist client to set up a system for remembering to take medications as prescribed (e.g., divided pill container, use of timer).

  - Emphasize the importance of taking only those medications that are prescribed, following the directions carefully, and keeping the physician informed of adverse effects experienced.

  - Provide client with a written schedule for any laboratory tests that are to be done to monitor the therapeutic effect or side effects of medications being taken.

RATIONALE

Informs client of what to observe for and what to do should adverse effects occur. It also improves adherence to medication regimen.

Facilitates assessment of the effects of medications on these systems

Helps to appropriately determine amount of medication client should receive and prevents drug toxicity

Provides an ongoing source of information about client's medications

Facilitates appropriate administration of client's medications

Prevents interaction between medications that may decrease or increase the potency of the client's medications

Facilitates client taking mediations at the appropriate times and what should be monitored

THERAPEUTIC INTERVENTIONS	RATIONALE
• Encourage client to get all of medications from one pharmacy and to provide that pharmacy with a complete medical history and list of medications being taken.	*Prevents potential drug interactions if client received multiple prescriptions from multiple pharmacies*
If signs and symptoms of drug toxicity occur, withhold dose and notify appropriate health care provider (e.g., physician, practitioner, pharmacist).	*Prevents further buildup of drug toxicity and allows for prompt intervention*
Dependent/Collaborative Actions Implement measures to prevent drug toxicity:	
• Consult appropriate resource (e.g., pharmacist, physician, drug book, geriatrician) for:	*Provides multidisciplinary approach to medication administration*
• Information about possible drug interactions of the medications client is taking	*Facilitates monitoring of drug toxicity effects*
• Appropriate dosages of medications for elderly clients	*The smallest effective dose of a medication should be ordered for elderly persons to reduce the risk of adverse effects.*
• Schedule for and order of administration of medications	*The absorption, distribution, metabolism, and excretion of many medications may be altered by other medications as well as the age-related changes in body function and the client's current illness.*
Administer central nervous system depressants judiciously.	*Central nervous system depressants decrease client's level of consciousness so that drug toxicity may be difficult to recognize.*

Nursing Diagnosis # INEFFECTIVE SEXUALITY PATTERN NDx

Definition: Expressions of concern regarding own sexuality

Related to:
• Fear of rejection associated with feelings of loss of physical attractiveness
• Inadequate opportunities for sexual expression associated with lack of available partner
• Misconceptions about sexual functioning in old age
• Fear of urinary incontinence
• Dyspareunia associated with vaginal changes (e.g., decreased vaginal lubrication, thinning and loss of elasticity of the vaginal wall, shortening and narrowing of the vagina) resulting from decreased estrogen levels
• Embarrassment associated with possible impotence (erections are usually less intense and slower in the elderly male and may be further affected by certain disease processes [e.g., diabetes, vascular disorders, chronic renal failure] and medications [e.g., thiazide diuretics, tricyclic antidepressants, certain antihypertensive agents])

CLINICAL MANIFESTATIONS

Subjective	Objective
Reports of sexual concerns; report of difficulties in performing sexual activities	N/A

RISK FACTORS
• Lack of interest and/or partner
• Medication regimen
• Chronic illness
• Changes in sexual response

DESIRED OUTCOMES

The client will demonstrate beginning adaptation to changes in sexuality patterns as evidenced by:
  a. Verbalization of a perception of self as sexually acceptable and adequate
  b. Statements reflecting ways to adjust to effects of aging on sexual functioning

NOC OUTCOMES

Psychosocial adjustment: life change; sexual identity

NIC NTERVENTIONS

Body image enhancement; sexual counseling

NDx = NANDA-I Diagnosis   **D** = Delegatable Action   ● = UAP   ✦ = LVN/LPN   ⊖▶ = Go to ⊖volve for animation

Continued...

NURSING ASSESSMENT	RATIONALE
Assess for symptoms of altered sexuality patterns (e.g., verbalization of sexual concerns, limitations, or difficulties; reports of changes in sexual activities or behaviors).	*Early recognition of signs and symptoms of altered sexuality patterns allows for prompt intervention.*
Determine client's perception of desired sexuality, usual pattern of sexual expression, recent changes in sexuality patterns, and knowledge of age-related changes in sexual functioning.	*Be aware that the client may be reluctant to express concerns because of the common stereotype that the elderly are not sexually active.*

THERAPEUTIC INTERVENTIONS	RATIONALE

Independent Actions

Implement measures to promote an optimal sexuality pattern:

- Educate client on the age-related changes in sexual functioning (e.g., sexual responses are slower and less intense, vaginal secretions are diminished, erections take longer to achieve, seminal fluid volume is reduced, erection is rapidly lost after orgasm, refractory time between orgasms is longer); encourage questions and clarify misconceptions.

  Provides client factual information about changes in sexual performance that client may not have known

- Facilitate communication between client and partner; focus on feelings shared by the couple and assist them to identify changes that may affect their sexual relationship.

  Allows client and significant other to discuss and make changes in a safe environment

- Discuss ways to be creative in expressing sexuality (e.g., massage, fantasies, cuddling).

  Client may not be aware of alternative methods of expressing sexuality.

- Arrange for uninterrupted privacy if desired by couple.

  Allows client and significant other to explore identified changes

- Perform actions to improve client's self-concept (e.g., limit negative self-reflection, assist client in identification of effective coping mechanisms).

  Positive self-esteem should have a positive effect on client's sexuality.

- If dyspareunia is a problem:
  - Encourage female client to use a water-soluble lubricant before sexual intercourse.

    Reduces vaginal dryness

  - Suggest experimentation with different positions during intercourse.

    Reduces the depth of penetration

- If impotence is a problem:
  - Encourage client to discuss it with physician.

    Impotence may be due to reversible factors such as medication therapy, alcohol, and poorly controlled chronic disease conditions.

  - Assure client that occasional episodes of impotence are normal.

    Assures client of normalcy

  - Suggest alternative methods of sexual gratification if appropriate.

    May improve sexual gratification

  - Encourage client to discuss various treatment options (e.g., penile prosthesis, sildenafil, vardenafil, intraurethral alprostadil pellet placement, external vacuum device) with physician if appropriate.

    Allows client to know there are options available to treat impotence and the appropriateness of discussing this with his physician

- Reinforce the importance of rest before sexual activity.

  Improves ability to perform sexually

- If incontinence of urine is a problem, encourage client to void just before intercourse and other sexual activity.

  Decreases incidence of incontinence during sexual activity

- Include partner in above discussions and encourage continued support of the client.

  Demonstrates support for client and partner and allows them to receive factual information

Dependent/Collaborative Actions

Implement measures to promote an optimal sexuality pattern:

- If dyspareunia is a problem:
  - Administer estrogen if ordered or provide client with information about estrogen therapy.

    Reduces vaginal dryness and thinning of vaginal epithelium

Consult appropriate health care provider (counselor, sex therapist, physician) if counseling appears indicated.

Allows for a multidisciplinary treatment plan

Nursing Diagnosis **RISK FOR LONELINESS** NDx

Definition: At risk for experiencing discomfort associated with a desire or need for more with others

Related to:
* Reduced opportunities for socialization associated with inadequate financial resources, death or disability of friends and family members, reluctance of others to include the elderly in activities, reluctance to establish new relationships and try new activities, and/or a move to a different location (e.g., family member's home, foster home, extended care facility)
* Decreased desire to communicate with others associated with an imbalance between the effort required to interact with others and the anticipated rewards of the interaction
* Decreased participation in usual activities associated with changes in sensory and motor function and fear of falls
* Withdrawal from others associated with fear of embarrassment resulting from functional changes such as incontinence or hearing loss

CLINICAL MANIFESTATIONS

Subjective	Objective
Expression of feelings of rejection; being different from others or being lonely	Sad, dull affect; hostility; uncommunicative and withdrawn; absence of supportive significant others

RISK FACTORS
* Chronic illness
* Sedentary lifestyle
* Loss of friends and/or family
* Lack of interest in interacting with others

DESIRED OUTCOMES

The client will not experience a sense of isolation and loneliness as evidenced by:
   a. Maintenance of relationships with significant others
   b. No expression of feelings of isolation and loneliness

NOC OUTCOMES

Social support; psychosocial adjustment: life change; quality of life

NIC INTERVENTIONS

Socialization enhancement; visitation facilitation; support system enhancement

NURSING ASSESSMENT	RATIONALE
Assess for indications of isolation and loneliness (e.g., absence of supportive significant others; uncommunicative and withdrawn; expression of feelings of rejection, being different from others, or being lonely; hostility; sad, dull affect).	*Early recognition of signs and symptoms of loneliness allows for prompt intervention.*

THERAPEUTIC INTERVENTIONS	RATIONALE

Independent Actions
Implement measures to decrease isolation and reduce the risk for loneliness:
* Assist client to identify reasons for feeling isolated and alone; aid client in developing a plan of action to reduce these feelings.
* Use touch to demonstrate acceptance of client. **D** ● ✦
* Encourage significant others to visit. **D** ● ✦
* Encourage client to maintain telephone contact with others. **D** ● ✦
* Schedule time each day to sit and talk with client. **D** ● ✦
* Assist client to identify a few persons he/she feels comfortable with and encourage interactions with them.
* Make objects such as telephone, TV, radio, newspapers, and greeting cards accessible to client. **D** ● ✦
* Have significant others bring client's favorite objects from home and place in room. **D** ● ✦
* Change room assignments, if necessary.

Helps clients to realize they have to be actively involved in changing feelings of loneliness

Decreases loneliness
Helps client to understand he/she is not alone
Helps client become actively engaged in decreasing feelings of loneliness
Demonstrates acceptance of client and shows client that having positive interactions with others is possible

Makes client feel more at home in the health care environment

Provide the client with a roommate with similar interests.

Continued...

THERAPEUTIC INTERVENTIONS	RATIONALE
• Encourage interaction between client and roommate.	*Demonstrates to client that others find client interesting and are willing to spend time with him/her*
• Emphasize the importance of maintaining active friendships and seeking out new relationships; encourage participation in support groups if appropriate.	*Encourages client to engage in interactions with others*
• Encourage client to participate in structured activity programs after discharge; provide information about community senior centers and the programs they offer.	*Provides for continuum of care postdischarge from the acute care facility*

Nursing Diagnosis INEFFECTIVE FAMILY THERAPEUTIC REGIMEN MANAGEMENT NDx

Definition: Pattern of regulating and integrating into family processes a program for treatment of illness and its sequelae that is unsatisfactory for meeting specific health goals

Related to:
• Lack of motivation, inadequate support and supervision, and insufficient financial resources
• Confusion about appropriate health care practices and a decreased level of trust associated with conflicting advice from multiple health care providers
• Conflicting values between client and health care providers
• Knowledge deficit regarding current diagnosis, medications and treatments prescribed, and consequences of failure to comply with treatment plan

CLINICAL MANIFESTATIONS

Subjective	Objective
Statements of inability to care for self at home; statements reflecting lack of understanding of self-care; statements reflect understanding of disease progression with or without treatment; statements of unwillingness to engage in required treatment regimen	Nonadherence to diet; refusing to be involved in treatment regimen

RISK FACTORS
• Chronic illness
• Medication regimen
• Lack of resources both social and financial

DESIRED OUTCOMES

The client will demonstrate the probability of effective management of therapeutic regimen as evidenced by:
    a. Willingness to learn about and participate in treatments and care
    b. Statements reflecting ways to modify personal habits and integrate treatments into lifestyle
    c. Statements reflecting an understanding of the implications of not following the prescribed treatment plan

NOC OUTCOMES

Knowledge: treatment regimen; knowledge: disease process; participation in health care decisions; compliance behavior; health beliefs: perceived resources

NIC INTERVENTIONS

Discharge planning; health system guidance; self-modification assistance; teaching: disease process; teaching: procedure/treatment; support group; values clarification; financial resource assistance

NURSING ASSESSMENT	RATIONALE
Assess for indications that the client may be unable to effectively manage the therapeutic regimen: • Statements reflecting inability to manage care at home • Failure to adhere to treatment plan (e.g., not adhering to dietary modifications, refusing medications, refusing to ambulate)	*Early recognition of signs and symptoms of ineffective therapeutic management allows for prompt intervention.*

NURSING ASSESSMENT	RATIONALE

- Statements reflecting a lack of understanding of the factors that will cause further progression of current illness and/or accelerate aging process
- Statements reflecting an unwillingness or inability to modify personal habits and integrate necessary treatments into lifestyle
- Statements reflecting view that situation is hopeless and that efforts to comply are useless

THERAPEUTIC INTERVENTIONS	RATIONALE

Independent Actions

Implement measures to promote effective management of the therapeutic regimen:

- Discuss with client the specific factors that may interfere with management of care (e.g., inadequate financial resources, religious or cultural conflicts, lack of support systems).

  Helps client identify underlying cause of ineffective treatment management

- Explain the aging process and current diagnosis in terms the client can understand; stress the fact that adherence to the treatment plan is necessary in order to delay and/or prevent complications associated with the diagnosis and minimize some of the changes that occur with aging.

  Helps client understand that some physiological changes are part of the aging process, but others require adherence to a treatment regimen

- Assist client to clarify values and to identify ways to incorporate the therapeutic goals and priorities into value system.

  Values clarification and lifestyle changes

- Encourage questions and clarify misconceptions the client has about aging and his/her diagnosis and effects of each.

  Ensures client's understanding

- Perform actions to promote trust in caregivers (e.g., validate conflicting advice, explain reasons for treatment plan).

  Helps improve adherence

- Encourage client to participate in treatment plan (e.g., take medications as prescribed, perform recommended exercises).

  Helps to improve client's self-confidence in ability to care for self

- Provide instruction regarding medications and treatments prescribed; allow time for return demonstration of procedures; determine areas of difficulty and misunderstanding and reinforce teaching as necessary.

  Knowledge of medications and how they impact the system improves client adherence to treatment regimen and understanding of the importance of adhering to the prescribed medication regimen. The client must be able to recognize alterations in functioning related to medication administration and what clinical manifestations that should be reported to the health care provider.

- Provide client with written instructions about medications and treatments.

  Provides a reference once discharged from the acute care facility

- Assist client to identify ways to incorporate treatments into lifestyle; focus on modifications of lifestyle rather than complete change if possible.

  Clients will adhere more closely to lifestyle modifications that they identify.

- Encourage client to discuss financial concerns; obtain a social service consult to assist client with financial planning and to obtain financial aid if indicated.

  Provides for ongoing support postdischarge from the acute care facility

- Provide information about and encourage use of community resources that can assist client to make necessary lifestyle changes if appropriate.

  Provides ongoing support and continuum of care postdischarge from the acute care facility

- Encourage client to attend follow-up educational classes if appropriate.

  Increases client's understanding of disease process and ongoing self-care

- Reinforce behaviors suggesting future compliance with the therapeutic regimen (e.g., statements reflecting plans for integrating treatments into lifestyle, active participation in exercise program, changes in personal habits).

  Improves client's self-confidence in abilities to adhere to treatment regimen and to care for self

Continued...

THERAPEUTIC INTERVENTIONS	RATIONALE
• Include significant others in explanations and teaching sessions and encourage their support; reinforce the need for client to assume responsibility for managing as much of care as possible.	*Provides ongoing support once the client is discharged from the acute care facility*
Dependent/Collaborative Actions	
Consult appropriate health care provider about referrals to community health agencies if continued instruction, support, or supervision is needed.	*Allows for multidisciplinary client care*

Nursing Diagnosis   INTERRUPTED FAMILY PROCESSES NDx

Definition: Change in family relationships and/or functioning

Related to:
• Financial, physical, and psychological stresses associated with family member's illness and/or progressive disability
• Inadequate knowledge about the normal aging process, client's current diagnosis, and necessary care
• Inadequate support services
• Decreased ability of client to fulfill usual family roles
• Guilt associated with need to change client's living situation resulting from family's inability to provide necessary care

CLINICAL MANIFESTATIONS

Subjective	Objective
Verbal reports of increased stress related to financial, physical, and/or psychological associated with disability.	Change in financial situations; change in psychological stress; change in communication patterns; changes in intimacy; changes in participation in problem-solving; changes in rituals; changes in satisfaction with family; changes in somatic behavior; changes in stress-reduction behavior

RISK FACTORS
• Chronic illness
• Sedentary lifestyle
• Changes in roles and responsibilities
• Poor self-esteem
• Poor social support system

DESIRED OUTCOMES

The family members* will demonstrate beginning adjustment to changes in functioning of family member and family roles and structure as evidenced by:
    a. Meeting client's needs
    b. Verbalization of ways to adapt to required role and lifestyle changes
    c. Active participation in decision-making and client's rehabilitation
    d. Positive interactions with one another

NOC OUTCOMES

Family coping; family functioning; family involvement promotion; family normalization; family resiliency

NIC INTERVENTIONS

Family integrity promotion; family process maintenance; family support

NURSING ASSESSMENT	RATIONALE
Assess for signs and symptoms of interrupted family processes (e.g., inability to meet client's needs, statements of not being able to accept client's disabilities or make necessary role and lifestyle changes, inability to make decisions, inability or refusal to participate in client's care and/or rehabilitation, negative family interactions).	*Early recognition of signs and symptoms of interrupted family processes allows for prompt intervention.*
Identify components of the family and their patterns of communication and role expectations.	

*The term "family members" is being used here to include client's significant others.

THERAPEUTIC INTERVENTIONS	RATIONALE

Independent Actions

Implement measures to facilitate family members' adjustment to age- or diagnosis-related changes in client and resultant changes in family roles and structure:

- Encourage family members to verbalize feelings about changes in client and the effect of these changes on family structure; actively listen to each family member and maintain a nonjudgmental attitude about feelings shared.

  Helps them work through their issues and concern related to changes in the family structure

- Instruct client and family about normal aging processes (e.g., sensory deficits, decreased muscle strength, reduced coordination).

  Provides client and family with factual information

- Reinforce physician's explanation of the effects of the current diagnosis and planned treatment and rehabilitation.

  Reinforcing important information allows the nurse to both summarize key concepts and further assess client's understanding of instructions.

- Assist family members to gain a realistic perspective of client's situation, conveying as much hope as appropriate.

  Improves family support and understanding of client's situation and the importance of their support

- Provide privacy so that family members and client can share their feelings with one another; stress the importance of and facilitate the use of good communication techniques.

  Allows for open communication between family members and client

- Assist family members to progress through their own grieving processes; explain that they may encounter times when they need to focus on meeting their own rather than the client's needs.

  Helps family members understand that a significant change has occurred and it is OK to grieve the changes

- Emphasize the need for family members to obtain adequate rest and nutrition and to identify and use stress management techniques.

  Assists them to deal emotionally and physically with the changes experienced

- Encourage and assist family members to identify coping strategies for dealing with client's age-related changes and changes in health status and their effect on the family.

  Helps them learn what mechanisms work best for them in dealing with client and family changes

- Assist family members to identify realistic goals and ways of reaching these goals.

  Helps to decrease disappointment when unrealistic goals are not met

- Include family members in decision-making about client's care; convey appreciation for their input and continued support of client.

  Helps family have some sense of control over the situation

- Encourage and allow family members to participate in client's care and rehabilitation; instruct family in any special procedures and allow them to practice with supervision before discharge of the client.

  Improves family's understanding of treatment regimen and their ability to support client

- Assist family members to identify resources that could assist them in coping with their feelings and meeting their immediate and long-term needs (e.g., counseling and social services; pastoral care; service, church, and support groups); initiate a referral if indicated.

  Provides for continuum of care once client is discharged from the acute care facility

Dependent/Collaborative Actions

Consult appropriate health care provider if family members continue to demonstrate difficulty adapting to changes in client's functioning, roles, and family structure.

Allows for multidisciplinary input into continuum of care

ADDITIONAL NURSING DIAGNOSES

DISTURBED SELF-CONCEPT* NDx
Related to:
- Changes in appearance and body functioning (e.g., graying and thinning of hair; sagginess of eyelids, earlobes, and breasts; dry, wrinkled skin; reduced height; increase in and change in distribution of body fat; reduction in lean body mass; decreased bladder control; diminished visual acuity and hearing)
- Increased dependence on others to meet basic needs
- Feelings of powerlessness
- Change in usual lifestyle and roles associated with decreased strength and endurance and disturbed sensory perception

FEAR AND ANXIETY NDx
Related to:
- Unfamiliar environment
- Signs and symptoms of current diagnosis

- Lack of understanding of diagnostic tests, diagnosis, and treatment plan
- Financial concerns
- Effects of diagnosis on health status, usual roles, and ability to live independently

RISK FOR POWERLESSNESS NDx
Related to:
- Increased dependence on others to meet basic needs
- Inability to pursue usual life activities and roles associated with age-related changes in body functioning, current diagnosis and its treatment, and inadequate financial resources
- Inability to control many of the changes that occur with aging

---

*This diagnostic label includes the nursing diagnoses of disturbed body image, low self-esteem, and ineffective role performance.

16

End-of-Life Nursing Care

This care plan focuses on care of the adult client who is expected to die soon. The information included is appropriate for clients in acute or extended care settings or in the home. The major goals of nursing care are to prevent or control physiological problems that could reduce the quality of the client's remaining life; facilitate the client's psychological adjustment to his/her imminent death; and assist the client to experience a peaceful, dignified death. The nurse also assists the significant others to understand the dying process, support the dying person, meet their own physical and emotional needs, and adjust to their loss of the client.

This care plan does not deal with any particular medical diagnosis. The nursing diagnoses included are those that are relatively common to all persons facing death. Care plans that pertain to the client's specific medical diagnosis will provide additional guidelines for nursing care during the terminal stages of that illness.

Use in conjunction with the Care Plan on Immobility and care plans that pertain to the client's medical diagnosis.

Nursing Diagnosis **IMPAIRED RESPIRATORY FUNCTION***

Definition: Inability of an individual to maintain adequate ventilation of the respiratory tract and perfusion of oxygen (O_2) and carbon dioxide (CO_2) between the lungs and vascular system to maintain adequate tissue oxygenation.

Ineffective breathing pattern NDx related to:
- Increased rate of respirations associated with fear, anxiety, and pain
- Decreased rate of respirations associated with the depressant effect of some medications (e.g., narcotic [opioid] analgesics, some antiemetics and antianxiety agents)
- Decreased depth of respirations associated with recumbent positioning (in this position, full expansion of the lungs is restricted by the bed surface and by the abdominal contents pushing up against the diaphragm), fear, anxiety, weakness, fatigue, and/or abdominal distention
- Altered function of the respiratory center (can occur as a result of the underlying disease process)

Ineffective airway clearance NDx related to:
- Stasis of secretions associated with:
  - Decreased mobility
  - Difficulty coughing up secretions resulting from diminished lung/chest wall expansion and presence of tenacious secretions if fluid intake is inadequate
- Fluid accumulation in the alveoli and bronchioles associated with pulmonary edema if present
- Airway obstruction associated with the underlying disease process and/or relaxation of the tongue (can occur with decreased level of consciousness and as a result of administration of central nervous system depressants)

Impaired gas exchange NDx related to:
- Loss of effective lung tissue (can occur as a result of the underlying disease process)
- A thickened alveolar-capillary membrane associated with stasis of pulmonary secretions and pulmonary edema if present
- Decreased oxygen availability associated with anemia (can result from decreased nutritional status and/or the underlying disease process)

CLINICAL MANIFESTATIONS

Subjective	Objective
Reports of feeling of suffocation or drowning; significant decrease in oximetry results	Rapid, shallow, slow, or irregular respirations; dyspnea, orthopnea; use of accessory muscles when breathing; adventitious breath sounds; diminished or absent breath sounds; restlessness, agitation; cough, gurgling or rattling respirations; confusion, somnolence

*This diagnostic label includes the following nursing diagnoses: ineffective breathing pattern, ineffective airway clearance, and impaired gas exchange.

NDx = NANDA-I Diagnosis   **D** = Delegatable Action   ● = UAP   ✦ = LVN/LPN   ⊝▶ = Go to ⊝volve for animation

Continued...

RISK FACTORS

- Immobility
- Inadequate fluid intake

DESIRED OUTCOMES

The client will not experience respiratory distress as evidenced by:
  a. Unlabored respirations
  b. Absence of restlessness and agitation
  c. Absence of gurgling or rattling respirations
  d. No reports of feeling of suffocation or drowning

NOC OUTCOMES

Respiratory status: ventilation; respiratory status: airway patency; respiratory status: gas exchange; comfortable death; comfort level

NIC INTERVENTIONS

Respiratory monitoring; airway management; oxygen therapy; anxiety reduction

NURSING ASSESSMENT

Assess for signs and symptoms of respiratory dysfunction:
- Reports of feeling of suffocation or drowning
- Significant decrease in oximetry results
- Rapid, shallow, slow, or irregular respirations
- Dyspnea, orthopnea
- Use of accessory muscles when breathing
- Adventitious breath sounds
- Diminished or absent breath sounds
- Restlessness, agitation
- Cough, gurgling or rattling respirations
- Confusion, somnolence

RATIONALE

Early recognition of signs and symptoms of respiratory dysfunction allows for prompt intervention.

THERAPEUTIC INTERVENTIONS

RATIONALE

Independent Actions
Implement measures to maintain an adequate respiratory status and prevent respiratory distress:
- Perform actions to reduce pain:
  - Provide for or assist with nonpharmacological methods for pain relief (e.g., massage; position change; diversional activities). **D** ✦ ●

- Perform actions to decrease accumulation of gastrointestinal gas and fluid (e.g., avoid intake of carbonated beverages and gas-producing foods).

- Perform actions to decrease fear and anxiety:
  - Encourage the client to breathe deeply and more slowly. **D** ✦

- Perform actions to reduce the risk for aspiration.
  - Perform oral hygiene/oropharyngeal suctioning as often as needed to remove excess secretions. **D** ✦ ●

- Place client in a semi- to high-Fowler's position unless contraindicated; position client with pillows. **D** ● ✦

- Instruct client to breathe slowly if hyperventilating.

- Assist client with position change at least every 2 hours. **D** ● ✦

- Perform actions to promote removal of secretions:
  - Instruct and assist client to deep breathe and cough or "huff" every 1 to 2 hours.

- Encourage activity as tolerated.

Actions help to prevent any change in the depth or rate of respirations that can occur in response to pain.

Actions help to decrease pressure on the diaphragm, facilitating adequate ventilation.

Decreasing fear and anxiety allows the client to focus on breathing more slowly and taking deeper breaths.

Aspiration of gastric contents can lead to the development of adult respiratory distress syndrome (ARDS).

Prevention of slumping is essential because slumping causes abdominal contents to be pushed up against the diaphragm and restricts lung expansion.

Hyperventilation is an ineffective breathing pattern that can lead to respiratory alkalosis.

Frequent repositioning promotes maximal chest wall and lung expansion.

Coughing or "huffing" accelerates airflow through the airways, which helps mobilize and clear mucus from the respiratory tract.

Activity helps to mobilize secretions and promotes deeper breathing.

THERAPEUTIC INTERVENTIONS	RATIONALE

Dependent/Collaborative Actions

Implement measures to maintain an adequate respiratory status and prevent respiratory distress:

- Perform actions to reduce pain:
  - Administer analgesics as ordered before activities and procedures. **D** ✦

  Pain reduction enables the client to increase activity and cough and deep breathe more effectively, which promote effective airway clearance.

- Perform actions to promote removal of secretions: **D** ✦
  - Implement measures to thin tenacious secretions and reduce dryness of the respiratory mucous membrane:
    (1) Encourage maximum fluid intake allowed and tolerated.
    (2) Humidify inspired air as ordered.

  Adequate hydration and humidified inspired air help thin secretions, which facilitates mobilization and expectoration.

  - Perform oral, pharyngeal, and/or tracheal suctioning if necessary (tracheal suctioning should be avoided during the final stage of dying).

  Suctioning removes secretions from large airways and stimulates coughing, which helps clear airways and promotes oxygenation.

- Maintain oxygen therapy as ordered. **D** ✦
- Administer the following medications if ordered:
  - Diuretics **D** ✦
  - Morphine sulfate
  - Bronchodilators

  - Anticholinergics

  Diuretics decrease fluid accumulation in the lungs.
  Morphine helps to reduce dyspnea.
  Bronchodilators dilate upper airway passages, facilitating ventilation.
  Anticholinergics help reduce bronchial secretions if frequent suctioning is necessary or the sound of excessive secretions is disturbing to significant others.

Consult appropriate health care provider (e.g., respiratory therapist, palliative care nurse, hospice nurse, physician) if the client is experiencing respiratory distress.

Consulting the appropriate health care provider allows for modification of the treatment plan.

Nursing Diagnosis ## RISK FOR ASPIRATION NDx

Definition: At risk for entry of gastrointestinal secretions, oropharyngeal secretions, solids, or fluids into the tracheobronchial tract

Related to:

- Decreased level of consciousness
- Absent or diminished gag reflex associated with the underlying disease process and/or the depressant effect of some medications (e.g., narcotic [opioid] analgesics, some antiemetics and antianxiety agents)
- Supine positioning
- Increased risk for gastroesophageal reflux associated with increased gastric pressure resulting from decreased gastrointestinal motility
- Impaired swallowing associated with dry mouth and absent or diminished swallowing reflex (can occur as a result of the underlying disease process)

CLINICAL MANIFESTATIONS

Subjective	Objective
Not applicable	Rhonchi; dull percussion note over affected lung area; cough; tachypnea; tachycardia; development of or increase in dyspnea; presence of tube feeding in tracheal aspirate; chest radiograph showing pulmonary infiltrate

Continued...

RISK FACTORS

- Delayed gastric emptying
- Impaired swallowing
- Decreased level of consciousness
- Tube feeding

DESIRED OUTCOMES

The client will not aspirate secretions or foods/fluids as evidenced by:
  a. Clear or usual breath sounds
  b. Resonant percussion note over lungs
  c. Absence of cough and tachypnea
  d. Absence of or no increase in dyspnea

NOC OUTCOMES

Aspiration prevention; respiratory status: gas exchange

NIC INTERVENTIONS

Respiratory monitoring; aspiration precautions; airway precautions

NURSING ASSESSMENT	RATIONALE

Assess for and report signs and symptoms of aspiration of secretions, vomitus, or foods/fluids:
- Rhonchi
- Dull percussion note over affected lung area
- Cough, tachypnea, tachycardia
- Development of or increase in dyspnea
- Presence of tube feeding in tracheal aspirate

Assess chest radiograph for evidence of pulmonary infiltrates.

Early recognition of signs and symptoms of aspiration allows for prompt intervention.

THERAPEUTIC INTERVENTIONS	RATIONALE

Independent Actions
Implement measures to reduce the risk for aspiration:
- Position client in side-lying or semi- to high-Fowler's position at all times. **D** ● ✦
- Perform actions to prevent nausea and vomiting:
  - Eliminate noxious sights/odors.
- Perform actions to reduce the accumulation of gastrointestinal gas and fluid (e.g., expel flatus, eructate).
- Withhold oral food/fluids if gag reflex is depressed or absent, client is not alert, or client is experiencing severe dysphagia.
- If client is receiving tube feedings:
  - Check tube placement before each feeding or on a routine basis if continuous feeding. **D** ✦

  - Maintain client in a high-Fowler's position during and for at least 30 minutes after feeding unless contraindicated. **D** ● ✦
  - Stop tube feeding and notify physician if residuals exceed established parameters.
- If client is taking foods/fluids orally:
  - Offer foods/fluids that promote an effective swallow (e.g., thick rather than thin fluids, moist rather than dry foods). **D** ✦
  - Encourage client to concentrate on eating and drinking and allow ample time for meals. **D** ✦

  - Instruct client to avoid talking or laughing when swallowing.

Reducing nausea and vomiting reduces the risk for aspiration.

Actions help to reduce the risk of gastric distention and gastro-esophageal reflux.

Risk for aspiration is high when mechanisms to protect the client's airway (e.g., gag reflex) are impaired.

Validation of appropriate location of feeding tube ensures that tube feeding solution goes into the alimentary tract and not the lungs.

Head-of-bed elevation facilitates movement of foods and fluid through the pharynx into the esophagus where the risk for aspiration is greatly reduced.

High residual volumes can lead to upward pressure placed on the lower esophagus, increasing the risk for regurgitation.

Thin fluids rapidly pass through the mouth and can pour over the back of the tongue without triggering an effective swallow, increasing the risk for aspiration.

If a client becomes distracted during meals or is rushed, swallowing and breathing attempts can become uncoordinated, increasing the risk for aspiration.

Laughing or talking results in the larynx remaining opened during eating and increases the risk of aspiration.

THERAPEUTIC INTERVENTIONS	RATIONALE
• Maintain client in high-Fowler's position during and for at least 30 minutes after meals and snacks unless contraindicated. **D** ● ✦	*A high-Fowler's position uses gravity to aid in the flow of fluids/ foods through the esophagus.*
• Assist client with oral hygiene after eating. **D** ● ✦	*Good oral hygiene after meals results in the removal of remaining food particles that could enter the larynx and be aspirated into the lungs.*

If signs and symptoms of aspiration occur:
* Perform tracheal suctioning.
* Withhold oral intake.
* Prepare client for chest radiograph if ordered.

Dependent/Collaborative Actions

Implement measures to reduce the risk for aspiration:
* Perform oropharyngeal suctioning and oral hygiene as often as needed.
* If client is receiving tube feedings:
  * Do not increase rate of continuous tube feeding unless allowed and tolerated; administer intermittent tube feedings slowly.

Oropharyngeal suctioning helps to remove excess secretions, vomitus, and food particles.

Nursing Diagnosis ## ACUTE/CHRONIC PAIN NDx

Definition: Unpleasant sensory and emotional experience arising from actual or potential tissue damage. *Acute:* sudden or slow onset of any intensity from mild to severe with an anticipated or predictable end and a duration of <6 months. *Chronic:* sudden or slow onset of any intensity from mild to severe; constant or recurs without an anticipated or predictable end and has a duration of >6 months.

Related to:
* The underlying disease process
* Muscle spasms or stiff joints associated with decreased mobility
* Reluctance to take pain medication associated with fear of loss of control and/or oversedation, feeling that taking medication is a sign of weakness or that pain has redemptive qualities, and/or need to be stoic

CLINICAL MANIFESTATIONS

Subjective	Objective
Verbalization of pain	Grimacing; reluctance to move; restlessness; diaphoresis; increased blood pressure (B/P); tachycardia

RISK FACTORS	DESIRED OUTCOMES
• Injury agents • Immobility • Chronic disability	The client will experience diminished pain as evidenced by: 　a. Verbalization of decrease in or absence of pain 　b. Relaxed facial expression and body positioning 　c. Stable vital signs

NOC OUTCOMES	NIC INTERVENTIONS
Comfort level; pain control	Analgesic administration; pain management; patient-controlled analgesia (PCA) assistance; environmental management: comfort; dying care

NURSING ASSESSMENT	RATIONALE
Assess for signs and symptoms of pain: • Grimacing • Reluctance to move • Restlessness • Diaphoresis • Increased B/P	*Early recognition of signs and symptoms of pain allows for prompt intervention.*

NDx = NANDA-I Diagnosis　　**D** = Delegatable Action　　● = UAP　　✦ = LVN/LPN　　⊖▶ = Go to ⊖volve for animation

Continued...

NURSING ASSESSMENT	RATIONALE

- Tachycardia
- Verbalization of pain

Assess client's perception of the severity of pain using a pain intensity rating scale.

Assess the client's pain pattern (e.g., location, quality, onset, duration, precipitating factors, aggravating factors, alleviating factors).

Ask the client to describe previous pain experiences and methods used to manage pain effectively.

THERAPEUTIC INTERVENTIONS	RATIONALE

Independent Actions

Implement measures to reduce pain:

- Perform actions to reduce fear and anxiety about the pain experience (e.g., assure client that the need for pain relief is understood, plan methods for achieving pain control with client).

  Actions help promote relaxation and subsequently increase the client's threshold and tolerance for pain.

- Perform actions to promote rest:
  - Cluster nursing care. **D** ● ✦

  Actions help reduce fatigue and subsequently increase the client's threshold and tolerance for pain.

- Plan methods for achieving pain control with client.

  Actions help assist client to maintain a sense of control over the pain experience.

- Provide or assist with nonpharmacological methods for pain relief (e.g., massage; position change; progressive relaxation exercise; restful environment; diversional activities such as watching television, reading, or conversing). **D** ✦

  Nonpharmacological pain management includes a variety of interventions. These interventions are believed to be effective because they stimulate closure of the gating mechanism in the spinal cord.

- If client has a PCA device, encourage client to use it as instructed.
- Maintain integrity of analgesia delivery system (e.g., epidural, intravenous, subcutaneous, transdermal).

Dependent/Collaborative Actions

Implement measures to reduce pain:

- Administer analgesics before activities and procedures that can cause pain and before pain becomes severe.

  Actions help to minimize pain that will be experienced.

- Administer the following medications as ordered to provide maximum pain relief with minimal side effects: **D** ✦
  - Narcotic (opioid) analgesics
  - Nonnarcotic (nonopioid) analgesics
  - Local anesthetics
  - Muscle relaxants

Consult appropriate health care provider (e.g., hospice nurse, palliative care nurse, pharmacist, physician, pain management specialist) if above measures fail to provide adequate pain relief.

Consulting the appropriate health care provider allows for modification of the treatment plan.

Nursing Diagnosis   ## NAUSEA   NDx

Definition: A subjective, unpleasant, wave-like sensation in the back of the throat, epigastrium, or abdomen that may lead to the urge or need to vomit

Related to: Stimulation of the vomiting center associated with:

- Stimulation of the visceral afferent pathways resulting from abdominal distention if present
- Stimulation of the cerebral cortex resulting from pain and stress
- Stimulation of the chemoreceptor trigger zone by some medications (e.g., morphine sulfate)

CLINICAL MANIFESTATIONS

Subjective	Objective
Verbal reports of nausea	Vomiting; retching

RISK FACTORS

- Excessive sputum production
- Medication regimen
- Chronic illness

DESIRED OUTCOMES

The client will experience relief of nausea and vomiting as evidenced by:
  a. Verbalization of relief of nausea
  b. Absence of vomiting

NOC OUTCOMES

Nausea and vomiting severity

NIC INTERVENTIONS

Nausea management; vomiting management

NURSING ASSESSMENT

Assess client for nausea and vomiting:
- Vomiting
- Retching
- Verbal reports of nausea

RATIONALE

Early recognition of signs and symptoms of nausea allows for prompt intervention.

THERAPEUTIC INTERVENTIONS

RATIONALE

Independent Actions
Implement measures to prevent nausea and vomiting:
- Perform actions to reduce accumulation of gastrointestinal gas and fluid:
  - Assist client with frequent position changes and ambulation as tolerated. **D** ● ✦

Activity stimulates peristalsis and expulsion of gas.

- Perform actions to reduce pain:
  - Administer analgesics before activities.
- Eliminate noxious sights and odors from the environment. **D** ● ✦

Noxious stimuli can cause stimulation of the vomiting center.

- Encourage client to take deep, slow breaths when nauseated. **D** ✦
- Instruct client to change positions slowly.

Rapid movement can result in stimulation of the chemoreceptor trigger zone and subsequent excitation of the vomiting center.

- Provide oral hygiene after each emesis. **D** ● ✦
- If oral intake is allowed and tolerated:
  - Avoid serving foods with an overpowering aroma; remove lids from hot foods before entering room.
  - Provide small, frequent meals; instruct client to ingest foods and fluids slowly.
  - Encourage client to eat dry foods (e.g., toast, crackers) and avoid drinking liquids with meals if nauseated.
  - Instruct client to avoid foods/fluids that irritate the gastric mucosa (e.g., spicy foods; caffeine-containing beverages such as coffee, tea, and colas).
- Instruct client to avoid foods high in fat.
- Instruct client to rest after eating with head of bed elevated.
- Administer medications known to cause gastric irritation (e.g., aspirin and aspirin-containing products, corticosteroids, ibuprofen) with or immediately after meals or snacks unless contraindicated. **D** ✦

Action helps to eliminate noxious tastes after emesis and promotes comfort.

Foods high in fat delay gastric emptying.

Dependent/Collaborative Actions
Implement measures to prevent nausea and vomiting:
- Administer medications ordered to control nausea and vomiting.

NDx = NANDA-I Diagnosis   **D** = Delegatable Action   ● = UAP   ✦ = LVN/LPN   ⊖▶ = Go to ⊖volve for animation

Continued...

THERAPEUTIC INTERVENTIONS	RATIONALE
If above measures fail to control nausea and vomiting: • Consult physician. • Be prepared to insert a nasogastric tube and maintain suction as ordered.	*Consulting the appropriate health care provider allows for modification of the treatment plan.*

Nursing Diagnosis **IMPAIRED COMFORT** NDx **(ABDOMINAL DISTENTION AND GAS PAIN)**

Definition: Perceived lack of ease, relief, and transcendence in physical, psychomotor, ent viront mental, and social dimensions

Related to: An accumulation of gas and fluid in the gastrointestinal tract associated with decreased gastrointestinal motility resulting from depressant effect of some medications (e.g., narcotic [opioid] analgesics) and decreased activity

CLINICAL MANIFESTATIONS

Subjective	Objective
Verbal reports of abdominal fullness or gas pain	Grimacing; clutching or guarding of abdomen; restlessness; reluctance to move; increasing abdominal girth

RISK FACTORS
• Immobility
• Narcotic administration

DESIRED OUTCOMES

The client will experience diminished abdominal distention and gas pain as evidenced by:
  a. Verbalization of decreased abdominal fullness and pain
  b. Relaxed facial expression and body positioning
  c. Decrease in abdominal girth

NOC OUTCOMES
Comfort level

NIC INTERVENTIONS
Flatulence reduction

NURSING ASSESSMENT	RATIONALE
Assess for signs and symptoms of abdominal distention and gas pain: • Grimacing • Clutching or guarding of abdomen • Restlessness • Reluctance to move • Increasing abdominal girth • Verbal reports of abdominal fullness or gas pain	*Early recognition of signs and symptoms of abdominal distention and gas pain allows for prompt intervention.*

THERAPEUTIC INTERVENTIONS	RATIONALE
Independent Actions Implement measures to reduce the accumulation of gastrointestinal gas and fluid: • Encourage and assist client with frequent position changes and ambulation as tolerated. **D** ● ✦ • Instruct client to avoid activities such as chewing gum and smoking. • Maintain patency of nasogastric tube if present. **D** ✦ • Maintain food and oral fluid restrictions if ordered. **D** ✦	*Activity stimulates peristalsis and expulsion of flatus.* *Avoiding such activities reduces air swallowing.* *Allows for optimal decompression of gastrointestinal tract.*

THERAPEUTIC INTERVENTIONS	RATIONALE

- Instruct client to avoid intake of carbonated beverages and gas-producing foods (e.g., cabbage, onions, beans). **D** = ✦
- Encourage client to eructate and expel flatus whenever the urge is felt.

Dependent/Collaborative Actions
Implement measures to reduce the accumulation of gastrointestinal gas and fluid:
- If appropriate, encourage the use of nonnarcotic analgesics rather than narcotic (opioid) analgesics for pain management.
- Administer the following medications if ordered: **D** ✦
  - Antiflatulents
  - Gastrointestinal stimulants
- Consult physician about insertion of a rectal tube or administration of a return-flow enema if indicated.
Consult appropriate health care provider (e.g., hospice nurse, palliative care nurse, physician) if signs and symptoms of abdominal distention or gas pain persist or worsen.

Antiflatulents help to reduce gas accumulation.
Gastrointestinal stimulants help to increase gastrointestinal motility.

Consulting the appropriate health care provider allows for modification of the treatment plan.

Nursing Diagnosis RISK FOR IMPAIRED TISSUE INTEGRITY NDx

Definition: Altered epidermis and/or dermis

Related to:
- Accumulation of waste products and decreased oxygen and nutrient supply to the skin and subcutaneous tissue associated with reduced blood flow from prolonged pressure on the tissues resulting from decreased mobility
- Damage to the skin and/or subcutaneous tissue associated with friction or shearing
- Frequent contact with irritants associated with incontinence of urine or stool
- Increased fragility of skin associated with inadequate nutritional status, dryness, and dependent edema

CLINICAL MANIFESTATIONS

Subjective	Objective
Verbalization of problem	Pallor; redness; obvious areas of skin breakdown

RISK FACTORS
- Immobility
- Shearing/pressure forces
- Impaired circulation
- Changes in fluid status

DESIRED OUTCOMES
The client will maintain tissue integrity as evidenced by:
a. Absence of redness and irritation
b. No skin breakdown

NOC OUTCOMES
Tissue integrity: skin and mucous membrane

NIC INTERVENTIONS
Skin surveillance; skin care: topical treatments; pressure ulcer prevention; positioning

NURSING ASSESSMENT	RATIONALE

Determine client's risk for skin breakdown using a risk assessment tool (e.g., Norton Scale, Braden Scale, Gosnell Scale).
Inspect the skin (especially bony prominences; dependent, edematous, and pruritic areas; and perianal area) for pallor, redness, and breakdown.

Early recognition of signs and symptoms of skin breakdown allows for prompt intervention.

Continued...

THERAPEUTIC INTERVENTIONS	RATIONALE

Independent Actions

Implement measures to prevent skin irritation resulting from incontinence of urine or stool in order to help prevent tissue breakdown:

- Perform actions to reduce the episodes of urinary and bowel incontinence:
  - Implement a bowel training program.
  - Offer assistance to defecate at regular intervals during the day. **D ●**
- Assist client to thoroughly cleanse and dry perineal area with soft tissue or cloth after each episode of incontinence; apply a protective ointment or cream. **D ● ✦**
- Apply a fecal incontinence pouch if bowel incontinence is a persistent problem. **D ✦**
- If use of absorbent products such as pads or undergarments is necessary, select those that effectively absorb moisture and keep it away from the skin.

Keeping skin dry and protected prevents breakdown.

Dependent/Collaborative Actions

If tissue breakdown occurs:

- Notify appropriate health care provider (e.g., wound care specialist, physician).
- Perform pressure ulcer care as ordered or per standard hospital procedure (extensiveness of treatment is usually limited to that necessary to maintain comfort).

Consulting the appropriate health care provider allows for modification of the treatment plan.

Nursing Diagnosis | ## IMPAIRED ORAL MUCOUS MEMBRANE NDx (DRYNESS AND IRRITATION)

Definition: Disruption of the lips and/or soft tissues of the oral cavity

Related to:

- Decreased salivation associated with decreased oral intake and some medications (e.g., tricyclic antidepressants, anticholinergics, narcotic [opioid] analgesics, phenothiazines)
- Deficient fluid volume associated with decreased fluid intake and increased fluid loss
- Prolonged oxygen therapy (especially if administered by mask)
- Mouth breathing
- Inadequate nutritional status

CLINICAL MANIFESTATIONS

Subjective	Objective
Reports of oral dryness and discomfort	Coated tongue; inflamed and/or ulcerated oral mucosa

RISK FACTOR

- Barriers to oral care

DESIRED OUTCOMES

The client will maintain a healthy oral cavity as evidenced by:
  a. Absence of inflammation and discomfort
  b. Moist, intact mucosa

NOC OUTCOMES	NIC INTERVENTIONS
Oral hygiene	Oral health maintenance; oral health restoration

NURSING ASSESSMENT	RATIONALE
Assess client for signs and symptoms of impaired oral mucous membrane: • Coated tongue • Inflamed and/or ulcerated oral mucosa • Reports of oral dryness and discomfort	*Early recognition of signs and symptoms of impaired oral mucosa allows for prompt intervention.*

THERAPEUTIC INTERVENTIONS	RATIONALE

Independent Actions

Implement measures to reduce dryness of the oral mucous membrane: • Assist client to perform oral hygiene as often as needed; avoid use of products that contain lemon and glycerin and mouthwashes containing alcohol. **D** ● ✦	*Agents have a drying and irritating effect on the oral mucous membrane.*
• Assist client to rinse mouth frequently with water. **D** ● ✦ • Lubricate client's lips frequently. **D** ● ✦	*Frequent rinsing of the mouth prevents dryness and assists with removal of food and debris that can harbor or promote the growth of organisms.*
• Encourage client to breathe through nose rather than mouth.	*Air inspired through the nose is humidified.*
• Encourage client not to smoke or chew tobacco. • Perform actions to prevent further fluid loss: • Implement measures to prevent nausea and vomiting if present: (1) Eliminate noxious odors. **D** ● ✦	*Smoking dries the mucosa; tobacco acts as an irritant to the oral mucosa.*
• Implement measures to reduce fever if present: (1) Administer antipyretics. **D** ✦	*A fever produces a hypermetabolic state that increases insensible fluid loss, leading to dehydration and drying of the mucous membranes.*
• Encourage fluid intake as allowed and tolerated; if client has difficulty drinking from a glass or through a straw:	*Adequate hydration keeps the oral mucosa moist. Actions help to stimulate salivation.*
• Give frequent sips of water or juice using a syringe. **D** ● ✦	*Actions help to lubricate the mucous membrane.*
• Use a spoon to provide small amounts of ice chips. **D** ● ✦ • Provide frozen juice bars if client desires.	
• Encourage client to suck on hard candy unless contraindicated. **D** ✦	*Sucking on hard candy can stimulate salivation.*
• Encourage client to use a saliva substitute such as Salivart if needed. **D** ✦	*Saliva substitutes lubricate oral mucosa in the absence of normal salivary flow.*
If oral mucosa is irritated or cracked, implement measures to relieve discomfort and promote healing: **D** ✦ • If client is alert and able to take nourishment by mouth, assist him/her to select soft, bland foods.	
• Instruct client to avoid foods/fluids that are extremely hot. • Use a soft bristle brush, gauze-wrapped tongue blade, sponge-tipped applicator, or low-pressure power spray for oral hygiene.	*Foods that are extremely hot or cold may cause thermal trauma to the oral mucosa.*

Dependent/Collaborative Actions

If oral mucosa is irritated or cracked, implement measures to relieve discomfort and promote healing: **D** ✦ • Administer topical anesthetics, oral protective agents, and analgesics if ordered.	*Topical anesthetics promote comfort for inflamed oral mucous membranes.*
Consult appropriate health care provider (e.g., hospice nurse, palliative care nurse, physician) if dryness, irritation, and/or discomfort persist.	*Consulting the appropriate health care provider allows for modification of the treatment plan.*

NDx = NANDA-I Diagnosis   **D** = Delegatable Action   ● = UAP   ✦ = LVN/LPN   ⊖▶ = Go to ⊖volve for animation

Nursing Diagnosis FUNCTIONAL URINARY INCONTINENCE NDx

Definition: Inability of usually continent person to reach toilet in time to avoid unintentional loss of urine

Related to:
* Decreased ability to respond to the urge to urinate associated with decreased level of consciousness and impaired physical mobility
* Decreased awareness of full bladder and poor urinary sphincter control associated with decreased level of consciousness and/or the underlying disease process

CLINICAL MANIFESTATIONS

Subjective	Objective
Verbal report of urgency	Leakage of urine during body movements

RISK FACTORS
* Immobility
* Impaired cognition

DESIRED OUTCOME

The client will experience urinary continence.

NOC OUTCOMES

Urinary continence

NIC INTERVENTIONS

Urinary incontinence care; self-care assistance: toileting; urinary catheterization

NURSING ASSESSMENT	RATIONALE
Assess for urinary incontinence: • Leakage of urine during body movements • Verbal report of urgency	*Early recognition of signs and symptoms of urinary incontinence allows for prompt intervention.*

THERAPEUTIC INTERVENTIONS	RATIONALE

Independent Actions

Implement measures to maintain or regain urinary continence:

Bladder training programs help to reduce the incidence of incontinence.

* Offer bedpan or urinal or assist client to bedside commode or bathroom every 2 to 4 hours if indicated. **D** ● ✦
* Allow client to assume a normal position for voiding unless contraindicated.
* Perform actions to reduce delays in toileting (e.g., have call signal within client's reach and respond promptly to requests for assistance; have bedpan, urinal, or bedside commode readily available to client; provide client with easy- to-remove clothing such as pajamas with Velcro closures or an elastic waistband). **D** ● ✦

Actions help to promote complete bladder emptying.

* If client has a good fluid intake, encourage him/her to space fluids evenly throughout the day rather than drinking a large quantity at one time.

Rapid filling of bladder can result in incontinence if client has decreased urinary sphincter control.

* Encourage client to avoid drinking alcohol and beverages containing caffeine.

Alcohol and caffeine have a mild diuretic effect and act as irritants; these factors may make urinary control more difficult.

If urinary incontinence persists:
* Provide client with or apply disposable undergarments (e.g., Depends, Attends) if indicated. **D** ● ✦

Helps prevent exposure of skin to urine, preventing skin breakdown.

Dependent/Collaborative Actions

If urinary incontinence persists:
* Consult physician about intermittent catheterization, insertion of indwelling catheter, or use of external collection device (e.g., condom catheter).

Consulting the appropriate health care provider allows for modification of the treatment plan.

Nursing Diagnosis RISK FOR CONSTIPATION NDx

Definition: At risk for a decrease in normal frequency of defecation accompanied by difficult or incomplete passage of stool and/or passage of excessively hard, dry stool

Related to:
- Diminished defecation reflex associated with decreased nervous system responses in terminal state, suppression of the urge to defecate because of reluctance to use bedpan, and decreased gravity filling of lower rectum resulting from horizontal positioning
- Decreased ability to respond to the urge to defecate associated with weakened abdominal muscles, impaired physical mobility, and decreased level of consciousness
- Decreased gastrointestinal motility associated with decreased activity, increased sympathetic nervous system activity that occurs with anxiety, and use of some medications (e.g., narcotic [opioid] analgesics, antacids containing aluminum or calcium)
- Decreased intake of fluids and foods high in fiber

CLINICAL MANIFESTATIONS

Subjective	Objective
Verbal reports of decrease in normal frequency of defecation; difficulty in passing stool	Passage of excessively hard, dry, stool

RISK FACTORS
- Dehydration
- Immobility

DESIRED OUTCOME

The client will maintain a bowel routine that provides optimal comfort.

NOC OUTCOMES

Bowel elimination

NIC INTERVENTIONS

Constipation/impaction management

NURSING ASSESSMENT	RATIONALE
Assess client for signs and symptoms of constipation: • Verbal reports of decrease in normal frequency of defecation • Difficulty in passing stool • Passage of excessively hard, dry, stool	*Early recognition of signs and symptoms of constipation allows for prompt intervention.*

THERAPEUTIC INTERVENTIONS	RATIONALE
Independent Actions Implement additional measures to prevent constipation: **D** ● ✦ • Assist client to toilet or place in high-Fowler's position or on bedside commode for bowel movements unless contraindicated.	*A sitting position aids in the expulsion of stool by taking advantage of gravity. A sitting position also facilitates performance of the Valsalva maneuver.*
Dependent/Collaborative Actions Implement additional measures to prevent constipation: • If client is taking antacids containing aluminum or calcium, consult appropriate health care provider (e.g., physician, hospice nurse, palliative care nurse) about alternating them with antacids containing magnesium.	*Consulting the appropriate health care provider allows for modification of the treatment plan.*

Nursing Diagnosis	**BOWEL INCONTINENCE** NDx

Definition: Change in normal bowel habits characterized by involuntary passage of stool

Related to:
- Decreased ability to respond to the urge to defecate associated with decreased level of consciousness and impaired physical mobility
- Decreased awareness of urge to defecate and poor anal sphincter control associated with decreased level of consciousness
- Fecal impaction if present (continuous stimulation of the defecation reflex by the fecal mass inhibits the internal anal sphincter and results in loss of ability to retain the mucus and fluid that collect proximal to and leak around the fecal mass)

CLINICAL MANIFESTATIONS

Subjective	**Objective**
Not applicable	Involuntary passage of stool

RISK FACTORS
- Immobility
- Impaired cognition
- Toileting self-care deficit

DESIRED OUTCOME

The client will maintain optimal bowel control as evidenced by absence of or decrease in episodes of incontinence.

NOC OUTCOMES

Bowel continence

NIC INTERVENTIONS

Bowel incontinence care; self-care assistance: toileting

NURSING ASSESSMENT	RATIONALE
Monitor for episodes of bowel incontinence: • Involuntary passage of stool	*Early recognition of signs and symptoms of bowel incontinence allows for prompt intervention.*

THERAPEUTIC INTERVENTIONS	RATIONALE

Independent Actions
Implement measures to reduce the risk of bowel incontinence: **D** ● ✦
- Perform bowel care routinely to promote emptying of the lower colon.
- Perform actions to reduce delays in toileting (e.g., have call signal within client's reach and respond promptly to requests for assistance; have bedpan or bedside commode readily available to client; provide client with easy-to-remove clothing such as pajamas with Velcro closures or an elastic waistband).

These actions help to promote regular bowel movements which can lead to a decreased level of incontinence.

If bowel incontinence persists:
- Provide client with disposable liners for underwear or disposable undergarments such as Attends or Depends.

Dependent/Collaborative Actions
Implement measures to reduce the risk of bowel incontinence:
- Consult physician regarding measures to remove fecal impaction if present (e.g., digital removal of stool, oil retention enema).

If bowel incontinence persists:
- Consult appropriate health care provider (e.g., hospice nurse, palliative care nurse, physician) about use of a fecal incontinence pouch.

Consulting the appropriate health care provider allows for modification of the treatment plan.

Nursing Diagnosis | DISTURBED THOUGHT PROCESSES NDx*

Definition: Disruption in cognitive operations and activities

Related to:
- Drug toxicity associated with organ failure
- Deficient fluid volume and imbalanced electrolytes associated with decreased oral intake and the underlying disease process
- Cerebral hypoxia, cerebral tissue damage, and/or metabolic changes associated with the underlying disease process
- Uncontrolled pain

CLINICAL MANIFESTATIONS

Subjective	**Objective**
Not applicable	Impaired memory; shortened attention span; slowed verbal response time; confusion

RISK FACTOR	**DESIRED OUTCOME**
• Impaired cerebral tissue, perfusion	The client will maintain optimal thought processes.

NOC OUTCOMES	**NIC INTERVENTIONS**
Cognitive orientation; communication	Reality orientation; hallucination management

NURSING ASSESSMENT	**RATIONALE**
Assess client for disturbed thought processes: • Impaired memory • Shortened attention span • Slowed verbal response time • Confusion	*Early recognition of signs and symptoms of disturbed thought processes allows for prompt intervention.*
Ascertain from significant others client's usual level of cognitive functioning.	*Obtaining a baseline assessment allows for future comparisons.*

THERAPEUTIC INTERVENTIONS | RATIONALE

Independent Actions
If client shows evidence of disturbed thought processes:

- Assess for possible causes (e.g., drug toxicity, pain, hypoxia, imbalanced fluid and electrolytes) and implement measures to treat them if appropriate.

  Side effects/toxic effects of medications as well as many metabolic processes may induce disturbed thought processes and should be ruled out as a cause.
- Reorient client to person, place, time, and others as necessary. **D** ● ✦

  Actions help to clarify reality for client and in addition, will help to reduce anxiety.
- Encourage significant others to bring in client's favorite items and place them within client's view. **D** ● ✦

  Items familiar to client can assist in orientation and help to create a calm and safe environment.
- Approach client in a slow, calm manner; allow adequate time for communication.

  Helps to reduce anxiety in a client who may be confused.
- Repeat instructions as necessary using clear, simple language and short sentences. **D** ● ✦
- Keep environmental stimuli to a minimum. **D** ● ✦

  Helps to create a calm, safe environment.
- Have client perform only one activity at a time and allow adequate time for performance of activities. **D** ● ✦
- If client is having vision-like experiences (e.g., hearing and talking to persons not in the room), affirm, rather than deny or argue about, the experience. **D** ● ✦
- Encourage significant others to spend time with and to be supportive of client; instruct them in methods of dealing with client's disturbed thought processes.

  Contacts with persons close to the client can assist with reorientation.
- Leave light on at night to facilitate client's orientation to surroundings. **D** ● ✦

  Actions help to create a calm, and safe environment.

*The diagnostic label of acute or chronic confusion may be more appropriate depending on the client's symptoms.

Nursing Diagnosis   DEATH ANXIETY NDx

Definition: A vague, uneasy feeling of discomfort or dread generated by perceptions of a real or imagined threat to one's existence

Related to:
- Concern about the well-being of caregivers and the impact of death on significant others
- Fear of loss of physical and mental capabilities during dying process
- Anticipated discomfort (e.g., pain, nausea, difficulty breathing) during dying process
- Feeling of powerlessness over issues related to death
- Feeling of doubt about existence of a God or higher being
- Unfinished business and unresolved conflicts
- Fear of abandonment and dying alone

CLINICAL MANIFESTATIONS

Subjective	Objective
Verbal report of a vague, uneasy feeling of discomfort or dread generated by perceptions of a real or imagined threat to one's existence	Not applicable

RISK FACTORS
- Uncertainty about a higher power
- Pain/suffering

DESIRED OUTCOMES

The client will experience a reduction in death anxiety as evidenced by:
   a. Verbalization of feeling less anxious
   b. Usual sleep pattern
   c. Relaxed facial expression and body movements
   d. Stable vital signs
   e. Statements reflecting resolution of unfinished business, conflicts, and concerns

NOC OUTCOMES

Anxiety self-control; fear self-control; dignified life closure; spiritual health

NIC INTERVENTIONS

Anxiety reduction; presence; emotional support; spiritual support; decision-making support; self-esteem enhancement

NURSING ASSESSMENT	RATIONALE
Assess client for signs and symptoms of a vague, uneasy feeling of discomfort or dread generated by perceptions of a real or imagined threat to one's existence.	*Early recognition of signs and symptoms of death anxiety allows for prompt intervention.*

THERAPEUTIC INTERVENTIONS	RATIONALE

Independent Actions
Implement additional measures to reduce fear and anxiety about dying:
- Perform actions to reduce discomfort:
  - Position client for comfort. **D** ✦ ●

Perform actions to improve respiratory status: **D** ✦ ●   *Actions help to relieve dyspnea if present and reduce anxiety.*
  - Change to position of comfort to facilitate breathing.
  - Encourage coughing and deep breathing.   *Helps to expand alveoli, increasing gas exchange and improving oxygenation.*

- Spend time with client.   *Action helps to reduce feelings of abandonment and aloneness.*
- Assist client to formulate plans for completing unfinished business and providing for care of significant others if appropriate.
- If appropriate, encourage and assist client to record (e.g., write, audiotape, videotape) information he/she would like others to know at the present time and after his/her death.

THERAPEUTIC INTERVENTIONS	RATIONALE
• Encourage significant others to stay with client and participate in care if their presence seems to relieve the client's fear and anxiety. • Perform actions to promote resolution of spiritual distress and a sense of spiritual well-being. • Perform actions to reduce feelings of powerlessness (e.g., provide information about advance directives, encourage participation in decisions about care and after-death arrangements, involve client in as much of self-care as possible).	

Nursing Diagnosis **GRIEVING** NDx

Definition: A normal, complex process that includes emotional, physical, spiritual, social, and intellectual responses and behaviors by which communities incorporate an actual, anticipated, or perceived loss into their daily lives

Related to: Loss of control over life and body functioning, changes in body image, loss of significant others, and imminent death

CLINICAL MANIFESTATIONS

Subjective	Objective
Expression of distress about terminal illness and dying; denial of impending death	Change in eating habits; inability to concentrate; insomnia; anger; sadness; withdrawal from significant others

RISK FACTOR	DESIRED OUTCOMES
• Anticipatory loss of body processes	The client will demonstrate progression through the grieving process as evidenced by: a. Verbalization of feelings about dying b. Usual sleep pattern c. Use of available support systems

NOC OUTCOMES	NIC INTERVENTIONS
Grief resolution	Grief work facilitation; emotional support; presence; support system enhancement; dying care

NURSING ASSESSMENT	RATIONALE
Assess for signs and symptoms of grieving: • Expression of distress about terminal illness and dying • Denial of impending death • Change in eating habits • Inability to concentrate • Insomnia • Anger • Sadness • Withdrawal from significant others	*Early recognition of signs and symptoms of grieving allows for prompt intervention.*

THERAPEUTIC INTERVENTIONS	RATIONALE
Independent Actions Implement measures to facilitate the grieving process: • Assist client to acknowledge that death is imminent. • Assess for factors that may hinder and facilitate acknowledgment.	*Acknowledgment of imminent death allows grief work to progress.*

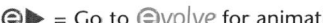

NDx = NANDA-I Diagnosis   **D** = Delegatable Action   ● = UAP   ✦ = LVN/LPN   ⊖▶ = Go to ⊖volve for animation

Continued...

THERAPEUTIC INTERVENTIONS	RATIONALE
• Discuss the grieving process and assist client to accept the phases of grieving as an expected response to anticipated losses and impending death.	
• Allow time for client to progress through the phases of grieving. Be aware that not every phase is expressed by all individuals, that phases do not necessarily occur in sequential order, and that recurrence of phases is common during the course of an illness and the dying process.	*Phases of grieving vary among theorists but progress from shock and alarm to acceptance.*
• Provide an atmosphere of care and concern (e.g., provide privacy, be available and nonjudgmental, display empathy and respect).	*Action helps client to feel free to express feelings.*
• Perform actions to promote trust (e.g., answer questions honestly, provide requested information).	
• Encourage the verbal expression of anger and sadness about anticipated losses; recognize displacement of anger and assist client to see the actual cause of angry feelings and resentment; establish limits on abusive behavior if demonstrated.	
• Encourage client to express feelings in whatever ways are comfortable (e.g., writing, drawing, conversation).	
• Assist client to identify and use techniques that have helped him/her cope in previous situations of loss.	
• If desired by client, assist with after-death arrangements (e.g., funeral, religious service, who should be called).	
• Perform actions to assist the client to maintain a positive self-concept and feel good about the life he/she has experienced:	
• Visit frequently and encourage verbalization about past events, life accomplishments, interests, and feelings.	
• Help client to focus on positive rather than negative aspects of his/her life experience.	
• Maintain a nonjudgmental attitude about the kind of life client has led and his/her beliefs.	
• Encourage participation in decisions about care.	
• Encourage and assist client with good physical hygiene and grooming; suggest use of personal rather than hospital clothing.	*Use of personal clothing helps client to maintain his/her identity.*
• Support behaviors suggesting successful grief work (e.g., verbalizing feelings about dying, statements reflecting that dying is difficult but a part of life, comfortable and realistic remembrances about significant relationships, use of available support systems).	
• Explain the phases of the grieving process to significant others; encourage their support and understanding.	
• Facilitate communication between the client and significant others; be aware that they may be in different phases of the grieving process.	
• Provide information about counseling services and support groups that might assist client and significant others in working through grief.	
• Perform actions to promote a sense of spiritual well-being.	

Dependent/Collaborative Actions

Consult appropriate health care provider (e.g., hospice nurse, palliative care nurse, psychiatric nurse clinician, physician) regarding a referral for counseling if signs of dysfunctional grieving (e.g., persistent denial of terminal state, excessive anger or sadness, emotional lability) occur.

Consulting the appropriate health care provider allows for modification of the treatment plan.

Nursing Diagnosis **RISK FOR SPIRITUAL DISTRESS** NDx

Definition: Impaired ability to experience and integrate meaning and purpose of life through connectedness with self, others, art, music, literature, nature, and/or a power greater than oneself

Related to:
- Challenged belief and value system as a result of intense or prolonged suffering and imminent death
- Separation from religious/cultural ties
- Overwhelming grief and sense of hopelessness

CLINICAL MANIFESTATIONS

Subjective	Objective
Verbalization of conflict about beliefs and relationship with deity; reports of anger toward God; questioning the purpose for suffering; verbalizing that illness and imminent death are a punishment	Refusal to participate in usual religious practices or to have visits from clergy; apathy; hostility; withdrawal

RISK FACTORS
- Active dying
- Chronic illness
- Pain
- Social alienation

DESIRED OUTCOMES

The client will not experience spiritual distress as evidenced by:
- a. Expression of a sense of spiritual well-being
- b. Participation in usual religious/spiritual practices when possible
- c. Maintaining connectedness with significant others

NOC OUTCOMES

Hope; spiritual health; dignified life closure

NIC INTERVENTIONS

Spiritual support; grief work facilitation; spiritual growth facilitation

NURSING ASSESSMENT	RATIONALE
Assess client's religious/spiritual beliefs and practices: • Verbalization of conflict about beliefs and relationship with deity • Reports of anger toward God • Questioning the purpose for suffering • Verbalizing that illness and imminent death are a punishment • Refusal to participate in usual religious practices or to have visits from clergy • Apathy, hostility, withdrawal	*Provides baseline understanding of client's beliefs.*
Assess for signs and symptoms of spiritual distress.	*Early recognition of signs and symptoms of spiritual distress allows for prompt intervention.*

THERAPEUTIC INTERVENTIONS	RATIONALE
Independent Actions Implement measures to promote a sense of spiritual well-being: • Give client permission to express feelings and concerns about his/her religious/spiritual beliefs. • Maintain a nonjudgmental attitude about client's beliefs and any inner conflicts client is experiencing. • Encourage client to use available spiritual resources (e.g., clergy, prayer, religious rituals) for support.	*Spirituality, whether it is religion or other beliefs, has been associated with decreased despair in patients at the end of life.*

NDx = NANDA-I Diagnosis   **D** = Delegatable Action   ● = UAP   ✦ = LVN/LPN   ⊖▶ = Go to ⊖volve for animation

Continued...

THERAPEUTIC INTERVENTIONS	RATIONALE
• Perform actions to facilitate the grieving process. Encourage verbalization of anger (e.g., allow time for client to progress through phases of grief). • Perform actions to reduce feelings of hopelessness. (e.g., allow client to exert control over activities as much as possible).	
Dependent/Collaborative Actions Consult appropriate resource (e.g., clergy, psychiatric nurse clinician, physician, palliative care nurse, hospice nurse) if signs and symptoms of spiritual distress occur and client's response is inappropriate and/or destructive.	*Consulting the appropriate health care provider allows for modification of the treatment plan.*

Nursing Diagnosis HOPELESSNESS NDx

Definition: A subjective state in which an individual sees limited or no alternatives or personal choices available and is unable to mobilize energy on own behalf

Related to: Deteriorating physical condition, feelings of abandonment, loss of belief in religious/cultural values, and inability to reach self-fulfillment associated with terminal state

CLINICAL MANIFESTATIONS

Subjective Statements of feeling hopeless	**Objective** Decreased response to significant others; decreased participation in self-care and decision-making; decreased verbalization; flat affect

RISK FACTORS
• Long-term stress
• Deteriorating physical condition

DESIRED OUTCOMES

The client will maintain hope as evidenced by:
  a. Verbal expression of same
  b. Maintenance of satisfying relationships with others
  c. Participation in self-care and decision-making as able
  d. Identification of realistic goals

NOC OUTCOMES	NIC INTERVENTIONS
Hope; decision-making; quality of life; dignified life closure; spiritual well-being	Decision-making support; presence; grief work facilitation; hope instillation

NURSING ASSESSMENT	RATIONALE
Assess client for signs and symptoms of hopelessness: • Decreased response to significant others • Decreased participation in self-care and decision-making • Decreased verbalization • Flat affect • Statements of feeling hopeless	*Early recognition of signs and symptoms of hopelessness allows for prompt intervention.*

THERAPEUTIC INTERVENTIONS	RATIONALE
Independent Actions Implement measures to assist client to reduce feelings of hopelessness: • Perform actions to facilitate the grieving process: • Provide an atmosphere of care and concern.	*Grieving occurs in phases or stages over time.* *Stages must be allowed to occur in order to reduce the risk for dysfunctional grieving.*

THERAPEUTIC INTERVENTIONS	RATIONALE
• Perform actions to promote a sense of spiritual well-being (e.g., encourage client to use available spiritual resources).	*Spiritual support can be a great source of strength and solace to the client and can facilitate resolution of grief.*
• Allow client to retain as much control as possible over activities of daily living; involve client in as much self-care and decision-making as feasible.	
• Assist client to identify goals that are achievable in the time that client has left, ways to continue working toward goals previously set even if not possible to achieve them totally, and the purpose remaining in client's life such as role model or advisor to significant others.	

Dependent/Collaborative Actions

Consult appropriate health care provider (e.g., palliative care nurse, hospice nurse, psychiatric nurse clinician, physician) if client demonstrates increased feelings of hopelessness.	*Consulting the appropriate health care provider allows for modification of the treatment plan.*

Nursing Diagnosis ## INTERRUPTED FAMILY PROCESSES NDx

Definition: Change in family relationships and/or functions

Related to: Excessive anxiety, grief, disorganization, and role changes within the family unit, inadequate support systems, and fatigue

CLINICAL MANIFESTATIONS

Subjective	Objective
Statements of not being able to accept client's imminent death or to make necessary role and lifestyle changes, verbalization of guilt	Inability to make decisions; infrequent visits; inappropriate response to client's situation; preoccupation with other aspects of life; negative family interactions

RISK FACTORS

- Situational crisis
- Shift in health status of family member

DESIRED OUTCOMES

The family members will demonstrate beginning adjustment to loss of client and changes in family roles and structure as evidenced by:
  a. Verbalization of ways to adapt to required role and lifestyle changes
  b. Active participation in decision-making and client's care
  c. Positive interactions with one another

NOC OUTCOMES

Family coping; family functioning; family resiliency; family normalization

NIC INTERVENTIONS

Family involvement promotion; family integrity promotion; family process maintenance; family support; caregiver support; support system enhancement

NURSING ASSESSMENT	RATIONALE
Assess for signs and symptoms of interrupted family processes:	*Early recognition of signs and symptoms of interrupted family processes allows for prompt intervention.*
• Statements of not being able to accept client's imminent death or to make necessary role and lifestyle changes	
• Verbalization of guilt	
• Inability to make decisions	
• Infrequent visits	
• Inappropriate response to client's situation	

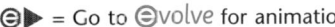

NDx = NANDA-I Diagnosis   **D** = Delegatable Action   ● = UAP   ✦ = LVN/LPN   ⊖▶ = Go to ⊖volve for animation

Continued...

NURSING ASSESSMENT	RATIONALE

- Preoccupation with other aspects of life
- Negative family interactions

Identify components of the family and their patterns of communication and role expectations.

THERAPEUTIC INTERVENTIONS	RATIONALE

Independent Actions

Implement measures to facilitate family members' adjustment to imminent loss of client and altered family roles and structure:

- Encourage and assist family members to verbalize feelings about the death of the client and the effect of it on their lifestyle and family structure; actively listen to each family member and maintain a nonjudgmental attitude about feelings shared.

  Client and family member must be given time to openly and honestly express feelings to facilitate the grieving process.

- Assist family members to confront the reality of the client's imminent death when they are ready; encourage them to imagine life after death of the client and to set some personal goals if appropriate.

- Provide privacy so that family members can share their feelings and grief with one another; stress the importance of and facilitate the use of good communication techniques.

  Discussion of feelings helps the client and family work through the grieving process.

- Explain the phases of grieving and assist family members to progress through their own grieving process; explain that they may encounter times when they need to focus on meeting their own rather than the client's needs.

- Emphasize the need for family members to obtain adequate rest and nutrition and to identify and use stress management techniques so that they are better able to emotionally and physically deal with the death of the client; assure them that the client will be well cared for in their absence.

- Encourage and assist family members to identify coping strategies for dealing with the client's death and its effect on those left behind.

- Include family members in decision-making about client and his/her care; convey appreciation of their input and continued support of the client.

- Encourage and allow family members to participate in client's care if desired by both client and family members.

- Assist family members to make necessary postmortem arrangements for or with the client (e.g., funeral home, burial place, clergy visitation).

  Assistance with funeral planning may be needed based on the coping abilities of the family.

- Provide information to family members about:
  - The current status of client
  - Behaviors to expect as the client progresses through terminal stages of disease and his/her own grieving
  - Physical signs and symptoms of approaching death (e.g., decrease in appetite and thirst; lack of interest in environment; withdrawal from relationships; disorientation; restlessness; agitation; vision-like experiences; "out-of-character" statements or requests; increased sleeping; incontinence; decreased level of consciousness; reduced urine output; cool, mottled extremities; respiratory sounds such as gurgling or rattling, labored breathing, or periods of no breathing)
  - Ways they can best assist in meeting client's needs

THERAPEUTIC INTERVENTIONS	RATIONALE
• When appropriate, help and encourage family members to "let go" of client and say goodbye.	*Family members must be given time to acknowledge sadness, forgive one another, and say goodbye.*
• Assist family members to identify resources that can assist them in coping with their feelings and in meeting their immediate and long-term needs (e.g., counseling and social services; pastoral care; service, bereavement, and church groups; hospice); initiate a referral if indicated.	
• Assist family members to contact appropriate persons (e.g., funeral home director, clergy) when death occurs.	
Dependent/Collaborative Actions	
Consult appropriate health care provider (e.g., hospice nurse, palliative care nurse, physician) if family members continue to demonstrate difficulty adjusting to the loss of the client and role changes within the family unit.	*Consulting the appropriate health care provider allows for modification of the treatment plan.*

ADDITIONAL NURSING DIAGNOSES

RISK FOR DEFICIENT FLUID VOLUME NDx
Related to:
• Decreased oral intake and increased fluid loss associated with vomiting and/or diaphoresis if client has a fever

IMPAIRED PHYSICAL MOBILITY NDx
Related to:
• Weakness and fatigue
• Dyspnea and/or sensory and motor deficits (can occur as a result of the underlying disease process)
• Reluctance to move associated with pain and nausea if present
• Decreased level of consciousness

SELF-CARE DEFICIT NDx
Related to:
• Weakness and fatigue
• Activity limitations associated with the underlying disease process

• Pain, nausea, dyspnea, and/or disturbed thought processes if present
• Decreased level of consciousness

DISTURBED SLEEP PATTERN NDx
Related to: Decreased physical activity, fear, anxiety, unfamiliar environment, discomfort, and inability to assume usual sleep position associated with orthopnea if present

RISK FOR FALLS NDx
Related to: Weakness, fatigue, and attempting activity unassisted because of agitation or confusion

Bibliography

GENERAL BIBLIOGRAPHY

Abrams A, Pennington S, & Lammon C: *Clinical drug therapy: Rationales for nursing practice*, ed 8, Philadelphia, 2007, Lippincott, Williams & Wilkins.

Ackley B, Ladwig G: *Nursing diagnosis handbook: An evidence-based guide to planning care*, ed 8, St Louis, 2008, Mosby-Elsevier.

Berman A, Snyder S, Jackson C: *Skills in clinical nursing*, ed 6, Upper Saddle River, NJ, 2008, Pearson Prentice Hall.

Berman AJ, Snyder S, Kosier B, Erb, G: *Fundamentals of nursing: Concepts, process, and process*, ed 8, Upper Saddle River, NJ, 2007, Prentice Hall.

Brashers V: *Clinical applications of pathophysiology: An evidence-based approach*, ed 3, St Louis, 2006, Mosby-Elsevier.

Bulechek GM, Butcher HK, Dochterman JM (Eds): *Nursing interventions classification (NIC)*, ed 5, St Louis, 2008, Mosby-Elsevier.

Carpenito-Moyet L: *Nursing care plans & documentation: Nursing diagnoses and collaborative problems*, ed 4, St Louis, 2004, Mosby-Elsevier.

Copstead L, Banasik J: *Pathophysiology*, ed 4, St Louis, 2010, Mosby-Elsevier.

Doenges M, Moorhouse M, Murr M: *Nursing diagnosis manual: Planning, individualizing, and documenting client care*, ed 2, Philadelphia, 2008, FA Davis.

Gulanick M, Myers J: *Nursing care plans: Nursing diagnosis and intervention*, ed 6, St Louis, 2007, Mosby-Elsevier.

Herdman T: *NANDA International Nursing Diagnosis: Definitions & classification 2009-2011*, Oxford, 2009, Wiley-Blackwell.

Huether S, McCance K: *Understanding pathophysiology*, ed 4, St Louis, 2008, Mosby-Elsevier.

Holloway NM: *Medical-surgical care planning*, ed 4, Philadelphia, 2004, Lippincott Williams & Wilkins.

Ignatavicius DD, Workman ML: *Medical-surgical nursing: Patient-centered collaborative care*, ed 5, Philadelphia, 2010, Saunders.

Jarvis C: *Physical examination & health assessment*, ed 5, St Louis, 2008, Saunders-Elsevier.

Lewis SL, Heitkemper MM, Dirksen SR, O'Brien PG, Bucher L: *Medical-surgical nursing: Assessment and management of clinical problems*, ed 7, St. Louis, 2007, Mosby-Elsevier.

McCance K, Huether S: *Pathophysiology: The biologic basis for disease in adults and children*, ed 5, St Louis, 2006, Mosby-Elsevier.

Moorhead S, Johnson M, Maas M, Swanson E: *Nursing Outcomes Classification (NOC)*, ed 4, St Louis, 2008, Mosby-Elsevier.

Newfield S, Hinz M, Tilley D, Sridaromont K, Maramba P: *Cox's clinical applications of nursing diagnosis*, ed 5, Philadelphia, 2007, FA Davis.

Page C, Curtis M, Walker M, Hoffman B: *Integrated pharmacology*, ed 3, St Louis. 2006, Mosby-Elsevier.

Pagana K, Pagana T: *Mosby's diagnostic and laboratory test references*, ed 9, St Louis, 2008, Mosby-Elsevier.

Perry A, Potter P: *Clinical nursing skills & techniques*, ed 7, St Louis, 2010, Mosby-Elsevier.

Potter A, Perry P: *Fundamentals of nursing*, ed 7, St Louis, 2009, Mosby-Elsevier.

Sole ML, Klein DG, Moseley MJ: *Introduction to critical care nursing*, ed 5, St Louis, 2008, Mosby-Elsevier.

Swearingen P: *All-in-one care planning resource*, ed 2, St Louis, 2008, Mosby-Elsevier.

Van Leeuwen A, Poelhuis-Leth D: *Davis's comprehensive handbook of laboratory and diagnostic tests with nursing implications*, ed 3, Philadelphia, 2009, Davis.

Wilcox C: Appendicitis, diverticulitis and miscellaneous intestinal inflammatory conditions. In Goldman L, Ausiello D (eds): *Cecil textbook of medicine*, ed 22, Philadelphia, 2004, Saunders.

CHAPTER-BY-CHAPTER BIBLIOGRAPHY

1 PRIORITIZATION, DELEGATION, AND CRITICAL THINKING IN CLIENT MANAGEMENT

Alfaro-Lefevre R: *Critical thinking and clinical judgment: a practical approach*, ed 3, St Louis, 2004, Saunders.

Hansten R, Jackson M: *Clinical delegation skills: a handbook for clinical practice*, ed 3, Sudbury, Mass, 2004, Jones and Bartlett.

LaCharity L, Kumagai C, Bartz B: Prioritization, delegation &
assignment: Practice exercises for medical-surgical nursing, St Louis, 2006, Mosby-Elsevier.

ANA & NCSBN Joint Statement on Delegation American Nurses Association (ANA) and the National Council of State Boards of Nursing (NCSBN), retrieved 2009, www.ncsbn.org/Joint_statement.pdf.

3 NURSING CARE OF THE CLIENT HAVING SURGERY

American Society of PeriAnesthesia Nurses. *2008-2010 Standards of perianesthesia nursing practice*, New Jersey, 2008, ASPAN.

Arbique JC: Stopping UTIs in their tracts, *Nursing 2003* 33(6):32hn1-32hn4, 2003.

Byrne B: Deep vein thrombosis prophylaxis: The effectiveness and implications of using below-knee or thigh-length graduated compression stockings, *J Vascular Nursing* 20(2): 53-59, 2002.

Capriotte T: Preventing nosocomial spread of MRSA is in your hands, *MEDSURG Nursing* 12(3):193-196, 2003.

Church V: Staying on guard for DVT and PE, *Nursing2000* 30(2):35-42, 2000.

Day MW: Recognizing and managing DVT, *Nursing2003* 33(5):37-41, 2003.

Dudek SG: Malnutrition in hospitals, *American Journal of Nursing* 100(4):36-42, 2000.

Epley O: Pulmonary emboli risk reductions, *Journal of Vascular Nursing* 18(2):61-70, 2000.

Godwin SA, Caro DA, Wolf SJ, Jagoda AS, Charles R, Marett BE, Moore J, American College of Emergency Physicians: Clinical policy: Procedural sedation and analgesia in the emergency department, *Annals of Emergency Medicine* 45(2):177-196, Feb 2005.

Hashmi S, Kelly E, Rogers SO, Gates J: Urinary tract infection in surgical patients, *American Journal of Surgery* 186(1):53-56, 2003.

Kleinpell RM: Shock states, *Nurseweek* 4(14):20-22, 2003.

Nagel CL, Markie MB, Richards KC, Taylor JL: Sleep promotion in hospitalized elders, *MEDSURG Nursing* 12(5):279-288, 2003.

Parini S, Myers F. Keeping up with hand hygiene recommendations, *Nursing2003* 33(2):17, 2003.

Schick L, Windle P (Eds): *PeriAnesthesia nursing core curriculum: Preprocedure phase I and phase II nursing,* ed 2, St Louis, 2009, Saunders.

Stratton MA, Anderson FA, Bussey HI, et al: Prevention of venous thromboembolism, *Archives of Internal Medicine* 160(3):334-340, 2000.

4 THE CLIENT WITH ALTERATIONS IN RESPIRATORY FUNCTION

Agnelli C, Prandoni P, Becattini C, et al: Extended oral anticoagulant therapy after a first episode of pulmonary embolism, *Annals of Internal Medicine* 139(10):19-25, 2003.

Altman E: Update on COPD: Today's strategies improve quality of life, *Advances in Nursing Practice* 12(3):49-54, 2004.

Bartley M: Keep venous thromboembolism at bay, *Nursing* 36(10):36-42, 2006.

Bauldoff G, Diaz P: Improving outcomes for COPD patients, *The Nurse Practitioner* 21(8):26-43, 2006.

Beck D: Venous thromboembolism (VTE) prophylaxis: implications for medical-surgical nurses, *Medsurg Nursing* 15(5):282-288, 2006.

Brooker R: Chronic obstructive pulmonary disease and the NICE guidelines, *Nursing Standard* 19(22):43-52, 2005.

Bruce M, McEnvoy P: COPD: Your role in early detection, *The Nurse Practitioner* 32(11):24-33, 2007.

Cantrell C, Ward K, Van Wicklin S: Translating research on venous thromboembolism into practice. *AORN Journal* 86(4):590-606, 2007.

Centers for Disease Control and Prevention: Cover your cough, 2006, www.cdc.gov/flu/protect/covercough.htm, accessed July 2008.

Centers for Disease Control and Prevention: *Trends in tuberculosis, 2006,* Atlanta, 2007, TB Elimination Division; available online: www.ded.gov/tb (accessed July, 2008).

Cohen S: Diagnosis and treatment of tuberculosis, *Journal for Nurse Practitioners* 2(6):390-396, 2006.

Conboy-Ellis K: Asthma: Pathogenesis and management, *The Nurse Practitioner* 31(11):24-37, 2006.

Conghlin A, Parchinsky C: Go with the flow of chest tube therapy, *Nursing2006* 36(3):36-41, 2006.

Copeland D, Gretzer M: Deep venous thrombosis, *Contemporary Urology* May, 48-54, 2006.

Coughlin A: Combating community-acquired pneumonia, *Nursing2007* 37(2):64hn1-64hn3, 2007.

Dresang L, Fontain P, Leeman L, King V: Venous thromboembolism during pregnancy, 72(12):1709-1716, 2008.

Forrest S: Learning and teaching: The reciprocal link, *Continuing Education for Nursing* 32(5):74-79, 2004.

Global Initiative for Chronic Obstructive Lung Disease (GOLD) *Global strategy of the diagnosis, management, and prevention of chronic obstructive pulmonary disease,* MCR Vision, Inc, 2007, www.gold.copd.org.

Graduated compression stockings for the prevention of post-operative venous thromboembolism, *Best Practice* 12(4):1-4, 2008.

Grap MJ, Munro CL: Preventing ventilator associated pneumonia: Evidenced based care. *Critical Care Nursing Clinics of North America* 16(3):349-358, 2004.

Halm M: TO strip or not to strip: Physiological effects of chest tube manipulation, *American Journal of Critical Care* 16(6):609-612, 2007.

Ignatavicius D, William M: *Medical-surgical nursing: Critical thinking for collaborative care,* ed 6, Philadelphia, 2005, Mosby-Elsevier.

International Council of Nurses: *TB guidelines for nurses in the care and control of tuberculosis and multi-drug resistant TB,* ed 2, Geneva, Switzerland, 2008, International Council of Nurses.

Kallus C: Building a solid understanding of mechanical ventilation, *Nursing* 39(6):22-29, 2009.

Kehl-Pruett W: Deep vein thrombosis in hospitalized patients: a review of evidence-based guidelines for prevention, *Dimensions of Critical Care Nursing* 25(2):53-61, 2006.

Koschel M: Pulmonary embolism: quick diagnosis can save a patient's life, *American Journal of Nursing* 104(6):46-50, 2004.

Lewis S, Heitkemper M, Dirksen S, O'Brien P, Bucher L: *Medical-surgical nursing: assessment and management of clinical problems,* ed 7, St Louis, 2007, Mosby-Elsevier.

Loveridge C: The effects of weather on COPD, *British Journal of Primary Care Nursing* 2(3):39-41, 2008.

MacIntyre NR: Evidenced based ventilator weaning and discontinuation, *Respiratory Care* 49(7):830-836, 2004.

Milner D: The physiological effects of smoking on the respiratory system, *Nursing Times* 100(4):56-59, 2004.

National Institutes of Health: *Guidelines for the diagnosis and management of asthma: Expert panel report 3,* Bethesda, Md, 2007, US Department of Health and Human Services.

O'Keefe-McCarthy S, Santiago C, Lau G: Ventilator-associated pneumonia bundled strategies: An evidenced based practice, *Worldviews on Evidenced Based Nursing,* 5(4):193-204, 2008.

Olinzock B: A model for assessing learning readiness for self-direction of care in individuals with spinal cord injuries: A qualitative study, *SCI Nurse* 21(2)69-74, 2004.

Perry A, Potter P: Closed chest drainage systems. In *Clinical nursing skills & techniques,* ed 6, St Louis, 2006, Mosby-Elsevier.

Perry A, Potter P: Preoperative and postoperative care. In *Clinical nursing skills & techniques,* ed 6, St Louis, 2006, Mosby-Elsevier.

Porth C: *Essentials of pathophysiology: Concepts of altered health states,* ed 2, Philadelphia, 2007, Lippincott Williams & Wilkins.

Pruitt W: Caring for a patient with asthma. *Nursing2005* 35(2), 48-51, 2005.

Roman M, Mercado D: Review of chest tube use, *MEDSURG Nursing* 15(1):41-43, 2006.

Roman M: Asthma, *MEDSURG Nursing* 16(3), 209-210, 2007.

Ruffolo DC: Pulmonary embolism: intervene quickly to halt the great masquerader, *Advances in Nursing Practice* 12(6):30-34, 2004.

Rushing J: Managing a water-seal chest drainage unit, *Nursing2007* 27(12):12, 2007.

Schleder BJ: Taking charge of hospital acquired pneumonia, *Nursing Practice* 29(3):50-53, 2004.

Simmons P, Simmons M: Informed nursing practice: the administration of oxygen to patients with COPD, *MEDSURG Nursing* 13(2):83-85, 2004.

Sole ML, Klein DG, Moseley MJ: *Introduction to Critical Care Nursing,* ed 5, St Louis, 2008, Mosby-Elsevier.

Wall M: Predictors of functional performance in community-dwelling people with COPD, *Journal of Nursing Scholarship* 39(3):222-228, 2007.

Warren M, Livesay S: Taking action against acute COPD, *American Nurse Today* 1(3):12-15, 2006.

Wenzel R, Covar S: Update in Asthma 2005, *American Journal of Respiratory and Critical Care Medicine* 173:698-706, 2005.

Wise R, Tashkin D: Optimizing treatment of chronic obstructive pulmonary disease: An assessment of current therapies, *American Journal of Medicine* 120(8 Suppl A):S4-S13, 2007.

5 THE CLIENT WITH ALTERATIONS IN CARDIOVASCULAR FUNCTION

Aquila A: Deep vein thrombosis, *Journal of Cardiovascular Nursing* 15(4):25-44, 2001.

Bither CJ, Apple S: Home management of the failing heart, *American Journal of Nursing* 101(12):41-47, 2001.

Branch WT, Schlant RC, Alexander RW, Hurst JW (editors): *Cardiology in primary care,* New York, 2000, McGraw-Hill.

Braunwald E, Zipes DP, Libby P: *Heart disease: a textbook of cardiovascular medicine,* ed 6, Philadelphia, 2001, Saunders.

Byrne B: Deep vein thrombosis prophylaxis: the effectiveness and implications of using below-knee or thigh-length graduated compression stockings, *Journal of Vascular Nursing* 20(2):53-59, 2002.

Cannon DS: Implantable cardioverter defibrillator trials: what's new? *Current Opinion in Cardiology* 17(1):29-35, 2002.

Caplan L. Protecting the brains of patients after heart surgery, *Archives of Neurology* 58(4):549-550, 2001.

Capriotti T: Pharmacologic implications of the new JNC 7 blood pressure guidelines, *MEDSURG Nursing* 12(5):325-330, 2003.

Chase SL, Hypertensive crisis, *RN* 63(6):62-68, 2000.

Chobanian AV, Bakris GL, Black HR, Cushman WC, et al: The seventh report of the Joint National Commission on Prevention, Detection, Evaluation, and Treatment of High Blood Pressure: the JNC 7 Report, *Journal of the American Medical Association* 289(19):2560-2572, 2003.

Church V: Staying on guard for DVT and PE, *Nursing2000* 30(2):34-42, 2000.

Cohen M: The role of low-molecular-weight heparin in the management of acute coronary syndromes, *Current Opinion in Cardiology* 16(6):384-389, 2001.

Criner JA, Appelt M, Loker C, et al: Rhabdomyolysis: the hidden killer, *MEDSURG Nursing* 11(3):58-63, 2002.

Cundy JB: Carotid artery stenosis and endarterectomy: *Association of Operating Room Nurses Journal* 75(2):309-310, 312, 314-324, 2002.

Davis S: How the heart failure picture has changed, *Nursing2002* 32(11):36-44, 2002.

Day MW: Recognizing and managing DVT, *Nursing2003* 33(5):37-41, 2003.

Ellenbogen KA, Kay GN, Wilkoff BL: *Clinical cardiac pacing and defibrillation,* ed 2, Philadelphia, 2000, Saunders.

Epley O: Pulmonary emboli risk reductions, *Journal of Vascular Nursing* 18(2):61-70, 2000.

Fahey VA: *Vascular nursing,* ed 4, Philadelphia, 2004, Saunders.

Fort CW: How to combat three deadly trauma complications, *Nursing2003* 33(3):58-63, 2003.

Fowler SB: Patient care following carotid endarterectomy, *MEDSURG Nursing* 8(1):47-52, 1999.

Fuster V, Alexander RW, O'Rourke RA, editors: *Hurst's the heart,* ed 10, New York, 2001, McGraw-Hill.

Gravlee G, et al. editors: *Cardiopulmonary bypass principles and practice,* ed 2, Philadelphia, 2000, Lippincott Williams & Wilkins.

Henke K, Eigsti J: After cardiopulmonary bypass: watching for complications, *Nursing2003* 33(3):32cc1-32cc4, 2003.

Hickey JV: *The clinical practice of neurological and neurosurgical nursing,* ed 5, Philadelphia, 2003, Lippincott Williams & Wilkins.

Hirsch AT, Criqui MH, Treat-Jacobson D, et al: Peripheral arterial disease detection, awareness, and treatment in primary care, *Journal of the American Medical Association* 286(11):1317-1324, 2001.

Hunt SA, Abraham WT, Chin MH, Feldman AM, Francis GS, Ganiats TG, et al: *ACC/AHA 2005 guideline update for the diagnosis and management of chronic heart failure in the adult: a report of the American College of Cardiology/American Heart Association Task Force on Practice Guidelines* [trunc], Bethesda, Md, Aug, 2005, American College of Cardiology Foundation.

Irwin RS, Rippe JM, editors: *Irwin and Rippe's intensive care medicine,* ed 5, Philadelphia, 2003, Lippincott Williams & Wilkins.

Krenzer ME: Unplugging the mystery of carotid endarterectomy patient care, *Critical Care Nursing Clinics of North America* 11(2):189-208, 1999.

McNamara RL, Bass EB, Miller MR, et al: *Management of new onset atrial fibrillation,* AHRQ Pub No 01-E026, Rockville, Md, 2001, Agency for Healthcare Research and Quality.

Meister J, Reddy D: Rhabdomyolysis: an overview, *American Journal of Nursing* 102(2):75-79, 2002.

Moore WS: *Vascular surgery: a comprehensive review,* ed 6, Philadelphia, 2002, Saunders.

National High Blood Pressure Education Program: *The seventh report of the Joint National Committee on Prevention, Detection, Evaluation, and Treatment of High Blood Pressure,* NIH Pub No 98-4080, Bethesda, Md, 2004. National Institutes of Health.

Parrillo JE, Dellinger RP: *Critical care medicine: principles of diagnosis and management in the adult,* ed 2, St Louis, 2001, Mosby.

Reynolds J, Apple S. A systemic approach to pacemaker assessment, *AACN Clinical Issues: Advanced Practice Acute Critical Care* 12(1):14-26, 2001.

Ridker P, et al: Long-term, low-intensity warfarin therapy for the prevention of recurrent venous thromboembolism, *New England Journal of Medicine* 348(15):1425-1434, 2003.

Rutherford RB: *Vascular surgery,* ed 5, Philadelphia, 2000, Saunders.

Sacks FM, Svetkey LP, Vollmer WM, Appel AJ, et al: Effects on blood pressure of reduced dietary sodium and the Dietary Approaches to Stop Hypertension (DASH) diet, *New England Journal of Medicine,* 344(1):3-10, 2001.

Stordahl NJ, Back MR: The efficacy of carotid endarterectomy: a vascular surgery perspective reducing hospital stay. *MEDSURG Nursing* 9(3):113121, 2000.

Stratton MA, Anderson FA, Bussey HI, et al: Prevention of venous thromboembolism, *Archives of Internal Medicine* 160(3):334-340, 2000.

Topol EJ: *Textbook of interventional cardiology,* ed 4, Philadelphia, 2003, Saunders.

Urden LD, Stacy KM, Lough ME. *Thelan's critical care nursing: diagnosis and management,* ed 5, St Louis, 2006, Mosby.

Wallace CJ. Diagnosing and treating pacemaker syndrome, *Critical Care Nurse* 21(1):24-31, 35-37, 2001.

Weber KT: Mechanisms of disease: aldosterone in congestive heart failure, *New England Journal of Medicine* 345(23):1689-1697, 2001.

White E: Patients with implantable cardioverter defibrillators: transition to home, *Journal of Cardiovascular Nursing* 14(3):42-52, 2000.

Woods SL, Froelicher ESS, Motzer SA: *Cardiac nursing,* ed 4, Philadelphia, 2000, Lippincott

6 THE CLIENT WITH ALTERATIONS IN NEUROLOGICAL FUNCTION

Abraham I, MacDonald K, Nadzam D: Measuring the quality of nursing care to Alzheimer's patients, *Nursing Clinics of North America* 41(1):95-104, March 2006. Retrieved November 10,

2008, from CINAHL Plus with Full Text database.

Ackerman R, Kedersha K, Vliet N: Every step of the way: care management of the patient with spinal cord injury, Care Management, 8(3):23-28, 2002.

Adams Jr, HP del Zoppo, G, Alberts MJ, Bhatt DL, Brass L, Furlan A, et al: Guidelines for the early management of adults with ischemic stroke: a guideline from the American Heart Association/American Stroke Association Stroke Council, Clinical Cardiology Council, Cardiovascular Radiology and Intervention Council, and the Atherosclerotic Peripheral Vascular Disease and Quality of Care Outcomes in Research Interdisciplinary Work Groups, *Stroke.* 38(5), 1655-1711, 2007.

Arnold FM, Filardi TZ, Strang RD, McMahon J K: Early neurologic assessment of the patient with spinal cord injury, *Topics in Spinal Cord Injury Rehabilitation* 12(1):38-48, 2006.

Backer J: The symptom experience of patients with Parkinson's disease, *Journal of Neuroscience Nursing* 38(1):51-57, Feb 2006.

Barker E: New hope for stroke patients, *RN* 68(2):38-42, 2005.

Barker E: SCI patients take a big step forward, *RN* 68(2):38-42, 2005.

Barker E, Saulino M: First ever guidelines for spinal cord injuries, *RN* 65(10):32-37, 2002.

Berlly M, Shem K: Respiratory management during the first five days after spinal cord injury, *Journal of Spinal Cord Medicine* 30(4):309-318, 2007.

Bingham V, Habermann B: The influence of spirituality on family management of Parkinson's disease, *Journal of Neuroscience Nursing* 38(6):422-427, Dec 2006.

Cifu D, Carne W, Brown R, Pegg P, Ong J, Qutubuddin A: Caregiver distress in parkinsonism, *Journal of Rehabilitation Research and Development* 43(4):499-508, Jul/Aug, 2006.

Cohen-Mansfield J, Jensen D, Malone T, et al: Dressing of cognitively impaired nursing home residents: description and analysis, *Gerontologist* 46(1):89-96, 2006.

Carpico B: Suspected cervical spine injury, *Nursing2007* 37(3):88, 2007.

Cortez R, Levi AD: Acute spinal cord injury, *Current Treatment Options in Neurology* 9(2):115-125, 2007.

Dolinak D, Balraj E: Autonomic dysreflexia and sudden death in people with traumatic spinal cord injury, *American Journal of Forensic Medicine and Pathology* 28(2):95-98, 2007.

Elliot S: Ejaculation and orgasm: sexuality in men with SCI, *Topics in Spinal Cord Injury Rehabilitation* 8(1):1-15, 2002.

Engleman K, Mathews R, Altus D: Restoring dressing independence in persons with Alzheimer's disease: a pilot study, *American Journal of Alzheimer's Disease and Other Dementias* 17(1):37-43, 2002.

Fisher C, Noonan V, Divorak M: Changing the face of spinal trauma care in North America, *Spine* 31(11 Suppl):S2-S8, 2006.

Fries J: Critical rehabilitation of the patient with spinal cord injury, *Critical Care Nurse Quarterly* 28(2):179-187, 2005.

Frizzell JP: Acute stroke: Pathophysiology, diagnosis and treatment, *AACN Clinical Issues: Advanced Practice in Acute Critical Care* 16(4):421-440, 2005.

Galvan TJ: Dysphagia: going down and staying down, *American Journal of Nursing* 101(1):37-42, 2001.

Gibson KL: Caring for a patient who lives with spinal cord injury, *Nursing2003* 33(7):36-42, 2003.

Ganzer C: Assessing Alzheimer's disease and dementia: best practices in nursing care, *Geriatric Nursing* 28(6):358-365, Nov 2007. Retrieved November 10, 2008, from CINAHL Plus with Full Text database.

Gibson K: Caring for a patient who lives with spinal cord injury, *Nursing2003* 33(7):26-42, 2003.

Goodwin VA, et al. The effectiveness of exercise interventions for people with Parkinson's disease: a systematic review and meta-analysis, *Movement Disorders* 23(5):631-640, 2008.

Gramitto M, Galitz D: Update on stroke: the latest guidelines, *The Nurse Practitioner* 33(1):39-47, 2008.

Habermann B, Davis L: Caring for family with Alzheimer's disease and Parkinson's disease, *Journal of Gerontological Nursing* 31(6):49-54, 2005.

Harris M, Sethi R: The initial assessment and management of the multiple trauma patient associated with spine injury, *Spine* 31(11 Suppl):S9-S15, 2006.

Hirsch M, Dunlin M, Hammond F: Exercise for management and treatment of Parkinson's disease, *American Family Physician* 79(12):1043, 2009.

Hinkle JL: Acute ischemic stroke review, *Journal of Neuroscience Nursing* 39(5):285-293, 310, 2007.

Kim J: How do I respond to autonomic dysreflexia? *Nursing2003* 33(2):18, 2003.

Latt M, Menz H, Fung V, Lord S: Acceleration patterns of the head and pelvis during gait in older people with Parkinson's disease: a comparison, Journal of Gerontology, 64A(6):700-706, 2009.

Lees A, Hardy J, Revesz T: Parkinson's disease, *Lancet* 373:2055-2066, 2009.

Leibowitz R: Sexual rehabilitation services after spinal cord injury: What do women want? *Sexuality and Disability* 23(2), 81-107, 2005.

McCaffery C: Quick! My patient is having an ischemic stroke, *Nursing2006* 36(7):56cc1-4, 2006.

Morrison K: Improving the care of stroke patients, *American Nurse Today* 2(4):38-44, 2007.

Miller J, Elmore S: Call a stroke code! *Nursing2005* 35(3):58-63, 2005.

Nair M: Alzheimer's disease: nursing management of the patient with Alzheimer's disease, *British Journal of Nursing (BJN)* 15(5):258-262, Mar 9, 2006. Retrieved November 10, 2008, from CINAHL Plus with Full Text database.

Noble C: Understanding Parkinson's disease, *Nursing Standard* 21(34):48-56, May 2-8, 2007.

Pretzer-Aboff I, Galik E, Resnick B: Parkinson's disease: barriers and facilitators to optimizing function, *Rehabilitation NURSING* 34(2):55-63, Mar-April 2009.

Rao S, Hofmann L, Shakil A: Parkinson's disease: diagnosis and treatment, *American Family Physician* 74(12): 2046-2054, 2006.

Rentz C: Alzheimer's disease: an elusive thief, *Nursing Management* 39(6):33-39, 2008.

Rees P, Fowler C, Maas C: Sexual dysfunction 2: sexual function in men and women with neurological disorders, *Lancet* 369:512-525, 2007.

Sadowski C, Jones C, Gordon B, Feeny D: Knowledge of risk factors for falling reported by patients with Parkinson disease, Journal of Neuroscience Nursing 39(6):336-342, 2007.

Singh R, Sharma S: Sexuality and women with spinal cord injury, *Sexuality and Disability* 23(1):21-33, 2005.

Sharer J: Tackling sundowning in a patient with Alzheimer's disease, *MEDSURG Nursing* 17(1):27-29, Feb 2008.

Sherwood P, Crago E, Spiro R, Okonkwo D: Cervical spine injuries: preserving function, improving outcomes, *American Nurse Today,* 2(9), 26-29, 2007.

Snyder C, Adler C:. The patient with Parkinson's disease: part I. Treating the motor symptoms, Journal of the

American Academy of Nurse Practitioners, 19(4):179-197, 2007.

Stewart D: NICE guideline for Parkinson's disease: *Age and Ageing* 36:240-242, 2007.

Vacca V: Acute paraplegia, *Nursing2007* 37(6):64, 2007.

7 THE CLIENT WITH ALTERATIONS IN HEMATOLOGIC AND IMMUNE FUNCTION

Bartlett J, Finkbeiner A: *The guide to living with HIV infection,* Baltimore, 2001, Johns Hopkins University Press.

Beutler E, Coller BS, Lichtman MA, Kipps TJ, editors: *Williams hematology,* ed 6, New York, 2001, McGraw-Hill.

Bradley-Springer L: HIV infection: what works? *American Journal of Nursing* 101:(6):45-50, 2001.

Centers for Disease Control and Prevention. *HIV/AIDS surveillance report,* 13(2):1-44, 2002.

Chettle CC: Sepsis: the body's overreaction to infection can prove deadly, *NurseWeek California* 16(4):19-21, 2003.

Coyne PJ, Lyne ME, Watson AC: Symptom management in people with AIDS, *American Journal of Nursing* 102(9):48-56, 2002.

Daughtry L, Bankston J, DeShotels J. HIV meds: keeping trouble at bay, *RN* 65(2):31-35, 2002.

Dellinger RP: Cardiovascular management of septic shock, *Critical Care Medicine* 31(3):946-955, 2003.

Destarac LA, et al: Sepsis in older patients: an emerging concern in critical care, *Advances in Sepsis* 2002. Available online at www.sepsis. remdica.com.

Dressler DK: DIC: coping with a coagulation crisis, *Nursing2004* 34(5):58-62, 2004.

Geiter H: Disseminated intravascular coagulopathy, *Dimensions of Critical Care Nursing* 22(33):108-116, 2003.

Gracia JS: Taking HAART: how to support patients with HIV/AIDS, *Nursing2001* 31(12):36-41, 2001.

Hoffman R, Benz EJ, Shattil SJ, et al: *Hematology: basic principles and practice,* ed 3,. New York, 2001, Churchill Livingstone.

Mandell GL, Bennett JE, Dolin R: *Mandell, Douglas, and Bennett's principles and practice of infectious diseases,* ed 5, New York, 2000, Churchill Livingstone.

McCoy C, Matthews SJ. Drotrecogin alfa (recombinant human activated protein C) for the treatment of severe sepsis. *Clinical Therapeutics,* 25(2):396-421, 2003.

Parrillo JE, Dellinger RP: *Critical care medicine: principles of diagnosis and management in the adult,* ed 2, St Louis, 2001, Mosby.

Piliero PJ, Colagreco JP: Clinical practice: simplified regimens for treating HIV infection and AIDS, *Journal of the American Academy of Nurse Practitioners* 15(7):305-312, 2003.

Schulman CS, Hare K: New thoughts on sepsis: the unifier of critical care, *Dimensions of Critical Care Nursing* 22(1):20-30, 2003.

Spleen removal. Available online at www. health.yahoo.com.

U.S. Department of Health and Human Services: *Guidelines for the prevention of opportunistic infections among HIV-infected persons,* 2002. Retrieved August 9, 2009 from http://aidsinfo. nih.gov/contentfiles/OIpreventionGL. pdf

Wenzel RP: Treating sepsis, *New England Journal of Medicine* 347(13):966-967, 2002.

Williams A: Adherence to HIV regimens: 10 vital lessons, *American Journal of Nursing* 101(6):37-44, 2001.

World Health Organization: *Antiretroviral therapy for HIV infection in adults and adolescents: recommendations for a public health approach,* 2006. Retrieved August 9, 2009 from www.who.int/ hiv/pub/guidelines/artadultguidelines. pdf.

8 THE CLIENT WITH ALTERATIONS IN METABOLIC FUNCTION

American Diabetes Association: Summary of revisions for the 2008 clinical practice recommendations, *Diabetes Care* 31(Suppl 1):S3-S4, 2008.

American Diabetes Association: Standards of medical care in diabetes, *Diabetes Care* 31(Suppl 1), S12-S54, 2008.

American Diabetes Association: Nutrition recommendations and interventions in diabetes, *Diabetes Care* 31(Suppl 1):S61-A78, 2008.

Austin M: AADE Position Statement: Self-monitoring of blood glucose: benefits and utilization, *The Diabetes Educator* 32(6):835-847, 2006.

Bloomgarden Z: Approaches to treatment of type 2 diabetes, *Diabetes Care* 31(8):1697-1703, 2008.

Bloomgarden Z: The diabetic foot, *Diabetes Care* 31(2):372-376, 2008.

Boulton A: Management of diabetic peripheral neuropathy, *Clinical Diabetes* 2:9-15, 2005.

Boulton A, Armstrong D, Albert S, Frykberg R, Hellman R, Kirkman S, et al: Comprehensive foot

examination and risk assessment, *Diabetes Care* 31:1679-1685, 2008.

Brent G, Larsn RR, Davies T: Hypothyroidism and thyroiditis. In H Kronenberg, S Melmed, K Polonsky, PR Larsen. (Eds.). *Williams' textbook of endocrinology, ed 11,* Philadelphia, 2008, Saunders.

Briscoe V, Davis S: Hypoglycemia in type I and type 2 diabetes: physiology, pathophysiology and management, *Clinical Diabetes* 24(3):115-121, 2006.

Ceriello A: Postprandial hyperglycemia and diabetes complications, *Diabetes* 54(1):1-7, 2005.

Clement S, Braithwaite SS, Magee MF, Ahmann A, Smith EP, Schafer RG et al: Management of diabetes and hyperglycemia in hospitals, *Diabetes Care* 27(2):553-591, 2004.

Corbett CF: Practical management of patients with peripheral neuropathy, *Diabetes Educator* 31(4):523-540, 2005.

Devdhar M, Ousman Y, Burman K: Hypothyroidism, *Endocrinology and Metabolism Clinics of North America* 36(4):595-615, 2007.

Fain J: Unlock the mysteries of insulin therapy, *Nursing* 34(3): 41-43, 2004.

Fain JA: Insulin pumps, *Nursing2003* 33(6):51-53, 2003.

Funnell M, Brown T, Childs B, Haas L, Hosey G, Jensen B, et al: National standards for Diabetes self-management education, *Diabetes Care* 31S:S97-S104, 2008.

Goolsby MJ, Blackwell J: Evaluation and treatment of hyperthyroidism and hypothyroidism, *Journal of the American Academy of Nurse Practitioners* 16(10):422-425, 2004.

Gross JL, De Azevedo MJ, Silveiro SP, Canani LH, Caramori ML, Zelmanovitz T: Diabetic nephropathy: diagnosis, prevention, and treatment, *Diabetes Care* 28(1):164-176, 2005.

Holcomb S: Detecting thyroid disease, *Nursing2005* 35(10), 4-8, 2005.

Horner B, Chase HP: Continuous glucose monitoring, *Practical Diabetology* 29(1):30-42, 2007.

Kumrow D, Dahlen R: Thyroidectomy: understanding the potential for complications, *MEDSURG Nursing* 11(5), 228-234, 2002.

Mauk K: Rooting out hypothyroidism in the elderly, *Nursing2005* 35(12):65-66, 2005.

Nayak B, Burman K: Thyrotoxicosis and thyroid storm, *Endocrinology and Metabolism Clinics of North America* 35(4):663-686, 2006.

Nayak B, Hodak S: Hyperthyroidism, *Endocrinology and Metabolism Clinics of North America* 5(4):617-656, 2006.

Noble K: Thyroid storm, *Journal of PeriAnesthesia Nursing* 21(2):119-125, 2006.

Reid J, Wheeler S: Hyperthyroidism: diagnosis and treatment, *American Family Physician* 72(4):623-630, 2005.

Nugent BW: Hyperosmolar hyperglycemic state, *Emergency Medicine Clinics of North America* 23(2):629-648, 2005.

Seley J, Weinger K: Executive summary: the state of the science on nursing best practices for diabetes self-management, *American Journal of Nursing* 107(6):73-78, 2007.

Sigal RJ, Kenny GP, Wasserman DH, Castaneda-Sceppa C, White RD: Physical activity/exercise and type 2 diabetes: a consensus statement from the American Diabetes Association, *Diabetes Care* 29(6):1433-1438, 2006.

Stoner GD: Hyperosmolar hyperglycemic state, *American Family Physician* 71(9):1723-1730, 2005.

Weeks B: Graves' disease: the importance of early diagnosis, *Nurse Practitioner* 30(11):34-45, 2005.

Wolpert H: The nuts and bolts of achieving end points with real-time continuous glucose monitoring, *Diabetes Care* 31(S146-S149), 2008.

9 THE CLIENT WITH ALTERATIONS IN THE GASTROINTESTINAL TRACT

Ables A, Simon I, Meoton E: Update on *Helicobacter pylori* treatment, *American Family Physician* 75(3):351-358, 2007.

American College of Emergency Physicians Clinical Policies Committee, Clinical Policies Subcommittee on Acute Blunt Abdominal Trauma: Clinical policy: critical issues in the evaluation of adult patients presenting to the emergency department with acute blunt abdominal trauma, *Annals of Emergency Medicine* 43(2), 278-290, 2004.

American Society of Parenteral and Enteral Nutrition Board of Directors and the Clinical Guidelines Task Force: Guidelines for the use of parenteral and enteral nutrition in adults and pediatric patients, *Journal of Parenteral and Enteral Nutrition* 26(2):144, 2002.

Barba K, Fitzgerald P, Wood S: Managing peptic ulcer disease, *Nursing2007* 37(7):56hn1-56hn4, 2007.

Barth M, Jenson C: Postoperative nursing care of gastric bypass patients,

American Journal of Critical Care 15(4):378-388, 2006.

Blank-Reid C: Abdominal trauma: dealing with the damage, *Nursing2004* 34(9):36-41, 2004.

Bourgault AM, Ipe L, Weaver J, Swartz S, O'Dea PJ: Development of evidenced-based guidelines and critical care nurses' knowledge of enteral feedings, *Critical Care Nurse* 27(4):17-48, 2007.

Bulechek GM, Butcher HK, Dochterman JM (Eds): *Nursing interventions classification (NIC)*, ed 5, St Louis, 2008, Mosby-Elsevier.

Carter M, Lobo A, Travis R, the Irritable Bowel Disease Section of the British Society of Gastroenterology: Guidelines for the management of inflammatory bowel disease in adults, *Gut* 53(Suppl V):V1-V16, 2004.

Cima RR, Pemberton JH: Ileostomy, colostomy, and pouches. In M Feldman et al (Eds): *Sleisenger and Fordtran's gastrointestinal and liver disease*, ed 8, vol 2, pp. 2549-2561, Philadelphia, 2006, Saunders-Elsevier.

Dooley TP, Curto EV, Reddy SP, Davis RL, Lambert GW, Wilborn TW et al: Regulation of gene expression in inflammatory bowel disease and correlation with IBD drugs: screening by DNA microassays, *Inflammatory Bowel Diseases* 10(1):1-14, 2004.

Eckert K: Penetrating and blunt abdominal trauma, *Critical Care Nurse* 25(1):41-50, 2005.

Freeman LC: Responding to small-bowel obstruction, *Nursing2007* 37(5):56hn1-56hn2, May 2007.

Grindle M, Grindle C: Nursing care of the person having bariatric surgery, *MEDSURG Nursing* 15(3):129-146, 2006.

Ide P, Fabar E, Lautz D: Perioperative nursing care of the bariatric surgical patient, *AORN Journal* 99(1):30-58, 2008.

Khan AN, MacDonald S, Howat JMT: Small bowel obstruction, *eMedicine*. Available online at www.emedicine.com/radio/topic781.htm, 2004. Accessed April 15, 2008.

Klonowski E, Masoodi J: The patient with Crohn's disease, *RN* 62(3):32-37, 1999.

Lewis SL, Heitkemper MM, Dirksen SR, O'Brien G, Bucher L: *Medical-surgical nursing: assessment and management of clinical problems*, ed 7, St Louis, 2007, Mosby-Elsevier.

MayoClinic.com. *Crohn's disease*. Retrieved November 10, 2008, from www.mayoclinic.com.

Mirtallo J, Canada T, Johnson D, Kumpf V, Petersen C et al: Safe practices for

parenteral nutrition, *Journal of Parenteral and Enteral Nutrition* 28(6S):S39-S71, 2004.

Metheny NA: Preventing respiratory complications of tube feedings: evidence based practice, *American Journal of Critical Care* 15(4):360-369, 2006.

Metheny NA: Residual volume measurement should be retained in enteral feeding protocols, *American Journal of Critical Care Nursing* 17(1):62-64, 2008.

Moorhead S, Johnson M, Maas ML, Swanson E (Eds): *Nursing outcomes classification (NOC)*, ed 4, St Louis, 2008, Mosby-Elsevier.

Pearson, C. (2004). Inflammatory bowel disease. *Nursing Times* 100(9), 86-90.

Persson E, Gustavsson G, Hellstrom A, Lappas G, Hulten L: Ostomy patients perceptions of quality of care, *Journal of Advanced Nursing* 49(1):51-58, 2004.

Ramakrishnan K, Salina R: Peptic ulcer disease, *American Family Physician* 76(7):1005-1012, 2007.

Rayhorn N, Rayhorn BS: Inflammatory bowel disease: symptoms in the bowel and beyond, *Nurse Practitioner* 27(11):3-16, 23-29, 2002.

Sands B: Inflammatory bowel disease: past, present, and future, *Journal of Gastroenterology* 42:16-25, 2007.

Sole ML, Klein DG, Moseley MJ: *Introduction to critical care nursing*, ed 5, St Louis, 2008, Mosby-Elsevier.

Trouble down below: understanding small bowel obstruction, *Nursing2005* 35(7):32cc4-32cc7, 2005.

Turnbull G: *Intimacy, sexuality, and an ostomy*, 2005, United Ostomy Association.

Twedell D: Crohn's disease and ulcerative colitis, *Journal of Continuing Education in Nursing* 39(4):151-152, 2008.

United Ostomy Association: *Ileostomy guide*, 2005, United Ostomy Association.

Walsh A, Albano H, Jones D: A perioperative team approach to treating patients undergoing laparoscopic bariatric surgery, *AORN Journal* 88(1):59:54, 2008.

Wound, Ostomy, and Continence Nurses Society: Basic ostomy skin care: a guide for patients and health care providers, Glenview, Ill, 2007, The Society.

Wound, Ostomy, and Continence Nurses Society: Discharge planning for a patient with a new ostomy: best practice for clinicians, Glenview, Ill, 2004, The Society.

Willcutts K, Scarano K, Eddins CW: Ostomies and fistulas: a collaborative approach, *Practical Gastroenterology* 29(11):63-79, 2005.

Williams J: Caring for the older ostomate, *Nursing & Residential Care* 10(2):64-67, 2008.

10 THE CLIENT WITH ALTERATIONS IN THE LIVER, BILIARY TRACT, AND PANCREAS

American Nephrology Nurses' Association: *ANNA nephrology nursing standards of practice and guidelines for care*, Pittman, NJ, 2005, The Association.

American Nephrology Nurses' Association: *Core curriculum for nephrology nurses*, ed 5, Pittman, NJ, 2008, The Association.

Amerine E: Get optimum outcomes for acute pancreatitis patients, *The Nurse Practitioner* 32(6):44-48, 2007.

Baltimore JL, Davidson J: Caring for a patient with acute cholecystitis, *Nursing2007* 37(3), 64hn1-4, 2007.

Befeler A, Herrine SK: Complications of cirrhosis—Clinical insights and implications for practice, Available online at www.medscape.com/viewprogram/8362_pnt. Retrieved November, 2008.

Bellows CF, Berger DH, Crass RA: Management of gallstones, *American Family Physician* 72(4):637-642, 2005.

Beitz M: Continent diversions: the new gold standards of ileoanal reservoir and neobladder, *Ostomy Wound Management* 50(9):26-35, 2004.

Brundage SC, Fitzpatrick AN: Hepatitis A, *American Family Physician* 73(12):2162-2168, 2006.

Burruss N, Holz S: Understanding acute pancreatitis, *Nursing2005* 35(3):32hn1-4, 2005.

Cole L: Unraveling the mystery of acute pancreatitis, *Nursing2001* 31(12):58-63, 2001.

Dougherty AS, Dreher HM: Hepatitis C: current treatment strategies for an emerging epidemic, *MEDSURG Nursing* 10(1):9-13, 2001.

Dugernier TL, Laterre PF, Wittebole X, et al: Compartmentalization of the inflammatory response during acute pancreatitis, *American Journal of Respiratory and Critical Care Medicine* 168(2):148-157, 2003.

Garcia-Tsao G, Sanyal AJ, Grace ND, Carey W, Practice Guidelines Committee of the American Association for the Study of Liver Diseases, Practice Parameters Committee of the American College of Gastroenterology: Prevention and management of gastroesophageal varices and variceal hemorrhage in cirrhosis, *Hepatology* 46(3) 922-938, 2007.

Gavaghan M: The pancreas: hermit of the abdomen, *AORN Journal* 75(6):1110-1114, 1117, 1119, 2002.

Glacken M, Coates V, Kernohan G, Hegarty J: The experience of fatigue for people living with hepatitis C, *Journal of Clinical Nursing* 12(2):244-252, 2003.

Hale AS, Moseley MJ, Warner SC: Treating pancreatitis in the acute care setting, *Dimensions of Critical Care Nursing* 19(4):15-21, 2000.

Harkness GA: Emerging infections: hepatitis C: the silent stalker: a rapidly mutating virus that's difficult to detect, *American Journal of Nursing* 103(9):24-25, 2003.

Herrine S: AASLD 2006: Complications of cirrhosis and portal hypertension-variceal bleeding: clinical insights and implications for practice, 2006. Available online at www.medscape.com/viewarticle/548129. Retrieved November 2008.

Holcomb SS: Stopping the destruction of acute pancreatitis, *Nursing2007* 37(6):43-48, 2007.

Ho J, Yoshida E: The extrahepatic consequences of cirrhosis, 2006. Available online at www.medscape.com/viewarticle/518096. Retrieved November, 2008.

Indar A, Beckingham I: Acute cholecystitis, *British Medical Journal* 325(Sept 21) 639-643, 2002.

Iosue K: Chronic hepatitis C: latest treatment options, *Nurse Practitioner* 27(4):32-49, 2002.

Kleinpell RM: Shock states, *NurseWeek* 4(14):20-22, 2003.

Matthews RE, McGuire BM, Estrada CA: Outpatient management of cirrhosis: a narrative review, *Southern Medical Association* 90(6):600-606, 2006.

Nathens A, Curtis J, Beale J, et al: Management of the critically ill patient with severe acute pancreatitis, *Critical Care Medicine* 32(12), 2524-2536, 2004.

Overstreet D, Sims T: Care of the patient undergoing radical cystectomy with a robotic approach, *Urologic Nursing* 26(2):117-123, 2006.

Parini S: Hepatitis C, *Nursing2003* 33(4):57-63, 2003.

Patel K, Muir AJ, McHutchinson JG: Diagnosis and treatment of chronic hepatitis C infection, *British Medical Journal* 332(7548):1013-1017, 2006.

Quillen SM: Identification of pancreatitis in the ambulatory setting, *Gastroenterology Nursing* 24(1):20-22, 2010.

11 THE CLIENT WITH ALTERATIONS IN THE KIDNEY AND URINARY TRACT

Al-Arabi S: Quality of life: subjective descriptions of challenges to patients with end stage renal disease, *Nephrology Nursing Journal* 33(3):285-293, 2006.

American Nephrology Nurses' Association: *ANNA nephrology nursing standards of practice and guidelines for care*, Pittman, NJ, 2005, ANNA.

American Nephrology Nurses' Association: *Core curriculum for nephrology nurses*, ed 5, Pittman, NJ, 2008, ANNA.

Beitz M: Continent diversions: the new gold standards of ileoanal reservoir and neobladder, *Ostomy Wound Management* 50(9):26-35, 2004.

Broscious S, Castagnola J: Chronic kidney disease: acute manifestations and role of critical care nurses, *Critical Care Nurse* 24(4):17-27, 2006.

Burrows-Hudson S: Chronic kidney disease: an overview, *American Journal of Nursing* 105(2):40-49, 2005.

Campbell D: How acute renal failure puts the brakes on kidney function, *Nursing2003* 33(10):59-64, 2003.

Campoy S, Elwell R: Pharmacology & CKD, *American Journal of Nursing* 105(9):60-71, 2005.

Castner D, Douglas C: Now onstage: chronic kidney disease, *Nursing2006* 35(12):58-63, 2005.

Dinwiddie L, Burrows-Hudson S, Peacock E: Stage 4 chronic kidney disease, *American Journal of Nursing* 106(9):40-51, 2006.

Holcomb S: Evaluating chronic kidney disease risk, *The Nurse Practitioner* 30(4):12-25, 2005.

Katz A: What have my kidneys got to do with my sex life? *American Journal of Nursing* 106(9):81-83, 2006.

Kopyt N: Management and treatment of chronic kidney disease, *The Nurse Practitioner* 32(11):14-23, 2007.

Legg V: Complications of chronic kidney disease, *American Journal of Nursing* 105(6):40-49, 2005.

Overstreet D, Sims T: Care of the patient undergoing radical cystectomy with a robotic approach, *Urologic Nursing* 26(2):117-123, 2006.

Rushing J: Caring for your patient's suprapubic catheter, *Nursing2006* 36(7):32, 2006.

Schneider V, Levesque LE, Zhang B, Hutchinson T, Brophy JM:

Association of selective and conventional nonsteroidal anti-inflammatory drugs with acute renal failure: a population-based nested case-control analysis, *American Journal of Epidemiology* 164(9):881-889, 2006.

Sclauzero P, Casarotto S, Martingano M, Morpurgo F, Rocconi I, Scala K, et al: Improving quality of assistance and outcome in critically ill patients with acute renal failure, *EDTNA/ERCA Journal* 32(3):181-185, 2006.

Thomas-Hawkins C, Zazworsky D: Self-management of chronic kidney disease, *American Journal of Nursing* 105(10):40-48, 2005.

12   THE CLIENT WITH ALTERATIONS IN MUSCULOSKELETAL FUNCTION

Bailey J: Getting a fix on orthopedic care, *Nursing2003* 33(6):5864, 2003.

Browner BD, Jupiter JB, Levine AM, Trafton PG: *Skeletal trauma: basic science, management, and reconstruction,* ed 3, Philadelphia, 2003, Saunders.

Canale ST (Ed): *Campbell's operative orthopaedics,* ed 10, St Louis, 2003, Mosby.

Chan KC, Gill GS: Cemented hemiarthroplasties for elderly patients with intertrochanteric fractures, *Clinical Orthopaedics* 371:206-215, 2000.

Chapman MW (Ed): *Chapman's orthopaedic surgery,* ed 3, Philadelphia, 2001, Lippincott Williams & Wilkins.

Church V: Staying on guard for DVT and PE, *Nursing2000* 30(2):34-42, 2000.

Feldt KS, Gunderson J: Treatment of pain for older hip fracture patients across setting, *Orthopaedic Nursing* 21(5):63-64, 66-71, 2002.

Ginsberg B: Pain management in knee surgery, *Orthopaedic Nursing* 20(2):37-44, 2001.

Maher A, Salmond SW, Pellino TA (Eds): *Orthopaedic nursing,* ed 3, Philadelphia, 2002, Saunders.

Nassif JM, Ritter MA, Medling JB, et al: The effect of intraoperative intravenous fixed-dose heparin during total joint arthroplasty on the incidence of fatal pulmonary emboli, *Journal of Arthroplasty* 15:16-21, 2000.

Parker MJ: Evidence-based case report: managing an elderly patient with a fractured femur, *British Medical Journal* 320:102-103, 2000.

Phantom Pain Options. Available at www.members.fortunecity.com.

Ragucci MV, Leali A, Moroz A, Fetto J: Comprehensive deep vein thrombosis

prevention strategy after total knee arthroplasty, *American Journal of Physical Medicine and Rehabilitation* 82(3):164-168, 2003.

Reed SJ: Managing phantom limb pain with drugs, *Nursing2000* 29(4):32hn1-32hn4, 2000.

Resnick D: *Diagnosis of bone and joint disorders,* ed 4, Philadelphia, 2002, Saunders.

Rutherford RB: *Vascular surgery,* ed 5, Philadelphia, 2000, Saunders.

Samana CM, Vray M, Barre J, Fiessinger J, et al: Extended venous thromboembolism prophylaxis after total hip replacement: a comparison of low-molecular-weight heparin with oral anticoagulants, *Archives of Internal Medicine* 162(19):2191-2196, 2002.

Schoen D (Ed): *Adult orthopaedic nursing,* Philadelphia, 2000, Lippincott Williams & Wilkins.

Schoen DC (Ed): *NAON core curriculum for orthopaedic nursing,* ed 4, Pitman, NJ, 2001, National Association of Orthopaedic Nurses.

Schuurmans MJ, Duursman SA, Shortridge-Baggett LM, et al: Elderly patients with a hip fracture: the risk for delirium, *Applied Nursing Research* 16(2):75-84, 2003.

Stern SH, Wixson RL, O'Connor D: Evaluation of the safety and efficacy of enoxaparin and warfarin for prevention of deep vein thrombosis after total knee arthroplasty, *Journal of Arthroplasty* 15(2):153-158, 2000.

Turpie AGG, Gallus AS, Hoek JA: A synthetic pentasaccharide for the prevention of deep vein thrombosis after total hip replacement, *New England Journal of Medicine* 344(9):619-625, 2001.

13   THE CLIENT WITH ALTERATIONS IN THE BREAST AND REPRODUCTIVE SYSTEM

Baron RH, Fey JV, Raboy S, et al: Eighteen sensations after breast cancer surgery: a comparison of sentinel lymph node biopsy and axillary node dissection, *Oncology Nursing Forum* 29(4):651-659, 2002.

Cancer Information Network. Available at www.cancerlinksusa.com.

DeVita VT Jr, Hellman S, Rosenberg SA (Eds): *Cancer: principles and practice of oncology,* ed 6, Philadelphia, 2001, Lippincott Williams & Wilkins.

Erickson VS, Pearson ML, Ganz PA, et al: Arm edema in breast cancer patients, *Journal of the National Cancer Institute* 93(2):96-111, 2001.

Held-Warmkessel J: What your patient needs to know about prostate cancer, *Nursing2002* 32(12):36-42, 2002.

Holmberg SK, Scott LL, Alexy W, et al: Relationship issues of women with breast cancer, *Cancer Nursing* 24(1):53-60, 2001.

Hoskins CN, Haber J: Adjusting to breast cancer, *American Journal of Nursing* 100(4):26-31, 2000.

Hull MM: Lymphedema in women treated for breast cancer, *Seminars in Oncology Nursing* 16(3):226-237, 2000.

MacDonald DJ: Women's decisions regarding management of breast cancer risks, *MEDSURG Nursing* 11(4):183-186, 2002.

Otto SE: *Oncology nursing,* ed 4, St Louis, 2001, Mosby.

Resnick B, Belcher AE: Breast reconstruction: options, answers, and support for patients making a difficult personal decision, *American Journal of Nursing* 102(4):26-33, 2002.

Rondorf-Klym LM, Colling J: Quality of life after radical prostatectomy, *Oncology Nursing Forum* 30(2):E24-32, 2003.

Sandau KE: Free TRAM flap breast reconstruction, *American Journal of Nursing* 102(4):36-43, 2002.

Therapies for the treatment of benign prostatic hyperplasia. Available at www.cpmcnet.columbia.edu/dept/urology/bphtherapy.

Thomas S, Greifzu SP: Oncology today: breast cancer, *RN* 63(4):40-47, 2000.

Walsh PC, Retik AB, Vaughn ED, Jr, et al (Eds): *Campbell's urology,* ed 8, Philadelphia, 2002, Saunders.

14   THE CLIENT RECEIVING TREATMENT FOR NEOPLASTIC DISORDERS

Abel L, Dafoe-Lambie J, Butler WM: Treatment outcomes and quality-of-life issues for patients treated with prostate brachytherapy, *Clinical Journal of Nursing Oncology* 7(1):48-54, 2003.

Abeloff MD, Armitage JD, Lichter A, Nierderhuber JE (Eds): *Clinical oncology,* ed 2, New York, 2000, Churchill Livingstone.

American Cancer Society. Available at www.cancer.org.

American Pain Society: *Principles of analgesic use in the treatment of acute pain and chronic cancer pain: a concise guide to medical practice,* ed 4, Skokie, Il, 1999, American Pain Society.

Borjeson S, Hursti TJ, Tishelman C, et al: Treatment of nausea and emesis during cancer chemo: discrepancies between antiemetic effect and well-being, *Journal of Pain and Symptom Management* 24(3):345-358, 2002.

Brown JK: A systematic review of the evidence on symptom management of cancer-related anorexia and cachexia, *Oncology Nursing Forum* 29(3):517-532, 2002.

Buchsel PC, Murph BS, Newton SA: Epoetin alpha: current and future indications and nursing implications, *Clinical Journal of Oncology Nursing* 6(5):261-267, 2002.

Cady J: Understanding opioid tolerance in cancer pain, *Oncology Nursing Forum* 28(10):1561-1568, 2001.

Cancer Information Network. Available at www.cancernetwork.com.

Chernecky C: Pulmonary complications in patients with cancer, *American Journal of Nursing* 101(5):24A, 24E, 24G-H, 2001.

Chu E, DeVita VT Jr: *Physicians' cancer chemotherapy drug manual*, 2003, Sudbury, Mass, 2003, Jones & Bartlett.

Colella J, Scrofine S: High dose brachytherapy for treating prostate cancer: nursing considerations, *Urological Nursing* 24(1):39-52.

Cunningham RS (Ed): Nutrition and cancer, *Seminars in Oncology Nursing* 16(2):1-173, 2000.

DeVita VT Jr, Hellman S, Rosenberg SA (Eds): Cancer *principles and practice of oncology*, ed Philadelphia, 2001, Lippincott Williams & Wilkins.

Ghen MJ, Cole F: Nutritional effects of cancer chemotherapy, *Natural Pharmacology* 6(3):1, 6-7, 21, 2002.

Gosselin TK, Waring JS: Nursing management of patients receiving brachytherapy for gynecologic malignancies, *Clinical Journal of Oncology Nursing* 5(2): 59-63.

Haskell CM: *Cancer treatment*, ed 5, Philadelphia, 2001, Saunders.

Hogle WP, Quinn AE, Heron DE: Advances in brachytherapy: new approaches to target breast cancer, *Clinical Journal of Oncology Nursing* 7(3):324-328, 2003.

Holland J: New treatment modalities in radiation therapy, *Journal of Intravenous Nursing* 24(2):95-101, 2001.

Janjan N: Radiation therapy: beating side effects, *Bottom Line/Health* 17(4):11-12, 2003.

Kufe DW, Pollock RE, Weichselbaum RR, et al (Eds): *Holland and Freis cancer medicine*, Hamilton, Ontario, 2003, BC Decker.

Kurtz ME, Kurtz JC, Stommel M, et al: Physical functioning and depression among older persons with cancer, *Cancer Practice* 9(1):11-18, 2001.

Letizia M: Addressing alopecia: helping patients with cancer deal with hair loss, *American Journal of Nursing* 101(40):24, 2001.

Lyne ME, Coyne PJ, Watson AC: Pain management issues for cancer survivors, *Cancer Practice* 10(1):S27-S32, 2002.

McCarthy D, Weihofen D: The effect of nutritional supplements on food intake in patients undergoing radiotherapy, *Oncology Nursing Forum* 26(5):897-900, 1999.

Mendelson FA, Divino CM, Reis ED, Kerstein MD: Wound care after radiation therapy, *Advances in Skin and Wound Care* 15(5):216, 218-224, 2002.

Nail LM: Fatigue in patients with cancer, *Oncology Nursing Forum* 29(3):537-546, 2002.

National Cancer Institute. Available at www.nci.nih.gov.

Otto SE: *Oncology nursing*, ed 4, St Louis, 2001, Mosby.

Pierce DN: Use of amifostine (ETHYOL) as a radioprotector, *Images* 22(1):7, 28, 2003.

Randall ME: Brachytherapy for gynecologic cancers, *Gynecological Oncology Nursing* 18(3):5-10, 2008.

Ratain JM, Tempero M, Skosey C: *Outline of oncology therapeutics*, Philadelphia, 2001, Saunders.

Ream E, Richardson A, Alexander-Dann C: Facilitating patients' coping with fatigue during chemotherapy, *Cancer Nursing* 25(4):300-308, 2002.

Rogers BB: Mucositis in the oncology patient, *Nursing Clinics of North America* 36(4):745-760, 2001.

Sadler GR, Stoudt A, Fullerton JT, et al: Managing the oral sequelae of cancer therapy, *MEDSURG Nursing* 12(1):28-36, 2003.

Schnell FM: Chemotherapy-induced nausea and vomiting: the importance of acute antiemetic control, *Oncologist* 8(2):187-198, 2003.

Shih A, Misakowski C, Dodd ML, et al: A research review of current treatment for radiation-induced oral mucositis in patients with head and neck cancer, *Oncology Nursing Forum* 29(7):1063-1080, 2002.

Swinburne C: Looking good, *Nursing Standard* 17(39):16-17, 2003.

Wagler RM, Baum BJ: Prophylactic treatment reduces the severity of xerostomia following radiation for oral cavity cancer, *Archives of Otolaryngology: Head and Neck Surgery* 129(2):247-250, 2003.

Watson AC, Coyne PJ: Recognizing the faces of cancer pain, *Nursing2003* 33(4):32hn1-32hn8, 2003.

Wickham R, Rehwaldt M, Defer C, et al: Taste changes experienced by patients receiving chemotherapy, *Oncology Nursing Forum* 26(4):697-706, 1999.

Wilkes GM, Ingwersen K, Barton-Burke M: *Oncology nursing drug handbook*, Sudbury, Mass, 2003, Jones & Bartlett.

Wilson RL: Optimizing nutrition for patients with cancer, *Clinical Journal of Oncology Nursing* 4(1):23-28, 2000.

Winningham ML, Barton-Burke M (Eds): *Fatigue in cancer: a multidisciplinary approach*, Sudbury, Mass, Jones & Bartlett, 2000.

Wojtaszek C: Management of chemotherapy-induced stomatitis, *Clinical Journal of Oncology Nursing* 4(1):263-270, 2000.

Yarbro CH, Frogge MH, Goodman M, Groenwald S (Eds): *Cancer nursing: principles and practice*, ed 5, Sudbury, Mass, 2000, Jones & Bartlett.

15 NURSING CARE OF THE ELDERLY CLIENT

Abrams WB, Beers MH, Berkow R: *Merck manual of geriatrics*, ed 3, Whitehouse Station, NJ, 2006, Merck & Company.

American Nurses Association: *Scope and standards of gerontological nursing practice*, ed 2, Washington, DC, 2001, American Nurses Publishing.

Burke MM, Laramie JA. *Primary care of the older adult: a multidisciplinary approach*, St Louis, 2000, Mosby.

Carlson D, Pfadt E: *Clinical coach for effective nursing care for older adults*, Philadelphia, 2009, FA Davis.

Cassell CK (Ed): *Geriatric medicine: an evidence-based approach*, ed 4, New York, 2003, Springer.

DeLaine C, Scammell J, Heaslip V: Continuing professional development: older people, *Primary Health Care* 13(1):43-50, 2003.

Ebersole P, Hess P: *Geriatric nursing and healthy aging*, St Louis, 2001, Mosby.

Ebersole P, Touhy T, Hess P, Jett K, Luggen A: *Toward health aging*, ed 7, St Louis, 2008, Mosby.

Eliopoulos C: *Gerontological nursing*, ed 8, Philadelphia, 2005, Lippincott Williams & Wilkins.

Fantl JA, Newman DK, Colling J, et al: *Managing acute and chronic urinary incontinence: clinical practice guideline*, AHCPR Pub. No. 96-0686, Rockville, Md, 1996 update, Agency for Health Care Policy and Research.

Halter J, Ouslander J, Tinetti M, Sudenski S, High K, Asthana S: *Hazzard's geriatric medicine & gerontology*, ed 6, New York, 2009, McGraw Hill.

Hogstell MO: *Gerontology: nursing care of the older adult,* Clifton Park, NY, 2001, Delmar.

Luekenotte A: *Gerontologic nursing,* ed 2, St Louis, 2005, Mosby.

Maas ML, Buckwalter KC, Hardy MD, et al: *Nursing care of older adults: diagnoses, outcomes, and interventions,* St Louis, 2001, Mosby.

Mauk K: *Gerontological nursing: competencies for care,* Sudbury, Mass, 2006, Jones & Bartlett.

Mayer BH (Ed): *Better elder care: a nurse's guide to caring for older adults,* Springhouse, Pa, 2002, Springhouse.

Meiner S, Lueckenott A: *Gerontologic nursing,* ed 3, St Louis, 2006, Mosby-Elsevier.

Mezey MD (Eds): *The encyclopedia of elder care,* New York, 2001, Springer.

Nagel CL, Markie MB, Richards KC, Taylor JL: Sleep promotion in hospitalized elders, *MEDSURG Nursing* 12(5):279-288, 2003.

Osterweil D, Brummel-Smith K, Beck JC: *Comprehensive geriatric assessment,* New York, 2000, McGraw-Hill.

Peate I: Medicines and the older person: principles of good practice, *British Journal of Nursing* 12(9):530-535, 2003

Stanley M, Blair K, Beare P: *Gerontological nursing: promoting successful aging with older adults,* ed 3, Philadelphia, 2005, FA Davis.

Tallis RC, Fillit HM (Eds): *Brocklehurst's textbook of geriatric medicine and gerontology,* ed 6, New York, 2003, Churchill Livingstone.

Watson RR (Eds): *Handbook of nutrition in the aged,* ed 3, Boca Raton, Fl, 2001, CRC Press.

16 END-OF-LIFE NURSING CARE

Ameling A, Povilonis M: Spirituality, meaning, mental health, and nursing, *Journal of Psychosocial Nursing and Mental Health Services* 39(4):14-20, 2002.

Block SD: Assessing and managing depression in the terminally ill patient, *Annals of Internal Medicine* 132(3):209-218, 2000.

Brenner ZR, Drenzer ME: Using complementary and alternative therapies to promote comfort at end of life, *Critical Care Nursing Clinics of North America* 15(3):355-362, 2003.

Easley MK, Elliott S: Managing pain at the end of life, *Nursing Clinics of North America* 36(4):779-794, 2001.

Egan KA, Arnold RL: Grief and bereavement care, *American Journal of Nursing* 103(9):42-52, 2003.

Ellershaw J, Ward C: Care of the dying patient: the last hours or days of life, *British Medical Journal* 326(7379):30-34, 2003.

Fetters MD, Churchill L, Danis M: Conflict resolution at the end of life, *Critical Care Medicine* 29(5):921-925, 2001.

Herman CP: Spiritual needs of dying patients: a qualitative study, *Oncology Nursing Forum* 21(91):67, 2001.

Kemp C: *Terminal illness: a guide to nursing care,* ed 2, Philadelphia, 1999, Lippincott Williams & Wilkins.

LaDuke S: Terminal dyspnea and palliative care, *American Journal of Nursing* 101(11):26-31, 2001.

Matzo ML, Sherman DW (Eds): *Palliative care nursing: quality care to the end of life,* New York, 2001, Springer.

Pimple C, Schmidt L, Tidwell S: Achieving excellence in end-of-life care, *Nurse Educator* 28(1):40-43, 2003.

Pitorak EF: Care at the time of death, *American Journal of Nursing* 103(7):42-52, 2003.

Plaisance L, Ellis JA: Opioid-induced constipation, *American Journal of Nursing* 102(3):72-73, 2002.

Poor B, Poirrier GP: *End of life nursing care,* Sudbury, Mass, 2001, Jones and Bartlett.

Radcliffe M: Dealing with death, *Nursing Times* 97(21):26, 2001.

Stewart M: Reflecting on the psychological care of patients with a terminal illness, *Professional Nurse* 18(7):402-405, 2003.

Werth JL Jr, Gordon JR, Johnson RR Jr: Psychosocial issues near the end of life, *Aging and Mental Health* 6(4):402-412, 2002.

Zerwekh J: End-of-life hydration: benefit or burden? *Nursing2003* 33(2):32hn1-32hn3, 2003.

Index